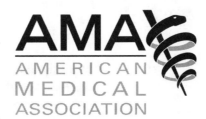

Health Care Careers QuickConsult

American Medical Association 312 464-5000
515 N State St, Chicago, IL 60654
www.ama-assn.org

Membership information 800 621-8335

Council on Ethical and Judicial Affairs 312 464-4823
www.ama-assn.org/go/ceja

Council on Medical Education 312 464-4515
www.ama-assn.org/go/councilmeded

Council on Science and Public Health 312 464-5046
www.ama-assn.org/go/csa

Allied Health 312 464-4635
www.ama-assn.org/go/alliedhealth

Adolescent Health 312 464-5315
www.ama-assn.org/go/adolescenthealth

Domestic Violence 312 464-5437
www.ama-assn.org/go/violence

Genetics and Molecular Medicine 312 464-4964
www.ama-assn.org/go/genetics

Health Disparities 312 464-4452
www.ama-assn.org/go/healthdisparities

Health Literacy 312 464-5357
www.amafoundation.org

Medical Education 312 464-4635
www.ama-assn.org/go/meded

Minority Affairs Section 312 464-5622
www.ama-assn.org/go/mac

Section on Medical Schools 312 464-4655
www.ama-assn.org/go/sms

Virtual Mentor 312 464-5260
www.virtualmentor.org

Health Care Careers Information

Anesthesiologist Assistant
American Academy of Anesthesiologists' Assistants
www.anesthetist.org

Art Therapy
American Art Therapy Association
www.arttherapy.org

Athletic Training
National Athletic Trainers' Association
www.nata.org

Audiology
American Speech-Language-Hearing Association
www.asha.org

Blindness and Visual Impairment Professions
Association for Education and Rehabilitation of the Blind and Visually Impaired
www.aerbvi.org

Blood Bank Technology, Specialist in
American Society for Clinical Pathology
www.ascp.org

Cardiovascular Technology
Society for Vascular Ultrasound
www.svunet.org

American Society of Echocardiography
www.asecho.org

Clinical Laboratory Science/Medical Technology
American Society for Clinical Laboratory Science
www.ascls.org

American Society for Clinical Pathology
www.ascp.org

Counseling
American Counseling Association
www.counseling.org

Cytotechnology
American Society of Cytopathology
www.cytopathology.org

Dance Therapy
American Dance Therapy Association
www.adta.org

Dentistry
American Dental Association
www.ada.org

Dental Assisting
American Dental Assistants Association
www.dentalassistant.org

Dental Hygiene

American Dental Hygienists' Association
www.adha.org

Dental Laboratory Technician

National Association of Dental Laboratories
www.nadl.org

Diagnostic Medical Sonography

Society of Diagnostic Medical Sonographers
www.sdms.org

Dietetics

American Dietetic Association
www.eatright.org

Electroneurodiagnostic Technology

American Society of Electroneurodiagnostic Technologists
www.aset.org

Emergency Medical Technician-Paramedic

National Association of Emergency Medical Technicians
www.naemt.org

Exercise Science

American Alliance for Health, Physical Education, Recreation, and Dance
www.aahperd.org

Genetic Counseling

National Society of Genetic Counselors
www.nsgc.org

Health Care Management

Association of University Programs in Health Administration
www.aupha.org

Health Information Management

American Health Information Management Association
www.ahima.org

Histotechnology

National Society for Histotechnology
www.nsh.org

Kinesiotherapy

American Kinesiotherapy Association
www.akta.org

Lactation Consultant

International Lactation Consultant Association
www.ilca.org

Massage Therapy

American Massage Therapy Association
http://www.amtamassage.org

Medical Assisting

American Association of Medical Assistants
www.aama-ntl.org

Medical Librarian

Medical Library Association
www.mlanet.org/career

Music Therapy

American Music Therapy Association
www.musictherapy.org

Nuclear Medicine Technology

Society of Nuclear Medicine—Technologist Section
www.snm.org

Nursing

National League for Nursing
www.nln.org

American Nurses Association
nursingworld.org

Occupational Therapy

American Occupational Therapy Association
www.aota.org

Ophthalmic Dispensing Optician

Opticians Association of America
www.opticians.org

Ophthalmic Medical Technician

Joint Commission on Allied Health Personnel in Ophthalmology
http://www.jcahpo.org

Optometrist

American Optometric Association
www.aoa.org

Orthoptist

American Orthoptic Council
www.orthoptics.org

Orthotist and Prosthetist

American Orthotic and Prosthetic Association
www.aopanet.org

Pathologists' Assisting

American Association of Pathologists' Assistants
www.pathologistsassistants.org

Perfusionist

American Society of Extra-Corporeal Technologists
www.amsect.org

Pharmacist

American Pharmacists Association
www.aphanet.org

Pharmacy Technician

American Association of Pharmacy Technicians
www.pharmacytechnician.com

Physical Therapy

American Physical Therapy Association
www.apta.org

Physician (allopathic)

American Medical Association
www.ama-assn.org/go/becominganmd

Physician (osteopathic)

American Osteopathic Association
www.osteopathic.org

Physician Assistant

American Academy of Physician Assistants
www.aapa.org

Podiatrist

American Podiatric Medical Association
www.apma.org/careers

Psychologist

American Psychological Association
www.apa.org/students

Radiologic Technology

American Society of Radiologic Technologists
www.asrt.org

Rehabilitation Counseling

National Council on Rehabilitation Education
www.rehabeducators.org

Respiratory Therapy

American Association for Respiratory Care
www.aarc.org

Sleep Technology

American Association of Sleep Technologists
www.aptweb.org

Speech-Language Pathology

American Speech-Language-Hearing Association
www.asha.org

Surgical Technology

Association of Surgical Technologists
www.ast.org

Recreational Therapist

American Therapeutic Recreation Association
www.atra-online.com/cms/

Veterinary Medicine, Veterinary Technology

American Veterinary Medical Association
www.avma.org

Other Sources for Health Care Careers Information

Alabama Health Careers

Alabama Hospital Association
www.AlabamaHealthCareers.com

Career Voyages

US Departments of Labor and Education
www.careervoyages.gov/healthcare-alliedhealth.cfm

Careers That Heal

St. Tammany Healthcare Alliance and Delgado Community College
(Louisiana)
www.careersthatheal.com

CareerZone, California

Carl Perkins, with funding from the California Department of
Education
www.cacareerzone.org

CareerZone, New York

New York State Department of Labor with a grant from the United
States Department of Labor
www.nycareerzone.org

Colorado Health Career Guide

Central Colorado AHEC and Workforce Boulder County
www.coloradohealthcareers.org/index.htm

Diagnostic Detectives

Michigan Department of Community Health
www.medlabcareers.msu.edu

ExploreHealthCareers.org

American Dental Education Association, with funding from the
Robert Wood Johnson Foundation
www.explorehealthcareers.org

Health Care Career Advisor

Cookeville Regional Medical Center Education Department,
Tennessee Hospital Association, and Putnam County Schools.
www.healthcareadvisortn.org

Health Care Careers Report

Labor Market Information Division, State of California
*www.labormarketinfo.edd.ca.gov/cgi/career/
?PAGEID=3&SUBID=169*

Health Careers Center, Mississippi Hospital Association
www.mshealthcareers.com

Health Occupations for Today and Tomorrow

Michigan Health Council
www.mihott.com

Health Opportunities for Today and Tomorrow

South Dakota Department of Health/Office of Rural Health
www.sdjobs.org/sdhott

H.O.T. Jobs: Health Opportunities in Texas

East Texas Area Health Education Center

West Texas Area Health Education Center

Center for South Texas Programs
www.texashotjobs.org

Iowa Health Careers Information Center

Iowa Department of Public Health
www.idph.state.ia.us/healthcareers

Labs are Vital

Abbott Diagnostics Division
www.labsarevital.com

LifeWorks

Office of Science Education, National Institutes of Health
http://science.education.nih.gov/lifeworks.nsf

Louisiana Health Careers Directory

The Governor's Office of the Workforce Commission and the four Louisiana Area Health Education Centers (AHECs):

- North Louisiana AHEC
- Central Louisiana AHEC
- Southwest Louisiana AHEC
- Southeast Louisiana AHEC

www.lahealthcareers.com

My First Day

Minnesota Hospital Association and Virginia Hospital Association
www.myfirstday.org

My Health Career

Northern Area Health Education Center
www.myhealthcareer.org

New York Health Careers

www.healthcareersinfo.net

Utah Directory of Health Professions Training Programs

Utah Center for Rural Health
www.suu.edu/ruralhealth/Health%20Careers%20Resources.htm

Vermont Health Care Careers Portal

University of Vermont College of Medicine AHEC Program
www.vthealthcareers.org

Accrediting Agencies

Accreditation Council for Education in Nutrition and Dietetics
www.eatright.org/acend

- Dietitian/nutritionist
- Dietetic technician

Accreditation Council for Occupational Therapy Education
www.aota.org

- Occupational therapist
- Occupational therapy assistant

Accreditation Council for Pharmacy Education
www.acpe-accredit.org

- Pharmacist

Accreditation Council on Optometric Education
www.aoa.org

- Optometrist, Optometric Technician

Accreditation Review Commission on Education for the Physician Assistant
www.arc-pa.org

- Physician assistant

American Academy of Professional Coders
www.aapc.com

- Medical coder

American Art Therapy Association
www.arttherapy.org

- Art therapist

American Board of Genetic Counseling
www.abgc.net

- Genetic counselor

American Dance Therapy Association
www.adta.org

- Dance therapist

American Orthoptic Council
www.orthoptics.org

- Orthoptist

American Psychological Association Committee on Accreditation
www.apa.org

- Psychologist

American Society of Health System-Pharmacists
www.ashp.org

- Pharmacy technician

American Veterinary Medical Association, Committee on Veterinary Technician Education and Activities
www.avma.org/education/cvea/

- Veterinary technologist

American Veterinary Medical Association, Council on Education
www.avma.org/education/cvea/

- Veterinarian

Association for Education and Rehabilitation of the Blind and Visually Impaired
www.aerbvi.org

- Orientation and mobility specialist
- Teacher of the visually impaired
- Rehabilitation teacher
- Low vision therapist

Association for Healthcare Documentation Integrity
www.ahdionline.org

- Medical transcriptionist

Association of University Programs in Health Administration
www.aupha.org

- Health care management

Commission on Accreditation for Health Informatics and Information Management Education
www.cahiim.org

- Health information administrator
- Health information technician

Commission on Accreditation for Respiratory Care
www.coarc.com

- Respiratory therapist

Commission on Accreditation in Physical Therapy Education
www.apta.org

- Physical therapist
- Physical therapist assistant

Commission on Accreditation of Athletic Training Education
www.caate.net

- Athletic trainer

Commission on Accreditation of Ophthalmic Medical Programs
www.jcahpo.org/coa-omp

- Ophthalmic medical technician

Commission on Accreditation of Allied Health Education Programs
www.caahep.org

- Anesthesia technologist/technician
- Anesthesiologist assistant
- Cardiovascular technologist
- Cytotechnologist
- Diagnostic medical sonographer
- Emergency medical technician-paramedic
- Exercise physiologist (applied and clinical)
- Exercise science professional
- Kinesiotherapist
- Lactation consultant
- Medical assistant
- Medical illustrator
- Neurodiagnostic technologist
- Orthotist/prosthetist
- Perfusionist
- Personal fitness trainer
- Polysomnographic technologist
- Recreational therapist
- Specialist in blood bank technology
- Surgical assistant
- Surgical technologist

Commission on Collegiate Nursing Education
www.aacn.nche.edu/accreditation

- Nurse

Commission on Dental Accreditation of the American Dental Association
www.ada.org

- Dentist
- Dental assistant
- Dental hygienist
- Dental laboratory technologist

Commission on Massage Therapy Accreditation
www.comta.org

- Therapeutic massage and bodywork

Commission on Opticianry Accreditation
www.COAccreditation.com

- Ophthalmic laboratory technician
Ophthalmic dispensing optician

Commission on Osteopathic College Accreditation
www.osteopathic.org

- Physician (osteopathic)

Council for Accreditation of Counseling and Related Educational Programs
www.cacrep.org

- Community counselor
- Marriage, couple, and family counselor/therapist
- Mental health counselor
- Student affairs practitioner
- School counselor

Council on Academic Accreditation in Audiology and Speech-Language Pathology
www.asha.org

- Audiologist
- Speech-language pathologist

Council on Chiropractic Education
www.cce-usa.org

- Chiropractor

Council on Podiatric Medical Education
www.cpme.org

- Podiatrist

Council on Rehabilitation Education
http://core-rehab.org

- Rehabilitation counselor

Joint Review Committee on Education in Radiologic Technology
www.jrcert.org

- Medical dosimetrist
- Magnetic resonance technologist
- Radiation therapist
- Radiographer

Joint Review Committee on Educational Programs in Nuclear Medicine Technology
www.jrcnmt.org

- Nuclear medicine technologist

Liaison Committee on Medical Education
www.lcme.org

- Physician (allopathic)

Medical Library Association
www.mlanet.org

- Medical librarian

National Accrediting Agency for Clinical Laboratory Sciences
www.naacls.org

- Clinical assistant
- Clinical laboratory scientist/medical technologist
- Clinical laboratory technician/medical lab technician
- Cytogenetic technologist
- Diagnostic molecular scientist
- Histotechnologist
- Pathologists' assistant
- Phlebotomist

National Association of Schools of Music
www.arts-accredit.org

- Music therapist

National Cancer Registrars Association
www.ncra-usa.org

- Cancer registrar
- Scholarship Information

Scholarship Information

Health Career Opportunity Program
Health Resources and Services Administration, Bureau of Health Professions
http://bhpr.hrsa.gov/diversity/hcop/default.htm

Federal Student Aid
US Department of Education
http://tinyurl.com/4tfej

College Is Possible
American Council on Education
www.collegeispossible.org

Key National Organizations

Association of Academic Health Centers
www.ahcnet.org

Association of Schools of Allied Health Professions
www.asahp.org

Health Occupations Students of America
www.hosa.org

Health Professions Network
www.healthpronet.org

National Association of Advisors for the Health Professions
www.naahp.org

National Commission for Certifying Agencies
www.noca.org/Resources/NCCAAccreditation/tabid/82/Default.aspx

National Network of Health Career Programs in Two-Year Colleges
www.nn2.org

National Society of Allied Health
www.nsah.org

Publication

Occupational Outlook Handbook
US Department of Labor, Bureau of Labor Statistics
www.bls.gov/oco

Contents

Preface

The *2012-2013 Health Care Careers Directory* encompasses
- 8,900 programs
- 2,700 sponsoring institutions
- 82 health care careers

Organization of the Directory

Section I: Health Care Careers and Educational Programs includes career descriptions, employment characteristics, and information about educational programs, such as length, curriculum, and educational standards, for the majority of the health care fields listed. Section I also provides sources for information on careers, certification, licensure, and registration.

This information is followed by a complete list of accredited/approved educational programs in alphabetical order by state, for each occupation. Most program listings include the educational program name and address and Web site address.

The list of programs is followed by a data chart showing class capacity (per start date or session), month(s) classes begin, program length(s), yearly tuition cost (resident and nonresident), yearly stipend (if any), academic award(s) granted, availability of evening/weekend courses, whether a program offers education/courses in medical/ health care terms in non-English languages, availability of distance education, and whether the program offers education in cultural competence or in patient communication. These data are shown only for those programs that completed the 2011 AMA Survey of Health Professions Education Programs.

Section II: Institutions Sponsoring Accredited Programs lists institutions (such as hospitals, colleges or universities, and academic medical centers) that sponsor the educational programs listed in Section I. Sponsoring institutions are listed by state and city in alphabetical order. The majority of entries for each institution include the name, address, telephone number, and email address of the chief executive officer and a list of the accredited health education programs for which the institution is a sponsor. Also included are the type of institution and its control status (eg, for-profit, government, nonprofit, etc).

Annual Survey of Health Professions Education Programs

The AMA uses an online survey to collect data on selected health professions education programs. Data collected on the annual survey are available to researchers, workforce analysts, policy makers, professional associations, career counselors, and students. Available data variables include:

Student data
- data on program enrollments, attrition, and graduates by gender and race/ethnicity

Program data
- tuition cost(s) (total for first-year student)
- class capacity (per start date or session)
- availability of evening/weekend classes
- program length(s), in months
- program start date(s)
- credential(s) awarded
- data on percentages of recent graduates (within last 6 months) finding employment or seeking additional education
- name, address, telephone/fax numbers, and email addresses of program officials.

For more information or to order, call (312) 464-4635 or email fred.lenhoff@ama-assn.org.

AMA MedEd Update

This monthly email newsletter covers educational trends and career-related issues in medical education and the health professions. To view the current issue, see http://www.ama-assn.org/go/amamededupdate; to subscribe, see http://www.ama-assn.org/ama/pub/news/subscribe-newsletters.page or email meded@ama-assn.org.

Disclaimer

The information on health care careers in the Directory is solely for information purposes and may not be construed as an acknowledgment of the therapeutic value or endorsement of these professions/organizations by the AMA.

Acknowledgments

The AMA gratefully acknowledges the cooperative relationships with the majority of health professions accrediting agencies listed in the Health Care Careers QuickConsult; these relationships and the hard work of accrediting agency staff throughout the year are essential for establishing the survey population and for providing information about and updates to accredited programs. The AMA also expresses its deep appreciation for the assistance of those program directors who provide updated information via the annual survey.

Acknowledgments are also due to Mike Jelsenik, Dave Badger, and Eric Fox of Dakota Systems for survey and database assistance; Rod Hill for production support; and AMA customer service staff for handling the questions generated by this product. In addition, thanks are due to the AMA staff listed on page ii.

Fred Donini-Lenhoff, MA, Editor
Elizabeth Unal, Editorial Assistant
Susan Skochelak, MD, MPH, Vice President, Medical Education

Section I

Health Care Careers and Educational Programs

Section I: *Health Care Careers and Educational Programs* offers descriptions and general information for 82 health care careers and includes listings for 8,900 accredited educational programs in all 50 states, Puerto Rico, Canadian provinces, and some other countries.

Each profession description contains many if not all of the following elements, identified by an icon:

 History describes the development of the profession over time, from the origin and evolution of each profession's key duties and responsibilities, and the establishment of the first sponsoring institutions and programs, to important convocations of decision-makers, accrediting bodies, and market forces that have shaped and defined the current state of the profession.

 Career Description details the general duties of the profession within the context of the health care environment in which it exists. Background information on the area of medical care that the profession supports (eg, laboratory testing, physical rehabilitation, surgery, administration, diet and nutrition) is also included. Also included is a more in-depth depiction of the day-to-day activities of each profession, including the duties and responsibilities that could be expected or assigned, depending on the facility, physical location, staff needs, and work environment.

 Employment Characteristics describes the workplace, facility, or physical location where the profession's duties are typically performed. Lengths of shifts, typical work weeks, and on-call status are also included, if available.

 Salary, from a variety of government, professional association, and industry survey sources, are provided if available. (For more information, refer to *www.ama-assn.org/go/hpsalary*.)

 Employment Outlook, if available, gives statistics or trend summaries from government, professional associations, and industry surveys about overall projections for demand, growth, and staffing needs within each profession's field of activity.

 Educational Programs offers general information regarding the length, prerequisites, typical coursework, and specific subjects of study for accredited educational programs in the chosen profession. This section also describes the various levels of educational attainment (eg, certificate, associate's degree, bachelor's degree, master's level) that are offered, as well as those that are required, to work in the selected profession.

 Licensure, Certification, and Registration specifies the legal and/or professional requirements, if any, for practicing in a chosen profession. Renewal cycles for certification and continuing education standards, as well as information on national and local accrediting bodies, may also be included.

 Inquiries lists names, addresses, and other contact information for national professional associations, accrediting bodies, and related information resources.

List of Programs. The lists of educational programs are in alphabetical order by state, then city, for each occupation. Most program listings include the name and address of the educational program and Web site address.

At the end of each profession's section is a data chart showing class capacity (per start date or session), month(s) classes begin, program length(s), yearly tuition cost (resident and nonresident), yearly stipend (if any), academic award(s) granted, availability of evening/weekend courses, whether a program offers education/courses in medical/health care terms in non-English languages, availability of distance education, and whether the program offers education in cultural competence or in patient communication. These data are shown only for those programs that completed the 2011 AMA Survey of Health Professions Programs.

Data Sources; Updates to Listings

The data in each of the program listings (Section I) and institution listings (Section II) are the product of two processes: The cooperative relationships between the AMA and the majority of health professions accrediting agencies, and the cooperation of program directors and institutional officials in responding to the Annual Survey of Health Professions Education Programs.

Program directors or institutional officials wishing to update the listings in Sections I or II should make the required changes on the annual survey, available by contacting *survey-admin@ama-hccd.org* or 312 324-3140. Updates can also be sent to the AMA at the following address:

American Medical Association
Medical Education Products
attn: Fred Donini-Lenhoff
515 North State Street
Chicago, IL 60654
312 464-4635
312 464-5830 Fax
E-mail: *fred.lenhoff@ama-assn.org*

Anesthesiologist Assistant

The anesthesiologist assistant (AA) is a skilled person qualified by advanced academic and clinical education to provide anesthetic care under the direction of a qualified anesthesiologist. The anesthesiologist, who is responsible for the AA is available to prescribe and direct particular therapeutic interventions in the operating room and the intensive care setting.

By virtue of the basic science education and clinical practice experience, the AA is skilled in the use of contemporary state-of-the-art patient monitoring techniques in anesthesia care environments. The AA performs complementary and supplementary anesthetic care and monitoring tasks, allowing the directing anesthesiologist to more efficiently and effectively use his or her own skills.

The anesthesiologist assistant is prepared to gather patient data, to assist in the evaluation of patients' physical and mental status, to record the surgical procedures planned, and to help the directing anesthesiologist administer the therapeutic plan that has been formulated for the anesthetic care of the patient. The tasks performed by AAs reflect regional variations in anesthesia practice and state regulatory factors.

Under the direction of the supervising anesthesiologist, in agreement with the guidelines established by the American Society of Anesthesiologists (ASA) statement on the Anesthesia Care Team (ACT), and in accordance with the American Academy of Anesthesiologist Assistants (AAAA) statement on the ACT, the anesthesiologist assistant's functions include, but are not limited to, the following:

- Obtain an appropriate and accurate preanesthetic health history, perform an appropriate physical examination, and record pertinent data in an organized and legible manner;
- Conduct diagnostic laboratory and related studies as appropriate, such as drawing arterial and venous blood samples;
- Establish noninvasive and invasive routine monitoring modalities, as delegated by the supervising anesthesiologist;
- Administer induction agents, maintain and alter anesthesia levels, administer adjunctive treatment, and provide continuity of anesthetic care into and during the post-operative recovery period;
- Apply and interpret advanced monitoring techniques, such as pulmonary artery catheterization, electroencephalographic spectral analysis, echocardiography, and evoked potentials;
- Use advanced life support techniques, such as high frequency ventilation and intra-arterial cardiovascular assist devices;
- Make post-anesthesia patient rounds by recording patient progress notes, compiling and recording case summaries, and by transcribing standing and specific orders;
- Evaluate and treat life-threatening situations, such as cardiopulmonary resuscitation, on the basis of established protocols (BLS, ACLS, and PALS);
- Perform duties in intensive care units, pain clinics, and other settings, as appropriate;

- Train and supervise personnel in the calibration, trouble shooting, and use of patient monitors;
- Delegate administrative duties in an anesthesiology practice or anesthesiology; department in such functions as the management of personnel, supplies and devices;
- Participate in the clinical instruction of others; and
- Perform and monitor regional anesthesia to include, but not limited to, spinal, epidural, IV regional, and other special techniques such as local infiltration and nerve blocks.

The AA may also be used in pain clinics or may participate in administrative and educational activities.

History
Anesthesiologist assistant educational programs began in 1969 at Case Western University in Cleveland, Ohio, and at Emory University in Atlanta, Georgia. Beginning with the National Academy of Sciences' original description of the physician assistant role in both general and specialty areas of medicine, these programs were created in response to task-analysis studies, which showed the increasing need for anesthetists with technical backgrounds. The functional relationship of graduates to the anesthesiologist is similar to that of physician assistants to the general medical as well as surgical specialties.

In 1975, the ASA took action in support of this new emerging profession on the basis of its review of the educational and clinical objectives. In 1976, the ASA petitioned the AMA Council on Medical Education (CME) for recognition of the anesthesiologist assistant as an emerging health profession. The CME's recognition followed in 1978.

In 1987, standards for the education of the AA were adopted by the AMA, and programs at Emory University and Case Western University were evaluated and initially accredited by the Committee on Allied Health Education and Accreditation (CAHEA) in 1988.

Career Description
In addition to the duties described in the occupational description above, anesthesiologist assistants provide other support according to established protocols. Such activities may include pretesting anesthesia delivery systems and patient monitors and operating special monitors and support devices for critical cardiac, pulmonary, and neurological systems. AAs may be involved in the operation of bedside electronic computer-based monitors and have supervisory responsibilities for laboratory functions associated with anesthesia and operating room care. They provide cardiopulmonary resuscitation in association with other anesthesia care team members, and in accordance with approved emergency protocols.

Employment Characteristics
Anesthesiologist assistants work as members of the anesthesia care team in any locale where they may be appropriately directed by legally responsible

anesthesiologists. The AAs most often work within organizations that also employ nurse anesthetists, and their responsibilities are identical. Experience to-date has been that AAs are most commonly employed in larger facilities that perform procedures such as cardiac surgery, neurosurgery, transplant surgery, and trauma care, given the training in extensive patient monitoring devices and complex patients and procedures, which are emphasized in AA educational programs. However, AAs are used in hospitals of all sizes and assist anesthesiologists in a variety of settings and for a wide range of procedures.

Salary

Starting salaries for 2006 graduates are $95,000 up to $120,000 for the 40-hour work week plus benefits and consideration of on-call activity. The high end of the salary range is around $160,000 to $180,000 for experienced anesthetists (including overtime). For more information, go to *www.ama-assn.org/go/hpsalary*.

Educational Programs

Length. These post baccalaureate programs are typically 24 to 28 months.

Prerequisites. The programs require an undergraduate premedical background (premedical courses in biology, chemistry, physics, and math) and a baccalaureate degree. Although any baccalaureate major is acceptable (if premedical requirements are met), typical majors are biology, chemistry, physics, mathematics, computer science, or one of the allied health professions, such as respiratory therapy, medical technology, or nursing.

Certification

The National Commission for Certification of Anesthesiologist Assistants (NCCAA), which was founded in 1989, provides the certification process for AAs in the United States. The Commission includes anesthesiologists and anesthesiologist assistants. NCCAA contracts with the National Board of Medical Examiners to assist with the certification process, including task analyses, development of content grids, item writing and editing, and administration of examinations. The certification process incorporates a 6-year cycle of certifying examination, examination for continued demonstration of qualifications, and registration of continuing medical education.

Inquiries

Careers

Curriculum inquiries should be directed to the individual programs. Inquiries regarding AA careers should be directed to:

American Academy of Anesthesiologist Assistants
2209 Dickens Road
Richmond, VA 23230-2005
804 565-6353
866 328-5858 Toll-free
804 282-0090 Fax
E-mail: *aaaa@societyhq.com*
www.anesthetist.org

Certification

National Commission for Certification of Anesthesiologist
   Assistants
1500 Sunday Drive, Suite 102
Raleigh, NC 27607
919 573-5439
877 558-0411 Toll-free
919 573-5440 Fax
E-mail: *business.office@aa-nccaa.org*
www.aa-nccaa.org

Program Accreditation

Commission on Accreditation of Allied Health Education Programs
   (CAAHEP)
1361 Park Street, Clearwater, FL 33756
727 210-2350
727 210-2354 Fax
E-mail: *mail@caahep.org*
www.caahep.org
in collaboration with:
Accreditation Review Committee for the Anesthesiologist Assistant
Jennifer Anderson Warwick, Executive Director
2027 Burnside Dr
Allen, TX 75013
469 656-1103
E-mail: *arcaamember@gmail.com*
www.caahep.org/Committees-On-Accreditation/?ID=AA

Anesthesiologist Assistant

Florida

Nova Southeastern University
Anesthesiologist Asst Prgm
3200 University Drive
Health Professions Division
Fort Lauderdale, FL 33328-2018
www.nova.edu/mhs/anesthesia

Nova Southeastern University - Tampa
Anesthesiologist Asst Prgm
9503 Princess Palm Ave
Tampa, FL 33619

Georgia

Emory University
Anesthesiologist Asst Prgm
57 Executive Park South, Ste 300
Atlanta, GA 30329
www.emory.edu
Prgm Dir: Richard G Brouillard, ScD
Tel: 404 727-3188   *Fax:* 404 727-3021
E-mail: richard.brouillard@emory.edu

South University
Cosponsor: Mercer University School of Medicine
Anesthesiologist Asst Prgm
709 Mall Blvd
Savannah, GA 31406
www.southuniversity.edu/
   anethesiologist-assistant-program.aspx

Missouri

University of Missouri - Kansas City
Anesthesiologist Asst Prgm
UMKC School of Medicine 2411 Holmes St
Kansas City, MO 64108

Ohio

Case Western Reserve University
Anesthesiologist Asst Prgm
Master of Science in Anesthesia Program
11100 Euclid Ave, Lakeside Rm 2532 LKS5007
University Hospitals Case Medical Center
Cleveland, OH 44106-1716
www.anesthesiaprogram.com
Prgm Dir: Joseph M Rifici, AA-C MEd
Tel: 216 844-8077   *Fax:* 216 844-7349
E-mail: info@anesthesiaprogram.com

Texas

Case Western Reserve University
Anesthesiologist Asst Prgm
University of Texas Professional Building (UTPB)
Suite 480
6410 Fannin St
Houston, TX 77030

Anesthesiologist Assistant

Programs*	Class Capacity	Begins	Length (months)	Award	Res. Tuition	Non-res. Tuition		Offers:† 1	2	3	4
Georgia											
Emory Univ (Atlanta)	50	Aug	24	MMSc							
Ohio											
Case Western Reserve Univ (Cleveland)	22	Jun	24	MS	$48,197	$48,197	total tuition			•	•

*Data are shown only for programs that completed the 2011 AMA Survey of Health Professions Education Programs.

†Key to Offers: 1: Evening or weekend classes; 2: Non-English instruction; 3: Cultural competence instruction; 4: Distance education component.

Anesthesia Technologist/Technician

Certified anesthesia technologists and technicians are vital members of the anesthesia patient care team. Their role is to assist licensed anesthesia providers in the acquisition, preparation and application of equipment, medications and supplies required for the monitoring and administration of anesthesia. In this role, they contribute to safe, efficient and cost-effective anesthesia care.

Career Description

Depending on individual knowledge, expertise and training, the tasks of the certified anesthesia technologist and technician may include:

- Support to the anesthesia providers for routine and complex surgical cases
- Equipment maintenance and servicing such as cleaning and sterilizing, assembling, calibrating and testing, troubleshooting, requisitioning and recording of inspections and maintenance
- Operating a variety of mechanical, pneumatic, and electronic equipment used to monitor the patient undergoing anesthesia.

With the appropriate training, the practitioner may also perform inspection, maintenance, and on-site repairs.

In addition, the anesthesia technologist or technician may be responsible for purchasing and distributing supplies and equipment as well as maintaining inventories and service records. Individuals functioning as anesthesia technologists or technicians should be capable of a level of self-direction and supervision commensurate with their training.

Certified Anesthesia Technologists are generally employed at a higher level of service and management including lead, supervisory and administrative positions. The technologist assists in the care of the patient at a higher level as well.

Educational Programs

The National Standard Curriculum of the American Society of Anesthesia Technologists and Technicians (ASATT) notes that students should receive instruction that encompasses:

I

  A. Didactic:800 hours

  B. Clinical: 800 hours

  C. Total Minimum Didactic and Clinical Hours required for AS Degree = 1,600 hours (includes General Education)

II

  A. Prerequisite Courses (General Education) for AS Degree: 30 units

  B. Anesthesia Technology Courses (Certificate of Achievement): 30 units

  C. Minimum required for completion = 60 units total

Certification

The ASATT offers the only nationally recognized certification for anesthesia technicians (Cer AT); the first examination was administered in May 1996.

A Certification Test Development and Test Writing Committee evaluates and develops ASATT certification standards and exams in conjunction with Applied Measurement Professionals (AMP), an organization that develops and administers certification exams. The Test Writing Committee consists of an anesthesiologist, certified registered nurse anesthetists, a professor of anesthesia education, a corporate representative, and certified anesthesia technicians and technologists. The ASATT is a member of the National Organization for Competency Assurance (NOCA), a nationally recognized organization that establishes standards for credentialing examination programs.

Effective July 15, 2015, the technician certification exam will no longer be available. In addition, after July 2015, all candidates seeking to take the technologist exam must have graduated from an approved program.

Certification is granted for a 2-year period. To maintain certification, a minimum of 20 continuing education contact hours (CE/CH) must be obtained and submitted to the ASATT Certification and Recertification Review Committee. At the end of each 2-year recertification period, certified anesthesia technicians must reapply for certification.

Certification for the technologist level has been offered since 2001, when the first exam was administered. The certified anesthesia technologist must submit 30 continuing education contact hours (CE/CH) relevant to the field of anesthesia technology at the end of each 2-year recertification period.

Inquiries

American Society of Anesthesia Technologists and Technicians

7044 South 13th Street

Oak Creek, WI 53154-1429

414 908-4942 ext 450

E-mail: *customercare@asatt.org*

www.asatt.org

Program Accreditation

Commission on Accreditation of Allied Health Education Programs (CAAHEP) in collaboration with:

Accreditation Review Committee for the Anesthesia Technologist/Technician

1361 Park Street, Clearwater, FL 33756

727 210-2350

727 210-2354 Fax

E-mail: *mail@caahep.org*

Anesthesia Technologist/Technician

Pennsylvania

Sanford-Brown Institute
Anesthesia Technologist/Technician Prgm
421 7th Ave
Pittsburgh, PA 15219
www.sanfordbrown.edu

Cardiovascular Technologist and Sonographer

The certified cardiovascular technologist and sonographer perform diagnostic examinations and/or therapeutic interventions of the heart and/or blood vessels at the request or direction of a physician in one or more of the following concentrations:

- Invasive cardiovascular technology—cardiac catheterization
- Adult echocardiography
- Pediatric echocardiography
- Noninvasive vascular study—vascular ultrasound
- Cardiac electrophysiology

History

In December 1981, the AMA Council on Medical Education (CME) officially recognized cardiovascular technology as an allied health profession. Subsequently, an initial draft of the proposed *Standards and Guidelines for the Accreditation of Educational Programs in Cardiovascular Technology* was finalized in 1983.

Career Description

The cardiovascular technologist is qualified by specific didactic, laboratory, and clinical technological education to perform diagnostic or therapeutic procedures in various cardiovascular or peripheral vascular procedures. Careers in cardiovascular technology include:

- *Invasive cardiovascular technologists* are responsible for maintaining the cardiac catheterization laboratory and assisting cardiologists in the catheterization procedures used to diagnose and treat the various diseases of the cardiovascular system.
- *Adult and pediatric echocardiographers* are cardiac sonographers who perform echocardiography examinations to evaluate heart function and physiology under the supervision of cardiologists to include cardiac stress testing and assist in trans-esophageal echocardiography. Echocardiography procedures are performed on adults and pediatric patients (infant through adolescence). .
- *Non-invasive vascular ultrasound sonographers* work under the direction of various clinical disciplines including vascular surgeons, interventional radiologists, or cardiologists to perform non-invasive vascular ultrasound and other non-ultrasonographic, procedures to evaluate the extra- and intracranial, peripheral and visceral vascular systems.
- *Cardiac electrophysiology technologists* are responsible for maintaining the cardiac electrophysiology laboratory and assisting cardiologists in the various procedures used to diagnose and treat patients with cardiac arrhythmias.

Employment Characteristics

Cardiovascular technologists provide diagnostic services to patients in medical settings under the supervision of a doctor of medicine (MD) or osteopathy (DO). The procedures performed by the cardiovascular technologist may be found in:

- Invasive cardiac catheterization or endovascular laboratories, where cardiac, electrophysiologic, and vascular catheterization procedures are performed;
- Noninvasive cardiac (Echocardiography) laboratories and hospital inpatient settings, where cardiac ultrasound and exercise stress tests are performed.

- Vascular laboratories and hospital inpatient settings, where peripheral vascular duplex ultrasound , segmental blood pressure , transcutaneous oxygen tension, transcranial Doppler and plethysmographic studies are performed.

Salary

Although salary may vary significantly depending on region and demographics, entry-level salaries range from $40,000 to $50,000. The overall average is $50,000 to $65,000, with the upper-level ranges from $75,000 plus.

Data from the US Bureau of Labor Statistics (*www.bls.gov/oes/current/oes292031.htm*) from May 2011 show that wages at the 10th percentile are $27,430, the 50th percentile (median) at $51,020, and the 90th percentile at $79,290.

In addition, the American Society of Echocardiography has a salary survey that includes data for cardiovascular sonographers, and is available at *www.asecho.org/i4a/ams/amsstore/category.cfm?category_id=19* .

For more information, go to *www.ama-assn.org/go/hpsalary*.

Employment Outlook

Employment of cardiovascular technologists and sonographers is expected to increase 29% through the year 2020, much faster than the average for all occupations, according to the BLS. Demand will stem from the prevalence of heart disease and an aging population, which has a higher incidence of heart disease and other complications of the heart and vascular system..

Educational Programs

Length. Programs are available in colleges, hospitals, medical centers, or branches of the United States Armed Forces. Program length ranges from 1 year (hospital certificate), 2 years (associate degree) to 4 years (baccalaureate degree).

Prerequisites. High school diploma or equivalent or qualifications in a clinically related allied health profession. Requirements are determined by institutional requirements and concentration(s) studied.

Curriculum. Curricula of accredited programs include didactic instruction, laboratory experiences, and patient-based clinical instruction. Suggested areas of instruction are outline in the National Education Curriculum for Sonography and the core curriculum include an introduction to the field of cardiovascular technology, general and/or applied sciences, human anatomy and physiology, basic pharmacology, and basic medical electronics and medical instrumentation. Emphasis, following the core curriculum, is given in the concentration(s) selected: invasive cardiology, noninvasive/ echocardiography, noninvasive peripheral vascular, and cardiac electrophysiology study. Both didactic instruction and clinical experiences are provided in these areas.

Inquiries

Careers/Curriculum
Society for Vascular Ultrasound
4601 Presidents Drive, Suite 260
Lanham, MD 20706-4831
301 459-7550 or 800 SVU-VEIN 800 788-8346
www.svunet.org

American Society of Echocardiography
2100 Gateway Centre Boulevard, Suite 310
Morrisville, NC 27560
919 861-5574
www.asecho.org

Society of Diagnostic Medical Sonography
2745 Dallas Pkwy Ste 350
Plano, TX 75093-8730
800 229-9506
www.sdms.org

Society of Invasive Cardiovascular Professionals
1500 Sunday Drive, Suite 102
Raleigh, NC 27607
919 861-4546
www.sicp.com

Certification/Registration
Cardiovascular Credentialing International
1500 Sunday Drive, Suite 102
Raleigh, NC 27607
800 326-0268
www.cci-online.org

American Registry for Diagnostic Medical Sonography
51 Monroe Street, Plaza East One
Rockville, MD 20850-2400
3 01 738-8401
www.ardms.org

Program Accreditation
Commission on Accreditation of Allied Health Education Programs (CAAHEP)
1361 Park Street, Clearwater, FL 33756
7 27 210-2350
7 27 210-2354 Fax
E-mail: *mail@caahep.org*
www.caahep.org

in collaboration with:
Joint Review Committee on Education in Cardiovascular Technology (JRC-CVT)
William W. Goding, Executive Director
6 Pine Knoll Drive
Beverly, MA 01915-1425
9 78 456-5594
E-mail: *office@jrccvt.org*
www.jrccvt.org

ALLIED HEALTH

Cardiovascular Technologist

California

Orange Coast College
Cardiovascular Tech (Invasive/Noninvasive) Prgm
2701 Fairview Rd
Costa Mesa, CA 92628-5005
www.orangecoastcollege.edu

Grossmont College
Cardiovascular Tech (Invasive/Vasc/Echo) Prgm
8800 Grossmont College Dr
Attn: CVT Program
El Cajon, CA 92020-1799
www.grossmont.edu/cvt
Prgm Dir: Andrew Biondo
Tel: 619 644-7302 *Fax:* 619 644-7961
E-mail: andy.biondo@gcccd.edu

Florida

Edison State College
Cardiovascular Tech (Invasive) Prgm
8099 College Pkwy SW
Fort Myers, FL 33906
www.edison.edu

Sanford-Brown Institute - Ft Lauderdale
Cardiovascular Tech (Echocardiography) Prgm
1201 West Cypress Creek Rd
Ft Lauderdale, FL 33309

Santa Fe College
Cardiovascular Tech (Invasive/Noninv/Vasc) Prgm
3000 NW 83rd St
Gainesville, FL 32606
www.santafe.cc.fl.us

Valencia College
Cardiovascular Tech (Invasive) Prgm
1800 S Kirkman Rd
Orlando, FL 32802

Central Florida Institute
Cardiovascular Tech (Invasive/Noninv/Vasc) Prgm
Invasive/Noninvasive/Cardiovascular Ultrasound Tracks
30522 US Hwy 19 N
Ste 300
Palm Harbor, FL 34684
www.cfinstitute.com

Polk State College
Cardiovascular Tech (Invasive) Prgm
999 Ave H NE Box 150
Winter Haven, FL 33881

Georgia

Darton College
Cardiovascular Tech (Invasive/Echo) Prgm
2400 Gillionville Rd
Albany, GA 31707

Augusta Technical College
Cardiovascular Tech (Invasive/Noninv/Vasc) Prgm
University Hospital
Harry T Harper Jr Sch of Cardiac & Vas Tech
1350 Walton Way
Augusta, GA 30915
www.augustatech.edu

Kentucky

Norton Healthcare
Cardiovascular Tech (Echocardiography) Prgm
One Audubon Plaza Drive
Louisville, KY 40217

Spencerian College
Cardiovascular Tech (Invasive) Prgm
4627 Dixie Hwy
Louisville, KY 40216
www.spencerian.edu

Louisiana

Cardiovascular Technology Training Inc
Cosponsor: The Louisiana Medical Center and Heart Hospital
Cardiovascular Technology Prgm
64040 Hwy 434, Ste 200
Lacombe, LA 70445
www.cardiovasculartechnologytraining.com

Louisiana State Univ Health Sciences Center
Cardiovascular Tech (Noninvasive) Prgm
1900 Gravier St
New Orleans, LA 70112
www.lsuhsc.edu

Maryland

Howard Community College
Cardiovascular Tech (Invasive) Prgm
10901 Little Patuxent Pkwy
Columbia, MD 21044
www.howardcc.edu

Michigan

Carnegie Institute
Cardiovascular Tech (Invasive/Vasc/Echo) Prgm
Noninvasive Peripheral Vascular, Invasive CVT & Non-InvEcho
550 Stephenson Hwy Suite 100
Troy, MI 48083
www.carnegie-institute.edu

Minnesota

Northland Community & Technical College
Cardiovascular Tech (Invasive) Prgm
2022 Central Ave NE
East Grand Forks, MN 56721
www.northlandcollege.edu

St Cloud Technical and Community College
Cardiovascular Tech (Invasive/Echo) Prgm
1540 Northway Dr
St Cloud, MN 56303
www.sctc.edu

Nebraska

BryanLGH College of Health Sciences
Cosponsor: BryanLGH Medical Center
Cardiovascular Tech (Invasive/Noninv/Vasc) Prgm
5035 Everett St
Lincoln, NE 68506-1398
www.bryanlghcollege.org

New Jersey

Atlantic Health - Morristown Memorial Hosp
Cardiovascular Tech (Invasive/Noninv/Vasc) Prgm
100 Madison Ave?Box 5
Morristown, NJ 07962-1956
www.morristownmemorialhospital.org

Univ of Medicine & Dent of New Jersey
Cardiovascular Tech (Vascular) Prgm
1776 Raritan Rd, Rm 545
Scotch Plains, NJ 07076
www.umdnj.edu

New York

Molloy College
Cardiovascular Tech (Invasive/Noninv/Vasc) Prgm
1000 Hempstead Ave
PO Box 5002
Rockville Centre, NY 11571-5002
www.molloy.edu
Prgm Dir: Michael J Hartman, MS RDMS RVT RT(R)
Tel: 516 678-5000, Ext 6958   *Fax:* 516 256-2252
E-mail: mhartman@molloy.edu

North Carolina

Central Piedmont Community College
Cardiovascular Tech (Invasive/Echo) Prgm
PO Box 35009
Charlotte, NC 28235

Ohio

Sanford-Brown College - Middleburg Heights
Cardiovascular Tech (Echocardiography) Prgm
17535 Rosbough Drive
Middleburg Heights, OH 44130

Pennsylvania

Geisinger Medical Center
Cardiovascular Tech (Invasive) Prgm
100 N Academy Ave, MS 2011
Danville, PA 17822-2011
www.geisinger.org

Gwynedd-Mercy College
Cardiovascular Tech (Invasive/Noninvasive) Prgm
1325 Sumneytown Pike, PO Box 901
Gwynedd Valley, PA 19437
www.gmc.edu

Harrisburg Area Community College
Cardiovascular Tech (Invasive/Noninvasive) Prgm
Invasive Cardiology, Non-Invasive Cardiology
1641 Old Philadelphia Pike
Office 207-D East Building
Lancaster, PA 17602
www.hacc.edu

Lancaster Gen Coll of Nursing & Hlth Sciences
Cardiovascular Tech (Invasive) Prgm
410 N Lime St
Lancaster, PA 17602
www.LancasterGeneral.org
Prgm Dir: Lee Ann Johnson,
Tel: 717 544-7543   *Fax:* 717 544-1185
E-mail: Lejohnso@lancastergeneral.org

South Carolina

Sister of Charity Providence Hospital
Cardiovascular Tech (Invasive/Noninv/Vasc) Prgm
School of Cardiovascular Diagnostics
Department 7195
2435 Forest Dr
Columbia, SC 29204
www.provhosp.com

South Dakota

Southeast Technical Institute
Cardiovascular Tech (Invasive/Noninv/Vasc) Prgm
2320 N Career Ave
Sioux Falls, SD 57107
www.southeasttech.com

Tennessee

Northeast State Community College
Cardiovascular Tech (Invasive) Prgm
PO Box 246, 2425 Hwy 75
Blountville, TN 37617-0246
www.NortheastState.edu

Texas

El Centro College
Cardiovascular Tech (Invasive) Prgm
Echocardiology Technology Program
Main and Lamar Sts
Dallas, TX 75202
www.elcentrocollege.edu

Sanford-Brown College - Dallas
Cardiovascular Tech (Echocardiography) Prgm
1250 W Mockingbird Lane
Dallas, TX 75247

Medical Education and Training Campus (METC)
Cardiovascular Tech (Invasive) Prgm
3085 Wilson Way
Fort Sam Houston, TX 78234
www.cs.amedd.army.mil/300y6/

Virginia

Geneva College
Cardiovascular Tech (Invasive) Prgm
INOVA Fairfax Hospital 3300 Gallows Rd
Falls Church, VA 22046

Sentara Norfolk General Hospital
Cardiovascular Tech (Invasive/Noninv/Vasc) Prgm
600 Gresham Dr
Norfolk, VA 23507
www.sentara.com

Washington

Spokane Community College
Cardiovascular Tech (Invasive/Noninvasive) Prgm
N 1810 Greene St MS 2090
Spokane, WA 99217-5499
www.scc.spokane.edu

Wisconsin

Milwaukee Area Technical College
Cardiovascular Tech (Invasive) Prgm
700 W State St
Milwaukee, WI 53233-1443
www.matc.edu

Cardiovascular Technologist

Programs*	Class Capacity	Begins	Length (months)	Award	Res. Tuition	Non-res. Tuition	Offers:† 1	2	3	4
California										
Grossmont College (El Cajon)	54	Aug	22	Dipl, AS	$1,500	per credit		•		
New York										
Molloy College (Rockville Centre)	17	Sep	24	AS					•	
Pennsylvania										
Lancaster Gen Coll of Nursing & Hlth Sciences	13	Jun	12, 24	AS					•	

*Data are shown only for programs that completed the 2011 AMA Survey of Health Professions Education Programs.

†Key to Offers: 1: Evening or weekend classes; 2: Non-English instruction; 3: Cultural competence instruction; 4: Distance education component.

Emergency Medical Technician-Paramedic

Emergency Medical Technicians (EMTs) and Paramedics are educated to provide prehospital emergency care to people who have suffered from an illness or an injury outside of the hospital setting. EMTs and Paramedics work under protocols approved by a physician medical director to recognize, assess, and manage medical emergencies and transport critically ill or injured patients to definitive medical care at a hospital. EMTs provide Basic Life Support (BLS), and EMT-Paramedics provide Advanced Life Support (ALS).

History

In 1975, the AMA recognized the Emergency Medical Technician-Paramedic as an allied health occupation for the purpose of accrediting entry-level educational programs in the profession, and the educational *Standards (Essentials)* to evaluate EMT-Paramedic programs seeking accreditation were adopted in 1978.

Today, programs are accredited by the Commission on Accreditation of Allied Health Education Programs (CAAHEP) in collaboration with the Committee on Accreditation of Educational Programs for the EMS Professions (CoAEMSP). The *Standards* were most recently revised in 2005.

Career Description

EMTs and Paramedics may be employed by a private ambulance company, fire department, police department, public EMS agency, private ambulance company, hospital, or combination of the above. EMS responders may be paid or serve as volunteers in the community.

EMTs must be proficient in Basic Life Support (BLS), and training is centered on recognizing and treating life-threatening conditions outside the hospital environment. EMTs learn the basics of how to handle cardiac and respiratory arrest, heart attacks, seizures, diabetic emergencies, respiratory problems, and other medical emergencies. They also learn how to manage traumatic injuries such as falls, fractures, lacerations, and burns. EMTs also are introduced into patient assessment, history taking, and vital signs.

EMTs perform CPR, artificial ventilations, oxygen administration, basic airway management, defibrillation using an Automated External Defibrillator (AED), spinal immobilization, vital signs, bandaging/splinting, and, under the direction of a physician, may administer Nitroglycerin, Glucose, Epinephrine, and Albuterol in special circumstances.

Paramedics perform all of the skills performed by an EMT. In addition, they perform advanced airway management, such as endotracheal intubation, under medical supervision and from a base station, usually in a hospital emergency department. They obtain and interpret electrocardiographs (ECGs), introduce intravenous lines, and administer numerous emergency medications. Paramedics assess ECG tracings and defibrillate. They have extensive education in patient assessment and are exposed to a variety of clinical and field experiences during their education.

Salary

Earnings of EMTs and Paramedics depend on the employment setting and geographic location as well as the individual's education and experience. Median annual earnings of EMTs and Paramedics were $30,000 in May 2010. The middle 50% earned between $23,650 and $39,250. The lowest 10% earned less than $19,880, and the highest 10% earned more than $53,050. Median annual earnings in the industries employing the largest numbers of EMTs and Paramedics in May 2010 were:

- Local government $38,400
- General medical and surgical hospitals $34,270
- Other ambulatory health care services $30,980

Note: These data may not accurately reflect compensation for both EMTs and EMT-Paramedics, as these fields have different training and education requirements and different salary levels as well. Combining salary data for EMTs and EMT-Paramedics may skew these data lower (or higher) than what may be occurring in the marketplace.

Those in Emergency Medical Services, who are part of fire or police departments, receive the same benefits as firefighters or police officers. For example, many are covered by pension plans that provide retirement at half pay after 20 or 25 years of service, or if the worker is disabled in the line of duty.

For more salary information, go to *www.ama-assn.org/go/hpsalary*.

Employment Outlook

The job opportunities for EMS professionals are expected to grow 33% from 2010-2020, about as fast as the average for all occupations, according to the US Department of Labor.

Educational Programs

In most locations in the United States, the minimum level of education that most EMS professionals have before entering the workforce is that of an EMT. Individuals who work as firefighters or police officers may perform some emergency medical work when trained as first responders. Some Paramedic programs provide an all-inclusive program that includes both EMT and Paramedic education in one program. All levels of EMS training are set by the federal government through the National Highway Traffic Safety Administration (NHTSA).

EMT training is offered at community colleges, technical schools, hospitals, and universities as well as EMS, fire, and police academies. Those interested in EMT training should contact their state's EMS Office. For those interested in Paramedic education, contact CAAHEP and the Committee on Accreditation of Educational Programs for the EMS Professionals (CoAEMSP). Both of these agencies can help potential students find local training and educational opportunities. Beginning in 2013, all paramedics must graduate from CAAHEP-accredited programs to be eligible for national certification from the National Registry of EMTs.

Length. EMT training varies from 2 to 6 months, depending on the training site and hours of class scheduled per week. There are training programs that have classes every day for several months for those interested in a quick completion. Longer programs are available to accommodate students who have family, a full-time job, or other responsibilities that limit their available time for education. Approximate educational requirements are:

- Emergency Medical Responder 40 hours of training
- EMT 110 hours of training
- Advanced EMT 200-400 hours of training
- Paramedic 1,000 or more hours of education

Prerequisites. An EMT student is expected to be a high school graduate or the equivalent (GED), and to meet the physical and mental demands of the occupation. Paramedic students must have completed their EMT education prior to enrollment in most paramedic education courses unless they are jointly enrolled in an EMT and paramedic program. Some paramedic education programs are part of the Associate of Applied Science (AAS) or Bachelor of Science (BS) degree programs offered at colleges and universities. A Certificate of Completion is generally offered to those who did not complete a college degree.

Curriculum. EMT and paramedic education programs are composed of in-classroom didactic instruction; in-hospital clinical practice; and a supervised field internship on an ambulance. Courses typically are competency-based and supported by performance assessments. Instruction provides students with knowledge of acute and critical changes in physiological, psychological, and clinical symptoms that they might encounter in an emergency medical situation.

Inquiries

Careers
National Association of Emergency Medical
Technicians (NAEMT)
PO Box 1400
Clinton, MS 39060-1400
800 34-NAEMT
www.naemt.org

Certification/Licensure
National Registry of Emergency Medical Technicians (NREMT)
Rocco V. Morando Bldg
Box 29233
6610 Busch Blvd
Columbus, OH 43229-0233
614 888-4484
www.nremt.org

Program Accreditation
Commission on Accreditation of Allied Health Education Programs
    (CAAHEP)
1361 Park Street, Clearwater, FL 33756
727 210-2350
727 210-2354 Fax
E-mail: *mail@caahep.org*
www.caahep.org

in collaboration with:
Committee on Accreditation of Educational Programs for the EMS
    Professions (CoAEMSP)
8301 Lakeview Parkway, Suite 111-312
Rowlett, TX 75088
Phone: 214-703-8445Fax: 214-703-8992
E-mail: *george@coaemsp.org*
www.coaemsp.org

Note: Adapted in part from the Bureau of Labor Statistics, US Department of Labor, *Occupational Outlook Handbook*, 2010-2011 Edition, Emergency Medical Technicians and Paramedics, at *www.bls.gov/oco/ocos101.htm*.

Emergency Medical Technician-Paramedic

Alabama

Lurleen B Wallace Community College
Emergency Med Tech-Paramedic Prgm
PO Box 1418
1000 Dannelly Blvd
Andalusia, AL 36420
www.lbwcc.edu

Jefferson State Community College
Emergency Med Tech-Paramedic Prgm
2601 Carson Rd
Birmingham, AL 35215

Calhoun Community College
Emergency Med Tech-Paramedic Prgm
PO Box 2216 Hwy 31 N
Decatur, AL 35609
www.calhoun.cc.al.us

Wallace Community College
Emergency Med Tech-Paramedic Prgm
1141 Wallace Dr
Dothan, AL 36303
www.wallace.edu

Gadsden State Community College
Emergency Med Tech-Paramedic Prgm
PO Box 227
1001 George Wallace Dr
Gadsden, AL 35902-0227
www.gadsdenstate.edu

James H Faulkner State Community College
Emergency Med Tech-Paramedic Prgm
3301 Gulf Shores Parkway
Gulf Shores, AL 36542
www.faulknerstate.edu

Wallace State Community College
Emergency Med Tech-Paramedic Prgm
801 Main St, PO Box 2000
Hanceville, AL 35077
www.wallacestate.edu

Bishop State Community College - Baker Gaines Central Campus
Emergency Med Tech-Paramedic Prgm
1365 Martin Luther King Ave
Mobile, AL 36603

University of South Alabama
Emergency Med Tech-Paramedic Prgm
2002 Old Bay Front Dr
Mobile, AL 36615
www.southalabama.edu

Trenholm State Technical College
Emergency Med Tech-Paramedic Prgm
1225 Air Base Blvd
Montgomery, AL 36108
www.trenholmtech.cc.al.us

Northwest-Shoals Community College
Emergency Med Tech-Paramedic Prgm
PO Box 2545
Muscle Shoals, AL 35662
www.nwscc.cc.al.us

Southern Union State Community College
Emergency Med Tech-Paramedic Prgm
1701 Lafayette Pkwy
Opelika, AL 36801
www.suscc.edu

Northeast Alabama Community College
Emergency Med Tech-Paramedic Prgm
PO Box 159
Rainsville, AL 35986-0159
www.nacc.edu

Bevill State Community College
Emergency Med Tech-Paramedic Prgm
PO Box 800 Sumiton
Sumiton, AL 35148
www.bscc.edu/mainsumiton.asp

Alaska

University of Alaska - Fairbanks Community & Technical College
Emergency Med Tech-Paramedic Prgm
Box 758120
Fairbanks, AK 99775

Arizona

Mohave Community College
Emergency Med Tech-Paramedic Prgm
1971 Jagerson Ave
Kingman, AZ 86401

Yavapai County Health Department
Emergency Med Tech-Paramedic Prgm
6955 Panther Path
Prescott, AZ 86314

Pima Community College
Emergency Med Tech-Paramedic Prgm
401 N Bonita Ave
Tucson, AZ 85709

Arkansas

Univ of Arkansas Comm Coll - Batesville
Emergency Med Tech-Paramedic Prgm
2005 White Dr, PO Box 3350
Batesville, AR 72501
www.uaccb.edu

NorthWest Arkansas Community College
Emergency Med Tech-Paramedic Prgm
1 College Dr
Bentonville, AR 72712
www.nwacc.edu
Prgm Dir: Jamin Snarr, NREMT-P BSEd
Tel: 479 619-4251 *Fax:* 479 619-4254
E-mail: jsnarr@nwacc.edu

Arkansas Northeastern College
Emergency Med Tech-Paramedic Prgm
I-55 and Hwy 148
Burdette, AR 72321
www.anc.edu

South Arkansas Community College
Emergency Med Tech-Paramedic Prgm
PO Box 7010
El Dorado, AR 71731

East Arkansas Community College
Emergency Med Tech-Paramedic Prgm
1700 Newcastle Rd
Forrest City, AR 72335
www.eacc.edu

North Arkansas College
Emergency Med Tech-Paramedic Prgm
1515 Pioneer Dr
Harrison, AR 72601
www.northark.edu

Univ of Arkansas Comm Coll - Hope
Emergency Med Tech-Paramedic Prgm
PO Box 140
Hope, AR 71801
www.uacch.edu

National Park Community College
Emergency Med Tech-Paramedic Prgm
101 College Dr
Hot Springs, AR 71913
www.npcc.edu

University of Arkansas for Medical Sciences
Emergency Med Tech-Paramedic Prgm
4301 W Markham St
CHRP, UAMS, #635
Little Rock, AR 72205
www.uams.edu

U of Arkansas at Monticello Coll of Tech
Emergency Med Tech-Paramedic Prgm
124 Sunset Lane
PO Box 747
McGehee, AR 71654-9329
www.uamont.edu

Arkansas Tech University - Ozark Campus
Emergency Med Tech-Paramedic Prgm
1700 Helberg Lane
Ozark, AR 72949
www.atuoc.atu.edu

Southeast Arkansas College
Emergency Med Tech-Paramedic Prgm
1900 Hazel St
Pine Bluff, AR 71603
www.seark.edu

Black River Technical College
Emergency Med Tech-Paramedic Prgm
PO Box 468
Pocahontas, AR 72455
www.blackrivertech.edu

Arkansas State University - Beebe
Emergency Med Tech-Paramedic Prgm
PO Box 909
Searcy, AR 72145
http://asub.edu

California

College of the Redwoods
Emergency Med Tech-Paramedic Prgm
220 F St
Arcata, CA 95521

Bakersfield College
Emergency Med Tech-Paramedic Prgm
1801 Panorama Dr
Bakersfield, CA 93305
www.bakersfieldcollege.edu

National College of Technical Instruction - Santa Barbara
Emergency Med Tech-Paramedic Prgm
240 E Highway 246 Suite 200
Buellton, CA 93427-9645

California State University - Chico
Emergency Med Tech-Paramedic Prgm
PO Box 906
Chico, CA 95927

Palomar Community College
Emergency Med Tech-Paramedic Prgm
1951 E Valley Pkwy
Escondido, CA 92026
www.palomar.edu

North Coast Emergency Medical Services
Cosponsor: College of the Redwoods
Emergency Med Tech-Paramedic Prgm
7351 Tompkins Hill Rd
Eureka, CA 95501
www.redwoods.edu/departments/paramedic

California EMS Academy Inc
Emergency Med Tech-Paramedic Prgm
1098 Foster City Blvd, Ste 106 PMB 708
Foster City, CA 94404
www.caems-academy.com

Fresno City College
Emergency Med Tech-Paramedic Prgm
1901 E Shields, Ste 250
Fresno, CA 93726
www.fccti.com

Fresno County Paramedic Program
Emergency Med Tech-Paramedic Prgm
1221 Fulton Mall
Fresno, CA 93721
www.fresnocitycollege.edu

Imperial Valley Community College
Emergency Med Tech-Paramedic Prgm
380 E Aten Rd
PO Box 158
Imperial, CA 92251
www.imperial.edu
Prgm Dir: Rick Goldsberry, Director of EMS Trainiig
Programs
Tel: 760 355-6275 *Fax:* 760 355-6346
E-mail: rick.goldsberry@imperial.edu

University of Antelope Valley (UAV)
Emergency Med Tech-Paramedic Prgm
44055 N Sierra Hwy
Lancaster, CA 93534

National College of Technical Instruction - Bay Area Counties
Emergency Med Tech-Paramedic Prgm
7543 Southfront Rd #A
Livermore, CA 94550
www.ncti-online.com

UCLA Medical Center, Department of Pathology
Emergency Med Tech-Paramedic Prgm
UCLA-Daniel Freeman Paramedic Education Program
Box 957367
405 Hilgard Ave
Los Angeles, CA 90095
www.uclahealth.org

Saddleback College
Emergency Med Tech-Paramedic Prgm
28000 Marguerite Pkwy
Mission Viejo, CA 92692
www.saddleback.edu

Napa Valley College
Emergency Med Tech-Paramedic Prgm
2277 Napa Vallejo Hwy
Napa, CA 94558

Butte College
Emergency Med Tech-Paramedic Prgm
3536 Butte Campus Dr
Oroville, CA 95965
www.butte.edu

Foothill College
Emergency Med Tech-Paramedic Prgm
4000 Middlefield Rd, Ste I
Palo Alto, CA 94303
www.foothill.edu

Moreno Valley College
Emergency Med Tech-Paramedic Prgm
Ben Clark Training Center 16888 Bundy Ave
Riverside, CA 92518

Riverside Comm Coll - Moreno Valley Campus
Emergency Med Tech-Paramedic Prgm
16888 Bundy Ave
Ben Clark Training Center
Riverside, CA 92518
www.rcc.edu

National College of Technical Instruction - Riverside
Emergency Med Tech-Paramedic Prgm
333 Sunrise Ave, Ste 500
Roseville, CA 95661
www.ncti-online.com

National College of Technical Instruction - Roseville
Emergency Med Tech-Paramedic Prgm
333 Sunrise Ave Suite 500
Roseville, CA 95661

American River College
Emergency Med Tech-Paramedic Prgm
4700 College Oak Dr
Sacramento, CA 95841-4217
www.arc.losrios.edu

California State University - Sacramento
Emergency Med Tech-Paramedic Prgm
3000 State University Drive East Napa Hall
Sacramento, CA 95819

Emergency Medical Sciences Training Institute
Emergency Med Tech-Paramedic Prgm
1104 Corporate Way
Sacramento, CA 95831

National College of Technical Instruction - San Diego
Emergency Med Tech-Paramedic Prgm
2655 Camino Del Rio North Suite 400
San Diego, CA 92108

Southwestern College
Emergency Med Tech-Paramedic Prgm
Higher Education Center, Otay Mesa
8100 Gigantic St 900 Otay Lakes Rd
San Diego, CA 91910
www.swccd.edu

City College of San Francisco
Emergency Med Tech-Paramedic Prgm
1860 Hayes St
San Francisco, CA 94117
www.ccsf.edu

WestMed College
Emergency Med Tech-Paramedic Prgm
3031 Tisch Way
San Jose, CA 95128
www.westmedtraining.com

Cuesta College
Emergency Med Tech-Paramedic Prgm
PO Box 8106
San Luis Obispo, CA 93403

Emergency Training Services Inc
Emergency Med Tech-Paramedic Prgm
3050 Paul Sweet Rd
Santa Cruz, CA 95065
www.emergencytraining.com

IEC Corporation
Emergency Med Tech-Paramedic Prgm
3050 Paul Sweet Rd
Santa Cruz, CA 95065

Los Angeles County EMS Agency
Cosponsor: El Camino College
Emergency Med Tech-Paramedic Prgm
10100 Pioneer Blvd, Suite 200
Santa Fe Springs, CA 90670
http://ems.dhs.lacounty.gov/

Emergency Medical Sciences Training Institute
Cosponsor: San Joaquin County EMS Agency
Emergency Med Tech-Paramedic Prgm
1801 E March Lane Suite 260
Stockton, CA 95210
www.emsti.com

Mendocino Community College
Emergency Med Tech-Paramedic Prgm
1000 Hensley Creek Rd
Ukiah, CA 95482
www.mendocino.edu

Ventura College
Emergency Med Tech-Paramedic Prgm
4667 Telegraph Rd
Ventura, CA 93003
www.venturacollege.edu

Victor Valley Community College District
Emergency Med Tech-Paramedic Prgm
18422 Bear Valley Rd
Victorville, CA 92395
www.vvc.edu

Mt San Antonio College
Emergency Med Tech-Paramedic Prgm
1100 N Grand Ave
Walnut, CA 91789
www.mtsac.edu

National College of Technical Instruction - Siskiyous County
Emergency Med Tech-Paramedic Prgm
800 College Ave
Weed, CA 96094

Santa Rosa Junior College
Emergency Med Tech-Paramedic Prgm
5743 Skylane Blvd
Windsor, CA 95492
www.santarosa.edu/ps

Crafton Hills College
Emergency Med Tech-Paramedic Prgm
11711 Sand Canyon Rd
Yucaipa, CA 92399
www.craftonhills.edu

Colorado

Pikes Peak Community College
Emergency Med Tech-Paramedic Prgm
5675 S Academy Blvd, CC-13
Colorado Springs, CO 80906
www.ppcc.edu

Centura Health-St Anthony Hospitals
Emergency Med Tech-Paramedic Prgm
4231 W 16th Ave, Ste 413
Denver, CO 80204
www.sahems.org

Community College of Aurora
Emergency Med Tech-Paramedic Prgm
9235 E 10th Drive, Room 118
Denver, CO 80230
www.ccaurora.edu/ems

Denver Health Medical Center
Emergency Med Tech-Paramedic Prgm
190 W 6th Ave
Mail Code 3652
Denver, CO 80204
www.denverhealth.org/education

Colorado Mountain College
Emergency Med Tech-Paramedic Prgm
150 Miller Ranch Rd
Edwards, CO 81632
http://coloradomtn.edu

HealthONE EMS
Cosponsor: Arapahoe Community College
Emergency Med Tech-Paramedic Prgm
333 W Hampden Ave #200
Englewood, CO 80110
www.healthONEcares.com
Prgm Dir: Patricia Tritt, RN MA
Tel: 303 788-6236   *Fax:* 303 788-7656
E-mail: patricia.tritt@healthonecares.com

Colorado Mesa University
Emergency Med Tech-Paramedic Prgm
1100 North Ave
Grand Junction, CO 81501
www.mesastate.edu

Mesa State College
Emergency Med Tech-Paramedic Prgm
1100 North Ave
Grand Junction, CO 81501

Aims Community College
Emergency Med Tech-Paramedic Prgm
5401 W 20th St PO Box 69
Greeley, CO 80632

Pueblo Community College
Emergency Med Tech-Paramedic Prgm
900 W Orman Ave
Pueblo, CO 81004
www.pueblocc.edu

Connecticut

Capital Community College
Emergency Med Tech-Paramedic Prgm
950 Main St
Hartford, CT 06103
www.ccc.commnet.edu
Prgm Dir: Terry DeVito, EdD RN EMT-P EMS I
Tel: 860 906-5153   *Fax:* 860 906-5148
E-mail: tdevito@ccc.commnet.edu

New Haven Sponsor Hospital
Emergency Med Tech-Paramedic Prgm
77-D Willow St
New Haven, CT 06511

Delaware

Delaware Technical Community College - Dover
Emergency Med Tech-Paramedic Prgm
100 Campus Dr
ETB 706 Terry Campus
Dover, DE 19904
www.dtcc.edu

Florida

Manatee Technical Institute
Emergency Med Tech-Paramedic Prgm
5520 Lakewood Ranch Blvd
Bradenton, FL 34211
www.manateetechnicalinstitute.org

Brevard Community College
Emergency Med Tech-Paramedic Prgm
1519 Clearlake Rd
Cocoa, FL 32922
www.brevardcc.edu

Broward College
Emergency Med Tech-Paramedic Prgm
3501 SW Davie Rd
Bldg 8
Davie, FL 33314
www.broward.edu

Daytona State College, Daytona Beach Campus
Emergency Med Tech-Paramedic Prgm
1200 W International Speedway Blvd
Building 320 - EMS
Daytona Beach, FL 32120-2811
www.daytonastate.edu

Lake Technical Center
Emergency Med Tech-Paramedic Prgm
2001 Kurt St
Eustis, FL 32726
www.laketech.org

Edison State College
Emergency Med Tech-Paramedic Prgm
8099 College Pkwy SW, PO Box 06210
Fort Myers, FL 33906-6210
www.edison.edu

Indian River State College
Emergency Med Tech-Paramedic Prgm
3209 Virginia Ave
Fort Pierce, FL 34981-5599
www.irsc.edu

Santa Fe College
Emergency Med Tech-Paramedic Prgm
3737 NE 39th Ave
Institute of Public Safety
Gainesville, FL 32609
www.sfcollege.edu/centers/kirkpatrick/ems/

Florida State College at Jacksonville
Emergency Med Tech-Paramedic Prgm
North Campus, 4501 Capper Rd
Jacksonville, FL 32218
www.fscj.edu
Prgm Dir: Marjorie Heatherington, MA EMT-P
Tel: 904 766-6513   *Fax:* 904 766-5573
E-mail: mheather@fscj.edu

Florida Gateway College
Emergency Med Tech-Paramedic Prgm
Emergency Medical Paramedic Program 149 SE College
  Place
Lake City, FL 32025

Palm Beach State College
Emergency Med Tech-Paramedic Prgm
4200 S Congress Ave, MS60
Lake Worth, FL 33461
www.pbcc.edu

Dade Medical College
Emergency Med Tech-Paramedic Prgm
Medical Center Campus
950 NW 20th St
Miami, FL 33127
www.mdc.edu

Pasco-Hernando Community College
Emergency Med Tech-Paramedic Prgm
10230 Ridge Rd
New Port Richey, FL 34654-5199
www.phcc.edu

College of Central Florida
Emergency Med Tech-Paramedic Prgm
PO Box 1388
3001 SW College Rd
Ocala, FL 34478
www.cfu.edu

Valencia College
Emergency Med Tech-Paramedic Prgm
PO Box 3028
1800 S Kirkman Rd
Orlando, FL 32811
www.valenciacc.edu

Gulf Coast State College
Emergency Med Tech-Paramedic Prgm
5230 W US Hwy 98
Panama City, FL 32401
www.gulfcoast.edu

Pensacola State College
Emergency Med Tech-Paramedic Prgm
Warrington Campus
5555 W Hwy 98
Pensacola, FL 32507-1097
www.pjc.edu

Seminole State College
Emergency Med Tech-Paramedic Prgm
100 Weldon Blvd
Sanford, FL 32773-6199
www.scc-fl.edu

Sarasota County Technical Institute
Emergency Med Tech-Paramedic Prgm
4748 Beneva Rd
Sarasota, FL 34233
www.SarasotaTech.org

St Petersburg College
Emergency Med Tech-Paramedic Prgm
Health Education Ctr
PO Box 13489
St Petersburg, FL 33733
www.spcollege.edu

First Coast Technical College
Emergency Med Tech-Paramedic Prgm
2980 Collins Ave
St. Augustine, FL 32084-1921

Tallahassee Community College
Emergency Med Tech-Paramedic Prgm
444 Appleyard Dr
Tallahassee, FL 32304
www.tcc.fl.edu

Hillsborough Community College
Emergency Med Tech-Paramedic Prgm
PO Box 30030
Tampa, FL 33630
www.hccfl.edu
Prgm Dir: William D Corso, RN EMT-P MA
Tel: 813 253-7454   *Fax:* 813 253-7464
E-mail: bcorso@hccfl.edu

Polk State College
Emergency Med Tech-Paramedic Prgm
999 Ave H NE
Winter Haven, FL 33881-4299
www.polk.edu

Georgia

Gwinnett County Fire and Emergency Services
Emergency Med Tech-Paramedic Prgm
3608 Braselton Hwy
Dacula, GA 30019

Gwinnett Technical College
Emergency Med Tech-Paramedic Prgm
5150 Sugarloaf Pkwy
Lawrenceville, GA 30043-5702
www.gwinnetttech.edu

Georgia Northwestern Technical College - Rome
Emergency Med Tech-Paramedic Prgm
One Maurice Culberson Drive
Rome, GA 30161

Idaho

Idaho State University
Emergency Med Tech-Paramedic Prgm
College of Technology
Box 8380
Pocatello, ID 83209-8380
www.isu.edu

Brigham Young University
Emergency Med Tech-Paramedic Prgm
Clarke Building 145-M
Rexburg, ID 83460

College of Southern Idaho
Emergency Med Tech-Paramedic Prgm
315 Falls Ave, PO Box 1238
Twin Falls, ID 83303
www.csi.edu/paramedic

Illinois

Advocate Good Samaritan Hospital
Emergency Med Tech-Paramedic Prgm
3815 Highland Ave
Downers Grove, IL 60515

Loyola University Medical Center
Emergency Med Tech-Paramedic Prgm
2160 S First Ave
Building 110LL, Room 0221
Maywood, IL 60153
www.lumc.edu

Swedish American Hospital
Emergency Med Tech-Paramedic Prgm
1401 East State St
Rockford, IL 61104

Indiana

St Francis Hospital & Health Centers
Emergency Med Tech-Paramedic Prgm
1600 Albany St
Beech Grove, IN 46107
www.ssfhs.org

Ivy Tech Community College - Bloomington
Emergency Med Tech-Paramedic Prgm
200 Daniels Way
Bloomington, IN 47404

Pelham - Ball Memorial Consortium
Emergency Med Tech-Paramedic Prgm
699 E Dillman Rd
Bloomington, IN 47401

Ivy Tech Community College - Columbus
Emergency Med Tech-Paramedic Prgm
4475 Central Ave
Columbus, IN 47203
www.ivytech.edu

Harrison County Hospital Paramedic Consortium
Emergency Med Tech-Paramedic Prgm
1141 Hospital Drive NW
Corydon, IN 47112

St Anthony Medical Center
Emergency Med Tech-Paramedic Prgm
1201 S Main St
Crown Point, IN 46307

Adams Memorial Hospital
Emergency Med Tech-Paramedic Prgm
1100 Mercer Ave
Decatur, IN 46733

Elkhart General Hospital
Emergency Med Tech-Paramedic Prgm
600 E Blvd
Elkhart, IN 46514
www.egh.org

Ivy Tech Community College
Cosponsor: St Mary's Medical Center and Deaconess
  Hospital
Emergency Med Tech-Paramedic Prgm
3501 First Ave
Evansville Paramedic Science Program
Evansville, IN 47710
www.ivytech.edu

Ivy Tech Community College - Northeast
Emergency Med Tech-Paramedic Prgm
3800 N Anthony Blvd
Fort Wayne, IN 46805
www.ivytech.edu

Methodist Hospitals Inc
Emergency Med Tech-Paramedic Prgm
Midlake Campus
2269 W 2269th Ave
Gary, IN 46404
www.methodisthospitals.org

Indiana University Health - Goshen Hospital
Emergency Med Tech-Paramedic Prgm
200 High Park Ave
Goshen, IN 46526

Community Health Network
Emergency Med Tech-Paramedic Prgm
1500 N Ritter Ave Lower Level-Bldg 3, Suite 3
Indianapolis, IN 46219

Indiana University
Emergency Med Tech-Paramedic Prgm
Paramedic Science Program Room 100
3930 Georgetown Rd
Indianapolis, IN 46254

Indiana University Health
Cosponsor: Methodist Hospital
Emergency Med Tech-Paramedic Prgm
Wile Hall Rm 631
1701 N Senate Blvd
Department of Emergency Medicine
Indianapolis, IN 46202
www.medicine.iu.edu

St Vincent Hosp & Health Care Ctr
Emergency Med Tech-Paramedic Prgm
2001 W 86th St
Indianapolis, IN 46260

Howard Regional Health System
Emergency Med Tech-Paramedic Prgm
3500 S Lafountain
Kokomo, IN 46902

Ivy Tech Community College - Kokomo
Emergency Med Tech-Paramedic Prgm
700 E Firmin St
PO Box 1373
Kokomo, IN 46903-1373
www.ivytech.edu

Ivy Tech Community College - North Central
Emergency Med Tech-Paramedic Prgm
220 Dean Johnson Blvd
South Bend, IN 46601-3415

Ivy Tech Community College
Emergency Med Tech-Paramedic Prgm
8000 S Education Dr
Terre Haute, IN 47802
www.ivytech.edu

Vincennes University
Emergency Med Tech-Paramedic Prgm
1002 First St, North
Vincennes, IN 47591

Iowa

Kirkwood Community College
Emergency Med Tech-Paramedic Prgm
6301 Kirkwood Blvd SW
PO Box 2068
Cedar Rapids, IA 52310
www.kirkwood.edu

Mercy Medical Center - Des Moines
Emergency Med Tech-Paramedic Prgm
207 Crocker, Ste 100
Des Moines, IA 50309
www.mchs.edu

University of Iowa Hospitals & Clinics
Emergency Med Tech-Paramedic Prgm
200 Hawkins Dr, S608-1 GH
EMS Learning Resources Center
Iowa City, IA 52242
www.uihealthcare.com

Indian Hills Community College
Emergency Med Tech-Paramedic Prgm
655 Indian Hills Drive Bldg 21
Ottumwa, IA 52501

Western Iowa Tech Community College
Emergency Med Tech-Paramedic Prgm
Box 5199
Sioux City, IA 51102

Southeastern Community College
Emergency Med Tech-Paramedic Prgm
1500 West Agency Rd
West Burlington, IA 52655

Kansas

Coffeyville Community College
Emergency Med Tech-Paramedic Prgm
400 W 11th St
Coffeyville, KS 67337
www.coffeyville.edu/emt

Flint Hills Technical College
Emergency Med Tech-Paramedic Prgm
3301 W 18th St
Emporia, KS 66801
www.fhtc.net

Garden City Community College
Emergency Med Tech-Paramedic Prgm
801 Campus Dr
John Collins Vocational Building
Garden City, KS 67846
www.gcccks.edu

Barton County Community College
Emergency Med Tech-Paramedic Prgm
245 NE 30th Rd
Great Bend, KS 67530
www.bartonccc.edu/instruction/programs/
    emergencyservices.html

Hutchinson Community College
Emergency Med Tech-Paramedic Prgm
1300 North Plum
Hutchinson, KS 67501

Kansas City Kansas Community College
Emergency Med Tech-Paramedic Prgm
7250 State Ave
Kansas City, KS 66112
www.kckcc.cc.ks.us

Johnson County Community College
Emergency Med Tech-Paramedic Prgm
12345 College Blvd
Department of Emergency Medical Science
Overland Park, KS 66210-1299
www.jccc.edu

Cowley County Community College
Emergency Med Tech-Paramedic Prgm
1406 E 8th St
Winfield, KS 67156
www.cowley.edu/departments/allied/ems/

Kentucky

Eastern Kentucky University
Emergency Med Tech-Paramedic Prgm
Dizney 225
521 Lancaster Ave
Richmond, KY 40475-3135
www.eku.edu

Louisiana

Louisiana State U Fire & Emergency Training I
Emergency Med Tech-Paramedic Prgm
6868 Nicholson Drive
Baton Rouge, LA 70820

Bossier Parish Community College
Emergency Med Tech-Paramedic Prgm
6220 E Texas St
Bossier City, LA 71111
www.bpcc.edu

National EMS Academy /South Louisiana Community College
Emergency Med Tech-Paramedic Prgm
2916 North University
Lafayette, LA 70507

Delgado Community College
Emergency Med Tech-Paramedic Prgm
615 City Park Ave
Bldg 4, Room 136
New Orleans, LA 70119
www.dcc.edu

Maryland

Anne Arundel Community College
Emergency Med Tech-Paramedic Prgm
101 College Pkwy
Arnold, MD 21012-1895
www.aacc.edu
Prgm Dir: Melanie Miller, MSN RN CCRN NREMT-P
Tel: 410 777-7385   *Fax:* 410 777-7099
E-mail: mkmiller@aacc.edu

Community College of Baltimore County
Emergency Med Tech-Paramedic Prgm
7201 Rossville Blvd
Baltimore, MD 21237
www.ccbcmd.edu

University of Maryland Baltimore County
Emergency Med Tech-Paramedic Prgm
1000 Hilltop Circle
316 AC IV
Academic IV, Room 316
Baltimore, MD 21250
www.umbc.edu/ehs

Howard Community College
Emergency Med Tech-Paramedic Prgm
10901 Little Patuxent Pkwy
Columbia, MD 21045
www.howardcc.edu

Associates in Emergency Care
Emergency Med Tech-Paramedic Prgm
PO Box 490
Damascus, MD 20872

Hagerstown Community College
Emergency Med Tech-Paramedic Prgm
11400 Robinwood Drive
Hagerstown, MD 21742

Massachusetts

Pro EMS Center for Medics
Emergency Med Tech-Paramedic Prgm
31 Smith Place
Cambridge, MA 02138

Michigan

Huron Valley Ambulance
Emergency Med Tech-Paramedic Prgm
1200 State Circle
Ann Arbor, MI 48108
www.hva.org
Prgm Dir: Shaun Pochik, BS EMTP
Tel: 734 477-6731   *Fax:* 734 477-6927
E-mail: spochik@hva.org

Kalamazoo Valley Community College
Emergency Med Tech-Paramedic Prgm
Texas Township Campus 6767 West O Ave, PO Box 4070
Kalamazoo, MI 49003

Lansing Community College
Emergency Med Tech-Paramedic Prgm
3100-HHPS Division
500 N Washington, PO Box 40010
Lansing, MI 48901-7210
www.lcc.edu

Minnesota

Northland Community & Technical College
Emergency Med Tech-Paramedic Prgm
2022 Central Ave NE
East Grand Forks, MN 56721
www.northlandcollege.edu

Mesabi Range Community and Technical College
Emergency Med Tech-Paramedic Prgm
1100 Industrial Park Drive
Eveleth, MN 55734

ER Training Assoc/Greater Minn Paramedic Cons
Cosponsor: Emergency Training Associates
Emergency Med Tech-Paramedic Prgm
PO Box 1014
214 East Junius Ave
Fergus Falls, MN 56537
www.emergencytrainingassociates.com

Inver Hills Community College
Emergency Med Tech-Paramedic Prgm
2500 E 80th St
Inver Grove Heights, MN 55076-3224
www.inverhills.edu

Hennepin County Medical Center
Emergency Med Tech-Paramedic Prgm
701 Park Ave, MC 825
Minneapolis, MN 55415

Ridgewater College - Willmar Campus
Emergency Med Tech-Paramedic Prgm
701 Park Ave #825
Minneapolis, MN 55415

South Central College
Emergency Med Tech-Paramedic Prgm
1920 Lee Blvd
North Mankato, MN 56003
www.southcentral.edu

Rochester Community & Technical College
Emergency Med Tech-Paramedic Prgm
851 30th Ave SE
Rochester, MN 55904
www.rctc.edu/program/icp/

St Cloud Technical and Community College
Emergency Med Tech-Paramedic Prgm
1540 Northway Dr
St Cloud, MN 56303
www.sctc.edu

Century College
Emergency Med Tech-Paramedic Prgm
3300 Century Ave N
White Bear Lake, MN 55110
www.century.edu/ems
Prgm Dir: Chris Caulkins,
Tel: 651 779-5743   *Fax:* 651 779-5797
E-mail: chris.caulkins@century.edu

Mississippi

East Central Community College
Emergency Med Tech-Paramedic Prgm
PO Box 129
Decatur, MS 39327
www.eccc.edu

Jones County Junior College
Emergency Med Tech-Paramedic Prgm
900 S Court St
Ellisville, MS 39437
www.jcjc.edu
Prgm Dir: Gregory M Cole, MPH NREMT-P CCEMT-P
   FP-C
Tel: 601 477-4074   *Fax:* 601 477-4152
E-mail: mike.cole@jcjc.edu

Itawamba Community College
Emergency Med Tech-Paramedic Prgm
602 W Hill St
Fulton, MS 38843
www.icc.cc.ms.us

Mississippi Gulf Coast Community College
Emergency Med Tech-Paramedic Prgm
2226 Switzer Rd
Gulfport, MS 39507
www.mgccc.edu

Hinds Community College - Jackson
Emergency Med Tech-Paramedic Prgm
1750 Chadwick Drive
Jackson, MS 39204

East Mississippi Community College
Emergency Med Tech-Paramedic Prgm
8731 South Frontage Rd
Mayhew, MS 39753

Holmes Community College
Emergency Med Tech-Paramedic Prgm
412 W Ridgeland Ave
Ridgeland, MS 39157
www.holmescc.edu

Northwest Mississippi Community College
Emergency Med Tech-Paramedic Prgm
4975 Hwy 51 N
Box 7020
Senatobia, MS 38668
www.northwestms.edu

Missouri

Cape Girardeau Career & Technology Center
Emergency Med Tech-Paramedic Prgm
1080 South Silver Springs Rd
Cape Girardeau, MO 63703

Grand River Technical School
Emergency Med Tech-Paramedic Prgm
235 Southwest Drive
Chillicothe, MO 64601

Ozarks Technical Community College
Emergency Med Tech-Paramedic Prgm
1001 East Chestnut Expressway
Springfield, MO 65802-3625

IHM Health Studies Center
Cosponsor: Washington University School of Medicine
Emergency Med Tech-Paramedic Prgm
2500 Abbott Pl
St Louis, MO 63143
www.ihmhealthstudies.com

South Howell County Ambulance District
Emergency Med Tech-Paramedic Prgm
1951 East State Rt K
West Plains, MO 65775

Montana

Montana State University Billings
Emergency Med Tech-Paramedic Prgm
3803 Central Ave
Billings, MT 59102
www.msubillings.edu/cot
Prgm Dir: David Gurchiek, PhD NREMT-P
Tel: 406 247-3076   *Fax:* 406 247-3026
E-mail: dgurchiek@msubillings.edu

Montana State Univ - Great Falls Coll of Tech
Emergency Med Tech-Paramedic Prgm
College of Technology 2100 16th Ave S
Great Falls, MT 59405

Nebraska

Central Community College
Emergency Med Tech-Paramedic Prgm
PO Box 4903
Grand Island, NE 68802

Creighton University
Emergency Med Tech-Paramedic Prgm
EMS Education
2514 Cuming St
Omaha, NE 68131
www.creighton.edu/ems/
Prgm Dir: Michael Miller, MS BS EMS RN NREMT-P
Tel: 402 280-1280   *Fax:* 402 280-1288
E-mail: mikemiller@creighton.edu

Metropolitan Community College - Omaha
Emergency Med Tech-Paramedic Prgm
Box 3777
Omaha, NE 68103

Nevada

College of Southern Nevada
Emergency Med Tech-Paramedic Prgm
6375 West Charleston Blvd W2B-204M
Las Vegas, NV 89146
www.csn.edu

New Hampshire

NHTI, Concord's Community College
Emergency Med Tech-Paramedic Prgm
31 College Dr
Concord, NH 03301
www.ccsnh.edu
Prgm Dir: Nancy L Brubaker, MEd EMT-P RN
Tel: 603 271-7157   *Fax:* 603 271-8650
E-mail: nbrubaker@ccsnh.edu

New England EMS Institute
Emergency Med Tech-Paramedic Prgm
One Elliot Way
Manchester, NH 03103
www.neemsi.org

New Jersey

Jersey City Medical Center EMS
Emergency Med Tech-Paramedic Prgm
415 Montgomery St
Union City, NJ 07302

New Mexico

Central New Mexico Community College
Emergency Med Tech-Paramedic Prgm
5600 Eagle Rock Ave
Albuquerque, NM 87113

University of New Mexico
Emergency Med Tech-Paramedic Prgm
School of Medicine
2700 Yale Blvd SE
Ste 100
Albuquerque, NM 87106
www.unm.edu

Dona Ana Community College
Emergency Med Tech-Paramedic Prgm
Box 30001, Dept 3DA
3400 South Espina, MSC 3DA
Las Cruces, NM 88003
http://dabcc.nmsu.edu
Prgm Dir: Joyce S Bradley, NREMT-P AAS BHCS
Tel: 575 527-7645   *Fax:* 575 528-7035
E-mail: jobradle@nmsu.edu

Eastern New Mexico University - Roswell
Emergency Med Tech-Paramedic Prgm
PO Box 6000
52 University Blvd
Roswell, NM 88202-6000
www.enmu.edu

Santa Fe Community College
Emergency Med Tech-Paramedic Prgm
6401 Richards Ave
Santa Fe, NM 87508

New York

New York Methodist Hospital
Emergency Med Tech-Paramedic Prgm
2009 85th St
Brooklyn, NY 11214

SUNY Cobleskill
Emergency Med Tech-Paramedic Prgm
State Route 7
Home Economics Bldg, Room 101
Cobleskill, NY 12043

Nassau Community College /Nassau County Fire Police EMS Academy at NUMC
Emergency Med Tech-Paramedic Prgm
2201 Hempstead Turnpike, Box 80 Bldg B, 2nd floor
East Meadow, NY 11554

St. John's University
Emergency Med Tech-Paramedic Prgm
Dr Andrew J Bartilucci Center 175-05 Horace Harding Expwy
Fresh Meadows, NY 11365

CUNY Borough of Manhattan Community Coll
Emergency Med Tech-Paramedic Prgm
199 Chambers St North
Dept of Allied Hlth Sciences
New York, NY 10007
www.bmcc.cuny.edu

Monroe Community College
Emergency Med Tech-Paramedic Prgm
1190 Scottsville Rd, Ste 216
MCC
Rochester, NY 14624
www.monroecc.edu

Hudson Valley Community College
Emergency Med Tech-Paramedic Prgm
80 Vandenburgh Ave
Troy, NY 12180
www.hvcc.edu

Faxton - St Luke's Healthcare
Emergency Med Tech-Paramedic Prgm
2521 Sunset Ave
Utica, NY 13502

Dutchess Community College
Emergency Med Tech-Paramedic Prgm
31 Marshall Rd
Wappingers Falls, NY 12590
www.sunydutchess.edu

North Carolina

Western Carolina University
Emergency Med Tech-Paramedic Prgm
122 Moore
Department of Health Sciences
Cullowhee, NC 28723
www.wcu.edu

Blue Ridge Community College
Emergency Med Tech-Paramedic Prgm
180 West Campus Drive
Flat Rock, NC 28731

Joint Special Operations Medical Training Ctr
Emergency Med Tech-Paramedic Prgm
Uniformed Services University of the Health Sciences
SWMG(A), USAJFKSWCS, AOJK-MED, Stop A
3004 Ardennes St
Fort Bragg, NC 28310

Catawba Valley Community College
Emergency Med Tech-Paramedic Prgm
2550 Hwy 70 SE
Hickory, NC 28602-9699
www.cvcc.edu
Prgm Dir: Tonja Pool, BS NREMT-P NCEMT-P
Tel: 828 327-7000, Ext 4167   *Fax:* 828 624-5250
E-mail: tpool@cvcc.edu

Southwestern Community College - Sylva
Emergency Med Tech-Paramedic Prgm
447 College Dr
Sylva, NC 28779

North Dakota

St Alexius Med Ctr/Bismarck State College
Emergency Med Tech-Paramedic Prgm
PO Box 5510
Bismarck, ND 58506-5510
www.bismarckstate.edu

F-M Ambulance-North Dakota State College of Sciences
Emergency Med Tech-Paramedic Prgm
2215 18th St South
Fargo, ND 58103
www.fmambulance.com

Ohio

Akron General Medical Center
Emergency Med Tech-Paramedic Prgm
400 Wabash Ave
Akron, OH 44307
www.agmc.org

Summa Health System
Emergency Med Tech-Paramedic Prgm
444 N Main St
Akron, OH 44310
www.summahealth.org

University of Cincinnati
Emergency Med Tech-Paramedic Prgm
9555 Plainfield Rd ML 0086
Cincinnati, OH 45236-0086
www.rwc.uc.edu

Columbus State Community College
Emergency Med Tech-Paramedic Prgm
550 E Spring St
Columbus, OH 43215
www.cscc.edu

Life Care EMS Training Academy /Lorain County CC Consortium
Emergency Med Tech-Paramedic Prgm
166 Railroad St
LaGrange, OH 44050

Owens Community College
Emergency Med Tech-Paramedic Prgm
PO Box 10000
Toledo, OH 43699

Youngstown State University
Emergency Med Tech-Paramedic Prgm
Department of Health Professions
One University Plaza
Youngstown, OH 44555-3327
www.ysu.edu
Notes: The program allows the EMS student to complete the Paramedic phase during the first year of college. After two more semesters, the AAS is awarded. Upon completion of two final years of classes, a 4 year degree in Health Professions is awarded.

Oklahoma

Great Plains Technology Center
Emergency Med Tech-Paramedic Prgm
4500 W Lee Blvd
Lawton, OK 73505

Oklahoma City Community College
Emergency Med Tech-Paramedic Prgm
7777 S May Ave
Oklahoma City, OK 73159
www.occc.edu

Kiamichi Technical Center
Emergency Med Tech-Paramedic Prgm
Box 825
Poteau, OK 74953

Gordon Cooper Technology Center
Emergency Med Tech-Paramedic Prgm
One John C Bruton Blvd
Shawnee, OK 74804

Oregon

Lane Community College
Emergency Med Tech-Paramedic Prgm
4000 E 30th Ave
Eugene, OR 97405

National College of Technical Instruction
Emergency Med Tech-Paramedic Prgm
College of Emergency Services 9800 SE McBrod #200
Milwaukie, OR 97222

Portland Community College
Emergency Med Tech-Paramedic Prgm
705 N Killingsworth St
Portland, OR 97280

Chemeketa Community College
Emergency Med Tech-Paramedic Prgm
4000 Lancaster Dr NE
PO Box 14007
Salem, OR 97309-7070
www.chemeketa.edu/programs/ems

Oregon Health & Science University
Cosponsor: Oregon Institute of Technology
Emergency Med Tech-Paramedic Prgm
12400 SW Tonquin Rd
Sherwood, OR 97140
www.oit.edu/paramedic

Pennsylvania

Lehigh Valley Hospital
Emergency Med Tech-Paramedic Prgm
2166 S 12th, Ground Floor
Allentown, PA 18103
www.lvh.com

Harrisburg Area Community College
Emergency Med Tech-Paramedic Prgm
One HACC Dr
Harrisburg, PA 17110-2999
www.hacc.edu

Conemaugh Valley Memorial Hospital
Emergency Med Tech-Paramedic Prgm
1086 Franklin St
Johnstown, PA 15905

Ctr for Emer Med of Western Pennsylvania
Emergency Med Tech-Paramedic Prgm
230 McKee Pl
Suite 500
Pittsburgh, PA 15213
www.centerem.com

Pennsylvania College of Technology
Emergency Med Tech-Paramedic Prgm
One College Ave
DIF105
Williamsport, PA 17701
www.pct.edu/schools/hs/paramedic

South Carolina

Trident Technical College
Emergency Med Tech-Paramedic Prgm
7000 Rivers Ave
PO Box 118067
Charleston, SC 29423-8067
www.tridenttech.edu
Notes: The program will be expanding to include
certifications at each EMT level: An initial EMT
paramedic program and an Advanced placement
program for currently certified paramedics who wish
to obtain their Associate's Degree.

Greenville Technical College
Emergency Med Tech-Paramedic Prgm
506 S Pleasantburg Dr 106D #702
PO Box 5616, Mailstop 1066
Greenville, SC 29606-5616
www.gvltec.edu

Horry - Georgetown Technical College
Emergency Med Tech-Paramedic Prgm
743 Hemlock Ave
Myrtle Beach, SC 29577

South Dakota

Avera McKennan Hospital
Emergency Med Tech-Paramedic Prgm
School of EMS
800 E 21st St
PO Box 5045
Sioux Falls, SD 57117
www.averamckennan.org

Lake Area Technical Institute
Emergency Med Tech-Paramedic Prgm
230 11th St NE
Watertown, SD 57201-0730

Tennessee

Northeast State Community College
Emergency Med Tech-Paramedic Prgm
PO Box 246
Blountville, TN 37617-0246

Chattanooga State Community College
Emergency Med Tech-Paramedic Prgm
4501 Amnicola Hwy
Chattanooga, TN 37406
www.chattanoogastate.edu

Columbia State Community College
Emergency Med Tech-Paramedic Prgm
PO Box 1315
1665 Hampshire Pike
Columbia, TN 38401
www.coscc.cc.tn.us

Tennessee Technological University
Emergency Med Tech-Paramedic Prgm
PO Box 5073
Cookeville, TN 38505

Volunteer State Community College
Emergency Med Tech-Paramedic Prgm
1480 Nashville Pike
Gallatin, TN 37066
www.volstate.edu

Jackson State Community College
Emergency Med Tech-Paramedic Prgm
2046 N Parkway St
Jackson, TN 38301-3797
www.jscc.edu

Roane State Community College
Emergency Med Tech-Paramedic Prgm
132 Hayfield Rd
Knoxville, TN 37922-2301
www.roanestate.edu

Southwest Tennessee Community College
Emergency Med Tech-Paramedic Prgm
PO Box 780
Memphis, TN 38101

Walters State Community College
Emergency Med Tech-Paramedic Prgm
500 S Davy Crockett Pkwy
Morristown, TN 37813-6899
www.ws.edu

Texas

Texas State Technical College - Abilene
Emergency Med Tech-Paramedic Prgm
650 E Hwy 80
Abilene, TX 79601

Austin Community College
Emergency Med Tech-Paramedic Prgm
3401 Webberville Rd
Austin, TX 78702
www.austincc.edu/health/emsp

Univ TX at Brownsville/TX Southmost Coll
Emergency Med Tech-Paramedic Prgm
80 Ft Brown
Brownsville, TX 78520
www.utb.edu

Blinn College
Emergency Med Tech-Paramedic Prgm
Texas A&M Health Science Center Clinical Building I
Suite 2500 8441 State Highway 47
Bryan, TX 77807
www.blinn.edu

Lone Star College-CyFair
Emergency Med Tech-Paramedic Prgm
9191 Barker Cypress Rd
Cypress, TX 77433

Univ of Texas Southwestern Med Ctr
Cosponsor: El Centro College
Emergency Med Tech-Paramedic Prgm
5323 Harry Hines Blvd
Dallas, TX 75390-9134
www.UTsouthwestern.edu

Grayson County College
Emergency Med Tech-Paramedic Prgm
6101 Grayson Drive
Denison, TX 75020

Brookhaven College
Emergency Med Tech-Paramedic Prgm
3939 Valley View Lane
Building X 1082
Farmers Branch, TX 75244
www.brookhavencollege.edu

Galveston College
Emergency Med Tech-Paramedic Prgm
4015 Ave Q
Galveston, TX 77550
www.gc.edu

Houston Community College
Emergency Med Tech-Paramedic Prgm
555 Community College Dr
Houston, TX 77013
www.hccs.edu

Lone Star College-North Harris
Emergency Med Tech-Paramedic Prgm
2700 W W Thorne Dr, Ste WN174
Houston, TX 77073
www.lonestar.edu

San Jacinto College North
Emergency Med Tech-Paramedic Prgm
5800 Uvalde Rd
Houston, TX 77049-4599
www.sjcd.edu
Prgm Dir: Joseph J Hamilton, MS LP EMS-C
Tel: 281 459-7151   *Fax:* 281 459-7603
E-mail: joe.hamilton@sjcd.edu

Tarrant County College
Emergency Med Tech-Paramedic Prgm
Northeast Campus
828 Harwood Rd
Hurst, TX 76054-3299
www.tccd.edu

Central Texas College
Emergency Med Tech-Paramedic Prgm
6200 W CTE
Killeen, TX 76549
www.ctcd.edu

Brazosport College
Emergency Med Tech-Paramedic Prgm
500 College Dr
Lake Jackson, TX 77566
www.brazosport.edu

South Plains College
Emergency Med Tech-Paramedic Prgm
1401 S College Ave
Levelland, TX 79336
www.southplainscollege.edu

South Plains College
Emergency Med Tech-Paramedic Prgm
516 Gilbert Drive, Building 2
Lubbock, TX 79416

Collin County Community College District
Emergency Med Tech-Paramedic Prgm
2200 West University Drive
McKinney, TX 75070-8001

Paris Junior College
Emergency Med Tech-Paramedic Prgm
2400 Clarksville St
Paris, TX 75460

San Jacinto College Central
Emergency Med Tech-Paramedic Prgm
8060 Spencer Hwy
PO Box 2007
Pasadena, TX 77501-2007
www.sjcd.us
Prgm Dir: Joseph J Hamilton, MS LP
Tel: 281 476-1501, Ext 1862   *Fax:* 713 478-2754
E-mail: Joe.Hamilton@sjcd.edu

San Antonio College
Emergency Med Tech-Paramedic Prgm
1300 San Pedro Ave
San Antonio, TX 782124299

UT Health Science Center - San Antonio
Emergency Med Tech-Paramedic Prgm
7703 Floyd Curl Dr
MC 7775
San Antonio, TX 78229-3900
www.uthscsa.edu/shp/ehs

Temple College
Emergency Med Tech-Paramedic Prgm
2600 South First St
Temple, TX 76504

College of the Mainland
Emergency Med Tech-Paramedic Prgm
1200 Amburn Rd
Texas City, TX 77591
www.com.edu

Weatherford College
Emergency Med Tech-Paramedic Prgm
225 College Park Drive
Weatherford, TX 76086

Wharton County Junior College
Emergency Med Tech-Paramedic Prgm
911 East Boling Highway
Wharton, TX 77488
www.wcjc.cc.tx.us

Utah

Weber State University
Emergency Med Tech-Paramedic Prgm
3902 University Circle
Ogden, UT 84408-3902
www.weber.edu
Prgm Dir: Jeffrey Grunow,
Tel: 801 626-6521   *Fax:* 801 626-6610
E-mail: jgrunow@weber.edu

Utah Valley University
Emergency Med Tech-Paramedic Prgm
3131 Mike Jense Parkway
FS-140
Provo, UT 84601
www.uvu.edu

Unified Fire Authority/Utah Valley University
Emergency Med Tech-Paramedic Prgm
3380 South 900 West
Salt Lake City, UT 84119
www.unitedfireauthority.org

University of Utah
Emergency Med Tech-Paramedic Prgm
Mt Nebo Training 1901 S Campus Drive Room 2068
Salt Lake City, UT 84112

Dixie State College of Utah
Emergency Med Tech-Paramedic Prgm
225 South 700 East
Taylor Bldg #250
St George, UT 84770
www.dixie.edu

Virginia

Piedmont Virginia Community College
Cosponsor: University of Virginia Dept of Emergency
    Medicine
Emergency Med Tech-Paramedic Prgm
501 College Dr
Charlottesville, VA 22902
www.pvcc.edu

Loudoun County Dept of Fire-Rescue
Emergency Med Tech-Paramedic Prgm
803 Sycolin Rd, Suite 104
Leesburg, VA 20175-5657
www.loudoun.gov/fire

Central Virginia Community College
Emergency Med Tech-Paramedic Prgm
3506 Wards Rd
Lynchburg, VA 24502

Southwest Virginia Community College
Cosponsor: MECC - VHCC - SWCC - WCC
Emergency Med Tech-Paramedic Prgm
PO Box SVCC
US Hwy 19
369 College Rd
Richlands, VA 24641
www.sw.edu/catalogs/AAS/emt.htm

J Sargeant Reynolds Community College
Emergency Med Tech-Paramedic Prgm
PO Box 85622
Richmond, VA 23285
www.reynolds.edu

Virginia Commonwealth Univ/Health System
Emergency Med Tech-Paramedic Prgm
PO Box 980044
Richmond, VA 23298-0044
www.vcu.edu

Jefferson College of Health Sciences
Emergency Med Tech-Paramedic Prgm
PO Box 13186
101 Elm Ave SE
Roanoke, VA 24013
www.jchs.edu

National College - (Salem) Roanoke Valley
Emergency Med Tech-Paramedic Prgm
1813 East Main St
Salem, VA 24153

Northern Virginia Community College
Emergency Med Tech-Paramedic Prgm
6699 Springfield Center Dr, Office 239
Springfield, VA 22150
www.nvcc.edu/medical/health/emt

Tidewater Community College
Emergency Med Tech-Paramedic Prgm
1700 College Crescent
Virginia Beach, VA 23456
www.tcc.edu

Washington

**Whatcom Medic One/Bellingham Fire Dept -
    Western Washington University**
Emergency Med Tech-Paramedic Prgm
1800 Broadway
Bellingham, WA 98225

Central Washington University
Emergency Med Tech-Paramedic Prgm
Dept of Nutrition, Exercise, and Health Sciences
400 E University Way
Ellensburg, WA 98926-7572
www.cwu.edu/~nehs/paramedics/

Columbia Basin College
Emergency Med Tech-Paramedic Prgm
2600 N 20th Ave
Mailstop R-2
Pasco, WA 99301
www.columbiabasin.edu

University of Washington
Emergency Med Tech-Paramedic Prgm
325 Ninth Ave, Mailbox 359727
Seattle, WA 98104
www.washington.edu

Spokane Community College
Emergency Med Tech-Paramedic Prgm
N 1810 Greene St, MS 2090
Spokane, WA 99217
www.scc.spokane.edu

Tacoma Community College
Emergency Med Tech-Paramedic Prgm
6501 S 19th St, Bldg 19
Tacoma, WA 98466
www.tacomacc.edu

Tacoma Fire Department
Cosponsor: Pierce College
Emergency Med Tech-Paramedic Prgm
2124 E Marshall Ave
Tacoma, WA 98421
www.tacomafiredepartment.org

West Virginia

Blue Ridge Community & Technical College
Emergency Med Tech-Paramedic Prgm
400 W Stephen St
Martinsburg, WV 25401

Wisconsin

Lakeshore Technical College
Emergency Med Tech-Paramedic Prgm
1290 North Ave
Cleveland, WI 53015

Waukesha County Technical College
Emergency Med Tech-Paramedic Prgm
800 Main St S-232
Pewaukee, WI 53072

Northcentral Technical College
Emergency Med Tech-Paramedic Prgm
1000 W Campus Drive
Wausau, WI 54401

Wyoming

Casper College
Emergency Med Tech-Paramedic Prgm
125 College Drive
Casper, WY 82601

Laramie County Community College
Emergency Med Tech-Paramedic Prgm
1400 East College Drive TC 109
Cheyenne, WY 82007

Emergency Medical Technician-Paramedic

Programs*	Class Capacity	Begins	Length (months)	Award	Res. Tuition	Non-res. Tuition		Offers:† 1	2	3	4
Arkansas											
NorthWest Arkansas Community College (Bentonville)	16	May	12, 24	Cert, AAS	$2,700	$6,000					
California											
Imperial Valley Community College	20	Jan	11	Cert, AS	$4,000						
Colorado											
HealthONE EMS (Englewood)	20	Jan Jun	6, 12	Cert, AAS	$6,800	$6,800	per year			•	
Connecticut											
Capital Community College (Hartford)	30	Aug Jan	13	AS	$4,600	$13,000		•		•	
Florida											
Florida State College at Jacksonville	24	Jan Sep	16, 24	Cert, AS	$4,164	$16,657		•			
Hillsborough Community College (Tampa)	40	Aug Jan May	10	AS, AAS	$5,000	$15,000					
Maryland											
Anne Arundel Community College (Arnold)	24	Jan	18, 24	Cert, AAS	$5,611	$8,619	per year			•	•
Michigan											
Huron Valley Ambulance (Ann Arbor)	30	Sep Jan	14		$5,075			•			
Minnesota											
Century College (White Bear Lake)	26	Aug Jan	14, 24	Dipl, AAS	$9,000	$9,000	per year	•		•	•
Mississippi											
Jones County Junior College (Ellisville)	15	Aug Jan	18	AAS							
Montana											
Montana State Univ Billings	18	Sep	24	AAS				•		•	•
Nebraska											
Creighton Univ (Omaha)	40	Mid Aug	12	Cert, BS EMS, AS EMS						•	•
New Hampshire											
NHTI, Concord's Community College	14	Sep 2	18	AS	$8,000	$18,000	per credit			•	•
New Mexico											
Dona Ana Community College (Las Cruces)	20	Jul	12, 36	Cert, AAS	$3,055	$9,306				•	
North Carolina											
Catawba Valley Community College (Hickory)	25	Aug	21	AAS	$1,586	$7,324	per year			•	•
Texas											
San Jacinto College Central (Pasadena)	60	Sep	19	AAS	$725	$1,050		•		•	•
San Jacinto College North (Houston)	30	Sep	19, 24	AAS	$725	$1,050		•		•	•
Utah											
Weber State Univ (Ogden)	48	Sep	9	Cert, AAS	$5,500	$16,500		•			•

*Data are shown only for programs that completed the 2011 AMA Survey of Health Professions Education Programs.

†Key to Offers: 1: Evening or weekend classes; 2: Non-English instruction; 3: Cultural competence instruction; 4: Distance education component.

ALLIED HEALTH

Exercise Science

Includes:
- Exercise physiology (clinical and applied)
- Exercise science
- Personal fitness training

History
In 2003, the American College of Sports Medicine (ACSM) petitioned the Commission on Accreditation of Allied Health Education Programs (CAAHEP) for inclusion of two new professions in the CAAHEP system. The petition envisioned a baccalaureate-level profession, tentatively designated as *health and fitness specialist*, and another at the master's degree level, as *clinical exercise specialist*. Both professions were voted unanimously to be eligible for participation in CAAHEP in April 2003. In April 2004, a Committee on Accreditation for the Exercise Sciences was voted admission into the CAAHEP system as a collaborating Committee on Accreditation with the American College of Sports Medicine as their sponsoring organization. Two sets of standards and Guidelines were formally approved by the CAAHEP Board of Directors in 2004, with the *health and fitness specialist*, now designated as the *exercise science professional* and the *clinical exercise specialist*, as the *exercise physiologist*. For exercise physiology, the standards laid out two tracks: applied and clinical.

Exercise Physiology

Career Description
Exercise physiology is a discipline that includes clinical exercise physiology and applied exercise physiology. Applied exercise physiologists manage programs to assess, design, and implement individual and group exercise and fitness programs for apparently healthy individuals and individuals with controlled disease. Clinical exercise physiologists work under the direction of a physician to apply physical activity and behavioral interventions in clinical situations, in which they have been scientifically proven to provide therapeutic or functional benefit.

Employment Characteristics
As a clinical part of the health and wellness team, exercise physiologists can work with personal fitness trainers, exercise science professionals, and physicians in cardiac rehabilitation, typically in a hospital or clinical setting. Exercise physiologists work with clients who have been diagnosed with a chronic metabolic, pulmonary, or cardiac disease.

Educational Programs
Length: Exercise physiologist programs can be completed in a 2-year master's degree level program.
Prerequisites: Applicants should have a high school diploma or equivalent, meet the specific institutional entrance requirements, and have a bachelor's degree in exercise science.
Curriculum: Exercise physiologist programs will include a comprehensive academic curriculum and at least one culminating internship experience.

Exercise Science

Career Description
Exercise science encompasses a wide variety of disciplines, including but not limited to, biomechanics, sports nutrition, sport psychology, motor control/development, and exercise physiology. The study of these disciplines is integrated into the academic preparation of exercise science professionals. Exercise science professionals work in the health and fitness industry, and are skilled in evaluating health behaviors and risk factors, conducting fitness assessments, writing appropriate exercise prescriptions, and motivating individuals to modify negative health habits and maintain positive lifestyle behaviors for health promotion.

Employment Characteristics
As an integral part of the health and wellness team, exercise science professionals can work with personal fitness trainers and exercise physiologists in a number of different settings, such as corporate, clinical, community, and commercial fitness and wellness centers. Exercise science professionals work with the apparently healthy population and clients with controlled disease, leading and demonstrating these clients in safe and effective methods of exercise. The exercise science professional can also assess risk factors and identify the health status of clients.

Educational Programs
Length. Exercise science programs can be completed in a 4-year bachelor's degree level program.
Prerequisites. Applicants should have a high school diploma or equivalent and meet the specific institutional entrance requirements.
Curriculum. Exercise science programs include a comprehensive academic curriculum and at least one culminating internship experience.

Personal Fitness Training

Career Description
Personal fitness trainers are skilled practitioners, who work with a wide variety of client demographics in one-to-one and small group environments. They are familiar with multiple forms of exercises, used to improve and maintain health-related components of physical fitness and performance. They are knowledgeable in basic assessment and development of exercise recommendations. In addition, they are proficient in leading and demonstrating safe and effective methods of exercise, and motivating individuals to begin and to continue with healthy behaviors. They consult with and refer to other appropriate allied health professionals when client conditions exceed the personal trainer's education, training, and experience.

Employment Characteristics

As an integral part of the health and wellness team, personal fitness trainers can work with exercise science professionals and exercise physiologists in a number of different settings, such as corporate, clinical, community, and commercial fitness and wellness centers. Personal fitness training involves working with apparently healthy population, and leading and demonstrating safe and effective methods of exercising to these clients.

Educational Programs

Length. Personal fitness training programs can be completed in a 1-year certificate program or in a 2-year associate's degree level program.

Prerequisites. Applicants should have a high school diploma or equivalent and meet the specific institutional entrance requirements.

Curriculum. Personal fitness training programs will include a comprehensive academic curriculum and at least one culminating internship experience.

Inquiries

Careers
American Kinesiotherapy Association (AKTA)
118 College Dr. #5142
Hattiesburg, MS 39406
800 296-2582
www.akta.org

Certification
American College of Sports Medicine (ACSM)
401 West Michigan Street
Indianapolis, IN 46202
317 637-9200
www.acsm.org

American Council on Exercise (ACE)
4851 Paramount Drive
San Diego, CA 92123
888 825-3636
www.acefitness.org

National Academy of Sports Medicine (NASM)
26632 Agoura Road
Calabasas, CA 91302
800 460-6276
www.nasm.org

The Cooper Institute
12330 Preston Road
Dallas, TX 75230
972 341-3200
www.cooperinst.org

Program Accreditation
Commission on Accreditation of Allied Health Education
    Programs (CAAHEP)
1361 Park Street, Clearwater, FL 33756
727 210-2350
727 210-2354 Fax
E-mail: *mail@caahep.org*
www.caahep.org

in collaboration with:
Committee on Accreditation of the Exercise Sciences (CoAES)
401 West Michigan Street
Indianapolis, IN 46202
317 637-9200 ext 147
www.coaes.org

Exercise Physiologist

Georgia

Georgia State University
Exercise Physiology - Applied Prgm
KH Department P O Box 3975
Atlanta, GA 30302

Louisiana

University of Louisiana at Monroe
Exercise Physiology - Clinical Prgm
Department of Kinesiology
700 University Ave
Monroe, LA 71209
www.ulm.edu

Massachusetts

Springfield College
Exercise Physiology - Clinical Prgm
263 Alden St
Springfield, MA 01109

North Carolina

Univ of North Carolina at Charlotte
Exercise Physiology - Clinical Prgm
Department of Kinesiology 9201 University City Blvd
Charlotte, NC 28223

Pennsylvania

Bloomsburg University
Exercise Physiology - Applied Prgm
Dept of Exercise Science and Athletics 124 Centennial
    Hall
Bloomsburg, PA 17815

East Stroudsburg University
Exercise Physiology - Applied Prgm
Exercise Physiology Program
Koehler Fieldhouse
East Stroudsburg, PA 18301
www.esu.edu

East Stroudsburg University
Exercise Physiology - Clinical Prgm
200 Prospect St
East Stroudsburg, PA 18301

Exercise Science Professional

Colorado

Metropolitan State College of Denver
Exercise Science Prgm
HPS Dept, Campus Box 25 PO Box 173361
Denver, CO 80217-3362

Connecticut

Southern Connecticut State University
Exercise Science Prgm
501 Crescent St Human Performance Lab - MFH
New Haven, CT 06515

Georgia

Georgia State University
Exercise Science Prgm
KH Department PO Box 3975
Atlanta, GA 30303

Indiana

University of Indianapolis
Exercise Science Prgm
1400 East Hanna Ave
Indianapolis, IN 46227

Exercise Science Professional

Programs*	Class Capacity	Begins	Length (months)	Award	Res. Tuition	Non-res. Tuition	Offers:† 1 2 3 4
North Dakota							
North Dakota State Univ (Fargo)	50	Fall semester	48	BS	$3,068	$3,209	

*Data are shown only for programs that completed the 2011 AMA Survey of Health Professions Education Programs.

†Key to Offers: 1: Evening or weekend classes; 2: Non-English instruction; 3: Cultural competence instruction; 4: Distance education component.

Louisiana

University of Louisiana at Monroe
Exercise Science Prgm
Department of Kinesiology
700 University Ave
Monroe, LA 71209
www.ulm.edu

Maine

University of Southern Maine
Exercise Science Prgm
37 College Ave
Gorham, ME 04038

Maryland

Salisbury University
Exercise Science Prgm
Maggs Physical Acitivity Center
Salisbury, MD 21801
www.salisbury.edu

Massachusetts

Springfield College
Exercise Science Prgm
208 AT/Exercise Complex 263 Alden St
Springfield, MA 01109

Westfield State College
Exercise Science Prgm
Department of Movement Sciences
577 Western Ave
Westfield, MA 01086
www.wsc.ma.edu/dept/mssls/

Minnesota

Saint Catherine University
Exercise Science Prgm
2004 Randolph Ave
St. Paul, MN 55105

Missouri

Missouri Baptist University
Exercise Science Prgm
One College Park Drive
St. Louis, MO 63141

North Carolina

Univ of North Carolina at Charlotte
Exercise Science Prgm
Department of Kinesiology 9201 University City Blvd
Charlotte, NC 28223

North Dakota

University of Mary
Exercise Science Prgm
7500 University Dr
Bismarck, ND 58504

North Dakota State University
Exercise Science Prgm
Bentson Bunker Fieldhouse
Fargo, ND 58105
www.ndsu.edu
Prgm Dir: Donna Terbizan, Professor and Coordinator
Tel: 701 231-7792   *Fax:* 701 231-8872
E-mail: d.terbizan@ndsu.edu

Ohio

Ohio Northern University
Exercise Science Prgm
106C King Horn Center
Dept of Human Performance and Sport Sciences
Ada, OH 45810

Kent State University
Exercise Science Prgm
162 Gym Annex
Kent, OH 44242

Oklahoma

University of Central Oklahoma
Exercise Science Prgm
100 N University Dr
Edmond, OK 73034

Pennsylvania

Bloomsburg University
Exercise Science Prgm
Dept of Exercise Science and Athletics 124 Centennial Hall
Bloomsburg, PA 17815

East Stroudsburg University
Exercise Science Prgm
Koehler Fieldhouse
Exercise Physiology Program
East Stroudsburg, PA 18301
www.esu.edu

Indiana University of Pennsylvania
Exercise Science Prgm
233 Zink Hall Room 202
Dept HPED
Indiana, PA 15705
www.iup.edu

Slippery Rock University of Pennsylvania
Exercise Science Prgm
128 E Gym, Stoner Complex
Exercise and Rehab Sciences
Slippery Rock, PA 16057
www.sru.edu

Eastern University
Exercise Science Prgm
McInnis Learning Center 122 1300 Eagle Rd
St. David's, PA 19087

West Chester University
Exercise Science Prgm
New St Sturzebecker Hall HSC 204
West Chester, PA 19383

Vermont

Lyndon State College
Exercise Science Prgm
1001 College Rd
Lyndonville, VT 05821

Virginia

Liberty University
Exercise Science Prgm
1971 University Blvd
Lynchburg, VA 24502

Lynchburg College
Exercise Science Prgm
Turner Gymnasium 1501 Lakeside Dr
Lynchburg, VA 24501

Old Dominion University
Exercise Science Prgm
140 HPE Bldg
Dept of Exercise Science, Sport and Physical
Norfolk, VA 23529
www.odu.edu

Personal Fitness Trainer

Ohio

Sinclair Community College
Personal Fitness Training Prgm
444 West Third St
Dayton, OH 45402

Kinesiotherapist

Kinesiotherapy is the application of scientifically based exercise principles to rehabilitation physical therapy, which is adapted to enhance the strength, endurance, and mobility of individuals with functional limitations or those requiring extended physical conditioning. The kinesiotherapist is academically and clinically prepared to provide rehabilitation exercise and education under the prescription of a licensed physician, physician's assistant, or nurse practitioner in an appropriate setting.

History

Kinesiotherapy (formerly Corrective Therapy) is an allied health profession that has been in existence since 1946, but the root of the profession began during World War II when the increased survival of troops who suffered from illness or injury led to a great demand to return soldiers to active duty. Therefore, corrective physical reconditioning units were established to enhance this process. Physical reconditioning specialists for the Armed Forces were established to employ exercise and mobility programs for the troops. As the demand for these specialists grew, the early leaders in rehabilitation saw the need to organize and accredit these new specialists, and in 1953 the American Corrective Therapy Association was formed. In 1987, the name Corrective Therapy was formally changed to Kinesiotherapy, and the national organization is now known as the American Kinesiotherapy Association (AKTA). In a continuing effort to meet and maintain the highest standards for rehabilitation, the Council on Professional Standards for Kinesiotherapy was formed. In 1995, Kinesiotherapy was formally recognized as an allied health profession by the Commission on Accreditation of Allied Health Education Programs (CAAHEP). In 1998, the *Standards and Guidelines for Accredited Educational Programs for Kinesiotherapy* was approved.

Career Description

Kinesiotherapists are qualified to implement exercise programs designed to reverse or minimize debilitation, and enhance the functional capacity of medically stable patients in a wellness, sub-acute, or extended care setting. The role of the kinesiotherapist demands intelligence, judgment, honesty, interpersonal skills, and the capacity to react to emergencies in a calm and reasoned manner. Expected attributes include an attitude of respect for self and others, adherence to the concepts of privilege and confidentiality, the ability to communicate with patients, and a commitment to the patient's welfare. At a minimum, a kinesiotherapist is educated in areas of basic exercise science and clinical applications of rehabilitation exercise. Training is received in orthopedic, neurological, psychiatric, pediatric, cardiovascular/pulmonary, and geriatric practice settings.

The kinesiotherapist, in collaboration with the client, determines the appropriate evaluation tools and interventions necessary to establish a goal-specific treatment plan. The intervention process includes developing and implementing a treatment plan, assessing progress toward goals, and modifications necessary to achieve goals and outcomes, as well as client education. The foundation of clinician-client rapport is based on education, instruction, demonstration, and mentoring of therapeutic techniques and behaviors to restore, maintain, and improve overall functional abilities.

The *Scope of Practice for Kinesiotherapy* reflects the evaluation procedures and treatment interventions for medically stable individuals who require extended physical conditioning, and it identifies the job tasks that registered kinesiotherapists are qualified to perform. The individual kinesiotherapist may obtain additional training and credentials in areas beyond the scope of practice. The *Standards of Practice for Registered Kinesiotherapists* serves as a guideline for practicing registered kinesiotherapists and provides a basis for assessment of kinesiotherapy practices.

Employment Characteristics

Registered kinesiotherapists are employed in Department of Veterans Affairs Medical Centers, public and private hospitals, medical fitness facilities, rehabilitation facilities, learning disability centers, schools, colleges and universities, and private practice, as well as exercise consultants.

The types of treatments carried out by kinesiotherapists focus on, but are not limited to:
- Therapeutic exercise
- Ambulation training
- Geriatric rehabilitation
- Aquatic therapy
- Adapted fitness and conditioning
- Prosthetic/orthotic rehabilitation
- Psychiatric rehabilitation
- Driver training
- Adapted exercise for the home setting

Salary

Depending on the particular job setting, the average projected starting salary for Registered Kinesiotherapists is $36,000 to $47,000 annually. The overall average is $60,000; upper-level salaries are in the range of $70,000-$90,000. For more information, go to *www.ama-assn.org/go/hpsalary*.

Educational Programs

Length. The kinesiotherapy program is four to five years. The total minimum requirements are 128 semester hours. Minimum requirements for years one and two are 59 semester hours and for years three and four are 67 semester hours.

Prerequisites. Applicants should have a high school diploma or equivalent and meet institutional entrance requirements.

Curriculum. The program has a comprehensive academic and clinical curriculum plan that fulfills or exceeds the minimum requirements for kinesiotherapy accreditation.

The curriculum plan includes an organized and sequential series of integrated learning experiences designed to achieve or exceed minimum competencies.

All academic and clinical courses are guided by written measurable behavioral objectives utilizing case-based, patient-centered, problem-solving activities.

The curriculum plan includes academic learning experiences, which lead to the attainment of all academic competencies listed in the *Minimum Core Competencies of Kinesiotherapists*. Students must complete the following content areas:
- Human anatomy

- Human physiology
- Exercise physiology
- Kinesiology/biomechanics
- Therapeutic exercise/adapted physical education
- Growth and development
- Motor learning/control/performance
- General psychology
- Organization and administration
- Tests and measurements
- Research methods or statistics
- First aid and cardiopulmonary resuscitation
- Introduction to Kinesiotherapy
- Pathophysiology
- Clinical neurology
- Rehabilitation procedures
- Patient assessment and management
- Therapeutic activities

Students are strongly encouraged to complete the following academic courses:
- Abnormal psychology or mental health
- Physiological psychology
- Exercise testing and prescription
- Gerontology
- Medical ethics
- Medical terminology
- Pharmacology
- Health/medical/functional outcomes management
- Health education
- Kinesiotherapy I and II

Center of Excellence Certificate Program

Length. The COE Kinesiotherapy Clinical Training Program is a 6 month program, requiring a minimum of 1000 clinical experience hours at an approved Kinesiotherapy Center of Excellence clinical training site.

Prerequisites. Applicants must have a Master's degree in exercise science or related field, an overall minimum GPA of 2.5 on a 4.0 scale, a minimum of 100 previous hours of rehabilitation clinical observation hours, and a grade of B or better in the following core coursework:
- Human anatomy
- Human physiology
- Exercise physiology
- Kinesiology/biomechanics
- Therapeutic exercise/adapted physical education
- Growth and development/motor learning
- General psychology
- Research methods or statistics
- First aid
- Pathophysiology/clinical neurology
- Organization and administration of Kinesiotherapy

Completion of the following classes is recommended:
- Abnormal psychology or mental health issues
- Physiological psychology
- Exercise testing and prescription
- Gerontology
- Medical ethics
- Medical terminology
- Pharmacology
- Health/medical/functional outcomes management
- Health education
- Cardiopulmonary resuscitation

Curriculum. The curriculum plan includes an organized and sequential series of integrated learning experiences designed to achieve or exceed minimum competencies. All clinical experiences are guided by written measurable behavioral objectives and competencies utilizing case-based, patient-centered, problem-solving activities.

Inquiries

Careers

American Kinesiotherapy Association
118 College Drive, #5142
Hattiesburg, MS 39406
800 296 2582
E-mail: *Melissa.ziegler@usm.edu* or *info@akta.org*

Credentialing

Board of Registration for Kinesiotherapy
University of Toledo
2801 West Bancroft
Toledo, OH 43606-2434
419 530-2731
E-mail: *doris.woods@utoledo.edu*

Program Accreditation

Commission on Accreditation of Allied Health Education Programs
  (CAAHEP)
1361 Park Street, Clearwater, FL 33756
727 210-2350
727 210-2354 Fax
E-mail: *mail@caahep.org*
www.caahep.org

in collaboration with:
Committee on Accreditation of Education Programs for
  Kinesiotherapy
University of Southern Mississippi
118 College Drive, #5142
Hattiesburg, MS 39406
601 266-5371
E-mail: *jerry.purvis@usm.edu*

Kinesiotherapist

California

California State University - Long Beach
Kinesiotherapy Prgm
1250 Bellflower Blvd
Long Beach, CA 90815
www.csulb.edu

San Diego State University
Kinesiotherapy Prgm
5500 Campanile Dr
Department of Exercise & Nutritional Sciences
San Diego, CA 92182-7251
www.sdsu.edu

Mississippi

University of Southern Mississippi
Kinesiotherapy Prgm
118 College Dr #5142
Hattiesburg, MS 39406-5142
www.usm.edu

North Carolina

Shaw University
Kinesiotherapy Prgm
118 E South St
Raleigh, NC 27601
www.shawu.edu

Ohio

University of Toledo
Kinesiotherapy Prgm
2801 W Bancroft St
HH 2505J, Main Campus, MS 119
Toledo, OH 43606-3390
www.utoledo.edu

Virginia

Norfolk State University
Kinesiotherapy Prgm
700 Park Ave
Norfolk, VA 23504
www.nsu.edu

Lactation Consultant

Occupational Description

Lactation consultants are health professionals with specialized knowledge and clinical expertise in breastfeeding and human lactation who educate women, families, health professionals, and the community.

Career Description

Lactation consultants advocate for breastfeeding as the child-feeding norm and educate and support parents and families to encourage informed decision-making about infant and child feeding. Lactation consultants:

- Provide holistic, evidence-based breastfeeding support and care from preconception to weaning for women and their families
- Provide anticipatory guidance to promote optimal breastfeeding practices and minimize the potential for breastfeeding problems or complications
- Provide positive feedback and emotional support for continued breastfeeding, especially in difficult or complicated circumstances
- Utilize a pragmatic problem-solving approach, sensitive to the learner's culture, questions, and concerns
- Share current evidence-based information and clinical skills in collaboration with other health professionals
- Advocate for policies that protect, promote, and support breastfeeding

Employment Characteristics

Lactation consultants work in a variety of settings, including hospitals, neonatal intensive care units and special care nurseries, lactation clinics, and maternal and child health services, as well as in private practice. The majority of lactation consultants are employed in hospitals and other maternity-care facilities.

Educational Programs

Length. Accredited programs are between one and four years (certificate, associate, and baccalaureate level), depending on program design, objectives, and the degree or certificate awarded. A student entering directly from high school would need about two years to complete the curriculum requirements. A student entering with previous college or with a health care license in another field may complete the requirements in one year.

Curriculum. Education in the lactation consultant profession ranges from 45-hour courses taught by independent educators to 4-year academic degree programs. Accreditation is a means to establish minimal criteria for the education of lactation consultants and is an avenue to moving formal education into academia.

Curriculum requirements for accredited programs correlate to the requirements for certification in the profession, which include specified general education in the health sciences, specified lactation education, and clinical experience in providing breastfeeding care.

Certification

The International Board of Lactation Consultant Examiners (IBLCE) develops and administers the certification examination for lactation consultants. While certification as an IBCLC is voluntary, it is the desired endpoint upon completion of an accredited program. Currently, licensure is not required in this field.

Inquiries

Careers

International Lactation Consultant Association
2501 Aerial Center Parkway, Suite 103
Morrisville, NC 27560
919 861-5577
www.ilca.org

Certification

International Board of Lactation Consultant Examiners
6402 Arlington Boulevard, Suite 350
Falls Church, VA 22042
703 560-7330
www.iblce.org

Program Accreditation

Commission on Accreditation of Allied Health Education Programs (CAAHEP)
1361 Park Street, Clearwater, FL 33756
727 210-2350
727 210-2354 Fax
E-mail: *mail@caahep.org*
www.caahep.org

in collaboration with:
Lactation Education Accreditation and Approval Review Committee
International Lactation Consultant Association
c/o 228 Park Lane
Chalfont PA 18914
215 822-5545
215 822-5545 Fax
E-mail: *judil@imiae.com*
www.aarclactation.org

Medical Assistant

Medical assisting is a multiskilled allied health profession; practitioners work primarily in ambulatory settings such as medical offices and clinics. Medical assistants function as members of the health care delivery team and perform administrative and clinical procedures.

Career Description

Medical assistants work under the supervision of physicians in their offices or other medical settings. In accordance with respective state laws, they perform a broad range of administrative and clinical duties:

Administrative Duties
- Scheduling and receiving patients
- Preparing and maintaining medical records
- Performing basic secretarial skills and medical transcription
- Handling telephone calls and writing correspondence
- Serving as a liaison between the physician and other individuals
- Managing practice finances

Clinical Duties
- Asepsis and infection control
- Taking patient histories and vital signs
- Performing first aid and CPR
- Preparing patients for procedures
- Assisting the physician with examinations and treatments
- Collecting and processing specimens
- Performing selected diagnostic tests
- Preparing/administering medications under physician direction
- Assisting with patient education

Both administrative and clinical duties involve maintenance of equipment and supplies for the practice. A medical assistant, who is sufficiently qualified by education and/or experience, may be responsible for supervising personnel, health coaching, developing and conducting public outreach programs to market the physician's professional services, and participating in the negotiation of leases and equipment and supply contracts.

Employment Characteristics

 More medical assistants are employed by practicing physicians than any other type of allied health personnel. Medical assistants are usually employed in physicians' offices and other ambulatory healthcare settings, in which they perform a variety of administrative and clinical tasks to facilitate the work of the physician.

The responsibilities of medical assistants vary, depending on whether they work in a clinic, hospital, large group practice, or small private office. The team model for improved patient-centered health care delivery is growing rapidly throughout the U.S. and medical assistants are regarded as vital members of these teams. Frequently, a major goal of these teams is to address the growing incidence of chronic conditions such as diabetes, hypertension, obesity, asthma, and depression. Treating these patients requires a health provision approach that includes patient self-management support, evidence-based decision support, clinical information systems to monitor outcomes, and community partnerships that provide patients with linkages to community resources. Such a model has considerable impact on medical assistant roles, including their greater involvement with health information management.

Salary

 According to the US Bureau of Labor Statistics (BLS), the median annual wages of wage-and-salary medical assistants were $29,100 in May 2011. The middle 50% earned between $24,670 and $35,080. The lowest 10% earned less than $20,880, and the highest 10% earned more than $40,810. For more information, refer to *www.bls.gov/oes/current/oes319092.htm*.

Employment Outlook

 With demand from more than 200,000 physicians, there are, and will probably continue to be, almost unlimited opportunities for formally educated medical assistants. According to the BLS, employment of medical assistants is expected to grow 31% from 2010 to 2020, much faster than the average for all occupations. As the health care industry expands because of technological advances in medicine and the growth and aging of the population, there will be an increased need for all health care workers. The increasing prevalence of certain conditions, such as obesity and diabetes, also will increase demand for health care services and medical assistants. Increasing use of medical assistants to allow doctors to care for more patients will further stimulate job growth.

Educational Programs

 Length. Programs grant an associate's degree, certificate, or diploma.

Prerequisites. High school diploma or equivalent is usually required.

Curriculum. The curricula of programs accredited by the Commission on Accreditation of Allied Health Education Programs (CAAHEP) must ensure achievement of the *Entry-Level Competencies for the Medical Assistant.* The curriculum must include anatomy and physiology, medical terminology, medical law and ethics, psychology, communications (oral and written), medical assisting administrative procedures, and medical assisting clinical procedures. Programs must include a practicum that provides practical experience in qualified physicians' offices, accredited hospitals, or other health care facilities.

Inquiries

 Careers
American Association of Medical Assistants
20 North Wacker Drive, Suite 1575
Chicago, IL 60606-2903
800 228-2262
312 899-1500
www.aama-ntl.org

American Medical Technologists
10700 West Higgins Road, Suite 150
Rosemont, IL 60018
847 823-5169
E-mail: *mail@amt1.com*
www.amt1.com

Certification
American Association of Medical Assistants
20 North Wacker Drive, Suite 1575
Chicago, IL 60606-2903
312 424-3100

American Medical Technologists
710 Higgins Road
Park Ridge, IL 60068-5765
847 823-5169
E-mail: *mail@amt1.com*
www.amt1.com

Program Accreditation
Commission on Accreditation of Allied Health Education Programs
 (CAAHEP)
1361 Park Street, Clearwater, FL 33756
727 210-2350
727 210-2354 Fax
E-mail: *mail@caahep.org*
www.caahep.org

in collaboration with:
Medical Assisting Education Review Board (MAERB)
20 North Wacker Drive, Suite 1575
Chicago, IL 60606-2963
312 899-1500
312899-1259 Fax
www.maerb.org
E-mail: *accreditation@maerb.org*

Note: Adapted in part from the Bureau of Labor Statistics, US Department of Labor, *Occupational Outlook Handbook,* Medical Assistants, at *www.bls.gov/oco/ocos164.htm* .

Medical Assistant

Alabama

Wallace Community College
Medical Assistant Prgm
1141 Wallace Dr
Dothan, AL 36303-0943
www.wallace.edu

Wallace State Community College
Medical Assistant Prgm
PO Box 2000
801 Main St
Hanceville, AL 35077-2000
www.wallacestate.edu

South University
Medical Assistant Prgm
5355 Vaughn Rd
Montgomery, AL 36116-1120
www.southuniversity.edu

Trenholm State Technical College
Medical Assistant Prgm
1225 Air Base Blvd
Montgomery, AL 36108-3105
www.trenholmtech.cc.al.us
Prgm Dir: Chandrika McQueen, RN MSN
Tel: 334 420-4425   *Fax:* 334 420-4335
E-mail: cmcqueen@trenholmstate.edu

Alaska

University of Alaska Anchorage
Medical Assistant Prgm
Allied Health Sciences Building Room 166
3211 Providence Dr
Anchorage, AK 99508-4630
www.uaa.alaska.edu

University of Alaska - Fairbanks
Medical Assistant Prgm
PO Box 758040
Fairbanks, AK 99701-8040
www.uaf.edu

Arizona

Central Arizona College
Medical Assistant Prgm
273 E Old West Hwy
Apache Junction, AZ 85248-6092

Kaplan College
Medical Assistant Prgm
13610 N Black Canyon Hwy, Ste 104
Phoenix, AZ 85029
www.kc-phoenix.edu

Arkansas

Arkansas Tech University
Medical Assistant Prgm
Dean Suite 201
402 West O St
Russellville, AR 72801-2222
www.atu.edu

California

Everest College - Alhambra
Medical Assistant Prgm
2215 Mission Rd
Alhambra, CA 91803
www.everest.edu/campus/alhambra

Everest College - Anaheim
Medical Assistant Prgm
511 N Brookhurst St, Ste 300
Anaheim, CA 92801-5229
www.everest.edu/campus/anaheim

Carrington College California - Antioch
Medical Assistant Prgm
2157 Country Hills Dr
Antioch, CA 94509
www.westerncollege.edu

Cabrillo College
Medical Assistant Prgm
6500 Soquel Dr
Aptos, CA 95003-3194
www.cabrillo.edu

Carrington College California - Citrus Heights Campus
Medical Assistant Prgm
7301 Greenback Lane, Ste A
Citrus Heights, CA 95621-5587
www.westerncollege.com

Heald College - Concord
Medical Assistant Prgm
5130 Commerical Circle
Concord, CA 94520-8522
www.heald.edu

Orange Coast College
Medical Assistant Prgm
2701 Fairview Rd
Costa Mesa, CA 92626-5561
www.orangecoastcollege.edu

Carrington College California - Emeryville
Medical Assistant Prgm
6001 Shellmound St, Ste 145
Emeryville, CA 94608
www.westerncollege.edu

Heald College - Fresno
Medical Assistant Prgm
255 W Bullard Ave
Fresno, CA 93704-1706
www.heald.edu

Everest College - Gardena
Medical Assistant Prgm
1045 W Redondo Beach Blvd, Ste 275
Gardena, CA 90247-4128
www.everest.edu

Chabot College
Medical Assistant Prgm
25555 Hesperian Blvd
Hayward, CA 94545-2447
www.chabotcollege.edu

Heald College - Hayward
Medical Assistant Prgm
25500 Industrial Blvd
Hayward, CA 94545-2352
www.heald.edu

Everest College - Los Angeles
Medical Assistant Prgm
3460 Wilshire Blvd, Ste 500
Los Angeles, CA 90010-2223
www.everest-college.com

Heald College - Milpitas
Medical Assistant Prgm
341 Great Mall Pkwy
Milpitas, CA 95035-8008
www.heald.edu
Prgm Dir: Nina Goloubeva,
Tel: 408 876-5122   *Fax:* 408 876-5202
E-mail: Nina_Goloubeva@heald.edu

Modesto Junior College
Medical Assistant Prgm
435 College Ave
Modesto, CA 95350-5800
www.mjc.edu
Prgm Dir: Shirley M Buzbee, CMA
Tel: 209 575-6377   *Fax:* 209 575-6593
E-mail: buzbees@mjc.edu

Pasadena City College
Medical Assistant Prgm
1570 E Colorado Blvd
Pasadena, CA 91106-2003
www.pasadena.edu

Carrington College California - Pleasant Hill
Medical Assistant Prgm
380 Civic Dr, Ste 300
Pleasant Hill, CA 94523
www.westerncollege.edu

Heald College - Rancho Cordova
Medical Assistant Prgm
2910 Prospect Park Dr
Rancho Cordova , CA 95670
www.heald.edu
Prgm Dir: Barbette Williams,
Tel: 916 414-2778, Ext 2778   *Fax:* 916 414-2678
E-mail: barbette_williams@heald.edu

Heald College - Roseville
Medical Assistant Prgm
7 Sierra Gate Plaza
Roseville, CA 95678-6602
www.heald.edu

Carrington College California - Sacramento
Medical Assistant Prgm
8909 Folsom Blvd
Sacramento, CA 95826-3203
www.westerncollege.edu

Cosumnes River Community College
Medical Assistant Prgm
8401 Center Pkwy
Sacramento, CA 95823-5704
www.crc.losrios.edu

Heald College - Salinas
Medical Assistant Prgm
1450 N Main St
Salinas, CA 93906-5100
www.heald.edu

Everest College - San Bernardino
Medical Assistant Prgm
217 North Club Center Dr
Suite A
San Bernardino, CA 92408
www.everest.edu/campus/san_bernadino

City College of San Francisco
Medical Assistant Prgm
1860 Hayes St
San Francisco, CA 94117-1220
www.ccsf.edu

Everest College - San Francisco
Medical Assistant Prgm
A Corinthian School Ste 500
814 Mission St, 5th Fl
San Francisco, CA 94103-3038
www.everest.edu

Heald College - San Francisco
Medical Assistant Prgm
350 Mission St
San Francisco, CA 94105-2206
www.heald.edu

Carrington College California - San Jose
Medical Assistant Prgm
6201 San Ignacio Ave
San Jose, CA 95119-1325
www.westerncollege.edu

Everest College - San Jose
Medical Assistant Prgm
1245 S Winchester, Ste 102
San Jose, CA 95128
www.everest.edu

Carrington College California - San Leandro
Medical Assistant Prgm
15555 E 14th St, Ste 500
San Leandro, CA 94578
www.westerncollege.edu

Carrington College California - Stockton
Medical Assistant Prgm
1313 W Robinhood Drive Suite B
Stockton, CA 95207-5509

Heald College - Stockton
Medical Assistant Prgm
1605 E March Ln
Stockton, CA 95210-5667

Southern California Regional Occupational Ctr
Medical Assistant Prgm
2300 Crenshaw Blvd
Torrance, CA 90501-3324
http://socalroc.com

East San Gabriel Valley ROP
Medical Assistant Prgm
Technical Center
1501 W Del Norte St
West Covina, CA 91790-2105
www.esgvrop.org

Colorado

Everest College
Medical Assistant Prgm
14280 E Jewell Ave, Ste 100
Aurora, CO 80012

Everest College
Medical Assistant Prgm
5125 N Academy Blvd
Colorado Springs, CO 80918-4001
www.national.edu

National American University-Colorado Springs
Medical Assistant Prgm
1915 Jamboree Dr, Ste 185
Colorado Springs, CO 80920

Community College of Denver
Medical Assistant Prgm
1070 Alton Way Building 849
Denver, CO 80230
www.ccd.edu

Everest College
Medical Assistant Prgm
9065 Grant St
North Campus-Thornton
Denver, CO 80229-4339
www.everest.edu/campus/thornton

National American University - Denver
Medical Assistant Prgm
1325 S Colorado Blvd, Ste100
Denver, CO 80222-3308

Westwood College
Medical Assistant Prgm
Institute of Health Careers
7350 N Broadway
North Campus
Denver, CO 80221-3610
www.westwood.edu

Red Rocks Community College
Medical Assistant Prgm
13300 Sixth Ave Campus Box 27
Lakewood, CO 80228-1213
www.rrcc.edu

Arapahoe Community College
Medical Assistant Prgm
5900 S Santa Fe Dr
PO Box 9002
Littleton, CO 80160-9002
www.arapahoe.edu

Front Range Comm College
Medical Assistant Prgm
2121 Miller Dr
Longmont, CO 80501-6743
www.frontrange.edu

Connecticut

Branford Hall Career Institute
Medical Assistant Prgm
One Summit Pl
Branford, CT 06405
www.branfordhall.com

St Vincent's College
Medical Assistant Prgm
2800 Main St
Bridgeport, CT 06606-4201
www.stvincentscollege.edu

Quinebaug Valley Community College
Medical Assistant Prgm
742 Upper Maple St
Danielson, CT 06239-1436
www.qvctc.commnet.edu

Goodwin College
Medical Assistant Prgm
745 Burnside Ave
East Hartford, CT 06108
http://goodwin.edu

Stone Academy
Medical Assistant Prgm
1315 Dixwell Ave
Hamden, CT 06514-4125
www.stoneacademy.com

Capital Community College
Medical Assistant Prgm
950 Main St
Hartford, CT 06103-1207
www.ccc.commnet.edu

Lincoln Tech Institute
Medical Assistant Prgm
200 John Downey Dr
New Britain, CT 06051
www.lincolntech.com

Ridley-Lowell Business & Technical Institute
Medical Assistant Prgm
470 Bank St
New London, CT 06320-5548
www.ridley.edu

Norwalk Community College
Medical Assistant Prgm
188 Richards Ave
Norwalk, CT 06854-1655
www.ncc.commnet.edu

Lincoln College of New England
Medical Assistant Prgm
2279 Mt Vernon Rd
Southington, CT 06489-1057
www.briarwood.edu

American Institute
Medical Assistant Prgm
99 South St
West Hartford, CT 06110-1922

Northwestern Connecticut Comm College
Medical Assistant Prgm
Park Place East, Office 218
Winsted, CT 06098
www.nwctc.commnet.edu

Delaware

Delaware Technical Community College
Medical Assistant Prgm
333 Shipley St
AH/SCI Department
Wilmington, DE 19801-2412
www.dtcc.edu/wilmington/ah

Florida

Manatee Technical Institute
Medical Assistant Prgm
5520 Lakewood Ranch Blvd
Bradenton, FL 34211
www.manateetechnicalinstitute.org

Brevard Community College
Medical Assistant Prgm
1519 Clearlake Rd
Cocoa, FL 32922-6597
www.brevardcc.edu
Prgm Dir: Kris A Hardy, AS CDF CMA
Tel: 321 433-7545   *Fax:* 321 634-3731
E-mail: hardyk@brevardcc.edu

McFatter Technical Center
Medical Assistant Prgm
6500 Nova Dr
Davie, FL 33317
www.mcfattertech.com

**Daytona State College, Daytona Beach
 Campus**
Medical Assistant Prgm
1200 W International Speedway Blvd
PO Box 2811
Daytona Beach, FL 32120-2811
www.daytonastate.edu

Keiser University
Medical Assistant Prgm
1800 Business Park Blvd
Daytona Beach, FL 32114-1229
www.keiseruniversity.edu

Broward College
Medical Assistant Prgm
3501 SW Davie Rd
Fort Lauderdale, FL 33314
www.broward.edu

Palm Beach State College
Medical Assistant Prgm
4200 S Congress Ave, ETA Bldg
Mail Station #60
Lake Worth, FL 33461-4796
www.palmbeachstate.edu
Prgm Dir: Barbara Kalfin, CMA(AAMA)
Tel: 561 868-3562   *Fax:* 561 868-3635
E-mail: kalfinb@palmbeachstate.edu

Everest Univ - Lakeland Campus
Medical Assistant Prgm
995 E Memorial Blvd, Ste 110
Lakeland, FL 33801
www.everest.edu/campus/lakeland

Everest Univ - Largo Campus
Medical Assistant Prgm
1199 East Bay Drive
Largo Campus
Largo , FL 33770-2556
www.everest.edu/campus/largo

Everest Univ - Melbourne Campus
Medical Assistant Prgm
2401 N Harbor City Blvd
Melbourne, FL 32935-6657
www.everest.edu/campus/melbourne

Robert Morgan Educational Center
Medical Assistant Prgm
18180 SW 122nd Ave
Miami, FL 33177-2407
rmec.dadeschools.net/Career%20Technical/
 healtheducation.htm

Florida Career Institute
Medical Assistant Prgm
5925 Imperial Pkwy, Ste 200
Mulberry, FL 33860
www.floridacareerinstitute.com

Fortis Institute
Medical Assistant Prgm
5925 Imperial Parkway Suite 200
Mulberry, FL 33860

Hodges University
Medical Assistant Prgm
2655 Northbrooke Drive
Naples, FL 34119-7932
www.hodges.edu

Lorenzo Walker Institute of Technology
Medical Assistant Prgm
3702 Estey Ave
Naples, FL 34104-4405
www.lwit.edu

**Community Technical & Adult Education
 Center**
Medical Assistant Prgm
1014 SW Seventh Rd
Ocala, FL 34471-0572
www.mcctae.com
Prgm Dir: Gail McPadden, Allied Health Coordinator
Tel: 352 671-4129   *Fax:* 352 671-7221
E-mail: gail.mcpadden@marion.k12.fl.us

Everest Univ - North Orlando Campus
Medical Assistant Prgm
5421 Diplomat Cir
Orlando, FL 32810-5600
www.everest.edu/campus/north_orlando

Everest University - Orlando College South
Medical Assistant Prgm
9200 South Park Center Loop
Orlando, FL 32819-8606
www.everest.edu/campus/south_orlando

Pensacola State College
Medical Assistant Prgm
Warrington Campus
5555 W Hwy 98
Pensacola, FL 32507-1015
www.pjc.edu

Indian River State College
Medical Assistant Prgm
500 NW California Blvd
Port St Lucie, FL 34986

First Coast Technical College
Medical Assistant Prgm
2980 Collins Ave
St Augustine, FL 32084-1921
www.fctc.edu

Lively Technical Center
Medical Assistant Prgm
500 Appleyard Dr
Tallahassee, FL 32304-2810
www.livelytech.com

Erwin Technical Center
Medical Assistant Prgm
2010 E Hillsborough Ave
Tampa, FL 33610-8255
www.erwin.edu

Everest Univ - Brandon Campus
Medical Assistant Prgm
3924 Coconut Palm Dr
Brandon Campus
Tampa, FL 33619-1354
www.everest.edu/campus/brandon

Everest Univ - Tampa
Medical Assistant Prgm
3319 W Hillsborough Ave
Hillsborough Campus
Tampa, FL 33614-5801
www.everest.edu/campus/tampa

Fortis College-Winter Park
Medical Assistant Prgm
1573 W Fairbanks Ave Ste 100
Winter Park, FL 32789-4601

Winter Park Tech
Medical Assistant Prgm
901 Webster Ave
Winter Park, FL 32789-3098
www.wpt.ocps.net

Georgia

**Chattahoochee Technical College
 North Metro - Acworth**
Medical Assistant Prgm
5198 Ross Rd
Acworth, GA 30102
www.northmetrotech.edu

Albany Technical College
Medical Assistant Prgm
1704 S Slappey Blvd
Albany, GA 31701-2648
www.albanytech.org

Atlanta Technical College
Medical Assistant Prgm
1560 Metropolitan Pkwy SW
Atlanta, GA 30310
www.atlantatech.org

Westwood College - Midtown
Medical Assistant Prgm
1100 Spring St NW Suite 200
Atlanta, GA 30309-2848

Westwood College - Northlake Campus
Medical Assistant Prgm
2309 Parklake Dr NE
Northlake Campus
Atlanta, GA 30345
www.westwood.edu

Augusta Technical College
Medical Assistant Prgm
3200 Augusta Tech Dr
900 Building
Augusta, GA 30906-8243
www.augustatech.edu

North Georgia Technical College - Blairsville Campus
Medical Assistant Prgm
434 Meeks Ave
Blairsville, GA 30512
www.northgatech.edu

North Georgia Technical College
Medical Assistant Prgm
PO Box 65
1500 Hwy 197 N
Clarkesville, GA 30523-0065
www.northgatech.edu

Georgia Piedmont Technical College
Medical Assistant Prgm
495 N Indian Creek Dr
Clarkston, GA 30021-2397

Georgia Piedmont Technical College
Medical Assistant Prgm
495 N Indian Creek Dr
Clarkston, GA 30021-2397
www.dekalbtech.org

Columbus Technical College
Medical Assistant Prgm
928 Manchester Expressway
Columbus, GA 31904-6535
www.columbustech.org

Lanier Technical College - Cumming
Medical Assistant Prgm
7745 Majors Rd Forsyth Campus
Cumming, GA 30041-7050

Dalton State College
Medical Assistant Prgm
650 College Dr
Dalton, GA 30720-3778
http://daltonstate.edu

Oconee Fall Line Technical College
Medical Assistant Prgm
560 Pinehill Rd
Dublin, GA 31021-1599
www.hgtc.org

Southern Crescent Technical College
Medical Assistant Prgm
501 Varsity Rd
Griffin, GA 30223-2042
www.griffintech.edu

Gwinnett Technical College
Medical Assistant Prgm
5150 Sugarloaf Pkwy
Lawrenceville, GA 30043-5702
www.gwinnetttech.edu

Chattahoochee Technical College
Medical Assistant Prgm
980 S Cobb Dr
Marietta, GA 30060-3300
www.chattcollege.com

Moultrie Technical College
Medical Assistant Prgm
361 Industrial Dr
Moultrie, GA 31768
www.moultrietech.edu

Lanier Technical College
Medical Assistant Prgm
2990 Landrum Education Dr
Oakwood, GA 30566-3405
www.laniertech.edu

Georgia Northwestern Technical College
Medical Assistant Prgm
265 Bicentennial Trail
PO Box 569
Rock Spring, GA 30739-0569
www.northwesterntech.edu

Georgia Northwestern Technical College
Medical Assistant Prgm
One Maurice Culberson Dr
Rome, GA 30161-7603
www.GNTC.edu

Savannah Technical College
Medical Assistant Prgm
5717 White Bluff Rd
Savannah, GA 31405-5521
www.savannahtech.edu

South University
Cosponsor: Educational Management Corporation
Medical Assistant Prgm
709 Mall Blvd
Savannah, GA 31406-4805
www.southuniversity.edu/campus/Savannah

Medix School
Medical Assistant Prgm
2108 Cobb Pkwy
Smyrna, GA 30080-7630
www.medixschool.edu

Ogeechee Technical College
Medical Assistant Prgm
One Joe Kennedy Blvd
Statesboro, GA 30458-3199
www.ogeecheetech.edu

Southwest Georgia Technical College
Medical Assistant Prgm
15689 US Hwy 19 N
Thomasville, GA 31792-2622
www.southwestgatech.edu
Prgm Dir: Glenda L Hatcher, BSN RN CMA (AAMA)
Tel: 229 225-5081 *Fax:* 229 225-5289
E-mail: ghatcher@southwestgatech.edu

Southeastern Technical College
Medical Assistant Prgm
3001 E First St
Vidalia, GA 30474
www.southeasterntech.org

West Georgia Technical College
Medical Assistant Prgm
176 Murphy Campus Blvd
Waco, GA 30182-2407
www.westcentraltech.edu

Okefenokee Technical College
Medical Assistant Prgm
1701 Carswell Ave
Waycross, GA 31503

Lanier Technical College
Medical Assistant Prgm
89 E Athens St
Winder, GA 30680
www.laniertech.edu

Guam

Guam Community College
Medical Assistant Prgm
PO Box 23069
Barrigada, GU 96921

Guam Community College
Medical Assistant Prgm
PO Box 23069
GMF Barrigada, GU 96921
www.guamcc.edu

Hawaii

Heald College - Honolulu Campus
Medical Assistant Prgm
1500 Kapiolani Blvd
Suite 201
Honolulu, HI 96814-3732
www.heald.edu

Kapiolani Community College
Medical Assistant Prgm
4303 Diamond Head Rd
Honolulu, HI 96816-4496
www.kcc.hawaii.edu

Idaho

Eastern Idaho Technical College
Medical Assistant Prgm
1600 S 25th E
Idaho Falls, ID 83404-5788
www.eitc.edu

Lewis-Clark State College
Medical Assistant Prgm
500 8th Ave
Lewison, ID 83501
www.lcsc.edu

Idaho State University
Medical Assistant Prgm
Campus Box 8380
College of Technology
Pocatello, ID 83209-0001
isu.edu
Prgm Dir: Norma J Bird, MEd BS CMA
Tel: 208 282-4370 *Fax:* 208 282-3975
E-mail: birdnorm@isu.edu
Notes: The program also offers three Bachelor's degree options: Bachelor of Applied Science, Bachelor of Applied Technology, and Bachelor of Science in Health Science.

Brigham Young University
Medical Assistant Prgm
200 Kimball Building
Rexburg, ID 83460-1690

College of Southern Idaho
Medical Assistant Prgm
PO Box 1238
315 Falls Ave
Twin Falls, ID 83303-1238
www.csi.edu

Illinois

Southwestern Illinois College
Medical Assistant Prgm
2500 Carlyle Rd
Belleville, IL 62221-5899
www.swic.edu

Northwestern College - Southwest Campus
Medical Assistant Prgm
7725 S Harlem Ave
Bridgeview, IL 60455
www.northwesternbc.edu

Everest College - Burr Ridge
Medical Assistant Prgm
6880 N Frontage Rd, Ste 400
Burr Ridge, IL 60527
www.everest.edu

Westwood College - Calumet City
Medical Assistant Prgm
80 River Oaks Center Suite 111
Calumet City, IL 60409

Kaplan University - Chicago
Medical Assistant Prgm
550 W Van Buren St 7th Floor
Chicago, IL 60607-3836

National Latino Education Institute
Medical Assistant Prgm
Bilingual MA Prgm
2011 West Pershing Rd
Chicago, IL 60609
www.nlei.org

Northwestern College
Medical Assistant Prgm
4811 North Milwaukee Ave
Chicago, IL 60630
www.northwesternbc.edu

Robert Morris University
Medical Assistant Prgm
401 S State St
Chicago, IL 60605-1229
www.robertmorris.edu

Westwood College - Chicago
Medical Assistant Prgm
8501 W Higgins Rd
Suite 100
Chicago, IL 60631-2810
www.westwood.edu

Illinois Central College
Medical Assistant Prgm
201 SW Adams St
East Peoria, IL 61635-0001

Highland Community College
Medical Assistant Prgm
2998 West Pearl City Rd
Freeport, IL 61032-9973

College of DuPage
Medical Assistant Prgm
425 Fawell Blvd
Glen Ellyn, IL 60137
www.cod.edu/academic/acadprog/occ_voc/MedAsst.htm

College of Lake County
Medical Assistant Prgm
19351 W Washington St
Grayslake, IL 60030-1198

Northwestern College
Medical Assistant Prgm
Naperville Campus
1809 N Mill St
Suite F
Naperville, IL 60563
www.northwesternbc.edu

Everest College - North Aurora
Medical Assistant Prgm
150 S Lincolnway #100
North Aurora, IL 60542-1838
www.everest-college.com

Harper College
Medical Assistant Prgm
1200 W Algonquin Rd, HC
Health Careers X250
Palatine, IL 60067-7373
www.HarperCollege.edu
Prgm Dir: Geri Kale-Smith, MS CMA
Tel: 847 925-6444   *Fax:* 847 925-6047
E-mail: gkalesmi@harpercollege.edu

Moraine Valley Community College
Medical Assistant Prgm
9000 W College Parkway
B 150
Palos Hills, IL 60465-0937
www.morainevalley.edu

Midstate College
Medical Assistant Prgm
411 W Northmoor Rd
Peoria, IL 61614-3558
www.midstate.edu

Rockford Career College
Medical Assistant Prgm
730 N Church
Rockford, IL 61103-6917

Everest College - Skokie
Medical Assistant Prgm
9811 Woods Dr, Ste 200
Skokie, IL 60077
www.everestcollege.edu

South Suburban College
Medical Assistant Prgm
15800 S State St, Rm 4453
Nursing Department Room 4120
South Holland, IL 60473-1200
www.southsuburbancollege.edu

Midwest Technical Institute - Springfield
Medical Assistant Prgm
2731 Farmer Market Rd
Springfield, IL 62707
www.midwesttech.edu

Robert Morris University - Springfield
Medical Assistant Prgm
3101 Montvale Dr
Springfield, IL 62704-4260
www.robertmorris.edu

Waubonsee Community College
Medical Assistant Prgm
Route 47 at Waubonsee Dr, Akerlow 230
Health Career Occupations
Sugar Grove, IL 60554
www.wcc.cc.il.us

Indiana

Harrison College - Anderson
Medical Assistant Prgm
140 E 53rd St
Anderson, IN 46013-1717
www.harrison.edu

Ivy Tech Community College - Anderson
Medical Assistant Prgm
104 W 53rd St
Anderson, IN 46013-1502
www.ivytech.edu

Harrison College - Columbus
Medical Assistant Prgm
2222 Poshard Dr
Columbus, IN 47203-1843
www.harrison.edu

Ivy Tech Community College - Columbus
Medical Assistant Prgm
4475 Central Ave
Columbus, IN 47203-1868
www.ivytech.edu/columbus
Prgm Dir: Katherine Hawkins, MS CMA (AAMA)
Tel: 812 374-5163   *Fax:* 812 372-0311
E-mail: khawkins@ivytech.edu

Harrison College - Elkhart
Medical Assistant Prgm
56075 Parkway Ave
Elkhart, IN 46516-9325

Harrison College - Evansville
Medical Assistant Prgm
4601 Theater Dr
Evansville, IN 47715-3901
www.harrison.edu

Brown Mackie College - Fort Wayne
Medical Assistant Prgm
3000 E Coliseum Blvd
Fort Wayne, IN 46805
www.brownmackie.edu

Harrison College - Fort Wayne
Medical Assistant Prgm
6413 N Clinton St
Fort Wayne, IN 46825
www.harrison.edu

International Business College - Ft Wayne
Medical Assistant Prgm
5699 Coventry Ln
Fort Wayne, IN 46804-7145
www.ibcfortwayne.edu

Ivy Tech Community College - Fort Wayne
Cosponsor: Brown Mackie College Ft. Wayne
Medical Assistant Prgm
3000 East Coliseum Blvd
Fort Wayne, IN 46805
www.brownmackie.edu

Ivy Tech Community College - Northeast
Medical Assistant Prgm
3800 N Anthony Blvd
Fort Wayne, IN 46805-1430
www.ivytech.edu

Medtech College-Fort Wayne
Medical Assistant Prgm
7230 Engle Rd, Suite 200
Fort Wayne, IN 46804

MedTech College-Greenwood
Medical Assistant Prgm
1500 American Way
Greenwood, IN 46221

Harrison College - Downtown (Indianapolis)
Medical Assistant Prgm
550 E Washington St
Indianapolis, IN 46204
www.harrison.edu

Harrison College - Indianapolis
Medical Assistant Prgm
8150 Brookville Rd
Indianapolis, IN 46239
www.harrison.edu

International Business Coll - Indianapolis
Medical Assistant Prgm
7205 Shadeland Station
Indianapolis, IN 46256-3997
www.ibcindianapolis.edu
Prgm Dir: Judy D Mackey, CMA AAS
Tel: 317 813-2304   *Fax:* 317 841-6419
E-mail: jmackey@ibcindianapolis.edu

Ivy Tech Community College - Central Indiana Region
Medical Assistant Prgm
9301 E 59th St
Indianapolis, IN 46216-2236

Ivy Tech Community College - Lawrence Campus
Medical Assistant Prgm
9301 E 59th St
Indianapolis, IN 46216-2236
www.ivytech.edu

Kaplan College
Medical Assistant Prgm
7302 Woodland Dr
Indianapolis, IN 46278-1736
www.kaplan.edu

MedTech College-Indianapolis
Medical Assistant Prgm
6612 E 75th St Suite 300
Indianapolis, IN 46250

National College - Indianapolis
Medical Assistant Prgm
6060 Castleway West Dr
Indianapolis, IN 46250-1930

Ivy Tech Community College - Kokomo
Medical Assistant Prgm
700 E Firmin St
PO Box 1373
Kokomo, IN 46902-2395
ivytech.edu/kokomo

Harrison College - Lafayette
Medical Assistant Prgm
4705 Meijer Court
Lafayette, IN 47905
www.harrison.edu

Ivy Tech Community College - Lafayette
Medical Assistant Prgm
3101 S Creasy Ln
PO Box 6299
Lafayette, IN 47905-5241
www.ivytech.edu

Ivy Tech Community College - Lawrenceburg
Medical Assistant Prgm
50 Walnut St
Lawrenceburg, IN 47025
www.ivytech.edu
Prgm Dir: Theresa I Disch, BS BA LPN CMA
Tel: 812 537-4010, Ext 5234   *Fax:* 812 537-0993
E-mail: tdisch@ivytech.edu

Ivy Tech Community College - Madison
Medical Assistant Prgm
590 Ivy Tech Dr
Madison, IN 47250
www.ivytech.edu/madison

Harrison College - Marion
Medical Assistant Prgm
830 N Miller Ave
Marion, IN 46952
www.harrison.edu
Notes: Program closing in December 2010.

Ivy Tech Community College - Marion
Medical Assistant Prgm
1015 E 3rd St
Marion, IN 46952
www.ivytech.edu

Ivy Tech Community College - Michigan City
Medical Assistant Prgm
3714 Franklin St
Michigan City, IN 46360-7311
www.ivytech.edu

Ivy Tech Community College - Muncie
Medical Assistant Prgm
4301 S Cowan Rd
Muncie, IN 47302

Ivy Tech Community College - Richmond
Medical Assistant Prgm
2325 Chester Blvd
Richmond, IN 47374
www.ivytech.edu

Ivy Tech Community College - Sellersburg
Medical Assistant Prgm
8204 Hwy 311
Sellersburg, IN 47172
www.ivytech.edu/sellersburg

Brown Mackie College - Fort Wayne (South Bend)
Medical Assistant Prgm
3454 Douglas Rd
South Bend, IN 46635
www.brownmackie.edu

Ivy Tech Community College - South Bend
Medical Assistant Prgm
220 Dean Johnson Blvd
South Bend, IN 46601-3415
www.ivytech.edu

Harrison College - Terre Haute
Medical Assistant Prgm
1378 South State Rd 46
Terre Haute, IN 47803
www.harrison.edu

Ivy Tech Community College - Terre Haute
Medical Assistant Prgm
8000 S Education Dr
Terre Haute, IN 47802-4845
www.ivytech.edu

Iowa

Des Moines Area Community College
Medical Assistant Prgm
2006 S Ankeny Blvd
Health Sciences Building
Bldg 9 9-15
Ankeny, IA 50023-8995
www.dmacc.edu

Kaplan University - Cedar Falls
Medical Assistant Prgm
7009 Nordic Dr
Cedar Falls, IA 50613-6309

Kaplan University - Cedar Rapids
Medical Assistant Prgm
3165 Edgewood Pkwy SW
Cedar Rapids, IA 52404-7826

Kirkwood Community College
Medical Assistant Prgm
6301 Kirkwood Blvd SW, PO Box 2068
221 Linn Hall
Cedar Rapids, IA 52404-5260
www.kirkwood.edu

Iowa Western Community College
Medical Assistant Prgm
2700 College Rd, PO Box 4C
Council Bluffs, IA 51503-1057
www.iwcc.cc.ia.us

Kaplan University - Council Bluffs
Medical Assistant Prgm
1751 Madison Ave Suite 750
Council Bluffs, IA 51503

Kaplan University, Davenport Campus
Medical Assistant Prgm
1801 E Kimberly Rd, Ste 1
Suite 100
Davenport, IA 52807-2095
www.kaplan.edu

Mercy College of Health Sciences
Medical Assistant Prgm
928 6th Ave
Des Moines, IA 50309-1225
www.mchs.edu

Iowa Central Community College
Medical Assistant Prgm
One Triton Circle
Fort Dodge, IA 50501
www.iowacentral.edu

Ellsworth Community College
Medical Assistant Prgm
1100 College Ave
Iowa Falls, IA 50126-1163

Kaplan University - Mason City
Medical Assistant Prgm
2570 4th St SW
Mason City, IA 50401

North Iowa Area Community College
Medical Assistant Prgm
500 College Dr
Mason City, IA 50401-7213
www.niacc.edu

Western Iowa Tech Community College
Medical Assistant Prgm
4647 Stone Ave PO Box 5199
Sioux City, IA 51102-5199

Iowa Lakes Community College
Medical Assistant Prgm
1900 N Grand
Suite 8
Spencer, IA 51301-2200
www.iowalakes.edu

Kaplan University - Des Moines
Medical Assistant Prgm
4655 121st St
Urbandale, IA 50323

Southeastern Community College
Medical Assistant Prgm
1500 West Agency Rd
West Burlington, IA 52655-1695
www.scciowa.edu
Prgm Dir: Debra S Shaffer, RN
Tel: 319 208-5213   *Fax:* 319 752-4957
E-mail: dshaffer@scciowa.edu

Kansas

Coffeyville Community College
Medical Assistant Prgm
700 Roosevelt
Coffeyville, KS 67337

Northwest Kansas Technical College
Medical Assistant Prgm
1209 Harrison St, PO Box 668
Goodland, KS 67735-3441
www.nwktc.org

National American University - Overland Park
Medical Assistant Prgm
10310 Mastin St
Overland Park, KS 66212-5451

Wichita Area Technical College
Medical Assistant Prgm
3639 N Comotara St
324 N Emporia
Wichita, KS 67202-2512
www.watc.edu

Kentucky

National College - Danville
Medical Assistant Prgm
115 E Lexington Ave
Danville, KY 40422-1517
www.ncbt.edu

National College - Florence
Medical Assistant Prgm
7627 Ewing Blvd
Florence, KY 41042-1812
www.national-college.edu

Henderson Community College
Medical Assistant Prgm
2660 S Green St
Henderson, KY 42420-4623
www.hencc.kctcs.edu

Bluegrass Community and Technical College
Medical Assistant Prgm
308 Vo-Tech Rd
Lexington, KY 40511

National College - Lexington
Medical Assistant Prgm
2376 Sir Barton Way
Lexington, KY 40509
www.national-college.edu

Spencerian College - Lexington
Cosponsor: Sullivan University Systems
Medical Assistant Prgm
1575 Winchester Rd
Lexington, KY 40505
www.spencerian.edu

Sullivan University - Lexington
Medical Assistant Prgm
2355 Harrodsburg Rd
Lexington, KY 40504
www.sullivan.edu

Georgetown College (Louisville)
Medical Assistant Prgm
4205 Dixie Hwy
Louisville, KY 40216-3801
www.national-college.edu

Jefferson Community and Technical College
Medical Assistant Prgm
727 W Chestnut St
Louisville, KY 40203-2074
www.jefferson.kctcs.edu

National College - Louisville
Medical Assistant Prgm
4205 Dixie Hwy
Louisville, KY 40216-3801
www.ncbt.edu

Spencerian College
Medical Assistant Prgm
4627 Dixie Hwy
Louisville, KY 40216-2605
www.spencerian.edu

Maysville Comm & Tech College
Medical Assistant Prgm
609 Viking Dr
Morehead, KY 40351

National College - Pikeville
Medical Assistant Prgm
50 National College Blvd
Pikeville, KY 41501
www.ncbt.edu

National College - Richmond
Medical Assistant Prgm
125 S Killarney Ln
Richmond, KY 40475
www.national-college.edu

Louisiana

Bossier Parish Community College
Medical Assistant Prgm
6220 E Texas St
Bossier City, LA 71111
www.bpcc.edu

Career Technical College
Medical Assistant Prgm
2319 Louisville Ave
Monroe, LA 71201
www.careertc.com

Career Technical College
Medical Assistant Prgm
1227 Shreveport-Barksdale Hwy
Shreveport, LA 71105
www.careertc.com/shreveportwelcome.html

Maine

Beal College
Medical Assistant Prgm
99 Farm Rd
Bangor, ME 04401-6831
www.bealcollege.edu

Eastern Maine Community College
Medical Assistant Prgm
354 Hogan Rd
Bangor, ME 04401-4206

Washington County Technical College
Medical Assistant Prgm
One College Drive
Calais, ME 04619

Kennebec Valley Community College
Medical Assistant Prgm
92 Western Ave
Fairfield, ME 04937-1367
www.kvcc.me.edu

Maryland

Anne Arundel Community College
Medical Assistant Prgm
101 College Pkwy
Arnold, MD 21012-1895
www.aacc.edu/default.cfm

Harford Community College
Medical Assistant Prgm
401 Thomas Run Rd
Bel Air, MD 21015

Allegany College of Maryland
Medical Assistant Prgm
12401 Willowbrook Rd SE
Cumberland, MD 21502-2559
www.allegany.edu

Kaplan College - Hagerstown
Medical Assistant Prgm
18618 Crestwood Dr
Hagerstown, MD 21742-2752
www.kaplancollege.com

Cecil Community College
Medical Assistant Prgm
1 Seahawk Dr
North East, MD 21901-1900
www.cecilcc.edu

Fortis College - Towson
Medical Assistant Prgm
700 York Rd
Towson, MD 21204-2503
www.medixschool.edu

Massachusetts

American Career Institute
Medical Assistant Prgm
725 Granite St
Braintree, MA 2184

Massasoit Community College
Medical Assistant Prgm
900 Randolph St
Ctr for Careers & Technology
Canton, MA 02021-1372
www.massasoit.mass.edu

Porter and Chester Institute - Chicopee
Medical Assistant Prgm
134 Dulong Circle
Chicopee, MA 01022-1153
porterchester.com
Prgm Dir: Elizabeth Murphy, Director of Education
Tel: 413 593-3339   *Fax:* 413 593-6439
E-mail: emurphy@porterchester.com

North Shore Community College
Medical Assistant Prgm
One Ferncroft Rd
PO Box 3340
Danvers, MA 01923-4017
www.northshore.edu

Bristol Community College
Medical Assistant Prgm
777 Elsbree St
Fall River, MA 02720-7399
www.bristol.mass.edu

Mount Wachusett Community College
Medical Assistant Prgm
444 Green St
Gardner, MA 01440-1395
www.mwcc.mass.edu

Northern Essex Community College
Medical Assistant Prgm
45 Franklin St
Lawrence, MA 01840-1121
www.necc.mass.edu

Middlesex Community College
Medical Assistant Prgm
33 Kearney Square
Lowell, MA 01852-1901
www.middlesex.mass.edu

Charles H McCann Technical School
Medical Assistant Prgm
70 Hodges Cross Rd
North Adams, MA 01247-3940
www.mccanntech.org

Southeastern Technical Institute
Medical Assistant Prgm
250 Foundry St
Code 2411
South Easton, MA 02375-1780
www.southeasterntech.org

Springfield Technical Community College
Medical Assistant Prgm
Armory Square, Suite 1 PO Box 9000
Springfield, MA 01102-9000

Cape Cod Community College
Medical Assistant Prgm
2240 Iyanough Rd
West Barnstable, MA 02668-1532
www.capecod.edu

The Salter School
Medical Assistant Prgm
184 W Boylston
Suite 1
West Boylston, MA 01583-1756
www.saltercollege.com

Quinsigamond Community College
Medical Assistant Prgm
670 W Boylston St
Admin Bldg Rm 403-A
Worcester, MA 01606-2031
www.qcc.edu

Michigan

Baker College of Allen Park
Medical Assistant Prgm
4500 Enterprise Dr
Allen Park, MI 48101-3033

Alpena Community College
Medical Assistant Prgm
665 Johnson St
Alpena, MI 49707-1495
www.alpena.cc.mi.us

Baker College of Auburn Hills
Medical Assistant Prgm
1500 University Dr
Auburn Hills, MI 48326-2642
www.baker.edu

Davenport University - Battle Creek
Medical Assistant Prgm
200 Van Buren St W
Battle Creek Career Center
Battle Creek, MI 49017-3007
www.davenport.edu

Baker College of Cadillac
Medical Assistant Prgm
9600 E 13th St
Cadillac, MI 49601-9600
www.baker.edu

Davenport University - Caro
Medical Assistant Prgm
1231 Cleaver Rd
Caro, MI 48723-9376
www.davenport.edu

Glen Oaks Community College
Medical Assistant Prgm
62249 Shimmel Rd
Centreville, MI 49032-9784
www.glenoaks.cc.mi.us

Baker College of Clinton Township
Medical Assistant Prgm
34950 Little Mack Ave
Clinton Township, MI 48035-4701
www.baker.edu

Macomb Community College
Medical Assistant Prgm
Health and Human Services
44575 Garfield Rd
Clinton Township, MI 48038-1139
www.macomb.edu

Henry Ford Community College
Medical Assistant Prgm
5101 Evergreen Rd
Dearborn, MI 48128-1495
www.hfcc.edu

Baker College of Flint
Medical Assistant Prgm
G 1050 W Bristol Rd
Flint, MI 48507-5508
www.baker.edu

Schoolcraft College
Medical Assistant Prgm
1751 Radcliff St
Garden City, MI 48135-1197
www.schoolcraft.edu

**Davenport University - Grand Rapids
(Fulton St)**
Medical Assistant Prgm
415 E Fulton St E
Grand Rapids, MI 49503
www.davenport.edu

Mid Michigan Community College
Medical Assistant Prgm
1375 S Clare Ave
Harrison, MI 48625
www.midmich.edu
Prgm Dir: Janice Noteboom, Faculty Coordinator of
Allied Health
Tel: 989 386-6622, Ext 315 *Fax:* 989 386-6666
E-mail: jnoteboom@midmich.edu

Baker College of Jackson
Medical Assistant Prgm
2800 Springport Rd
Jackson, MI 49202-1230
www.baker.edu

Jackson Community College
Medical Assistant Prgm
2111 Emmons Rd
Jackson, MI 49201-8395
www.jccmi.edu

Kalamazoo Valley Community College
Medical Assistant Prgm
PO Box 4070, 6767 West O Ave
Kalamazoo, MI 49003-4070
www.kvcc.edu

Davenport University - Lansing
Medical Assistant Prgm
220 E Kalamazoo St
Lansing, MI 48933-2110
www.davenport.edu

Baker College of Muskegon
Medical Assistant Prgm
1903 Marquette Ave
Muskegon, MI 49442-1453
www.baker.edu

Baker College of Owosso
Medical Assistant Prgm
1020 S Washington St
Owosso, MI 48867-8956
www.baker.edu

Baker College of Port Huron
Medical Assistant Prgm
3403 Lapeer Rd
Port Huron, MI 48060-2597

Montcalm Community College
Medical Assistant Prgm
2800 College Dr
Sidney, MI 48885-9723
www.montcalm.cc.mi.us

Everest Institute-Southfield
Medical Assistant Prgm
21107 Lahser Rd
Southfield, MI 48033

National Institute of Technology
Medical Assistant Prgm
26111 Evergreen Rd, Ste 201
21107 Lahser Rd
Southfield, MI 48033
www.everest.edu/campus/southfield

Carnegie Institute
Medical Assistant Prgm
550 Stephenson Hwy, Ste 100
Troy, MI 48083
www.carnegie-institute.edu

Oakland Community College
Medical Assistant Prgm
7350 Cooley Lake Rd
HL HH206
Waterford, MI 48327-4187
www.oaklandcc.edu

Minnesota

Anoka Technical College
Medical Assistant Prgm
1355 W Hwy 10
Anoka, MN 55303-1590
www.anokatech.edu

Academy College
Medical Assistant Prgm
1101 E 78th St
Bloomington, MN 55420

Rasmussen College - Brooklyn Park
Medical Assistant Prgm
8301 93rd Ave N
Brooklyn Park, MN 55445-1512
www.rasmussen.edu

Herzing University
Medical Assistant Prgm
5700 W Broadway Ave
Crystal, MN 55428

Duluth Business University
Medical Assistant Prgm
4724 Mike Colalillo Dr
Duluth, MN 55807-2723
www.dbumn.edu

Lake Superior College
Medical Assistant Prgm
2101 Trinity Rd
Duluth, MN 55811-3349
www.lsc.edu

Argosy University Twin Cities Campus
Medical Assistant Prgm
1515 Central Parkway
Eagan, MN 55121
www.argosyu.edu

Rasmussen College - Eagan
Medical Assistant Prgm
3500 Federal Dr
Eagan, MN 55122-1346

Northland Community & Technical College
Medical Assistant Prgm
2022 Central Ave NE
East Grand Forks, MN 56721-2702
www.northlandcollege.edu

Hennepin Technical College
Medical Assistant Prgm
13100 Collegeview Drive
Eden Prairie, MN 55347-2600

Rasmussen College - Eden Prairie
Medical Assistant Prgm
7905 Golden Triangle Dr Ste 100
Eden Prairie, MN 55344-7220

Rasmussen College - Lake Elmo
Medical Assistant Prgm
8565 Eagle Point Circle
Lake Elmo, MN 55042-8637

Minnesota West Comm & Tech College
Medical Assistant Prgm
311 N Spring St
Luverne, MN 56156
www.mnwest.edu

Rasmussen College - Mankato
Medical Assistant Prgm
130 Saint Andrews Drive
Mankato, MN 56001-8658
www.rasmussen.edu

Rasmussen College - Moorhead
Medical Assistant Prgm
1250 29th Ave South
Moorhead, MN 56560-5058

Dakota County Technical College
Medical Assistant Prgm
1300 E 145th St
County Rd 42
Rosemount, MN 55068-2932
www.dctc.edu

Minneapolis Business College
Medical Assistant Prgm
1711 W County Rd B
Suite 100N
Roseville, MN 55113-4024
www.minneapolisbusinesscollege.edu
Prgm Dir: Caryn M Ziegler, CMA
Tel: 651 636-7406   *Fax:* 651 636-8185
E-mail: cziegler@minneapolisbusinesscollege.edu

National American University - Roseville
Medical Assistant Prgm
1550 Highway 36 W
Roseville, MN 55113-4035

Rasmussen College - St Cloud
Medical Assistant Prgm
226 Park Ave S
St Cloud, MN 56301-3713
www.rasmussen.edu

Central Lakes College
Medical Assistant Prgm
1830 Airport Rd
Staples, MN 56479

Century College
Medical Assistant Prgm
3300 Century Ave N
White Bear Lake, MN 55110-1842
www.century.edu
Prgm Dir: Michelle Blesi, CMA (AAMA) AA BA MA
Tel: 651 748-2610   *Fax:* 651 747-4077
E-mail: michelle.blesi@century.edu

Ridgewater College - Willmar Campus
Medical Assistant Prgm
2101 15th Ave NW, PO Box 1097
Willmar, MN 56201-3096
www.ridgewater.edu

Mississippi

Northeast Mississippi Community College
Medical Assistant Prgm
101 Cunningham Blvd
Booneville, MS 38829-1726
www.nemcc.edu

Hinds Community College
Medical Assistant Prgm
3805 Hwy 80 E
Pearl, MS 39208-4295
www.hindscc.edu

Missouri

National American University
Medical Assistant Prgm
3620 Arrowhead Ave
Independence, MO 64057

Everest College - Springfield Campus
Medical Assistant Prgm
1010 W Sunshine St
Springfield, MO 65807-2446
www.everest.edu

Montana

Montana State Univ - Great Falls Coll of Tech
Medical Assistant Prgm
2100 16th Ave S
Great Falls, MT 59406-6010

Flathead Valley Community College
Medical Assistant Prgm
777 Grandview Dr
Kalispell, MT 59901-2699
www.fvcc.edu

Nebraska

Central Community College
Medical Assistant Prgm
Hastings Campus, 550 S Technical Blvd
East Highway 6
Hastings, NE 68902-1024
www.cccneb.edu
Prgm Dir: Michel K McKinney, CMA (AAMA)
Tel: 402 461-2405   *Fax:* 402 460-2138
E-mail: mmckinney@cccneb.edu

Kaplan University - Lincoln
Medical Assistant Prgm
1821 K St
Lincoln, NE 68508-2668

Southeast Community College
Medical Assistant Prgm
8800 O St
Lincoln, NE 68520-1227
www.southeast.edu

Kaplan University - Omaha
Medical Assistant Prgm
3350 N 90th St
Omaha, NE 68134-4710
www.hamiltonomaha.edu

Metropolitan Community College - Omaha
Medical Assistant Prgm
810 N 96th St
Omaha, NE 68114

Nebraska Methodist College
Medical Assistant Prgm
720 N 87th St
Omaha, NE 68114-2852
www.methodistcollege.edu

Nevada

College of Southern Nevada
Medical Assistant Prgm
6375 W Charleston Blvd, W4K
West Charleston Campus
Las Vegas, NV 89146-1164
www.csn.edu

New Hampshire

White Mountains Community College
Medical Assistant Prgm
2020 Riverside Drive
Berlin, NH 03570

River Valley Community College
Medical Assistant Prgm
One College Dr
Claremont, NH 03743-9707
www.claremont.nhctc.edu

Hesser College
Medical Assistant Prgm
3 Sundial Ave
Manchester, NH 03103-7230
www.hesser.edu

Manchester Community College
Medical Assistant Prgm
1066 Front St
Manchester, NH 03102-8528

New Jersey

Raritan Valley Community College
Medical Assistant Prgm
118 Lamington Rd
Branchburg, NJ 08876

Dover Business College - Clifton
Medical Assistant Prgm
600 Getty Ave
Clifton, NJ 07011-2108

Sussex County Community College
Medical Assistant Prgm
Health Sciences Department
One College Hill Building A
Newton, NJ 07860
www.sussex.edu

Bergen Community College
Medical Assistant Prgm
Medical Office Assistant Program
400 Paramus Rd
Paramus, NJ 07652-1595
www.bergen.edu
Prgm Dir: Steven W Toth, MS CMA RMA
Tel: 201 612-5490   *Fax:* 201 612-3876
E-mail: stoth@bergen.edu

Warren County Community College
Medical Assistant Prgm
445 Marshall St
Phillipsburg, NJ 08865
www.warren.edu
Prgm Dir: Marianne Van Deursen, MSEd CMA (AAMA)
    MLT
Tel: 908 835-2430   *Fax:* 908 878-0170
E-mail: vandeursen@warren.edu

Mercer County Technical Schools
Medical Assistant Prgm
1070 Klockner Rd
Health Careers Center
Trenton, NJ 08619-3027
www.mctec.net

Fortis Institute
Medical Assistant Prgm
201 Willowbrook Blvd
2nd Floor
Wayne, NJ 07470-7041
www.fortisinstitute.com
Prgm Dir: Lisa M Maldonado, RMA
Tel: 973 837-1818   *Fax:* 973 256-0816
E-mail: lmaldonado@edaff.com

Fortis Institute - Wayne
Medical Assistant Prgm
201 Willowbrook Blvd Second Floor
Wayne, NJ 07470-7041

New Mexico

National American University-Albuquerque
Medical Assistant Prgm
4775 Indian School Rd NE Ste 200
Albuquerque, NM 87110-3976

Eastern New Mexico University - Roswell
Medical Assistant Prgm
PO Box 6000
52 University Blvd
Roswell, NM 88203-8435
www.enmu.edu

Santa Fe Community College
Medical Assistant Prgm
6401 Richards Ave
Santa Fe, NM 87508-4887

New York

Bryant & Stratton College - Albany
Medical Assistant Prgm
1259 Central Ave
Albany, NY 12205-5230
www.bryantstratton.edu

Broome Community College
Medical Assistant Prgm
Decker Bldg, PO Box 1017
907 Upper Front St
Binghamton, NY 13902-1017
www.sunybroome.edu

Ridley-Lowell Business & Technical Institute
Medical Assistant Prgm
116 Front St
Binghamton, NY 13905-3102
www.ridley.edu

ASA Institute of Business & Computer Tech
Medical Assistant Prgm
81 Willoughby St
Brooklyn, NY 11201-5291
www.asa.edu

Bryant & Stratton College - Buffalo
Medical Assistant Prgm
465 Main St, Ste 400
Buffalo, NY 14203-1700
www.bryantstratton.edu

Trocaire College
Medical Assistant Prgm
360 Choate Ave
Buffalo, NY 14220-2094
www.trocaire.edu
Prgm Dir: Nicole Miller,
Tel: 716 827-2560   *Fax:* 716 828-6107
E-mail: millern@trocaire.edu

Elmira Business Institute
Medical Assistant Prgm
303 N Main St
Satellite campus: 4100 Vestal Rd, Vestal, NY 13850
Elmira, NY 14901
www.ebi-college.edu

Plaza College
Medical Assistant Prgm
74-09 37th Ave
Jackson Heights, NY 11372-6300
www.plazacollege.edu

Wood Tobe'-Coburn School
Medical Assistant Prgm
8 E 40th St
Room 201
New York, NY 10016-0190
www.woodtobecoburn.edu
Prgm Dir: Janette M Rodriguez,
Tel: 212 897-0153   *Fax:* 212 686-9171
E-mail: jrodriguez@woodtobecoburn.edu

Ridley-Lowell Business & Technical Institute
Medical Assistant Prgm
26 S Hamilton St
Poughkeepsie, NY 12601-3328
www.ridley.edu

Bryant & Stratton College - Rochester
Medical Assistant Prgm
Henrietta Campus, 1225 Jefferson Rd
Greece Campus, 150 Bellwood Dr
Rochester, NY 14625
www.bryantstratton.edu
Prgm Dir: Jean Arlauckas
Tel: 585 292-5627, Ext 148   *Fax:* 585 292-6015
E-mail: jarlauckas@bryantstratton.edu

Everest Institute
Medical Assistant Prgm
1630 Portland Ave
Rochester, NY 14621-3007
www.everest-institute.com

Niagara County Community College
Medical Assistant Prgm
3111 Saunders Settlement Rd
Sanborn, NY 14132-9460
www.niagaracc.suny.edu

Bryant & Stratton College - Syracuse
Medical Assistant Prgm
953 James St
Syracuse, NY 13203-2555
www.bryantstratton.edu

Erie Community College - North Campus
Medical Assistant Prgm
6205 Main St
Bldg B - North Campus
Williamsville, NY 14221-8402
www.ecc.edu

North Carolina

Stanly Community College
Medical Assistant Prgm
141 College Dr
Albemarle, NC 28001-7458
www.Stanly.edu

Asheville-Buncombe Technical Comm College
Medical Assistant Prgm
340 Victoria Rd
Asheville, NC 28801-4816

South College - Asheville
Medical Assistant Prgm
29 Turtle Creek Dr
Asheville, NC 28803
www.southcollegenc.com

Miller-Motte College - Cary
Medical Assistant Prgm
2205 Walnut St
Cary, NC 27518-9209
www.miller-motte.edu

Brookstone College of Business
Medical Assistant Prgm
10125 Berkeley Place Dr
Charlotte, NC 28262

Central Piedmont Community College
Medical Assistant Prgm
PO Box 35009
Charlotte, NC 28235-5009
www.cpcc.edu

King's College
Medical Assistant Prgm
322 Lamar Ave
Charlotte, NC 28204-2436
www.kingscollegecharlotte.edu

Haywood Community College
Medical Assistant Prgm
185 Freelander Dr
Clyde, NC 28721-9441
www.haywood.edu

Cabarrus College of Health Sciences
Medical Assistant Prgm
401 Medical Park Dr
Concord, NC 28025-3959
www.cabarruscollege.edu

Gaston College
Medical Assistant Prgm
201 Hwy 321 S
Dallas, NC 28034-1499
www.gaston.edu
Prgm Dir: Betty D Jones, MA RN CMA
Tel: 704 922-6465   *Fax:* 704 922-2333
E-mail: jones.betty@gaston.edu

Surry Community College
Medical Assistant Prgm
630 S Main St
PO Box 304
Dobson, NC 27017-8432
www.surry.edu
Prgm Dir: Jean L Mosley, BS CMA (AAMA)
Tel: 336 386-3407   *Fax:* 336 386-3497
E-mail: mosleyj@surry.edu

Durham Technical Community College
Medical Assistant Prgm
1637 E Lawson St
Durham, NC 27703-5023

College of The Albemarle
Medical Assistant Prgm
1208 N Rd St
PO Box 2327
Elizabeth City, NC 27906-2327
www.albemarle.edu

Wayne Community College
Medical Assistant Prgm
Caller Box 8002
3000 Wayne Memorial Dr
Goldsboro, NC 27533-8002
www.waynecc.edu

Alamance Community College
Medical Assistant Prgm
PO Box 8000
1247 Jimmie Kerr Rd
Graham, NC 27253-8000
www.alamancecc.edu

Pamlico Community College
Medical Assistant Prgm
PO Box 185
5049 Highway 306 South
Grantsboro, NC 28529-0185
www.pamlicocc.edu

Pitt Community College
Medical Assistant Prgm
PO Drawer 7007, Hwy 11 S
Greenville, NC 27835-7007
www.pittcc.edu

Richmond Community College
Medical Assistant Prgm
1042 W Hamlet Ave
PO Box 1189
Hamlet, NC 28345-1189
www.richmondcc.edu

Guilford Technical Community College
Medical Assistant Prgm
601 High Point Rd, PO Box 309
Jamestown, NC 27282-8572
www.gtcc.cc.nc.us

James Sprunt Community College
Medical Assistant Prgm
PO Box 398
Hwy 11 S
133 James Sprunt Dr
Kenansville, NC 28349-0398
www.jamessprunt.com

Lenoir Community College
Medical Assistant Prgm
PO Box 188
231 Hwy 58S
Kinston, NC 28502-0188
www.lenoircc.edu/Academic_Programs/
medassistA45400.htm
Prgm Dir: Linda Susan Johnson, CMA (AAMA) CPC
Tel: 252 527-6223, Ext 815   *Fax:* 252 520-9598
E-mail: ljohnson@lenoircc.edu

Davidson County Community College
Medical Assistant Prgm
PO Box 1287
297 DCCC Rd
Lexington, NC 27293-1287
www.davidsonccc.edu

Central Carolina Community College - Harnett County
Medical Assistant Prgm
1075 E Cornelius Harnett Blvd
Lillington, NC 27546
www.cccc.edu

Vance-Granville Community College
Medical Assistant Prgm
PO Box 777
8100 NC 56 Hwy W
Louisburg, NC 27549-0777
www.vgcc.edu

Mitchell Community College
Medical Assistant Prgm
219 N Academy St
Mooresville, NC 28115-3106
www.mitchellcc.edu
Prgm Dir: Mary M Marks, FNP-C MSN
Tel: 704 978-5424   *Fax:* 704 663-5239
E-mail: mmarks@mitchellcc.edu

Carteret Community College
Medical Assistant Prgm
3505 Arendell St
Morehead City, NC 28557-2905
www.carteret.edu

Western Piedmont Community College
Medical Assistant Prgm
1001 Burkemont Ave
Morganton, NC 28655-4511
www.wp.cc.nc.us

Tri-County Community College
Medical Assistant Prgm
4600 Hwy 64 East
Murphy, NC 28906
www.tricountycc.edu

Craven Community College
Medical Assistant Prgm
800 College Court
E149
New Bern, NC 28562-4984
www.craven.cc.nc.us/

Central Carolina Community College - Pittsboro
Medical Assistant Prgm
764 West St
Pittsboro, NC 27312
www.cccc.edu

South Piedmont Community College
Medical Assistant Prgm
PO Box 126
680 Highway 74 West
Polkton, NC 28135-0126
www.spcc.edu

Miller-Motte College - Raleigh
Medical Assistant Prgm
3901 Capital Blvd Suite 151
Raleigh, NC 27604-3488

Wake Technical Community College
Medical Assistant Prgm
9101 Fayetteville Rd
HS Medical Assisting Dept
Raleigh, NC 27603-5655
www.waketech.edu

Nash Community College
Medical Assistant Prgm
522 North Old Carriage Rd PO Box 7488
Rocky Mount, NC 27804-0488

Piedmont Community College
Medical Assistant Prgm
PO Box 1197
Roxboro, NC 27573

Johnston Community College
Medical Assistant Prgm
PO Box 2350
245 College Rd
Smithfield, NC 27577-2350
www.johnstoncc.edu

Mayland Community College
Medical Assistant Prgm
PO Box 547
200 Mayland Drive
Spruce Pine, NC 28777
www.mayland.edu

Southwestern Community College - Sylva
Medical Assistant Prgm
447 College Drive
Sylva, NC 28779

Edgecombe Community College
Medical Assistant Prgm
2009 W Wilson St
Tarboro, NC 27886
www.edgecombe.edu

Montgomery Community College
Medical Assistant Prgm
1011 Page St
PO Box 787
Troy, NC 27371-8387
www.montgomery.cc.nc.us

Wilkes Community College
Medical Assistant Prgm
PO Box 120
1328 S Collegiate Dr
Wilkesboro, NC 28697-0120
www.wilkescc.edu

Martin Commuity College
Medical Assistant Prgm
1161 Kehukee Park Rd
Williamston, NC 27892-8307
www.martin.cc.nc.us

Miller-Motte College - Wilmington
Medical Assistant Prgm
5000 Market St
Wilmington, NC 28405-3430
www.miller-motte.com

Forsyth Technical Community College
Medical Assistant Prgm
2100 Silas Creek Pkwy
Winston-Salem, NC 27103-5197
www.forsythtech.edu

Living Arts Institute at School of Comm Arts
Medical Assistant Prgm
1100 South Stratford Rd Suite 200
Winston-Salem, NC 27103-3217

Ohio

Akron Institute of Herzing College
Medical Assistant Prgm
1600 South Arlington
Suite 100
Akron, OH 44306-3958
www.akroninstitute.com

Brown Mackie College - Akron
Medical Assistant Prgm
755 White Pond Dr
Suite 101
Akron, OH 44320-4221
www.brownmackie.edu
Prgm Dir: Esther Brown, Dept Chair Allied Health
Tel: 330 869-3658   *Fax:* 330 869-3670
E-mail: eebrown@brownmackie.edu

The University of Akron
Medical Assistant Prgm
Polsky 124C
Summit College
Akron, OH 44325-3702
www.uakron.edu

Northwest State Community College
Medical Assistant Prgm
22600 State Route 34
Archbold, OH 43502-9517
www.northweststate.edu

Ashland County - West Holmes Career Center
Medical Assistant Prgm
1783 State Route 60
Ashland, OH 44805-9377
www.acwhcc-jvs.k12.oh.us

Univ of Cincinnati - Clermont College
Medical Assistant Prgm
4200 Clermont College Drive
Batavia, OH 45103

Mahoning County Career & Technical Center
Medical Assistant Prgm
7300 N Palmyra Rd
Canfield, OH 44406-9710
www.mahoningctc.com

Canton City Schools
Medical Assistant Prgm
Adult Community Education Center
116 McKinley Ave NW, Room 209
Canton, OH 44702-1710
www.ccsdistrict.org
Prgm Dir: Sherrell Wimer, CLPN AAS CNAC CMA-AAMA
Tel: 330 438-2556, Ext 100   *Fax:* 330 454-6767
E-mail: n8oog@yahoo.com

Stark State College
Medical Assistant Prgm
6200 Frank Ave NW
Canton, OH 44720
www.starkstate.edu

Fairfield Career Center (EVSD)
Medical Assistant Prgm
4000 Columbus-Lancaster Rd
Carroll, OH 43112-9563
www.ncacasi.org

Fortis College- Centerville
Medical Assistant Prgm
555 E Alex Bell Rd
Centerville, OH 45459-2712

Pickaway Ross Joint Vocational School
Medical Assistant Prgm
17273 St Rt 104 Bldg 4
VA Medical Center Bldg 4
Chillicothe, OH 45601-8608
www.pickawayross.com
Prgm Dir: Faye Vermillion, RN BSN M Ed
Tel: 740 642-1450   *Fax:* 740 642-1454
E-mail: faye.vermillion@pickawayross.com

Brown Mackie College - Cincinnati
Medical Assistant Prgm
1011 Glendale-Milford Rd
Cincinnati, OH 45215-1107
www.brownmackie.edu

Cincinnati State Tech & Comm College
Medical Assistant Prgm
3520 Central Pkwy
Cincinnati, OH 45223-2690
www.cincinnatistate.edu

National College - Cincinnati
Medical Assistant Prgm
6871 Steger Dr
Cincinnati, OH 45237
www.national-college.edu

University of Cincinnati
Medical Assistant Prgm
Raymond Walters College
9555 Plainfield Rd
Cincinnati, OH 45236-1007
www.rwc.uc.edu

Miami Valley Career Technology Center
Medical Assistant Prgm
6800 Hoke Rd
Clayton, OH 45315-8975
www.mvctc.com

Cuyahoga Community College
Medical Assistant Prgm
Metro Campus
2900 Community College Ave
Health Careers and Science, Room 106-A
Cleveland, OH 44115-3123
www.tri-c.edu
Prgm Dir: Sherry Brewer, BS CMA-AC(AAMA)
Tel: 216 987-4439   *Fax:* 216 987-4285
E-mail: Sherry.brewer@tri-c.edu

American School of Technology
Medical Assistant Prgm
4599 Morse Center Rd
Columbus, OH 43229-6689
www.ast.edu

Bradford School
Medical Assistant Prgm
2469 Stelzer Rd
Columbus, OH 43219-3129
www.bradfordschoolcolumbus.edu

Columbus State Community College
Medical Assistant Prgm
550 E Spring St
Columbus, OH 43216
www.cscc.edu

Ohio Business College
Medical Assistant Prgm
1880 E Dublin Granville Rd Ste 100
Columbus, OH 43229-3523

Kaplan College - Dayton
Medical Assistant Prgm
2800 East River Rd
Dayton, OH 45439

Miami-Jacobs Career College
Medical Assistant Prgm
110 N Patterson Blvd
Dayton, OH 45402

Ohio Institute of Photography & Technology
Medical Assistant Prgm
Division of Allied Health
2029 Edgefield Rd
Dayton, OH 45439
www.oipt.com

Sinclair Community College
Medical Assistant Prgm
444 W Third St
Dayton, OH 45402-1421
www.sinclair.edu

Ohio Valley College of Technology
Medical Assistant Prgm
16808 St Clair Ave, PO Box 7000
East Liverpool, OH 43920-9139
www.ovct.edu

Lorain County Community College
Medical Assistant Prgm
1005 N Abbe Rd
Elyria, OH 44035-1613
www.lorainccc.edu

Portage Lakes Career Center
Medical Assistant Prgm
4401 Shriver Rd
PO Box 248
Green, OH 44232-0248
http://portagelakescareercenter.org

Southern State Community College
Medical Assistant Prgm
100 Hobart Dr
Hillsboro, OH 45133-9487
www.sscc.edu

National College - Kettering
Medical Assistant Prgm
1837 Woodman Center Dr
Kettering, OH 45420
www.ncbt.edu

Lakeland Community College
Medical Assistant Prgm
7700 Clocktower Dr
Kirtland, OH 44094-5198
http://lakelandcc.edu/ACADEMIC/SH/MedAsst/MedAsst.htm

Ohio University - Lancaster
Medical Assistant Prgm
1570 Granville Pike
Lancaster, OH 43130-1037
www.ohio.edu

Apollo Career Center
Medical Assistant Prgm
3325 Shawnee Rd
Lima, OH 45806-1497
www.apollocareercenter.com

University of Northwestern Ohio
Medical Assistant Prgm
1441 N Cable Rd
Lima, OH 45805-1409
www.unoh.edu

Washington County Career Center
Medical Assistant Prgm
21740 State Route 676
Marietta, OH 45750
www.mycareerschool.com

Marion Technical College
Medical Assistant Prgm
1467 Mt Vernon Ave
Marion, OH 43302-5694
www.mtc.edu

Stautzenberger College
Medical Assistant Prgm
1796 Indian Wood Cir
Maumee, OH 43537
www.sctoday.edu

Medina County Career Center
Medical Assistant Prgm
1101 W Liberty St
Medina, OH 44256-1346
www.mccc-jvsd.org

Polaris Career Center
Medical Assistant Prgm
7285 Old Oak Blvd
Middleburg Heights, OH 44130-3342
www.polaris.edu

EHOVE Ghrist Adult Career Center
Medical Assistant Prgm
316 W Mason Rd
Milan, OH 44846-9500
www.ehove.net

Knox County Career Center
Medical Assistant Prgm
308 Martinsburg Rd
Mount Vernon, OH 43050-4298
www.knoxcc.org
Prgm Dir: Kimberly Williams, LPN RMA
Tel: 740 393-2933, Ext 1102   *Fax:* 740 393-1659
E-mail: kwilliams@knoxcc.org

Hocking College
Medical Assistant Prgm
3301 Hocking Pkwy
Nelsonville, OH 45764-9582
www.hocking.edu

Lorain Cnty Joint Voc School - Adult Career
Medical Assistant Prgm
15181 State Route 58
Oberlin, OH 44074-9753
www.loraincounty.comjvadult

Bryant & Stratton College - Parma
Medical Assistant Prgm
12955 Snow Rd
Cleveland West Campus
Parma, OH 44130-1013
www.bryantstratton.edu
Prgm Dir: Brina Hollis, Healthcare Programs Director
Tel: 216 265-3151, Ext 255   *Fax:* 216 265-0325
E-mail: bmhollis@bryantstratton.edu

Edison Community College
Medical Assistant Prgm
1973 Edison Dr
Piqua, OH 45356
www.edisonohio.edu/medicalassistant

Ohio Business College
Medical Assistant Prgm
5095 Waterford Drive
Sheffield Village, OH 44035-0701

Wayne County Schools Career Center
Medical Assistant Prgm
518 West Prospect
Smithville, OH 44677

Clark State Community College
Medical Assistant Prgm
570 E Leffel Ln
Springfield, OH 45505-4749

Belmont Technical College
Medical Assistant Prgm
120 Fox-Shannon Pl
St Clairsville, OH 43950-8751
http://btc.edu

Eastern Gateway Community College
Medical Assistant Prgm
4000 Sunset Blvd
Steubenville, OH 43952-3598
www.jefferson.kctcs.edu

National College - Stow
Medical Assistant Prgm
3855 Fishcreek Rd
Stow, OH 44224-4305

Davis College
Medical Assistant Prgm
4747 Monroe St
Toledo, OH 43623-4307
www.daviscollege.edu

Owens Community College
Medical Assistant Prgm
PO Box 10000 Oregon Rd
Toledo, OH 43699-1947

Trumbull Career & Technical Center
Medical Assistant Prgm
528 Educational Hwy
Warren, OH 44483
www.tctcadulttraining.org

Mount Vernon Nazarene University
Cosponsor: National College
Medical Assistant Prgm
3487 Belmont Ave
Youngstown, OH 44505
www.national-college.edu

National College - Stow - Youngstown
Medical Assistant Prgm
3487 Belmont Ave
Youngstown, OH 44505

Youngstown State University
Medical Assistant Prgm
Medical Assisting Technology Program
Dept of Health Professions
One University Plaza
Youngstown, OH 44555-0001
www.ysu.edu

Zane State College
Medical Assistant Prgm
1555 Newark Rd
Zanesville, OH 43701-2626
www.zanestate.edu
Prgm Dir: Shanna L Morgan,
Tel: 740 588-1283   *Fax:* 740 454-0035
E-mail: smorgan@zanestate.edu

Oklahoma

Moore Norman Technology Center
Medical Assistant Prgm
PO Box 4701
Norman, OK 73070-4701
www.mntechnology.com

Francis Tuttle Technology Center
Medical Assistant Prgm
12777 N Rockwell Ave
Oklahoma City, OK 73142-2710
www.francistuttle.com

Metro Tech Health Careers Center
Medical Assistant Prgm
1720 Springlake Dr
Oklahoma City, OK 73111-5296
www.metrotech.org

Tulsa Community College
Medical Assistant Prgm
909 S Boston Ave
Tulsa, OK 74119-2095
www.tulsacc.edu

Oregon

Linn-Benton Community College
Medical Assistant Prgm
6500 SW Pacific Blvd
Albany, OR 97321-3755
http://linnbenton.edu

Central Oregon Community College
Medical Assistant Prgm
2600 NW College Way
Bend, OR 97701-5933
www.cocc.edu

Lane Community College
Medical Assistant Prgm
4000 E 30th Ave
Family and Health Careers
Eugene, OR 97405-0640
www.lanecc.edu

Mt Hood Community College
Medical Assistant Prgm
26000 SE Stark St
Allied Health Dept
Gresham, OR 97030-3300
www.mhcc.edu

Clackamas Community College
Medical Assistant Prgm
7738 SE Harmony Rd
Milwaukie, OR 97222
www.clackamas.edu

Concorde Career College - Portland
Medical Assistant Prgm
1425 NE Irving St
Suite 300
Portland, OR 97232-4203
www.concorde.edu

Everest College
Medical Assistant Prgm
425 SW Washington St
Portland, OR 97204-2241
www.everest.edu

Heald College
Medical Assistant Prgm
6035 NE 78th Court
Portland, OR 97218
www.heald.edu

Portland Community College
Medical Assistant Prgm
705 N Killlingsworth
Cascade Campus, Building JH, Room 208A
Portland, OR 97217-2332
www.pcc.edu

Brown Mackie College
Medical Assistant Prgm
400 E Scenic Dr
The Dalles, OR 97058

Pennsylvania

Greater Altoona Career & Technology Center
Medical Assistant Prgm
1500 Fourth Ave
Altoona, PA 16602-3616
www.gactc.com/cont-ed

Butler County Community College
Medical Assistant Prgm
PO Box 1203
Oak Hill Campus - College Drive
Butler, PA 16003-1203
www.bc3.edu

Mount Aloysius College
Medical Assistant Prgm
7373 Admiral Peary Hwy
Cresson, PA 16630-1999
www.mtaloy.edu

McCann School of Business and Technology - Dickson City
Medical Assistant Prgm
2227 Scranton Carbondale Highway
Dickson City, PA 18508

Fortis Institute-Erie
Medical Assistant Prgm
5757 W 26th St
Erie, PA 16506-1013

Harrisburg Area Community College
Medical Assistant Prgm
One HACC Dr, PC-333
Harrisburg, PA 17110-2999
www.hacc.edu

Kaplan Career Institute - Harrisburg
Medical Assistant Prgm
5650 Derry St
Harrisburg, PA 17111-3571

McCann School of Business and Technology - Hazleton
Medical Assistant Prgm
370 Maplewood Drive
Hazle Township, PA 18202
www.mccanschool.edu

YTI Career Institute
Medical Assistant Prgm
3050 Hempland Rd
Lancaster, PA 17601
www.yti.edu

Delaware County Community College
Medical Assistant Prgm
Rte 252 Allied Health & Nursing Dept
901 S Media Line Rd
Media, PA 19063-1027
www.dccc.edu
Prgm Dir: Jennifer E DeCaro, MPH BS CMA (AAMA)
Tel: 610 359-5289   *Fax:* 610 359-7350
E-mail: jdecaro@dccc.edu

Pittsburgh Technical Institute
Medical Assistant Prgm
1111 McKee Rd
Oakdale, PA 15071-3211
www.pti.edu

Community College of Philadelphia
Medical Assistant Prgm
1700 Spring Garden St
W2-5E
Philadelphia, PA 19130-3936
www.ccp.edu

Kaplan Institute - Philadelphia
Medical Assistant Prgm
3010 Market St Floor 1
Philadelphia, PA 19104

Bradford School - Pittsburgh
Medical Assistant Prgm
125 West Station Square Dr, Ste 129
Pittsburgh, PA 15219-2601
www.bradfordpittsburgh.edu
Prgm Dir: Cynthia Boles, CMA MBA MT(ASCP)
Tel: 412 391-6339   *Fax:* 412 471-6714
E-mail: cboles@bradfordpittsburgh.edu

Everest Institute
Medical Assistant Prgm
100 Forbes Ave, Ste 1200
Kossman Building
Pittsburgh, PA 15222-1320
www.everest.edu/campus/pittsburgh

Kaplan Career Institute - ICM Campus
Medical Assistant Prgm
10 Wood St
Pittsburgh, PA 15222-1918
www.kci-pittsburgh.com

Central Pennsylvania Institute of Sci & Tech
Medical Assistant Prgm
540 N Harrison Rd
Pleasant Gap, PA 16823
www.cpi.edu

Montgomery County Community College
Medical Assistant Prgm
101 College Dr
340 DeKalb Pike
Pottstown and Blue Bell, PA 19464
www.mc3.edu

McCann School of Business and Technology - Pottsville
Medical Assistant Prgm
2650 Woodglen Rd
Pottsville, PA 17901-1335
www.mccannschool.edu

Lehigh Carbon Community College
Medical Assistant Prgm
4525 Education Park Dr
Schnecksville, PA 18078-2598
www.lccc.edu

Central Pennsylvania College
Medical Assistant Prgm
College Hill and Valley Roads
Summerdale, PA 17093-0309
www.cenralpenn.edu

McCann School of Business and Technology - Sunbury
Medical Assistant Prgm
1147 N Fourth St
Sunbury, PA 17801-1221
www.mccannschool.com

Penn Commercial Inc
Medical Assistant Prgm
242 Oak Spring Rd
Washington, PA 15301-2871
www.penncommercial.edu

Community College of Allegheny County
Medical Assistant Prgm
1750 Clairton Rd
West Mifflin, PA 15122
www.ccac.edu

Berks Technical Institute
Medical Assistant Prgm
2205 Ridgewood Rd
Wyomissing, PA 19610-1168
www.berkstech.com

Westmoreland County Community College
Medical Assistant Prgm
400 Armbrust Rd
Youngwood, PA 15697-1895

South Carolina

Aiken Technical College
Medical Assistant Prgm
PO Drawer 696
US Highway 1 and 78 South
Aiken, SC 29802-0696
www.atc.edu

Forrest College
Medical Assistant Prgm
601 E River St
Anderson, SC 29624-2405
www.forrestcollege.edu

Miller-Motte Technical College
Medical Assistant Prgm
8085 Rivers Ave Ste E
Charleston, SC 29406-9239
www.mmtccharleston.com

Trident Technical College
Medical Assistant Prgm
7000 Rivers Ave
PO Box 118067
Charleston, SC 29423-8067
www.tridenttech.edu

South University
Medical Assistant Prgm
9 Science Court
Columbia, SC 29203-9344
www.southuniversity.edu

Greenville Technical College
Medical Assistant Prgm
PO Box 5616
216 S Pleasantburg Dr
Buck Mickel Center, BMC 173
Greenville, SC 29606-5616
www.gvltec.edu

Piedmont Technical College
Medical Assistant Prgm
PO Box 1467
620 N Emerald Rd
Greenwood, SC 29648-1467
www.ptc.edu

Orangeburg Calhoun Technical College
Medical Assistant Prgm
3250 Saint Matthews Rd NE
Orangeburg, SC 29118-8222
www.octech.edu

Tri-County Technical College
Medical Assistant Prgm
PO Box 587
7900 Hwy 76
Pendleton, SC 29670
www.tctc.edu

Spartanburg Community College
Medical Assistant Prgm
PO Box 4386
Business Interstate 85 at New Cut Rd
Spartanburg, SC 29305-4386
www.sccsc.edu

Central Carolina Technical College
Medical Assistant Prgm
506 N Guignard Dr
Sumter, SC 29150-2468
www.cctech.edu

Midlands Technical College
Medical Assistant Prgm
Airport Campus
1260 Lexington Dr
West Columbia, SC 29170
www.midlandstech.edu
Prgm Dir: Dorothy Bouldrick, MBA
Tel: 803 822-3398   *Fax:* 803 822-3417
E-mail: bouldrickd@midlandstech.edu

South Dakota

Presentation College
Medical Assistant Prgm
1500 N Main St
Aberdeen, SD 57401-1280
www.presentation.edu

Mitchell Technical Institute
Medical Assistant Prgm
1800 East Spruce
Michell, SD 57301
www.mitchelltech.edu
Prgm Dir: Cori Hoffman, RN BSN CMA
Tel: 605 995-7160   *Fax:* 605 996-3299
E-mail: cori.hoffman@mitchelltech.edu

Colorado Technical University
Medical Assistant Prgm
3901 W 59th St
Sioux Falls, SD 57108-2272
www.sf.coloradotech.edu

National American University
Medical Assistant Prgm
5801 S Corporate Pl
Sioux Falls, SD 57108
www.national.edu

Lake Area Technical Institute
Medical Assistant Prgm
230 11th St NE
PO Box 730
Watertown, SD 57201-0730
www.lakeareatech.edu

Tennessee

National College of Business and Technology
Medical Assistant Prgm
5760 Stage Rd
Bartlett, TN 38134-4516

Chattanooga State Community College
Medical Assistant Prgm
4501 Amnicola Hwy
Chattanooga, TN 37406-1018
www.chattanoogastate.edu

Miller-Motte Technical College - Chattanooga
Medical Assistant Prgm
6020 Shallowford Rd
Chattanooga, TN 37421-7226
www.miller-motte.com

Miller-Motte Technical College - Clarksville
Medical Assistant Prgm
1820 Business Park Dr
Clarksville, TN 37040-6023
http://miller-motte.com/clarksville-index.htm

Cleveland State Community College
Medical Assistant Prgm
PO Box 3570
3535 Adkisson Dr
Cleveland, TN 37320-3570
www.clevelandstatecc.edu
Prgm Dir: Karmon L Kingsley, CMA (AAMA) BS
Tel: 423 614-8702, Ext 702   *Fax:* 423 478-6258
E-mail: kkingsley@clevelandstatecc.edu

South College
Medical Assistant Prgm
3904 Lonas Dr
Knoxville, TN 37909-3323
www.southcollegetn.edu

Tennessee Technology Center - Knoxville
Medical Assistant Prgm
1100 Liberty St
Knoxville, TN 37919-2327
www.knoxville.tec.tn.us

National College of Business and Technology - Madison
Medical Assistant Prgm
900 Madison Square
Madison, TN 37115-4614

Tennessee Technology Center - McMinnville
Medical Assistant Prgm
241 Vo-Tech Dr
McMinnville, TN 37110
www.mcminnville.tec.tn.us

National College of Business and Technology - Memphis
Medical Assistant Prgm
3545 Lamar Ave
Memphis, TN 38118

National College of Business and Technology - Nashville
Medical Assistant Prgm
1638 Bell Rd
Nashville, TN 37211

Texas

Cisco College
Medical Assistant Prgm
717 E Industrial Blvd
Abilene, TX 79602-8115
www.cisco.edu

Lone Star College-CyFair
Medical Assistant Prgm
9191 Barker Cypress Rd
Suite HSC
Cypress, TX 77433-1383
www.nhmccd.edu

El Centro College
Medical Assistant Prgm
801 Main St
Dallas, TX 75202-3605
www.elcentrocollege.edu

Richland College
Medical Assistant Prgm
12800 Abrams Rd
Dallas, TX 75243-2199
www.rlc.dcccd.edu

Westwood College
Medical Assistant Prgm
8390 LBJ Freeway
Executive Center One, Suite 100
Dallas, TX 75243-1215
www.westwood.edu

El Paso Community College
Medical Assistant Prgm
PO Box 20500
100 W Rio Grande Ave
El Paso, TX 79902-3914
www.epcc.edu

Kaplan College
Medical Assistant Prgm
8360 Burnham Rd Suite 100
El Paso, TX 79907-1500

Vista College
Medical Assistant Prgm
6101 Montana Ave
El Paso, TX 79925-2021

Westwood College - Fort Worth
Medical Assistant Prgm
4232 North Freeway
Fort Worth, TX 76137

Texas School of Business - Friendswood
Medical Assistant Prgm
3208 W Parkwood Ave
FM 528
Friendswood, TX 77546
www.tbc.edu

Texas State Technical College - Harlingen
Medical Assistant Prgm
1902 N Loop 499
Harlingen, TX 78550-3697
www.harlingen.tstc.edu

Houston Community College
Medical Assistant Prgm
1900 Pressler Dr, Ste 434
Coleman Health Sciences Center
Houston, TX 77030-3717
www.hccs.edu

Lone Star College-North Harris
Medical Assistant Prgm
Health Professions Building 17200 Red Oak, #200E
Houston, TX 77090

San Jacinto College North
Medical Assistant Prgm
5800 Uvalde Rd
Houston, TX 77049-4513
www.sjcd.edu

Texas School of Business - East Campus
Medical Assistant Prgm
12030 I-10 East Freeway
Houston, TX 77029
www.tsb.edu

Texas School of Business - North Campus
Medical Assistant Prgm
711 E Airtex
North Campus
Houston, TX 77073
www.tsb.edu

Texas School of Business - Southwest Campus
Medical Assistant Prgm
6363 Richmond Ave, Suite 300
Houston, TX 77057
www.tsb.edu

Westwood College - Houston
Medical Assistant Prgm
7322 Southwest Fwy Suite 110 South Campus
Houston, TX 77074-2082

College of the Mainland
Medical Assistant Prgm
150 Parker Ct
League City, TX 77573-1970

Northeast Texas Community College
Medical Assistant Prgm
2886 FM 1735 Chapel Hill Rd P O Box 1307
Mount Pleasant, TX 75456

Hallmark College of Technology
Medical Assistant Prgm
10401 IH - 10 West
San Antonio, TX 78230-1737
www.hallmarkcollege.edu

Kaplan College - San Antonio
Medical Assistant Prgm
7142 San Pedro Ave Suite 100
San Antonio, TX 78216-6255

San Antonio College
Medical Assistant Prgm
1300 San Pedro Ave
134J
San Antonio, TX 78212-4201
www.alamo.edu/sac/alldhlth/medasst
Notes: In 1969, we became the first accredited medical
assisting program in the US. Our graduates are highly
sought after by employers in this area.

Utah

Davis Applied Technology College
Medical Assistant Prgm
550 East 300 South
Kaysville, UT 84037-2699
www.datc.edu

Bridgerland Applied Technology College
Medical Assistant Prgm
1301 North 600 West
Logan, UT 84321-2292
http://batc.edu

Stevens-Henager College
Medical Assistant Prgm
755 S Main St
Logan, UT 84321-5402
www.stevenshenager.edu

Ogden-Weber Applied Technology College
Medical Assistant Prgm
200 N Washington Blvd
Ogden, UT 84404-4089
www.owatc.edu

Stevens-Henager College
Medical Assistant Prgm
PO Box 9428
1890 South 1350 West
Ogden, UT 84401
http://stevenshenager.edu

Stevens-Henager College
Medical Assistant Prgm
1476 S Sandhill Rd
Orem, UT 84058-7310

Latter Day Saints Business College
Medical Assistant Prgm
95 North 300 West
Salt Lake City, UT 84101-3500
www.ldsbc.edu

Broadview University
Medical Assistant Prgm
1902 W 7800 S
West Jordan, UT 84088-4021

Salt Lake Community College
Medical Assistant Prgm
3491 Wight Fort Rd
PO Box 30808
West Jordan, UT 84088
www.slcc.edu

Everest College - West Valley City
Medical Assistant Prgm
3280 W 3500 S
West Valley City, UT 84119-2668

Virginia

National College - Charlottesville
Medical Assistant Prgm
1819 Emmet St
Charlottesville, VA 22901
www.national-college.edu

National College - Danville
Medical Assistant Prgm
336 Old Riverside Dr
Danville, VA 24540
www.ncbt.edu

National College - Harrisonburg
Medical Assistant Prgm
1515 Country Club Rd
Harrisonburg, VA 22801
www.national-college.edu

Miller-Motte Technical College
Medical Assistant Prgm
1011 Creekside Lane
Lynchburg, VA 24502-4353
www.miller-motte.com/lynchburg-index.htm

National College - Lynchburg
Medical Assistant Prgm
104 Candlewood Court
Lynchburg, VA 24502
www.national-college.edu

National College - Martinsville
Medical Assistant Prgm
905 N Memorial Blvd
Martinsville, VA 24112
www.national-college.edu

Bryant & Stratton College - Richmond
Medical Assistant Prgm
8141 Hull St Rd
Richmond, VA 23235-6411
www.bryantstratton.edu

Washington

National College - Roanoke Valley
Medical Assistant Prgm
1813 E Main St
Roanoke Valley Campus
Salem, VA 24153
www.national-college.edu

Bryant & Stratton College - Virginia Beach
Medical Assistant Prgm
301 Centre Pointe Dr
Virginia Beach, VA 23462-4417
www.bryantstratton.edu

Tidewater Community College
Medical Assistant Prgm
1700 College Crescent
Virginia Beach, VA 23453-1999
www.tcc.edu

Washington

Whatcom Community College
Medical Assistant Prgm
237 W Kellogg Rd
Bellingham, WA 98226-8033
www.whatcom.ctc.edu

Everest College - Bremerton
Medical Assistant Prgm
155 Washington Ave, Ste 200
Bremerton, WA 98337
www.everest.edu
Prgm Dir: Lisa L Cook, CMA (AAMA) AS
Tel: 360 473-1120, Ext 133 *Fax:* 360 792-2404
E-mail: lcook@cci.edu

Olympic College
Medical Assistant Prgm
1600 Chester Ave
Bremerton, WA 98337-1600
www.olympic.edu

Highline Community College
Medical Assistant Prgm
PO Box 98000
Des Moines, WA 98198-9800
http://flightline.highline.edu/medassist

Everest College - Everett
Medical Assistant Prgm
906 SE Everett Mall Way, Ste 600
Everett, WA 98208
www.everest.edu/campus/everett

Everett Community College
Medical Assistant Prgm
2000 Tower St
Everett, WA 98201-1390
www.everettcc.edu

Lake Washington Institute of Technology
Medical Assistant Prgm
11605 132nd Ave NE
Kirkland, WA 98034-8505
www.lwtc.edu

Clover Park Technical College
Medical Assistant Prgm
4500 Steilacoom Blvd SW
Bldg 14
Lakewood, WA 98499-4044
www.cptc.edu

Lower Columbia College
Medical Assistant Prgm
1600 Maple St
Longview, WA 98632-3907
www.lowercolumbia.edu

Skagit Valley College
Medical Assistant Prgm
2405 E College Way
Mount Vernon, WA 98273-5899
www.skagit.edu

South Puget Sound Community College
Medical Assistant Prgm
2011 Mottman Rd SW
Olympia, WA 98512-6218
www.spscc.ctc.edu

Columbia Basin College
Medical Assistant Prgm
2600 North 20th Ave
Pasco, WA 99301

Everest College - Renton
Medical Assistant Prgm
981 Powell Ave SW, Ste 200
Renton, WA 98055-2990
www.everest.edu

Renton Technical College
Medical Assistant Prgm
3000 NE Fourth St
Renton, WA 98056-4195
www.rtc.edu

North Seattle Community College
Medical Assistant Prgm
9600 College Way N
Seattle, WA 98103-3514
www.northseattle.edu/health/medasst
Prgm Dir: Michaelann Marie Allen, MAEd CMA
Tel: 206 527-5667 *Fax:* 206 527-3715
E-mail: mallen@sccd.ctc.edu

Seattle Vocational Institute
Medical Assistant Prgm
2120 S Jackson St
Seattle, WA 98144-2219
www.sviweb.sccd.ctc.edu
Prgm Dir: Richard St Clare,
Tel: 206 934-4910 *Fax:* 206 934-4939
E-mail: Richard.StClare@SeattleColleges.edu

Spokane Community College
Medical Assistant Prgm
1810 N Greene St
Spokane, WA 99217-5399
www.scc.spokane.edu

Clark College
Medical Assistant Prgm
1800 E McLoughlin Blvd
Vancouver, WA 98663-3598
www.clark.edu

Everest College - Vancouver
Medical Assistant Prgm
120 NE 136 Ave, Ste 130
Vancouver, WA 98684
www.everest.edu

Wenatchee Valley College
Medical Assistant Prgm
1300 Fifth Ave
Wenatchee, WA 98801-1741
www.wvc.edu

Yakima Valley Community College
Medical Assistant Prgm
PO Box 22520
South 16th Ave & Nob Hill Blvd
Yakima, WA 98907-2520
www.yvcc.edu

West Virginia

Mountain State University
Medical Assistant Prgm
PO Box 9003
609 S Kanawha St
Beckley, WV 25802-9003
www.mountainstate.edu

Benjamin Franklin Career & Technical Ed Ctr
Medical Assistant Prgm
500 28th St
Dunbar, WV 25064-1622
www.bfcc.kana.tec.wv.us

Huntington Junior College
Medical Assistant Prgm
900 Fifth Ave
Huntington, WV 25701-2004
www.huntingtonjuniorcollege.edu

Mountwest Community & Technical College
Medical Assistant Prgm
1 John Marshall Drive
Huntington, WV 25755
www.marshall.edu/ctc

National College
Medical Assistant Prgm
421 Hilltop Dr
Princeton, WV 24740
www.national-college.edu

West Virginia Northern Community College
Medical Assistant Prgm
1704 Market St
Wheeling, WV 26003
www.wvncc.edu/CresapD/MASoptions.htm

Wisconsin

Chippewa Valley Technical College
Medical Assistant Prgm
Health Education Center
620 W Clairemont Ave
Eau Claire, WI 54701-6162
www.cvtc.edu

Gateway Technical College - Elkhorn
Medical Assistant Prgm
400 County Rd H
Elkhorn, WI 53121-2035
www.gtc.edu

Southwest Wisconsin Technical College
Medical Assistant Prgm
1800 Bronson Blvd
Fennimore, WI 53809-9778
www.swtc.edu

Moraine Park Technical College
Medical Assistant Prgm
235 North National Ave
Fond du Lac, WI 54935-2897
www.morainepark.edu

Northeast Wisconsin Technical College
Medical Assistant Prgm
2740 W Mason St, PO Box 19042
Green Bay, WI 54303-4966
www.nwtc.edu

Rasmussen College - Green Bay
Medical Assistant Prgm
904 South Taylor Suite 100
Green Bay, WI 54302-2349

Lac Courte Oreills Ojibwa Community College
Medical Assistant Prgm
13466 W Trepania Rd
Hayward, WI 54843-2181
www.lco.edu

Blackhawk Technical College
Medical Assistant Prgm
6004 Prairie Rd, PO Box 5009
Janesville, WI 53547-5009
www.blackhawk.edu

Western Technical College
Medical Assistant Prgm
400 7th St North, PO Box C-908
La Crosse, WI 54602-0908
www.westerntc.edu

Madison Area Technical College
Medical Assistant Prgm
3550 Anderson St
Madison, WI 53791-9674
http://matcmadison.edu

Mid-State Technical College - Marshfield
Medical Assistant Prgm
2600 W Fifth St
Marshfield, WI 54449
www.mstc.edu

Bryant & Stratton College - Milwaukee
Medical Assistant Prgm
310 W Wisconsin Ave
Suite 500 East
Milwaukee, WI 53203-2213
www.bryantstratton.edu

Concordia University Wisconsin
Medical Assistant Prgm
1127 S 35th St
South Center
Milwaukee, WI 53215-1409
www.cuw.edu

Milwaukee Area Technical College
Medical Assistant Prgm
700 W State St
Milwaukee, WI 53233-1443
www.matc.edu

Wisconsin Indianhead Technical College
Medical Assistant Prgm
1019 S Knowles Ave
New Richmond, WI 54017-1738
www.witc.edu

Fox Valley Technical College
Medical Assistant Prgm
150 N Campbell Rd
PO Box 2217
Oshkosh, WI 54902-3480
www.fvtc.edu

Waukesha County Technical College
Medical Assistant Prgm
800 Main St
Pewaukee, WI 53072-4601
www.wctc.edu/web/areas/health/ma/ma.php

Nicolet Area Technical College
Medical Assistant Prgm
PO Box 518
Rhinelander, WI 54501-0518
www.nicoletcollege.edu

Wisconsin Indianhead Technical College - Superior
Medical Assistant Prgm
600 N 21st St
Superior, WI 54880-5207
www.witc.edu
Prgm Dir: Luci Gunderson, RN MS MA
Tel: 715 394-6677 *Fax:* 715 934-3771
E-mail: luci.gunderson@witc.edu

Northcentral Technical College
Medical Assistant Prgm
1000 W Campus Dr
Wausau, WI 54401
www.ntc.edu

Medical Assistant

Programs*	Class Capacity	Begins	Length (months)	Award	Res. Tuition	Non-res. Tuition		Offers:† 1	2	3	4
Alabama											
Trenholm State Technical College (Montgomery)	30	Aug Jan May	18	AAT	$7,810	$7,810				•	
California											
Heald College - Milpitas	30	Every quarter	18	AAS				•		•	
Heald College - Rancho Cordova	25	Every quarter	18	AAS				•		•	•
Modesto Junior College	25	Aug	7	Cert, , AS Degree						•	
Florida											
Brevard Community College (Cocoa)	32	Open	12	Cert	$6,000			•		•	•
Community Technical & Adult Education Center (Ocala)	24	Jan Jul	12	Cert	$3,055	$12,220	per year				
Palm Beach State College (Lake Worth)	24	May Aug	13	Cert	$3,351	$13,130	per year			•	•
Georgia											
Southwest Georgia Technical College (Thomasville)	24	Each semester	15, 18	Dipl, AAS	$3,375	$6,750	per year	•		•	•
Idaho											
Idaho State Univ (Pocatello)	18	Aug	24	AAS	$4,968	$14,770	per year				•
Illinois											
Harper College (Palatine)	30	Aug Jan Jun	12, 24	Cert	$4,200	$13,400	per credit	•		•	•
Indiana											
International Business Coll - Indianapolis	48	Sep Mar	10, 14	Dipl, AAS						•	
Ivy Tech Community College - Columbus	20	Aug Jan May	18, 24	Cert, TC, AAS	$3,000	$6,000		•		•	•
Ivy Tech Community College - Lawrenceburg	50	Aug Jan May	18, 24	Cert, TC, AAS	$3,137	$6,641	per year	•		•	•
Iowa											
Southeastern Community College (West Burlington)	20	Aug	11	Dipl						•	
Massachusetts											
Porter and Chester Institute - Chicopee	80	Jan Apr Jul Oct	9, 13	Dipl				•			•
Michigan											
Mid Michigan Community College (Harrison)	20	Aug	24	Dipl, AAS	$6,013	$7,638				•	
Minnesota											
Century College (White Bear Lake)	20	Aug Jan	14, 24	Dipl				•		•	•
Minneapolis Business College (Roseville)	160	Fall	10, 14	Dipl, AAS	$14,040	$14,040				•	
Nebraska											
Central Community College (Hastings)	30	Fall	12, 24	Dipl, AAS						•	•
New Jersey											
Bergen Community College (Paramus)	25	Sep	24	AAS	$4,420	$8,840	per year	•		•	
Fortis Institute (Wayne)		Every 6 wks	9					•		•	
Warren County Community College (Phillipsburg)	30	Aug Jan	7	Cert, AAS	$5,199	$5,199		•		•	
New York											
Bryant & Stratton College - Rochester	200	Jan May Sep	16	AAS	$8,000	$8,000		•		•	•
Trocaire College (Buffalo)	65	Sep	24	AAS							
Wood Tobe'-Coburn School (New York)	104	Sep Mar	14	Dipl, AD							

*Data are shown only for programs that completed the 2011 AMA Survey of Health Professions Education Programs.

†Key to Offers: 1: Evening or weekend classes; 2: Non-English instruction; 3: Cultural competence instruction; 4: Distance education component.

Medical Assistant

Programs*	Class Capacity	Begins	Length (months)	Award	Res. Tuition	Non-res. Tuition		Offers:† 1	2	3	4
North Carolina											
Gaston College (Dallas)	45	Aug	21	AAS	$2,712	$11,928	per year				
Lenoir Community College (Kinston)	20	Aug	21	AAS	$3,238	$12,070	per year	•		•	•
Mitchell Community College (Mooresville)	20	Aug	12	Dipl	$67	$245	per credit			•	•
Surry Community College (Dobson)	20	Aug	21	AAS	$1,808	$7,952					•
Ohio											
Brown Mackie College - Akron	300	Monthly	24, 12	Dipl, AAS	$14,064			•			
Bryant & Stratton College - Parma	20	Jan May Sep	18, 24	AAB				•		•	
Canton City Schools	14	Sep	10	Cert	$6,500	$6,500	per year	•			
Cuyahoga Community College (Cleveland)	20	Aug Jan	9, 18	Cert, AAS	$2,775			•		•	
Knox County Career Center (Mount Vernon)	20	Sep	10	Cert	$8,760	$8,760	per year	•			
Pickaway Ross Joint Vocational School (Chillicothe)	24	Aug	10	Cert	$6,300			•			
Zane State College (Zanesville)	50	Sep	18, 21	AAS	$1,128	$2,256					
Pennsylvania											
Bradford School - Pittsburgh	70	Jul Sep	10, 14	Dipl, ASB	$14,980	$14,980	per year	•			
Delaware County Community College (Media)	24	Sep	1, 24	Cert, AAS			per year	•		•	•
South Carolina											
Midlands Technical College (West Columbia)	20	Aug	12	Cert	$10,000	$15,000				•	•
South Dakota											
Mitchell Technical Institute (Michell)	20	Aug	18	AAS							•
Tennessee											
Cleveland State Community College	20	Aug	24	AAS				•			
Washington											
Everest College - Bremerton	24	Every 4 wks	8	Dipl				•			
North Seattle Community College	100	Sep Jan Mar Jun	18, 15	Cert, AAS	$3,760	$10,680	per year	•		•	•
Seattle Vocational Institute	30	Sep Jan Apr Jun	12	Dipl, Cert				•			
Wisconsin											
Wisconsin Indianhead Technical College - Superior	22	Jan	10	Dipl						•	•

*Data are shown only for programs that completed the 2011 AMA Survey of Health Professions Education Programs.

†Key to Offers: 1: Evening or weekend classes; 2: Non-English instruction; 3: Cultural competence instruction; 4: Distance education component.

Medical Illustrator

Medical illustrators specialize in the visual transformation, display, and communication of scientific information. Their graduate level training in biomedical science, art, design, visual technology, education, and communication enables them to understand and visualize scientific data and concepts to teach the general public and professionals in the fields of health care, research, pharmaceuticals, biotechnology, and demonstrative evidence. Medical illustrations are used in medical textbooks, medical advertisements, professional journals, instructional animations, computer-assisted learning programs, scientific exhibits, lecture presentations, general magazines, and courtroom presentations. Depending on the intended use, medical illustrations can be highly realistic and anatomically precise, or they can be thematic, interpretive, abstract, or even wildly conceptual. Although medical illustration is commonly seen in print and electronic media, medical illustrators also work in three-dimensional medium, creating anatomical teaching models, models for simulated medical procedures, and prosthetic parts for patients.

History

Formal educational programs for the medical illustrator date back to the early 1900s, with Max Broedel's school at Johns Hopkins University. The Association of Medical Illustrators (AMI) was established in 1945. Under the auspices of the AMI, standards were developed, with accredited medical illustration programs in existence in the United States since 1967.

In 1986, the AMI expressed a desire to have educational programs for the medical illustrator accredited by the Committee on Allied Health Education and Accreditation (CAHEA) of the AMA. This desire stemmed from the recognition that professional medical illustrator programs were more closely related to allied health than to the visual arts.

An ad hoc committee on outside accreditation of the AMI worked with AMA staff to modify the existing *Standards* to comply with the format recommended by the CAHEA. The resulting *Essentials and Guidelines of an Accredited Educational Program for the Medical Illustrator* was adopted by the AMI and the AMA Council on Medical Education (CME) in 1987. Today, the *Standards* are adopted by CAAHEP in collaboration with the AMI.

Career Description

Medical illustrators work closely with clients to interpret their needs and create visual solutions for them through effective problem solving. While some medical illustrators specialize in a single art medium or work primarily for one medical specialty, the majority handle an ever-changing variety of assignments from different clients, involving a variety of biomedical content, and requiring a variety of media solutions. In addition to design and production roles, medical illustrators may function as consultants, art directors, supervisors, and administrators within the field of biocommunications.

Employment Characteristics

Many medical illustrators are employed in medical schools and large medical centers that have teaching and research programs. Other medical artists are employed by hospitals, clinics, dental schools, or schools of veterinary medicine. Some institutional medical illustrators work alone, whereas, others are part of large multimedia departments. Other medical illustrators choose to target specific markets such as medical publishers, pharmaceutical companies, advertising agencies, animation studios, physicians, or attorneys. Some work independently on a freelance basis; others set up small companies designed to provide illustration services to various targeted markets.

The employment outlook for medical illustrators is good. This is in part due to the relatively few medical illustrators who graduate each year, and in part due to the growth in medical research that continually reveals new treatments and technologies that require medical illustrations. A growing demand by patients to better understand their own bodies and medical options has expanded the need for medical illustration aimed at the public. In addition, increased need for medical illustrations and models to educate juries during courtroom presentations has also expanded the medical-legal subspecialty of medical illustration.

Salary

Earnings vary according to (1 the experience and ability of the artist, 2 the type of work, and 3) the area of the country where one works. The title "Medical Illustrator" is a broad term. Depending on the type of employer and services provided, job skills may include animation, multimedia, interactive development, illustration, or web and graphic design. In general, medical illustrators with diverse skills and more responsibility for concept development command higher salaries. Based on 2006 survey data, the average starting salary in a university or institutional setting for a medical illustrator is around $44,000 to $55,000 per year plus benefits. Those who specialize in animation and multimedia typically earn a higher salary. Mid-level salaried medical illustrators 6 -15 years) usually earn between $54,000 and $74,000 per year. Administrators and those with faculty appointments may earn between $70,000 and $150,000 per year. About 43% of salaried illustrators often supplement their income with freelance work.

Self-employed (freelance) medical illustrators may have set-prices for particular kinds of art, but most establish fees based on usage rights granted and project complexity. Based on 2006 survey data, sole proprietors earn on average from $65,000 up to $225,000 per year. Although the earnings of self-employed medical illustrators may be more erratic than those of salaried illustrators, the highest earnings are generally made by those whose art and professionalism keep them in constant demand.

In addition to earnings from salary or freelance projects, some medical artists have royalty, coauthor, and reuse arrangements with publishers and clients, which can provide an additional, and sometimes significant, source of income.

For more information, refer to *www.ama-assn.org/go/hpsalary*.

Educational Programs

Length. Accredited programs generally last two years resulting in a master's degree.

Prerequisites. All current medical illustrator programs are at an advanced level and are based on a master's model. Although admission requirements to accredited programs vary, a bachelors degree with an emphasis on art and science is preferred.

In addition, a portfolio of artwork and a personal interview are required.

Curriculum. While the area of emphasis may vary from program to program, the curriculum includes the following courses: an advanced course in human anatomy with dissection and courses in other biomedical sciences such as embryology, histology, neuro-anatomy, cell biology, molecular biology, physiology, pathology, immunology, pharmacology, and genetics. Art and theory courses include anatomical drawing, illustration techniques in line, tone, and color (hand-rendered and computer-generated), surgical illustration, graphic design, computer graphics and multimedia, instructional design, motion media production, three-dimensional models and exhibits, management and business practices, and professional ethics.

Inquiries

Careers/Curriculum
Association of Medical Illustrators
PO Box 1897
Lawrence, KS 66044
866 393-4264
E-mail: *hq@ami.org*
www.ami.org

Program Accreditation
Commission on Accreditation of Allied Health Education Programs (CAAHEP)
1361 Park Street
Clearwater, FL 33756
727 210-2350
727 210-2354 Fax
E-mail: *mail@caahep.org*
www.caahep.org

in collaboration with:
Accreditation Review Committee for the Medical Illustrator

Medical Illustrator

Georgia

Georgia Health Sciences University
Medical Illustrator Prgm
Allied Hlth and Grad Studies, Ste CJ-1101
1120 15th St
Augusta, GA 30912-0300
www.mcg.edu

Illinois

University of Illinois at Chicago
Medical Illustrator Prgm
Dept of Biomed Visualization (MC-527
College of Applied Health Sciences
1919 W Taylor St
Chicago, IL 60612
www.uic.edu

Maryland

Johns Hopkins School of Medicine
Medical Illustrator Prgm
Dept of Art Applied to Med
1830 E Monument St/Suite 7000
Baltimore, MD 21205
www.hopkinsmedicine.org/medart/

Ontario, Canada

University of Toronto
Medical Illustrator Prgm
1 King's College Circle
Medical Sciences Bldg, Rm 2356
Toronto, ON M5S 1A8
www.bmc.med.utoronto.ca/BMC

Texas

Univ of Texas Southwestern Med Ctr
Medical Illustrator Prgm
Biomedical Communications Graduate Program
5323 Harry Hines Blvd
Dallas, TX 75390-8881
www.UTsouthwestern.edu

Neurodiagnostic Technologist

Neurodiagnostic technology (also known as neurodiagnostics) is the allied health care profession centered around recording, monitoring, and analyzing nervous system function to promote the effective treatment of pathologic conditions.

Neurodiagnostic professionals:

- are credentialed;
- have met a minimum education level and related educational and performance standards;
- meet continuing education requirements;
- perform within a code of ethics and defined scope of practice;
- are recognized by physicians, employers, the public, governmental agencies, payers, and other health care professionals;
- form a national society whose activities include advocating for the profession; and
- contribute to the advancement of knowledge in neuroscience.

History

The AMA's involvement in the evaluation and accreditation of educational programs in electroencephalographic (EEG) technology began in 1972 with the AMA's recognition of EEG technology as an allied health profession. Subsequently, AMA staff worked with representatives of the professional organizations representing this clinical discipline (including the American Clinical Neurophysiology Society [then the American EEG Society], the American Medical EEG Association, and the American Society of Electroneurodiagnostic Technologists [then the American Society of EEG Technologists]) to develop the *Standards (Essentials) of an Accredited Educational Program for the Electroencephalographic Technologist.*

In 1987, evoked potential (EP) techniques were included in *Standards* for programs desiring recognition in both EEG and EP techniques. In 1995, polysomnography (PSG) techniques were included for programs desiring recognition in EEG, EP, and PSG techniques. In 2008, Intraoperative Neuromonitoring (IONM), Long Term Monitoring (LTM), and Nerve Conduction Studies (NCS) techniques were included in the *Standards* for programs desiring recognition in IONM, LTM and NCS. The *Standards*, which were revised most recently in 2008, include a companion document of graduate competencies required for a neurodiagnostic program and EP, IONM, LTM, NCS, and PSG add-ons.

Career Description

Technologists record electrical activity from the brain, spinal cord, peripheral nerves, and somatosensory or motor nerve systems using a variety of techniques and instruments. Technologists prepare data and documentation for interpretation by a physician. Considerable individual initiative, reasoning skill, and sound judgment are all expected of the neurodiagnostic professional. The most common neurodiagnostic procedures include:

- Electroencephalogram (EEG)
- Intraoperative Neuromonitoring (IONM)
- Long Term Monitoring for Epilepsy (LTME)
- Polysomnogram/Sleep Studies (PSG)
- Evoked Potential (EP)
- Nerve Conduction Studies (NCS)
- Continuous EEG Monitoring in the ICU
- ICU Monitoring

Employment Characteristics

Neurodiagnostic personnel work primarily in neurology-related departments of hospitals, but many also work in clinics and the private offices of neurologists and neurosurgeons. Growth in employment within the profession is expected to be greater than average, owing to the increased use of EEG and EP techniques in surgery; in diagnosing and monitoring patients with epilepsy; continuous EEG monitoring in the intensive care unit; and in diagnosing sleep disorders. Technologists generally work a 40-hour week, but may work 12-hour days for sleep studies and be on-call for emergencies and intraoperative monitoring.

Salary

According to the ASET – The Neurodiagnostic Society, 2011 entry-level salaries average $43,000; mid-range salaries average $61,000, and the upper range of salaries is an average of $97,000.

For more information, go to *www.ama-assn.org/go/hpsalary*.

Educational Programs

Length. Programs may be 12 to 24 months, and are typically integrated into a community college-sponsored program leading to an associate degree.

Prerequisites. High school diploma or equivalent.

Curriculum. The curriculum includes anatomy, physiology, and neuroanatomy (with major emphasis on the brain), as well as instrumentation, personal and patient safety, recording techniques, clinical neurodiagnostics, and correlations. Clinical rotations are conducted in medical centers.

Certification/Registration

The American Board of Registration of Electroencephalographic and Evoked Potential Technologists (ABRET) offers four credentials in Neurodiagnostics:

- R. EEG T. (Registered EEG Technologist)
- R. EP T. (Registered Evoked Potential Technologist)
- CNIM (Certification in Neurophysiologic Intraoperative Monitoring)
- CLTM (Certification in Long Term Monitoring)

In addition, the American Association of Electrodiagnostic Technologists (AAET) offers the R.NCS.T. credential (Registered Nerve Conduction Studies Technologist), and the Board of Registered Polysomnographic Technologists (BRPT) offers the RPSGT credential (Registered Polysomnographic Technologist) and the CPSGT (Certified Polysomnographic Technician).

Inquiries

Careers

ASET – The Neurodiagnostic Society
402 E. Bannister Rd. Suite A
Kansas City, MO 64131
816 931-1120
E-mail: *info@aset.org*
www.aset.org

Certification/Registration (Credentials R. EEG T., R. EP T., CNIM, CLTM)
American Board of Registration of Electroencephalographic and
    Evoked Potential Technologists (ABRET)
2509 West Iles Avenue, Suite 102
Springfield, IL 62704
217 726-7980
E-mail: *abreteo@att.net*
www.abret.org

Certification/Registration (Credentials R.NCS.T)
American Association of Electrodiagnostic Technologists (AAET)
PO Box 2770
Cedar Rapids, IA 52406
877 333-2238
E-mail: *aaet@aaet.info*
www.aaet.info

Certification/Registration (Credentials RPSGT, CPSGT)
The Board of Registered Polysomnographic Technologists (BRPT)
8400 Westpark Drive, Second Floor
McLean, VA 22102
703 610-9020
E-mail: *info@brpt.org*
www.brpt.org

Program Accreditation
Commission on Accreditation of Allied Health Education Programs
(CAAHEP)
1361 Park Street, Clearwater, FL 33756
7 27 210-2350
7 27 210-2354 Fax
E-mail: *mail@caahep.org*
www.caahep.org

in collaboration with:
Committee on Accreditation for Education in Neurodiagnostic
Technology (CoA-NDT)
6654 South Sycamore Street
Littleton, CO 80120
3 03 738-0770
E-mail: *office@coa-ndt.org*
www.coa-ndt.org

Neurodiagnostic Technologist

Arizona

GateWay Community College - Phoenix
Neurodiagnostic Tech Prgm
108 North 40th St
Phoenix, AZ 85034

California

Orange Coast College
Neurodiagnostic Tech Prgm
2701 Fairview Rd, PO Box 5005
Costa Mesa, CA 92626-5005
www.orangecoastcollege.edu
Prgm Dir: Walter Banoczi, R EEG/EP T CNIM RPSGT
    CLTM BVE
Tel: 714 432-5591   *Fax:* 714 432-5534
E-mail: wbanoczi@cccd.edu

Florida

Erwin Technical Center
Neurodiagnostic Tech Prgm
2010 E Hillsborough Ave
Tampa, FL 33610
www.erwin.edu

Illinois

St John's Hospital
Cosponsor: Lincoln Land Community College
Neurodiagnostic Tech Prgm
School of ENDT
800 E Carpenter St
Springfield, IL 62769
www.st-johns.org

Indiana

Indiana University Health
Neurodiagnostic Tech Prgm
Wile Hall Room 604
I-65 at 21st St
Indianapolis, IN 46206-1367
www.clarian.org

Iowa

Scott Community College
Neurodiagnostic Tech Prgm
500 Belmont Rd
Bettendorf, IA 52722
www.eicc.edu/scc

Kirkwood Community College
Cosponsor: Univ of Iowa Hosp and Clinics/Kirkwood
    Community College
Neurodiagnostic Tech Prgm
Dept of Neurology
6301 Kirkwood Blvd SW, PO Box 2068
Cedar Rapids, IA 52406-9973
www.kirkwood.edu
Prgm Dir: Marjorie Tucker, R EEG/EPT CNIM CLTM
Tel: 319 356-8768   *Fax:* 319 351-1209
E-mail: marjorie-tucker@uiowa.edu

Maryland

Institute of Health Sciences
Neurodiagnostic Tech Prgm
1300 York Rd Suite 190-D
Timonium, MD 21093

Massachusetts

Laboure College
Neurodiagnostic Tech Prgm
2120 Dorchester Ave
Boston, MA 02124
www.laboure.edu

Michigan

Carnegie Institute
Neurodiagnostic Tech Prgm
550 Stephenson Hwy, Suites 100-110
Troy, MI 48083
www.carnegie-institute.edu

Minnesota

Minneapolis Community & Technical College
Neurodiagnostic Tech Prgm
1501 Hennepin Ave
Minneapolis, MN 55403

Mayo School of Health Sciences
Neurodiagnostic Tech Prgm
Clinical Neurophysiology Technology Program
Mayo Clinic
200 First St SW
Rochester, MN 55905
www.mayo.edu/mshs

New Jersey

DeVry University
Neurodiagnostic Tech Prgm
Forough Ghahramani 630 US Highway One
North Brunswick, NJ 08902-3362

North Carolina

Pamlico Community College
Neurodiagnostic Tech Prgm
PO Box 185
5049 Hwy 306 S
Grantsboro, NC 28529-0185
www.pamlicocc.edu
Prgm Dir: Marc Williams
Tel: 252 249-1851, Ext 3043   *Fax:* 252 249-1807
E-mail: mwilliams@pamlicocc.edu

Catawba Valley Community College
Neurodiagnostic Tech Prgm
2550 Hwy 70 SE
Hickory, NC 28602
www.cvcc.edu

Ohio

Cuyahoga Community College
Neurodiagnostic Tech Prgm
11000 Pleasant Valley Rd
Parma, OH 44130
www.tri-c.edu

Pennsylvania

Harcum College
Neurodiagnostic Tech Prgm
750 Montgomery Ave
Bryn Mawr, PA 19010-3476

Crozer-Keystone Medical Center
Neurodiagnostic Tech Prgm
One Medical Ctr Blvd
Upland, PA 19013
www.crozer.org
Prgm Dir: Violet Long, Director Neurology Services
Tel: 610 447-2915   *Fax:* 610 447-2696
E-mail: violet.long@crozer.org

South Dakota

Southeast Technical Institute
Neurodiagnostic Tech Prgm
Terrence Sullivan Health Science Center
2320 North Career Ave
Sioux Falls, SD 57107

Texas

Alvin Community College
Neurodiagnostic Tech Prgm
3110 Mustang Rd
Alvin, TX 77511

Medical Education and Training Campus (METC)
Neurodiagnostic Tech Prgm
METC 3085 Wilson Way
Ft. Sam Houston, TX 78234-6402

McLennan Community College
Neurodiagnostic Tech Prgm
1400 College Dr
Waco, TX 76708
www.mclennan.edu

Neurodiagnostic Technologist

Programs*	Class Capacity	Begins	Length (months)	Award	Res. Tuition	Non-res. Tuition		Offers:† 1	2	3	4
California											
Orange Coast College (Costa Mesa)	24	Aug (even yrs)	22	Dipl, AS	$1,500	$3,000					
Iowa											
Kirkwood Community College (Cedar Rapids)	20	Aug (odd yrs)	21	AAS	$6,750	$7,550					
North Carolina											
Pamlico Community College (Grantsboro)	30	Aug	24	AAS	$922	$3,994				•	•
Pennsylvania											
Crozer-Keystone Medical Center (Upland)	12	Oct	18	Cert	$9,000	$9,000	per year			•	•

*Data are shown only for programs that completed the 2011 AMA Survey of Health Professions Education Programs.

†Key to Offers: 1: Evening or weekend classes; 2: Non-English instruction; 3: Cultural competence instruction; 4: Distance education component.

Orthopaedic Physician's Assistant

The certified Orthopaedic Physician's Assistant is a professional physician extender who has met the criteria set forth by the National Board for Certification of Orthopaedic Physician's Assistants (NBCOPA) and has successfully passed the certification examination as such, and maintains certification by complying with the bylaws of the NBCOPA. The Certified Orthopaedic Physician's Assistant may use the short title OPA-C.

These guidelines are designed to direct and cue the Certified Orthopaedic Physician's Assistant to assist the orthopaedic physician complete assessment of signs, symptoms, analysis, treatment and care for the orthopaedic patient. Passage of the certification examination signifies an entry level of knowledge of the following categories in the specialty of orthopaedic medicine and surgery: Anatomy and Physiology; Pharmacology: Assessment and Treatment of Adult and Pediatric Orthopaedic Diseases and Injuries; Principals and Techniques of Operative Procedures; Functions and Application of Instrumentation and Equipment Utilized in Operative Orthopedic Procedures; Principals and Techniques of Traction, Casting and Splint Applications; Evaluation and Interpretation of Laboratory, Radiological and other Diagnostic Studies; Clinical History and Physical Assessment.

Career Description

In addition to the duties described in the occupational description above, the OPA-C shall function in practice under the authority of the supervising orthopaedic physician. Functions shall include performing skilled services and procedures within the clinical setting, out-patient and in-patient facilities where privileges have been granted accordingly. The OPA-C may function as a part of the whole patient treatment and management team. Services may be performed by the OPA-C in primary orthopaedic care, pre-operative care, intra-operative care, and post-operative care for the orthopaedic patient in accordance with established policies and procedures. The OPA-C reports to the supervising orthopaedic physician the complete patient status and shall notify accordingly of any abnormal findings, problems or complaints regarding the whole care of the patient.

Employment Characteristics

OPA-Cs work as members of the orthopaedic care team in any locale where legally responsible board certified orthopaedic physicians may appropriately direct them. OPA-Cs most often work within orthopaedic organizations that also employ general allied health professionals. OPA-Cs are commonly employed in private practice settings, with solo practicing surgeons, within hospital organizations and within surgical assisting groups. The practice of an OPA-C is often diverse given the nature of practice or hospital employed and many have subspecialty training within the field of orthopaedic medicine.

Educational Program

OPA Masters Program through University of St. Augustine

Length. The OPA Masters program is a two-year program.

The program combines a year of classroom/online learning with a full-year of orthopaedic-specific clinical rotations. The master's

program requires an undergraduate baccalaureate degree from an accredited institution. The following prerequisite courses are as follows: Medical Terminology; General College Chemistry I & II, Cell Biology; Microbiology; General Physics I & II; Anatomy & Physiology I & II; and Social Sciences. Visit *www.usa.edu* for all requirements and further information.

Certification

The National Board for Certification of Orthopaedic Physician's Assistants (NBCOPA), provides the certification process for OPAs in the United States. NBCOPA focuses on continued professional development and education of OPAs. The certification process incorporates a 4-year cycle of recertification and registration of continuing medical education.

Inquiries

American Society of Orthopaedic Physician's Assistants (ASOPA)

8365 Keystone Crossing, Suite 107
Indianapolis, IN 46240
Phone: 800 824-3044
Fax: 317 205-9481
E-mail: *asopa@hp-assoc.com*
www.asopa.org

Certification

National Board for Certification of Orthopaedic Physician's Assistants (NBCOPA)
c/o Melody Raymond, AAOS Special Society Services
6300 North River Road, Suite 727
Rosemont, IL 60018
847 698-1698
Fax: 847 823-0536
E-mail: *raymond@aaos.org*
www.asopa.org/sections/certification.php

Educational Program (School)

University of St. Augustine
1 University Boulevard
St. Augustine, FL 32086
800 241-1027
www.usa.edu

Orthotist and Prosthetist

Career Description

Orthotics and prosthetics is a specialized health care profession that combines a unique blend of clinical and technical skills. Orthotists and prosthetists evaluate patients and custom-design, fabricate, and fit orthoses and prostheses. Orthotic patients have neuromuscular and musculoskeletal disorders, and prosthetic patients have a partial or total absence of a limb. Orthotists and prosthetists give their patients the ability to lead more active and independent lives by working with physicians and members of the rehabilitation team to create a treatment plan and custom device. This work requires substantial clinical and technical skill and judgment

The principles of biomechanics, pathomechanics, gait analysis, kinesiology, anatomy and physiology are crucial to the practitioner's ability to provide comprehensive patient care and a positive clinical outcome. Patient assessment, treatment, and education are part of the practitioner's responsibility, all of which requires collaborative communication skills.

The practice of an orthotist and/or prosthetist includes evaluating the patient, formulating a treatment plan, designing and fabricating the prosthesis or orthosis, fitting and modifying the prosthesis or orthosis, and follow-up treatment care and practice management.

Patient evaluation may include, but is not limited to, the following:
- Skin integrity
- Pain
- Biomechanics
- Gait analysis, including temporal and spatial assessment
- Range of motion
- Muscle strength
- Posture and balance
- Activities of daily living
- Environmental barriers including social, home and work reintegration
- The need for physical and occupational therapy modalities

Formulation of a treatment plan based on a comprehensive assessment includes, but is not limited to:
- Evaluation of prescription/documentation
- A needs assessment based on patient and/or caregiver input
- Development of functional goals
- Analysis of structural and design requirements
- Assessment of potential physical and occupational therapy requirements
- Consultation with and/or referral to other health care professionals

Implementation of the orthotic and/or prosthetic treatment plan includes, but is not limited to:
- Preparatory care
- Material selection
- Fabrication of orthoses and/or prostheses
- Prototype development including evaluative wear
- Structural evaluation
- Diagnostic fitting
- Gait training
- Patient education and instruction
- Supervision of the provision of care

Follow-up treatment planning, which ensures successful orthotic and/or prosthetic outcomes, patient health, and quality of life, includes, but is not limited to:
- Documentation of functional changes
- Formulation of modifications to ensure successful outcomes
- Reassessment of patient expectations
- Reassessment of treatment objectives
- Development of long-term treatment plan
- Confirmation of patient education and instruction
- Evidence-based practice

Practice management involves the development and documentation of policies and procedures ensuring patient protection that includes, but is not limited to:
- Adherence to applicable local, state, and federal laws and regulations
- Following patient care guidelines and procedures
- Maintaining a safe and professional environment for patient care
- Understanding of claims development and submission

History

The practice of orthotics and prosthetics has its history in the artisans and other skilled craftsmen of the past. Many of the developments in both professions are a result of the two world wars and the polio epidemics of the 1950s. Today's practitioners work in a variety of settings and use innovative materials and techniques to restore function and provide relief for various impairments.

The American Orthotic & Prosthetic Association (AOPA) originated in 1917 as the Artificial Limb Manufacturers and Brace Association (ALMBA). Anticipating that World War I casualties would require orthotic and prosthetic treatment, the Council of National Defense and artificial limb and brace manufacturers met to prepare the industry to meet those needs.

Between the world wars, ALMBA's focus changed. Its members began to view themselves as clinicians and professionals, who care for patients, rather than craftspeople and blacksmiths hammering on leather and metal. Furthermore, the rehabilitation of people with disabilities was also becoming a priority.

Through World War II and the Korean conflict, O&P practitioners realized a need for more research in the field and, through the Association, interested the government in funding studies. During these years, membership expanded and the Association assumed more duties. It also changed its name to the Orthopedic Appliance and Limb Manufacturers Association (OALMA) and established a national office in Washington, DC to work more effectively with the federal government. Through the years, AOPA has changed its scope and evolved to become the unified voice of the O&P profession and industry.

The American Academy of Orthotists and Prosthetists (AAOP) was founded in 1970 to further the scientific and educational achievements of professional practitioners in the disciplines of orthotics and prosthetics. The American Academy of Orthotists and Prosthetists is dedicated to promoting professionalism and advancing the standards of patient care through education, literature, research, advocacy, and collaboration. Voting, membership in the Academy is restricted to individuals who have been certified in orthotics or prosthetics by and who remain in good standing with the American Board for Certification in Orthotics, Prosthetics and Pedorthies, Inc (ABC). Other membership categories exist to ensure that every professional in the O&P field has access to the latest research and the best continuing education, although these members are non-voting.

The ABC was established in 1948 by a group of practitioners who were concerned about patient care and wanted to develop standards to ensure that patients treated by certified practitioners at accredited facilities would receive the best care possible. ABC continues to set clinical and organizational standards, furthering professionalism and establishing the orthotics ,prosthetics, and pedorthics practitioner as a valuable member of the allied health care community. ABC certifications and registrations are considered the profession's highest standards for professionals providing patient care and technical services. These credentials are awarded to individuals who have met ABC's education, experience, and competency assessment (examination) requirements. The individuals who have achieved these certifications and registrations have passed specific examinations based on a comprehensive practice analysis of the orthotic, prosthetic and pedorthic professions.

Employment Characteristics

The practice of orthotics and prosthetics is carried out in many settings, including orthotic and prosthetic facilities, hospitals, specialty clinics, acute care facilities, rehabilitation facilities, university and research facilities, rural outreach clinics, home health settings, and skilled nursing facilities.

Salary

According to the American Orthotic and Prosthetic Association (AOPA), salaries for board-certified orthotists and prosthetists averages between $69,800 and $88,700, depending on the certification type and work setting.

For more information, refer to *www.ama-assn.org/go/hpsalary*. Data from the US Bureau of Labor Statistics (*http://www.bls.gov/oes/current/oes292091.htm*) from May 2011 show that wages at the 10th percentile are $34,580, the 50th percentile (median) at $65,250, and the 90th percentile at $112,680.

Employment Outlook

Data from the US Bureau of Labor Statistics indicate that projected 2010-2020 employment of orthotists and prosthetists is expected to grow faster than average, compared to other occupations.

Educational Programs

Length. Individuals interested in an education in orthotics and prosthetics attend schools with curriculum specific programs accredited by the Commission on Accreditation of Allied Health Education Programs (CAAHEP) and the National Commission on Orthotic and Prosthetic Education (NCOPE). The education is at the entry-level master's. Post-graduate clinical experience is required through a structured residency program. NCOPE-accredited residency sites provide the orthotic and prosthetic resident with qualified experience that extends the education and training process into the patient management setting.

Prerequisites. Applicants for the master's level program requires appropriate course work in life sciences/biology with lab, chemistry with lab, physics with lab, human anatomy and physiol-

ogy, human growth and development or abnormal psychology and statistics.

Curriculum. The professional curriculum includes formal instruction in:
- Advanced clinical and applied technology
- Applied clinical skills
- Applied technical skills
- Behavioral sciences
- Bioethics
- Biomechanics
- Clinical pathology
- Clinical pharmacology
- Communication skills
- Diagnostic studies
- Evidence-based practice
- Gait analysis/pathomechanics
- Health care economics
- Human anatomy and physiology
- Kinesiology
- Materials science
- Models of disablement
- Neuroscience
- Practice management
- Professional issues
- Rehabilitation science
- Research methods
- Measurement
- Impression taking
- Model rectification
- Diagnostic fitting
- Definitive fitting
- External powered technology
- Static and dynamic alignment of sockets related to various amputation levels
- Fitting and alignment of orthoses for lower limb, upper limb, and spine.

The curriculum also includes a structured clinical experience.

Certification

The American Board for Certification in Orthotics, Prosthetics and Pedorthics, Inc (ABC) is the certifying and accrediting body for the orthotic, prosthetic, and pedorthic professions. The certification process includes a written exam, written simulation exam, and hands-on clinical patient management exam. Exams are given three times a year at nationwide sites, with the exception of the Clinical Patient Management Exams, which are given twice a year at two specific locations.

Inquiries

Careers
Information on careers in orthotics and prosthetics is available at *www.opcareers.org*.

Education
Information on colleges and universities offering master's degree programs is available from:
National Commission on Orthotic and Prosthetic Education (NCOPE)
330 John Carlyle Street, Suite 200
Alexandria, VA 22314
703 836-7114
E-mail: *info@ncope.org*
www.ncope.org

Certification

American Board for Certification in Orthotics, Prosthetics and
    Pedorthics, Inc. (ABC)
330 John Carlyle Street, Suite 210
Alexandria, VA 22314
703 836-7114
E-mail: *info@abcop.org*
www.abcop.org

Program Accreditation

Commission on Accreditation of Allied Health Education Programs
    (CAAHEP)
1361 Park Street, Clearwater, FL33756
727 210-2350
727 210-2354 Fax
E-mail: *mail@caahep.org*
www.caahep.org

in collaboration with:
National Commission on Orthotic and Prosthetic Education

Orthotist/Prosthetist

California

California State University - Dominguez Hills
Orthotist/Prosthetist Prgm
5901 East 7th St
Building 149, Suite 130
Long Beach, CA 90822
www.csudh.edu/oandp

Connecticut

University of Hartford
Orthotist/Prosthetist Prgm
200 Bloomfield Ave
West Hartford, CT 06117

Florida

St Petersburg College
Orthotist/Prosthetist Prgm
PO Box 13489
St. Petersburg, FL 33733

Georgia

Georgia Institute of Technology
Orthotist/Prosthetist Prgm
281 Ferst Drive
Atlanta, GA 30332-0356
www.ap.gatech.edu/mspo
Prgm Dir: Christopher Hovorka
Tel: 404 385-2895   *Fax:* 404 894-9982
E-mail: chris.hovorka@ap.gatech.edu

Illinois

Northwestern University
Orthotist/Prosthetist Prgm
680 North Lake Shore Drive, Suite 1100
Chicago, IL 60611-4496
www.northwestern.edu

Michigan

Eastern Michigan University
Cosponsor: University of Michigan Orthotic-Prosthetic
    Center
Orthotist/Prosthetist Prgm
318 Porter Bldg
Ypsilanti, MI 48197
www.emich.edu/hphp/orthotics_index.html

Minnesota

Century College
Orthotist/Prosthetist Prgm
3300 Century Ave N
White Bear Lake, MN 55110
www.century.edu

Pennsylvania

University of Pittsburgh
Orthotist/Prosthetist Prgm
5043 Forbes Tower
Pittsburgh, PA 15260

Texas

Univ of Texas Southwestern Med Ctr
Orthotist/Prosthetist Prgm
6011 Harry Hines Blvd, Suite V.5.400
Dallas, TX 75235-9091
www.utsouthwestern.edu/po
Prgm Dir: Susan Kapp, MEd CPO LPO
Tel: 214 648-1580   *Fax:* 214 645-8258
E-mail: susan.kapp@utsouthwestern.edu

Washington

University of Washington
Orthotist/Prosthetist Prgm
1959 NE Pacific St
Box 356490
Seattle, WA 98195-6490
www.rehab.washington.edu/education/degree/po/

Orthotist/Prosthetist

Programs*	Class Capacity	Begins	Length (months)	Award	Res. Tuition	Non-res. Tuition	Offers:† 1	2	3	4
Georgia										
Georgia Institute of Technology (Atlanta)	12	Aug	2	MSPO	$12,488	$35,616			•	
Texas										
Univ of Texas Southwestern Med Ctr (Dallas)	14	May	19	Dipl, MPO	$14,914	$31,879			•	

*Data are shown only for programs that completed the 2011 AMA Survey of Health Professions Education Programs.
†Key to Offers: 1: Evening or weekend classes; 2: Non-English instruction; 3: Cultural competence instruction; 4: Distance education component.

Perfusionist

A perfusionist is a skilled person, qualified by academic and clinical education, who operates extracorporeal circulation equipment during any medical situation in which it is necessary to support or temporarily replace the patient's circulatory or respiratory function. The perfusionist is knowledgeable concerning the variety of equipment available to perform extracorporeal circulation functions and is responsible, in consultation with the physician, for selecting the appropriate equipment and techniques to be used.

History
The field of cardiovascular perfusion emerged in the mid-1960s, with most of its practitioners trained on the job until the mid-1970s. Trainees often come from other disciplines: nursing, respiratory therapy, biomedical engineering, surgical technology, monitoring technicians, and the laboratory sciences.

In 1972, the American Society of Extra-Corporeal Technologists (AmSECT) began a program of certification for perfusionists. In 1975, this program was turned over to a new agency established to conduct certification as an independent activity: the American Board of Cardiovascular Perfusion (ABCP). The ABCP also adopted minimum standards for training programs as developed by AmSECT and began evaluation and accreditation activities. The following year, the AMA Council on Medical Education (CME) granted recognition of the occupation.

The *Standards (Essentials) and Guidelines for an Accredited Educational Program for the Perfusionist* was adopted in 1980, and accreditation of programs began in 1981. The *Standards* was recently revised in 2005.

Career Description
A perfusionist is a skilled allied health professional, trained and educated specifically as a member of an open-heart, surgical team responsible for the selection, setup, and operation of a mechanical device, commonly referred to as the heart-lung machine.

During open heart surgery, when the patient's heart is immobilized and cannot function in a normal fashion while the operation is being performed, the patient's blood is diverted and circulated outside the body through the heart-lung machine and returned again to the patient. In effect, the machine assumes the function of both the heart and lungs.

The perfusionist is responsible for operating the machine during surgery, closely monitoring the altered circulatory process, taking appropriate corrective action when abnormal situations arise, and keeping both the surgeon and anesthesiologist fully informed.

In addition to the operation of the heart-lung machine during surgery, perfusionists often function in supportive roles for other medical specialties in operating mechanical devices to assist in the conservation of blood and blood products during surgery, and provide extended, long-term support of patients' circulation outside of the operating room environment.

Employment Characteristics
Perfusionists primarily work in the operating room during cardiac surgery procedures, and may be employed by the hospital, by surgeons, or as employees of a contract independent group practice. The majority of procedures are performed during regular weekly work hours. As a critical member of the clinical team, perfusionists are required to take call and be available for emergency procedures, which can occur at any time. The call schedule depends on the number of perfusionists employed by the institution.

Salary
Perfusionists are well compensated for their services. According to the American Society of Extra-Corporeal Technology (AmSECT), the average base salary range for practicing perfusionists is as follows:
- Recently graduated perfusionist: $60,000-$75,000
- Perfusionist with 2 to 5 years experience: $70,000-$90,000
- Perfusionist with 6 to 10 years experience: $80,000-$100,000
- Perfusionist managers: over $100,000

For more information, refer to *www.ama-assn.org/go/hpsalary*.

Educational Programs
Length. Programs are generally one to four years, depending on the program design, objectives, prerequisites, and student qualifications. Certificate programs require that applicants have a bachelor's degree.

Prerequisites. Prerequisites vary depending on the length and design of the program. Most programs require college-level science and mathematics. A background in medical technology, respiratory therapy, or nursing is suggested for some programs.

Curriculum. Curricula of accredited programs include courses covering heart-lung bypass for adult, pediatric, and infant patients undergoing heart surgery; long-term supportive extracorporeal circulation; monitoring of patients undergoing extracorporeal circulation; autotransfusion; and special applications of the technology. Curricula include clinical experience, which incorporates and requires performance of an adequate number and variety of circulation procedures.

Inquiries
Careers
American Society of Extra Corporeal Technology (AmSECT) National Office
2209 Dickens Road
Richmond, VA 23230-2005
804 565-6363
E-mail: *amsect@amsect.org*
www.amsect.org

American Academy of Cardiovascular Perfusion
515A East Main Street
Annville, PA 17003
717 867-1485
E-mail: *officeAACP@aol.com*
www.theaacp.com

Certification
American Board of Cardiovascular Perfusion
207 North 25th Avenue
Hattiesburg, MS 39401
601 582-2227
E-mail: *abcp@abcp.org*
www.abcp.org

Program Accreditation
Commission on Accreditation of Allied Health Education Programs
   (CAAHEP)
1361 Park Street, Clearwater, FL 33756
727 210-2350
727 210-2354 Fax
E-mail: *mail@caahep.org*
www.caahep.org

in collaboration with:
Accreditation Committee - Perfusion Education
6654 South Sycamore Street
Littleton, CO 80120
303 738-0770
E-mail: *ac-pe@msn.com*
www.ac-pe.org

Perfusionist

Arizona

Midwestern University - Glendale Campus
Perfusion Prgm
19555 N 59th Ave
Glendale, AZ 85308
www.midwestern.edu

University of Arizona College of Medicine
Perfusion Prgm
1501 N Campbell Ave
Room 4402
Arizona Health Sciences Center
Tucson, AZ 85724
www.arizona.edu

Connecticut

Quinnipiac University
Perfusion Prgm
275 Mount Carmel Ave, EC-RSP
EC-BMS
Hamden, CT 06518
www.quinnipiac.edu/x810.xml

District of Columbia

Walter Reed National Military Med Ctr
Perfusion Prgm
6900 Georgia Ave NW
Building 2 Room C-405
Washington, DC 20037-5001
www.wramc.amedd.army.mil

Florida

Barry University
Perfusion Prgm
11300 NE 2nd Ave
Miami Shores, FL 33161
www.barry.edu/cvp

Illinois

Rush University
Cosponsor: Rush University Medical Center
Perfusion Prgm
600 S Paulina, Ste 1021 D
Chicago, IL 60612
www.rush.edu

Iowa

University of Iowa Hospitals & Clinics
Perfusion Prgm
200 Hawkins Drive, SE 545 GH
Iowa City, IA 52242-1062
www.uihealthcare.com

Nebraska

University of Nebraska Medical Center
Perfusion Prgm
985155 Nebraska Medical Center
Omaha, NE 68198-5155
www.unmc.edu

New Jersey

Cooper University Hospital
Perfusion Prgm
3 Cooper Plaza Suite 411
310 Sarah Cooper Bldg
Camden, NJ 08103
www.cooperhealth.org

New York

North Shore University Hospital
Cosponsor: LIU CW Post
Perfusion Prgm
School of Cardiovascular Perfusion
225 Community Dr South Entrance
Great Neck, NY 11021
www.northshorelij.com

SUNY Upstate Medical University
Perfusion Prgm
750 E Adams St
Syracuse, NY 13210
www.upstate.edu

Ohio

Cleveland Clinic Foundation
Perfusion Prgm
School of Perfusion
9500 Euclid Ave/J4-604
Cleveland, OH 44195-5130
www.clevelandclinic.org
Prgm Dir: Clifford O Ball
Tel: 216 444-3895   *Fax:* 216 445-2725
E-mail: ballc@ccf.org

Pennsylvania

UPMC Presbyterian Shadyside
Perfusion Prgm
5230 Centre Ave
Pittsburgh, PA 15232
www.upmc.com

South Carolina

Medical University of South Carolina
Perfusion Prgm
College of Health Professions, Cardiovascular Perfusion
151 B Rutledge Ave
PO Box 250964
Charleston, SC 29425
www.musc.edu/cp
Prgm Dir: Joseph J Sistino, CCP
Tel: 843 792-2298   *Fax:* 843 792-4417
E-mail: sistinoj@musc.edu

Tennessee

Vanderbilt University Medical Center
Perfusion Prgm
Vanderbilt Heart and Vascular Institute
1215 21st Ave S
Nashville, TN 37232-8802
www.mc.vanderbilt.edu/cvpt

Texas

Texas Heart Institute
Perfusion Prgm
PO Box 20345
Mail Code 1 - 224
Houston, TX 77225
www.texasheart.org/perfusion

Wisconsin

Milwaukee School of Engineering
Perfusion Prgm
1025 N Broadway St
Perfusion Program
Milwaukee, WI 53202-3109
www.msoe.edu/academics/academic_departments/eecs/
  msp/
Prgm Dir: Ron Gerrits, PhD
Tel: 414 277-7561   *Fax:* 414 277-7465
E-mail: gerrits@msoe.edu

Perfusionist											
Programs*	Class Capacity	Begins	Length (months)	Award	Res. Tuition	Non-res. Tuition		Offers:† 1	2	3	4
Ohio											
Cleveland Clinic Foundation	6	Jan	18	Cert	$20,000	$20,000	per year				
South Carolina											
Medical Univ of South Carolina (Charleston)	16	Aug	21	BS	$16,870	$27,934	per year				
Wisconsin											
Milwaukee School of Engineering	8	Sep	21	MSP	$21,000	$21,000	per year				

*Data are shown only for programs that completed the 2011 AMA Survey of Health Professions Education Programs.

†Key to Offers: 1: Evening or weekend classes; 2: Non-English instruction; 3: Cultural competence instruction; 4: Distance education component.

Polysomnographic Technologist

Polysomnographic technologists perform sleep tests and work with physicians to provide information needed for the diagnosis and treatment of sleep disorders. The technologist monitors brain waves, eye movements, muscle activity, multiple breathing variables, and blood oxygen levels during sleep using specialized recording equipment. The technologist interprets the recording as it happens and responds appropriately to emergencies. Technologists provide support services related to the treatment of sleep-related problems, including helping patients use devices for the treatment of breathing problems during sleep and helping individuals develop good sleep habits.

History

In 2002, the Association of Polysomnographic Technologists (APT) was voted into the Commission on Accreditation of Allied Health Education Programs (CAAHEP) as an associate member organization. In 2004, the Committee on Accreditation for Polysomnographic Technology was approved, along with three sponsoring organizations: the American Academy of Sleep Medicine, the Association of Polysomnographic Technologists (now the American Association of Sleep Technologists), and the Board of Registered Polysomnographic Technologists. Accreditation standards were formally approved by the CAAHEP Board of Directors the same year.

Career Description

Polysomnographic technologists use sleep technology as part of a team, under the general supervision of a licensed physician, by applying a unique body of knowledge and methodological skills involving the education, evaluation, treatment and follow-up of sleep disorders in patients of all ages. The polysomnographic technologist performs polysomnography and tests such as the Multiple Sleep Latency Test, Maintenance of Wakefulness Test, Actigraphy, and others used by a physician to diagnose and treat sleep disorders. These tests involve recording, monitoring, and analyzing EEG (electroencephalography), EOG (electrooculography), EMG (electromyography), ECG (electrocardiography), and multiple breathing variables, including capnometry and oximetry, during sleep and wakefulness. Testing procedures may involve applying and adjusting therapeutic modalities such as supplemental oxygen or positive airway pressure and include applying techniques, equipment, and procedures that are safe, aseptic, preventive, and restorative. Interpretive knowledge is required to recognize and respond to respiratory, cardiac, or behavioral events that may occur during testing procedures. Technologists also provide supportive services related to the ongoing treatment of sleep-related problems. The professional realm of this support includes patient instruction on the use of devices for the treatment of breathing problems during sleep and helping individuals develop sleeping habits that promote good sleep hygiene.

Employment Characteristics

Most polysomnographic technologists work in sleep disorders centers. Sleep disorders centers may be located within or affiliated with a hospital, or "freestanding" (in a physician's office or professional building). Some senior technologists may spend all or part of their time scoring sleep recordings, performing daytime tests, and managing a center, but most of the polysomnographic technologist's work is done at night. Typical shifts are three to four 10- to 12-hour shifts per week. The recommended workload is two patients per night. Salaries and benefits are competitive with other allied health professions.

Educational Programs

Length. A two-year program leading to an associate's degree is preferred. However, some programs provide a certificate after a year of training.

Curriculum. The curriculum of an accredited program focuses on correct performance of polysomnographic procedures, therapeutic intervention, and patient safety. Students learn principles of physiological monitoring and the pathophysiology of sleep disorders. Through lecture and observation, they gain experience with study protocols.

Certification

There are two polysomnographic technologist credentials: the Registered Polysomnographic Technologist (RPSGT) and the Certified Polysomnographic Technician (CPSGT). The RPSGT is an internationally recognized certification credential for health professionals who clinically assess patients with sleep disorders; more than 17,000 practitioners worldwide have earned the RPSGT credential.

The CPSGT is an entry-level certification earned by individuals new to the sleep field. The CPSGT is time-limited; certificate holders must earn the RPSGT credential within three years or lose the CPSGT designation. The Board of Registered Polysomnographic Technologists (BRPT), an independent non-profit certification board, develops and administers both the RPSGT and CPSGT exams.

Inquiries

Careers
American Association of Sleep Technologists (AAST)
2510 North Frontage Road
Darien, IL 60561
630 737-9704
630 737-9788 Fax
E-mail: *aast@aastweb.org*

Certification
John Ganoe, CAE, Executive Director
Board of Registered Polysomnographic Technologists (BRPT)
8400 Westpark Drive, 2nd Floor
McLean, VA 22102
703 610-9020
703 610-0229 Fax
E-mail: *info@brpt.org*

Program Accreditation
Commission on Accreditation of Allied Health Education Programs (CAAHEP)
1361 Park Street, Clearwater, FL 33756
727 210-2350
727 210-2354 Fax
E-mail: *mail@caahep.org*
www.caahep.org

in collaboration with:
Committee on Accreditation for Polysomnographic Technologist
Education (CoA PSG)
Florence Tate, CoA, PSG, Executive Director
133 College Road
Concord, MA 01742-1526
774 855-4100
E-mail: *office@coapsg.org*
www.coapsg.org

Polysomnographic Technologist

Alabama

Wallace State Community College
Polysomnographic Technology Prgm
801 Main St NW PO Box 2000
Hanceville, AL 35077-2000

Arizona

GateWay Community College - Phoenix
Polysomnographic Technology Prgm
108 N 40th St
Phoenix, AZ 85034

Arkansas

Baptist Health Schools Little Rock
Polysomnographic Technology Prgm
11900 Colonel Glenn Rd
Little Rock, AR 72210

California

Orange Coast College
Polysomnographic Technology Prgm
2701 Fairview Rd, PO Box 5005
Costa Mesa, CA 92626-5005
www.orangecoastcollege.edu
Prgm Dir: Walt Banoczi, REEG/EP T CNIM RPSGT
  CLTM BVE
Tel: 714 432-5591   *Fax:* 714 432-5534
E-mail: wbanoczi@cccd.edu

Colorado

Pueblo Community College
Polysomnographic Technology Prgm
900 West Orman Ave
Pueblo, CO 81004

Florida

Central Florida Institute - Palm Harbor
Polysomnographic Technology Prgm
30522 US Highway 19 North
Palm Harbor, FL 34684

Illinois

Moraine Valley Community College
Polysomnographic Technology Prgm
9000 W College Parkway
Palos Hills, IL 60465
www.morainevalley.edu

Iowa

Mercy College of Health Sciences
Polysomnographic Technology Prgm
928 6th Ave
Des Moines, IA 50309-1239
www.mchs.edu

Kansas

Johnson County Community College
Polysomnographic Technology Prgm
12345 College Blvd
Overland Park, KS 66210

Kentucky

Bowling Green Technical College
Polysomnographic Technology Prgm
1845 Loop Dr
Bowling Green, KY 42101

Bluegrass Community and Technical College
Polysomnographic Technology Prgm
330F Oswald Bldg 407 Cooper Drive
Lexington, KY 40506

West Kentucky Community & Technical College
Polysomnographic Technology Prgm
PO Box 7380 4810 Alben Barkley Drive
Paducah, KY 42002

Maryland

Community College of Baltimore County
Polysomnographic Technology Prgm
7400 Sollers Point Rd
Dundalk, MD 21222
www.ccbcmd.edu

Montgomery County Community College
Polysomnographic Technology Prgm
7600 Takoma Ave HSC 358
Takoma Park, MD 20912

Massachusetts

Northern Essex Community College
Polysomnographic Technology Prgm
45 Franklin St
Lawrence, MA 01841
www.necc.mass.edu

Michigan

Beaumont Sleep Evaluation Svcs - Berkley Ctr
Polysomnographic Technology Prgm
1949 W 12 Mile Rd
Berkley, MI 48072

Baker College of Flint
Polysomnographic Technology Prgm
1050 W Bristol Rd
Health Science Department
Flint, MI 48507-5508
www.baker.edu

Minnesota

Minneapolis Community & Technical College
Polysomnographic Technology Prgm
1501 Hennepin Ave
Minneapolis, MN 55403

Mississippi

Coahoma Community College
Polysomnographic Technology Prgm
3240 Friars Point Rd
Clarksdale, MS 38614

Missouri

Sanford-Brown College - Fenton
Polysomnographic Technology Prgm
1345 Smizer Mill Rd
Fenton, MO 63026

Nebraska

Southeast Community College
Polysomnographic Technology Prgm
8800 O St
Lincoln, NE 68520

New Jersey

Thomas Edison State College
Polysomnographic Technology Prgm
The Center for Sleep Medicine 1401
  Whitehorse-Mercerville Rd
Hamilton, NJ 08619

New York

Genesee Community College
Polysomnographic Technology Prgm
One College Rd
Batavia, NY 14020

Stony Brook University
Polysomnographic Technology Prgm
School of Health Technology and Management
Health Science Ctr Level 2, Rm 449
Stony Brook, NY 11794

North Carolina

Central Carolina Community College
Polysomnographic Technology Prgm
10 Scottish Lane
Durham, NC 27707

Pitt Community College
Polysomnographic Technology Prgm
PO Drawer 7007
Greenville, NC 27835-7007
www.pittcc.edu

Catawba Valley Community College
Polysomnographic Technology Prgm
2550 US Hwy 70 SE
Hickory, NC 28602
www.cvcc.edu

Lenoir Community College
Polysomnographic Technology Prgm
231 Highway 58 South
Kinston, NC 28502

Sandhills Community College
Polysomnographic Technology Prgm
3395 Airport Rd
Pinehurst, NC 28374

Ohio

Sleep Care Inc
Polysomnographic Technology Prgm
7634 Rivers Edge Dr
Columbus, OH 43235
www.sleepcareinc.com

Cuyahoga Community College
Polysomnographic Technology Prgm
11000Pleasant Valley Rd
Parma, OH 44130

Mercy College of Northwest Ohio
Polysomnographic Technology Prgm
2221 Madison Ave
Toledo, OH 43604

Oregon

Linn-Benton Community College
Polysomnographic Technology Prgm
6500 SW Pacific Blvd
Albany, OR 97321

Oregon Institute of Technology
Polysomnographic Technology Prgm
3201 Campus Drive Mail Stop OW 143
Klamath Falls, OR 97601

Tennessee

Miller-Motte Technical College - Clarksville
Polysomnographic Technology Prgm
1820 Business Park Dr
Clarksville, TN 37040-6023

East Tennessee State University
Polysomnographic Technology Prgm
1000 Jason Witten Way
Elizabethton, TN 37643
www.etsu.edu

Volunteer State Community College
Polysomnographic Technology Prgm
1420 Nashville Pike
Gallatin, TN 37066-3188
www.volstate.edu

Roane State Community College
Polysomnographic Technology Prgm
132 Hayfield Rd
Knoxville, TN 37922
www.roanestate.edu

Texas

Alvin Community College
Polysomnographic Technology Prgm
3110 Mustang Rd
Alvin, TX 77511

TSSMT/STRC Consortium for Polysom Edu
Polysomnographic Technology Prgm
Texas School of Sleep Medicine & Technology
5290 Medical Dr
San Antonio, TX 78229

Virginia

J Sargeant Reynolds Community College
Polysomnographic Technology Prgm
PO Box 85622
Richmond, VA 23285

Washington

Highline Community College
Polysomnographic Technology Prgm
2400 S 240th St
Des Moines, WA 98198

Polysomnographic Technologist

Programs*	Class Capacity	Begins	Length (months)	Award	Res. Tuition	Non-res. Tuition		Offers:† 1	2	3	4
California											
Orange Coast College (Costa Mesa)	24	Aug (odd yrs)	22	AS	$1,380	$2,740	per year				

*Data are shown only for programs that completed the 2011 AMA Survey of Health Professions Education Programs.

†Key to Offers: 1: Evening or weekend classes; 2: Non-English instruction; 3: Cultural competence instruction; 4: Distance education component.

Respiratory Therapist

History

In 1957, a resolution to develop schools of inhalation therapy was introduced to the AMA House of Delegates by the Medical Society of New York. Following approval, the resolution was referred to the AMA Council on Medical Education (CME), which subsequently resulted in the *Standards (Essentials) for an Approved School of Inhalation Therapy Technicians*, which was formally approved by the AMA House of Delegates in 1962. The *Standards* was revised in 1967 and it included the requirements of an 18-month program.

In 1970, the Board of Schools was reorganized and incorporated as the Joint Review Committee for Inhalation Therapy Education. In 1972, the Standards underwent a third revision, and additional standards were developed and approved for a shorter educational program for training individuals to function as technicians. Revised *Standards* was recently approved in 2003.

In 1997, the review committee's name was changed to the Committee on Accreditation for Respiratory Care (CoARC).

In 2009, the Committee on Accreditation for Respiratory Care formally separated from the Commission on Accreditation of Allied Health Education Programs (CAAHEP) and became a freestanding accreditation agency, the Commission on Accreditation for Respiratory Care.

Career Description

Respiratory therapists work in a wide variety of settings to evaluate, treat, and manage patients of all ages with respiratory illnesses and other cardiopulmonary disorders. The advanced respiratory therapist participates in clinical decision-making and patient education, develops and implements respiratory care plans, applies patient-driven protocols, utilizes evidence-based clinical practice guidelines, and participates in health promotion, disease prevention, and disease management. The advanced-level respiratory therapist may be required to exercise considerable independent judgment either under the supervision of a physician or in the respiratory care of patients.

In fulfillment of the advanced therapist role, the respiratory therapist may perform the following procedures:

- Acquiring and evaluating clinical data
- Assessing the cardiopulmonary status of patients
- Performing and assisting in the performance of prescribed diagnostic studies, such as obtaining blood samples, blood gas analysis, pulmonary function testing, and polysomnography
- Evaluating data to assess the appropriateness of prescribed respiratory care
- Establishing therapeutic goals for patients with cardiopulmonary disease
- Participating in the development and modification of respiratory care plans
- Performing case management of patients with cardiopulmonary and related diseases
- Initiating prescribed respiratory care treatments, evaluating and monitoring patient responses to such therapy, and modifying the prescribed therapy to achieve the desired therapeutic objectives
- Initiating and conducting prescribed pulmonary rehabilitation

- Providing patient, family, and community education
- Promoting cardiopulmonary wellness, disease prevention, and disease management
- Participating in life support activities as required and promoting evidence-based medicine, research, and clinical practice guidelines

Employment Characteristics

Respiratory therapists are employed in a variety of settings that include acute, chronic, subacute, and extended care, such as rehabilitation facilities; educational institutions; clinics; physician's offices; home care; sleep labs; diagnostic and research labs; and industry.

Salary

The 2009 Human Resources Study from the American Association for Respiratory Care (AARC) indicated that advanced level respiratory therapists with a Registered Respiratory Therapist (RRT) credential earned a median annual income of $60,000 in 2008. Data from this study shows that annual income for registered respiratory therapists was $37,000 at the 10th percentile and $90,000 at the 90th percentile.

May 2011 data from the US Bureau of Labor Statistics show that wages are $40,660 at the 10th percentile, $55,250 at the 50th percentile (median), and $74,400 at the 90th percentile (*www.bls.gov/oes/current/oes291126.htm*). *Note:* These data reflect salary information for all respiratory therapists, including those who have not yet earned the RRT credential, in various job venues and metropolitan statistical areas.

For more information, refer to *www.ama-assn.org/go/hpsalary*.

Educational Programs and Credentialing

Length, Award. Respiratory therapists complete two or more years of formal training and education, leading to an associate, baccalaureate, or graduate degree. Credentialing exists at the entry and advanced levels; to qualify for the advanced credentialing examinations (RRT), graduates must first earn the entry-level credential (CRT). All educational programs prepare students for advanced level exam eligibility.

Curriculum. The knowledge and skills for performing these functions are achieved through formal college- or university-based programs of classroom, laboratory, and clinical preparation. Biological and physical sciences required include anatomy, physiology, chemistry, physics, microbiology, computer science, pharmacology, and pathophysiology. Coursework may also be required in mathematics, communications, psychology, medical ethics, and the social sciences. Professional coursework may include:

- Patient assessment, monitoring, and evaluation
- Diagnostic and therapeutic procedures
- Airway management and mechanical ventilatory support
- Infection control
- Basic and advanced life support
- Patient and caregiver education
- Rehabilitation and disease management
- Health promotion/disease prevention

Clinical training in all aspects of respiratory care applicable to pediatric, adult, and geriatric patients is also provided.

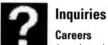

Inquiries

Careers
American Association for Respiratory Care
9425 North MacArthur Blvd, Suite 100
Irving, TX 75063-4706
972 243-2272
http://www.aarc.org/career/be_an_rt/

Licensure/Certification/Registration
National Board for Respiratory Care
18000 West 105th Street
Olathe, KS 66061-7543
913 895-4900
www.nbrc.org

Program Accreditation
Commission on Accreditation for Respiratory Care (CoARC)
1248 Harwood Road
Bedford, TX 76021-0244
817 283-2835
www.coarc.com

Respiratory Therapist

Alabama

University of Alabama at Birmingham
Respiratory Care Prgm
RMSB 486
1705 University Blvd
Birmingham, AL 35294-1212
www.uab.edu/rt

Wallace Community College
Respiratory Care Prgm
1141 Wallace Dr
Dothan, AL 36303
www.wallace.edu

Wallace State Community College
Respiratory Care Prgm
PO Box 2000
Hanceville, AL 35077-2000
www.wallacestate.edu

University of South Alabama
Respiratory Care Prgm
1504 Springhill Ave, Ste 2545
Mobile, AL 36604
www.usouthal.edu

Shelton State Community College
Respiratory Care Prgm
3401 M L King Jr Blvd
Tuscaloosa, AL 35401

Arizona

Pima Medical Institute - Mesa
Respiratory Care Prgm
957 S Dobson Rd
Mesa, AZ 85202
www.pmi.edu

GateWay Community College
Respiratory Care Prgm
108 N 40th St
Phoenix, AZ 85034

Kaplan College
Respiratory Care Prgm
13610 N Black Canyon Hwy, Ste 104
Phoenix, AZ 85029
www.KC-Phoenix.com

Pima Community College
Respiratory Care Prgm
2202 W Anklam Rd/HRP 242
Tucson, AZ 85709-0080
www.pima.edu
Prgm Dir: Jody Kosanke, MEd RRT-NPS
Tel: 520 206-3107   *Fax:* 520 206-3027
E-mail: Jody.Kosanke@pima.edu

Pima Medical Institute - Tucson
Respiratory Care Prgm
3350 E Grant Rd
Tucson, AZ 85716

Arkansas

NorthWest Arkansas Community College
Respiratory Care Prgm
One College Dr
Bentonville, AR 72712
www.nwacc.edu

University of Arkansas for Medical Sciences
Cosponsor: Central Arkansas Veterans Healthcare
  Services
Respiratory Care Prgm
CHRP
4301 W Markham St, Slot 704 (14B/NLR)
Little Rock, AR 72205
www.uams.edu/chrp/resp.htm

Southeast Arkansas College
Respiratory Care Prgm
1900 Hazel St
Pine Bluff, AR 71603
www.seark.edu

Black River Technical College
Respiratory Care Prgm
PO Box 468
Hwy 304 East
Pocahontas, AR 72455
www.blackrivertech.org

University of Arkansas for Medical Sciences
Respiratory Care Prgm
UAMS AHEC-Southwest
300 E 6th St
Texarkana, AR 71854
www.uams.edu
Notes: Program is transitioning to a satelite program,
  with final graduating class in 2011.

California

San Joaquin Valley College - Bakersfield
Respiratory Care Prgm
201 New Stine Rd
Bakersfield, CA 93309
www.sjvc.edu

Pima Medical Institute - Chula Vista
Respiratory Care Prgm
780 Bay Blvd
Chula Vista, CA 91910
www.pmi.edu

Orange Coast College
Respiratory Care Prgm
2701 Fairview Rd, PO Box 5005
Costa Mesa, CA 92626
www.orangecoastcollege.edu
Prgm Dir: Daniel S Adelmann, MS RRT
Tel: 714 432-5541   *Fax:* 714 432-5534
E-mail: dadelmann@occ.cccd.edu

Grossmont College
Respiratory Care Prgm
8800 Grossmont College Dr
El Cajon, CA 92020-1799
www.grossmont.edu/healthprofessions
Prgm Dir: Lorenda Seibold-Phalan, MA RRT-NPS RCP
Tel: 619 644-7448   *Fax:* 619 644-7961
E-mail: lorenda.seibold-phalan@gcccd.edu

Ohlone College
Respiratory Care Prgm
43600 Mission Blvd, PO Box 3909
Fremont, CA 94539
www.ohlone.cc.ca.us/instr/resp_ther

Fresno City College
Respiratory Care Prgm
1101 E University Ave
Fresno, CA 93741
www.fresnocitycollege.edu

Loma Linda University
Respiratory Care Prgm
Nichol Hall, Room 1926
Loma Linda, CA 92350
www.llu.edu

Foothill College
Respiratory Care Prgm
12345 El Monte Rd
Los Altos Hills, CA 94022
www.foothill.edu/bio/programs/respther

Modesto Junior College
Respiratory Care Prgm
435 College Ave
Modesto, CA 95350

East Los Angeles College
Respiratory Care Prgm
1301 Avenida Cesar Chavez
Monterey Park, CA 91754
www.elac.edu

Napa Valley College
Respiratory Care Prgm
2277 Napa Vallejo Hwy
Napa, CA 94558
www.napavalley.edu

Concorde Career College - North Hollywood
Respiratory Care Prgm
12412 Victory Blvd
North Hollywood, CA 91606

Butte College
Respiratory Care Prgm
3536 Butte Campus Dr
Oroville, CA 95965
www.butte.edu/departments/careertech/
    healthoccupations/rt/
Prgm Dir: Donna Davis, BS RRT
Tel: 530 895-2827   *Fax:* 530 895-2472
E-mail: davisdo@butte.edu

**San Joaquin Valley College - Rancho
    Cucamonga**
Respiratory Care Prgm
10641 Church St
Rancho Cucamonga, CA 91730

American River College
Respiratory Care Prgm
4700 College Oak Dr
Sacramento, CA 95841
www.arc.losrios.edu

Kaplan College - Salida
Respiratory Care Prgm
5172 Kiernan Ct
Salida, CA 95368
www.maricollege.edu

Skyline College
Respiratory Care Prgm
3300 College Dr
San Bruno, CA 94066
Prgm Dir: Raymond Hernandez,
Tel: 650 738-4457   *Fax:* 650 738-4299
E-mail: hernandezr@smccd.net

California College San Diego
Respiratory Care Prgm
2820 Camino Del Rio S
San Diego, CA 92108
www.cc-sd.edu

Simi Valley Adult School
Respiratory Care Prgm
3192 Los Angeles Ave
Simi Valley, CA 93065

El Camino College
Respiratory Care Prgm
16007 S Crenshaw Blvd
Torrance, CA 90506
www.elcamino.edu/respiratorycare

Los Angeles Valley College
Respiratory Care Prgm
5800 Fulton Ave
Valley Glen, CA 91401-4096
www.lavc.edu/restherapy

Victor Valley Community College District
Respiratory Care Prgm
18422 Bear Valley Rd
Victorville, CA 92392-5849
www.vvc.edu

San Joaquin Valley College - Visalia
Respiratory Care Prgm
8400 W Mineral King
Visalia, CA 93291
www.sjvc.edu

Mt San Antonio College
Respiratory Care Prgm
1100 N Grand Ave
Walnut, CA 91789
www.mtsac.edu

Crafton Hills College
Respiratory Care Prgm
11711 Sand Canyon Rd
Yucaipa, CA 92399
www.craftonhills.edu

Colorado

T H Pickens Technical Center
Respiratory Care Prgm
500 Airport Blvd
Aurora, CO 80011-9307

Pima Medical Institute - Denver
Respiratory Care Prgm
7475 Dakin St
Denver, CO 80221

Pueblo Community College
Respiratory Care Prgm
900 W Orman Ave
Pueblo, CO 81004
www.pueblocc.edu

Connecticut

Quinnipiac University
Respiratory Care Prgm
Mt Carmel Ave
Hamden, CT 06518

Manchester Community College
Respiratory Care Prgm
Great Path, PO Box 1046
Manchester, CT 06045-1046
www.mcc.commnet.edu

**Norwalk Hospital/Norwalk Community
    College**
Respiratory Care Prgm
24 Maple St
Norwalk, CT 06856
www.norwalkhealth.org

Naugatuck Valley Community College
Respiratory Care Prgm
750 Chase Pkwy
Waterbury, CT 06708
www.nvcc.commnet.edu

University of Hartford
Respiratory Care Prgm
200 Bloomfield Ave
West Hartford, CT 06117
www.hartford.edu
Prgm Dir: Peter W Kennedy, PhD RRT
Tel: 860 768-4823   *Fax:* 860 768-5706
E-mail: pkennedy@hartford.edu

Delaware

**Delaware Technical Community College -
    Owens Campus**
Respiratory Care Prgm
PO Box 610
Georgetown, DE 19947
www.dtcc.edu

Delaware Technical Community College
Cosponsor: Christiana Care Health Services
Respiratory Care Prgm
Ste 101, Medical Arts Complex
700 W Lea Blvd
Wilmington, DE 19802

District of Columbia

University of the District of Columbia
Respiratory Care Prgm
4200 Connecticut Ave NW
Washington, DC 20008
www.udc.edu

Florida

Broward College
Respiratory Care Prgm
1000 Coconut Creek Blvd
Coconut Creek, FL 33066
www.broward.edu

**Daytona State College, Daytona Beach
    Campus**
Respiratory Care Prgm
PO Box 2811
1200 W Internatonal Speedway Blvd
Daytona Beach, FL 32114
www.daytonastate.edu

Edison State College
Respiratory Care Prgm
8099 College Pkwy SW
PO Box 60210
Fort Myers, FL 33906-6210
www.edison.edu

Indian River State College
Respiratory Care Prgm
3209 Virginia Ave
Fort Pierce, FL 34981

Florida State College at Jacksonville
Respiratory Care Prgm
North Campus, 4501 Capper Rd
Jacksonville, FL 32218
www.fccj.org

ATI Health Education Centers
Respiratory Care Prgm
1395 NW 167th St, Ste 200
Miami, FL 33169

Dade Medical College
Respiratory Care Prgm
Medical Center Campus
950 NW 20th St
Miami, FL 33127
www.mdc.edu/medical/academic_programs/respiratory/
    respiratory.htm

University of Central Florida
Respiratory Care Prgm
Dept of Health Professions
HPA II-206, PO Box 162205
Orlando, FL 32816-2205

Valencia College
Respiratory Care Prgm
PO Box 3028
Orlando, FL 32802-9961
http://valenciacc.edu

Palm Beach State College
Respiratory Care Prgm
3160 PGA Blvd
Palm Beach Gardens, FL 33410-2893

St Petersburg College
Respiratory Care Prgm
7200 66th St N
Pinellas Park, FL 33781

Seminole State College
Respiratory Care Prgm
100 Weldon Blvd
Sanford, FL 32773
www.scc-fl.edu/respiratory/

Florida A&M University
Respiratory Care Prgm
Ware-Rhaney Extension
Suite 328
Tallahassee, FL 32307

Tallahassee Community College
Respiratory Care Prgm
444 Appleyard Dr
Tallahassee, FL 32304
www.tcc.fl.edu

Hillsborough Community College
Respiratory Care Prgm
PO Box 30030
4001 Tampa Bay Blvd
Tampa, FL 33630-3030
www.hccfl.edu

Georgia

Darton College
Respiratory Care Prgm
2400 Gillionville Rd
Albany, GA 31707
www.darton.edu
Prgm Dir: William F Thomas, MS RRT
Tel: 229 317-6896 *Fax:* 229 317-6682
E-mail: william.thomas@darton.edu

Athens Technical College
Respiratory Care Prgm
800 US Hwy 29 N
Athens, GA 30601-1500
www.athenstech.edu

Georgia State University
Respiratory Care Prgm
PO Box 4019
Atlanta, GA 30302-4019
chhs.gsu.edu/rt

Augusta Technical College
Respiratory Care Prgm
3200 Augusta Tech Dr
Augusta, GA 30906
www.augustatech.edu
Prgm Dir: Rita Waller, MSN RRT
Tel: 706 771-4194 *Fax:* 706 771-4181
E-mail: rwaller@augustatech.edu

Georgia Health Sciences University
Respiratory Care Prgm
815 St Sebastian Way, Rm HM-143
Augusta, GA 30912-0850

Oconee Fall Line Technical College
Respiratory Care Prgm
560 Pinehill Rd
Dublin, GA 31021
www.heartofgatech.edu/ncontacts.htm

Southern Crescent Technical College
Respiratory Care Prgm
501 Varsity Rd
Griffin, GA 30223
www.griffintech.edu

Gwinnett Technical College
Respiratory Care Prgm
5150 Sugarloaf Pkwy
Lawrenceville, GA 30043-5702
www.gwinnetttech.edu

Macon State College
Respiratory Care Prgm
100 College Station Dr
Macon, GA 31297
www.maconstate.edu

Georgia Northwestern Technical College
Respiratory Care Prgm
One Maurice Culberson Dr
Rome, GA 30161

Armstrong Atlantic State University
Respiratory Care Prgm
11935 Abercorn St
Savannah, GA 31419
www.armstrong.edu

Southwest Georgia Technical College
Respiratory Care Prgm
15689 US Highway 19 North
Thomasville, GA 31792
www.southwestgatech.edu
Prgm Dir: Tammy A Miller, MEd CPFT RRT
Tel: 912 225-5094 *Fax:* 912 225-5289
E-mail: tmiller@southwestgatech.edu

Hawaii

Kapiolani Community College
Respiratory Care Prgm
4303 Diamond Head Rd
Honolulu, HI 96816

Idaho

Boise State University
Respiratory Care Prgm
College of Health Sciences
1910 University Dr/Rm HSR 207
Boise, ID 83725
http://hs.boisestate.edu/respcare/
Prgm Dir: Jody Lester, MA RRT
Tel: 208 426-3383 *Fax:* 208 426-4093
E-mail: jlester@boisestate.edu

Illinois

Southwestern Illinois College
Respiratory Care Prgm
St Elizabeth's Hospital
211 S Third St
Belleville, IL 62222
www.swic.edu

Southern Illinois University Carbondale
Respiratory Care Prgm
School of Allied Health, 1365 Douglas Dr
College of Applied Sciences & Arts, MC6615
Carbondale, IL 62901
Notes: Currently inactive

Kaskaskia College
Respiratory Care Prgm
27210 College Rd
Centralia, IL 62801
www.kaskaskia.edu

Parkland College
Respiratory Care Prgm
2400 W Bradley Ave
Champaign, IL 61821
www.parkland.edu

Malcolm X College
Respiratory Care Prgm
1900 W Van Buren St
Chicago, IL 60612-3197
http://malcolmx.ccc.edu

Olive Harvey College
Respiratory Care Prgm
10001 W Woodlawn Ave, Rm 3317
Chicago, IL 60628

St Augustine College
Respiratory Care Prgm
1333-45 W Argyle
Chicago, IL 60640

Illinois Central College
Cosponsor: OSF St. Francis Medical Center
Respiratory Care Prgm
Health Careers Department
One College Drive
East Peoria, IL 61615
www.icc.edu

Kankakee Community College
Respiratory Care Prgm
100 College Dr
Kankakee, IL 60901-6505

Moraine Valley Community College
Respiratory Care Prgm
9000 W College Dr Room B 150
Palos Hills, IL 60465
www.morainevalley.edu/programs/2008-2009/2008-2009_
fall/1241_course.htm

Triton College
Respiratory Care Prgm
2000 N Fifth Ave
River Grove, IL 60171

Rock Valley College
Respiratory Care Prgm
4151 Samuelson Rd
Rockford, IL 61109-3272
www.rockvalleycollege.edu

St John's Hospital
Cosponsor: Lincoln Land Community College
Respiratory Care Prgm
School of Respiratory Care
800 E Carpenter St
Springfield, IL 62769
www.st-johns.org

Indiana

University of Southern Indiana
Respiratory Care Prgm
8600 University Blvd
Evansville, IN 47712

Ivy Tech Community College - Northeast
Respiratory Care Prgm
3800 N Anthony Blvd
Fort Wayne, IN 46805
www.ivytech.edu

Indiana University Northwest
Respiratory Care Prgm
3400 Broadway NW Campus
Hawthorne Hall
Gary, IN 46408
www.iun.edu

Indiana University
Respiratory Care Prgm
1140 W Michigan St, CF 224
Indianapolis, IN 46202
www.indiana.edu

Indiana University Health
Cosponsor: Indiana Respiratory Therapy Education
Consortium
Respiratory Care Prgm
1701 N Senate Blvd
Wile Hall 631
Indianapolis, IN 46202
www.iuhealth.org

Ivy Tech Community College
Respiratory Care Prgm
Central Indiana Region
9301 E 59th St
Indianapolis, IN 46216
www.ivytech.edu

Ivy Tech Community College - Lafayette
Respiratory Care Prgm
3101 S Creasy Ln
Lafayette, IN 47903

Ivy Tech Community College
Respiratory Care Prgm
3714 Franklin St
Michigan City, IN 46360

Ivy Tech Community College
Respiratory Care Prgm
8204 Hwy 311
Sellersburg, IN 47172

Ivy Tech Community College
Respiratory Care Prgm
8000 S Education Dr
Terre Haute, IN 47802

Iowa

Des Moines Area Community College
Respiratory Care Prgm
2006 S Ankeny Blvd
Ankeny, IA 50023
www.dmacc.edu/programs/respiratorytherapy/welcome.
htm

Kirkwood Community College
Respiratory Care Prgm
6301 Kirkwood Blvd SW, PO Box 2068
Cedar Rapids, IA 52406-9973

Northeast Iowa Community College
Respiratory Care Prgm
10250 Sundown Rd
Peosta, IA 52068

St. Luke's College/St. Luke's Regl Med Ctr
Respiratory Care Prgm
2720 Stone Park Blvd
Sioux City, IA 51104

Hawkeye Community College
Respiratory Care Prgm
1501 E Orange Rd
PO Box 8015
Waterloo, IA 50704-8015
www.hawkeye.cc.ia.us

Southeastern Community College
Respiratory Care Prgm
1500 West Agency PO 180
PO Box 180
West Burlington, IA 52655-0180
www.scciowa.edu

Kansas

Kansas City Community College
Respiratory Care Prgm
7250 State Ave
Kansas City, KS 66112
www.kckcc.edu

University of Kansas Medical Center
Respiratory Care Prgm
3901 Rainbow Blvd, 4006 Delp, Mail Stop 1013
Kansas City, KS 66160
www.kumc.edu/SAH/resp_care
Prgm Dir: Barbara A Ludwig, MA RRT
Tel: 913 588-4634   *Fax:* 913 588-4631
E-mail: bludwig@kumc.edu

Seward County Community College
Respiratory Care Prgm
PO Box 1137
Liberal, KS 67901-1137
http://sccc.edu

Johnson County Community College
Respiratory Care Prgm
Respiratory Care, 12345 College Blvd
Overland Park, KS 66210
www.jccc.net/home/depts/001256

Labette Community College
Respiratory Care Prgm
200 S 14th St
Parsons, KS 67357
www.labette.edu

Washburn University
Respiratory Care Prgm
1700 SW College Ave
Topeka, KS 66621
www.washburn.edu/respiratory
Prgm Dir: Rusty Taylor, MEd RRT
Tel: 785 670-2172   *Fax:* 785 670-1027
E-mail: rusty.taylor@washburn.edu

Newman University
Respiratory Care Prgm
3100 McCormick Ave
Wichita, KS 67213-2097
www.newmanu.edu
Prgm Dir: Meg Trumpp, MEd RRT AE-C
Tel: 316 942-4291, Ext 2344   *Fax:* 316 942-4483
E-mail: trumppm@newmanu.edu

Kentucky

Bowling Green Technical College
Respiratory Care Prgm
1845 Loop Dr
Bowling Green, KY 42101
www.bowlinggreen.kctcs.edu

Northern Kentucky University
Respiratory Care Prgm
Nunn Dr, AHC-225
Highland Heights, KY 41099-8002
Prgm Dir: Debra Kasel, MEd RRT CPFT AE-C
Tel: 859 572-5608   *Fax:* 859 572-1314
E-mail: kaseld@nku.edu

Bluegrass Community and Technical College
Cosponsor: University of Kentucky
Respiratory Care Prgm
Rm 330 Oswald Bldg, Cooper Dr
Lexington, KY 40506-0235
www.bluegrass.kctcs.edu/LCC/RCP/

Jefferson Community and Technical College
Respiratory Care Prgm
109 E Broadway St
Louisville, KY 40202
www.jefferson.kctcs.edu

Madisonville Community College
Respiratory Care Prgm
Health Campus
750 N Laffoon St
Madisonville, KY 42431

Maysville Comm & Tech College
Respiratory Care Prgm
609 Viking Dr
Morehead, KY 40351

Laurel Technical College - Rockcastle
Respiratory Care Prgm
PO Box 275
Mount Vernon, KY 40456

West Kentucky Community & Technical College
Respiratory Care Prgm
4810 Alben Barkley Dr, PO Box 7380
Paducah, KY 42002-7380

Big Sandy Community & Technical College
Respiratory Care Prgm
Mayo Campus
513 Third St
Paintsville, KY 41240
www.bigsandy.kctcs.edu
Prgm Dir: Melissa Skeens, BA RRT-NPS RPFT
Tel: 606 789-5321, Ext   *Fax:* 606 789-9753
E-mail: melissa.skeens@kctcs.edu

Southeast Kentucky Comm & Tech College
Respiratory Care Prgm
3300 US Highway 25E S
Pineville, KY 40977

Louisiana

Our Lady of the Lake College
Cosponsor: LSU Health Sciences Center
Respiratory Care Prgm
7434 Perkins Rd
Baton Rouge, LA 70808
www.ololcollege.edu

Bossier Parish Community College
Respiratory Care Prgm
6220 E Texas St
Bossier City, LA 71111
www.bpcc.edu
Prgm Dir: Ashley Dulle,
Tel: 318 813-2935   *Fax:* 318 813-2915
E-mail: adulle@lsuhsc.edu

Louisiana State University at Eunice
Respiratory Care Prgm
PO Box 1129
Eunice, LA 70535
www.lsue.edu

Acadiana Technical College - West Jefferson Campus
Respiratory Care Prgm
475 Manhattan Blvd
Harvey, LA 70058
www.dcc.edu

Nicholls State University
Respiratory Care Prgm
235 Civic Center Blvd
Houma, LA 70360
www.nicholls.edu_respiratory_therapy

Delgado Community College
Respiratory Care Prgm
615 City Park Ave
New Orleans, LA 70119

Louisiana State Univ Health Sciences Center
Respiratory Care Prgm
1900 Gravier St
New Orleans, LA 70112
http://alliedhealth.lsuhsc.edu/Cardiopulmonary
Prgm Dir: John Zamjahn, PhD RRT
Tel: 504 568-4228   *Fax:* 504 599-0410
E-mail: jzamja@lsuhsc.edu

Our Lady of Holy Cross College
Cosponsor: Alton Ochsner School of Allied Health Sciences
Respiratory Care Prgm
4123 Woodland Dr
New Orleans, LA 70131
www.ochsner.org

LSU Health Science Center Shreveport
Respiratory Care Prgm
1501 Kings Hwy
Shreveport, LA 71130
www.lsuhsc.edu

Southern Univ at Shreveport
Respiratory Care Prgm
3050 Martin Luther King Jr Dr
Shreveport, LA 71107

Maine

Kennebec Valley Community College
Respiratory Care Prgm
92 Western Ave
Fairfield, ME 04937-1367
www.kvcc.me.edu

Southern Maine Community College
Respiratory Care Prgm
Two Fort Rd
South Portland, ME 04106
www.smccme.edu

Maryland

Baltimore City Community College
Respiratory Care Prgm
2901 Liberty Heights Ave
Baltimore, MD 21215
www.bccc.edu

Community College of Baltimore County -
   Essex Campus
Respiratory Care Prgm
7201 Rossville Blvd
Baltimore, MD 21237
www.ccbcmd.edu

Allegany College of Maryland
Respiratory Care Prgm
12401 Willowbrook Rd SE
Cumberland, MD 21502-2596
www.allegany.edu

Frederick Community College
Respiratory Care Prgm
7932 Opossumtown Pike
Frederick, MD 21702

Prince George's Community College
Respiratory Care Prgm
301 Largo Rd
Largo, MD 20774
www.pgcc.edu

Salisbury University
Respiratory Care Prgm
1101 Camden Ave
Salisbury, MD 21801
www.salisbury.edu

Washington Adventist University
Respiratory Care Prgm
7600 Flower Ave
Health Science Building #106
Takoma Park, MD 20912
www.wau.edu
Prgm Dir: Vicki Rosette, RRT RPFT
Tel: 301 891-4187   *Fax:* 301 891-4181
E-mail: vrosette@wau.edu

Massachusetts

Northeastern University
Respiratory Care Prgm
249 Ryder Hall
360 Huntington Ave
Boston, MA 02115
www.spcs.neu.edu/ms_respther/

Massasoit Community College
Respiratory Care Prgm
One Massasoit Blvd
Brockton, MA 02301
www.massasoit.mass.edu

North Shore Community College
Respiratory Care Prgm
One Ferncroft Rd, PO Box 3340
Danvers, MA 01923-0840
www.northshore.edu

Northern Essex Community College
Respiratory Care Prgm
45 Franklin St
Lawrence, MA 01841
www.necc.mass.edu

Berkshire Community College
Respiratory Care Prgm
1350 West St
Pittsfield, MA 01201
http://Berkshirecc.edu

Springfield Technical Community College
Respiratory Care Prgm
One Armory Sq
Springfield, MA 01105
www.stcc.edu

Quinsigamond Community College
Respiratory Care Prgm
670 W Boylston St
Worcester, MA 01606-2092
www.qcc.mass.edu

Michigan

Ferris State University
Respiratory Care Prgm
200 Ferris Dr, VFS 210A
Big Rapids, MI 49307-2740
www.ferris.edu

Macomb Community College
Respiratory Care Prgm
44575 Garfield Rd, East Bldg Rm 219
Clinton Township, MI 48038-1139
www.macomb.edu

Henry Ford Community College
Respiratory Care Prgm
Health Careers Education Center
5101 Evergreen Rd
Dearborn, MI 48128-1495

Mott Community College
Respiratory Care Prgm
1401 E Court St
Flint, MI 48503
www.mcc.edu/indexmain.shtml

Kalamazoo Valley Community College
Respiratory Care Prgm
Texas Township Campus
6767 West O Ave, PO Box 4070
Kalamazoo, MI 49003-4070

Monroe County Community College
Respiratory Care Prgm
1555 S Raisinville Rd
Monroe, MI 48161
www.monroeccc.edu

Muskegon Community College
Respiratory Care Prgm
221 S Quarterline Rd
Muskegon, MI 49442
http://muskegon.cc.mi.us/~devriesd/resp-home.htm

Oakland Community College
Respiratory Care Prgm
22322 Rutland Dr
Southfield, MI 48075
www.oaklandcc.edu

Delta College
Respiratory Care Prgm
1961 Delta Rd
University Center, MI 48710
www.delta.edu/health/rt
Prgm Dir: Earl B Gregory, MS RRT
Tel: 989 686-9489   *Fax:* 989 667-2230
E-mail: ebgregor@delta.edu

Minnesota

Lake Superior College
Respiratory Care Prgm
2101 Trinity Rd
Duluth, MN 55811
www.lsc.edu

Northland Community & Technical College
Respiratory Care Prgm
2022 Central Ave NE
East Grand Forks, MN 56721
www.northlandcollege.edu
Prgm Dir: Anthony Sorum, BA RRT
Tel: 218 773-4791, Ext 2628   *Fax:* 218 793-2842
E-mail: tony.sorum@northlandcollege.edu

Saint Catherine University - Minneapolis
Respiratory Care Prgm
601 25th Ave S
Minneapolis, MN 55454
www.stkate.edu/RC

Mayo School of Health Sciences
Respiratory Care Prgm
200 First St SW
1012 Siebens
Rochester, MN 55905

Saint Paul College
Respiratory Care Prgm
235 Marshall Ave
St Paul, MN 55102
www.sptc.mnscu.edu

Mississippi

Northeast Mississippi Community College
Respiratory Care Prgm
101 Cunningham Blvd
Booneville, MS 38829
www.nemcc.edu

Itawamba Community College
Respiratory Care Prgm
602 W Hill St
Fulton, MS 38843
iccms.edu
Prgm Dir: James Newell, MPA RRT
Tel: 602 862-8347   *Fax:* 601 862-8350
E-mail: jwnewell@iccms.edu

Mississippi Gulf Coast Community College
Respiratory Care Prgm
PO Box 100
Gautier, MS 39553

Pearl River Community College
Respiratory Care Prgm
Forrest County Voc-Tech Ctr
5448 US Hwy 49 S
Hattiesburg, MS 39401
www.prcc.edu

Hinds Community College
Respiratory Care Prgm
1750 Chadwick Dr
Jackson, MS 39204
www.hindscc.edu

Meridian Community College
Respiratory Care Prgm
910 Hwy 19 N
Meridian, MS 39307
www.meridiancc.edu

Copiah-Lincoln Community College
Respiratory Care Prgm
Natchez Campus Career and Technical
30 Campus Dr
Natchez, MS 39120-5398
www.colin.edu

Northwest Mississippi Community College
Respiratory Care Prgm
5197 WE Ross Pkwy
Southaven, MS 38671

Missouri

Cape Girardeau Career & Technology Center
Cosponsor: Mineral Area College
Respiratory Care Prgm
1080 S Silver Spring Rd
Cape Girardeau, MO 63703
www.cape.k12.mo.us/cc

University of Missouri
Respiratory Care Prgm
605 Lewis Hall
Columbia, MO 65211
www.umshp.org/rt
Prgm Dir: Shawna Strickland, PhD RRT-NPS AE-C
FAARC
Tel: 573 882-9722   *Fax:* 573 884-1490
E-mail: stricklandsl@health.missouri.edu

Sanford-Brown College
Respiratory Care Prgm
1345 Smizer Mill Rd
Fenton, MO 63026
www.sanford-brown.edu

Hannibal Career & Technical Center
Cosponsor: Hannibal LaGrange College
Respiratory Care Prgm
4550 McMasters Ave
Hannibal, MO 63401
www.hannibal.k12.mo.us

Concorde Career College - Kansas City
Respiratory Care Prgm
3239 Broadway Blvd
Kansas City, MO 64111
www.concordecareercolleges.com

Rolla Technical Center
Respiratory Care Prgm
500 Forum Dr
Rolla, MO 65401

Ozarks Technical Community College
Respiratory Care Prgm
1001 E Chestnut Expressway
Springfield, MO 65802
www.otc.edu

St Louis Community College - Forest Park
Respiratory Care Prgm
5600 Oakland Ave
St Louis, MO 63110
www.stlcc.edu

Missouri State University
Respiratory Care Prgm
128 Garfield
West Plains, MO 65775

Montana

Montana State Univ - Great Falls Coll of Tech
Respiratory Care Prgm
2100 16th Ave S
Great Falls, MT 59405
www.msugf.edu

University of Montana
Respiratory Care Prgm
909 S Ave W
Missoula, MT 59801

Nebraska

Southeast Community College
Respiratory Care Prgm
8800 O St
Lincoln, NE 68520-1299
www.southeast.edu/programs/resp

Alegent Health
Cosponsor: Midland University/University Nebraska
Kearney
Respiratory Care Prgm
6901 N 72nd St
Omaha, NE 68122
http://Alegent.com
Prgm Dir: Todd Klopfenstein, BS RRT
Tel: 402 572-2312   *Fax:* 402 572-2249
E-mail: todd.klopfenstein@alegent.org

Metropolitan Community College
Respiratory Care Prgm
PO Box 3777
Omaha, NE 68103

Nebraska Methodist College
Respiratory Care Prgm
720 N 87th St
Omaha, NE 68114
www.methodistcollege.edu

Nevada

College of Southern Nevada
Respiratory Care Prgm
6375 W Charleston Blvd, W1B
Las Vegas, NV 89146-1124

Pima Medical Institute
Respiratory Care Prgm
3333 E Flamingo Rd
Las Vegas, NV 89121

New Hampshire

River Valley Community College
Respiratory Care Prgm
One College Dr
Claremont, NH 03743

New Jersey

Brookdale Community College
Respiratory Care Prgm
765 Newman Springs Rd
Lincroft, NJ 07738
www.brookdalecc.edu
Prgm Dir: Carol Schedel, MA RRT
Tel: 732 224-2692   *Fax:* 732 224-2998
E-mail: cschedel@brookdalecc.edu

Univ of Medicine & Dent of New Jersey
Respiratory Care Prgm
School of Health Related Professions
65 Bergen St
Newark, NJ 07101

Bergen Community College
Respiratory Care Prgm
400 Paramus Rd
Paramus, NJ 07652
www.bergen.edu/academics/respiratory_therapy/

Northwest NJ Consortium Resp Care Educ
Respiratory Care Prgm
County College of Morris
214 Center Grove Rd
Randolph, NJ 07869

Univ of Medicine & Dent of New Jersey
Respiratory Care Prgm
Sch of Hlth Related Professions
UEC 40 East Laurel Rd
Stratford, NJ 08084
http://shrp.umdnj.edu

New Mexico

Central New Mexico Community College
Respiratory Care Prgm
525 Buena Vista SE
Albuquerque, NM 87106
www.cnm.edu

Pima Medical Institute - Albuquerque
Respiratory Care Prgm
7 Ariel Court
Albuquerque, NM 87043
www.pmi.edu

Dona Ana Community College
Respiratory Care Prgm
Box 30001, Dept 3DA
3400 S Espina St
Las Cruces, NM 88003-0001
http://dabcc.nmsu.edu

Eastern New Mexico University
Respiratory Care Prgm
PO Box 6000
52 University Blvd
Roswell, NM 88202-6000
www.roswell.enmu.edu

New York

Genesee Community College
Respiratory Care Prgm
1 College Rd
Batavia, NY 14020-1519
www.genesee.edu

Long Island University - Brooklyn Campus
Respiratory Care Prgm
University Plaza
Brooklyn, NY 11201
www.liu.edu

Nassau Community College
Respiratory Care Prgm
One Education Dr
Garden City, NY 11530
http://ncc.edu

CUNY Borough of Manhattan Community Coll
Respiratory Care Prgm
199 Chambers St
New York, NY 10007
www.bmcc.cuny.edu/j2ee/index.jsp

Molloy College
Respiratory Care Prgm
1000 Hempstead Ave
PO Box 5002
Rockville Centre, NY 11571-5002
www.molloy.edu

Stony Brook University
Respiratory Care Prgm
Sch of Health Tech and Management
Stony Brook, NY 11794-8203
www.hsc.stonybrook.edu/shtm/rc/index.cfm

Onondaga Community College
Respiratory Care Prgm
4585 W Seneca Turnpike
Syracuse, NY 13215
www.sunyocc.edu

SUNY Upstate Medical University
Respiratory Care Prgm
750 E Adams St
Syracuse, NY 13210
www.upstate.edu/chp/csrc/

Hudson Valley Community College
Respiratory Care Prgm
80 Vandenburgh Ave
Troy, NY 12180
www.hvcc.edu

Mohawk Valley Community College
Respiratory Care Prgm
1101 Sherman Dr
Utica, NY 13501
www.mvcc.edu

Westchester Community College
Respiratory Care Prgm
75 Grasslands Rd
Valhalla, NY 10595
www.sunywcc.edu

Erie Community College - North Campus
Respiratory Care Prgm
6205 Main St
Williamsville, NY 14221

North Carolina

Stanly Community College
Respiratory Care Prgm
141 College Dr
Albemarle, NC 28001

Central Piedmont Community College
Respiratory Care Prgm
PO Box 35009
Charlotte, NC 28235-5009
www.cpcc.edu
Prgm Dir: Brian Stearns, RRT
Tel: 704 330-6274   *Fax:* 704 330-6131
E-mail: brian.stearns@cpcc.edu

Durham Technical Community College
Respiratory Care Prgm
1637 Lawson St/Drawer 11307
Durham, NC 27703
www.durhamtech.edu

Fayetteville Technical Community College
Respiratory Care Prgm
2201 Hull Rd
Fayetteville, NC 28303

Pitt Community College
Respiratory Care Prgm
PO Drawer 7007
Greenville, NC 27835
www.pittcc.edu

Catawba Valley Community College
Respiratory Care Prgm
2550 Hwy 70 SE
Hickory, NC 28602
www.cvcc.edu
Prgm Dir: Catherine A Bitsche, MA RRT
Tel: 828 327-7000, Ext 4391   *Fax:* 828 327-7276
E-mail: cbitsche@cvcc.edu

Robeson Community College
Respiratory Care Prgm
PO Box 1420
Lumberton, NC 28359

Carteret Community College
Respiratory Care Prgm
3505 Arendell St
Morehead City, NC 28557
www.carteret.edu

Sandhills Community College
Respiratory Care Prgm
3395 Airport Rd
Pinehurst, NC 28374
www.sandhills.edu

Edgecombe Community College
Respiratory Care Prgm
225 Tarboro St
Rocky Mount, NC 27801
www.edgecombe.edu

Southwestern Community College
Respiratory Care Prgm
447 College Dr
Sylva, NC 28779-9578

Rockingham Community College
Respiratory Care Prgm
PO Box 38
Wentworth, NC 27375-0038
www.rockinghamcc.edu

Forsyth Technical Community College
Respiratory Care Prgm
2100 Silas Creek Pkwy
302A Bob Greene Hall
Winston-Salem, NC 27103-5197
www.forsythtech.edu

North Dakota

University of Mary/St Alexius Medical Ctr
Respiratory Care Prgm
900 E Broadway/PO Box 5510
Bismarck, ND 58502
http://st.alexius.org

NDSU/Sanford Health Consortium
Respiratory Care Prgm
Sanford Medical Center
PO Box 2010
Fargo, ND 58122-0207
www.ndsu.edu/rc
Prgm Dir: Robyn Urlacher, BS RRT
Tel: 701 234-6147   *Fax:* 701 234-6942
E-mail: robyn.urlacher@sanfordhealth.org

Ohio

The University of Akron
Respiratory Care Prgm
Akron, OH 44325-3702
http://uakron.edu

Collins Career Center
Cosponsor: Marshall Community and Technical College
Respiratory Care Prgm
11627 State Route 243
Chesapeake, OH 45619
www.collins-cc.k12.oh.us

Cincinnati State Tech & Comm College
Cosponsor: UC Clermont
Respiratory Care Prgm
3520 Central Pkwy
Cincinnati, OH 45223
www.cincinnatistate.edu
Prgm Dir: Debra Lierl, MEd RRT
Tel: 513 569-1690   *Fax:* 513 569-1559
E-mail: debra.lierl@cincinnatistate.edu

Columbus State Community College
Respiratory Care Prgm
550 E Spring St
Columbus, OH 43215
www.cscc.edu/Respiratory/

The Ohio State University
Respiratory Care Prgm
431 Atwell Hall
453 W Tenth Ave
Columbus, OH 43210
amp.osu.edu/RT

Sinclair Community College
Respiratory Care Prgm
444 W Third St
Dayton, OH 45402
Prgm Dir: Cynthia Beckett, PhD RRT RPFT
Tel: 937 512-2849   *Fax:* 937 512-2058
E-mail: cynthia.beckett@sinclair.edu

Bowling Green State University
Respiratory Care Prgm
One University Dr
Huron, OH 44839-9791
www.firelands.bgsu.edu/programs/rt
Prgm Dir: Rod C Roark, MS RRT
Tel: 419 433-5560, Ext   *Fax:* 419 372-0755
E-mail: rroark@bgsu.edu

Kettering College of Medical Arts
Respiratory Care Prgm
3737 Southern Blvd
Kettering, OH 45429
www.kcma.edu

Lakeland Community College
Respiratory Care Prgm
7700 Clocktower Dr
Kirtland, OH 44094-5198
www.lakelandcc.edu

Rhodes State College
Respiratory Care Prgm
4240 Campus Dr
Lima, OH 45804
www.rhodesstate.edu
Prgm Dir: Pamela Halfhill, BS RRT
Tel: 419 995-8366   *Fax:* 419 995-8818
E-mail: halfhill.p@rhodesstate.edu

North Central State College
Respiratory Care Prgm
2441 Kenwood Circle, PO Box 698
Mansfield, OH 44901
www.ncstatecollege.edu
Prgm Dir: Robert A Slabodnick, MEd BS RRT/NPS
Tel: 419 755-4891, Ext 4891   *Fax:* 419 755-5630
E-mail: rslabod@ncstatecollege.edu

Washington State Community College
Respiratory Care Prgm
710 Colegate Dr
Marietta, OH 45750
www.wscc.edu

Stark State College
Respiratory Care Prgm
6200 Frank Ave NW
North Canton, OH 44720-7299
www.starkstate.edu

Cuyahoga Community College
Respiratory Care Prgm
11000 Pleasant Valley Rd
Parma, OH 44130
www.tri-c.edu/programs/healthcareers/respiratory/Pages

Shawnee State University
Respiratory Care Prgm
940 Second St
Portsmouth, OH 45662
www.shawnee.edu

Eastern Gateway Community College
Respiratory Care Prgm
4000 Sunset Blvd
Steubenville, OH 43952
www.jcc.edu

University of Toledo
Respiratory Care Prgm
Judith Herb College of Edu, Health Science & Human Services
2801 W Bancroft St, Mail Stop 119
Toledo, OH 43606
www.utoledo.edu/hshs/respiratorycare/

Youngstown State University
Respiratory Care Prgm
One University Plaza
Youngstown, OH 44555
www.ysu.edu

Oklahoma

Great Plains Technology Center
Respiratory Care Prgm
4500 W Lee Blvd
Lawton, OK 73505

Rose State College Rose State College
Respiratory Care Prgm
6420 SE 15th St
Midwest City, OK 73110-2704
www.rose.edu/respiratory-therapist
Prgm Dir: Kathe Rowe, BSEd RRT-NPS
Tel: 405 733-7571   *Fax:* 405 736-0338
E-mail: krowe@rose.edu

Francis Tuttle Technology Center
Cosponsor: Oklahoma City Community College
Respiratory Care Prgm
12777 N Rockwell Ave
Oklahoma City, OK 73142-2789
www.francistuttle.com

Tulsa Community College
Respiratory Care Prgm
909 S Boston Ave
Tulsa, OK 74119
www.tulsacc.edu

Oregon

Lane Community College
Respiratory Care Prgm
4000 E 30th Ave
Eugene, OR 97405-0640
www.lanecc.edu
Prgm Dir: Norma Driscoll, BS RRT
Tel: 541 463-3176   *Fax:* 541 463-4151
E-mail: driscolln@lanecc.edu

Mt Hood Community College
Respiratory Care Prgm
26000 SE Stark St
Gresham, OR 97030

Oregon Institute of Technology
Respiratory Care Prgm
202 S Riverside Ave
Medford, OR 97501
www.oit.edu/rcp

Pennsylvania

West Chester University
Cosponsor: Bryn Mawr Hospital
Respiratory Care Prgm
130 South Bryn Mawr Ave
Bryn Mawr, PA 19010
www.wcupa.edu/_academics/Healthsciences/health/resp
care/
Prgm Dir: Brian Kellar, MS MEd RRT-NPS RPFT
Tel: 484 337-3347   *Fax:* 484 337-3821
E-mail: kellarb@mlhs.org

Gannon University
Respiratory Care Prgm
109 University Square
Erie, PA 16541
www.gannon.edu/departmental/resp

Gwynedd-Mercy College
Respiratory Care Prgm
1325 Sumneytown Pike, PO Box 901
Gwynedd Valley, PA 19437
www.gmc.edu

Harrisburg Area Community College
Respiratory Care Prgm
One HACC Dr
Harrisburg, PA 17110
www.hacc.edu
Prgm Dir: Bradley A Leidich, RRT MSEd FAARC
Tel: 717 780-2315   *Fax:* 717 780-1165
E-mail: baleidic@hacc.edu

University of Pittsburgh - Johnstown
Respiratory Care Prgm
227 Krebs Hall
450 Schoolhouse Rd
Johnstown, PA 15904
www.upj.pitt.edu/372/

Millersville University of Pennsylvania
Cosponsor: Lancaster Regional Medical Center
Respiratory Care Prgm
PO Box 1002
Millersville, PA 17551-0302
www.millersville.edu/rtp
Prgm Dir: John M Hughes
Tel: 717 291-8457   *Fax:* 717 390-3804
E-mail: muprt@comcast.net

Luzerne County Community College
Respiratory Care Prgm
1333 S Prospect St
Nanticoke, PA 18634
www.luzerne.edu
Prgm Dir: Christopher Tino, BS RRT
Tel: 570 740-0467   *Fax:* 570 740-0526
E-mail: ctino@luzerne.edu

Community College of Philadelphia
Respiratory Care Prgm
1700 Spring Garden St
Philadelphia, PA 19130
www.ccp.edu

Community College of Allegheny County
Respiratory Care Prgm
808 Ridge Ave
Pittsburgh, PA 15212
www.ccac.edu

Indiana University of Pennsylvania
Cosponsor: West Penn Hospital School of Respiratory
    Care
Respiratory Care Prgm
4800 Friendship Ave
Pittsburgh, PA 15224

Reading Area Community College
Respiratory Care Prgm
Ten S Second St, PO Box 1706
Reading, PA 19603
www.racc.edu
Prgm Dir: Maria Dodson, MSA RRT
Tel: 610 372-4721, Ext 5435   *Fax:* 610 236-3948
E-mail: mdodson@racc.edu
Notes: Currently inactive

Mansfield University
Cosponsor: Robert Packer Hospital
Respiratory Care Prgm
One Guthrie Square
Sayre, PA 18840
www.guthrie.org/content/respiratory-therapy-program
Prgm Dir: Larry Vosburgh, BS RRT
Tel: 570 887-4513   *Fax:* 570 887-6509
E-mail: vosburgh_larry@guthrie.org

Crozer-Keystone Medical Center
Cosponsor: Delaware County Community College
Respiratory Care Prgm
One Medical Center Blvd
Upland, PA 19013
Prgm Dir: Patti L Curran, MEd RRT RPFT
Tel: 610 447-2440   *Fax:* 610 447-6353
E-mail: Patti.Curran@Crozer.org

York College of Pennsylvania
Cosponsor: York Hospital
Respiratory Care Prgm
1001 S George St
York, PA 17405
www.wellspan.org
Prgm Dir: Mark Simmons, MSEd RPFT RRT-NPS
Tel: 717 851-2464   *Fax:* 717 851-2934
E-mail: msimmons@wellspan.org

Rhode Island

Community College of Rhode Island
Respiratory Care Prgm
1762 Louisquisset Pike
Lincoln, RI 02865-4585
www.ccri.edu/alliedhealth

South Carolina

Trident Technical College
Respiratory Care Prgm
PO Box 118067
7000 Rivers Ave
Charleston, SC 29423
www.tridenttech.edu

Midlands Technical College
Respiratory Care Prgm
PO Box 2408
Columbia, SC 29202
www.midlandstech.edu

Florence-Darlington Technical College
Respiratory Care Prgm
PO Box 100548
Florence, SC 29501-0548
www.fdtc.edu

Greenville Technical College
Respiratory Care Prgm
PO Box 5616
Greenville, SC 29606
www.gvltec.edu

Piedmont Technical College
Respiratory Care Prgm
PO Box 1467, Emerald Rd
Greenwood, SC 29647
www.ptc.edu

Tri-County Technical College
Respiratory Care Prgm
PO Box 587
Pendleton, SC 29670
www.tctc.edu

Spartanburg Community College
Respiratory Care Prgm
PO Drawer 4386
Spartanburg, SC 29305-4386
www.stcsc.edu

South Dakota

Dakota State University
Respiratory Care Prgm
Science Center
Madison, SD 57042-1799
www.dsu.edu
Prgm Dir: Bruce Feistner, MSS RRT
Tel: 605 322-8613   *Fax:* 605 322-6666
E-mail: bruce.feistner@dsu.edu

Tennessee

Chattanooga State Community College
Respiratory Care Prgm
4501 Amnicola Hwy
Chattanooga, TN 37406

Columbia State Community College
Respiratory Care Prgm
1665 Hampshire Pike
Columbia, TN 38402
www.columbiastate.edu

East Tennessee State University
Respiratory Care Prgm
1000 West E St, ETSU Nave Center
Elizabethton, TN 37643
www.etsu.edu

Volunteer State Community College
Respiratory Care Prgm
1480 Nashville Pike
Gallatin, TN 37066-3188
www.volstate.edu

Roane State Community College
Respiratory Care Prgm
276 Patton Ln
Harriman, TN 37748
www.roanestate.edu

Jackson State Community College
Respiratory Care Prgm
2046 N Parkway St
Jackson, TN 38301-3797
www.jscc.edu

Baptist College of Health Sciences
Respiratory Care Prgm
1003 Monroe Ave
Memphis, TN 38104
www.bchs.edu

Concorde Career College - Memphis
Respiratory Care Prgm
5100 Poplar Ave, Ste 132
Memphis, TN 38137
www.concorde.edu

Walters State Community College
Respiratory Care Prgm
500 S Davy Crockett Pkwy
Morristown, TN 37813
www.ws.edu

Tennessee State University
Respiratory Care Prgm
3500 John A Merritt Blvd
Nashville, TN 37209

Texas

SWT/HMC Respiratory Care School Consortium
Respiratory Care Prgm
1900 Pine St
Abilene, TX 79601

Alvin Community College
Respiratory Care Prgm
3110 Mustang Rd
Alvin, TX 77511
www.alvincollege.edu

Amarillo College
Respiratory Care Prgm
PO Box 447
Amarillo, TX 79178
www.actx.edu/respiratory

Lamar Institute of Technology
Respiratory Care Prgm
PO Box 10061
Beaumont, TX 77710
www.lit.edu

Univ TX at Brownsville/TX Southmost Coll
Respiratory Care Prgm
80 Ft Brown
Brownsville, TX 78520

Del Mar College
Respiratory Care Prgm
101 Baldwin
Corpus Christi, TX 78404

ATI-Career Training
Respiratory Care Prgm
10003 Technology Blvd W
Dallas, TX 75220
www.aticareertraining.com

El Centro College
Respiratory Care Prgm
Main and Lamar Sts
Dallas, TX 75202

Medical Education and Training Campus (METC)
Cosponsor: Thomas Edison State University-AMEDD Consortium
Respiratory Care Prgm
Department of Medical Science
Physician's Extender Branch Bldg 1151, 2651 McIdoe Rd
Fort Sam Houston, TX 78234
www.cs.amedd.army.mil/dms/91v

Tarrant County College
Respiratory Care Prgm
245 E Belknap
Fort Worth, TX 76102
Prgm Dir: John D Hiser, MEd RRT FAARC
Tel: 817 515-2401   *Fax:* 817 515-0640
E-mail: john.hiser@tccd.edu

University of Texas Medical Branch
Respiratory Care Prgm
School of Health Professions
301 University Blvd
Galveston, TX 77555-1146
www.sahs.utmb.edu/programs/rc/
Prgm Dir: Jon Nilsestuen, PhD RRT FAARC
Tel: 409 772-5693   *Fax:* 409 772-3014
E-mail: jnilsest@utmb.edu

Houston Community College
Respiratory Care Prgm
1900 Pressler Dr
Houston, TX 77030

Texas Southern University
Respiratory Care Prgm
3100 Cleburne Ave
Houston, TX 77004
www.tsu.edu

Lone Star College - Kingwood
Respiratory Care Prgm
20,000 Kingwood Dr
Kingwood, TX 77339
www.lonestar.edu

South Plains College
Respiratory Care Prgm
Reese Center
819 Gilbert Dr
Lubbock, TX 79416
www.southplainscollege.edu

Angelina College
Respiratory Care Prgm
PO Box 1768
Lufkin, TX 75902-1768

Collin College
Respiratory Care Prgm
2200 W University Dr
McKinney, TX 75071
www.collincollege.edu/rcp

Midland College
Respiratory Care Prgm
3600 N Garfield
Midland, TX 79705
www.midland.edu

San Jacinto College Central
Respiratory Care Prgm
8060 Spencer Hwy, PO Box 2007
Pasadena, TX 77505-2007
http://sjcd.edu

UT Health Science Center - San Antonio
Respiratory Care Prgm
7703 Floyd Curl Dr MC6248
San Antonio, TX 78229-3900

Texas State University - San Marcos
Respiratory Care Prgm
601 University Dr
Health Professions Bldg Rm 350A
San Marcos, TX 78666-4616
www.health.txstate.edu/RC
Prgm Dir: S Gregory Marshall, PhD RRT RPSGT RST
Tel: 512 245-8243   *Fax:* 512 245-7978
E-mail: sm10@txstate.edu

USAF School of Health Care Sciences
Respiratory Care Prgm
USAF Cardiopulmonary Lab Technologist Program
383 TRS/XUFC- 939 Missile Rd
Sheppard AFB, TX 76311

Temple College
Respiratory Care Prgm
2600 S First St
Temple, TX 76504
www.templejc.edu

Tyler Junior College
Respiratory Care Prgm
PO Box 9020
Tyler, TX 75711

Victoria College
Respiratory Care Prgm
2200 E Red River
Victoria, TX 77901
www.victoriacollege.edu

Weatherford College
Respiratory Care Prgm
225 College Park Drive
Weatherford, TX 76086

Midwestern State University
Respiratory Care Prgm
3410 Taft Blvd
Wichita Falls, TX 76308
http://hs2.mwsu.edu/respiratory/index.asp?LL=802
Prgm Dir: Ann Medford, MA RRT
Tel: 940 397-4653   *Fax:* 940 397-4513
E-mail: ann.medford@mwsu.edu

Utah

Stevens-Henager College
Respiratory Care Prgm
383 W Vine St
5831 S Royalton Dr
Murray, UT 84107
http://stevenshenager.edu

Weber State University
Respiratory Care Prgm
3904 University Circle
Ogden, UT 84408-3904
http://weber.edu/dchp.xml
Prgm Dir: Paul Eberle, PhD RRT
Tel: 801 626-6840   *Fax:* 801 626-7075
E-mail: peberle@weber.edu

Vermont

Vermont Technical College
Respiratory Care Prgm
201 Lawrence Place
Box 1A
Williston, VT 05495
www.vtc.edu

Virginia

Mountain Empire Community College
Respiratory Care Prgm
3441 Mountain Empire Rd
Big Stone Gap, VA 24219
www.me.vccs.edu/programs/aas-degrees/respiratory.pdf

Central Virginia Community College
Respiratory Care Prgm
3506 Wards Rd
Lynchburg, VA 24502
www.cvcc.vccs.edu

Southwest Virginia Community College
Respiratory Care Prgm
Box SVCC
Richlands, VA 24641-1101
www.sw.edu/sarc

J Sargeant Reynolds Community College
Respiratory Care Prgm
PO Box 85622
Richmond, VA 23285-5622
www.reynolds.edu

Jefferson College of Health Sciences
Respiratory Care Prgm
101 Elm St, SE
Roanoke, VA 24013-2222
www.jchs.edu
Prgm Dir: Chase Poulsen, MA RRT-NPS
Tel: 540 985-8490   *Fax:* 540 224-4785
E-mail: crpoulsen@jchs.edu

Northern Virginia Community College
Respiratory Care Prgm
6699 Springfield Center Dr
Springfield, VA 22150
www.nvcc.edu/medical/health/respiratory/

Tidewater Community College
Respiratory Care Prgm
1700 College Crescent
Virginia Beach, VA 23456
www.tcc.edu

Shenandoah University
Respiratory Care Prgm
1775 N Sector Ct
Winchester, VA 22601-5195
www.su.edu

Washington

Highline Community College
Respiratory Care Prgm
2400 S 240th St
Des Moines, WA 98198-9800
www.highline.edu/home/home.htm

Seattle Central Community College
Respiratory Care Prgm
1701 Broadway, 2BE3210
Seattle, WA 98122
www.sccd.ctc.edu

Spokane Community College
Respiratory Care Prgm
N 1810 Greene St MS 2090
Spokane, WA 99217
www.scc.spokane.edu/?resp

Tacoma Community College
Respiratory Care Prgm
6501 S 19th St
Tacoma, WA 98466
www.tacomacc.edu
Prgm Dir: Greg Carter, BS RRT
Tel: 253 566-5231   *Fax:* 253 566-5273
E-mail: gcarter@tacomacc.edu

West Virginia

Carver Career Center
Respiratory Care Prgm
4799 Midland Dr
Charleston, WV 25306

West Virginia Northern Community College
Respiratory Care Prgm
1704 Market St
Wheeling, WV 26003
www.wvncc.edu

Wheeling Jesuit University
Respiratory Care Prgm
316 Washington Ave
Wheeling, WV 26003
www.wju.edu

Wisconsin

Chippewa Valley Technical College
Respiratory Care Prgm
620 W Clairemont Ave
Eau Claire, WI 54701

Northeast Wisconsin Technical College
Respiratory Care Prgm
2740 W Mason St, PO Box 19042
Green Bay, WI 54307
www.nwtc.edu

Western Technical College
Respiratory Care Prgm
400 7th St N
La Crosse, WI 54602-0908
www.westerntc.edu

Madison Area Technical College
Respiratory Care Prgm
3550 Anderson St
Madison, WI 53704
www.matcmadison.edu

Mid-State Technical College
Respiratory Care Prgm
2600 W 5th St
Marshfield, WI 54449
www.mstc.edu
Prgm Dir: Barbara Hughes, MS RRT
Tel: 715 389-7053   *Fax:* 715 389-2864
E-mail: barbara.hughes@mstc.edu

Milwaukee Area Technical College
Respiratory Care Prgm
700 W State St
Milwaukee, WI 53233

Respiratory Therapist

Programs*	Class Capacity	Begins	Length (months)	Award	Res. Tuition	Non-res. Tuition		Offers:† 1	2	3	4
Arizona											
Pima Community College (Tucson)	32	Aug	22	Dipl, AAS	$11,500	$16,000				•	
California											
Butte College (Oroville)	40	Aug	22	Dipl, Cert, AS						•	
Grossmont College (El Cajon)	45	Aug	18	Dipl, AS	$700	$5,000	per year			•	
Orange Coast College (Costa Mesa)	30	Aug	22	AS							
Skyline College (San Bruno)	25	Aug	24	Cert, AS	$1,400	$8,000				•	
Connecticut											
Univ of Hartford (West Hartford)	15	Sep	48	Cert, BS	$29,440	$29,440				•	
Georgia											
Augusta Technical College	18	Aug	28	AAS	$3,093	$6,186				•	•
Darton College (Albany)	20	Aug	21	AS					•	•	
Southwest Georgia Technical College (Thomasville)	24	Fall	24	AAS	$3,000	$6,000					•
Idaho											
Boise State Univ	26	Aug	45	BS	$5,200	$14,800	per year			•	
Kansas											
Newman Univ (Wichita)	20	Aug	28	ASHS	$19,872	$19,872	per year			•	
Univ of Kansas Medical Center (Kansas City)	18	Aug	22	BS	$8,600	$23,000					•
Washburn Univ (Topeka)	18	Aug	22	AS	$216	$489					•

*Data are shown only for programs that completed the 2011 AMA Survey of Health Professions Education Programs.

†Key to Offers: 1: Evening or weekend classes; 2: Non-English instruction; 3: Cultural competence instruction; 4: Distance education component.

Respiratory Therapist

Programs*	Class Capacity	Begins	Length (months)	Award	Res. Tuition	Non-res. Tuition		Offers:† 1	2	3	4
Kentucky											
Big Sandy Community & Technical College (Paintsville)	25	Aug	24	Cert, AAS	$3,900	$13,950		•		•	
Northern Kentucky Univ (Highland Heights)	20	Aug	21	AAS	$7,800	$15,000	per year			•	
Louisiana											
Bossier Parish Community College (Bossier City)	30	May	15	Dipl, AAS	$2,652	$5,460				•	
Louisiana State Univ Health Sciences Center (New Orleans)	15	May	24	BS	$6,741	$11,344				•	
Maryland											
Washington Adventist Univ (Takoma Park)	20	Aug	22	AAS	$18,200	$18,200	per year			•	
Michigan											
Delta College (Univ Center)	17	Aug Sep	21	Dipl, Cert, AAS	$2,640	$5,470				•	
Minnesota											
Northland Community & Technical College (East Grand Forks)	24	Aug	27	AAS	$5,889	$5,889				•	
Mississippi											
Itawamba Community College (Fulton)	16	Aug	18	AAS	$1,700	$3,400	per year			•	
Missouri											
Univ of Missouri (Columbia)	24	Aug	24	BHS	$10,372	$16,913				•	•
Nebraska											
Alegent Health (Omaha)	15	Aug	11	BS	$21,000	$21,000				•	•
New Jersey											
Brookdale Community College (Lincroft)	30	Sep	18	AAS	$3,800	$7,200				•	
North Carolina											
Catawba Valley Community College (Hickory)	15	Aug	21	AAS	$2,300					•	
Central Piedmont Community College (Charlotte)	25	Aug	21	AAS	$2,600	$8,300	per year				
North Dakota											
NDSU/Sanford Health Consortium (Fargo)	12	Aug	15	Cert, BS	$5,600	$7,000				•	•
Ohio											
Bowling Green State Univ (Huron)	30	Aug	28	AAS	$5,800	$15,000				•	•
Cincinnati State Tech & Comm College	25	Aug	20	AAS	$5,000	$10,000				•	
North Central State College (Mansfield)	24	Sep	21	AAS	$4,908	$9,817	per year				
Rhodes State College (Lima)	39	Jun	24	AAS		$5,800		•		•	•
Sinclair Community College (Dayton)	50	Sep	21	AAS	$2,100		per year				
Oklahoma											
Rose State College Rose State College (Midwest City)	24	Aug	12	AAS	$5,288	$11,768				•	•
Oregon											
Lane Community College (Eugene)	30	Sep	21	AAS	$3,276	$8,307	per year	•		•	•
Pennsylvania											
Crozer-Keystone Medical Center (Upland)	16	Sep	22	Cert, AAS	$11,630	$19,510	per year	•		•	•
Harrisburg Area Community College	25	May Aug	28, 24	AS	$4,505	$7,650					
Luzerne County Community College (Nanticoke)	28	Jun	24	AAS	$3,200	$6,400	per year				
Mansfield Univ (Sayre)	14	Aug	24	AAS	$6,240	$15,600	per year				
Millersville Univ of Pennsylvania	15	May		Cert, BS Biology, BSAH	$5,804	$7,255				•	•
Reading Area Community College	24	Aug	24	AAS	$3,000	$6,000			•		•
West Chester Univ (Bryn Mawr)	25	Aug	48	BS	$5,804	$14,510			•		
York College of Pennsylvania	14	Sep	36, 48	AS, BS	$7,000	$7,000	per year				
South Dakota											
Dakota State Univ (Madison)	36	Sep Jun	21, 44	AS, BS	$4,560	$6,675	per year			•	•
Texas											
Midwestern State Univ (Wichita Falls)	24	Jul	45	BS	$7,630	$8,710					•
Tarrant County College (Fort Worth)	26	Aug	21	AAS	$1,872	$2,736					
Texas State Univ - San Marcos	40	Sep	48	BSRC, Post-bacc Cert	$11,000	$22,000				•	•
Univ of Texas Medical Branch (Galveston)	25	Aug	24	BSRC	$10,372	$22,283	per year			•	•
Utah											
Weber State Univ (Ogden)	72	May Aug Jan	21, 33	AAS, BS	$4,548	$12,260				•	
Virginia											
Jefferson College of Health Sciences (Roanoke)	38	Aug	22	AAS RT, BSRT	$19,750	$19,750				•	
Washington											
Tacoma Community College	24	Sep	24	AAS	$12,000					•	
Wisconsin											
Mid-State Technical College (Marshfield)	24	Aug	22	AS	$4,500	per year				•	•

*Data are shown only for programs that completed the 2011 AMA Survey of Health Professions Education Programs.

†Key to Offers: 1: Evening or weekend classes; 2: Non-English instruction; 3: Cultural competence instruction; 4: Distance education component.

Surgical Assistant

Surgical assistants provide aid in exposure, hemostasis, closure, and other intraoperative technical functions that help the surgeon carry out a safe operation with optimal results for the patient. The surgical assistant performs these functions under the direction and supervision of that surgeon and in accordance with hospital policy and appropriate laws and regulations.

Career Description

The surgeon determines the exact position for the best exposure for the surgical procedure, and the surgical assistant carries out this order. The surgical assistant will ensure that points of pressure are padded, including elbows, heels, knees, eyes, face, and the axillary region. Surgical assistants also verify that circulation is not impaired, and nerves are protected from damage. Surgical assistants and anesthesia personnel discuss the patient's temperature and identify the particular methods that will be implemented to maintain the desired temperature. Surgical assistants are knowledgeable about common patient positions as they relate to the surgical procedure and are able to utilize the necessary equipment (fracture tables, head stabilizers, body stabilizers, C-arm extensions, and other equipment as needed) to provide that position. When the procedure has been completed, surgical assistants evaluate the patient for any possible damage resulting from that position, including assessment of the skin. The surgical assistant reports any abnormal condition to the surgeon and may assist with any treatment and documentation.

The surgical assistant provides visualization of the operative site by appropriately placing and securing retractors, with or without padding; packing with sponges; digitally manipulating tissue; suctioning, irrigating, or sponging; manipulating suture materials (loops, tags, running sutures); and employing the proper use of body mechanics to prevent obstruction of the surgeon's view.

Surgical assistants utilize appropriate permanent or temporary techniques to help achieve hemostasis by
- Clamping and/or cauterizing vessels or tissue
- Tying and/or ligating clamped vessels or tissue
- Applying hemostatic clips
- Applying local hemostatic agents
- Applying tourniquets
- Applying vessel loops, noncrushing clamps, and direct digital pressure

Surgical assistants participate in volume replacement or autotransfusion techniques when appropriate. Surgical assistants employ appropriate techniques to assist with the closure of body planes, including utilizing running or interrupted subcutaneous sutures; utilizing subcuticular closure technique; closing skin as directed by the surgeon; and administering subcutaneously postoperative injections of local anesthetics when directed by the surgeon. Surgical assistants select and apply appropriate wound dressings, including liquid or spray occlusive materials; absorbent material; and immobilizing dressing. Surgical assistants secure drainage systems to tissue.

Employment Characteristics

Many surgical assistants work in hospitals and physician clinics; a substantial number are self-employed.

Salary

According to the 2011 Association of Surgical Assistants salary survey, salaries for surgical assistants range from $40,000 to $67,000. Self-employed surgical assistants may earn substantially more income.

For more information, refer to *www.ama-assn.org/go/hpsalary*.

Employment Outlook

There are approximately 5,000 surgical assistants currently working. The forecast for this career is for positive growth due to the increasing demand for surgery.

Educational Programs

Length. Programs are 12 to 24 months.

Prerequisites. Programs establish prerequisites for entry into a surgical assisting program. However, as stated in the *Standards and Guidelines for the Accreditation of Educational Programs in Surgical Assisting* of the Commission on Accreditation of Allied Health Education Programs (CAAHEP), programs that do not require previous operating room experience or credentials that are specific to operating room practice must include in the program introductory operating room curriculum.

Curriculum. Accreditation standards require didactic and lab instruction and supervised clinical practice. Subject areas include:
- Advanced microbiology
- Advanced pathology
- Surgical pharmacology
- Anesthesia methods and agents
- Bioscience: wound management, wound closure, fluid replacement therapy
- Professional ethics, legal responsibilities, communication, and interpersonal skills
- Role of the surgical assistant in positioning, draping, and monitoring the patient
- Role of the surgical assistant in managing surgical complications and emergencies
- Use and application of equipment and supplies in care of the surgical patient
- Clinical rotation completing 135 documented surgical procedures performing in the role of the surgical assistant to the surgeon

Credentialing

The National Board for Surgical Technology and Surgical Assisting (NBSTSA) offers the Certified Surgical First Assistant (CSFA) credential, and the National Surgical Assistant Association (NSAA) offers a Certified Surgical Assistant (CSA) credential. To be eligible for NBSTSA testing, individuals must be graduates of a CAAHEP-accredited surgical assistant program or a CST with current certification who meets a number of other eligibility requirements. Criteria for eligibility to sit for the certification examination given by the NSAA includes graduates from CAAHEP-accredited programs; military trained personnel; foreign trained and US trained medical doctors with surgical training equal to 2,250 hours of surgical assisting; allied health personnel—RN, PA, CSFA, SA-C—who have been trained in surgical assisting and have 2,250 hours of surgical assisting experience in the past 3 years.

Clinical Preceptorship Training

Prerequisite. Certified Surgical Technologist credential.

Description. Completion of 350 documented surgical procedures performing the role of the surgical assistant under the supervision of the surgeon(s) who serve as preceptor(s) and documentation of experience as a surgical assistant for 2 years during the last 4 years. (This describes the NBSTSA alternate pathway to CSFA eligibility but is not a current requirement for accredited surgical assisting programs.)

Inquiries

Careers/Curriculum
Association of Surgical Assistants
6 West Dry Creek Circle, Suite 200
Littleton, CO 80120
800 637-7433 or 303 694-9130
www.surgicalassistant.org

National Surgical Assistant Association
2615 Amesbury Road
Winston Salem, NC 27103
888 633-0479 or 336 768-4443
www.nsaa.net

Certification/Registration

Inquiries regarding certification as a Certified Surgical First Assistant CSFA) may be addressed to:
National Board of Surgical Technology and Surgical Assisting
6 West Dry Creek Circle, Suite 100
Littleton, CO 80120
800 707-0057
www.nbstsa.org

Program Accreditation

Commission on Accreditation of Allied Health Education Programs (CAAHEP) in collaboration with:
Accreditation Review Council on Education in Surgical Technology and Surgical Assisting
6 West Dry Creek Circle, Suite 110
Littleton, CO 80120
303 694-9262
www.arcst.org

Surgical Assistant

Idaho

College of Southern Idaho
Surgical Assistant Prgm
315 Falls Ave HSHS Building 135
Twin Falls, ID 83301

Kentucky

Madisonville Community College
Surgical Assistant Prgm
Health Campus
750 N Laffoon St
Madisonville, KY 42431
www.madisonville.kctcs.edu

Michigan

Wayne County Community College District
Surgical Assistant Prgm
9555 Haggerty Rd
Belleville, MI 48111
www.wcccd.edu

Ohio

Univ of Cincinnati - Clermont College
Surgical Assistant Prgm
1981 James Sauls Sr Drive
Batavia, OH 45103

Tennessee

Meridian Institute of Surgical Assisting
Surgical Assistant Prgm
PO Box 758
1264 Jackson Felts Rd
Joelton, TN 37080
www.meridian-institute.com

Virginia

Eastern Virginia Medical School
Surgical Assistant Prgm
651 Colley Ave
ERB, Room 320
Norfolk, VA 23507-1607
www.evms.edu
Prgm Dir: R Clinton Crews, MPH
Tel: 757 446-6165   *Fax:* 757 446-6179
E-mail: crewsrc@evms.edu

Surgical Assistant

Programs*	Class Capacity	Begins	Length (months)	Award	Res. Tuition	Non-res. Tuition	Offers:† 1	2	3	4
Virginia										
Eastern Virginia Medical School (Norfolk)	24	Aug	22	Cert	$13,646	$14,495			•	

*Data are shown only for programs that completed the 2011 AMA Survey of Health Professions Education Programs.

†Key to Offers: 1: Evening or weekend classes; 2: Non-English instruction; 3: Cultural competence instruction; 4: Distance education component.

Surgical Technologist

Surgical technologists are allied health professionals working with surgeons and other medical practitioners providing surgical care to patients in a variety of settings as integral members of the health care team.

History

The profession of surgical technology was developed during World War II, when there was a critical need for assistance in performing surgical procedures and a shortage of qualified personnel to meet that need. Individuals were specifically educated to assist in surgical procedures and to function in the operative theater.

The Association of Surgical Technologists (AST) was organized in July 1969, with an advisory board of representatives from the American College of Surgeons (ACS), the Association of Operating Room Nurses (AORN), the American Hospital Association (AHA), and the American Medical Association (AMA).

In December 1972, the AMA's Council on Medical Education adopted the recommended educational standards for this field, and the Accreditation Review Committee on Education in Surgical Technology (ARC-ST) was formed. On August 1, 2009, the ARC-ST formally changed its name to the Accreditation Review Council on Education in Surgical Technology and Surgical Assisting (ARC/STSA), to more accurately reflect the full scope of accreditation services provided in both surgical technology and surgical assisting. The ARC/STSA is jointly sponsored by the AST and ACS. Updated standards were approved in 2010.

Career Description

Surgical technologists work under the supervision of the surgeon to ensure that the operating room or environment is safe, equipment functions properly, and operative procedure is conducted under conditions that maximize patient safety.

Surgical technologists possess expertise in the theory and application of sterile and aseptic technique combined with the knowledge of human anatomy, surgical procedures, and implementation tools and technologies to facilitate a physician's performance of invasive therapeutic and diagnostic procedures.

In the first scrub role, the surgical technologist handles the instruments, supplies, and necessary equipment during the surgical procedure. The surgical technologist understands the procedure being performed and anticipates the needs of the surgeon. The surgical technologist has the necessary knowledge and ability to ensure quality patient care during the operative procedure, and is always vigilant in the maintenance of a sterile field.

The surgical technologist checks supplies and equipment needed for the surgical procedure. The surgical technologist scrubs, gowns, and gloves himself/herself and sets up the sterile table with the necessary instruments, supplies, equipment, and medications/solutions. After other members of the surgical team have scrubbed, the surgical technologist will gown and glove them. The surgical technologist performs appropriate counts with the circulator prior to the operation and before the incision is closed. The scrub surgical technologist helps in draping the sterile field and passes instruments to the surgeon and maintains the highest standard of sterile technique during the procedure. The surgical technologist prepares sterile dressings; cleans and prepares instru-

ments for terminal sterilization; assists other members of the team with terminal cleaning of the room; and assists in prepping the room for the next patient.

In the assistant circulating role, the surgical technologist assists in obtaining additional instruments, supplies, and equipment necessary while the surgical procedure is in progress. The assistant circulating surgical technologist monitors conditions in the operating room and constantly reassesses the needs of the patient and surgical team. The assistant circulating surgical technologist obtains necessary sterile and nonsterile items; opens sterile supplies; checks the patient's chart; identifies the patient; verifies the type of surgical procedure with consent forms; and brings the patient to the assigned operating room. The assistant circulating surgical technologist also assists in transferring the patient to the operating room table; assesses comfort and safety measures; assists anesthesia personnel; assists in positioning the patient using the appropriate equipment; applies electrosurgical grounding pads, tourniquets, monitors, etc, before the procedure begins; and prepares the patient's skin prior to draping by the surgical team. The assistant circulating surgical technologist performs appropriate counts with the scrub surgical technologist prior to the operation and before the incision is closed. The assistant circulating surgical technologist also anticipates any additional supplies needed during the procedure; keeps accurate records throughout the procedure; properly cares for specimens; secures dressings after closure of the incision; helps transport the patient to the recovery room; and assists in cleaning the room and preparing it for the next patient.

In the second assisting role, the surgical technologist assists the surgeon and/or surgical assistant during the operative procedure by carrying out technical tasks other than cutting, clamping, and suturing of tissue. The second assisting surgical technologist may hold retractors or instruments as directed by the surgeon; sponge or suction the operative site; apply electrocautery to clamps on bleeders; cut suture material as directed by the surgeon; connect the drain to the suction apparatus; and apply dressings to the closed wound.

Employment Characteristics

The majority of surgical technologists work in hospitals, principally in the surgical suite, but also in emergency rooms and other settings that call for knowledge of and ability in maintaining asepsis, such as material management and central service. A number of surgical technologists work in a wide variety of settings and arrangements, including outpatient surgicenters, and private employment by physicians, or as self-employed technologists.

Workers in hospitals and other institutional settings are usually expected to work rotating shifts or to accommodate on-call assignments to ensure adequate staffing for emergency surgical procedures during evening, night, weekend, and holiday hours. Otherwise, surgical technologists follow a standard hospital workday.

Salary

Salaries vary depending on the experience and education of the individual, the economy of a given region, the responsibilities of the position, and the working hours. May 2011 data from the US Bureau of Labor Statistics (BLS) show that wages at the 10th percentile were $28,860, $40,950 at the 50th percentile (median), and $59,150 at the 90th percentile (*www.bls.gov/oes/current/oes292055.htm*).

For more information, refer to *www.ama-assn.org/go/hpsalary*.

Employment Outlook

According to BLS projections, employment of surgical technologists is expected to grow 19% between 2010 and 2020, faster than the average for all occupations, as the volume of surgeries increases. The number of surgical procedures is expected to continue to rise as the population grows and ages. Older people, including the baby-boom generation, which generally requires more surgical procedures, will continue to account for a larger portion of the US population. In addition, technological advances, such as fiber optics, robotics and laser technology, have allowed an increasing number of new surgical procedures to be performed and have allowed surgical technologists to assist with a greater number of procedures.

Educational Programs

Length. Programs range from 12 to 24 months.

Prerequisites. High school diploma or equivalent.

Curriculum. Accreditation standards require didactic and lab instruction and supervised clinical practice. Subject areas include:

- Medical terminology, professional ethics, and legal aspects of surgical patient care
- Anatomy and physiology, microbiology, anesthesia, and pharmacology
- Sterilization methods and aseptic technique
- Instruments, supplies, and equipment used in surgery
- Surgical patient care and safety precautions
- Operative procedures and biomedical sciences
- Supervised clinical practice in the operating room must include commonly performed procedures in general surgery, obstetrics and gynecology, ophthalmology, otorhinolaryngology, plastic surgery, urology, orthopedics, neurosurgery, thoracic surgery, and cardiovascular and peripheral vascular surgery.

Inquiries

Careers/Curriculum

Association of Surgical Technologists
6 West Dry Creek Circle, Suite 200
Littleton, CO 80120
800 637-7433 or 303 694-9130
www.ast.org

Certification/Registration

Inquiries regarding certification as a Certified Surgical Technologist (CST) or Certified Surgical First Assistant (CSFA) may be addressed to:

National Board for Surgical Technology and Surgical Assisting
6 West Dry Creek Circle, Suite 100
Littleton, CO 80120
800 707-0057
www.nbstsa.org

Program Accreditation

Commission on Accreditation of Allied Health Education Programs (CAAHEP) in collaboration with:
Accreditation Review Council on Education in Surgical Technology and Surgical Assisting
6 West Dry Creek Circle, Suite 110
Littleton, CO 80120
303 694-9262
www.arcst.org

Note: Adapted in part from the Bureau of Labor Statistics, US Department of Labor, *Occupational Outlook Handbook,* Surgical Technologists, at *www.bls.gov/oco/ocos106.htm*.

Surgical Technologist

Alabama

James H Faulkner State Community College
Surgical Technology Prgm
1900 Hwy 31 S
Bay Minette, AL 36507
www.faulknerstate.edu

Virginia College - Birmingham
Surgical Technology Prgm
PO Box 19249
488 Palisades Blvd
Birmingham, AL 35209
www.vc.edu

Calhoun Community College
Surgical Technology Prgm
PO Box 2216
6250 Highwa 31 North
Decatur, AL 35609-2216
www.calhoun.cc.al.us

Flowers Hospital
Surgical Technology Prgm
Home Health Bldg
4370 W Main St, Suite 1
PO Box 6907
Dothan, AL 36305
www.flowershospital.com

Virginia College - Mobile
Surgical Technology Prgm
2970 Cottage Hill Rd
Mobile, AL 36606
www.vc.edu

Virginia College - Montgomery
Surgical Technology Prgm
6200 Atlanta Hwy
Montgomery, AL 36117

Southern Union State Community College
Surgical Technology Prgm
1701 Lafayette Pkwy
Opelika, AL 36801
www.suscc.edu

Lurleen B Wallace Community College
Surgical Technology Prgm
MacArthur Campus 1708 N Main St
Opp, AL 36467

Bevill State Community College
Surgical Technology Prgm
PO Box 800
Sumiton, AL 35148
www.bscc.edu/mainsumiton.asp

Arizona

Mohave Community College
Surgical Technology Prgm
1977 W Acoma Blvd
Lake Havasu City, AZ 86403
www.mohave.cc.az.us

East Valley Institute of Technology
Surgical Technology Prgm
1601 West Main St
Mesa, AZ 85201

GateWay Community College
Surgical Technology Prgm
108 N 40th St
Phoenix, AZ 85015
www.gatewaycc.edu

Pima Community College
Surgical Technology Prgm
5901 S Calle Santa Cruz
Center for Training and Development
Tucson, AZ 85709-6350
www.pima.edu

Arkansas

South Arkansas Community College
Surgical Technology Prgm
300 South West Ave
El Dorado, AR 71731-7010

University of Arkansas - Fort Smith
Surgical Technology Prgm
PO Box 3649
5210 Grand Ave
Fort Smith, AR 72913
www.uafs.edu
Prgm Dir: Sydney Fulbright, PhD MSN RN CNOR
Tel: 479 788-7855   *Fax:* 479 788-7153
E-mail: sydney.fulbright@uafs.edu

North Arkansas College
Surgical Technology Prgm
1515 Pioneer Dr
Harrison, AR 72601
www.northark.edu

Baptist Health Schools Little Rock
Cosponsor: Baptist Health Medical Center
Surgical Technology Prgm
11900 Colonel Glenn Rd, Ste 1000
Little Rock, AR 72210-2820
www.bhslr.edu

University of Arkansas for Medical Sciences
Surgical Technology Prgm
4301 W Markham Slot 737
Little Rock, AR 72205
www.uams.edu/chrp
Prgm Dir: Gennie Castleberry, MEd CST
Tel: 501 526-4490   *Fax:* 501 526-4491
E-mail: castleberrygennier@uams.edu

Southeast Arkansas College
Surgical Technology Prgm
1900 Hazel St
Pine Bluff, AR 71603
www.seark.edu

Northwest Technical Institute
Surgical Technology Prgm
PO Box 2000
709 S Old Missouri Rd
Springdale, AR 72765
www.nti.tec.ar.us

California

American Career College - Anaheim
Surgical Technology Prgm
1200 N Magnolia Ave
Anaheim, CA 92801

San Joaquin Valley College - Bakersfield
Surgical Technology Prgm
201 New Stine Rd
Bakersfield, CA 93309
www.sjvc.edu

Southwestern College
Surgical Technology Prgm
900 Otay Lakes Rd
Chula Vista, CA 91910
www.swc.cc.ca.us

Carrington College California - Citrus Heights
Surgical Technology Prgm
7301 Greenback Lane, Ste A
Citrus Heights, CA 95621
www.westerncollege.com

Mt Diablo Adult Education
Surgical Technology Prgm
1266 San Carlos Ave
Concord, CA 94518
www.mdusd.k12.ca.us/adulted

Fresno City College
Surgical Technology Prgm
1101 E University Ave
Fresno, CA 93741
www.fresnocitycollege.edu

San Joaquin Valley College - Fresno
Surgical Technology Prgm
295 East Sierra Ave
Fresno, CA 93710
www.sjcv.edu
Prgm Dir: Teri Junge, MEd CSFA CST FAST
Tel: 559 448-8282, Ext 302   *Fax:* 559 448-8250
E-mail: terij@sjvc.edu

Glendale Career College
Surgical Technology Prgm
1015 Grandview Ave
Glendale, CA 91201
www.success.edu
Prgm Dir: Matti Maya, CST
Tel: 818 956-4915   *Fax:* 818 243-6028
E-mail: mmaya@success.edu

Premiere Career College
Surgical Technology Prgm
12901 Ramona Blvd Suite D
Irwindale, CA 91706
www.premierecollege.edu
Prgm Dir: Antonio Torres, BS MEd CST CRCST
Tel: 626 814-2080   *Fax:* 626 814-3242
E-mail: drtorres@prodigy.net

American Career College - Los Angeles
Surgical Technology Prgm
4021 Rosewood Ave
Los Angeles, CA 90004

Concorde Career College - North Hollywood
Surgical Technology Prgm
12412 Victory Blvd
North Hollywood, CA 91606
www.concorde.edu/hollywood
Prgm Dir: Julian Hortz
Tel: 818 766-8151, Ext 251   *Fax:* 818 766-1587
E-mail: jhortz@concorde.edu

MiraCosta College
Surgical Technology Prgm
One Barnard Drive
Oceanside, CA 92056

Career Networks Institute
Surgical Technology Prgm
986 Town and Country Rd
Orange, CA 92868
www.cnicollege.edu

Everest College - Reseda
Surgical Technology Prgm
18040 Sherman Way Suite 400
Reseda, CA 91335
www.everest.edu

Career Colleges of America - San Bernardino
Surgical Technology Prgm
184 W Club Center Dr
Suite K
San Bernardino, CA 92408
www.careercolleges.edu

Concorde Career College - San Bernardino
Surgical Technology Prgm
201 E Airport Dr, Ste A
San Bernardino, CA 92408
www.concorde.edu

Skyline College
Surgical Technology Prgm
3300 College Dr
San Bruno, CA 94066
www.skylinecollege.edu
Prgm Dir: Alice Erskine, CST MSN CNOR
Tel: 650 738-4470   *Fax:* 650 738-4299
E-mail: erskine@smccd.edu

Concorde Career College - San Diego
Surgical Technology Prgm
4393 Imperial Ave
Suite 100
San Diego, CA 92113
www.concorde.edu

Carrington College California - San Jose
Surgical Technology Prgm
6201 San Ignacio Ave
San Jose, CA 95119
www.westerncollege.edu

Newbridge College
Surgical Technology Prgm
1840 E 17th St, Ste 140
Santa Ana, CA 92705
www.newbridgecollege.edu

Simi Valley Adult School
Surgical Technology Prgm
20044 Tanager Ct Canyon Country
Simi Valley, CA 93065
www.simi.tec.ca.us

Career Colleges of America - South Gate
Surgical Technology Prgm
5612 E Imperial Hwy
South Gate, CA 90280
www.careercolleges.edu

North-West College
Surgical Technology Prgm
2101 West Garvey Ave, North
West Covina, CA 91790

Colorado

Concorde Career College - Aurora
Surgical Technology Prgm
111 N Havana St
Aurora, CO 80016
www.concorde.edu

Aims Community College
Surgical Technology Prgm
5401 W 20th St PO Box 69
Greeley, CO 80632

Colorado Technical University
Surgical Technology Prgm
1025 West 6th St
Pueblo, CO 81003

Everest College
Surgical Technology Prgm
9065 Grant St
Thornton, CO 80229
www.everest.edu/campus/thornton

Colorado Technical Univ - Denver North
Surgical Technology Prgm
1865 W 121st Ave
Westminster, CO 80234

Connecticut

Bridgeport Hospital
Surgical Technology Prgm
200 Mill Hill Ave
Bridgeport, CT 06610
www.bridgeporthospital.org/bhsn

Danbury Hospital
Surgical Technology Prgm
24 Hospital Ave
Danbury, CT 06810
www.danhosp.org

Eli Whitney Technical High School
Surgical Technology Prgm
71 Jones Rd
Hamden, CT 06401
www.cttech.org/whitney

A I Prince Technical High School
Surgical Technology Prgm
401 Flatbush Ave
Hartford, CT 06106
www.cttech.org/prince
Prgm Dir: Elia Acosta, CST BA MS
Tel: 860 951-7112, Ext 5174   *Fax:* 860 951-1529
E-mail: Elia.Acosta@ct.gov

Manchester Community College
Surgical Technology Prgm
PO Box 46 Great Path
Manchester, CT 06045- 104
www.mcc.commnet.edu

Florida

Manatee Technical Institute
Surgical Technology Prgm
5520 Lakewood Ranch Blvd
Bradenton, FL 34211

High Tech North-Lee County
Surgical Technology Prgm
360 Santa Barbara Blvd North
Cape Coral, FL 33993

Brevard Community College
Surgical Technology Prgm
1519 Clearlake Rd
Cocoa, FL 32922-6597
www.brevardcc.edu

Daytona State College, Daytona Beach Campus
Surgical Technology Prgm
PO Box 2811
1200 W International Speedway Blvd
Building 320/Room 428
Daytona Beach, FL 32114 ?
www.daytonastate.edu

Indian River State College
Surgical Technology Prgm
3209 Virginia Ave
Fort Pierce, FL 34981
www.irsc.edu

Santa Fe College
Surgical Technology Prgm
Health Sciences Building 3000 North West 83rd St W-201
Gainesville, FL 32606-6200

Keiser Career College - Greenacres
Surgical Technology Prgm
6812 Forest Hill Blvd, Ste D-1
Greenacres, FL 33413
www.keisercareer.edu

Everest Institute-Hialeah Campus
Surgical Technology Prgm
530 West 49th St
Hialeah, FL 33012

Sheridan Technical Center
Surgical Technology Prgm
5400 Sheridan St
Hollywood, FL 33021
www.sheridantechnical.com

Concorde Career Institute - Jacksonville
Surgical Technology Prgm
7960 Arlington Expressway
Suite 120
Jacksonville, FL 32211
www.concorde.edu

Florida State College at Jacksonville
Surgical Technology Prgm
4501 Capper Rd
North Campus
Jacksonville, FL 32218
www.fccj.edu

Virginia College-Jacksonville
Surgical Technology Prgm
5940 Beach Blvd
Jacksonville, FL 32207

Palm Beach State College
Surgical Technology Prgm
4200 S Congress Ave, MS60
MS 65 Toni Crowley
Lake Worth, FL 33461
www.pbcc.edu

Traviss Career Center
Surgical Technology Prgm
3225 Winter Lake Rd
Lakeland, FL 33803
www.travisstech.org

MedVance Institute - Lauderdale Lakes
Surgical Technology Prgm
4850 Oakland Park Blvd
Lauderdale Lakes, FL 33313
www.medvance.edu

Suwannee-Hamilton Technical Center
Surgical Technology Prgm
415 SW Pinewood Drive
Live Oak, FL 32064

Everest Institute-Kendall Campus
Surgical Technology Prgm
9020 Southwest 137th Ave
Miami, FL 33186

Lindsey Hopkins Tech Education Center
Surgical Technology Prgm
750 NW 20th St
Miami, FL 33127
www.lindsey.dadeschools.net

Keiser Career College - Miami Lakes
Surgical Technology Prgm
17395 NW 59th Ave
Miami Lakes, FL 33015
www.keisercareer.edu

Concorde Career Institute - Miramar
Surgical Technology Prgm
10933 Marks Way
Miramar, FL 33025

Lorenzo Walker Institute of Technology
Surgical Technology Prgm
3702 Estey Ave
Naples, FL 34104
www.lwit.edu

College of Central Florida
Surgical Technology Prgm
PO Box 1388
3001 SW College Rd
Ocala, FL 34474-4415
www.cfu.edu

Fortis College-Orange Park
Surgical Technology Prgm
560 Wells Rd
Orange Park, FL 32073

Orlando Tech
Surgical Technology Prgm
301 W Amelia St
Orlando, FL 32801
www.ocps.net

Central Florida Institute
Surgical Technology Prgm
30522 US 19th N, Ste 310
Suite 200/300
Palm Harbor, FL 34684
www.cfinstitute.com

MedVance Institute - West Palm Beach
Surgical Technology Prgm
1630 S Congress Ave
Suite 300
Palm Springs, FL 33461
www.medvance.edu

Gulf Coast State College
Surgical Technology Prgm
5230 W US Hwy 98
Panama City, FL 32401
www.gulfcoast.edu

Pensacola State College
Surgical Technology Prgm
5555 Hwy 98 W
Pensacola, FL 32507
www.pjc.edu

Virginia College at Penascola
Surgical Technology Prgm
19 W Garden St
Pensacola, FL 32501
www.vc.edu/site/campus.cfm?campus=pensacola

Keiser University - Port St Lucie
Surgical Technology Prgm
10330 South Federal Highway
Port St Lucie, FL 34952
www.keiseruniversity.edu

Sarasota County Technical Institute
Surgical Technology Prgm
4748 Beneva Rd
Sarasota, FL 34233-1798
www.SarasotaTech.org
Notes: Currently inactive

Keiser Career College - St Petersburg
Surgical Technology Prgm
11208 Danka Blvd
St Petersburg, FL 33716
www.keisercareer.edu

Pinellas Technical Education Centers - St Petersburg Campus
Surgical Technology Prgm
901 34th St South
St Petersburg, FL 33711
www.myptec.org
Prgm Dir: Peggy Gould, CST
Tel: 727 893-2500, Ext 1077   *Fax:* 727 893-2776
E-mail: gouldpe@pcsb.org

Concorde Career Institute - Tampa
Surgical Technology Prgm
4202 W Spruce St
Tampa, FL 33607

Everest Univ - Brandon Campus
Surgical Technology Prgm
3924 Coconut Palm Dr
Tampa, FL 33619
www.everest.edu/campus/brandon

Georgia

Chattahoochee Technical College
Surgical Technology Prgm
5198 Ross Rd
Acworth, GA 30102
www.ChattahoocheeTech.edu

Albany Technical College
Surgical Technology Prgm
1704 S Slappey Blvd
Albany, GA 31701-3514
www.albanytech.edu

Athens Technical College
Surgical Technology Prgm
800 US Hwy 29 N
Athens, GA 30601-1500
www.athenstech.edu

Augusta Technical College
Surgical Technology Prgm
3200 Augusta Tech Dr, 900 Bldg
Bldg 900
Augusta, GA 30906
www.augustatech.edu
Prgm Dir: L Gene Burke, Director of Surgical
    Technology
Tel: 706 771-4191   *Fax:* 706 771-4181
E-mail: lburke@augustatech.edu

Virginia College-Augusta
Surgical Technology Prgm
2807 Wylds Rd Suite B
Augusta, GA 30909

Columbus Technical College
Surgical Technology Prgm
928 Manchester Expressway
Columbus, GA 31904-6572
www.columbustech.edu

Southern Crescent Technical College
Surgical Technology Prgm
501 Varsity Rd
Griffin, GA 30223
www.griffintech.edu

Gwinnett Technical College
Surgical Technology Prgm
5150 Surgarloaf Pkwy
Lawrenceville, GA 30043-5702
www.gwinnetttech.edu

Central Georgia Technical College
Surgical Technology Prgm
3300 Macon Tech Dr
Macon, GA 31206
www.cgtcollege.org

Everest College-Marietta
Surgical Technology Prgm
1600 Terrell Mill Rd Suite G
Marietta, GA 30067

Lanier Technical College
Surgical Technology Prgm
2990 Landrum Education Dr
Oakwood, GA 30566
www.laniertech.edu

Georgia Northwestern Technical College
Surgical Technology Prgm
265 Bicentennial Trail
Rock Spring, GA 30739-2306
www.northwesterntech.edu

Savannah Technical College
Surgical Technology Prgm
5717 White Bluff Rd
Savannah, GA 31405
www.savannahtech.edu

Ogeechee Technical College
Surgical Technology Prgm
1 Joe Kennedy Blvd
Statesboro, GA 30458
www.ogeecheetech.edu

Southwest Georgia Technical College
Surgical Technology Prgm
15689 US Hwy 19 N
Thomasville, GA 31792
www.southwestgatech.edu

Moultrie Technical College
Surgical Technology Prgm
52 Tech Dr
Tifton, GA 31794
www.moultrietech.edu

Wiregrass Georgia Technical College
Surgical Technology Prgm
4089 Val Tech Rd
Valdosta, GA 31602

Southeastern Technical College
Surgical Technology Prgm
3001 E First St
Vidalia, GA 30474
www.southeasterntech.edu
Prgm Dir: Deborah Smith, RN CNOR
Tel: 912 538-3182   *Fax:* 912 538-3106
E-mail: dsmith@southeasterntech.edu

West Georgia Technical College
Surgical Technology Prgm
176 Murphy Campus Blvd
Waco, GA 30182
www.westcentraltech.edu

Middle Georgia Technical College
Surgical Technology Prgm
80 Cohen Walker Dr
Warner Robins, GA 31088
www.middlegatech.edu

Okefenokee Technical College
Surgical Technology Prgm
1701 Carswell Ave
Waycross, GA 31501
www.okefenokeetech.edu
Prgm Dir: Sally M Smith, RN MEd
Tel: 912 287-5839   *Fax:* 912 287-5839
E-mail: smsmith@okefenokeetech.edu

Hawaii

Kapiolani Community College
Surgical Technology Prgm
4303 Diamond Head Rd
Kopiko Building, Room 201
Honolulu, HI 96816
www.kcc.hawaii.edu

Idaho

College of Western Idaho
Surgical Technology Prgm
1910 University Drive
Boise, ID 83725-2005

Eastern Idaho Technical College
Surgical Technology Prgm
1600 S 25th E
Idaho Falls, ID 83404-5788
www.eitc.edu

College of Southern Idaho
Surgical Technology Prgm
315 Falls Ave, Aspen Bldg 158
PO Box 1238
Twin Falls, ID 83301 ????
www.csi.edu

Illinois

Parkland College
Surgical Technology Prgm
2400 W Bradley Ave
Room L147
Champaign, IL 61821-1899
www.parkland.edu

Malcolm X College
Surgical Technology Prgm
1900 W Van Buren St
Chicago, IL 60612
www.malcolmx.ccc.edu

Robert Morris University
Surgical Technology Prgm
401 S State St
Chicago, IL 60605-1229
www.robertmorris.edu/healthstudies/index.html

Prairie State College
Surgical Technology Prgm
202 S Halsted St
Chicago Heights, IL 60411
www.prairiestate.edu

Richland Community College
Surgical Technology Prgm
1 College Park
Decatur, IL 62521-8512
www.richland.edu
Prgm Dir: Katherine Lee, MS CST RST FAST
Tel: 217 875-7200, Ext 763   *Fax:* 217 875-7220
E-mail: klee@richland.edu

Elgin Community College
Surgical Technology Prgm
1700 Spartan Dr
Elgin, IL 60123
www.elgin.edu

College of DuPage
Surgical Technology Prgm
425 Fawell Blvd
Glen Ellyn, IL 60137
www.cod.edu

College of Lake County
Surgical Technology Prgm
19351 W Washington St
Grayslake, IL 60030-1198
www.clcillinois.edu

Southern Illinois Collegiate Common Market
Surgical Technology Prgm
3213 South Park Ave
Herrin, IL 62948
www.siccm.com

Illinois Central College
Surgical Technology Prgm
Peoria Campus Div
201 SW Adams St
Peoria, IL 61635-0001
www.icc.edu

John Wood Community College
Surgical Technology Prgm
1301 S 48th St
Quincy, IL 62305
www.jwcc.edu

Triton College
Surgical Technology Prgm
2000 N Fifth Ave
River Grove, IL 60171
www.triton.edu

Trinity College of Nursing & Health Sciences
Surgical Technology Prgm
2122 25th Ave
Rock Island, IL 61201-1216
www.trinityqc.edu

Rock Valley College
Surgical Technology Prgm
3301 N Mulford Rd
Rockford, IL 61114-5699

Waubonsee Community College
Surgical Technology Prgm
Rte 47 at Waubonsee Dr
Sugar Grove, IL 60554-9448
www.wcc.cc.il.us

Indiana

Ivy Tech Community College - Columbus
Surgical Technology Prgm
4475 Central Ave
Columbus, IN 47203-1868
www.ivytech.edu

Ivy Tech Community College - Evansville
Surgical Technology Prgm
3501 N First Ave
Evansville, IN 47710-3398
www.ivytech.edu

Brown Mackie College - Fort Wayne
Surgical Technology Prgm
3000 East Coliseum Blvd
Fort Wayne, IN 46805

Harrison College - Fort Wayne
Surgical Technology Prgm
6413 North Clinton St
Fort Wayne, IN 46825-4911

University of Saint Francis
Surgical Technology Prgm
2701 Spring St
Fort Wayne, IN 46808
www.sf.edu/sf/surgicaltech
Prgm Dir: Elizabeth Slagle, MS RN CST
Tel: 260 399-7700, Ext 8577   *Fax:* 260 399-8188
E-mail: eslagle@sf.edu

Harrison College - Indianapolis East Campus
Surgical Technology Prgm
8150 Brookvillle Rd
Indianapolis, IN 46239

Indiana University Health
Surgical Technology Prgm
PO Box 1367
White Hall Room 625
Indianapolis, IN 46206-1367
www.clarian.org

Ivy Tech Community College - Central Indiana Region
Surgical Technology Prgm
9301 E 59th St
Indianapolis, IN 46216
www.ivytech.edu

National College
Surgical Technology Prgm
6060 Castleway West Dr
Indianapolis, IN 46250
www.ncbt.edu

Ivy Tech Community College - Kokomo
Surgical Technology Prgm
700 E Firmin St
Kokomo, IN 46902
www.ivytech.edu

Ivy Tech Community College - Lafayette
Surgical Technology Prgm
3101 S Creasy Ln, PO Box 6299
Lafayette, IN 47905
www.ivytech.edu
Prgm Dir: Dorothy S McClannen, MSN RN CST
Tel: 765 269-5208   *Fax:* 765 269-5248
E-mail: dmcclannen@ivytech.edu

Brown Mackie College - Merrillville
Surgical Technology Prgm
1000 E 80th Place Suite 205M
Merrillville, IN 46410

Everest College
Surgical Technology Prgm
707 E 80th Pl, Ste 46410
Suite 200
Merrillville, IN 46410
www.everest.edu

Brown Mackie College - Fort Wayne (Michigan City)
Surgical Technology Prgm
325 E US Hwy 20
Michigan City, IN 46360
www.brownmackie.edu

Ivy Tech Community College - Muncie
Surgical Technology Prgm
4301 S Cowan Rd
Muncie, IN 47302

Ivy Tech Community College - Terre Haute
Surgical Technology Prgm
8000 S Education Drive
Terre Haute, IN 47802

Ivy Tech Community College - Northwest Region
Surgical Technology Prgm
3100 Ivy Tech Drive
Valparaiso, IN 46383
www.ivytech.edu

Vincennes University
Surgical Technology Prgm
1002 N First St, WAB-1
Vincennes, IN 47591
www.vinu.edu
Prgm Dir: Chris Keegan, MS CST FAST
Tel: 812 888-5893   *Fax:* 812 888-4550
E-mail: ckeegan@vinu.edu

Iowa

Kirkwood Community College
Surgical Technology Prgm
6301 Kirkwood Blvd SW
PO BOX 2068
Cedar Rapids, IA 52406
www.kirkwood.edu

Iowa Western Community College
Surgical Technology Prgm
2700 College Rd Box 4 C
Council Bluffs, IA 51502

Des Moines Area Community College
Surgical Technology Prgm
1100 7th St, Bldg 2 Room 102
Des Moines, IA 50314
www.dmacc.edu

Mercy College of Health Sciences
Surgical Technology Prgm
928 Sixth Ave
Des Moines, IA 50309-1239
www.mchs.edu

Western Iowa Tech Community College
Surgical Technology Prgm
4647 Stone Ave
PO Box 5199
Sioux City, IA 51106-5199
www.witcc.edu

Iowa Lakes Community College
Surgical Technology Prgm
1900 N Grand Ave, Ste 8
Clay County Center
Spencer, IA 51301-2294
www.iowalakes.edu

Kansas

Hutchinson Community College
Surgical Technology Prgm
815 N Walnut, Davis Hall
Davis Hall
Hutchinson, KS 67501
www.hutchcc.edu

Seward County Community College
Surgical Technology Prgm
PO Box 1137
1801 N Kansas Ave
Liberal, KS 67901
www.sccc.edu

Washburn University
Cosponsor: Washburn Institute of Technology
Surgical Technology Prgm
5724 Huntoon St
Topeka, KS 66604
www.washburntech.edu

Wichita Area Technical College
Surgical Technology Prgm
4501 E 47th St S
Southside Education Center
Wichita, KS 67210
www.watc.edu

Kentucky

Ashland Technical and Community College
Surgical Technology Prgm
4818 Roberts Dr
1400 College Drive
Ashland, KY 41101
www.ashland.kctcs.edu

Bowling Green Technical College
Surgical Technology Prgm
1845 Loop Dr
Bowling Green, KY 42101-3601
www.bowlinggreen.kctcs.edu/Academics/
    Programs_of_Study/Surgical_Technology.aspx

National College - Florence
Surgical Technology Prgm
7627 Ewing Blvd
Florence, KY 41042
www.national-college.edu

Brown Mackie College - Northern Kentucky
Surgical Technology Prgm
309 Buttermilk Pike
Fort Mitchell, KY 41017

Hazard Community & Technical College
Surgical Technology Prgm
One Community College Drive
Hazard, KY 41701

Bluegrass Community and Technical College
Surgical Technology Prgm
164 Opportunity Way
Building A-138
Lexington, KY 40511
www.bluegrass.kctcs.edu

National College - Lexington
Surgical Technology Prgm
2376 Sir Barton Way
Lexington, KY 40509

Brown Mackie College - Louisville
Surgical Technology Prgm
3605 Fern Valley Rd
Louisville, KY 40220

Jefferson Community and Technical College
Surgical Technology Prgm
800 W Chestnut St
Louisville, KY 40203
www.jefferson.kctcs.edu

National College - Louisville
Surgical Technology Prgm
4205 Dixie Hwy
Louisville, KY 40216
www.ncbt.edu

Spencerian College
Surgical Technology Prgm
4627 Dixie Hwy
Louisville, KY 40216
www.spencerian.edu

Madisonville Community College
Surgical Technology Prgm
750 N Laffoon St
Madisonville, KY 42431
www.madisonville.kctcs.edu

Maysville Comm & Tech College
Surgical Technology Prgm
1755 US 68
Maysville, KY 41056
www.maycc.kctcs.edu
Prgm Dir: Connie L Tucker, CST Assoc Professor
Tel: 606 759-7141, Ext   *Fax:* 606 759-7176
E-mail: connie.tucker@kctcs.edu

Owensboro Community & Technical College
Surgical Technology Prgm
4800 New Hartford Rd
Owensboro, KY 42303

West Kentucky Community & Technical College
Surgical Technology Prgm
4810 Alben Barkley Dr, PO Box 7408
Paducah, KY 42002-7380
www.westkentucky.kctcs.edu

Southeast Kentucky Comm & Tech College
Surgical Technology Prgm
10350 US Highway 25E
Pineville, KY 40977
www.southeast.kctcs.edu

Somerset Community College
Surgical Technology Prgm
808 Monticello St
Somerset, KY 42501
www.somerset.kctcs.edu

St Catharine College
Surgical Technology Prgm
2735 Bardstown Rd
St. Catharine, KY 40061

Louisiana

Fortis College
Surgical Technology Prgm
9255 Interline Ave
Baton Rouge, LA 70809
www.medvance.edu

Our Lady of the Lake College
Surgical Technology Prgm
7434 Perkins Rd
Baton Rouge, LA 70808
www.ololcollege.edu

Bossier Parish Community College
Surgical Technology Prgm
6220 E Texas St
c/o Allied Health Division
Bossier City, LA 71111
www.bpcc.edu

Acadiana Technical College - Lafayette
Surgical Technology Prgm
1101 Bertrand Drive
Lafayette, LA 70506

Career Technical College
Surgical Technology Prgm
2319 Louisville Ave
Monroe, LA 71201
www.careertc.com

Delgado Community College
Surgical Technology Prgm
615 City Park Ave
New Orleans, LA 70119-4399
www.dcc.edu

Southern Univ at Shreveport
Surgical Technology Prgm
610 Texas St, Ste 328
Shreveport, LA 71107
www.susla.edu

Acadiana Technical College - Lafourche Campus
Surgical Technology Prgm
1425 Tiger Dr
Thibodaux, LA 70301
scl.edu
Notes: The campus now offers all courses needed to complete the AAS degree in Surgical Technology. All pre-req courses must be successfully completed before acceptance into the program.

Maine

Eastern Maine Community College
Surgical Technology Prgm
354 Hogan Rd
Bangor, ME 04401
www.emtc.org

Maine Medical Center
Surgical Technology Prgm
School of Surgical Technology
Fort Rd 22 Bramhall St
Portland, ME 04102
www.mmc.org

Maryland

Baltimore City Community College
Surgical Technology Prgm
2901 Liberty Heights Ave
Baltimore, MD 21215-7893
www.bccc.edu

Community College of Baltimore County - Essex Campus
Surgical Technology Prgm
7201 Rossville Blvd
Baltimore, MD 21237-3899
www.ccbcmd.edu

Fortis Institute - Woodlawn
Surgical Technology Prgm
6901 Security Blvd, Ste 21
Baltimore, MD 21244

Frederick Community College
Surgical Technology Prgm
7932 Opossumtown Pike
Frederick, MD 21702
www.frederick.edu

Montgomery College
Surgical Technology Prgm
7600 Takoma Ave
Takoma, MD 20912
www.montgomerycollege.edu

Chesapeake College
Surgical Technology Prgm
PO Box 8
Wye Mills, MD 21679
www.chesapeake.edu

Massachusetts

Bunker Hill Community College
Surgical Technology Prgm
175 Hawthorne St, Room 114
Chelsea Campus
Chelsea, MA 02150-2917
www.bhcc.edu

North Shore Community College
Surgical Technology Prgm
1 Ferncroft Rd
PO Box 3340
Danvers, MA 01923-0840
www.northshore.edu

Massachusetts Bay Community College
Surgical Technology Prgm
19 Flagg Dr
Framingham, MA 01702
www.massbay.edu

Charles H McCann Technical School
Surgical Technology Prgm
70 Hodges Cross Rd
North Adams, MA 01247
www.mccanntech.org

Quincy College
Surgical Technology Prgm
24 Saville Ave
Quincy, MA 02169
www.quincycollege.edu

Springfield Technical Community College
Surgical Technology Prgm
One Armory Sq
PO Box 9000
Springfield, MA 01101
www.stcc.edu

Quinsigamond Community College
Surgical Technology Prgm
670 W Boylston St
Worcester, MA 01606-2092
www.qcc.edu

Michigan

Baker College of Allen Park
Surgical Technology Prgm
4500 Enterprise Dr
Allen Park, MI 48101
www.baker.edu/career-explorer/career/
    surgical-technologist/

Wayne County Community College District - Western Campus
Surgical Technology Prgm
9555 Haggerty Rd
Belleville, MI 48111

Baker College of Cadillac
Surgical Technology Prgm
9600 E 13th St
Cadillac, MI 49601-9169
www.baker.edu

Baker College of Clinton Township
Surgical Technology Prgm
34950 Little Mack Ave
Clinton Township, MI 48035-4701
www.baker.edu

Macomb Community College
Surgical Technology Prgm
44575 Garfield Rd
Clinton Township, MI 48038-1139
www.macomb.edu

Henry Ford Community College
Surgical Technology Prgm
5101 Evergreen Rd
Dearborn, MI 48128
www.hfcc.edu

Wayne County Community College District
Surgical Technology Prgm
8200 W Outer Dr
Detroit, MI 48219
www.wcccd.edu

Baker College of Flint
Surgical Technology Prgm
1050 W Bristol Rd
Flint, MI 48507-5508
www.baker.edu

Baker College of Jackson
Surgical Technology Prgm
2800 Springport Rd
Jackson, MI 49202
www.baker.edu

Lansing Community College
Surgical Technology Prgm
3400 Human Health & Public Service
PO Box 40010
422 N Grand Ave
Lansing, MI 48933
www.lcc.edu

Northern Michigan University
Surgical Technology Prgm
1401 Presque Isle Ave
3515 West Science Building
Marquette, MI 49855
www.nmu.edu

Baker College of Muskegon
Surgical Technology Prgm
1903 Marquette Ave
Muskegon, MI 49442
www.baker.edu

Baker College of Port Huron
Surgical Technology Prgm
3403 Lapeer Rd
Port Huron, MI 48060
www.baker.edu

Oakland Community College
Cosponsor: William Beaumont Hospital
Surgical Technology Prgm
3601 W 13 Mile Rd
Royal Oak, MI 48073

Delta College
Surgical Technology Prgm
1961 Delta Rd
University Center, MI 48710
www.delta.edu

Minnesota

Anoka Technical College
Surgical Technology Prgm
1355 W Hwy 10
Anoka, MN 55303
www.anokatech.edu
Prgm Dir: Rita M Schutz, RN
Tel: 763 576-4974   *Fax:* 763 576-4715
E-mail: rschutz@anokatech.edu

Rasmussen College - Brooklyn Park
Surgical Technology Prgm
8301 93rd Ave North
Brooklyn Park, MN 55445-1512

Lake Superior College
Surgical Technology Prgm
2101 Trinity Rd
Duluth, MN 55811
www.lsc.edu

Northland Community & Technical College
Surgical Technology Prgm
2022 Central Ave NE
East Grand Forks, MN 56721
www.northlandcollege.edu
Prgm Dir: Ruth LeTexier, CST BSN
Tel: 218 793-2525   *Fax:* 218 793-2842
E-mail: ruth.letexier@northlandcollege.edu

Minnesota West Comm & Tech College
Surgical Technology Prgm
311 N Spring St
Luverne, MN 56156

Saint Mary's University of Minnesota
Surgical Technology Prgm
2500 Park Ave
Minneapolis, MN 55404-4403
www.smumn.edu

Rasmussen College - Moorhead
Surgical Technology Prgm
1250 29th Ave South
Moorhead, MN 56560

Rochester Community & Technical College
Surgical Technology Prgm
851 30th Ave SE
Rochester, MN 55904
www.rctc.edu

St Cloud Technical and Community College
Surgical Technology Prgm
1540 Northway Dr
St Cloud, MN 56303
www.sctcc.edu
Prgm Dir: Laurie Green-Quayle, CST
Tel: 320 308-5921   *Fax:* 320 308-5960
E-mail: lgreenquayle@sctcc.edu

Rasmussen College - St. Cloud
Surgical Technology Prgm
226 Park Ave South
St. Cloud, MN 56301-3713

Mississippi

East Central Community College
Surgical Technology Prgm
PO Box 129
275 W Broad St
Decatur, MS 39327
www.eccc.edu

Holmes Community College
Surgical Technology Prgm
1060 Avent Dr
Grenada Center
Grenada, MS 38901
www.holmescc.edu
Prgm Dir: Jessica Elliott, RN CST FAST
Tel: 662 227-2310   *Fax:* 662 227-2296
E-mail: jelliott@holmescc.edu

Pearl River Community College
Surgical Technology Prgm
5448 US Hwy 49 S
Hattiesburg, MS 39401
www.prcc.edu

Hinds Community College
Surgical Technology Prgm
1750 Chadwick Dr
Jackson, MS 39204
www.hindscc.edu

Mississippi Gulf Coast Community College
Surgical Technology Prgm
PO Box 77
11203 Old Hwy 63 South
George County Center
Lucedale, MS 39452
http://mgccc.edu

Meridian Community College
Surgical Technology Prgm
910 Hwy 19 N
Meridian, MS 39307
www.meridiancc.edu

Itawamba Community College
Surgical Technology Prgm
2176 S Eason Blvd
Tupelo, MS 38804
www.iccms.edu
Prgm Dir: Tonya Davis, RN BSN
Tel: 662 620-5121   *Fax:* 662 620-5077
E-mail: tldavis@iccms.edu

Missouri

Southeast Missouri Hospital Coll of Nursing College of Nursing and Health Sciences
Surgical Technology Prgm
2001 William St
College of Nursing and Health Sciences
Cape Girardeau, MO 63703
www.southeastmissourihospital.com/college

Columbia Public Schools
Cosponsor: Columbia Area Career Center
Surgical Technology Prgm
1818 W Worley St
Health Sciences Center 4203 S Providence Rd
Columbia, MO 65203-6100
www.columbia.k12.mo.us

Lincoln University
Surgical Technology Prgm
820 Chestnut Elliff Hall-Tammy Mangold
Jefferson City, MO 65101

Franklin Tech Ctr/Missouri Southern St Univ
Surgical Technology Prgm
3950 E Newman Rd
Joplin Schools
Joplin, MO 64801-1595
www.ftcjoplin.com

Metropolitan Community College - Penn Valley
Surgical Technology Prgm
2700 E 18th St
Kansas City, MO 64127
www.mcckc.edu

Colorado Technical University
Surgical Technology Prgm
520 East 19th Ave
N. Kansas City, MO 64116

Rolla Technical Center
Surgical Technology Prgm
500 Forum Dr
Rolla, MO 65401
www.rolla.k12.mo.us/schools/rtirtc/
Prgm Dir: Nicole Claussen CST, BS
Tel: 573 458-0160, Ext   *Fax:* 573 458-0164
E-mail: nclaussen@rolla.k12.mo.us

Ozarks Technical Community College
Surgical Technology Prgm
1001 E Chestnut Expressway
Springfield, MO 65802-3625
www.otc.edu

Hillyard Technical Center
Surgical Technology Prgm
3434 Faraon St
St Joseph, MO 64506
www.sjsd.k12.mo.us

St Louis Community College - Forest Park
Surgical Technology Prgm
5600 Oakland Ave
St Louis, MO 63110
www.stlcc.edu
Prgm Dir: Diane Gerardot, CST MA
Tel: 314 644-9340   *Fax:* 314 951-9412
E-mail: dgerardot@stlcc.edu

South Central Career Center
Surgical Technology Prgm
1009 Jackson St
West Plains, MO 65775
http://wphs.k12.mo.us/sccc

Montana

Montana State Univ - Great Falls Coll of Tech
Surgical Technology Prgm
2100 16th Ave S
Great Falls - COT
Great Falls, MT 59405
www.msugf.edu

Flathead Valley Community College
Surgical Technology Prgm
777 Grandview Dr
Kalispell, MT 59901
www.fvcc.edu

University of Montana
Surgical Technology Prgm
College of Technology
909 South Ave W
Missoula, MT 59801
www.umt.edu

Nebraska

Southeast Community College
Surgical Technology Prgm
8800 O St
Lincoln, NE 68520-1299
www.southeast.edu

Nebraska Methodist College
Surgical Technology Prgm
720 N 87th St
Omaha, NE 68114
www.methodistcollege.edu

Nevada

College of Southern Nevada
Surgical Technology Prgm
6375 W Charleston Blvd
Sort Code: W4K
Las Vegas, NV 89146-1139
www.csn.edu

Nevada Career Institute
Surgical Technology Prgm
3231 N Decatur Blvd
Suite 119
Las Vegas, NV 89130
www.nevadacareerinstitute.com

New Hampshire

Concord Hospital
Surgical Technology Prgm
250 Pleasant St
Concord, NH 03301
www.crhc.org

Dartmouth Hitchcock Medical Center
Surgical Technology Prgm
One Medical Center Dr
Lebanon, NH 03756-0001
www.dhmc.org/goto/sst

Great Bay Community College
Surgical Technology Prgm
320 Corporate Drive
Portsmouth, NH 03801

New Jersey

Atlantic Cape Community College
Surgical Technology Prgm
Worthington Atlantic City Center
1535 Bacharach Blvd
Atlantic City, NJ 08401
www.atlantic.edu

Dover Business College - Clifton
Surgical Technology Prgm
600 Getty Ave
Clifton, NJ 07011

Sanford-Brown Institute
Surgical Technology Prgm
675 US 1 South
2nd Floor
Iselin, NJ 08830
www.sb-nj.com

Sussex County Community College
Surgical Technology Prgm
1 College Hill Rd Building A
Newton, NJ 07860
www.sussex.edu

Bergen Community College
Surgical Technology Prgm
400 Paramus Rd
Paramus, NJ 07652
www.bergen.edu

Eastwick College
Surgical Technology Prgm
10 South Franklin Turnpike
Ramsey, NJ 07446

New Mexico

Central New Mexico Community College
Surgical Technology Prgm
525 Buena Vista SE
Albuquerque, NM 87106
www.cnm.edu

San Juan College
Surgical Technology Prgm
4601 College Blvd
Farmington, NM 87402

New York

Kingsborough Community College
Surgical Technology Prgm
2001 Oriental Blvd
Brooklyn, NY 11235
www.kingsborough.edu

Long Island University - Brooklyn Campus
Surgical Technology Prgm
Center for Health Science Technologies
School of Health Professions
1 University Plaza (M-315
Brooklyn, NY 11201
www.liu.edu

Trocaire College
Surgical Technology Prgm
360 Choate Ave
Buffalo, NY 14220-2094
www.trocaire.edu

Nassau Community College
Surgical Technology Prgm
One Education Dr
Dept AHS
Garden City, NY 11530-6793
www.ncc.edu/surgicaltechnology
Prgm Dir: Caroline Kaufmann, Asst Professor RN CNOR
Tel: 516 572-7918   *Fax:* 516 572-7565
E-mail: caroline.kaufmann@ncc.edu

Bronx Lebanon Hospital
Surgical Technology Prgm
275 7th Ave, 16th Fl
The Consortium for Worker Education
New York, NY 10001
www.cwe.org

NYU Langone Medical Center
Surgical Technology Prgm
660 1st Ave, 2nd Floor
New York, NY 10016
www.surgical-technology.med.nyu.edu

Western Suffolk BOCES
Surgical Technology Prgm
152 Laurel Hill Rd
Northport, NY 11768
www.wsboces.org

Ulster County Board of Cooperative Ed Service
Surgical Technology Prgm
PO Box 601, Rte 9W
Port Ewen, NY 12466
www.ulsterboces.org

Niagara County Community College
Surgical Technology Prgm
3111 Saunders Settlement Rd
Sanborn, NY 14132
www.niagaracc.suny.edu

Onondaga Community College
Surgical Technology Prgm
4585 Onondaga Rd
Syracuse, NY 13215
www.sunyocc.edu

North Carolina

Asheville-Buncombe Technical Comm College
Surgical Technology Prgm
340 Victoria Rd
Asheville, NC 28801
www.abtech.edu

South College - Asheville
Surgical Technology Prgm
29 Turtle Creek Dr
Asheville, NC 28803
www.southcollegenc.com

Miller-Motte College - Cary
Surgical Technology Prgm
2205 Walnut St
Cary, NC 27511
www.miller-motte.edu

Carolinas College of Health Sciences
Cosponsor: Carolinas Health Care System
Surgical Technology Prgm
1200 Blythe Rd, PO Box 32861
Charlotte, NC 28232-2861
www.carolinascollege.edu

Central Piedmont Community College
Surgical Technology Prgm
Central Campus, PO Box 35009
Belk Bldg 3134
Charlotte, NC 28235
www.cpcc.edu
Prgm Dir: Eugene Pease, RN MSN CNOR
Tel: 704 330-6716   *Fax:* 704 330-6410
E-mail: gene.pease@cpcc.edu

Cabarrus College of Health Sciences
Surgical Technology Prgm
401 Medical Park Dr
Concord, NC 28025
www.cabarruscollege.edu

Durham Technical Community College
Surgical Technology Prgm
1637 Lawson St
Durham, NC 27703-5023
www.durhamtech.edu

College of The Albemarle
Surgical Technology Prgm
1208 N Rd St, PO Box 2327
Elizabeth City, NC 27906-2327
www.albemarle.edu

Fayetteville Technical Community College
Surgical Technology Prgm
PO Box 35236
2201 Hull Rd
Fayetteville, NC 28303
www.faytechcc.edu

Blue Ridge Community College
Surgical Technology Prgm
180 W Campus Drive
Flat Rock, NC 28731-9624
www.brcc.edu

Catawba Valley Community College
Surgical Technology Prgm
2550 Hwy 70 SE
Hickory, NC 28602
www.cvcc.edu
Prgm Dir: Carol Harrison, RN
Tel: 828 327-7000, Ext 4332   *Fax:* 828 327-7176
E-mail: charrison@cvcc.edu

Coastal Carolina Community College
Surgical Technology Prgm
444 Western Blvd
Jacksonville, NC 28546-6816
www.coastal.cc.nc.us

Guilford Technical Community College
Surgical Technology Prgm
601 High Point Rd, PO Box 309
Jamestown, NC 27282-0309
www.gtcc.cc.nc.us

Lenoir Community College
Surgical Technology Prgm
PO Box 188
Kinston, NC 28502-0188
www.lenoircc.edu
Prgm Dir: Jimi Spears, RN ADN CST
Tel: 252 527-6223, Ext 802   *Fax:* 252 520-9598
E-mail: jespears39@lenoircc.edu

Robeson Community College
Surgical Technology Prgm
5160 Fayetteville Rd
PO Box 1420
Lumberton, NC 28360
www.robeson.cc.nc.us

Sandhills Community College
Surgical Technology Prgm
3395 Airport Rd
Pinehurst, NC 28374
www.sandhills.edu

South Piedmont Community College
Surgical Technology Prgm
PO Box 126
US Highway 74
Polkton, NC 28135
www.spcc.edu

Wake Technical Community College
Surgical Technology Prgm
9109 Fayetteville Rd
Raleigh, NC 27603-5696
www.waketech.edu

**Foothills Surgical Technology Consortium
/Cleveland Community College**
Surgical Technology Prgm
137 South Post Rd
Shelby, NC 28152

Edgecombe Community College
Surgical Technology Prgm
2009 W Wilson St
Tarboro, NC 27886
www.edgecombe.edu

Rockingham Community College
Surgical Technology Prgm
PO Box 38
Wentworth, NC 27375-0038
www.rockinghamcc.edu

Cape Fear Community College
Surgical Technology Prgm
411 N Front St
Wilmington, NC 28401
http://cfcc.edu/sur/

Miller-Motte College - Wilmington
Surgical Technology Prgm
5000 Market St
Wilmington, NC 28405
www.miller-motte.com/wilmington-index.htm

Wilson Technical Community College
Surgical Technology Prgm
902 Herring Ave
PO Box 4305
Wilson, NC 27893
www.wilsontech.cc.nc.us

North Dakota

Bismarck State College
Surgical Technology Prgm
PO Box 5587
1500 Edwards Ave
Bismarck, ND 58506-5587
www.bismarckstate.edu

Ohio

Brown Mackie College - Akron
Surgical Technology Prgm
755 White Pond Drive, Suite 101
Akron, OH 44320
www.brownmackie.edu/Akron/Programs/default.aspx?di
    scID=71&ProgramId=279&OutComeLevelId=3&Loca

The University of Akron
Surgical Technology Prgm
225 South Main St
Akron, OH 44325-3702
www.commtech.uakron.edu/current/departments/allied
    health

Univ of Cincinnati - Clermont College
Surgical Technology Prgm
4200 Clermont College Dr
Batavia, OH 45103
www.ucclermont.edu

Collins Career Center
Surgical Technology Prgm
11627 State Route 243
Chesapeake, OH 45619
www.collins-cc.k12.oh.us

Brown Mackie College - Cincinnati
Surgical Technology Prgm
1011 Glendale-Milford Rd
Cincinnati, OH 45215-1107

Brown Mackie College - Findlay
Surgical Technology Prgm
6871 Steger Dr
Cincinnati, OH 45237-3055
www.ncbt.edu/programs/medical/srg.htm

Cincinnati State Tech & Comm College
Surgical Technology Prgm
3520 Central Pkwy
Cincinnati, OH 45223
www.cincinnatistate.edu

National College - Cincinnati
Surgical Technology Prgm
6871 Steger Drive
Cincinnati, OH 45237

Cuyahoga Community College
Surgical Technology Prgm
2900 Community College Ave
Health Careers & Sciences, 126-H
Attn: Beth Stokes
Cleveland, OH 44115-3196
www.tri-c.edu/programs/healthcareers/surgical

Columbus State Community College
Surgical Technology Prgm
550 E Spring St, PO Box 1609
Columbus, OH 43216-1609
www.cscc.edu
Prgm Dir: Dennis Murphy, BS CST
Tel: 614 287-2514, Ext 2514   *Fax:* 614 287-6080
E-mail: dmurphy@cscc.edu

Miami-Jacobs Career College
Surgical Technology Prgm
110 N Patterson Blvd
Dayton, OH 45402
www.miamijacobs.edu

Sinclair Community College
Surgical Technology Prgm
444 W Third St
Room 3340 Surgical Technology
Dayton, OH 45402-1460
www.sinclair.edu

Lorain County Community College
Surgical Technology Prgm
1005 N Abbe Rd
HS 223
Elyria, OH 44035-1691
www.lorainccc.edu

National College
Surgical Technology Prgm
1837 Woodman Center Dr
Kettering, OH 45420
www.ncbt.edu

Lakeland Community College
Surgical Technology Prgm
7700 Clocktower Dr
H211b
Kirtland, OH 44094
www.lakelandcc.edu
Prgm Dir: Nancymarie Phillips, RN PhD CNOR RNFA
Tel: 440 525-7016   *Fax:* 440 525-4733
E-mail: nphillips@lakelandcc.edu

Scioto County Career Technical Center
Surgical Technology Prgm
951 Vern Riffe Dr
Lucasville, OH 45648
www.sciototech.org

Washington County Career Center
Surgical Technology Prgm
21740 State Route 676
Marietta, OH 45750

EHOVE Ghrist Adult Career Center
Surgical Technology Prgm
316 W Mason Rd
Milan, OH 44846
ehove.net

Central Ohio Technical College
Surgical Technology Prgm
1179 University Dr
Newark, OH 43055-1797
www.cotc.edu

Buckeye Hills Career Center
Surgical Technology Prgm
351 Buckeye Hills Rd
PO Box 157
Rio Grande, OH 45674
www.buckeyehillscareercenter.com

National College - Stow
Surgical Technology Prgm
3855 Fishcreek Rd
Stow, OH 44224-4305

Owens Community College
Surgical Technology Prgm
PO Box 10,000, Oregon Rd
Toledo, OH 43699-1947
www.owens.edu
Prgm Dir: Kristine Flickinger, RN MAOM CNOR
Tel: 567 661-7000, Ext 7310   *Fax:* 567 661-7665
E-mail: kristine_flickinger@owens.edu

Fortis College-Westerville
Surgical Technology Prgm
4151 Executive Parkway Suite 120
Westerville, OH 43081

Choffin Career & Technical Center
Cosponsor: Youngstown City Schools
Surgical Technology Prgm
200 E Wood St
Youngstown, OH 44503
www.youngstown.k12.oh.us/choffin
Prgm Dir: Carole DuBose, LPN/CST
Tel: 330 744-8723   *Fax:* 330 744-8705
E-mail: Carole.Dubose@Youngstown.k12.oh.us

National College - Youngstown
Surgical Technology Prgm
3487 Belmont Ave
Youngstown, OH 44505

Oklahoma

Canadian Valley Technology Center
Surgical Technology Prgm
1401 Michigan Ave
Chickasha, OK 73018
www.cvtech.org

Central Technology Center
Surgical Technology Prgm
3 Ct Circle
Drumright, OK 74030
www.centraltech.edu

Autry Technology Center
Surgical Technology Prgm
1201 W Willow
Enid, OK 73703-2506
www.autrytech.com

Great Plains Technology Center
Surgical Technology Prgm
4500 W Lee Blvd
Lawton, OK 73505
www.gptech.org

Indian Capital Technology Center
Surgical Technology Prgm
2043 N 41st St East
Muskogee, OK 74403

Moore Norman Technology Center
Surgical Technology Prgm
4701 12th Ave NW
PO Box 4701
Norman, OK 73069-8399
http://mntechnology.com

Metro Tech Health Careers Center
Surgical Technology Prgm
Health Careers Center
1720 Springlake Dr
Oklahoma City, OK 73111
www.metrotech.org

Platt College - Oklahoma City
Surgical Technology Prgm
309 South Ann Arbor
Oklahoma City, OK 73128

Community Care College
Surgical Technology Prgm
4242 South Sheridan Rd
Tulsa, OK 74145
www.communitycarecollege.edu
Prgm Dir: Andrea Caygill, Department Head
Tel: 918 610-0027, Ext 2048   *Fax:* 918 610-0029
E-mail: acaygill@communitycarecollege.edu

Tulsa Technology Center
Surgical Technology Prgm
3350 S Memorial Dr
PO Box 477200
Tulsa, OK 74145-1390
www.tulsatech.org

Wes Watkins Technology Center District 25
Surgical Technology Prgm
7892 Hwy 9
Wetumka, OK 74883
www.wwtech.org

Oregon

Mt Hood Community College
Surgical Technology Prgm
26000 SE Stark St
Gresham, OR 97030
www.mhcc.edu

Concorde Career College - Portland
Surgical Technology Prgm
1425 NE Irving St, Building 300
Portland, OR 97232
www.concorde.edu

Pennsylvania

Northampton Community College
Surgical Technology Prgm
3835 Green Pond Rd
511 East Third St
Bethlehem, PA 18020
www.northampton.edu

St Luke's Hospital
Cosponsor: St Luke's University Health Network
Surgical Technology Prgm
801 Ostrum St
Bethlehem, PA 18015
www.slhn.org
Prgm Dir: Julie Bailey,
Tel: 484 526-4466, Ext 4466   *Fax:* 484 526-6097
E-mail: baileyj@slhn.org

Mount Aloysius College
Surgical Technology Prgm
7373 Admiral Peary Hwy
Cresson, PA 16630-1999
www.mtaloy.edu
Prgm Dir: Amanda Minor, BS CST
Tel: 814 886-6340   *Fax:* 814 886-6419
E-mail: aminor@mtaloy.edu

**McCann School of Business and Technology -
Dickson City**
Surgical Technology Prgm
2227 Scranton Carbondale Highway
Dickson City, PA 18519

Great Lakes Institute of Technology
Surgical Technology Prgm
5100 Peach St
Erie, PA 16509
www.glit.edu
Prgm Dir: Jacob Muth, CST BA
Tel: 814 864-6666, Ext 434   *Fax:* 814 868-1717
E-mail: Jacobm@glit.edu

**Harrisburg Area Community College -
Harrisburg**
Surgical Technology Prgm
349 Wiconisco St
One HACC Dr
Harrisburg, PA 17110
www.hacc.edu

McCann School of Business and Technology
Surgical Technology Prgm
370 Maplewood Drive
Humboldt Industrial Park
Hazelton, PA 18202
www.mccannschool.edu

Conemaugh Valley Memorial Hospital
Surgical Technology Prgm
1086 Franklin St
Johnstown, PA 15905-4398
www.conemaugh.org
Prgm Dir: Patricia Pavlikowski, MA RN CNOR CST
Tel: 814 534-9772 *Fax:* 814 534-9945
E-mail: Ppavlik@conemaugh.org
Notes: Tuition is subject to change every August as
  students pay tuition to the University of Pittsburgh at
  Johnstown. Tuition depends on state subsidy. A $300
  clinical fee is charged by Memorial Medical Center.

Lancaster Gen Coll of Nursing & Hlth Sciences
Surgical Technology Prgm
410 N Lime St
Lancaster, PA 17602
www.lancastergeneralcollege.edu
Prgm Dir: Connie Corrigan, Chair
Tel: 717 544-1283 *Fax:* 717 544-5970
E-mail: cmcorrig@lancastergeneralcollege.edu
Notes: Students entering the Diploma Program must
  have a degree from an institution of higher learning
  and have successfully completed A&P 1 and 2 prior to
  entering the program.

Delaware County Community College
Surgical Technology Prgm
901 S Media Line Rd
Media, PA 19063-1094
www.dccc.edu

Community College of Allegheny County
Surgical Technology Prgm
595 Beatty Rd
Boyce Campus
Monroeville, PA 15146-1395
www.ccac.edu

Luzerne County Community College
Surgical Technology Prgm
1333 S Prospect St
Nanticoke, PA 18634
www.luzerne.edu

Pittsburgh Technical Institute
Surgical Technology Prgm
1111 McKee Rd
Oakdale, PA 15071

Sanford-Brown Institute - Pittsburgh
Surgical Technology Prgm
777 Penn Center Blvd Building 7 - Suite 111
Pittsburgh, PA 15235

Montgomery County Community College
Surgical Technology Prgm
101 College Dr
Pottstown, PA 19464
www.mc3.edu

Reading Hospital & Medical Center
Cosponsor: The Reading Hospital School of Health
  Sciences
Surgical Technology Prgm
PO Box 16052
Reading, PA 19612-6052
www.readinghospital.org

McCann School of Business and Technology
Surgical Technology Prgm
1147 N Fourth St
Sunbury, PA 17801
www.mccannschool.com/

Lackawanna College
Surgical Technology Prgm
1 Progress Plaza
Towanda, PA 18848

Pennsylvania College of Technology
Surgical Technology Prgm
One College Ave
DIF 14
Williamsport, PA 17701
www.pct.edu

Rhode Island

New England Institute of Technology
Surgical Technology Prgm
2500 Post Rd
Warwick, RI 02886-2251
www.neit.edu

South Carolina

Technical College of the Lowcountry
Surgical Technology Prgm
PO Box 1288
Beaufort, SC 29901
www.tcl.edu

Midlands Technical College
Surgical Technology Prgm
PO Box 2408
Columbia, SC 29202
www.midlandstech.edu/surgtech
Prgm Dir: Kathy Patnaude, CST AOT BS
Tel: 803 822-3438 *Fax:* 803 822-3417
E-mail: patnaudek@midlandstech.edu

Florence-Darlington Technical College
Surgical Technology Prgm
PO Box 100548
320 W Cheves St
Florence, SC 29501-0548
www.fdtc.edu

Horry - Georgetown Technical College
Surgical Technology Prgm
4003 S Fraser St
Georgetown, SC 29440-9620
www.hgtc.edu

Aiken Technical College
Surgical Technology Prgm
2276 Jefferson Davis Highway
PO Box 696
Graniteville, SC 29829
www.atc.edu

Greenville Technical College
Surgical Technology Prgm
PO Box 5616
Greenville, SC 29606-8616
www.greenvilletech.com

Virginia College of Greenville
Surgical Technology Prgm
78 Global Drive Suite 200
Greenville, SC 29607

Piedmont Technical College
Surgical Technology Prgm
PO Box 1467, Emerald Rd
Greenwood, SC 29648
www.ptc.edu

Miller-Motte Technical College
Surgical Technology Prgm
8085 Rivers Ave
Suite E
North Charleston, SC 29406
www.mmtccharleston.com

Tri-County Technical College
Surgical Technology Prgm
PO Box 587
7900 Hwy 76
Pendleton, SC 29670-0587
www.tctc.edu

York Technical College
Surgical Technology Prgm
452 S Anderson Rd
Rock Hill, SC 29730
www.yorktech.com

Spartanburg Community College
Surgical Technology Prgm
PO Drawer 4386
Business Interstate 85 at New Cut Rd
Spartanburg, SC 29305
http://sccsc.edu

Central Carolina Technical College
Surgical Technology Prgm
506 N Guignard Dr
Bldg 600
Sumter, SC 29150
www.cctech.edu

South Dakota

Presentation College
Surgical Technology Prgm
1500 N Main St
Aberdeen, SD 57401
www.presentation.edu

Western Dakota Technical Institute
Surgical Technology Prgm
800 Mickelson Dr
Rapid City, SD 57703
www.westerndakotatech.org

Southeast Technical Institute
Surgical Technology Prgm
2320 N Career Ave
Sioux Falls, SD 57107
www.southeasttech.edu

Tennessee

Northeast State Community College
Surgical Technology Prgm
PO Box 246, 2425 Hwy 75
Blountville, TN 37617-0246
www.northeaststate.edu

Chattanooga State Community College
Surgical Technology Prgm
4501 Amnicola Hwy
Chattanooga, TN 37406-1097
www.chattanoogastate.edu

Miller-Motte Technical College - Chattanooga
Surgical Technology Prgm
6020 Shallowford Rd
Suite 100
Chattanooga, TN 37421
www.miller-motte.com

Miller-Motte Technical College - Clarksville
Surgical Technology Prgm
1820 Business Park Dr
Clarksville, TN 37040
http://miller-motte.com/clarksville-index.htm

Fortis Institute
Surgical Technology Prgm
1025 Highway 111
Cookeville, TN 38501
www.medvance.org

Tennessee Technology Center - Crossville
Surgical Technology Prgm
910 Miller Ave
PO Box 2959
Crossville, TN 38555
www.crossville.tec.tn.us

Tennessee Technology Center - Hohenwald
Surgical Technology Prgm
813 W Main St
Hohenwald, TN 38462-2201
www.hohenwald.tec.tn.us

Tennessee Technology Center - Jackson
Surgical Technology Prgm
2468 Technology Center Dr
Jackson, TN 38301
www.jackson.tec.tn.us

Tennessee Technology Center - Knoxville
Surgical Technology Prgm
1100 Liberty St
Knoxville, TN 37919
www.knoxville.tec.tn.us

Concorde Career College - Memphis
Surgical Technology Prgm
5100 Poplar Ave, Ste 132
Memphis, TN 38137
www.concorde.edu

National College of Business and Technology
Surgical Technology Prgm
3545 Lamar Ave
Memphis, TN 38118

Tennessee Technology Center - Murfreesboro
Surgical Technology Prgm
1303 Old Fort Pkwy
Murfreesboro, TN 37129
www.murfreesboro.tec.tn.us

Fortis Institute - Nashville
Surgical Technology Prgm
3354 Perimeter Hill Drive Suite 105
Nashville, TN 37211

Nashville State Community College
Surgical Technology Prgm
120 White Bridge Rd
Nashville, TN 37209
www.nscc.edu

Texas

Cisco College
Surgical Technology Prgm
717 E Industrial Blvd
Abilene, TX 79602
www.cisco.edu

Amarillo College
Surgical Technology Prgm
PO Box 447
Amarillo, TX 79178
www.actx.edu
Prgm Dir: Lisa Holdaway, RN CST
Tel: 806 356-3663   *Fax:* 806 354-6076
E-mail: leholdaway@actx.edu

Concorde Career Institute - Arlington
Surgical Technology Prgm
600 E Lamar Blvd
Suite 200
Arlington, TX 76011
www.concorde.edu

Iverson Business School
Surgical Technology Prgm
1600 E Pioneer Parkway Suite 200
Arlington, TX 76010

Austin Community College
Surgical Technology Prgm
3401 Webberville Rd
Austin, TX 78702
www.austincc.edu/health/srgt
Prgm Dir: Pedro Barrera III, CST
Tel: 512 223-5804   *Fax:* 512 223-5901
E-mail: pbarrera@austincc.edu

Virginia College at Austin
Surgical Technology Prgm
6301 E Hwy 290
Suite 200
Austin, TX 78723
www.vc.edu

North Central Texas College
Surgical Technology Prgm
1500 N Corinth St
1525 West California Gainesville, TX 76240
Corinth, TX 76208-5408
www.nctc.edu

Del Mar College
Surgical Technology Prgm
101 Baldwin Blvd
Corpus Christi, TX 78404-3897
www.delmar.edu
Prgm Dir: Warren Glenn Madden, Asst Professor
Tel: 361 698-2839   *Fax:* 361 698-2811
E-mail: wgmadden@delmar.edu

El Centro College
Surgical Technology Prgm
801 Main St
301 N Market St P305
Dallas, TX 75202-3604
www.elcentrocollege.edu

El Paso Community College
Surgical Technology Prgm
PO Box 20500
El Paso, TX 79998
www.epcc.edu
Prgm Dir: Cynthia Rivera, RN BSN
Tel: 915 831-4086   *Fax:* 915 831-4114
E-mail: criver32@epcc.edu

Medical Education and Training Campus (METC)
Surgical Technology Prgm
Attn: MCCS-ZD-M 2480 Garden Way, Bldg B
Ft. Sam Houston, TX 78234-1200

Tarrant County College
Surgical Technology Prgm
245 E Belknap
Ft. Worth, TX 76102
www.tccd.edu
Prgm Dir: Don Braziel, CST BS
Tel: 817 515-2404   *Fax:* 817 515-0772
E-mail: donnie.braziel@tccd.edu

Galveston College
Surgical Technology Prgm
4015 Ave Q
Galveston, TX 77550
www.gc.edu

Fortis Institute - Grand Prairie
Surgical Technology Prgm
401 E Palace Parkway Suite 100
Grand Prairie, TX 75050

Texas State Technical College - Harlingen
Surgical Technology Prgm
1409 N Loop 499
Harlingen, TX 78550-3653
www.harlingen.tstc.edu/surgtech
Prgm Dir: Robert Sanchez, BSN CST RN
Tel: 956 364-4805   *Fax:* 956 364-5227
E-mail: robert.sanchez@harlingen.tstc.edu

Academy of Health Care Professions
Surgical Technology Prgm
240 Northwest Mall
Houston, TX 77092
www.ahcp.edu

Fortis Institute - Houston North
Surgical Technology Prgm
450 N Sam Houston Pkwy Ste 200
Houston, TX 77060

Fortis Institute - Houston South
Surgical Technology Prgm
6220 Westpark, Ste 180
Houston, TX 77057
www.medvance.edu

Houston Community College
Surgical Technology Prgm
1900 Pressler Dr
Houston, TX 77030
www.hccs.edu

Sanford-Brown College - Houston
Surgical Technology Prgm
10500 Forum Place Dr #200
Houston, TX 77036
www.sbhouston.com

Sanford-Brown College - North Loop
Surgical Technology Prgm
2627 North Loop West, Suite 100
Houston, TX 77008

Trinity Valley Community College
Surgical Technology Prgm
Health Science Ctr, 800 Hwy 243 W
Kaufman, TX 75142
www.tvcc.edu/healthscience/surgtech.htm

Kilgore College
Surgical Technology Prgm
1100 Broadway
Kilgore, TX 75662
www.kilgore.edu

Covenant Medical Center
Surgical Technology Prgm
3615 19th
Lubbock, TX 79410

South Plains College
Surgical Technology Prgm
Reese Center
819 Gilbert Drive, Bldg 5
Lubbock, TX 79416
www.southplainscollege.edu

Angelina College
Surgical Technology Prgm
3500 S First St
Lufkin, TX 75904
www.angelina.edu/health/surgical_technology.html
Prgm Dir: Tonya LaForge, RN BSN CST
Tel: 936 633-5275   *Fax:* 936 633-5241
E-mail: tlaforge@angelina.edu

Collin County Community College District
Surgical Technology Prgm
2200 West University Drive
McKinney, TX 75070

Paris Junior College
Surgical Technology Prgm
2400 Clarksville St
Paris, TX 75460
www.parisjc.edu

San Jacinto College Central
Surgical Technology Prgm
8060 Spencer Hwy, PO Box 2007
Pasadena, TX 77501-2007
www.sjcd.us

Lamar State College - Port Arthur
Surgical Technology Prgm
PO Box 310
Port Arthur, TX 77641-0310
www.lamarpa.edu

Howard College
Surgical Technology Prgm
3501 N US Hwy 67
San Angelo, TX 76905
www.howardcollege.edu

Baptist Health System
Surgical Technology Prgm
School of Health Professions
8400 Datapoint Dr
San Antonio, TX 78229-3234
www.bshp.edu

St Philip's College
Surgical Technology Prgm
1801 Martin Luther King Dr
San Antonio, TX 78203-2098
http://accd.edu/spc

Temple College
Surgical Technology Prgm
2600 S First St
Temple, TX 76504
www.templejc.edu

Lone Star College - Tomball
Surgical Technology Prgm
700 Graham Rd
Tomball, TX 77375-4036

Tyler Junior College
Surgical Technology Prgm
PO Box 9020
1530 SSW Loop 323 (Zip 75701
1400 E Fifth St
Tyler, TX 75798
www.tjc.edu

McLennan Community College
Surgical Technology Prgm
1400 College Dr
Waco, TX 76708

Wharton County Junior College
Surgical Technology Prgm
911 Boling Hwy
Wharton, TX 77488
www.wcjc.cc.tx.us

Vernon College
Surgical Technology Prgm
4105 Maplewood Ave
Wichita Falls, TX 76308
www.vernoncollege.edu/surgtech

Utah

Davis Applied Technology College
Surgical Technology Prgm
550 East 300 South
Kaysville, UT 84037
www.datc.net

Stevens-Henager College
Surgical Technology Prgm
1890 South 1350 West
PO Box 9428
Ogden, UT 84401-0428
www.stevenshenager.edu

Ameritech College
Surgical Technology Prgm
1675 N Freedom Blvd, Ste 3B
Provo, UT 84604
www.ameritech.edu

Dixie State College of Utah
Surgical Technology Prgm
225 South 700 East
St George, UT 84770
www.dixie.edu

Salt Lake Community College
Surgical Technology Prgm
9301 S Wights Fort Rd
West Jordan, UT 84020
www.slcc.edu

Everest College
Surgical Technology Prgm
3280 West 3500 South
West Valley City, UT 84119
http://mwc.career-edu.net/start.htm#tab8_

Virginia

Piedmont Virginia Community College
Surgical Technology Prgm
501 College Dr
Charlottesville, VA 22902
www.pvcc.edu

Sentara Norfolk General Hospital /Sentara College of Health Sciences
Surgical Technology Prgm
1441 Crossways Blvd Ste 105
Chesapeake, VA 23320

National College - Danville
Surgical Technology Prgm
336 Old Riverside Drive
Danville, VA 24541

National College - Harrisonburg
Surgical Technology Prgm
1515 Country Club Rd
Harrisonburg, VA 22802

Miller-Motte Technical College
Surgical Technology Prgm
1011 Creekside Lane
Lynchburg, VA 24502
www.miller-motte.com

Riverside School of Health Careers
Surgical Technology Prgm
316 Main St
Newport News, VA 23601
www.riversideonline.com

Fortis College - Richmond
Surgical Technology Prgm
2000 Westmoreland St Suite A
Richmond, VA 23230

Washington

Bellingham Technical College
Surgical Technology Prgm
3028 Lindbergh Ave
Bellingham, WA 98225-1599
www.btc.ctc.edu

Clover Park Technical College
Surgical Technology Prgm
4500 Steilacoom Blvd SW
Lakewood, WA 98499
www.cptc.edu

Columbia Basin College
Surgical Technology Prgm
2600 North 20th Ave MS-R2
Pasco, WA 99301

Renton Technical College
Surgical Technology Prgm
3000 NE Fourth St
Box 103
Renton, WA 98056-4195
www.rtc.edu

Seattle Central Community College
Surgical Technology Prgm
1701 Broadway
Allied Health Division
Seattle, WA 98122
www.seattlecentral.org

Spokane Community College
Surgical Technology Prgm
N 1810 Greene St
Spokane, WA 99217-5399
www.scc.spokane.edu

Yakima Valley Community College
Surgical Technology Prgm
PO Box 22520
16th Ave and Nobhill Blvd
Yakima, WA 98907-2520
www.yvcc.edu

West Virginia

Carver Career Center
Surgical Technology Prgm
4799 Midland Dr
Charleston, WV 25306

James Rumsey Technical Institute
Surgical Technology Prgm
3274 Hedgesville Rd
Martinsburg, WV 25403
www.jamesrumsey.net

Monongalia County Tech Education Center
Cosponsor: Monongalia County Board of Education
Surgical Technology Prgm
1000 Mississippi St
Morgantown, WV 26501
www.mtecwv.edu

Southern West Virginia Comm & Tech College
Surgical Technology Prgm
PO Box 2900
Dempsey Branch Rd
Mount Gay, WV 25637
www.southern.wvnet.edu

West Virginia University - Parkersburg
Surgical Technology Prgm
300 Campus Dr
Parkersburg, WV 26101
www.wvup.edu

West Virginia Northern Community College
Surgical Technology Prgm
Hazel Atlas Building
1704 Market St
Wheeling, WV 26003
www.northern.wvnet.edu

Wisconsin

Chippewa Valley Technical College
Surgical Technology Prgm
620 W Clairemont Ave
Eau Claire, WI 54701-6162
www.cvtc.edu

Moraine Park Technical College
Surgical Technology Prgm
235 North National Ave
Fond du Lac, WI 54935-2897
www.morainepark.edu/programs-and-courses/programs-
    of-study/Surgical+Technology

Northeast Wisconsin Technical College
Surgical Technology Prgm
2740 W Mason St, PO Box 19042
Green Bay, WI 54307-9042
www.nwtc.edu

Gateway Technical College
Surgical Technology Prgm
3520 30th Ave
Kenosha, WI 53144-1690
http://gtc.edu

Western Technical College
Surgical Technology Prgm
400 7th St North, PO Box C-908
La Crosse, WI 54602-0908
www.westerntc.edu

Madison Area Technical College
Surgical Technology Prgm
Center for Health and Safety Education
3550 Anderson St
Madison, WI 53704
www.matcmadison.edu

Mid-State Technical College
Surgical Technology Prgm
2600 W Fifth St
Marshfield, WI 54449
www.mstc.edu
Prgm Dir: Kelly Altmann, RN BSN CNOR
Tel: 715 387-2538   *Fax:* 715 389-2864
E-mail: Kelly.altmann@mstc.edu

Milwaukee Area Technical College
Surgical Technology Prgm
700 W State St
Milwaukee, WI 53233
www.matc.edu

Waukesha County Technical College
Surgical Technology Prgm
800 Main St
Pewaukee, WI 53072
www.wctc.edu
Prgm Dir: Sharon A Corrao, RN BSN MEd CNOR CST
Tel: 262 691-5407   *Fax:* 262 691-5241
E-mail: scorrao@wctc.edu

Northcentral Technical College
Surgical Technology Prgm
1000 Campus Dr
Wausau, WI 54401
www.ntc.edu

Wyoming

Laramie County Community College
Surgical Technology Prgm
1400 E College Dr
Cheyenne, WY 82007
www.lccc.wy.edu

Surgical Technologist

Programs*	Class Capacity	Begins	Length (months)	Award	Res. Tuition	Non-res. Tuition		Offers:† 1	2	3	4
Arkansas											
Univ of Arkansas - Fort Smith	18	Aug	18	AAS	$13,147	$21,547				•	
Univ of Arkansas for Medical Sciences (Little Rock)	16	Aug	10, 20	AS	$9,953	$20,843	per year				
California											
Concorde Career College - North Hollywood	24	Jan Apr Jul Oct	13	Dipl	$26,203	$26,203					
Glendale Career College	20	Every 12 wks	16	Dipl	$26,040	per year					
Premiere Career College (Irwindale)		Jan May Aug	13	Dipl							
San Joaquin Valley College - Fresno	16	Every 33 wks	14	AS						•	
Skyline College (San Bruno)	25	Jun	12	Cert, AS	$1,380	$7,740				•	
Connecticut											
A I Prince Technical High School (Hartford)	12	Aug	10	Cert	$3,350	$3,350	per year			•	
Florida											
Pinellas Technical Education Centers - St Petersburg Campus	20	Aug Jun	14	Cert	$3,753	$15,076	per year			•	
Georgia											
Augusta Technical College	20	Aug	12	Dipl	$6,974	$13,489					•
Okefenokee Technical College (Waycross)	15	Fall quarter	24, 15	Dipl, AAS	$1,265	$2,530	per year	•			
Southeastern Technical College (Vidalia)	18	Jan	18		$3,561	$7,122	total				
Illinois											
Richland Community College (Decatur)	15	Aug	21	AAS	$5,212	$21,070				•	
Indiana											
Ivy Tech Community College - Lafayette	20	Aug	24	AAS							
Univ of Saint Francis (Fort Wayne)	22	Aug	20	AS	$23,900	$23,900	per year	•	•	•	•
Vincennes Univ	20	Aug	11, 24	Cert, CG, AD	$5,988	$14,544				•	•
Kentucky											
Maysville Comm & Tech College	12	Aug Jan	18		$3,509	$4,524	per year				
Minnesota											
Anoka Technical College	20	Aug Jan	13	Dipl, AAS	$11,703	$23,406	per year	•			•
Northland Community & Technical College (East Grand Forks)	28	Sep	18	AAS	$6,318	$6,318	per year	•		•	•
St Cloud Technical and Community College	24	Aug	12, 19	Dipl, AAS	$196	$196	per credit			•	
Mississippi											
Holmes Community College (Grenada)	12	Aug	12, 24	Cert, AAS	$2,330	$3,500	per year				
Itawamba Community College (Tupelo)	16	Aug	12, 24	Cert, AAS	$2,400	$5,145	per year				
Missouri											
Rolla Technical Center	20	Aug	12	Cert, AAS	$8,917	$8,917	per year			•	
St Louis Community College - Forest Park	24	Aug	12	Dipl, Cert	$5,300	$8,832	per year			•	
New York											
Nassau Community College (Garden City)	32	Sep	24	AAS	$1,866	$3,732	per year	•			•
North Carolina											
Catawba Valley Community College (Hickory)	20	Aug	12	Dipl	$4,000	$15,000				•	
Central Piedmont Community College (Charlotte)	20	Aug	24	AAS	$1,700	$8,500	per year	•	•	•	•
Lenoir Community College (Kinston)	20	Aug	12	Dipl	$2,573	$9,483	per year				

*Data are shown only for programs that completed the 2011 AMA Survey of Health Professions Education Programs.

†Key to Offers: 1: Evening or weekend classes; 2: Non-English instruction; 3: Cultural competence instruction; 4: Distance education component.

Programs*	Class Capacity	Begins	Length (months)	Award	Res. Tuition	Non-res. Tuition		Offers:† 1	2	3	4
Ohio											
Choffin Career & Technical Center (Youngstown)	25	Aug	10	Cert	$7,500	$7,500	per year			•	
Columbus State Community College	24	Autumn Q (Sep)	12, 18	Cert, Assoc	$2,844	$3,636	per credit	•	•	•	
Lakeland Community College (Kirtland)	14	Aug	22	AAS	$8,000	$12,000				•	
Owens Community College (Toledo)	24	Aug	20	AAS						•	
Oklahoma											
Community Care College (Tulsa)	90	Jul	13, 20	Dipl, AOS							•
Pennsylvania											
Conemaugh Valley Memorial Hospital (Johnstown)	20	Aug	12, 24	Cert, , Associate	$19,007	$33,439	per year			•	
Great Lakes Institute of Technology (Erie)	12	Aug	17	Dipl	$23,762	$23,762	per year				
Lancaster Gen Coll of Nursing & Hlth Sciences	15	Aug	12, 24	Cert, AAS	$17,000	$17,000	per year		•	•	
Mount Aloysius College (Cresson)	24	Aug	24	AS	$17,930	$17,930	per year			•	
St Luke's Hospital (Bethlehem)	12	Aug	11	Cert	$9,000	$9,000	per year			•	
South Carolina											
Midlands Technical College (Columbia)	24	Aug	12	Dipl						•	
Texas											
Amarillo College	25	Jun	11, 24	Cert, AAS	$3,300	$5,200	per year				•
Angelina College (Lufkin)	12	Jan	1	Cert	$4,500	$5,000				•	
Austin Community College	40	Aug Jan	16, 24	Cert, AAS	$4,090	$10,894				•	
Del Mar College (Corpus Christi)	20	May	12, 24	Cert, AAS	$1,978	$4,066				•	
El Paso Community College	12	Jun	12, 24	Cert, AAS	$3,517	$6,907	per year		•	•	
Tarrant County College (Ft. Worth)	30	Aug	11	Cert	$4,000					•	
Texas State Technical College - Harlingen	20	Aug	24	AAS	$11,376	$21,933					•
Wisconsin											
Mid-State Technical College (Marshfield)	20	Jun	12	Dipl	$4,258	$6,987	per year				
Waukesha County Technical College (Pewaukee)	14	Aug	24	AAS	$8,027	$11,775					

*Data are shown only for programs that completed the 2011 AMA Survey of Health Professions Education Programs.

†Key to Offers: 1: Evening or weekend classes; 2: Non-English instruction; 3: Cultural competence instruction; 4: Distance education component.

ALLIED HEALTH

Communication Sciences

Includes:
- Audiologist
- Speech-language pathologist

Audiologist

Career Description

Audiologists are professionals who work with people that exhibit hearing, balance, and related communication problems. They evaluate individuals of all ages and identify those with the symptoms of hearing loss and other auditory, balance, and related neural problems. They then assess the nature and extent of the problems and help the individuals manage them. Using clinical skills and technology, audiologists measure the loudness at which a person begins to hear sounds, the ability to distinguish between sounds, and the impact of hearing loss or balance problems on an individual's communication ability that impacts their daily life. Audiologists interpret these results and may coordinate them with medical, speech-language, educational, and psychological information to make a diagnosis and determine a course of treatment. Audiologists must effectively communicate diagnostic test results, interpretation, and proposed treatment in a manner easily understood by patients/clients and their families/caregivers as well as other professionals.

Hearing, balance, and related communication disorders can result from a variety of causes, including head trauma, viral infections, genetic disorders, exposure to loud noise, certain medications, or aging. Treatment may include examining and cleaning the ear canal, fitting and dispensing hearing aids and other hearing assistive technology, fitting and programming cochlear implants, and providing auditory rehabilitation. Auditory rehabilitation emphasizes counseling on adjusting to hearing loss, training on the use of hearing aids and other technology, and teaching communication strategies for use in a variety of listening environments. Audiologists also make recommendations on amplification systems for large areas and alerting devices for public spaces and classrooms. In addition, audiologists assess individuals with balance disorders and provide vestibular rehabilitation.

Some audiologists specialize in work with the elderly and others with very young children. Others develop and implement ways to protect workers' hearing from on-the-job exposure to loud noise. Audiologists measure noise levels in workplaces and conduct hearing protection programs in factories. They also administer hearing screening programs for newborns before they leave the hospital, as well as in schools and communities.

A graduate degree is necessary to practice as an audiologist in all states. A doctoral degree (AuD, ScD, PhD) is required for work in some settings. A clinical doctoral degree is required as the minimum educational requirement for new clinicians beginning in 2012.

Audiologists specialize in the study of:
- Normal and impaired hearing and balance
- Prevention of hearing loss
- Identification and assessment of hearing and balance problems

- Rehabilitation of persons with hearing and balance disorders

In addition, audiologists may:
- prepare future professionals in colleges and universities;
- manage agencies, clinics, or private practices;
- engage in research to enhance knowledge about normal hearing, and the evaluation and treatment of hearing disorders; and
- design hearing instruments and testing equipment.

Employment Characteristics

Audiologists may work in a wide range of settings, including schools, hospitals, rehabilitation centers, private practice, skilled nursing facilities, government health facilities, community clinics, geriatric facilities, health maintenance organizations (HMOs), public health departments, research laboratories, or industrial corporations.

Salary

Salaries of audiologists depend on educational background, specialty, and experience, along with the geographical location and type of setting in which they work. Beginning in 2010, salary data were separated into three sources: base salary, commissions, and bonuses. The median annual base salary in 2010 for audiologists certified by the American Speech-Language-Hearing Association (ASHA) was $70,000. Persons in supervisory positions—for example, administrators, supervisors, and directors—earned a median salary of $92,531. While the 2010 median starting annual salary for certified audiologists with one to three years of experience was $60,000, the median annual salary for certified audiologists with clinical doctorate degrees was $70,000, compared with $96,097 for those with research doctorates. In addition to base salaries, audiologists reported median commissions of $14,000 and median bonuses of $1,500. Good benefits packages, such as insurance programs and leave, are usually available to audiologists. For more information, see *www.ama-assn.org/go/hpsalary*, or refer to salary information on ASHA's website at *www.asha.org/research/memberdata/AudiologySurvey.htm*.

Employment Outlook

Employment of audiologists is expected to grow much faster than the average for all occupations through the year 2020 (*www.bls.gov/oco/ocos085.htm#outlook*). Because hearing loss is strongly associated with aging, the rapid growth in population aged 55 and older will cause the number of persons with hearing impairment to increase markedly. Members of the Baby Boom generation are now entering middle age, when the possibility of neurological disorders and associated hearing impairments increases. Medical advances are also improving the survival rate of premature infants and trauma and stroke victims, who need assessments and possible treatments. Most states now require that all newborns be screened for hearing loss and receive appropriate early intervention services. Opportunities in research and higher education are expected to increase as professionals currently in these positions retire. Greater awareness of the importance of early identification and diagnosis of speech, language, and hearing disorders in young children also will increase employment.

Education Programs

Approximately 72 universities in the United States offer accredited graduate education programs in audiology at the clinical doctoral degree level. Beginning in 2012, the clinical doctoral degree is the entry-level degree required to enter into independent professional practice. Although master's degree programs had been the prominent degree programs for preparation for professional practice since 1965, clinical doctoral degree programs have replaced the master's programs in the US. Most programs can be identified as Doctor of Audiology programs or AuD programs; some clinical doctoral programs have chosen to use other degree designations such as Clinical PhD or Doctor of Science (ScD). Research doctoral degree programs are also available as advanced degree programs for further study of audiology and hearing science.

Length. Most clinical doctoral programs are designed to be completed in 4 years (including summers) for full-time study, and include clinical training designed to meet requirements for state licensure and national certification.

Prerequisites. Knowledge of the biological sciences, physical sciences, mathematics/statistics, and behavioral or social sciences is required for the ASHA Certificate of Clinical Competence in Audiology. Undergraduate programs in communication sciences and disorders will provide a background in the sciences, linguistics, phonetics, psychology, normal speech, and language development, and introductory course work in audiology. Excellent oral and written communication skills are expected.

Curriculum. Graduate programs should offer a curriculum to allow a student to meet the knowledge and skills necessary to enter independent practice in audiology. A typical graduate program of study includes, among others, courses in genetics; normal and abnormal communication development; auditory, balance, and neural systems assessment and treatment; diagnosis and treatment; pharmacology; and ethics. Opportunities to work in a variety of different clinical settings and with a broad range of clients are provided during the graduate program of study.

Licensure and Certification

All 50 states and the District of Columbia require audiologists to comply with state regulatory (licensure) standards and/or have state teacher certification to practice in specific settings. Earning a graduate degree and passing a national examination are typically required to achieve the credentials. Individuals should contact the appropriate state licensure board or teacher certification agency for more information about the requirements. ASHA's Certificate of Clinical Competence in Audiology (CCC-A), a nationally recognized credential, offers certificate holders ease in qualifying for state credentials because those requirements are similar or identical to ASHA's CCC requirements, recognition as a "highest qualified provider" of audiology services for reimbursement, and increased opportunities for employment or promotion, as certain positions in hospitals, educational programs, or private practices may require ASHA certification. In 2012, a doctoral degree will be required by ASHA to award certification in audiology. Furthermore, some states already require a clinical doctoral degree for licensure.

Inquiries

For information about a specific program, contact the director of the audiology program in care of the institution listed. Program information can be accessed on ASHA's web site at: *www.asha.org/students/academic/EdFind*.

For additional information about the profession or program accreditation, contact:
American Speech-Language-Hearing Association (ASHA)
2200 Research Blvd.
Rockville, MD 20850
800 498-2071
www.asha.org

Note: Adapted in part from the Bureau of Labor Statistics, US Department of Labor, *Occupational Outlook Handbook*, Audiologists, at *www.bls.gov/oco/ocos085.htm*.

Audiologist

Alabama

Auburn University
Audiologist Prgm
Dept of Comm Disorders
1199 Haley Center
Auburn University, AL 36849-5232
www.auburn.edu

University of South Alabama
Audiologist Prgm
Dept of Speech Pathology and Audiology
2000 University Commons
Mobile, AL 36688-0002
www.southalabama.edu/alliedhealth/speechandhearing

Arizona

AT Still University of Health Sciences
Audiologist Prgm
Department of Audiology
5850 E Still Cir
Mesa, AZ 85206
www.atsu.edu

Arizona State University
Audiologist Prgm
Dept of Speech and Hearing
PO Box 870102
Tempe, AZ 85287-0102
www.asu.edu/clas/shs/pg-aud.html

University of Arizona
Audiologist Prgm
Speech, Language, and Hearing Sciences
PO Box 210071
Tucson, AZ 85721
www.slhs.arizona.edu

Arkansas

University of Arkansas at Little Rock
Audiologist Prgm
Coll of Related Health Profs
5820 Asher Ave Univ Plz Ste 600
Little Rock, AR 72204-1099
www.uams.edu/chrp/audiospeech

California

California State University - Los Angeles
Audiologist Prgm
Dept of Communication Disorders
5151 State University Dr
Los Angeles, CA 90032
www.calstatela.edu

San Diego State University
Cosponsor: University of California San Diego
Audiologist Prgm
School of Speech, Language, and Hearing Sciences
5500 Campanile Dr MC-1518
San Diego, CA 92182-1518
http://chhs.sdsu.edu/slhs/audmain.php

Colorado

University of Colorado at Boulder
Audiologist Prgm
2501 Kittredge Loop Rd
UCB 409
Boulder, CO 80309-0409
www.colorado.edu/slhs

University of Northern Colorado
Audiologist Prgm
Audiology and Speech Language Sciences
Gunter 1400, Box 140
Greeley, CO 80639-0030
www.unco.edu/nhs/asls

Connecticut

University of Connecticut
Audiologist Prgm
Communication Sciences
850 Bolton Rd, Unit 1085
Storrs, CT 06268-1085

District of Columbia

Gallaudet University
Audiologist Prgm
Audiology and Speech-Lang Path
800 Florida Ave NE
Washington, DC 20002-3695
www.gallaudet.edu

Florida

Nova Southeastern University
Audiologist Prgm
3200 S University Dr
Fort Lauderdale, FL 33328
www.nova.edu/aud

University of Florida
Audiologist Prgm
Communication Processes and Disorders
335 Dauer Hall, PO Box 117420
Gainesville, FL 32611-7420
www.clas.ufl.edu/cpd

University of South Florida
Audiologist Prgm
Communication Sciences and Disorders
4202 E Fowler Ave PCD 1017
Tampa, FL 33620-8150
www.usf.edu

Idaho

Idaho State University
Audiologist Prgm
Communication Sciences & Disorders and Education of
   the Deaf
Box 8116
Pocatello, ID 83209-0009
www.isu.edu/csed

Illinois

Univ of Illinois at Urbana-Champaign
Audiologist Prgm
220 Speech and Hearing Sci Bldg
901 S 6th St
Champaign, IL 61820
www.shs.uiuc.edu

Rush University Medical Center
Audiologist Prgm
Comm Disorders and Sciences
1653 W Congress Pkwy
Chicago, IL 60612
www.rushu.rush.edu/health/dept.html

Northern Illinois University
Audiologist Prgm
Communicative Disorders
DeKalb, IL 60115-2899
www.chhs.niu.edu/comd

Northwestern University
Audiologist Prgm
Comm Sciences and Disorders
2240 Campus Dr
Evanston, IL 60208-3540
www.northwestern.edu/csd

Illinois State University
Audiologist Prgm
Speech Pathology and Audiology
Fairchild Hall #204
Normal, IL 61790-4720
www.ilstu.edu

Indiana

Indiana University - Bloomington
Audiologist Prgm
Speech and Hearing Sciences
200 S Jordan Ave
Bloomington, IN 47405-7002
www.indiana.edu/~sphs/

Ball State University
Audiologist Prgm
Speech Pathology and Audiology
2000 University Ave
Muncie, IN 47306
www.bsu.edu/spaa

Purdue University
Audiologist Prgm
Speech, Language, and Hearing Sciences
500 Oval Dr
West Lafayette, IN 47907-2038
www.sla.purdue.edu/academic/aus

Iowa

University of Iowa
Audiologist Prgm
Speech Pathology and Audiology
119 SHC
Iowa City, IA 52242
www.shc.uiowa.edu

Kansas

University of Kansas
Audiologist Prgm
Intercampus Program in Communicative Disorders
3901 Rainbow Blvd
Kansas City, KS 66160-7605
www.ukans.edu/~splh/
Prgm Dir: John Ferraro, PhD
Tel: 913 588-5937   *Fax:* 913 588-5923
E-mail: jferraro@kumc.edu

Wichita State University
Audiologist Prgm
Communication Sciences and Disorders
1845 N Fairmount
Wichita, KS 67260-0075
www.wichita.edu/csd

Kentucky

University of Louisville
Audiologist Prgm
Surgery/Graduate Program in Communicative Disorders
Health Sciences Center, Myers Hall
Louisville, KY 40292
www.louisville.edu/medschool/surgery/com-disorders

Louisiana

Louisiana State Univ Health Sciences Center
Audiologist Prgm
Communication Disorders
1900 Gravier St
New Orleans, LA 70112
www.alliedhealth.lsuhsc.edu

Louisiana Tech University
Audiologist Prgm
Dept of Speech
PO Box 3165
Ruston, LA 71272
www.latech.edu/slp-aud

Maryland

Univ of Maryland at College Park
Audiologist Prgm
Hearing and Speech Science
Le Frak Hall
College Park, MD 20742
www.bsos.umd.edu/hesp/

Towson University
Audiologist Prgm
Audiology, Speech Language Pathology and Deaf Studies
8000 York Rd
Towson, MD 21252
www.towson.edu

Massachusetts

University of Massachusetts - Amherst
Audiologist Prgm
Communication Disorders
715 N Pleasant St
Amherst, MA 01003-9304
www.umass.edu/sphhs/comdis

Northeastern University
Audiologist Prgm
Speech-Language Pathology and Audiology
106 Forsyth Bldg, 360 Huntington Ave
Boston, MA 02115
www.neu.edu

Michigan

Wayne State University
Audiologist Prgm
Communication Sciences and Disorders
207 Rackham Building
Detroit, MI 48202
www.clas.wayne.edu/CSD

Western Michigan University
Audiologist Prgm
Speech Pathology and Audiology
Kalamazoo, MI 49008-5355
www.wmich.edu/hhs/sppa

Central Michigan University
Audiologist Prgm
Communication Disorders
Health Professions Bldg 1183
Mount Pleasant, MI 48859
www.cmich.edu/chp/x1468.xml
Prgm Dir: Gerald Church, PhD CCC-A
Tel: 989 774-7301   *Fax:* 989 774-2799
E-mail: churc1g@cmich.edu

Minnesota

University of Minnesota
Audiologist Prgm
115 Shevlin Hall
164 Pillsbury Dr SE
Minneapolis, MN 55455
www.slhs.umn.edu

Mississippi

University of Southern Mississippi
Audiologist Prgm
Dept of Speech and Hearing Sciences
PO Box 5092
Hattiesburg, MS 39406-5092
www.usm.edu/shs

Missouri

Missouri State University
Audiologist Prgm
Communication Disorders
901 S National Ave
Springfield, MO 65897-0095
www.missouristate.edu/csd/

Washington University
Audiologist Prgm
Program in Audiology and Communication Sciences
660 S Euclid Ave, Campus Box 8042
St Louis, MO 63110
http://pacs.wustl.edu
Prgm Dir: William Clark, Professor
Tel: 314 747-0101   *Fax:* 314 747-0105
E-mail: clarkw@wustl.edu

Nebraska

University of Nebraska - Lincoln
Audiologist Prgm
Dept of Special Education and Communication
    Disorders
301 Barkley Center
Lincoln, NE 68583-0234
www.unl.edu/Barkley/audiology

New Jersey

Montclair State University
Audiologist Prgm
Dept of Communication Sciences and Disorders
Upper Montclair, NJ 07043

New York

University at Buffalo - SUNY
Audiologist Prgm
Dept of Communicative Disorders and Sciences
122 Cary Hall
Buffalo, NY 14214-3005
http://cdswebserver.med.buffalo.edu/drupal/

Adelphi University Long Island AuD Consortium
Cosponsor: Hofstra/St John's Universities
Audiologist Prgm
Hy Weinberg Ctr
158 Cambridge Ave
Garden City, NY 11530
http://education.adelphi.edu/audiology/

CUNY Hunter College
Cosponsor: Brooklyn College
Audiologist Prgm
Clinical Doctoral Programs
365 Fifth Ave
New York, NY 10016
www.gc.cuny.edu

Syracuse University
Audiologist Prgm
Dept of Communication Sciences and Disorders
805 S Crouse Ave
Syracuse, NY 13244-2280
http://thecollege.syr.edu/depts/csd

North Carolina

University of North Carolina - Chapel Hill
Audiologist Prgm
Division of Speech and Hearing Sciences
CB 7190 Wing D Medical School
Chapel Hill, NC 27599-7190
www.med.unc.edu/ahs/sphs

East Carolina University
Audiologist Prgm
Dept of Communication Sciences and Disorders
College of Allied Health Sciences
Health Sciences Bldg
Greenville, NC 27858-4353
www.ecu.edu/csd/

Ohio

Kent State University Northeast Ohio AuD Consortium
Cosponsor: University of Akron
Audiologist Prgm
225 S Main St
Akron, OH 44308
www.kent.edu/aud

Ohio University
Audiologist Prgm
School of Hearing, Speech and Language Sciences
Grover Center W218
Athens, OH 45701-2979
www.cats.ohiou.edu/hearingspeech

University of Cincinnati
Audiologist Prgm
Communication Sciences and Disorders
Mail Station 379
Cincinnati, OH 45221-0379
www.uc.edu/csd

The Ohio State University
Audiologist Prgm
Dept of Speech and Hearing Sciences
110 Pressey Hall, 1070 Carmack Rd
Columbus, OH 43210-1002
www.osu.edu/sphs

Oklahoma

Univ of Oklahoma Health Sciences Center
Audiologist Prgm
Communication Sciences and Disorders
825 NE 14th, PO Box 26901
Oklahoma City, OK 73190
www.ah.ouhsc.edu/csd

Pennsylvania

Bloomsburg University
Audiologist Prgm
Dept of Audiology and Speech Pathology
400 E 2nd St, Centennial Hall
Bloomsburg, PA 17815-1301
www.bloomu.edu

Salus University
Audiologist Prgm
George S Osborne Coll of Aud
8360 Old York Rd
Elkins Park, PA 19027
www.salus.edu/audiology/

University of Pittsburgh
Audiologist Prgm
Communication Science and Disorders
4033 Fobes Tower, 3600 Atwood St
Pittsburgh, PA 15260
www.shrs.pitt.edu/csd/

South Dakota

University of South Dakota
Audiologist Prgm
Dept of Communication Disorders
414 E Clark St
Vermillion, SD 57069-2390
www.usd.edu/dcom

Tennessee

East Tennessee State University
Audiologist Prgm
Dept of Communicative Disorders
PO Box 70643
Johnson City, TN 37614-0643
www.etsu.edu/cpah/commdis

University of Tennessee - Knoxville
Audiologist Prgm
Audiology and Speech Pathology
578 S Stadium Hall
Knoxville, TN 37996-0740
http://web.utk.edu/~aspweb

University of Memphis
Audiologist Prgm
School of Audiology and Speech-Language Pathology
807 Jefferson Ave
Memphis, TN 38105
www.ausp.memphis.edu

Vanderbilt University Medical Center
Audiologist Prgm
Hearing and Speech Sciences
1215 21st Ave S, Rm 8310
Nashville, TN 37232-8718
http://vanderbiltbillwilkersoncenter.com/dhss.html

Texas

University of Texas at Austin
Audiologist Prgm
Communication Sciences and Disorders
1 University Station, A1100
Austin, TX 78712-1089
http://csd.utexas.edu/graduate.html

Lamar University
Audiologist Prgm
Dept of Communication
Box 10076, Lamar Station
Beaumont, TX 77710
www.lamar.edu

COMMUNICATION SCIENCES

University of Texas at Dallas
Audiologist Prgm
Program in Communication Disorders
1966 Inwood Rd
Dallas, TX 75235-7298
http://bbs.utdallas.edu

University of North Texas
Audiologist Prgm
Dept of Speech and Hearing Sciences
PO Box 305010
Denton, TX 76203-5010
www.unt.edu

Texas Tech Univ Health Sciences Center
Audiologist Prgm
Dept of Speech, Language, and Hearing Sciences
Stop 6073 - 3601 4th St
Lubbock, TX 79430
www.ttuhsc.edu/SAH

Utah

Utah State University
Audiologist Prgm
Comm Disorders and Deaf Educ
1000 Old Main Hill
Logan, UT 84322-1000
www.usu.edu

University of Utah
Audiologist Prgm
390 South 1530 East
Rm 1201 BEH SCI
Salt Lake City, UT 84112-0252
www.health.utah.edu/csd/

Virginia

James Madison University
Audiologist Prgm
Communication Sciences and Disorders
MSC 4304
Harrisonburg, VA 22807
www.jmu.edu

Washington

University of Washington
Audiologist Prgm
Speech and Hearing Sciences
1417 NE 42nd St
Seattle, WA 98105-6246

West Virginia

West Virginia University
Audiologist Prgm
Speech Pathology and Audiology
805 Allen Hall, Box 6122
Morgantown, WV 26506-6122
www.wvu.edu/~speechpa

Wisconsin

University of Wisconsin - Madison
Cosponsor: University of Wisconsin - Stevens Point
Audiologist Prgm
Communicative Disorders
1975 Willow Dr, Goodnight Hall
Madison, WI 53706
www.comdis.wisc.edu

Audiologist

Programs*	Class Capacity	Begins	Length (months)	Award	Res. Tuition	Non-res. Tuition	Offers:† 1	2	3	4
Kansas										
Univ of Kansas (Kansas City)	10	Jun Aug Jan	48	Dipl, AuD, PhD	$9,414	$21,000	•		•	•
Michigan										
Central Michigan Univ (Mount Pleasant)	40	Aug	48	AuD	$19,368	$30,600			•	
Missouri										
Washington Univ (St Louis)	12	Aug	48	Dipl, AuD	$31,500	$31,500			•	

*Data are shown only for programs that completed the 2011 AMA Survey of Health Professions Education Programs.

†Key to Offers: 1: Evening or weekend classes; 2: Non-English instruction; 3: Cultural competence instruction; 4: Distance education component.

Career Description
Speech-language pathologists are professionals who are educated in the study of human communication, its development, and its disorders. Speech-language pathologists work with people with reduced speech intelligibility; with speech rhythm and fluency problems, such as stuttering; with voice quality problems, such as inappropriate pitch or harsh voice; with problems understanding and producing spoken and written language; with cognitive communication impairments, such as attention, memory, and problem-solving disorders; and with hearing loss for people who use hearing aids or cochlear implants, in order to develop auditory skills and improve communication. They also work with people who have swallowing difficulties and those who do not have communication disorders but who would like to improve their presentation skills or modify an accent.

Speech and language difficulties can result from a variety of causes, including stroke, brain injury, or other neurologic conditions, developmental delays, autism, cerebral palsy, cleft palate, voice pathology, hearing impairment, or social/behavioral disorders. Speech-language pathologists use written and oral tests, observation and a variety of formative and summative assessments as well as special instruments, to diagnose the nature and extent of impairment and to record and analyze speech, language, and swallowing irregularities. For individuals with little or no speech production, speech-language pathologists may select augmentative or alternative communication methods, including manual and electronic communication systems, and teach their use. They help patients to develop, or recover, functional communication skills so patients can fulfill their educational, vocational, and social roles.

Speech-language pathologists often collaborate as a member of a multidisciplinary team with other education and health care professionals, such as teachers, physicians, social workers, and psychologists. They counsel individuals and their families concerning communication disorders and how to cope with the stress and misunderstanding that often accompany them. They also work with family members to recognize and change behavior patterns that impede communication and treatment and to show them communication-enhancing techniques to use at home.

A master's degree is required to work as a speech-language pathologist. A doctoral degree (PhD) is preferred in some career paths, such as college teaching and research.

Working with an understanding of the full range of human communication and its disorders, speech-language pathologists:
- Evaluate and diagnose speech, language, and swallowing disorders in individuals of all ages, from infants to the elderly
- Treat speech, language, and swallowing disorders
- Provide consultation for those who may be at risk for communication disorders
In addition, speech-language pathologists may:
- Prepare future professionals in colleges and universities
- Engage in research to enhance knowledge about human communication processes and investigate behavioral patterns associated with communication disorders

Employment Characteristics
Speech-language pathologists may work in a wide range of settings, including schools, universities, hospitals, rehabilitation centers, skilled nursing facilities, community clinics, geriatric facilities, home health care services, and public health departments, or in private practice.

Salary
Salaries of speech-language pathologists depend on educational background, specialty, and experience, along with the geographical location and type of setting in which they work. According to the ASHA 2010 Schools Survey Annual Salary Report, the median salary for ASHA-certified speech-language pathologists was $58,000 for those employed on an academic year (i.e., 9- to 10-month) basis and $65,000 for those on a calendar year (i.e., 11- to 12-month) basis. The 2010 median starting salary for certified speech-language pathologists in school settings with 1 to 3 years of experience in the professions was $45,200 for an academic year appointment. The median calendar year salary for management positions was $83,000.

According to the ASHA 2011 Health Care Survey Salary Report, the mean salary for ASHA-certified speech-language pathologists was $70,000. The 2011 median salary for certified speech-language pathologists in health care settings with four to six years' experience was $63,000. The median calendar-year salary for management positions was $90,000. Good benefits packages, such as insurance programs and leave, are usually available to speech-language pathologists.

Employment Outlook
The combination of growth in the occupation and an expected increase in retirements over the coming years should create excellent job opportunities for speech-language pathologists. Employment is expected to grow by 23 percent from 2010 to 2020, faster than the average for all occupations (*www.bls.gov/oco/ocos099.htm*). More frequent recognition of problems in preschool and school-age children by teachers and parents, combined with the increased number of older citizens and medical advances, have created a growing need for speech and language services. In addition, opportunities for employment in research and higher education are expected to increase as baby boomers currently in these positions retire. Clinical opportunities will be especially strong for those with bilingual and multicultural expertise. There are shortages of qualified personnel in some areas of the country, especially in inner city, rural, and less populated areas. Job opportunities in medically related areas are expected to grow at an above-average rate. Many states now require that all newborns be screened for hearing loss and receive appropriate early intervention services. Greater awareness of the importance of early identification and diagnosis of speech, language, swallowing, and hearing disorders will also increase employment opportunities.

Educational Programs
Approximately 250 accredited universities in the United States offer graduate education programs in speech-language pathology that prepare students for entry into independent professional practice. A master's degree is the entry-level degree required for practice. Clinical and research doctoral degree programs also are available as advanced degree programs for further study of speech-language pathology and speech or language science.

COMMUNICATION SCIENCES

Length. Full-time study typically takes 2 years (including summers) to complete a master's degree program in speech-language pathology. Graduate education in speech-language pathology requires a combination of academic and clinical course work as well as clinical internships.

Prerequisites. Knowledge of the biological sciences, physical sciences, mathematics, and behavioral or social sciences are required for the ASHA Certificate of Clinical Competence in Speech-Language Pathology. Undergraduate programs in communication sciences and disorders will provide a background in the sciences, linguistics, phonetics, psychology, normal speech, and language development, and introductory course work in speech-language pathology. Students without an undergraduate degree in communication sciences and disorders may be required to complete prerequisite course work. Excellent oral and written communication skills are expected.

Curriculum. Graduate programs should offer a curriculum to allow a student to meet the knowledge and skills necessary to enter practice in speech-language pathology. A typical graduate program of study will provide a curriculum that is sufficient for students to acquire and demonstrate knowledge of basic human communication and swallowing processes, including their biological, neurological, acoustic, psychological, developmental, and linguistic and cultural bases that includes articulation, fluency, voice and resonance, receptive and expressive language, hearing (including the impact on speech and language) swallowing, cognitive aspects of communication, and social aspects of communication. Coursework also includes principles and methods of prevention, assessment and intervention, standards of ethical conduct, processes and integration of research principles into evidence-based clinical practice, and contemporary professional issues. Opportunities to work in a variety of clinical settings and with a diverse range of clients should be provided during the graduate program of study.

Licensure and Certification

In most states, speech-language pathologists must comply with state regulatory (licensure) standards and/or have state teacher certification to practice in specific educational settings. Forty-eight states and the District of Columbia require speech-language pathologists to have a license to practice. Fifteen states currently require a license to practice in any work setting.

A graduate degree, completion of a 36-week full-time supervised clinical experience, and passage of a national examination are typically required to achieve the credentials. Individuals should contact the appropriate state licensure board or teacher certification agency for more information about requirements. ASHA's Certificate of Clinical Competence in Speech-Language Pathology (CCC-SLP), a nationally recognized credential, offers certificate holders ease in qualifying for state credentials. Although the CCC-SLP is not typically required for state licensure, the requirements leading to the CCC are generally required. Possession of the CCC-SLP qualifies individuals for certain employment opportunities, promotions, and salary supplements, and typically required for reimbursement of services provided by public and private insurance.

Inquiries

For information about a specific program, contact the director of the speech-language pathology program in care of the institution listed. Program information can be accessed on ASHA's web site at: *www.asha.org/students/academic/EdFind*.

For additional information about the profession or academic program accreditation, contact:

American Speech-Language-Hearing Association (ASHA)
2200 Research Boulevard
Rockville, MD 20850
800 498-2071
www.asha.org

Speech-Language Pathologist

Alabama

Auburn University
Speech-Language Pathology Prgm
Dept of Communication
1199 Haley Center
Auburn University, AL 36849-5232
www.auburn.edu

University of South Alabama
Speech-Language Pathology Prgm
Dept of Speech Pathology and Audiology
2000 University Commons
Mobile, AL 36688-0002
www.southalabama.edu/alliedhealth/speechandhearing

University of Montevallo
Speech-Language Pathology Prgm
Comm Science and Disorders
Station 6720
Montevallo, AL 35115-6720
www.montevallo.edu

Alabama A&M University
Speech-Language Pathology Prgm
Dept of Special Education
PO Box 580
Normal, AL 35762
www.aamu.edu

University of Alabama
Speech-Language Pathology Prgm
Dept of Comm Disorders
PO Box 870242
Tuscaloosa, AL 35487-0242
www.as.ua.edu/comdis/

Arizona

Northern Arizona University
Speech-Language Pathology Prgm
Communication Sciences and Disorders
NAU Box 15045
Flagstaff, AZ 86011-5045
http://jan.ucc.nau.edu/~csd-p/index.php

Arizona State University
Speech-Language Pathology Prgm
Speech and Hearing Science
PO Box 870102
Tempe, AZ 85287-0102
www.asu.edu/clas/shs

University of Arizona
Speech-Language Pathology Prgm
Dept of Speech and Hearing
PO Box 210071
Tucson, AZ 85721-0071
http://slhs.arizona.edu

Arkansas

University of Central Arkansas
Speech-Language Pathology Prgm
Box 4985
Conway, AR 72035-0001
www.uca.edu/chas

University of Arkansas
Speech-Language Pathology Prgm
Program in Communication Disorders
410 Arkansas Ave
Fayetteville, AR 72701
www.uark.edu/depts/coehp/cdis.html

University of Arkansas at Little Rock
Speech-Language Pathology Prgm
Coll of Related Health Profs
5820 Asher Ave Univ Plz Ste 600
Little Rock, AR 72204-1099
www.uams.edu/chrp/audiospeech

Harding University
Speech-Language Pathology Prgm
Dept of Comm and Sciences and Disorders
HU Box 10872
Searcy, AR 72149
www.harding.edu/cd

Arkansas State University
Speech-Language Pathology Prgm
PO Box 910
State University, AR 72467-0904
http://conhp.astate.edu/communicationdisorders/

California

California State University - Chico
Speech-Language Pathology Prgm
Dept of Communication
1st and Normal Sts
Chico, CA 95929-0350
www.csuchico.edu/cmas

California State University - Fresno
Speech-Language Pathology Prgm
Dept of Communicative Sci and Disorder
5048 N Jackson
Fresno, CA 93740-8022
www.csufresno.edu/csd

California State University - Fullerton
Speech-Language Pathology Prgm
Dept of Human Communication Studies
800 N State College Blvd
Fullerton, CA 92834
www.fullerton.edu

California State University - East Bay
Speech-Language Pathology Prgm
Communicative Sciences and Disorders
25800 Carlos Bee Blvd
Hayward, CA 94542-3065
http://class.csueastbay.edu/commsci

Loma Linda University
Speech-Language Pathology Prgm
Nichol Hall, Rm A804
Loma Linda, CA 92350
http://llu.edu

California State University - Long Beach
Speech-Language Pathology Prgm
Communicative Disorders
1250 Bellflower Blvd
Long Beach, CA 90840-2501
www.csulb.edu/cdweb

California State University - Los Angeles
Speech-Language Pathology Prgm
Communication Disorders
5151 State University Dr
Los Angeles, CA 90032
www.calstatela.edu

California State University - Northridge
Speech-Language Pathology Prgm
Dept of Communicative Disorders
18111 Nordhoff St
Northridge, CA 91330-8279
www.csun.edu

Chapman University
Speech-Language Pathology Prgm
College of Educational Studies Comm Sci and Disorders
One University Drive
Orange, CA 92666
www.chapman.edu/soe

University of Redlands
Speech-Language Pathology Prgm
Truesdail Center for Communication Disorders
PO Box 3080, 1200 E Colton Ave
Redlands, CA 92373-0999
www.redlands.edu

California State University - Sacramento
Speech-Language Pathology Prgm
Dept of Speech Pathology and Audiology
6000 J St
Sacramento, CA 95819-6071
www.csus.edu

San Diego State University
Speech-Language Pathology Prgm
School of Speech, Language, and Hearing Sciences
5500 Campanile Dr
San Diego, CA 92182-1518
http://chhs.sdsu.edu/SLHS/

San Francisco State University
Speech-Language Pathology Prgm
1600 Holloway Ave
Burk Hall Rm 104
San Francisco, CA 94132-4158
www.sfsu.edu/~spedcd

San Jose State University
Speech-Language Pathology Prgm
Speech and Hearing Ctr
One Washington Square
San Jose, CA 95192-0079
www.sjsu.edu

California State University - San Marcos
Speech-Language Pathology Prgm
Communicative Sci & Disorders
UH 323
333 S Twin Oaks Valley Rd
San Marcos, CA 92096
http://csusm.edu/coe/

University of the Pacific
Speech-Language Pathology Prgm
Dept of Speech-Language Pathology
3601 Pacific Ave
Stockton, CA 95211
www.pacific.edu

Colorado

University of Colorado at Boulder
Speech-Language Pathology Prgm
2501 Kittredge Loop Rd
Campus Box 409
Boulder, CO 80309-0409
www.colorado.edu/slhs

University of Northern Colorado
Speech-Language Pathology Prgm
Audiology and Speech-Language Sciences
Gunter 1400, Box 140
Greeley, CO 80639-0030

Connecticut

Southern Connecticut State University
Speech-Language Pathology Prgm
Communication Disorders
501 Crescent St
New Haven, CT 06515
www.southernct.edu/dept

University of Connecticut
Speech-Language Pathology Prgm
Communication Sciences
850 Bolton Rd, Unit 1085
Storrs, CT 06269-1085

District of Columbia

Gallaudet University
Speech-Language Pathology Prgm
Audiology and Speech-Lang Path
800 Florida Ave NE
Washington, DC 20002-3695
www.gallaudet.edu

George Washington University
Speech-Language Pathology Prgm
Dept of Speech and Hearing Science
1922 F St NW
Washington, DC 20052
www.gwu.edu/sphr

Howard University
Speech-Language Pathology Prgm
Communication Sciences and Disorders
525 Bryant St NW
Washington, DC 20059
www.howard.edu

University of the District of Columbia
Speech-Language Pathology Prgm
Communication Sciences
4200 Connecticut Ave NW
Washington, DC 20008
www.udc.edu

Florida

Florida Atlantic University
Speech-Language Pathology Prgm
Communication Sciences and Disorders
777 Glades Rd, PO Box 3091
Boca Raton, FL 33431-0991
www.coe.fau.edu/csd/spa.htm

University of Florida
Speech-Language Pathology Prgm
Comm Processes and Disorders
335 Dauer Hall, PO Box 117420
Gainesville, FL 32611-7420
www.clas.ufl.edu/cpd

Florida International University
Speech-Language Pathology Prgm
HLS 143, University Park
Miami, FL 33199
http://chua2.fiu.edu/csd

Nova Southeastern University
Speech-Language Pathology Prgm
Communication Sciences and Disorders
1750 NE 167th St
North Miami, FL 33162-3017
www.fgse.nova.edu/slp

University of Central Florida
Speech-Language Pathology Prgm
Communicative Disorders
PO Box 162215
Orlando, FL 32826-2215
www.ucf.edu

Florida State University
Speech-Language Pathology Prgm
Communication Disorders
107 RRC (R-89
Tallahassee, FL 32306-1200
www.fsu.edu/~commdis

University of South Florida
Speech-Language Pathology Prgm
Comm Sciences and Disorders
4202 E Fowler Ave PCD 1017
Tampa, FL 33620-8150
www.usf.edu

Georgia

University of Georgia
Speech-Language Pathology Prgm
Comm Sciences and Disorders
516 Aderhold Hall
Athens, GA 30602
www.uga.edu

Georgia State University
Speech-Language Pathology Prgm
Communication Disorders
33 Gilmer St SE
Atlanta, GA 30303-3086
www.gsu.edu

University of West Georgia
Speech-Language Pathology Prgm
Dept Spec Educ and Spch Lang Path
1601 Maple St
Carrollton, GA 30118
http://coe.westga.edu/sedslp/

Armstrong Atlantic State University
Speech-Language Pathology Prgm
11935 Abercorn St
Savannah, GA 31419-1997
www.armstrong.edu

Valdosta State University
Speech-Language Pathology Prgm
Dept of Special Education
1500 N Patterson St
Valdosta, GA 31698-0102
www.valdosta.edu

Hawaii

University of Hawaii at Manoa
Speech-Language Pathology Prgm
Dept of Speech Pathology and Audiology
1410 Lower Campus Dr
Honolulu, HI 96822
www.hawaii.edu

Idaho

Idaho State University
Speech-Language Pathology Prgm
Communication Sciences & Disorders and Education of
    the Deaf
650 Memorial Dr, Bldg 68, Box 8116
Pocatello, ID 83209-8116
www.isu.edu/departments/spchpath

Illinois

Southern Illinois University Carbondale
Speech-Language Pathology Prgm
Comm Disorders and Sciences
1025 Lincoln Dr, Rehn Hall #308
Carbondale, IL 62901-4609
www.siu.edu/~rehab

Univ of Illinois at Urbana-Champaign
Speech-Language Pathology Prgm
220 Speech and Hearing Sci Bldg
901 S 6th St
Champaign, IL 61820
www.shs.uiuc.edu

Eastern Illinois University
Speech-Language Pathology Prgm
Comm Disorders and Sciences
600 Lincoln Ave
Charleston, IL 61920-3099
www.eiu.edu/~commdis/

Rush University Medical Center
Speech-Language Pathology Prgm
Communication Disorders and Sciences
1653 W Congress Pkwy
Chicago, IL 60612
www.rushu.rush.edu/health/dept.html

Saint Xavier University
Speech-Language Pathology Prgm
Comm Disorders and Sciences
3700 W 103rd St
Chicago, IL 60655
www.sxu.edu

Northern Illinois University
Speech-Language Pathology Prgm
Communicative Disorders
DeKalb, IL 60115-2899
www.comd.niu.edu

Southern Illinois University Edwardsville
Speech-Language Pathology Prgm
Founders Hall, Rm 1300
Campus Box 1147
Edwardsville, IL 62026-1147

Northwestern University
Speech-Language Pathology Prgm
Comm Sciences and Disorders
2240 Campus Dr
Evanston, IL 60208
www.communication.northwestern.edu/csd/

Western Illinois University
Speech-Language Pathology Prgm
Dept of Communication
121 Memorial Hall
Macomb, IL 61455-1390
www.wiu.edu/users/micom/wiu/csd/csd.htm

Illinois State University
Speech-Language Pathology Prgm
Speech Pathology and Audiology
Fairchild Hall #204
Normal, IL 61790-4720
www.ilstu.edu

Governors State University
Speech-Language Pathology Prgm
Communication Disorders
University Park, IL 60466
www.govst.edu

Indiana

Indiana University - Bloomington
Speech-Language Pathology Prgm
Speech and Hearing Sciences
200 S Jordan Ave
Bloomington, IN 47405-7002
www.indiana.edu/~sphs/

Ball State University
Speech-Language Pathology Prgm
Speech Pathology and Audiology
2000 University Ave
Muncie, IN 47306
www.bsu.edu/csh/spa

Indiana State University
Speech-Language Pathology Prgm
Department of Communication Disorders
8th & Sycamore St
Terre Haute, IN 47809
counseling.indstate.edu

Purdue University
Speech-Language Pathology Prgm
Audiology and Speech Sciences
500 Oval Dr
West Lafayette, IN 47907-2038
www.sla.purdue.edu/academic/aus

Iowa

University of Northern Iowa
Speech-Language Pathology Prgm
Communicative Disorders
Cedar Falls, IA 50614-0356
www.uni.edu/comdis

St Ambrose University
Speech-Language Pathology Prgm
Colg of Educ and Hlth Sci
518 West Locust St
Davenport, IA 52803
www.sau.edu/Academic_Programs/
    Master_of_Speech-Language_Pathology.html

University of Iowa
Speech-Language Pathology Prgm
Speech Pathology and Audiology
Iowa City, IA 52242
www.shc.uiowa.edu

Kansas

Fort Hays State University
Speech-Language Pathology Prgm
Communication Disorders
600 Park St
Hays, KS 67601
www.fhsu.edu/commdis/

University of Kansas
Speech-Language Pathology Prgm
Intercampus Program in Communicative Disorders
3001 Dole Center
1000 Sunnyside Ave
Lawrence, KS 66045
www.ku.edu/~splh/ipcd

Kansas State University
Speech-Language Pathology Prgm
Comm Sciences and Disorders
Justin Hall 303
Manhattan, KS 66506-1403
www.ksu.edu/humec/fshs/fshs.htm

Wichita State University
Speech-Language Pathology Prgm
Communication Sciences and Disorders
1845 N Fairmount
Wichita, KS 67260-0075
www.wichita.edu/csd

Kentucky

Western Kentucky University
Speech-Language Pathology Prgm
1 Big Red Way
TPH, Rm 113
Bowling Green, KY 42101-3576
www.wku.edu

University of Kentucky
Speech-Language Pathology Prgm
Communication Disorders
900 S Limestone St, Suite 124G
Lexington, KY 40504-0200
www.uky.edu

University of Louisville
Speech-Language Pathology Prgm
Surgery/Graduate Program in Communicative Disorders
Health Sciences Center, Myers Hall
Louisville, KY 40292
www.louisville.edu/medschool/surgery/com-disorders

Murray State University
Speech-Language Pathology Prgm
Communication Disorders
125 Alexander Hall
Murray, KY 42071-3340
www.murraystate.edu

Eastern Kentucky University
Speech-Language Pathology Prgm
Communication Disorders
245 Wallace Bldg
521 Lancaster Ave
Richmond, KY 40475-3102
www.specialed.eku.edu/CD
Prgm Dir: Charlotte Hubbard, PhD CCC-SLP
Tel: 859 622-4442   *Fax:* 859 622-4443
E-mail: charlotte.hubbard@eku.edu

Louisiana

Louisiana State Univ and A&M College
Speech-Language Pathology Prgm
Communication Disorders
Music & Dramatic Arts Bldg, Rm 163
Baton Rouge, LA 70803-2606
www.lsu.edu

Southern Univ and A&M College
Speech-Language Pathology Prgm
Speech Pathology and Audiology
PO Box 11295
Baton Rouge, LA 70813
www.subr.edu

Southeastern Louisiana University
Speech-Language Pathology Prgm
Department of Communication Sciences and Disorders
PO Box 10879 - SLU
Hammond, LA 70402
www.selu.edu/csd

University of Louisiana at Lafayette
Speech-Language Pathology Prgm
Department of Communicative Disorders
PO Box 43170
Lafayette, LA 70504
http://speechandlanguage.louisiana.edu
Prgm Dir: Nancye Roussel, PhD
Tel: 337 482-6721   *Fax:* 337 482-6195
E-mail: ncroussel@louisiana.edu

University of Louisiana at Monroe
Speech-Language Pathology Prgm
Department of Communicative Disorders
College of Health Sciences
700 University Ave
Monroe, LA 71209-1032
www.ulm.edu/codi

Louisiana State Univ Health Sciences Center
Speech-Language Pathology Prgm
Communication Disorders
1900 Gravier St
New Orleans, LA 70112
www.alliedhealth.lsuhsc.edu

Louisiana Tech University
Speech-Language Pathology Prgm
Dept of Speech
PO Box 3165
Ruston, LA 71272
www.latech.edu

LSU Health Science Center Shreveport
Speech-Language Pathology Prgm
Mollie E Webb Speech and Hearing Center
3735 Blair Dr
Shreveport, LA 71106
www.sh.lsuhsc.edu/ah

Maine

University of Maine - Orono
Speech-Language Pathology Prgm
Communication Sciences and Disorders
5724 Dunn Hall
Orono, ME 04469-5724
www.umaine.edu/comscidis/

Maryland

Loyola University Maryland
Speech-Language Pathology Prgm
Speech-Language Pathology and Audiology
4501 N Charles St
Baltimore, MD 21210
www.loyola.edu/Clinics

Univ of Maryland at College Park
Speech-Language Pathology Prgm
Hearing and Speech Science
Le Frak Hall
College Park, MD 20742
www.bsos.umd.edu/hesp/

Towson University
Speech-Language Pathology Prgm
Audiology, Speech Language Pathology and Deaf Studies
8000 York Rd
Towson, MD 21252-0001
www.towson.edu

Massachusetts

University of Massachusetts - Amherst
Speech-Language Pathology Prgm
Communication Disorders
715 N Pleasant St
Amherst, MA 01003-9304
www.umass.edu/sphhs/comdis

Boston University
Speech-Language Pathology Prgm
Sargent Coll of Hlth and Rehab Sciences
635 Commonwealth Ave
Boston, MA 02215
www.bu.edu/sargent

Emerson College
Speech-Language Pathology Prgm
Communication Disorders
120 Beacon St
Boston, MA 02116-4624
www.emerson.edu

MGH Institute of Health Professions
Speech-Language Pathology Prgm
Comm Sciences and Disorders
36 1st Ave
Charlestown Navy Yard
Boston, MA 02129-4557
www.mghihp.edu

Northeastern University
Speech-Language Pathology Prgm
Speech-Language Pathology and Audiology
106 Forsyth Bldg, 360 Huntington Ave
Boston, MA 02115

Worcester State College
Speech-Language Pathology Prgm
Communication Disorders
486 Chandler St
Worcester, MA 01602-2597
www.worcester.edu

Michigan

Wayne State University
Speech-Language Pathology Prgm
Communication Sciences and Disorders
207 Rackham Building
Detroit, MI 48202
www.clas.wayne.edu/CSD

Michigan State University
Speech-Language Pathology Prgm
101 Oyer Bldg
East Lansing, MI 48824-1220
www.msu.edu

Calvin College
Speech-Language Pathology Prgm
Div Arts Lang & Ed
Spch Path & Aud
1810 E Beltline SE
Grand Rapids, MI 49546
www.calvin.edu

Western Michigan University
Speech-Language Pathology Prgm
Speech Pathology and Audiology
Kalamazoo, MI 49008-5355
www.wmich.edu/hhs/sppa

Central Michigan University
Speech-Language Pathology Prgm
Communication Disorders
HPB 2187
Mount Pleasant, MI 48859
www.cmich.edu

Eastern Michigan University
Speech-Language Pathology Prgm
110 Porter Bldg
Ypsilanti, MI 48197
www.emich.edu/public/speced/speced.html

Minnesota

University of Minnesota - Duluth
Speech-Language Pathology Prgm
Communicative Disorders
1207 Ordean Court, 221 Bohannon Hall
Duluth, MN 55812
www.d.umn.edu/csd

Minnesota State University - Mankato
Speech-Language Pathology Prgm
Communication Disorders
103 Armstrong Hall
Mankato, MN 56001
http://ahn.mnsu.edu/cd/

University of Minnesota
Speech-Language Pathology Prgm
115 Shevlin Hall
164 Pillsbury Dr SE
Minneapolis, MN 55455
www.slhs.umn.edu

Minnesota State University - Moorhead
Speech-Language Pathology Prgm
Speech-Language-Hearing Sciences
1104 7th Ave S
Moorhead, MN 56563
www.mnstate.edu/slhs

St Cloud State University
Speech-Language Pathology Prgm
A216 Education Bldg
720 4th Ave S
St Cloud, MN 56301
www.stcloudstate.edu/csd

Mississippi

Mississippi University for Women
Speech-Language Pathology Prgm
Speech-Language Pathology/Audiology
PO Box W-1340
Columbus, MS 39701
www.muw.edu/speech_hear/slp.htm

University of Southern Mississippi
Speech-Language Pathology Prgm
Dept of Speech and Hearing Sciences
PO Box 5092
Hattiesburg, MS 39406-5092
www.usm.edu/shs

Jackson State University
Speech-Language Pathology Prgm
Dept of Communication Disorders
University Center, 3825 Ridgewood Rd, Box 23
Jackson, MS 39211-6453
www.jsums.edu

University of Mississippi
Speech-Language Pathology Prgm
Communicative Disorders
PO Box 1848
University, MS 38677
www.olemiss.edu/depts/comm_disorders

Missouri

Southeast Missouri State University
Speech-Language Pathology Prgm
Dept of Communication Disorders
One University Plaza
Cape Girardeau, MO 63701-4799
www.semo.edu

University of Missouri
Speech-Language Pathology Prgm
Communication Science and Disorders
303 Lewis Hall
Columbia, MO 65211
http://shp.missouri.edu/csd/
Prgm Dir: Barbara McLay, MA CCC-A
Tel: 573 882-3873   *Fax:* 573 884-8686
E-mail: mclayb@health.missouri.edu

Rockhurst University
Speech-Language Pathology Prgm
Communication Sciences and Disorders
1100 Rockhurst Rd
Kansas City, MO 64110
www.rockhurst.edu

Truman State University
Speech-Language Pathology Prgm
Communication Disorders
Barnett Hall 222
Kirksville, MO 63501
http://comdis.truman.edu

Missouri State University
Speech-Language Pathology Prgm
Communication Disorders
901 S National Ave
Springfield, MO 65804-0095
www.missouristate.edu/csd

Fontbonne University
Speech-Language Pathology Prgm
Communication Disorders and Deaf Education
6800 Wydown Blvd
St Louis, MO 63105
www.fontbonne.edu

Saint Louis University
Speech-Language Pathology Prgm
Communication Sciences & Disorders
3570 Lindell Blvd
McGannon 23
St Louis, MO 63108
www.slu.edu/x10651.xml

University of Central Missouri
Speech-Language Pathology Prgm
Speech Pathology and Audiology
Martin Bldg 41
Warrensburg, MO 64093
www.cmsu.edu

Montana

University of Montana
Speech-Language Pathology Prgm
School of Edu, Dept of Communicative Sci ad Disorders
32 Campus Drive, Curry Health Center
Missoula, MT 59812

Nebraska

University of Nebraska - Kearney
Speech-Language Pathology Prgm
Communication Disorders Department
College of Education
Kearney, NE 68849-4597
www.unk.edu/departments/cdis

University of Nebraska - Lincoln
Speech-Language Pathology Prgm
Dept of Special Education and Communication
   Disorders
301 Barkley Center
Lincoln, NE 68583-0738
www.unl.edu/barkley/

University of Nebraska - Omaha
Speech-Language Pathology Prgm
Special Education and Communication Disorders
6001 Dodge St
Omaha, NE 68182-0054

Nevada

University of Nevada - Reno
Speech-Language Pathology Prgm
Dept of Speech Pathology and Audiology
Redfield Bldg/152
Reno, NV 89557-0046
www.medicine.nevada.edu/spa
Prgm Dir: Thomas Watterson, PhD
Tel: 775 784-4887   *Fax:* 775 784-4095
E-mail: twatterson@medicine.nevada.edu

New Hampshire

University of New Hampshire
Speech-Language Pathology Prgm
Dept of Communication Sciences and Disorders
4 Library Way, Hewitt Hall
Durham, NH 03824
www.unh.edu/communication-disorders

New Jersey

Richard Stockton College of New Jersey
Speech-Language Pathology Prgm
School of Health Sciences
Communication Disorders
101 Vera King Farris Dr
Galloway, NJ 08240
www2.stockton.edu

Seton Hall University
Speech-Language Pathology Prgm
400 S Orange Ave
South Orange, NJ 07079-2689
www.shu.edu

Kean University
Speech-Language Pathology Prgm
Dept of Communication Disorders and Deafness
1000 Morris Ave
Union, NJ 07083
www.kean.edu/~keangrad/grad_CE_slp.htm

Montclair State University
Speech-Language Pathology Prgm
Dept of Communication Sciences and Disorders
Speech Bldg
Upper Montclair, NJ 07043
www.montclair.edu

William Paterson Univ of New Jersey
Speech-Language Pathology Prgm
Communication Disorders
300 Pompton Rd
Wayne, NJ 07470
www.wpunj.edu

New Mexico

University of New Mexico
Speech-Language Pathology Prgm
Dept of Speech and Hearing Sciences
MSC01 1195, 1 Univ of New Mexico, 1700 Lomas Blvd NE
Albuquerque, NM 87131-0001
www.unm.edu/~sphrsci/

New Mexico State University
Speech-Language Pathology Prgm
Dept of Special Education/Communication Disorders
PO Box 30001/MSC 3SPE
Las Cruces, NM 88003
http://web.nmsu.edu/~nmsucd

Eastern New Mexico University
Speech-Language Pathology Prgm
Dept of Communicative Disorders
Station 3
Portales, NM 88130
www.enmu.edu

New York

College of St Rose
Speech-Language Pathology Prgm
Communication Disorders Dept
432 Western Ave, Box 100
Albany, NY 12203-1490
www.strose.edu

CUNY Herbert H Lehman College
Speech-Language Pathology Prgm
Dept of Speech-Language-Hearing Sciences
250 Bedford Park Blvd W
Bronx, NY 10468-1589
www.cuny.edu

CUNY Brooklyn College
Speech-Language Pathology Prgm
Speech-Language Pathology and Audiology
2900 Bedford Ave
Brooklyn, NY 11210
http://http//www.brooklyn.cuny.edu

Long Island University - Brooklyn Campus
Speech-Language Pathology Prgm
Dept of Communication Sciences and Disorders
One University Plaza
Brooklyn, NY 11201-8423
www.liu.edu

Touro College
Speech-Language Pathology Prgm
1610 E 19th St
Brooklyn, NY 11229
www.touro.edu/gsp/coursesforMS.asp

Long Island University - C W Post Campus
Speech-Language Pathology Prgm
Communication Sciences and Disorders
720 Northern Blvd
Brookville, NY 11548-1300
www.liunet.edu

Buffalo State, SUNY
Speech-Language Pathology Prgm
208 Ketchum Hall
1300 Elmwood Ave
Buffalo, NY 14222
www.buffalostate.edu/speech

University at Buffalo - SUNY
Speech-Language Pathology Prgm
Dept of Communicative Disorders and Sciences
122 Cary Hall
Buffalo, NY 14214-3005
www.wings.buffalo.edu/cds

Mercy College
Speech-Language Pathology Prgm
555 Broadway, Main Hall, Rm G15
Dobbs Ferry, NY 10522

CUNY Queens College
Speech-Language Pathology Prgm
Division of Arts & Humanities
Dept of Linguistics & Comm Disor
Speech-Lang-Hear Ctr/65-30 Kisse
Flushing, NY 11367
http://qcpages.qc.cuny.edu/lcd/csd

SUNY Fredonia
Speech-Language Pathology Prgm
Dept of Speech Pathology and Audiology
W123 Thompson Hall
Fredonia, NY 14063
www.fredonia.edu

Adelphi University
Speech-Language Pathology Prgm
Comm Sciences and Disorders
Hy Weinberg Center, Rm 001
Garden City, NY 11530
www.adelphi.edu
Prgm Dir: Robert Goldfarb, PhD
Tel: 516 877-4785   *Fax:* 516 877-4783
E-mail: goldfarb2@adelphi.edu

SUNY College of Geneseo
Speech-Language Pathology Prgm
Dept of Communicative Disorders and Sciences
1 College Circle, 218 Sturgis
Geneseo, NY 14454
www.geneseo.edu/~cds/CDS-Parts/CDS_Grad_Program.
   html

Hofstra University
Speech-Language Pathology Prgm
Dept of Speech-Language-Hearing Sciences
110 Hofstra University
Hempstead, NY 11550
www.hofstra.edu

Ithaca College
Speech-Language Pathology Prgm
Speech Pathology and Audiology
953 Danby Rd
Ithaca, NY 14850-7185
http://departments.ithaca.edu/slpa/

SUNY at New Paltz
Speech-Language Pathology Prgm
Dept of Communication Disorders
600 Hawk Dr
New Paltz, NY 12561-2499
www.newpaltz.edu

Columbia University Teachers College
Speech-Language Pathology Prgm
Speech and Language Pathology and Audiology
525 W 120th St, Box 206
New York, NY 10027

CUNY Hunter College
Speech-Language Pathology Prgm
Communication Sciences Program
425 E 25th St
New York, NY 10010-2590
www.hunter.cuny.edu/schoolhp/comsc

New York University
Speech-Language Pathology Prgm
Dept of Speech-Language Pathology and Audiology
719 Broadway, Suite 200
New York, NY 10003
www.nyu.edu/education/speech/

SUNY College at Plattsburgh
Speech-Language Pathology Prgm
Dept of Communication Disorders and Sciences
224 Sibley Hall, 101 Broad St
Plattsburgh, NY 12901
www2.plattsburgh.edu/cds

St John's University
Speech-Language Pathology Prgm
Speech and Hearing Ctr
8000 Utopia Pkwy
Queens, NY 11439
www.stjohns.edu

Nazareth College of Rochester
Speech-Language Pathology Prgm
Dept of Comm Sci and Disorder Speech-Lang Pathology
4245 East Ave
Rochester, NY 14618-3790
www.naz.edu/dept/speech

Molloy College
Speech-Language Pathology Prgm
Division of Natural Sciences
Comm Arts & Scis/Speech-Lang
1000 Hempstead Ave PO Box 5002
Rockville Centre, NY 11571-5002

Syracuse University
Speech-Language Pathology Prgm
Dept of Communication Sciences and Disorders
805 S Crouse Ave
Syracuse, NY 13244-2280
http://thecollege.syr.edu/depts/csd

New York Medical College
Speech-Language Pathology Prgm
School of Public Health
Valhalla, NY 10595
www.nymc.edu/slp

North Carolina

Appalachian State University
Speech-Language Pathology Prgm
Dept of Language, Reading and Exceptionalities
124 Edwin Duncan Hall, Box 32085
Boone, NC 28608-2085
www.lre.appstate.edu/gr-cd/1gr-intro.html

University of North Carolina - Chapel Hill
Speech-Language Pathology Prgm
Division of Speech and Hearing Sciences
CB 7190 Wing D Medical School
Chapel Hill, NC 27599-7190
www.med.unc.edu/ahs/sphs

Western Carolina University
Speech-Language Pathology Prgm
Human Services, Communication Sciences and
   Disorders
Killian 204, G30 McKee Bldg
Cullowhee, NC 28723-9043
www.ceap.wcu.edu/commdis/cd.html

North Carolina Central University
Speech-Language Pathology Prgm
Department of Communication Disorders
712 Cecil St
Durham, NC 27707
http://web.nccu.edu/soe/

University of North Carolina - Greensboro
Speech-Language Pathology Prgm
Communication Sciences and Disorders
300 Ferguson Bldg/UNCG, Box 26170
Greensboro, NC 27402-6170
www.uncg.edu/csd

East Carolina University
Speech-Language Pathology Prgm
Dept of Communication Sciences and Disorders
College of Allied Health Science
Greenville, NC 27858-4353
www.ecu.edu/csd

North Dakota

University of North Dakota
Speech-Language Pathology Prgm
Dept of Communication Sciences and Disorders
PO Box 8040
Grand Forks, ND 58202-8040
www.und.edu

Minot State University
Speech-Language Pathology Prgm
Dept of Communication Disorders
500 University Ave W
Minot, ND 58707
www.minotstateu.edu

Ohio

The University of Akron
Speech-Language Pathology Prgm
School of Speech-Language and Audiology
Polsky Building, Rm 188K
Akron, OH 44325-3001
www.uakron.edu/sslpa

Ohio University
Speech-Language Pathology Prgm
School of Hearing, Speech and Language Sciences
Grover Center W218
Athens, OH 45701-2979
www.ohiou.edu/hearingspeech

Bowling Green State University
Speech-Language Pathology Prgm
Dept of Communication Disorders
200 Health Center
Bowling Green, OH 43403-0149
www.bgsu.edu/departments/cdis

University of Cincinnati
Speech-Language Pathology Prgm
Communication Sciences and Disorders
Mail Station 379
Cincinnati, OH 45221-0379
www.uc.edu/csd

Case Western Reserve University
Speech-Language Pathology Prgm
Dept of Communication Sciences
11206 Euclid Ave
Cleveland, OH 44106-7154
www.case.edu/artsci/cosi

Cleveland State University
Speech-Language Pathology Prgm
Dept of Speech and Hearing
2121 Euclid Ave, MC 430
Cleveland, OH 44115
www.csuohio.edu/speech

The Ohio State University
Speech-Language Pathology Prgm
Dept of Speech and Hearing Sciences
110 Pressey Hall, 1070 Carmack Rd
Columbus, OH 43210-1002
www.osu.edu/sphs

Kent State University
Speech-Language Pathology Prgm
School of Speech Pathology and Audiology
A104 Music & Speech Bldg
Kent, OH 44242
http://dept.kent.edu/spa

Miami University
Speech-Language Pathology Prgm
Dept of Speech Pathology and Audiology
2 Bachelor Hall
Oxford, OH 45056-3414
http://casnov1.cas.muohio.edu/spa

University of Toledo
Speech-Language Pathology Prgm
Public Health and Rehabilitative Services
2801 W Bancroft St
Toledo, OH 43606
www.utoledo.edu

Oklahoma

University of Central Oklahoma
Speech-Language Pathology Prgm
Special Services, Speech-Language Pathology
100 N University Dr
Edmond, OK 73034
www.educ.ucok.edu

Univ of Oklahoma Health Sciences Center
Speech-Language Pathology Prgm
Communication Disorders
825 NE 14th, PO Box 26901
Oklahoma City, OK 73190
www.ouhsc.edu

Oklahoma State University
Speech-Language Pathology Prgm
Dept of Communication Sciences and Disorders
110 Hanner Bldg
Stillwater, OK 74078-5062
www.cas.okstate.edu/cdis

Northeastern State University
Speech-Language Pathology Prgm
600 N Vinita, Special Services Bldg
Tahlequah, OK 74464-7051
www.nsuok.edu

University of Tulsa
Speech-Language Pathology Prgm
Department of Communication Disorders
600 S College Ave
Tulsa, OK 74104-3189
www.utulsa.edu

Oregon

University of Oregon
Speech-Language Pathology Prgm
Communication Disorders and Sciences
5284 University of Oregon
Eugene, OR 97403-5284
http://education.uoregon.edu/cds

Portland State University
Speech-Language Pathology Prgm
Speech and Hearing Sciences
PO Box 751
Portland, OR 97207-0751
www.sphr.pdx.edu

Pennsylvania

Bloomsburg University
Speech-Language Pathology Prgm
Dept of Audiology and Speech Pathology
400 E 2nd St, Centennial Hall
Bloomsburg, PA 17815-1301
www.bloomu.edu

California University of Pennsylvania
Speech-Language Pathology Prgm
Dept of Communication Disorders
250 University Ave
California, PA 15419
www.cup.edu

Clarion University of Pennsylvania
Speech-Language Pathology Prgm
Dept of Communication Sciences and Disorders
840 Wood St, 118 Keeling Health Center
Clarion, PA 16214-1232
www.clarion.edu

Misericordia University
Speech-Language Pathology Prgm
Dept Speech Language Pathology
100 Lake St
Rm 231
Dallas, PA 18612
www.misericordia.edu/slp

East Stroudsburg University
Speech-Language Pathology Prgm
Speech Pathology and Audiology
LaRue Hall
East Stroudsburg, PA 18301-2999
www.esu.edu

Edinboro University of Pennsylvania
Speech-Language Pathology Prgm
Speech, Language and Hearing Department
115A Compton Hall
Edinboro, PA 16444
www.edinboro.edu

Indiana University of Pennsylvania
Speech-Language Pathology Prgm
Special Education and Clinical Svcs
203 Davis Hall, 570 S 11th St
Indiana, PA 15705
www.iup.edu

La Salle University
Speech-Language Pathology Prgm
1900 W Olney Ave
Philadelphia, PA 19141
www.lasalle.edu/speech

Temple University
Speech-Language Pathology Prgm
Communication Sciences
1701 N 13th St, 109 Weiss Hall
Philadelphia, PA 19122
www.temple.edu/commsci

Duquesne University
Speech-Language Pathology Prgm
600 Forbes Ave
Pittsburgh, PA 15282
www.slp.duq.edu

University of Pittsburgh
Speech-Language Pathology Prgm
Communication Science and Disorders
4033 Fobes Tower, Atwood St
Pittsburgh, PA 15260
www.shrs.pitt.edu/csd/

Marywood University
Speech-Language Pathology Prgm
Dept of Communication Sciences and Disorders
McGowan Center, 2300 Adams Ave
Scranton, PA 18509-1598
www.marywood.edu

Penn State University
Speech-Language Pathology Prgm
Dept of Communication Sciences and Disorders
110 Moore Bldg
University Park, PA 16802-3100
http://csd.hhdev.psu.edu/grad

West Chester University
Speech-Language Pathology Prgm
Dept of Communicative Disorders
201 Carter Dr
West Chester, PA 19383
www.wcupa.edu/_academics/sch_shs.spp

Puerto Rico

Universidad Del Turabo
Speech-Language Pathology Prgm
School of Health Sciences
PO Box 3030
Gurabo, PR 00778
www.suagm.edu/ut

Carlos Albizu University
Speech-Language Pathology Prgm
Speech Language Pathology Dept
PO Box 9203711
San Juan, PR 00902

University of Puerto Rico
Speech-Language Pathology Prgm
School of Health Related Professions
PO Box 365067, Med Sci Campus
San Juan, PR 00936-5067
www.rcm.upr.edu

Rhode Island

University of Rhode Island
Speech-Language Pathology Prgm
Dept of Communicative Disorders
Independence Sq, Suite 1
25 W Independence Way
Kingston, RI 02881-0821
www.uri.edu

South Carolina

University of South Carolina
Speech-Language Pathology Prgm
Dept of Communication Sciences and Disorders
Columbia, SC 29208
www.sph.sc.edu/comd/

South Carolina State University
Speech-Language Pathology Prgm
Speech Pathology and Audiology
300 College St NE, PO Box 7427
Orangeburg, SC 29117
www.scsu.edu

South Dakota

University of South Dakota
Speech-Language Pathology Prgm
Dept of Communication Disorders
414 E Clark St
Vermillion, SD 57069-2390
www.usd.edu/dcom

Tennessee

East Tennessee State University
Speech-Language Pathology Prgm
Dept of Communicative Disorders
PO Box 70643
Johnson City, TN 37614-0643
www.etsu.edu/cpah/commdis

University of Tennessee - Knoxville
Speech-Language Pathology Prgm
Dept of Audiology and Speech
578 S Stadium Hall
Knoxville, TN 37996-0740
http://web.utk.edu/~aspweb

University of Memphis
Speech-Language Pathology Prgm
School of Audiology and Speech-Language Pathology
807 Jefferson Ave
Memphis, TN 38105
www.ausp.memphis.edu

Tennessee State University
Speech-Language Pathology Prgm
330 10th Ave N, Ste A
PO Box 131
Nashville, TN 37203-3401
www.tnstate.edu

Vanderbilt University Medical Center
Speech-Language Pathology Prgm
Hearing and Speech Sciences
1114 19th Ave S
Nashville, TN 37212
http://vanderbiltbillwilkersoncenter.com/dhss.html

Texas

Abilene Christian University
Speech-Language Pathology Prgm
ACU Box 28058
Abilene, TX 79699-8058
www.acu.edu/academics/cehs/programs/
    comm_disorders/

University of Texas at Austin
Speech-Language Pathology Prgm
Communication Sciences and Disorders
1 University Station A1100
Austin, TX 78712-1089
http://csd.utexas.edu/graduate.html

Lamar University
Speech-Language Pathology Prgm
Dept of Speech and Hearing Sciences
Box 10076, Lamar Station
Beaumont, TX 77710
dept.lamar.edu/cofac/cmds/

West Texas A&M University
Speech-Language Pathology Prgm
PO Box 60757
Canyon, TX 79016-0001
www.wtamu.edu

University of Texas at Dallas
Speech-Language Pathology Prgm
Program in Communication Disorders
1966 Inwood Rd
Dallas, TX 75235-7298
http://bbs.utdallas.edu

Texas Woman's University
Speech-Language Pathology Prgm
Comm Sciences and Disorders
Box 425737, TWU Station
Denton, TX 76204-5737
www.twu.edu

University of North Texas
Speech-Language Pathology Prgm
Dept of Speech and Hearing Sciences
PO Box 305010
Denton, TX 76203-5010
www.sphs.unt.edu

Univ of Texas - Pan American
Speech-Language Pathology Prgm
Health Science and Human Services West 1.264
1201 W University Dr
Edinburg, TX 78541
www.panam.edu/dept/commdisorder

University of Texas at El Paso
Speech-Language Pathology Prgm
1101 N Campbell St
El Paso, TX 79902
www.utep.edu

Texas Christian University
Speech-Language Pathology Prgm
Dept of Communication Sciences and Disorders
TCU Box 297450
Fort Worth, TX 76129
www.csd.tcu.edu

University of Houston
Speech-Language Pathology Prgm
Communication Disorders
100 Clinical Research Services
Houston, TX 77204-6018
www.class.uh.edu/comd

Texas A&M University - Kingsville
Speech-Language Pathology Prgm
Communication Sciences and Disorders
MSC 177A, 700 University Blvd
Kingsville, TX 78363
www.tamu.edu

Texas Tech Univ Health Sciences Center
Speech-Language Pathology Prgm
Dept of Speech, Language, and Hearing Sciences
Stop 6073 - 3601 4th St
Lubbock, TX 79430
www.ttuhsc.edu/SAH

Stephen F Austin State University
Speech-Language Pathology Prgm
Communication Sciences and Disorders Program
PO Box 13019 SFA
Nacogdoches, TX 75962
www.sfasu.edu

Our Lady of the Lake University
Speech-Language Pathology Prgm
Comm and Learning Disorders
411 S 24th St
San Antonio, TX 78207
www.ollusa.edu

Texas State University - San Marcos
Speech-Language Pathology Prgm
Department of Communication Disorders
Health Professions Bldg, 601 University Dr
San Marcos, TX 78666-4616
www.health.txstate.edu/cdis/cdis.html

Baylor University
Speech-Language Pathology Prgm
Dept of Communication Sciences and Disorders
One Bear Place #97332
Waco, TX 76798
www.baylor.edu/communication_disorders

Utah

Utah State University
Speech-Language Pathology Prgm
Comm Disorders and Deaf Educ
1000 Old Main Mill
Logan, UT 84322-1000
www.usu.edu

Brigham Young University
Speech-Language Pathology Prgm
Communication Disorders
136 John Taylor Bldg
Provo, UT 84602-8641
www.byu.edu/mse/

University of Utah
Speech-Language Pathology Prgm
390 South 1530 East
Rm 1201 BEH SCI
Salt Lake City, UT 84112-0252
www.health.utah.edu/csd/

Vermont

University of Vermont
Speech-Language Pathology Prgm
Communication Sciences
Pomeroy Hall, 489 Main St
Burlington, VT 05405
http://http:/www.uvm.edu/~cmsi/

Virginia

University of Virginia
Speech-Language Pathology Prgm
Communication Disorders
2205 Fontaine Ave, Suite 202
Charlottesville, VA 22908-0781
http://curry.edschool.virginia.edu/commdis

Longwood University
Speech-Language Pathology Prgm
Dept of Social Work
Communication Sci & Disorders
201 High St
Farmville, VA 23909
www.longwood.edu/socialworkcsds/9283.htm

Hampton University
Speech-Language Pathology Prgm
Dept of Communicative Sciences and Disorders
Hampton, VA 23668
www.hamptonu.edu

James Madison University
Speech-Language Pathology Prgm
Communication Sciences and Disorders
Harrisonburg, VA 22807
www.csd.jmu.edu

Old Dominion University
Speech-Language Pathology Prgm
Speech Pathology and Audiology
Child Study Ctr
Norfolk, VA 23529-0136
www.odu.edu

Radford University
Speech-Language Pathology Prgm
Dept of Communication Sciences and Disorders
PO Box 6961
Radford, VA 24142
www.radford.edu

Washington

Western Washington University
Speech-Language Pathology Prgm
Dept of Communication Sciences and Disorders
Parks Hall 17, MS 9078
Bellingham, WA 98225-9078
www.wwu.edu/~csd

Washington State University
Speech-Language Pathology Prgm
Dept of Speech and Hearing Sciences
201 Daggy Hall, Box 642420
Pullman, WA 99164-2420
www.wsu.edu/~shsweb

COMMUNICATION SCIENCES

University of Washington
Speech-Language Pathology Prgm
Speech and Hearing Sciences
Seattle, WA 98195-6246
http://depts.washington.edu/sphsc

Eastern Washington University
Speech-Language Pathology Prgm
Dept of Communication Disorders
310 N Riverpoint Blvd, Box V
Spokane, WA 99202
www.ewu.edu/commdisorders

West Virginia

Marshall University
Speech-Language Pathology Prgm
Communication Disorders
400 Hal Greer Blvd
Huntington, WV 25755-2675
www.marshall.edu/commdis

West Virginia University
Speech-Language Pathology Prgm
Department of Speech Pathology and Audiology
805 Allen Hall, Box 6122
Morgantown, WV 26506-6122
www.wvu.edu/~speechpa

Wisconsin

University of Wisconsin - Eau Claire
Speech-Language Pathology Prgm
Dept of Communication Sciences and Disorders
105 Garfield Ave
Eau Claire, WI 54702-4004
www.uwec.edu

University of Wisconsin - Madison
Speech-Language Pathology Prgm
Communicative Disorders
475 Goodnight Hall
Madison, WI 53706
www.comdis.wisc.edu

Marquette University
Speech-Language Pathology Prgm
Dept of Speech-Language Pathology and Audiology
PO Box 1881
Milwaukee, WI 53201-1881
www.marquette.edu/chs/speech

University of Wisconsin - Milwaukee
Speech-Language Pathology Prgm
Dept of Communication Sciences and Disorders
PO Box 413
Milwaukee, WI 53201-0413
http://cfprod.imt.uwm.edu/chs/ugp/csd/graduatestudent
s.html

University of Wisconsin - River Falls
Speech-Language Pathology Prgm
Communicative Disorders
401 S Third St
River Falls, WI 54022-5001
www.uwrf.edu/comm-dis/

University of Wisconsin - Stevens Point
Speech-Language Pathology Prgm
Communicative Disorders
1901 4th Ave
Stevens Point, WI 54481-3897
www.uwsp.edu/commD/

University of Wisconsin - Whitewater
Speech-Language Pathology Prgm
Communicative Disorders
1011 Roseman Bldg, 800 W Main St
Whitewater, WI 53190-1790
http://academics.uww.edu/commdis

Wyoming

University of Wyoming
Speech-Language Pathology Prgm
Division of Communication Disorders
Dept 3311, 1000 E University Ave
Laramie, WY 82071
www.uwyo.edu/comdis

Speech-Language Pathologist

Programs*	Class Capacity	Begins	Length (months)	Award	Res. Tuition	Non-res. Tuition	Offers:† 1	2	3	4
Kentucky										
Eastern Kentucky Univ (Richmond)	40	Summer semester	24	MA	$13,134	$26,301			•	
Louisiana										
Univ of Louisiana at Lafayette	30	Aug	16, 30	MS, PhD						
Missouri										
Univ of Missouri (Columbia)	20	Summer session	24	Dipl, MHS					•	
Nevada										
Univ of Nevada - Reno				MS, PhD						
New York										
Adelphi Univ (Garden City)	200	Sep	2	MS			•		•	

*Data are shown only for programs that completed the 2011 AMA Survey of Health Professions Education Programs.

†Key to Offers: 1: Evening or weekend classes; 2: Non-English instruction; 3: Cultural competence instruction; 4: Distance education component.

Complementary and Alternative Medicine and Therapies

Includes:
- Acupuncture and Oriental medicine
- Chiropractic
- Massage therapist

Definition of Complementary and Alternative Medicine

The National Center for Complementary and Alternative Medicine (NCCAM), a component of the National Institutes of Health (NIH), is the federal government's lead agency for scientific research on complementary and alternative medicine (CAM). NCCAM's mission is to explore CAM healing practices in the context of rigorous science, train CAM researchers, and disseminate authoritative information to the public and professionals.

CAM is defined by the NCCAM as "a group of diverse medical and health care systems, practices, and products that are not presently considered to be part of conventional medicine. Complementary medicine is used together with conventional medicine, and alternative medicine is used in place of conventional medicine." The NCCAM also notes that "the list of what is considered to be CAM

changes continually, as those therapies that are proven to be safe and effective become adopted into conventional health care and as new approaches to health care emerge."

NCCAM groups CAM practices into the following domains:
- Whole medical systems, which are built upon complete systems of theory and practice. Examples include homeopathic medicine, and naturopathic medicine, traditional Chinese medicine, and Ayurveda.
- Mind-body medicine, which uses a variety of techniques to enhance the mind's capacity to affect bodily function and symptoms. Examples include meditation, prayer, mental healing, and therapies drawing on the creative arts, such as art, dance, or music. (*Note:* Art, dance, and music therapy programs are listed in the "Expressive/Creative Arts Therapies" section).
- Biologically based practices, which encompasses use of substances found in nature, such as herbs, foods, and vitamins. Some examples include dietary supplements, herbal products, and the use of other so-called natural but as yet scientifically unproven therapies.

Acupuncture and Oriental Medicine

Career Description
The practice of Acupuncture and Oriental Medicine (AOM) is an ancient and empirical system based on the concept of *Qi* (pronounced "chee"), which is usually translated as energy. Acupuncturists, also known as Oriental Medicine Practitioners, assess a patient's syndrome or pattern of disharmony by using questioning, palpitation, visual inspection, and olfactory-auditory data collection. An acupuncturist then determines the treatment principle and strategy to prompt the patient back to functional harmony. This approach is based on a conceptual framework that is unlike conventional modern medicine. The particular intervention is chosen from among several traditional methods. These interventions include acupuncture, electro-acupuncture, cupping, manual therapies such as acupressure and moxibustion, and exercises such as *tai chi* or *qi gong*, as well as Chinese herbal preparations and dietary therapy.

Employment Characteristics
Acupuncturists may be employed in a wide variety of health care workplaces such as community clinics, integrative practices, hospitals, disaster-relief teams, and/or private practice. Acupuncturists work an average 35-40 hours per week. Independent practitioners may set their own hours and may work evenings/weekends to accommodate patients. Practitioners in private practice also have the business responsibilities of running a practice. In a large practice, acupuncturists may employ office managers/assistants. Currently, more than 90% of licensed acupuncturists work as solo practitioners.

Salary
Salaries vary widely, depending on the type of practice (solo practitioner or employed in a clinic or hospital).

A 2008 study by the National Certification Commission for Acupuncture and Oriental Medicine (NCCAOM) found that certified acupuncturists and Oriental medicine practitioners earned on average $60,000 per year.

Educational Programs
Programs in acupuncture or Oriental medicine are accredited by the Accreditation Commission for Acupuncture and Oriental Medicine (ACAOM). ACAOM is recognized by the US Department of Education (USDE) as an authority in assessing master's degree and master's level certificate and diploma programs in acupuncture and Oriental medicine.

Length. Acupuncture and Oriental medicine programs are typically three to four academic years (90 to 120 instructional weeks), consisting of a minimum of 105 semester credits (1,905 hours) for an acupuncture program and 146 semester credits (2,625 hours) for an Oriental medicine program.

Prerequisites. Satisfactory completion of at least two academic years (60 semester credits/90 quarter credits) of education at the baccalaureate level that is appropriate preparation for graduate level work, or the equivalent, from an institution accredited by an agency recognized by the US Secretary of Education.

Curriculum

Acupuncture
- 47 semester credits (705 hours) in Oriental medical theory, diagnosis and treatment techniques in acupuncture and related studies
- 22 semester credits (660 hours) in clinical training
- 30 semester credits (450 hours) in biomedical clinical sciences

- 6 semester credits (90 hours) in counseling, communication, ethics, and practice management

Oriental Medicine:

- 47 semester credits (705 hours) in Oriental medical theory, diagnosis and treatment techniques in acupuncture, and related studies
- 30 semester credits (450 hours) in didactic Oriental herbal studies
- 29 semester credits (870 hours) in integrated acupuncture and herbal clinical training
- 34 semester credits (510 hours) in biomedical clinical sciences
- 6 semester credits (90 hours) in counseling, communication, ethics, and practice management

Licensure/Certification/Registration

Forty-three states and the District of Columbia either license, certify, or register comprehensively trained non-physician practitioners, thus statutorily recognizing the practice of acupuncture. In most states where statutory regulation exists, acupuncturists have independent status as practitioners, although there are a few states where practitioners must have supervision, prior referral, or initial diagnosis by a medical doctor. The administrative structure for regulating the profession in the states varies, with a number of states having an independent board composed of acupuncturists or a state medical board assisted by an acupuncture advisory board or committee. Other administrative arrangements may include regulation of the profession by a joint board composed of various conventional and complementary and alternative health care professions, regulation by another profession, or by a larger administrative division within a state department or agency, usually with the assistance of an acupuncture advisory body.

Certification by the National Certification Commission for Acupuncture and Oriental Medicine (NCCAOM) is the only nationally recognized certification available to qualified practitioners of acupuncture and Oriental medicine. Candidates who pass the examination are awarded the Dipl Ac (NCCAOM) (Diplomate in Acupuncture) designation. NCCAOM certification is a requirement for licensure in most states. Many third-party payers recognize NCCAOM certification as a criterion for reimbursement, and employers may require NCCAOM certification as a condition for hiring or promotion.

Inquiries

Careers

American Association of Acupuncture and Oriental Medicine
PO Box 162340
Sacramento, CA 95816
866 455-7999 or 916 443-4770
E-mail: *info@aaaomonline.org*
www. aaaomonline.org

Council of Colleges of Acupuncture and Oriental Medicine
3909 National Drive, Suite 125
Burtonsville, MD 20866
301 476-7791
E-mail: *executivedirector@ccaom.org*
www.ccaom.org

Licensure/Certification/Registration

National Certification Commission for Acupuncture and Oriental Medicine
76 South Laura Street, Suite 1290
Jacksonville, FL 32202
904 598-1005
E-mail: *kwardcook@nccaom.org*
www.nccaom.org

Federation of Acupuncture & Oriental Medicine Regulatory Agencies
Maryland Board of Acupuncture
4201 Patterson Avenue
Baltimore, MD 21215
410 764-4766
E-mail: *contact@faomra.com*
www.faomra.com

Program Accreditation

Accreditation Commission for Acupuncture and Oriental Medicine
Maryland Trade Center #3
7501 Greenway Center Drive, Suite 760
Greenbelt, MD 20770
301 313-0855
E-mail: *coordinator@acaom.org*
www.acaom.org

Research

Society for Acupuncture Research
PO Box 33015
Portland, OR 97292
E-mail: *rposner@acupunctureresearch.org*
www.acupunctureresearch.org

Acupuncture and Oriental Medicine

Arizona

Eastern School of Acupuncture and Traditional Oriental Medicine
301 E. Bethany Home Road, Suite A-100
Phoenix, AZ 85012
www.pihma.com
E-mail: contactus@pihma.edu

Swedish Institute School of Acupuncture and Oriental Medicine
3131 N. Country Club Road, Suite 100
Tucson, AZ 85716
www.asianinstitute.edu
E-mail: info@asianinstitute.edu

Southwest Acupuncture College
4646 East Fort Lowell Rd., Suite 104
Tucson, AZ 85712
www.asaom.edu
E-mail: asaom@dakotacom.net

California

Five Branches University: Graduate School of Traditional Chinese Medicine
Master of Science in Acupuncture and Oriental Medicine Prgm
1126 N. Brookhurst St.
Anaheim, CA 92801-1701
www.southbaylo.edu
E-mail: admin@southbaylo.edu

Seattle Institute of Oriental Medicine
Acupuncture & Integrative Medicine College, Berkeley Prgm
Master of Science in Oriental Medicine Prgm
2550 Shattuck Ave.
Berkeley, CA 94704
www.aimc.edu
E-mail: info@aimc.edu

Pacific College of Oriental Medicine
Master of Acupuncture and Traditional Chinese Medicine Prgm
13315 West Washington Blvd.
Los Angeles, CA 90066
www.Yosan.edu
E-mail: info@yosan.edu

Finger Lakes School of Acupuncture and Oriental Medicine
Master of Science in Acupuncture and Oriental Medicine Prgm
1541 Wilshire Blvd., 3rd floor
Los Angeles, CA 90017
http://www.scalu.com
E-mail: info@scalu.com

Emperor's College of Traditional Oriental Medicine
Master of Science in Oriental Medicine Prgm
1730 W. Olympic Blvd., 3rd Floor
Los Angeles, CA 90015
www.samra.edu
E-mail: info@samra.edu

University of Bridgeport College of Chiropractic
Master of Science in Oriental Medicine Prgm
440 South Shatto Place
Los Angeles, CA 90020
www.dru.edu
E-mail: info@dru.edu

Phoenix Institute of Herbal Medicine & Acupuncture
Academy of Chinese Culture and Health Sciences Prgm
Master of Science in Traditional Chinese Medicine Prgm
1601 Clay Street
Oakland, CA 94612
www.acchs.edu
E-mail: info@acchs.edu

East West College of Natural Medicine
Master of Science in Traditional Oriental Medicine Prgm
7445 Mission Valley Rd., Suite 105
San Diego, CA 92108
www.pacificcollege.edu
E-mail: admissions-sd@pacificcollege.edu

Southwest Acupuncture College
American College of Traditional Chinese Medicine Prgm
Master of Science in Traditional Chinese Medicine Prgm
455 Arkansas Street
San Francisco, CA 94107
www.actcm.edu
E-mail: info@actcm.edu

Colorado School of Traditional Chinese Medicine
Master of Traditional Chinese Medicine Prgm
3031 Tisch Way, Suite 605
San Jose, CA 95128
www.fivebranches.edu
E-mail: sjreceptionist@fivebranches.edu

Yo San University of Traditional Chinese Medicine
Master of Traditional Oriental Medicine Prgm
1807 B. Wilshire Boulevard
Santa Monica, CA 90403
www.emperors.edu
E-mail: admissions@emperors.edu

New York College of Traditional Chinese Medicine
Master of Science in Traditional Chinese Medicine Prgm
970 W. El Camino Real
Sunnyvale, CA 94087
www.uewm.edu
E-mail: info@uewm.edu

Florida College of Integrative Medicine
Master of Acupuncture and Oriental Medicine Prgm
16200 E. Amber Valley Drive, PO Box 1166
Whittier, CA 90604
www.scuhs.edu
E-mail: admissions@scuhs.edu

Colorado

Jung Tao School of Classical Chinese Medicine
6620 Gunpark Dr.
Boulder, CO 80301
www.acupuncturecollege.edu
E-mail: boulder@acupuncturecollege.edu

Traditional Chinese Medical College of Hawaii
1441 York Street, Suite 202
Denver, CO 80206-2127
www.cstcm.edu
E-mail: admin@cstcm.edu

Acupuncture & Massage College
325 W. South Boulder Road, Suite 2
Louisville, CO 80027
www.itea.edu
E-mail: info@itea.edu

Connecticut

New York College of Health Professions
Master of Science in Acupuncture Prgm
60 Lafayette Street
Bridgeport, CT 6601
www.bridgeport.edu
E-mail: acup@bridgeport.edu

Florida

Tai Sophia Institute
100 E. Broward Blvd., Suite 100
Fort Lauderdale, FL 33301
www.atom.edu
E-mail: atom@atom.edu

Pacific College of Oriental Medicine
Master of Acupuncture Prgm
305 SE 2nd Avenue
Gainesville, FL 32601
www.acupuncturist.edu
E-mail: info@acupuncturist.edu

University of East West Medicine
1000 NE 16th Avenue, Building F
Gainesville, FL 32601
www.dragonrises.edu
E-mail: info@dragonrises.edu

South Baylo University
Acupuncture & Massage College Prgm
Master of Science in Oriental Medicine Prgm
10506 North Kendall Drive
Miami, FL 33176
www.amcollege.edu
E-mail: admissions@amcollege.edu

Academy of Oriental Medicine at Austin
Master of Science in Oriental Medicine Prgm
7100 Lake Ellenor Drive
Orlando, FL 32809
www.fcim.edu
E-mail: info@fcim.edu

WON Institute of Graduate Studies
Master of Science in Oriental Medicine Prgm
3808 N Tamiami Trail
Sarasota, FL 34234
www.ewcollege.org
E-mail: registrar@ewcollege.org

Hawaii

Pacific College of Oriental Medicine
1110 University Avenue, Suite 308
Honolulu, HI 96826
www.acupuncture-hi.com
E-mail: worldmedicine@cs.com

Acupuncture & Integrative Medicine College
Master of Science in Oriental Medicine Prgm
Chinatown Cultural Plaza 100 North Beretania Street, Suite 2
Honolulu, HI 96817
www.orientalmedicine.edu
E-mail: info@orientalmedicine.edu

National College of Natural Medicine
Master of Science in Oriental Medicine Prgm
65-1206 Mamalohoa Highway
Building 3, Suite 9
Kamuela, HI 96743
www.tcmch.edu
E-mail: tcmch@tcmch.edu

Illinois

American College of Traditional Chinese Medicine
Master of Science in Oriental Medicine Prgm
4334 North Hazel, Suite 206
Chicago, IL 60613
www.acupuncture.edu

Dongguk University - Los Angeles
3646 North Broadway, 2nd Floor
Chicago, IL 60613
www.pacificcollege.edu
E-mail: admissions-sd@pacificcollege.edu

Maryland

Midwest College of Oriental Medicine
Master of Acupuncture Prgm
7750 Montpelier Road
Laurel, MD 20723
www.tai.edu
E-mail: admissions@tai.edu

Massachusetts

Asian Institute of Medical Studies
150 California Street, 3rd Floor
Newton, MA 2458
www.nesa.edu
E-mail: info@nesa.edu

Minnesota

American Institute of Alternative Medicine
Master of Acupuncture and Oriental Medicine Prgm
Northwestern Health Sciences University
2501 West 84th Street
Bloomington, MN 55431
www.nwhealth.edu
Tel: 952 885-5435 Fax: 952 887-1398
E-mail: mmckenzie@nwhealth.edu

Southern California University (SOMA)
American Academy of Acupuncture and Oriental Medicine Prgm
Master of Science in Acupuncture and Oriental Medicine Prgm
1925 West County Road B2
Roseville, MN 55113
www.aaaom.org
Tel: 651 631-0204 Fax: 651 631-0361
E-mail: tcmhealth@aol.com

New Jersey

World Medicine Institute
427 Bloomfield Avenue, Suite 301
Montclair, NJ 7042
www.easternschool.com
E-mail: easternschoolacup@earthlink.net

New Mexico

Institute of Taoist Education and Acupuncture
Master of Science in Oriental Medicine Prgm
7801 Academy Blvd. North Towne Bldg. #1, NE
Albuquerque, NM 87109
www.acupuncturecollege.edu
Tel: 505 888-8898 Fax: 505 888-1380
E-mail: abq@acupuncturecollege.edu

Institute of Clinical Acupuncture and Oriental Medicine
Master of Science in Oriental Medicine and Acupuncture Prgm
1622 Galisteo Street
Santa Fe, NM 87505
www.acupuncturecollege.edu
Tel: 505 438-8884 Fax: 505 438-8883
E-mail: sfe@acupuncturecollege.edu

New York

Bastyr University
Master of Science in Acupuncture and Oriental Medicine Prgm
155 First Street
Mineola, NY 11501
www.nyctcm.edu
E-mail: admissions@nyctcm.edu

New England School of Acupuncture
Master of Science in Acupuncture and Oriental Medicine Prgm
80 8th Ave., Suite 400
New York, NY 10011
www.tsca.edu
E-mail: inquiry@tsca.edu

Dragon Rises College of Oriental Medicine
Master of Science in Acupuncture and Traditional Oriental Medicine Prgm
915 Broadway, 2nd Floor
New York, NY 10010
www.pacificcollege.edu
E-mail: admissions-ny@pacificcollege.edu

Midwest College of Oriental Medicine
Master of Science in Acupuncture Prgm
226 West 26th Street, P.O. Box 11130
New York, NY 10001
www.swedishinstitute.org
E-mail: acupuncture@swedishinstitute.edu

Academy of Chinese Culture and Health Science
Master of Science in Acupuncture and Oriental Medicine Prgm
2360 State Route 89
Seneca Falls, NY 13148-0800
www..nycc.edu

Atlantic Institute of Oriental Medicine
Master of Science in Acupuncture and Oriental Medicine Prgm
6801 Jericho Turnpike
Syosset, NY 11791-4465
www.nycollege.edu
E-mail: info@nycollege.edu

North Carolina

Tri-State College of Acupuncture
382 Montford Avenue
Asheville, NC 28801
www.daoisttraditions.com
E-mail: daoist@bellsouth.net

American Academy of Acupuncture and Oriental Medicine
207 Dale Adams Road
Sugar Grove, NC 28679
www.jungtao.edu
E-mail: info@jungtao.edu

Ohio

Southwest Acupuncture College
Professional Master's Level Acupuncture Prgm
6685 Doubletree Avenue
Columbus, OH 43229
www.aiam.edu
E-mail: info@aiam.edu

Oregon

Daoist Traditions College of Chinese Medical
10525 SE Cherry Blossom Dr
Portland, OR 97216
www.ocom.edu
E-mail: admissions@ocom.edu

Arizona School of Acupuncture and Oriental Medicine
049 S.W. Porter
Portland, OR 97201
www.ncnm.edu
E-mail: admissions@ncnm.edu

Pennsylvania

Oregon College of Oriental Medicine
Master of Acupuncture Prgm
137 S. Easton Road
Glenside, PA 19038
www.woninstitute.org
Tel: 215 884-8942 Fax: 215 884-9002
E-mail: info@woninstitute.org

Texas

Samra University of Oriental Medicine
Master of Acupuncture and Oriental Medicine Prgm
2700 West Anderson Lane, Suite 204
Austin, TX 78757
www.aoma.edu
E-mail: info@aoma.edu

Minnesota College of Acupuncture and Oriental Medicine
4005 Manchaca Road, Suite 200
Austin, TX 78704
www.texastcm.edu
E-mail: texastcm@texastcm.edu

Southern California Univ of Health Sciences
Master of Acupuncture and Oriental Medicine Prgm
9100 Park West Drive
Houston, TX 77063
www.acaom.edu
E-mail: info@acaom.edu

Washington

Texas College of Traditional Chinese Medicine
Master of Science in Acupuncture and Oriental Medicine Prgm
14500 Juanita Drive, NE
Kenmore, WA 98028
www.bastyr.edu
Tel: 425 823-1300 Fax: 425 823-6222
E-mail: admiss@bastyr.edu

Five Branches University: Graduate School of Traditional Chinese Medicine
Master of Acupuncture and Oriental Medicine Prgm
916 NE 65th St.
Seattle, WA 98115
www.siom.edu
E-mail: info@siom.edu

Wisconsin

American College of Acupuncture and Oriental Medicine
6232 Bankers Road, Suites 5 & 6
Racine, WI 53403
www.acupuncture.edu
E-mail: info@acupuncture.edu

Chiropractic

The goal of chiropractic care is to enhance overall health and wellness and provide functional improvement without the use of drugs or surgery.

Career Description

Chiropractors practice a drug-free and hands-on form of care, which may include manual therapies (i.e., manipulation/adjustments); nutrition, dietary, and lifestyle counseling; physiotherapy; and physical medicine and rehabilitative exercises. For neuromusculoskeletal conditions, such as lower back pain, the care provided by a chiropractor may be the primary method of treatment. When other health conditions exist, chiropractors may work in conjunction with medical treatment.

Chiropractors assess patients to determine which treatments are best suited for a patient's condition. Chiropractors refer patients to other health care providers when chiropractic care is not suitable for the patient's condition.

Employment Characteristics and Outlook

Nearly 92% of chiropractors are in full-time practice, with the average chiropractor working between 30 and 39 hours per week. The majority (66.1%) work in solo practice.

Chiropractors determine their individual working hours and are able to arrange these hours by appointment. Job prospects for new chiropractors are expected to be good. In this occupation, replacement needs arise from retirement, and acute shortages exist in some areas of the United States. The U.S. Bureau of Labor Statistics projects that employment of chiropractors is expected to increase by 28% between 2010 and 2020—much faster than the average for all occupations.

Salary

May 2011 data from the US Bureau of Labor Statistics show that wages for chiropractors at the 10th percentile are $31,120, the 50th percentile (median) at $66,060, and the 90th percentile at $142,570. (*http://www.bls.gov/oes/current/oes291011.htm*).

In chiropractic, as in other types of independent practice, earnings are relatively low in the beginning and increase as the practice grows.

Educational Programs

Length. Chiropractors complete education in an accredited chiropractic college; four to five academic years of professional study are standard.

Prerequisites. The typical applicant at a chiropractic college has already acquired four years of undergraduate college education.

Curriculum. Chiropractic students study clinical subjects, including anatomy, physiology, rehabilitation, nutrition, and public health. Because of the hands-on nature of chiropractic, a significant portion of time is spent in clinical training.

Licensure/Certification/Registration

Chiropractors are required to be licensed in all 50 states and the District of Columbia, and all chiropractors are required to complete a comprehensive national board examination, which is administered by the National Board of Chiropractic Examiners (NBCE).

Inquiries

Careers
American Chiropractic Association (ACA)
1701 Clarendon Blvd
Arlington, VA 22209
703 276-8800
E-mail: *memberinfo@acatoday.org*
www.acatoday.org

For a listing of resources regarding a career in chiropractic, visit *www.acatoday.org/career*

Certification/Registration
For a listing of state boards overseeing chiropractic licensure, visit: *www.acatoday.org/content_css.cfm?CID=753*

Program Accreditation
The Council on Chiropractic Education (CCE), an agency accredited by the U.S. Department of Education, currently recognizes 15 chiropractic programs at 18 different locations. For a listing of chiropractic colleges, visit *www.acatoday.org/career*. For the CCE, visit *www.cce-usa.org*.

Note: Adapted in part from the Bureau of Labor Statistics, U.S. Department of Labor, *Occupational Outlook Handbook,* Chiropractors, at *www.bls.gov/oco/ocos071.htm*.

Chiropractic

California

Life Chiropractic College West
Chiropractic Prgm
25001 Industrial Blvd
Hayward, CA 94545
www.lifewest.edu

Cleveland Chripractic College of Los Angeles
Chiropractic Prgm
590 N Vermont Ave
Los Angeles, CA 90004
www.cleveland.edu

Palmer College of Chiropractic West
Chiropractic Prgm
90 E Tasman Dr
San Jose, CA 95134
www.palmer.edu

Southern California Univ of Health Sciences
Chiropractic Prgm
16200 E Amber Valley Dr
Whittier, CA 90604
www.scuhs.edu

Connecticut

University of Bridgeport
Chiropractic Prgm
126 Park Ave
Bridgeport, CT 06604
www.bridgeport.edu/chiro

Florida

Palmer College of Chiropractic
Chiropractic Prgm
4777 City Center Pkwy
Port Orange, FL 32129
www.palmer.edu/PCCF/

Georgia

Life University
Chiropractic Prgm
1269 Barclay Circle SE
Marietta, GA 30060
www.life.edu

Illinois

National University of Health Sciences
Chiropractic Prgm
200 E Roosevelt Rd
Lombard, IL 60148
www.nuhs.edu

Iowa

Palmer College of Chiropractic
Chiropractic Prgm
1000 Brady St
Davenport, IA 52803
www.palmer.edu

Kansas

Cleveland Chiropractic College of Kansas City
Chiropractic Prgm
10850 Lowell Ave
Overland Park, KS 66210
www.cleveland.edu

Minnesota

Northwestern Health Science University
Chiropractic Prgm
2501 West 84th St
Bloomington, MN 55431
www.nwhealth.edu

Missouri

Logan College of Chiropractic
Chiropractic Prgm
1851 Schoettler Rd
Chesterfield, MO 63017
www.logan.edu

New York

D'Youville College
Chiropractic Prgm
320 Porter Ave
Buffalo, NY 14201
www.dyc.edu

New York Chiropractic College
Chiropractic Prgm
2360 State Route 89
Seneca Falls, NY 13148
www.nycc.edu

Oregon

Western State Chiropractic College
Chiropractic Prgm
2900 NE 132nd Ave
Portland, OR 97230
www.wschiro.edu

South Carolina

Sherman College of Straight Chiropractic
Chiropractic Prgm
2020 Springfield Rd
Spartanburg, SC 29304
www.sherman.edu

Texas

Parker College of Chiropractic
Chiropractic Prgm
2500 Walnut Hill Lane
Dallas, TX 75229
www.parkercc.edu

Texas Chiropractic College
Chiropractic Prgm
5912 Spencer Hwy
Pasadena, TX 77505
www.txchiro.edu

COMPLEMENTARY & ALTERNATIVE MEDICINE & THERAPIES

Massage Therapist

History

Massage has its roots in the far reaches of human history. Rubbing a sore muscle or stroking another person for comfort is a natural response. The first written records that refer to massage date back more than 4,000 years to China. In ancient Greece, Hippocrates, the father of modern medicine, wrote, "The physician must be experienced in many things, but most assuredly in rubbing."

Massage comes from both Western and Eastern traditions. Western traditions date back to ancient Greece and Rome. Modern Western massage owes a great deal to the work of Peter Henrik Ling, a 19th-century educator and athlete from Sweden. His approach, which combined hands-on techniques with active movements, became known as Swedish Massage, probably the most common therapeutic massage modality in the West.

Eastern traditions can be traced back to the folk medicine of China and the Ayurvedic medicine of India. Shiatsu, acupressure, reflexology, and many other contemporary techniques have their roots in these sources.

The incorporation of massage into health care was fairly well-established in the 19th century, but those connections decreased through most of the 20th century. A growing body of clinical research on the efficacy and value of massage as part of integrated health care, as well as a rapid acceptance and adoption of use of massage in recent years, has fueled a renewed collaboration between massage therapists and other health professionals. Use of massage in the hospital setting has increased as well, and growth in the consumer acceptance of massage over the last three decades has been substantial.

Career Description

Leading professional massage associations have defined massage as systems of structured palpation or movement of the soft tissue of the body, including holding, causing movement, and/or applying pressure to the body. Massage therapy is a profession in which the practitioner applies manual techniques (by use of hand or body), and may apply adjunctive therapies, with the intention of positively affecting the health and well-being of the client.

An increasing body of research shows massage reduces heart rate, can help lower blood pressure, increases blood circulation and lymph flow, relaxes muscles, improves range of motion, and increases endorphins. Recent studies indicate massage enhances the functioning of the immune system. Although therapeutic massage does not increase muscle strength, it can stimulate weak, inactive muscles and, thus, partially compensate for the lack of exercise and inactivity resulting from illness or injury. It also can hasten and lead to a more complete recovery from exercise or injury. Further, a significant amount of research indicates that massage therapy can relieve stress and aid in pain relief and management, including post-operative pain.

Some of the most common types of massage include:

- Swedish massage
- Deep-tissue massage
- Shiatsu-acupressure
- Neuromuscular
- Trigger point
- Sports massage

Employment Characteristics

Massage therapists work in many different environments. The majority work at least some of their hours in private practice, and many combine that practice with part-time work in hospitals, physician or chiropractor offices, nursing homes, pain clinics, resorts, cruise ships, shopping malls, airports, spas, and salons. A significant percentage travel to clients' homes or to business offices. Onsite chair massage has become a very popular form of massage because of its convenience of use in a variety of settings, such as corporate offices. Some therapists focus exclusively on massage for stress relief and relaxation, while others specialize in such modalities as massage for pain relief, sports massage, pregnancy massage, massage to reduce lymphedema after cancer surgery, and hot stone massage among other specialties. With the proliferation of massage modalities in recent years, many therapists combine several to create unique offerings.

Massage therapy can be strenuous work at times. Practitioners must use correct body mechanics to prevent injury and fatigue. If the therapist travels to give massage, they transport either a massage table or massage chair and all supplies necessary to give a massage. The profession requires good listening skills and the ability to make clients comfortable and relaxed. Massage therapists often adopt massage practice as a second or third career and many enjoy the freedom of part-time work and independent practice.

In addition to the actual massage, massage therapists market their practices, keep financial and client records, maintain supplies and equipment, educate their clients about massage and inform them of any physical irregularities they discover, and work with health insurance companies to receive fees. Practitioners take basic medical histories on clients and discuss with the client their current health. During massage, therapists pay close attention to how the client is responding and discuss levels of massage pressure with the client. They also must be aware of medical conditions that might contraindicate massage and advise clients when massage is not appropriate. They may need to obtain physician approval before providing massage to someone under medical care.

Salary

Earnings among massage therapists vary widely, depending on where the therapist practices, their level of experience, the number of client-contact hours, and their ability to establish and sustain an independent business. Responsibilities in addition to massage include practice management, billing, marketing, etc.

Many massage therapists work part time and, therefore, yearly earnings can vary considerably, depending on the therapist's schedule. On average, massage therapists earn between $31 and $41 per hour and are paid for an average of 15 hours per week, earning them annual massage-related incomes between $20,000 and $30,000. A full-time practice for massage therapy is about 26 hours a week.

Another survey, reflecting prevalent part-time and private-practice models, shows that practitioners earn an average salary of $20,000 (as independent therapists); $23,750 (therapists working as employees); and $22,600 (combined independent and employed work). The average annual median salary, based on all three of these categories, was $21,000.

May 2011 data from the US Bureau of Labor Statistics show that wages for massage therapists at the 10th percentile are $18,300, the 50th percentile (median) at $35,830, and the 90th percentile at $69,070. (*http://www.bls.gov/oes/current/oes319011.htm*).

Employment Outlook

Projections from the US Bureau of Labor Statistics indicate that employment of massage therapists is expected to increase by 20 percent from 2010 to 2020, faster than the average for all occupations.

Educational Programs

Minimum entry-level standards for massage therapy training vary greatly, based on state or local requirements, professional association standards, or insurance requirements. State regulatory requirements for massage practice range from a minimum of 500 in-class hours at a recognized massage schools—the most prevalent standard—to 1,000 in-class hours of massage training in accredited massage programs.

Massage therapy training programs and schools can voluntarily seek accreditation from seven accrediting agencies recognized by the US Department of Education. Only 30 percent of state-approved massage therapy training programs have received such accreditation. The Commission on Massage Therapy Accreditation (COMTA) is one of these agencies and is the only agency dedicated solely to accreditation for massage therapy. Students are eligible for federal Title IV funding at 57 percent of massage programs in the US.

The two major professional massage organizations are the American Massage Therapy Association (a non-profit professional association first established in 1943) and the for-profit company Associated Bodywork & Massage Professionals (the largest of the two). As a condition of membership, both require the completion of a minimum number of classroom hours and state licensing in states where licensing has been enacted.

Licensure

Currently, 43 states and Washington, DC, regulate massage therapy. Some states license massage therapists, while others have title protection or certification. Regulation of massage therapy by the states has increased in recent years, with two thirds enacting regulation in the last two decades.

Entry Examination and Certification

Some states require passage of an exam before granting a license. In 2007, the Federation of State Massage Therapy Boards introduced the Massage and Bodywork Licensing Exam (MBLEx), which is designed to assess a massage therapist's readiness to practice safely and competently. Some states also accept, for entry purposes, a passing score on the test component involved in securing voluntary professional certification from the National Certification Board for Therapeutic Massage & Bodywork.

Inquiries

Massage Careers, Organizational Memberships
American Massage Therapy Association
500 Davis Street, Suite 900
Evanston, IL 60201-4695
847 864-0123
E-mail: *info@amtamassage.org*
www.amtamassage.org

Associated Bodywork & Massage Professionals
25188 Genesee Trail Road, Suite 200
Golden, CO 80401
800 458-2267
E-mail: *expectmore@abmp.com*
www.abmp.com

Entry Examination

Federation of State Massage Therapy Boards
7111 W 151st Street, Suite 356
Overland Park, KS 66223
888 703-7682
E-mail: *info@fsmtb.org*
www.fsmtb.org

Certification

National Certification Board for Therapeutic Massage & Bodywork
1901 S. Meyers Road, Suite 240
Oakbrook Terrace, IL 60181-5243
800 296-0664
E-mail: *info@ncbtmb.com*
www.ncbtmb.com

Program Accreditation

Commission on Massage Therapy Accreditation
5335 Wisconsin Ave NW, Suite 440
Washington, DC 20015
202 895-1518
E-mail: *info@comta.org*
www.comta.org

COMPLEMENTARY & ALTERNATIVE MEDICINE & THERAPIES

Massage Therapist

California

Mueller College of Holistic Studies
Massage Therapy Prgm
6160 Mission Gorge Rd
San Diego, CA 92120
www.mueller.edu

Colorado

Massage Therapy Institute of Colorado
Massage Therapy Prgm
1441 York St, Ste 301
Denver, CO 80206

Academy of Natural Therapy
Massage Therapy Prgm
123 Elm Ave
PO Box 237
Eaton, CO 80615
www.natural-therapy.com

Connecticut

Connecticut Center for Massage Therapy
Massage Therapy Prgm
1154 Poquonnock Rd
Groton, CT 06340
www.ccmt.com

Connecticut Center for Massage Therapy
Massage Therapy Prgm
75 Kitts Ln
Newington, CT 06111
www.ccmt.com

Connecticut Center for Massage Therapy
Massage Therapy Prgm
25 Sylvan Rd S
Westport, CT 06880
www.ccmt.com

Delaware

National Massage Therapy Institute
Massage Therapy Prgm
1601 Concord Pike, Ste 82-84
Wilmington, DE 19803
www.studymassage.com

District of Columbia

Potomac Massage Training Institute
Massage Therapy Prgm
5028 Wisconsin Ave NW - LL
Washington, DC 20016-4118
www.pmti.org

Florida

Florida College of Natural Health
Massage Therapy Prgm
616 67th St Circle E
Bradenton, FL 34208
www.fcnh.com

Florida School of Massage
Massage Therapy Prgm
6421 SW 13th St
Gainesville, FL 32608
www.floridaschoolofmassage.com

Florida College of Natural Health
Massage Therapy Prgm
2600 Lake Lucien Dr, Ste 140
Maitland, FL 32751
www.fcnh.com

Educating Hands School of Massage
Massage Therapy Prgm
120 SW 8th St
Miami, FL 33130-3513
www.educatinghands.com

Florida College of Natural Health
Massage Therapy Prgm
7925 NW 12th St, Ste 201
Miami, FL 33126
www.fcnh.com

Florida College of Natural Health
Massage Therapy Prgm
2001 W Sample Rd, Ste 100
Pompano Beach, FL 33064
www.fcnh.com

Sarasota School of Massage Therapy
Massage Therapy Prgm
1932 Ringling Blvd
Sarasota, FL 34236
www.sarasotaschoolofmassagetherapy.edu

Illinois

Chicago School of Massage Therapy
Cosponsor: Cortiva Institute
Massage Therapy Prgm
17 N State St, 5th Fl
Chicago, IL 60602
www.cortiva.com/locations/csmt

Morton College
Massage Therapy Prgm
3801 S Central Ave
Cicero, IL 60804
www.morton.edu

Chicago School of Massage Therapy
Cosponsor: McHenry County College Satellite
Massage Therapy Prgm
100 S Main St
Crystal Lake, IL 60014
www.csmt.com/csmt/

Elgin Community College
Massage Therapy Prgm
1700 Spartan Dr
Elgin, IL 60123-7193
www.elgin.edu

National University of Health Sciences
Massage Therapy Prgm
200 E Roosevelt Rd
Lombard, IL 60148
www.nuhs.edu

Kishwaukee College
Massage Therapy Prgm
21193 Malta Rd
Malta, IL 60150-9699
www.kishwaukeecollege.edu

Indiana

Alexandria School of Scientific Therapeutics
Massage Therapy Prgm
809 S Harrison
PO Box 287
Alexandria, IN 46001
www.assti.com

Iowa

Carlson College of Massage Therapy
Massage Therapy Prgm
11809 County Rd X-28
Anamosa, IA 52205
www.carlsoncollege.com

Louisiana

Blue Cliff College - Baton Rouge
Massage Therapy Prgm
6160 Perkins Rd, Ste 200
Baton Rouge, LA 70808-4191

Maine

New Hampshire Institute for Therapeutic Arts
Massage Therapy Prgm
27 Sandy Creek Rd
Bridgton, ME 04009
www.nhita.com

Downeast School of Massage
Massage Therapy Prgm
PO Box 24
99 Moose Meadow Ln
Waldoboro, ME 04572-0024
www.downeastschoolofmassage.net

Manitoba, Canada

Massage Therapy College of Manitoba
Massage Therapy Prgm
691 Wolseley Ave, 2nd Fl
Winnipeg, MB R3G 1C3
www.massagetherapycollege.com

Maryland

Allegany College of Maryland
Massage Therapy Prgm
12401 Willowbrook Rd SE
Cumberland, MD 21502
www.allegany.edu

Baltimore School of Massage
Massage Therapy Prgm
517 Progress Dr
Suite A-L
Linthicum, MD 21090
www.bsom.com

Massachusetts

Mount Wachusett Community College
Massage Therapy Prgm
444 Green St
Gardner, MA 01440
www.mwcc.edu

Stillpoint Program - Greenfield Comm Coll
Massage Therapy Prgm
270 Main St
Greenfield, MA 01301
www.gcc.mass.edu

Springfield Technical Community College
Massage Therapy Prgm
Dept of Myofascial
One Amory Square
Springfield, MA 01105
www.stcc.edu

Cortiva Institute - Muscular Therapy Inst
Massage Therapy Prgm
103 Morse St
Watertown, MA 02472
www.cortiva.com/

Michigan

Ann Arbor Institute of Massage Therapy
Massage Therapy Prgm
180 Jackson Plaza
Suite 100
Ann Arbor, MI 48103
www.aaimt.edu

Lakewood School of Therapeutic Massage
Massage Therapy Prgm
1102 6th St
Port Huron, MI 48060
www.lakewoodschool.com

Minnesota

**Northwestern Health Science University
School of Massage Therapy**
Massage Therapy Prgm
2501 W 84th St
Bloomington, MN 55431
www.nwhealth.edu

Mississippi

Mississippi School of Therapeutic Massage
Massage Therapy Prgm
5140 Galaxie Dr
Jackson, MS 39206-4339
www.mstm.info

Montana

Health Works Institute
Massage Therapy Prgm
111 S Grand Annex 3
Bozeman, MT 59715
www.healthworksinstitute.com

Nevada

College of Southern Nevada
Massage Therapy Prgm
College of Southern Nevada Massage Specialist Program
Sort Code W1A
6375 W Charleston Blvd
Las Vegas, NV 89146-1164
www.csn.edu

New Hampshire

New Hampshire Institute for Therapeutic Arts
Massage Therapy Prgm
153 Lowell Rd
Hudson, NH 03051
www.nhita.com

New Jersey

Institute for Therapeutic Massage - Browns Mills
Massage Therapy Prgm
200 Trenton Rd
Browns Mills, NJ 08015
www.massageprogram.com

National Massage Therapy Institute
Massage Therapy Prgm
6712 Washington Ave, Ste 302
Egg Harbor, NJ 08234

Academy of Massage Therapy
Massage Therapy Prgm
321 Main St, 2nd Fl
Hackensack, NJ 07601
www.academyofmassage.com

Academy of Massage Therapy
Massage Therapy Prgm
75 Montgomery St, 4th Floor
Jersey City, NJ 07302
www.academyofmassage.com

Institute for Therapeutic Massage - Morristown
Massage Therapy Prgm
95 Mount Kemble Ave
Morristown, NJ 07962
www.massageprogram.com

Institute for Therapeutic Massage - University of Medicine & Dentistry
Massage Therapy Prgm
150 Bergen St
Newark, NJ 07103
www.massageprogram.com

Omega Institute
Massage Therapy Prgm
7050 Rte 38 E
Pennsauken, NJ 08109

Cortiva Inst, Somerset Sch of Massage Therapy - Piscataway
Massage Therapy Prgm
180 Centennial Ave
Piscataway, NJ 08854
www.cortiva.com/

Institute for Therapeutic Massage - Pompton Lakes
Massage Therapy Prgm
125 Wanaque Ave
Pompton Lakes, NJ 07442
www.massageprogram.com

Institute for Therapeutic Massage
Massage Therapy Prgm
99 Hwy 37 W
Toms River, NJ 08755
www.massageprogram.com

National Massage Therapy Institute - Turnersville
Massage Therapy Prgm
108-L Greentree Rd and Black Horse Pike
Turnersville, NJ 08012

Cortiva Inst, Somerset Sch of Massage Therapy - Wall Township
Massage Therapy Prgm
1985 Hwy 34
Wall Township, NJ 07719
www.cortiva.com/locations/ssmt/

Healing Hands Institute for Massage Therapy
Massage Therapy Prgm
41 Bergenline Ave
Westwood, NJ 07675
www.healinghandsinstitute.com

New Mexico

Crystal Mountain Sch of Therapeutic Massage
Massage Therapy Prgm
4775 Indian School Rd NE
Suite 102
Albuquerque, NM 87110
www.crystalmtnmassage.com

North Carolina

Body Therapy Institute
Massage Therapy Prgm
300 Southwind Rd
Siler City, NC 27344
www.massage.net

Ohio

Cincinnati School of Medical Massage
Massage Therapy Prgm
11250 Cornell Park Dr, Ste 203
Cincinnati, OH 45242
www.massageschools.com

Dayton School of Medical Message
Massage Therapy Prgm
4457 Far Hills Ave
Dayton, OH 45429
www.massageschools.com

Dayton School of Medical Message
Massage Therapy Prgm
Apollo Career Center
3325 Shawnee Rd
Lima, OH 45806
www.massageschools.com

Cleveland Institute of Medical Massage
Massage Therapy Prgm
18334-D E Bagley Rd
Middleburg Heights, OH 44130
www.massageschools.com

Oregon

East-West Coll of the Healing Arts
Massage Therapy Prgm
525 NE Oregon St
Portland, OR 97232
www.eastwestcollege.com

Pennsylvania

Synergy Healting Arts Center & Massage School
Massage Therapy Prgm
13593 Monterey Ln
Blue Ridge Summit, PA 17214
www.synergymassage.com

Cortiva Inst - Penn School of Muscle Therapy
Massage Therapy Prgm
1173 Egypt Rd, PO Box 400
Oaks, PA 19456-0400
www.psmt.com

National Massage Therapy Institute
Massage Therapy Prgm
Division of PSB
10050 Roosevelt Blvd
Philadelphia, PA 19116

Baltimore School of Massage
Massage Therapy Prgm
170 Red Rock Rd
York, PA 17402
www.bsmyork.com

Rhode Island

Community College of Rhode Island
Massage Therapy Prgm
One John H Chafee Blvd
Newport, RI 02840
www.ccri.edu

Tennessee

Roane State Community College
Massage Therapy Prgm
Somatic Massage Therapy Program
701 Briarcliff Ave
Oak Ridge, TN 37830
www.rscc.cc.tn.us

Virginia

Virginia School of Massage
Massage Therapy Prgm
2008 Morton Dr
Charlottesville, VA 22903
www.vasom.com

National Massage Therapy Institute
Massage Therapy Prgm
803 W Broad St, Ste 110
Falls Church, VA 22046

Cayce/Reilly School of Massotherapy
Massage Therapy Prgm
215 67th St
Virginia Beach, VA 23451
www.are-cayce.com

Washington

Cortiva Institute - Seattle
Massage Therapy Prgm
425 Pontius Ave N, Ste 100
Seattle, WA 98109
www.cortiva.com

West Indies

Trinidad & Tobago Coll of Therapeutic Massage
Massage Therapy Prgm
68 Market St
Trinidad, West Indies, WN

West Virginia

Mountain State School of Massage
Massage Therapy Prgm
601 50th St
Charleston, WV 25304
www.mtnstmassage.com

Wisconsin

Blue Sky School of Professional Massage
Massage Therapy Prgm
220 American Blvd
De Pere, WI 54155
www.blueskymassage.com

Blue Sky School of Professional Massage
Massage Therapy Prgm
220 Oak St
Grafton, WI 53024
www.blueskymassage.com

Blue Sky School of Professional Massage
Massage Therapy Prgm
2122 Luann Ln
Madison, WI 53713
www.blueskymassage.com

Lakeside School of Massage Therapy -
  Milwaukee
Massage Therapy Prgm
1726 N 1st St, Ste 200
Milwaukee, WI 53212
www.lakeside.edu

Counseling

Includes:
- Counselor
- Genetic counselor
- Rehabilitation counselor

Counselor

History

In 1968, Robert Stripling, often called "the father of accreditation in counselor accreditation," commented that counseling had begun to realize its "obligation to protect society, insofar as possible, from poorly prepared counselors…through accrediting of counselor education programs." At the time, many institutions of higher learning had already developed counseling courses and programs in counseling at the undergraduate and graduate levels. With the adoption of standards both during the 1960s and in a broadened, refined form in the early 1970s, voluntary and developmental self-evaluation of counselor education programs began to gain the interest of a small but growing number of programs. This movement resulted in the creation in 1981 of the Council for Accreditation of Counseling and Related Educational Programs (CACREP), which accredits counseling education programs.

Career Description

The counseling profession differs from other human service professions in its developmental approach to problem solving. Counselors deal with human development concerns through support, therapeutic approaches, consultation, evaluation, teaching, and research. Simply stated, counseling is the art of helping people grow.

Employment Characteristics

Professional counselors can be found in a variety of settings, including:
- private practice
- elementary, middle, and secondary schools
- colleges/universities
- hospitals
- health maintenance organizations
- insurance firms
- drug and alcohol abuse rehabilitation agencies
- mental health agencies
- correctional institutions
- career development and vocational training facilities

Success in the counseling field requires motivation, a commitment to service, and skills in communication. Counselors will be faced with numerous challenges and opportunities in the future, including drug abuse, homelessness, disaster recovery, and the "graying of America" with an increasing percentage of Americans who are senior citizens. The foundations of the counseling profession have been intertwined with both social and educational reform movements in this century and will continue to be so in the future.

Salary

May 2011 data from the US Bureau of Labor Statistics show that wages for educational vocational, and school counselors at the 10th percentile are \$32,130, the 50th percentile (median) at \$54,130, and the 90th percentile at \$87,020 (*www.bls.gov/oes/current/oes211012.htm*).

As with most professions, pay scales differ based on education, prior experience, and geographical location.

For more information, refer to *www.ama-assn.org/go/hpsalary*.

Educational Programs

Length. Career Counseling, College Counseling, Community Counseling, Gerontological Counseling, School Counseling, and Student Affairs programs are a minimum of 48 semester hours or 72 quarter hours. Mental Health Counseling and Marital, Couple and Family Counseling/Therapy programs are a minimum of 60 semester hours or 90 quarter hours.

Curriculum. Curricular experiences and demonstrated knowledge in each of the eight common core areas are required of all counseling students:
1. Professional Identity
2. Social and Cultural Diversity
3. Human Growth and Development
4. Career Development
5. Helping Relationships
6. Group Work
7. Assessment
8. Research and Program Evaluation

Clinical Requirements. Students must complete supervised practicum experiences that total a minimum of 100 clock hours. The practicum provides for the development of counseling skills under supervision. The student's practicum includes the following:
1. Forty hours of direct service with clients, including experience in individual counseling and group work.
2. Weekly interaction with an average of one hour per week of individual and/or triadic supervision, which occurs regularly over the course of one academic term by a programs faculty member or a supervisor working under the supervision of a program faculty member.
3. An average of one-and-a-half hours per week of group supervision, provided on a regular schedule over the course of the student's practicum by a program faculty member or a supervisor under the supervision of a program faculty member.
4. Evaluation of the student's performance throughout the practicum, including a formal evaluation after the student completes the practicum.

The program requires students to complete a supervised internship of 600 clock hours after successful completion of the student's practicum. The internship provides an opportunity for the student to perform, under supervision, a variety of counseling activities that a professional counselor is expected to perform. The student's internship includes all of the following:

1. Two hundred and forty hours of direct service with clients appropriate to the programs of study.
2. Weekly interaction with an average of one hour per week of individual and/or triadic supervision, throughout the internship, usually performed by the on-site supervisor.
3. An average of one-and-a-half hours per week of group supervision provided on a regular schedule throughout the internship, usually performed by a program faculty member.
4. The opportunity for the student to become familiar with a variety of professional activities in addition to direct service (e.g., recordkeeping, supervision, information and referral, in-service and staff meetings).
5. The opportunity for the student to develop program-appropriate audio and/or videotapes of the student's interactions with clients for use in supervision.
6. The opportunity for the student to gain supervised experience in the use of a variety of professional resources, such as assessment instruments, technologies, print and nonprint media, professional literature, and research.
7. A formal evaluation of the student's performance during the internship by a program faculty member, in consultation with the site supervisor.

Certification

Some counselors elect to be nationally certified by the National Board for Certified Counselors, Inc (NBCC), which grants the general practice credential "National Certified Counselor." To be certified, a counselor must hold a master's degree with a concentration in counseling from a regionally accredited college or university; must have at least two years of supervised field experience in a counseling setting (graduates from counselor education programs accredited by CACREP are exempted); must provide two professional endorsements, one of which must be from a recent supervisor; and must have a passing score on the NBCC's National Counselor Examination for Licensure and Certification (NCE). This national certification is voluntary and is distinct from state licensing. However, in some states, those who pass the national exam are exempted from taking a state certification exam. NBCC also offers specialty certifications in school, clinical mental health, and addiction counseling, which supplement the national certified counselor designation. These specialty certifications require passage of a supplemental exam. To maintain their certification, counselors retake and pass the NCE or complete 100 credit hours of acceptable continuing education every five years.

Inquiries

Careers
American Counseling Association
5999 Stevenson Avenue
Alexandria, VA 22304
703 823-9800
www.counseling.org

Certification
National Board for Certified Counselors
3 Terrace Way, Suite D
Greensboro, NC 27403
336 547-0607
www.nbcc.org

Program Accreditation
Council for Accreditation of Counseling and Related Educational Programs
1001 North Fairfax Street, Suite 510
Alexandria, VA 22314
703 535-5990
www.cacrep.org

Note: Adapted in part from the Bureau of Labor Statistics, U.S. Department of Labor, *Occupational Outlook Handbook,* Counselors, at *www.bls.gov/oco/ocos067.htm*.

The following programs are coded as follows:
- Career counselor (CrC)
- College counselor (CIC)
- Community counselor (CC)
- Gerontological counseling (GC)
- Marital, couple and family counseling/therapy (MFC/T)
- Mental health counselor (MHC)
- School counselor (SC)
- Student affairs (SA)
- Student affairs-college counseling (SACC)
- Student affairs-professional practice (SAPP)
- Counselor education and supervision (CE)

As of July 1, 2009, the Council for Accreditation of Counseling and Related Educational Programs (CACREP) implemented new accreditation standards that combined Community Counseling (CC) and Mental Health Counseling (MHC) into Clinical Mental Health Counseling (CMHC). These standards also added Addiction Counseling (AC) and eliminated Gerontological Counseling (GC). As programs apply for new accreditation and reapply for renewed accreditation, these new titles will be added to the *Directory*. (CACREP does not accredit programs in genetic counseling or rehabilitation counseling.)

- Addiction Counseling
- Career Counseling
- Clinical Mental Health Counseling

Alabama

Auburn University
Counseling Prgm
2084 Haley Center
Auburn University, AL 36849-5222
www.auburn.edu/coun

University of Montevallo
Counseling Prgm
CC, SC Programs
College of Education, Station 6380
Montevallo, AL 35115
www.montevallo.edu

Troy University
Counseling Prgm
CC, MHC, SC Programs
One University Place
Phenix City, AL 36869
phenix.troy.edu

Troy University
Counseling Prgm
CC, SC Programs
10 McCartha Hall
Troy, AL 36082
www.troy.edu

University of Alabama
Counseling Prgm
CC, SC, CE Programs
PO Box 870231
Tuscaloosa, AL 35487-0231
www.ua.edu

Arizona

Northern Arizona University
Counseling Prgm
CC, SC Programs
Educational Psychology, PO Box 5774 - COE
Flagstaff, AZ 86011-5774

University of Phoenix
Counseling Prgm
CC Program
4635 E Elwood St, CJA 201
Phoenix, AZ 85040
www.phoenix.edu

Arizona State University
Counseling Prgm
CC Program
PO Box 870611
Payne Hall Rm 302
Tempe, AZ 85287-0611

Arkansas

Henderson State University
Counseling Prgm
PO Box 7774
Arkadelphia, AR 71999-0001

University of Arkansas
Counseling Prgm
CC, SC, CE Programs
136 Graduate Education Bldg
Fayetteville, AR 72701
www.uark.edu

Arkansas State University
Counseling Prgm
SC Program
PO Box 1560
State University, AR 72467-1560
www.clt.astate.edu/psycoun/
    eds-psychology_&_counseling.htm

British Columbia, Canada

Trinity Western University
Counseling Prgm
CC Program
7600 Glover Rd
Langley, BC V2Y 1Y1
www.twu.ca/cpsy

California

California State University - Fresno
Counseling Prgm
MFC/T Program
5005 N Maple Ave, M/S3
Fresno, CA 93740-8025
http://caracas.soehd.csufresno.edu

California State University - Los Angeles
Counseling Prgm
MFC/T, SC Programs
5151 State University Dr
King Hall C-1065
Los Angeles, CA 90032
www.calstatela.edu/academic/ccoe/

California State University - Northridge
Counseling Prgm
CrC, MFC/T, SACC, SC Programs
18111 Nordhoff St
Northridge, CA 91330-8265
www.csun.edu/edpsy

Sonoma State University
Counseling Prgm
CC, SC Programs
1801 E Cotati Ave, Rm N220
Rohnert Park, CA 94928
www.sonoma.edu/counseling

San Francisco State University
Counseling Prgm
Dept of Counseling
1600 Holloway Ave
Burk Hall Rm 524
San Francisco, CA 94132

Colorado

Adams State College
Counseling Prgm
CC, SC Programs
Dept of Psychology
ES309-Box J
Alamosa, CO 81102
www.adams.edu

University of Colorado at Colorado Springs
Counseling Prgm
4120 Austin Bluffs Pkwy
PO Box 7150
Colorado Springs, CO 80933-7150
www.uccs.edu/coegen

Regis University
Counseling Prgm
3333 Regis Blvd, L-16
Denver, CO 80221-1099
www.regis.edu

University of Colorado at Denver
Counseling Prgm
Campus Box 106
PO Box 173364 UDHSC
Denver, CO 80217-3364
www.ucdenver.edu/academics/colleges/schoolofeducatio
    n/academics/Pages

University of Colorado Denver - Anschutz MC
Counseling Prgm
CC, MFC/T, SC Programs
Health Sciences Center, Campus Box 106
PO Box 173364
Denver, CO 80217-3364

Colorado State University
Counseling Prgm
CrC, CC, SC Programs
Education 215
Counseling & Career Development
Fort Collins, CO 80523-1588

University of Northern Colorado
Counseling Prgm
CC, MFC/T, SC, CE Programs
Division of Professional Psychology
McKee Hall #248
Greeley, CO 80639
www.unco.edu

Denver Seminary
Counseling Prgm
CC Program
Counseling Division
6399 S Santa Fe Dr
Littleton, CO 80120

Connecticut

Western Connecticut State University
Counseling Prgm
CC, SC Programs
Education Dept
Westside Campus
Danbury, CT 06810
www.wcsu.ctstateu.edu

Fairfield University
Counseling Prgm
CC, SC Programs
Graduate School of Ed & Allied Prof
Fairfield, CT 06430-7524
www.fairfield.edu

Southern Connecticut State University
Counseling Prgm
CC, SC Programs
Counseling & School Psychology Dept
501 Crescent St
New Haven, CT 06515
www.southernct.edu

University of Connecticut
Counseling Prgm
249 Glenbrook Rd Unit 2064
Storrs, CT 06269-2064
www.education.uconn.edu/departments/epsy/

Delaware

Wilmington College
Counseling Prgm
31 Read's Way
Wilson Graduate Center
31 Read's Way
New Castle, DE 19720
www.wilmcoll.edu

District of Columbia

Gallaudet University
Counseling Prgm
MHC, SC Programs
800 Florida Ave NE
Washington, DC 20002
www.gallaudet.edu

George Washington University
Counseling Prgm
Graduate School of Edu and Human Dev
2134 G St NW
Washington, DC 20052
www.gwu.edu/~chaos

Florida

Florida Atlantic University
Counseling Prgm
MHC, SC Programs
777 Glades Rd
Bldg 47, Rm 270
Boca Raton, FL 33431
www.fau.edu/index.php

Stetson University
Counseling Prgm
MFC/T, MHC, SC Programs
421 N Woodland Blvd, Unit 8389
Deland, FL 32720
www.stetson.edu/artsci/counselor

Florida Gulf Coast University
Counseling Prgm
MHC, SC Programs
10501 FGCU Blvd S
Fort Myers, FL 33965-6565
coe.fgcu.edu

University of Florida
Counseling Prgm
Marriage and Family Counseling Program
Department of Counselor Education
1215 Norman Hall, Box 117046
Gainesville, FL 32611-7046
http://education.ufl.edu/counselor

University of Florida
Counseling Prgm
Counselor Education Dept
1215 Norman Hall, PO Box 117046
Gainesville, FL 32611-7046
http://education.ufl.edu/counselor

University of Florida
Counseling Prgm
Mental Health Counseling
Department of Counselor Education
1215 Norman Hall, Box 117046
Gainesville, FL 32611-7046
http://education.ufl.edu/counselor

University of North Florida
Counseling Prgm
MHC, SC Programs
4567 St Johns Bluff Rd S
Jacksonville, FL 32224-2645
www.unf.edu

Florida International University
Counseling Prgm
MHC, SC Programs
FIU University Park Campus
ZEB 214A
Miami, FL 33119
www.fiu.edu

Barry University
Counseling Prgm
MHC, SC, MFC/T Programs
11300 NE 2nd Ave
Miami Shores, FL 33161-6695
www.barry.edu

University of Central Florida
Counseling Prgm
MHC, SC, CE programs
400 Central Blvd
Orlando, FL 32816

Florida State University
Counseling Prgm
CrC, MHC, SC Programs
215 Stone Bldg
College of Education
Tallahassee, FL 32306
www.epls.fsu.edu

University of South Florida
Counseling Prgm
CrC, MHC, SC Programs
4202 E Fowler Ave EDU 162
Tampa, FL 33620-5650
www.coedu.usf.edu/deptpsysoc/ce/eds.htm

Rollins College
Counseling Prgm
MHC, SC Programs
1000 Holt Ave, PO Box 2726
Winter Park, FL 32789-4499
www.rollins.edu

Georgia

University of Georgia
Counseling Prgm
CC, SC Programs
402 Aderhold Hall
Athens, GA 30602-7142
www.coe.uga.edu/chds

Georgia State University
Counseling Prgm
CC, SC, CE programs
Professional Counseling Prgm
University Plaza
Atlanta, GA 30303-3083
www.gsu.edu

University of West Georgia
Counseling Prgm
CC, SC Programs
Dept of Counseling and Educational Psychology
Education Center Annex #237
Carrollton, GA 30118-5170
coe.westga.edu/cep

Columbus State University
Counseling Prgm
CC, SC Programs
4225 University Ave
Columbus, GA 31907-5645
www.colstate.edu

Idaho

Boise State University
Counseling Prgm
Counseling Dept Ed Bldg, Rm 612
1910 University Dr
Boise, ID 83725-1710
education.boisestate.edu/counselored

University of Idaho
Counseling Prgm
SC, CE programs
College of Education, Rm 206
Moscow, ID 83844-3083

Northwest Nazarene University
Counseling Prgm
CC, SC, MFC Programs
623 Holly St
Nampa, ID 83686
www.nnu.edu/counseloreducation

Idaho State University
Counseling Prgm
MHC, SC, SACC, CE, MFC/T Programs
PO Box 8120
Pocatello, ID 83209-8120
www.isu.edu/departments/counsel/homepage

Illinois

Southern Illinois University Carbondale
Counseling Prgm
CC, MFC/T, SC, CE Programs
Wham Bldg, Rm 223
Campus Mail Code 4618
Carbondale, IL 62901-4618
www.siu.edu/departments/coe/epse

Southern Illinois University Edwardsville
Counseling Prgm
Wham Building 223
Carbondale, IL 62901-4618
www.siu.edu/departments/coe/epse/

Eastern Illinois University
Counseling Prgm
CC, SC programs
2102 Buzzard Hall
600 Lincoln Ave
Charleston, IL 61920

Chicago State University
Counseling Prgm
CC, SC Programs
9501 S King Dr
Harold Washington Hall 328
Chicago, IL 60629
www.csu.edu/psychology/grad.htm

Northeastern Illinois University
Counseling Prgm
CC, SC, MFC/T Programs
5500 N St Louis Ave
Chicago, IL 60625-4699
www.neiu.edu

Roosevelt University
Counseling Prgm
CC, MHC Programs
Department of Counseling and Human Services
430 S Michigan Ave
Chicago, IL 60605
www.roosevelt.edu

Northern Illinois University
Counseling Prgm
CC, SC, CE Programs
Graham Hall 223
DeKalb, IL 60115-2854
www.niu.edu

Western Illinois University
Counseling Prgm
CC, SC Programs
Quad Cities Counselor Education Department
3561 60th St
Moline, IL 61265-5881
www.win.edu

Bradley University
Counseling Prgm
1501 W Bradley Ave
Westlake Hall
Peoria, IL 61625

Concordia University
Counseling Prgm
CC, SC Programs
Psychology Dept
7400 Augusta
River Forest, IL 60305-1499
www.cuchicago.edu

University of Illinois at Springfield
Counseling Prgm
CC, SC Programs
One University Plaza
BRK 332
Springfield, IL 62703
www.uis.edu

Governors State University
Counseling Prgm
CC, MFC/T, SC Programs
College of Education
University Park, IL 60466
www.govst.edu

Indiana

Indiana University - Bloomington
Counseling Prgm
School of Education 4003
201 N Rose Ave
Bloomington, IN 47405-1006
www.indiana.edu/~counsel/ccepro.html

Indiana University Health
Counseling Prgm
SC Program
4600 Sunset Dr
Indianapolis, IN 46208
www.butler.edu

Indiana Wesleyan University
Counseling Prgm
CC, MFC/T Programs
4201 S Washington St
Marion, IN 46953
www.graduatecounseling.indwes.edu

Ball State University
Counseling Prgm
CC, SC Programs
Teachers College, Rm 622
Muncie, IN 47306-0585
www.bsu.edu/counselingpsychology/

Indiana University South Bend
Counseling Prgm
CC, SC Programs
1700 Mishawaka Ave
South Bend, IN 46634
www.iusb.edu

Indiana State University
Counseling Prgm
MHC, SC Programs
School of Education, Rm 1517
Terre Haute, IN 47809
http://counseling.indstate.edu

Purdue University
Counseling Prgm
SC Program
Dept of Educational Studies
100 N University St
West Lafayette, IN 47907-2098

Iowa

University of Northern Iowa
Counseling Prgm
MHC, SC Programs
508 Schindler Education Center
Cedar Falls, IA 50614-0604
www.uni.edu

University of Iowa
Counseling Prgm
CC, CE, SC Programs
N338 Lindquist Center N
Iowa City, IA 52242-1529

Kansas

Emporia State University
Counseling Prgm
MHC, SC, SA Programs
Campus Box 4036
1200 Commercial
Emporia, KS 66801-5087
www.emporia.edu/counre/

Pittsburg State University
Counseling Prgm
CC Program
Dept of Psychology and Counseling
Pittsburg, KS 66762-7551

Kentucky

Western Kentucky University
Counseling Prgm
MFC/T, MHC Programs
1906 College Heights Blvd
51031 TPH 409
Bowling Green, KY 42101
www.wku.edu

Lindsey Wilson College
Counseling Prgm
MHC Program
210 Lindsey Wilson St
Columbia, KY 42728
www.lindseycounseling.org/

Eastern Kentucky University
Counseling Prgm
MHC, SC Programs
521 Lancaster Ave
Richmond, KY 40475
www.education.eku.edu/cel

Louisiana

Louisiana State University
Counseling Prgm
CC, SC Programs
122 Peabody Hall
Baton Rouge, LA 70803
www.lsu.edu

Southeastern Louisiana University
Counseling Prgm
CC, SC, MFC/T Programs
SLU Box 10863
Hammond, LA 70402
www.selu.edu

University of Louisiana at Monroe
Counseling Prgm
CC, MFC/T, SC Programs
700 University Ave
Monroe, LA 71209-0230
www.ulm.edu

Northwestern State University
Counseling Prgm
CIC, SA Programs
College of Education
Student Personnel Services Prgm
Natchitoches, LA 71497
www.nsula.edu

Loyola University New Orleans
Counseling Prgm
CC Program
6363 St Charles Ave, Camp Box 66
New Orleans, LA 70118
www.loyno.edu/education/counseling

Our Lady of Holy Cross College
Counseling Prgm
MFC/T, CC Programs
4123 Woodland Dr
New Orleans, LA 70131

University of New Orleans
Counseling Prgm
CC, CE, SC Programs
348 Education Bldg
New Orleans, LA 70148-2515
www.uno.edu

Maine

University of Southern Maine
Counseling Prgm
MHC, SC Programs
400D Bailey Hall
Gorham, ME 04038-1083
www.usm.maine.edu/cehd/counselor-education

Maryland

Loyola University Maryland
Counseling Prgm
4501 N Charles St
Baltimore, MD 21210
www.loyola.edu

Univ of Maryland at College Park
Counseling Prgm
CE, SC Programs
College of Education
3124 Benjamin Bldg
College Park, MD 20742
www.education.umd.edu/EDCP

Loyola University Maryland
Counseling Prgm
Pastoral Counseling Department
8890 McGaw Rd, Suite 380
Columbia, MD 21045
www.loyola.edu/pastoralcounseling

Massachusetts

Bridgewater State University
Counseling Prgm
34 Park Ave
Bridgewater, MA 02325
www.bridgew.edu/CounselingPrograms/

Michigan

Andrews University
Counseling Prgm
Bell Hall 159
Berrien Springs, MI 49104-0104
www.educ.andrews.edu

University of Detroit Mercy
Counseling Prgm
CC, SC Programs
444 Manning Hall
8200 W Outer Dr
Detroit, MI 48219-0900
www.udmercy.edu

Wayne State University
Counseling Prgm
CC, SC, CE Programs
311 Education Bldg
5425 Gullen Mall
Detroit, MI 48202
www.wayne.edu

Michigan State University
Counseling Prgm
438 Erickson Hall
East Lansing, MI 48824
http://ed-web3.educ.msu.edu/macounsel/

Western Michigan University
Counseling Prgm
CC, CE, CIC, SC Programs
3102 Sangren Hall
Kalamazoo, MI 49008-5195
www.wmich.edu/cecp

Oakland University
Counseling Prgm
CC, SC Programs
Dept of Counseling, 491B Pawley Hall
School of Education and Human Services
Rochester, MI 48309-4494

Eastern Michigan University
Counseling Prgm
CC, SACC, SC Programs
304 Porter Bldg
Ypsilanti, MI 48197
www.emich.edu/coe/leadcons/

Minnesota

Minnesota State University - Mankato
Counseling Prgm
CC, SAPP, SC Programs
107 Armstrong Hall
Mankato, MN 56002-2423
www.mnsu.edu

Minnesota State University - Moorhead
Counseling Prgm
CC, SACC, SAPP Programs
Counseling & Student Affairs
209H Lommen Hall
Moorhead, MN 56563
www.mnstate.edu/cnsa

Winona State University
Counseling Prgm
CC, SC Programs
University Center-Rochester
Hwy 14 E - 859 30th Ave SE
Rochester, MN 55904
www.winona.edu

St Cloud State University
Counseling Prgm
SC Program
720 4th Ave S
St Cloud, MN 56301
www.stcloudstate.edu/ceep

Mississippi

Delta State University
Counseling Prgm
CC, SC Programs
Ewing 335
PO Box 3142
Cleveland, MS 38733
www.deltast.edu/academics/educ/behavsci/public_html

Mississippi College
Counseling Prgm
MFC/T, MHC, SC Programs
PO Box 4013
Clinton, MS 39058
www.mc.edu

University of Southern Mississippi
Counseling Prgm
CC Program
Southern Station Box 05025
Hattiesburg, MS 39406-5025
www.usm.edu

Jackson State University
Counseling Prgm
PO Box 17122
Jackson, MS 39712-0122
www.jsums.edu

Mississippi State University
Counseling Prgm
CC, SACC, SC, CE Programs
PO Box 9727
Mississippi State, MS 39762
www.msstate.edu

University of Mississippi
Counseling Prgm
CC, SC, CE Programs
Suite 200, School of Education
PO Box 1848
University, MS 38677-1848
www.olemiss.edu

Missouri

Southeast Missouri State University
Counseling Prgm
CC, SC Programs
Mail Stop 5550
One University Plaza
Cape Girardeau, MO 63701-4799
www4.semo.edu/counsel

University of Missouri - St Louis
Counseling Prgm
469 Marillac Hall
1 University Blvd
St Louis, MO 63121-4400

Montana

Montana State University
Counseling Prgm
MFC/T, MHC, SC Programs
218 Herrick Hall
Bozeman, MT 59717
www.montana.edu/wwwhhd

University of Montana
Counseling Prgm
MHC, SC Programs
32 Campus Dr
Missoula, MT 59812-6356
www.soe.umt.edu/edldc

Nebraska

University of Nebraska - Kearney
Counseling Prgm
Dept of Counseling and School Psychology
College of Education Bldg
Kearney, NE 68849
www.unk.edu/acad.csp

University of Nebraska - Omaha
Counseling Prgm
CC, SC Programs
Kayser Hall 421
Omaha, NE 68182-0167
www.coe.unomaha.edu/couns/

Nevada

University of Nevada - Las Vegas
Counseling Prgm
CC, MFC/T, SC Programs
4505 S Maryland Pkwy
PO Box 453045
Las Vegas, NV 89154-3003
www.unlv.edu

University of Nevada - Reno
Counseling Prgm
CC, SACC, SC, CE Programs
1664 N Virginia St
MS 281
Reno, NV 89557-0213
www.unr.edu/educ/cep/cepindex.html

New Hampshire

Antioch University New England
Counseling Prgm
40 Avon St
Keene, NH 03431

Plymouth State University
Counseling Prgm
17 High St MSC #11
Plymouth, NH 03264
www.plymouth.edu/graduate/counseling/

New Jersey

The College of New Jersey
Counseling Prgm
CC, SC Programs
Forcina Hall 322 / PO Box 7718
Ewing, NJ 08620-0718
www.tcnj.edu/%7educat/counselor/

Rider University
Counseling Prgm
2083 Lawrenceville Rd
Lawrenceville, NJ 08648-3099
www.rider.edu

Montclair State University
Counseling Prgm
UN 3169 1 Normal Ave
Montclair, NJ 07043
http://cehs.montclair.edu/academics/counseling/

Univ of Medicine & Dent of New Jersey
Counseling Prgm
1776 Raritan Rd
Scotch Plains, NJ 07076
http://shrp.umdnj.edu/programs/msrehabcoun/

Kean University
Counseling Prgm
CC, SC Programs
1000 Morris Ave
Union, NJ 07083
www.kean.edu

William Paterson Univ of New Jersey
Counseling Prgm
Dept of Special Education and Counseling
300 Pompton Rd, Raubinger Hall
Wayne, NJ 07170

Monmouth University
Counseling Prgm
400 Cedar Ave, E148B
West Long Beach, NJ 07764
www.monmouth.edu/academics/
  psychological_counseling/default.asp

New Mexico

University of New Mexico
Counseling Prgm
CC, SC, CE Programs
College of Education, Simpson Hall
Albuquerque, NM 87131-1246
www.unm.edu/~divbse/couns/counselor.htm

New Mexico State University
Counseling Prgm
MHC Program
PO Box 30001
MSC 3CEP
Las Cruces, NM 88003
education.nmsu.edu/cep

New York

SUNY The College at Brockport
Counseling Prgm
350 New Campus Dr
Brockport, NY 14420-2953
http://brockport.edu

Long Island University - C W Post Campus
Counseling Prgm
MHC, SC Programs
Library Rm 320
720 Northern Blvd
Brookville, NY 11548-2814
www.cwpost.liu.edu/cwis/cwp

Canisius College
Counseling Prgm
2001 Main St
Buffalo, NY 14208-1098
www.canisius.edu/counselor_ed/

St John's University
Counseling Prgm
SC Program
Jamaica & Staten Island Campus
8000 Utopia Pkwy
Jamaica, NY 11439
www.stjohns.edu

SUNY College at Plattsburgh
Counseling Prgm
CC, SA, SC Programs
101 Broad St
Ward Hall - Draper Ave
Plattsburgh, NY 12901
http://web.plattsburgh.edu/academics/counselored

St John Fisher College
Counseling Prgm
3690 East Ave Murphy Hall - Room 145
Rochester, NY 114618
www.sjfc.edu/academics/nursing/departments/
    mentalhealth/

University of Rochester
Counseling Prgm
MHC, SC, CE Programs
Dewey Hall 1-314
Rochester, NY 14627
www.rochester.edu/Warner/

Syracuse University
Counseling Prgm
SACC, SC, CE, CC Programs
Counseling and Human Services
259 Huntington Hall
Syracuse, NY 13244-3240
http://soe.syr.edu/academics/grad/
    counseling_human_services/

North Carolina

Gardner-Webb University
Counseling Prgm
PO Box 7315
Boiling Springs, NC 28017
www.psychology.gardner-webb.edu/gwu.htm

Appalachian State University
Counseling Prgm
CC, SC, CIC Programs
Boone, NC 28608
www.hpc.appstate.edu

University of North Carolina - Chapel Hill
Counseling Prgm
SC Program
CB 3500 Peabody Hall
Chapel Hill, NC 27599-3500
www.unc.edu/depts/ed/med_sch_counseling

Univ of North Carolina at Charlotte
Counseling Prgm
CC, CE, SC Programs
9201 University City Blvd
Charlotte, NC 28223-0001
education.uncc.edu/counseling

Western Carolina University
Counseling Prgm
CC, SC Programs
204 Killiam Bldg
Cullowhee, NC 28723
www.ceap.wcu.edu/counseling

North Carolina Central University
Counseling Prgm
School of Education
712 Cecil St
Durham, NC 27707
www.nccucounseling.com

North Carolina A&T State University
Counseling Prgm
CC, SC Programs
Human Development & Services
212 Hudgin Hall
Greensboro, NC 27411-1066
prometheus.educ.ncat.edu/users/advsv

University of North Carolina - Greensboro
Counseling Prgm
CC, CE, GC, MFC/T, SACC, SC Programs
PO Box 26171
228 Curry Bldg
Greensboro, NC 27402-6170
www.uncg.edu/ced

North Carolina State University
Counseling Prgm
CC, SC, CIC, CE Programs
520 Poe Hall
PO Box 7801
Raleigh, NC 27695-7801

Wake Forest University
Counseling Prgm
CC, SC Programs
PO Box 7406
Reynolda Station
Winston-Salem, NC 27109
http://wfu.edu/counseling

North Dakota

North Dakota State University
Counseling Prgm
CC, SC Programs
School of Education, 210 FLC
Fargo, ND 58105-5057
www.ndsu.nodak.edu/ndsu/counsed

Ohio

The University of Akron
Counseling Prgm
Marriage and Family Therapy Programs
    (masters/doctoral)
127 Carroll Hall
Akron, OH 44325-5007
www.uakron.edu/colleges/educ/Counseling/

Ohio University
Counseling Prgm
CC, SC, CE Programs
201 McCracken Hall
Athens, OH 45701
www.coe.ohiou.edu

University of Cincinnati
Counseling Prgm
PO Box 210002
Cincinnati, OH 45221
www.uc.edu/counselingprogram

Xavier University
Counseling Prgm
3800 Victory Pkwy
Cincinnati, OH 45207-6612
www.xavier.edu

Cleveland State University
Counseling Prgm
CC, SC Programs
1983 E 24th St
1419 Rhodes Tower
Cleveland, OH 44115
www.csuohio.edu/casal

John Carroll University
Counseling Prgm
20700 N Park Blvd
University Heights
Cleveland, OH 44118-4581
www.jcu.edu/Graduate

University of Dayton
Counseling Prgm
300 College Park
Dayton, OH 45469
www.udayton.edu/education/cehs/

Wright State University
Counseling Prgm
CC, SC, MHC Programs
M052 Creative Arts Center
Dayton, OH 45435-0001
www.wright.edu

Kent State University
Counseling Prgm
CC, SC, CE Programs
310 White Hall
Kent, OH 44242-0001
www.kent.edu

Walsh University
Counseling Prgm
2020 East Maple St
North Canton, OH 44720
www.walsh.edu/counseling

University of Toledo
Counseling Prgm
Counselor Education and School Psychology
Mail Stop 119
Toledo, OH 43606-3390
http://cesp.utoledo.edu

Youngstown State University
Counseling Prgm
CC, SC Programs
Department of Counseling, BCOE Rm 3305
One University Plaza
Youngstown, OH 44555-0001
www.ysu.edu/counseling

Oklahoma

Oklahoma State University
Counseling Prgm
CC, SC Programs
421 Willard Hall
Stillwater, OK 74078
www.okstate.edu/education/sahep/cpsy

COUNSELING

Oregon

Oregon State University
Counseling Prgm
CC, SC, CE Programs
New School of Education
100 Education Hall
Corvallis, OR 97331
oregonstate.edu/education/counselor.html

Portland State University
Counseling Prgm
CC, SC Programs
PO Box 751
Portland, OR 97207-0751
www.ed.pdx.edu/spedcoun/counpgrm.html

Pennsylvania

Neumann University
Counseling Prgm
One Neumann Dr
Aston, PA 19014
www.neumann.edu

Geneva College
Counseling Prgm
3200 College Ave
Beaver Falls, PA 15010
www.geneva.edu/page/grad_counseling

California University of Pennsylvania
Counseling Prgm
250 University Ave Box 13
California, PA 15419-1394
www.cup.edu/graduate/counsed

Edinboro University of Pennsylvania
Counseling Prgm
SACC, SAPP, SC, CC Programs
128 Butterfield Hall
Edinboro, PA 16444
departments.edinboro.edu/education/professionalstudie
s/counseling

Gannon University
Counseling Prgm
Community Counseling Program
109 University Square
Erie, PA 16541
www.gannon.edu/departmental/cc

Indiana University of Pennsylvania
Counseling Prgm
206 Stouffer Hall
Indiana, PA 15705-1087
www.iup.edu/ce/

Duquesne University
Counseling Prgm
CC, MFC/T, SC Programs
School of Education
Canevin Hall
Pittsburgh, PA 15282
www.education.duq.edu/counselored

Marywood University
Counseling Prgm
MHC, SC Programs
2300 Adams Ave
Scranton, PA 18509
www.marywood.edu

University of Scranton
Counseling Prgm
CC, SC Programs
Dept of Counseling and Human Services
Scranton, PA 18510-4523
academic.scranton.edu/department/chs/

Shippensburg University
Counseling Prgm
CC, MHC, SC, CIC, SA Programs
1871 Old Main Dr, Rm 115
Shippensburg, PA 17257

Slippery Rock University of Pennsylvania
Counseling Prgm
CC Program
006 McKay Education Bldg
Slippery Rock, PA 16057
www.sru.edu

Penn State University
Counseling Prgm
Counselor Education
331 Cedar Bldg
University Park, PA 16828
www.ed.psu.edu/cned/ced.asp

West Chester University
Counseling Prgm
West Chester, PA 19383
www.wcupa.edu/_academics/coed/
AcademicDept/Counseling/

South Carolina

Clemson University
Counseling Prgm
CC, SACC, SAPP, SC Programs
Education and Human Development
330 Tillman Hall, Box 340710
Clemson, SC 29634-0710
www.hehd.clemson.edu/schoolofed/
g-comm_counsel.htm

University of South Carolina
Counseling Prgm
MFC/T, SC, CE Programs
Family Counseling Program
253 Wardlaw Hall
Columbia, SC 29208
edpsych.ed.sc.edu/ce/openpage.htm

South Carolina State University
Counseling Prgm
SC Program
300 College St NE
Orangeburg, SC 29177
www.scsu.edu

Winthrop University
Counseling Prgm
CC, SC Programs
143 Withers Bldg
Oakland Ave
Rock Hill, SC 29733
www.winthrop.edu

South Dakota

South Dakota State University
Counseling Prgm
CC, SACC, SC Programs
PO Box 507
Wenona Hall
Brookings, SD 57007-0095
www.sdstate.edu

University of South Dakota
Counseling Prgm
Delzell School of Education
414 E Clark St
Vermillion, SD 57069
www.usd.edu/cpe

Tennessee

University of Tennessee - Chattanooga
Counseling Prgm
CC, SC Programs
615 McCallie Ave
Dept 4154
Chattanooga, TN 37403
www.utc.edu

East Tennessee State University
Counseling Prgm
CC, SC Programs
PO Box 70548
College of Education
Johnson City, TN 37614-0548
www.etsu.edu/counseling

University of Tennessee - Knoxville
Counseling Prgm
MHC, SC, CE Programs
College of Education
439 Claxton
Knoxville, TN 37996-3400
cehhs.utk.edu

University of Memphis
Counseling Prgm
Ball Hall, Rm 100
Memphis, TN 38152-0001
coe.memphis.edu/cepr

Middle Tennessee State University
Counseling Prgm
SC Program
PO Box 87
Murfreesboro, TN 37132
www.mtsu.edu/~psych/counsel.htm

Vanderbilt University
Counseling Prgm
CC, SC Programs
PO Box 322-GPC
Nashville, TN 37203
www.vanderbilt.edu

Texas

University of Mary Hardin-Baylor
Counseling Prgm
900 College St
Belton, TX 76513
www.umhb.edu

Texas A&M University - Commerce
Counseling Prgm
202 Education North
Commerce, TX 75429
www.tamu-commerce.edu/counseling

Texas A&M University - Commerce
Counseling Prgm
202 Education North
Commerce, TX 75429-3011
www7.tamu-commerce.edu/counseling

Texas A&M University - Corpus Christi
Counseling Prgm
6300 Ocean Drive, Unit 5834
Corpus Christi, TX 78412
http://education.tamucc.edu/counseling/index.html

Texas A&M University - Corpus Christi
Counseling Prgm
CC, CE, MFC/T, SC Programs
6300 Ocean Dr
Corpus Christi, TX 78412
www.tamu.edu

Texas Woman's University
Counseling Prgm
CC, SC Programs
Dept of Family Sciences
PO Box 425769
Denton, TX 76204-5769
www.twu.edu/cope/famsci/index.htm

University of North Texas
Counseling Prgm
CC, SC, CIC, CE Programs
PO Box 310829
Denton, TX 76203-0829
www.coe.unt.edu/che/coun

Sam Houston State University
Counseling Prgm
PO Box 2119
Huntsville, TX 77341-2119
www.shsu.edu/~edu_elc/counseling/

Texas Tech University
Counseling Prgm
CC, SC, CE Programs
PO Box 41071
Lubbock, TX 79409-1071
www.educ.ttu.edu/edce

Stephen F Austin State University
Counseling Prgm
CC, SC Programs
Department of Human Services
PO Box 13019
Nacogdoches, TX 75962-3019
www.sfasu.edu/hs/counseli.htm

St Mary's University
Counseling Prgm
CC, CE, MHC Programs
One Camino Santa Maria
San Antonio, TX 78228-8527
www.stmarytx.edu

Texas State University - San Marcos
Counseling Prgm
CC, MFC/T, SACC, SC Programs
601 University Dr
San Marcos, TX 78666-4615
www.txstate.edu

Utah

University of Phoenix - Utah
Counseling Prgm
MHC Program
5373 S Green St
Salt Lake City, UT 84123

Vermont

University of Vermont
Counseling Prgm
Mann Hall
208 Colchester Ave
Burlington, VT 05405-1757
www.uvm.edu/~cslgprog

Virginia

Argosy University
Counseling Prgm
1550 Wilson Blvd Suite 600
Arlington, VA 22209
www.argosy.edu

Marymount University
Counseling Prgm
CC, SC Programs
2807 N Glebe Rd
Arlington, VA 22207
www.marymount.edu

Virginia Polytechnic Inst & State Univ
Counseling Prgm
CC, SC, CE Programs
Counselor Education
308 E Eggleston, 0302
Blacksburg, VA 24061-0302
www.vt.edu

University of Virginia
Counseling Prgm
Counselor Ed-Ruffner Hall #160
405 Emmet St S, PO Box 400269
Charlottesville, VA 22904-2495
curry.edschool.virginia.edu/curry/dept/edhs

Eastern Mennonite University
Counseling Prgm
1200 Park Rd
Harrisonburg, VA 22802
www.emu.edu/graduatecounseling/

James Madison University
Counseling Prgm
Department of Graduate Psychology
MSC 7401
Harrisonburg, VA 22807
www.psyc.jmu.edu

Lynchburg College
Counseling Prgm
CC, SC Programs
1501 Lakeside Dr
Lynchburg, VA 24501-3199
www.lynchburg.edu

Old Dominion University
Counseling Prgm
CC, SC, SA Programs
College of Education
Norfolk, VA 23529
www.odu.edu

Radford University
Counseling Prgm
PO Box 6994
Radford, VA 24142
eduweb.education.radford.edu/counselored

Virginia Commonwealth University
Counseling Prgm
1015 West Main St PO Box 842020
Richmond, VA 23284-2020
www.soe.vcu.edu/departments/ce/

Regent University
Counseling Prgm
1000 Regent University Dr
Virginia Beach, VA 23464-9800
www.regent.edu/counseling

College of William & Mary
Counseling Prgm
CC, SC, CE Programs
PO Box 8795
Williamsburg, VA 23187-8795
www.wm.edu

Washington

Western Washington University
Counseling Prgm
Dept of Psychology
516 High St
Bellingham, WA 98225-9089
www.ac.wwu.edu/~psych/

Central Washington University
Counseling Prgm
400 E University Way Department of Psychology, MS 7575
Ellensburg, WA 98926-7575
www.cwu.edu/~counpsy/

Eastern Washington University
Counseling Prgm
MHC, SC Programs
705 W First Ave
Spokane, WA 99201
www.ewu.edu

Gonzaga University
Counseling Prgm
East 502 Boone Ave
Gonzaga University
Spokane, WA 99208-0025
www.gonzaga.edu/soe

West Virginia

West Virginia University
Counseling Prgm
CC, SC Programs
3040 University Ave
PO Box 6122
Morgantown, WV 26506-6122
www.hre.wvu.edu/crc/counseling/index.htm

Wisconsin

University of Wisconsin - Oshkosh
Counseling Prgm
CC, SC Pgm, Department of Counselor Education
Nursing Education Building 001
800 Algoma Blvd
Oshkosh, WI 54901
www.coehs.uwosh.edu/counselor_ed/

University of Wisconsin - Superior
Counseling Prgm
CC, SC Programs
McCaskill Hall, Rm 111
Belknap & Catlin Ave, PO Box 2000
Superior, WI 54880
www.uwsuper.edu

University of Wisconsin - Whitewater
Counseling Prgm
Counselor Educ Dept
800 W Main St
Whitewater, WI 53190

Wyoming

University of Wyoming
Counseling Prgm
CC, SC, SA, CE Programs
PO Box 3374
University Station
Laramie, WY 82071
www.uwyo.edu/cnsled/directory.asp

COUNSELING

Genetic Counselor

Genetic counselors are health care professionals who work at the crossroads of medicine, counseling, and technology. They facilitate the translation of genetic discoveries to everyday medical care by working with individuals and families seeking information about medical conditions that may have a genetic contribution.

Career Description

As health care professionals, genetic counselors interpret and provide clear and comprehensive information about the risk of any medical condition that may have a genetic contribution and assist individuals and families in adapting to this information. This involves collecting and interpreting family, medical, and psychosocial history information. Analysis of this history information together with an understanding of genetic principles and the knowledge of current technologies allows genetic counselors to provide individuals and their families with information about risk, prognosis, medical management, and diagnostic and prevention options. Genetic counselors facilitate an informed decision-making process that elicits and respects the spectrum of personal beliefs and values that exist in society.

Employment Characteristics

Genetic counselors practice as part of a health care team. The settings in which genetic counselors work include hospitals and medical centers, public health agencies, colleges and universities, diagnostic laboratories, biotechnology companies, research institutions, private practice, and governmental agencies.

According to the 2010 Professional Status Survey (PSS), conducted by the National Society of Genetic Counselors (NSGC), 33 percent of all genetic counselors work in university medical centers, 19 percent in private hospitals/medical facilities, and 14 percent in public hospitals/medical facilities.

Prenatal, cancer, and pediatrics are the most common specialty areas in which genetic counselors work, according to the PSS. Examples of other specialty areas include adult, neurogenetics, psychiatry, cardiology, infertility, laboratory testing/ screening, and disease-specific clinics.

In addition to health care, advances made by genetic and genomic discoveries have relevance in many other fields. As a result, genetic counselors apply their skills in areas such as research, industry, education, policy, public health, administration, and advocacy work.

Salary

According to the 2010 PSS, the average salary for clinical genetic counselors reported by survey respondents was $63,700 but ranged up to $150,000. Salaries vary by location (*www.nsgc.org/Portals/ 0/Publications/PSS 2010 Executive Summary FINAL.pdf*).

For more information, refer to *www.nsgc.org*

Educational Programs

Length. Genetic counselors earn a master's degree from a graduate program, accredited by the American Board of Genetic Counseling, specifically designed to prepare individuals for a career as a genetic counselor. The training is specialized and includes coursework and supervised clinical experiences.

Curriculum. The coursework includes instruction in the following general content areas:

- Human, medical, and clinical genetics
- Psychosocial theory and counseling techniques
- Social, ethical, and legal issues
- Health care delivery systems and public health principles
- Teaching techniques
- Research methods

The supervised clinical experiences provide students with diversified clinical training and give them experience working with individuals and families affected with a broad range of genetic disorders and counseling situations. Clinical training includes rotations in prenatal, cancer, and pediatric settings at minimum and is important in exposing students to the natural history and management of and psychosocial issues associated with common genetic conditions and birth defects. Students also obtain experience in teaching, laboratory methods, and research.

Inquiries

Careers
Meghan Carey, Executive Director
National Society of Genetic Counselors
401 North Michigan Avenue
Chicago, IL 60611
312 321-6834
E-mail: *nsgc@nsgc.org*
www.nsgc.org

Credentialing/ Program Accreditation
Sheila O'Neal, Executive Director
American Board of Genetic Counseling
18000 West 105th Street
Olathe, KS 66061
913 895-4617
E-mail: *info@abgc.net*
www.abgc.net

Genetic Counselor

Alabama

University of Alabama at Birmingham
Genetic Counseling Prgm
Birmingham, AL 35294

Arkansas

University of Arkansas for Medical Sciences
Genetic Counseling Prgm
College of Health Related Professions
4301 W Markham St, #836
Little Rock, AR 72205
www.uams.edu/chrp/genetics/

British Columbia, Canada

University of British Columbia
Genetic Counseling Prgm
Department of Medical Genetics, MSc Program
Children's & Women's Hlth Centre of BC
4500 Oak St, Room C234
Vancouver, BC
www.medgen.ubc.ca/education/mast_gen.htm
Prgm Dir: Stephanie Kieffer, MS CGC CCGC
Tel: 604 875-2000, Ext 5440 *Fax:* 604 875-3490
E-mail: skieffer@cw.bc.ca

California

University of CA - Irvine School of Medicine
Genetic Counseling Prgm
Div of Human Genetics
Dept of Pediatrics, UCIMC-ZOT 4482
Orange, CA 92868
www.ucihs.uci.edu/pediatrics/gcprogram

Stanford University School of Medicine
Genetic Counseling Prgm
Palo Alto, CA 94305

California State University - Stanislaus
Genetic Counseling Prgm
One University Circle
Turlock, CA 95382
www.extendeded.com/msgenetics/

Colorado

University of Colorado Denver - Anschutz MC
Genetic Counseling Prgm
Education 2 South, L28-4107
13121 E 17th Ave
Aurora, CO 80045
www.ucdenver.edu/geneticcounseling
Prgm Dir: Carol Walton, MS CGC
Tel: 303 724-2356 *Fax:* 720 777-7322
E-mail: Carol.Walton@childrenscolorado.org

District of Columbia

Howard University
Genetic Counseling Prgm
520 W St NW, Box 75
Washington, DC 20059
www.howard.edu

Georgia

Emory University
Genetic Counseling Prgm
1365-B Clifton Rd NE
Atlanta, GA 30322

Illinois

Northwestern University
Genetic Counseling Prgm
Feinberg School of Medicine
676 N St Clair St, #1280
Chicago, IL 60611

Indiana

Indiana University
Genetic Counseling Prgm
School of Medicine
Dept of Medical and Molecular Genetics
975 W Walnut St, IB-130
Indianapolis, IN 46202-5251

Maryland

University of Maryland, Baltimore
Genetic Counseling Prgm
660 W Redwood St, Ste 570
Baltimore, MD 21201
http://medschool.umaryland.edu/mgc/

Johns Hopkins University
Cosponsor: National Human Genome Research Institute
Genetic Counseling Prgm
Social and Behavioral Research Branch NHGRI/NIH
31 Center Dr Rm B1B36, MSC 2073
Bethesda, MD 20892
www.genome.gov/10001156

Massachusetts

Boston University
Genetic Counseling Prgm
Center for Human Genetics
715 Albany St, W408
Boston, MA 02118
www.bumc.bu.edu/hg

Brandeis University
Genetic Counseling Prgm
Biology Dept MS008
Waltham, MA 02454
www.bio.brandeis.edu/gc01/

Michigan

University of Michigan
Cosponsor: UM Rackham Graduate School
Genetic Counseling Prgm
Dept of Human Genetics
4909 Buhl
Ann Arbor, MI 48109-5618
www.hg.med.umich.edu

Wayne State University
Genetic Counseling Prgm
540 E Canfield, 3216 Scott Hall
Detroit, MI 48201
www.wayne.edu

Minnesota

University of Minnesota
Genetic Counseling Prgm
Department of Genetics, Cell Biology
MMC 485, 420 Delaware St, SE
Minneapolis, MN 55455
www.geneticcounseling-grad.umn.edu
Notes: Students are not guaranteed financial support,
 but most are offered a first year Teaching
 Assistantship (TA), which offers partial (50%) tuition
 remission and a living stipend.

New York

Sarah Lawrence College
Genetic Counseling Prgm
One Mead Way
Bronxville, NY 10708-5999
www.sarahlawrence.edu

Long Island University - C W Post Campus
Genetic Counseling Prgm
720 Northern Blvd
Brookville, NY 11548
www.liu.edu/CWPost/Academics/Schools/CLAS/Dept/
 Biology/Graduate-Programs/MS-Genetic.aspx

Mt Sinai School of Medicine
Genetic Counseling Prgm
Dept of Genetics and Genomic Sciences, Box 1497
One Gustave Levy Pl
New York, NY 10029
www.mssm.edu

North Carolina

University of North Carolina - Greensboro
Genetic Counseling Prgm
MS Prgm
119 McIver St
Greensboro, NC 27402
www.uncg.edu/gen

Ohio

Cincinnati Children's Hospital Medical Center
Cosponsor: University of Cincinnati
Genetic Counseling Prgm
Division of Human Genetics
3333 Burnet Ave, ML 4006
Cincinnati, OH 45229
www.geneticcounseling4u.org

Case Western Reserve University
Genetic Counseling Prgm
10900 Euclid Ave
Cleveland, OH 44106-4955
http://genetics.cwru.edu

Oklahoma

University of Oklahoma
Genetic Counseling Prgm
Norman, OK 73019-2071

Ontario, Canada

University of Toronto
Genetic Counseling Prgm
1 King's College Circle
Toronto, ON M5S 1A8
www.utoronto.ca/medicalgenetics/gencounshome.htm

Pennsylvania

Arcadia University
Genetic Counseling Prgm
450 S Easton Rd
Glenside, PA 19038

University of Pittsburgh
Genetic Counseling Prgm
Dept of Human Genetics
A300 Crabtree Hall, 130 DeSoto St
Pittsburgh, PA 15261
www.hgen.pitt.edu

COUNSELING

Quebec, Canada

McGill University
Genetic Counseling Prgm
1205 Dr Penfield Ave, Room N5/13
Montreal, QC H3G 1Y5
www.mcgill.ca/humangenetics/programs/mscgc/
    information/
Prgm Dir: Jennifer Fitzpatrick, MS
Tel: 514 398-3600   *Fax:* 514 398-2430
E-mail: jennifer.fitzpatrick@mcgill.ca

South Carolina

University of South Carolina
Genetic Counseling Prgm
Dept of OB/GYN
Two Medical Park
Ste 208
Columbia, SC 29203
http://geneticcounseling.med.sc.edu

Texas

Univ of Texas Medical School at Houston
Genetic Counseling Prgm
Graduate School of Biomedical Sciences
Dept of Pediatrics
PO Box 20708
Houston, TX 77225

Utah

University of Utah Health Science Center
Genetic Counseling Prgm
15 North 2030 East #2100
Salt Lake City, UT 84112
http://geneticcounseling.genetics.utah.edu

Virginia

Virginia Commonwealth Univ/Health System
Genetic Counseling Prgm
Dept of Human and Molecular Genetics
PO Box 980033
Richmond, VA 23298-0033
www.gen.vcu.edu

Wisconsin

University of Wisconsin - Madison
Genetic Counseling Prgm
Rm 333 Waisman Center, 1500 Highland Ave
Madison, WI 53705
www.genetics.wisc.edu

Genetic Counselor

Programs*	Class Capacity	Begins	Length (months)	Award	Res. Tuition	Non-res. Tuition		Offers:† 1	2	3	4
British Columbia, Canada											
Univ of British Columbia (Vancouver)	6	Sep	20	MSc						•	
Colorado											
Univ of Colorado Denver - Anschutz MC (Aurora)	6	Aug	21	MS	$11,500	$18,000	per year			•	
Quebec, Canada											
McGill Univ (Montreal)	4	Sep 1	20	MSc	$3,500	$7,000		•		•	

*Data are shown only for programs that completed the 2011 AMA Survey of Health Professions Education Programs.

†Key to Offers: 1: Evening or weekend classes; 2: Non-English instruction; 3: Cultural competence instruction; 4: Distance education component.

Rehabilitation Counselor

History

Initially, rehabilitation professionals were recruited from a variety of human service disciplines, including public health nursing, social work, psychology, and school counseling. Although educational programs began to appear in the 1940s, it was not until the availability of federal funding for rehabilitation counseling programs in 1954 that the profession began to grow and establish its own identity. Historically, rehabilitation counselors primarily served working-age adults with disabilities. Today, the need for rehabilitation counseling services extends to persons of all age groups who have disabilities. Rehabilitation counselors also may provide general and specialized counseling to people with disabilities in public human service programs and private practice settings.

Rehabilitation counseling has been recognized as a significant human service program in the United States. A major value of rehabilitation counseling has been the importance of assisting individuals with disabilities deal with the various issues that influence self-sufficiency and employment. The success of programs has been supported by federal legislation of many types since 1920. Legislation has been passed that extended services to individuals with intellectual disabilities and mental illness, funded academic preparation programs for rehabilitation counselors, established a national commission on architectural barriers, and established a national center for deaf-blind students. Legislation directed at the rights of individuals with disabilities has also been significant.

Career Description

Three of the key goals of rehabilitation counseling are to empower individuals to make informed choices, help individuals achieve positive mental health, and maximize opportunities for economic independence (obtain employment if possible). Rehabilitation counselors assist people with physical, mental, or emotional disabilities to become or remain self-sufficient, productive citizens. Working directly with an individual with a disability or their advocates, a rehabilitation counselor is a special type of professional counselor who helps evaluate and coordinate needed services to assist people with disabilities in coping with limitations caused by such factors as cognitive and learning difficulties, environmental and societal discrimination and barriers, psychological conflict/distress, or loss of physical/functional ability. They also provide services to individuals without disabilities who are experiencing stress and coping-difficulties, problems with living, career indecision, job displacement, and general mental health issues.

Disabilities may result from congenital disability, illness and disease, work-related injuries, automobile accidents, the stresses of war, work, daily life, and the aging process. Rehabilitation counselors help individuals with disabilities deal with societal and personal problems, plan careers, and find and keep satisfying jobs. They also may work with individuals, professional organizations, and advocacy groups to address the environmental and social barriers that create obstacles for people with disabilities. The rehabilitation counselor builds bridges between the often isolated world of people with disabilities and their families, communities, and work environments. They may also assist individuals in adjusting in society by helping them move from a position of dependence to independence.

Other responsibilities for the rehabilitation counselor include:
- Evaluating an individual's potential for independent living and employment and arranging for medical and psychological services and vocational assessment, training, and job placement.
- Evaluating medical and psychological reports and conferring with physicians and psychologists about the types of work individuals can perform
- Working with employers to identify or modify job responsibilities to accommodate individuals with disabilities

The rehabilitation counselor draws on knowledge from several fields, including counseling, psychology, medicine, sociology, social work, education, and law. Their specialized knowledge of disabilities and environmental factors that influence adjustment, as well as specific knowledge and skills, differentiate rehabilitation counselors from other types of counselors. Rehabilitation counseling is considered a specialized counseling profession.

Employment Characteristics

Reflecting this wide range of job opportunities, rehabilitation counselors are often employed in positions with different job titles, such as counselor, job placement specialist, substance abuse counselor, rehabilitation consultant, independent living specialist, or case manager. The roles and responsibilities of rehabilitation counselors have expanded greatly over the last ten years, further increasing the attractiveness of a career in the profession. Rehabilitation counselors, for example, have begun to determine, coordinate, and arrange for rehabilitation and transition services for children within school systems. In addition, rehabilitation counselors are providing geriatric rehabilitation services to older persons with health problems, and workers injured on the job are increasingly receiving rehabilitation services through private rehabilitation counseling companies and employers' disability management and employee assistance programs. They may also become life-care planners assisting individuals who will experience major long-term disability. Many former teachers, attorneys, nurses, physical therapists, occupational therapists, clergy, and business people have found second careers as professional rehabilitation counselors.

Salary

May 2011 data from the US Bureau of Labor Statistics (*www.bls.gov/oes/current/oes211015.htm*) show that wages at the 10th percentile are $20,910, the 50th percentile (median) $33,740, and the 90th percentile $58,480. Average salaries in states that require the master's degree or disability-specific knowledge and skills such as sign language may be considerably higher. Determining salary opportunities are complicated by the manner in which job requirements vary in various states. Salary requirements in most states require a master's degree, but some states only require a bachelor's degree, which decreases the overall national salary mean.

Many rehabilitation counselors will choose work in state or federal rehabilitation agencies or community rehabilitation programs. Others will seek opportunities in the private or for-profit sector of rehabilitation. Because all state rehabilitation agencies follow the same general procedures, a rehabilitation counselor has geographical mobility and can find employment throughout the United

COUNSELING

States and its territories. Other potential employers include comprehensive rehabilitation centers, universities and academic settings, insurance companies, substance abuse rehabilitation centers, correctional facilities, halfway houses, and independent living centers.

Employment Outlook

Rehabilitation counselors serve a large portion of the US population. An estimated 54 million Americans have physical, mental, or psychological disabilities that restrict their activities and prevent them from obtaining or maintaining jobs. Consequently, the employment outlook for the profession is excellent. Based on national employment outlook studies and regional and state surveys, hundreds of rehabilitation counselor positions are expected to be available in the coming years for qualified master's level professionals. Recent studies show that rehabilitation counselor education programs are not graduating sufficient numbers of qualified students to meet current and anticipated marketplace needs.

Education and Training

Length. Rehabilitation counselor education programs typically provide between 18 and 24 months of academic and field-based clinical training. Clinical training consists of a practicum and a minimum of 600 hours of supervised internship experience. Clinical field experiences are available in a variety of community, state, federal, and private rehabilitation-related programs. Most accredited master's-level programs require 60 graduate hours of coursework. This allows graduates to become CRCs or LPCs in most states. Most public sector and private sector rehabilitation programs require the master degree.

Prerequisites. Although no formal requirements exist, most rehabilitation counseling graduate students have undergraduate degrees in rehabilitation services, psychology, sociology, or other human services-related fields.

Curriculum. Rehabilitation counselors are trained in
- Counseling theory, skills, and techniques
- Individual and group counseling
- Environmental assessment
- Psychosocial and medical aspects of disability, including human growth and development
- Social and cultural diversity
- Principles of psychiatric rehabilitation
- Case management and rehabilitation planning
- Issues and ethics in rehabilitation service delivery
- Technological adaptation
- Vocational evaluation and work adjustment
- Career counseling
- Research and program evaluation
- Job development and placement

In addition, students may enroll in courses that address content such as:
- Marriage and family counseling
- Substance abuse rehabilitation
- Juvenile and adult offender rehabilitation
- Intellectual disabilities
- Communication disorders
- Sign language
- Stress management
- Psychological testing
- Conflict management
- Crisis counseling

- DSM diagnosis and treatment planning
- Rehabilitation administration

Licensure, Certification, and Registration

Certification and licensure of rehabilitation counselors help protect the public and provide a means of identifying those individuals who possess the minimum training and meet supervised work experience standards established by professional groups and governmental agencies.

Certification. The Commission on Rehabilitation Counselor Certification (CRCC), an independent credentialing body incorporated in 1974, certifies rehabilitation counselors throughout the United States and in Canada who meet educational and work experience requirements, pass an examination, and maintain certification by completing 100 hours of acceptable continuing education credit every five years.

Licensure. A counseling license is a credential authorized by a state legislature that regulates the title and/or practice of professional counselors. Rehabilitation counselors are eligible for licensure as professional counselors in nearly all states that regulate counselors; licensure requirements include passing an examination, acquiring needed supervised counseling experience, and, in some states, completing specified coursework.

Registration. A number of state workers' compensation laws or regulations specify education, training, and/or credentials requirements for people providing rehabilitation counseling services to workers with disabilities. In these states, rehabilitation counselors pay a fee and provide proof of education and/or certification to register with the state workers' compensation agency. Many states also require the certified rehabilitation counselor (CRC) credential, although the permitted scope of services may vary from one state to the next.

Inquiries

Careers
National Council on Rehabilitation Education
1099 E. Champlain Drive, Suite A
PMB 137
Fresno, CA 93740
559 906-0787
www.ncre.org
E-mail: *info@ncre.org*

Certification
Commission on Rehabilitation Counselor Certification
Cindy Chapman, Executive Director
1699 East Woodfield Road, Suite 300
Schaumburg, IL 60173
847 944-1325
www.crccertification.com

Program Accreditation
Council on Rehabilitation Education
1699 East Woodfield Road, Suite 300
Schaumburg, IL 60173
847 944-1345
www.core-rehab.org

Alabama

Auburn University
Rehabilitation Counseling Prgm
Rehabilitation and Special Education
1228 Haley Center
Auburn University, AL 36849
www.auburn.edu/rse

University of Alabama at Birmingham
Rehabilitation Counseling Prgm
School of Education, Rm 157
901 S 13th St
Birmingham, AL 35294-1250
www.ed.uab.edu/counseloreducation/index.htm

Alabama A&M University
Rehabilitation Counseling Prgm
PO Box 580
Normal, AL 35762
www.aamu.edu

Troy University
Rehabilitation Counseling Prgm
College of Education
228 General Academic Bldg
Troy, AL 36082
www.troy.edu

University of Alabama
Rehabilitation Counseling Prgm
318 Graves Hall, PO Box 870231
Tuscaloosa, AL 35487-0231

Arizona

University of Arizona
Rehabilitation Counseling Prgm
Dept of Special Educ and Rehab
College of Education
Tucson, AZ 85721
www.arizona.edu

Arkansas

University of Arkansas
Rehabilitation Counseling Prgm
Rehabilitation Education and Research Program
100 Graduate Education Bldg
Fayetteville, AR 72701
www.uark.edu/depts/coehp/RHAB.htm

University of Arkansas at Little Rock
Rehabilitation Counseling Prgm
2801 S University Ave
Little Rock, AR 72204
www.ualr.edu/rc

Arkansas State University
Rehabilitation Counseling Prgm
Dept of Psychology and Counseling
PO Box 1560
State University, AR 72467
www.clt.astate.edu/mrcprogram

California

California State University - Fresno
Rehabilitation Counseling Prgm
5005 N Maple Ave, MS ED 3
Fresno, CA 93740
http://education.csufresno.edu/cser/

California State University - Los Angeles
Rehabilitation Counseling Prgm
5151 State University Dr, King Hall C1064
Los Angeles, CA 90032
www.calstatela.edu

California State University - Sacramento
Rehabilitation Counseling Prgm
College of Education
6000 J St
Sacramento, CA 95819-6079
www.csus.edu

California State University - San Bernardino
Rehabilitation Counseling Prgm
School of Education
5500 University Pkwy
San Bernardino, CA 92407

San Diego State University
Rehabilitation Counseling Prgm
Dept of Adm Rehab and Postsecondary Ed
3590 Camino del Rio, North
San Diego, CA 92108-1716
www.interwork.sdsu.edu

San Francisco State University
Rehabilitation Counseling Prgm
Dept of Counseling
1600 Holloway Ave
San Francisco, CA 94132
www.sfsu.edu

Colorado

University of Northern Colorado
Rehabilitation Counseling Prgm
School of Human Sciences
Gunter 1250, Box 132
Greeley, CO 80639
www.unco.edu/HHS/hs/hs.htm

Connecticut

Central Connecticut State University
Rehabilitation Counseling Prgm
165 Stanley St
New Britain, CT 06050
www.ccsu.edu

District of Columbia

George Washington University
Rehabilitation Counseling Prgm
Dept of Counseling, Human/Org Studies
2134 G St NW, 3rd Fl
Washington, DC 20052
www.gwu.edu/~chaos

Florida

Florida Atlantic University
Rehabilitation Counseling Prgm
777 Glades Rd
Boca Raton, FL 33431
www.fau.edu

University of Florida
Rehabilitation Counseling Prgm
Dept of Rehabilitation Counseling
PO Box 100175
Gainesville, FL 32610-0175
www.ufrehabcounseling.com

Florida State University
Rehabilitation Counseling Prgm
205 Stone Bldg
Tallahassee, FL 32306
www.coe.fsu.edu/cerds/programs/RehabCounsel.html

University of South Florida
Rehabilitation Counseling Prgm
Dept of Rehabilitation and Mental Health Counseling
4202 E Fowler Ave, SOC 107
Tampa, FL 33620-8100
www.cas.usf.edu/rehab_counseling

Georgia

Georgia State University
Rehabilitation Counseling Prgm
Counseling and Psych Services Dept
PO Box 3980
Atlanta, GA 30302-3980
http://education.gsu.edu/aae/ms/rehl

Fort Valley State University
Rehabilitation Counseling Prgm
1005 State College Dr
PO Box 31030-4313
Fort Valley, GA 31030-4313
www.fvsu.edu

Thomas University
Rehabilitation Counseling Prgm
Division of Counseling
1501 Millpond Rd
Thomasville, GA 31792
www.thomasu.edu

Hawaii

University of Hawaii at Manoa
Rehabilitation Counseling Prgm
Dept of Counselor Education
1776 University Ave, WA2-221
Honolulu, HI 96822
www.hawaii.edu

Idaho

University of Idaho
Rehabilitation Counseling Prgm
Counseling, Sch Psychology, Special Education, &
   Education
College of Education Rm 206
Moscow, ID 83844-3083

Illinois

Southern Illinois University Carbondale
Rehabilitation Counseling Prgm
Rehabilitation Institute
Suite 308
Carbondale, IL 62901-4609

Univ of Illinois at Urbana-Champaign
Rehabilitation Counseling Prgm
1206 S 4th, 121 Hoff
Champaign, IL 61820
www.uiuc.edu

Illinois Institute of Technology
Rehabilitation Counseling Prgm
Inst of Psych, Rm 252 Life Science Bldg
3105 S Dearborn St
Chicago, IL 60616
www.iit.edu/colleges/psych/

Northeastern Illinois University
Rehabilitation Counseling Prgm
5500 N St Louis Ave
Chicago, IL 60625
www.neiu.edu/~counsedu

Northern Illinois University
Rehabilitation Counseling Prgm
Dept of Communicative Disorders
DeKalb, IL 60115
www.niu.edu/index.shtml

Indiana

Ball State University
Rehabilitation Counseling Prgm
Dept of Counseling Psychology and Guidance Services
TC 622
Muncie, IN 47306-0585
www.bsu.edu

Iowa

Drake University
Rehabilitation Counseling Prgm
Counseling, Leadership, and Adult Development
3206 University
Des Moines, IA 50311
www.drake.edu

University of Iowa
Rehabilitation Counseling Prgm
N338 Lindquist Center
Iowa City, IA 52242-1529
www.coe164.education.uiowa.edu:8180/crsd/rehab
Prgm Dir: John Wadsworth, PhD CRC
Tel: 319 335-5246   *Fax:* 319 335-5291
E-mail: john-s-wadsworth@uiowa.edu

Kansas

Emporia State University
Rehabilitation Counseling Prgm
Campus Box 4036, 1200 Commerical
Emporia, KS 66801
www.emporia.edu/counre/

Kentucky

University of Kentucky
Rehabilitation Counseling Prgm
224 Taylor Education Bldg
Lexington, KY 40506
http://education.uky.edu/EDSRC/content/rcwelcome
Prgm Dir: Ralph Crystal, PhD CRC LPC
Tel: 859 257-3834   *Fax:* 859 257-3835
E-mail: crystal@uky.edu

Louisiana

Southern Univ and A&M College
Rehabilitation Counseling Prgm
229 Blanks Hall
Baton Rouge, LA 70813
www.subr.edu/science/rehabcounsel

Louisiana State Univ Health Sciences Center
Rehabilitation Counseling Prgm
School of Allied Health Professions
1900 Gravier St, Suite 8A1
New Orleans, LA 70112-2262

Maine

University of Southern Maine
Rehabilitation Counseling Prgm
400 Bailey Hall
Gorham, ME 04038

Maryland

Coppin State University
Rehabilitation Counseling Prgm
2500 W North Ave
Baltimore, MD 21216

University of Maryland, Baltimore
Rehabilitation Counseling Prgm
Counseling and Personnel Services Dept
Coll of Education, Benjamin Bldg Rm 3214
College Park, MD 20742
www.umd.edu

University of Maryland Eastern Shore
Rehabilitation Counseling Prgm
Ste 1062, Hazel Hall
Princess Anne, MD 21853
www.umes.edu/rehab

Massachusetts

University of Massachusetts - Boston
Rehabilitation Counseling Prgm
Counseling and School Psychology
Graduate College of Education
Boston, MA 02125-3393
www.umb.edu

Springfield College
Rehabilitation Counseling Prgm
Rehabilitation and Disability Studies Dept
263 Alden St
Springfield, MA 01109-3797
www.spfldcol.edu

Assumption College
Rehabilitation Counseling Prgm
Inst for Social and Rehab Services
500 Salisbury St
Worcester, MA 01609-1296
www.assumption.edu

Michigan

Wayne State University
Rehabilitation Counseling Prgm
Theoretical and Behavioral Foundation
323 College of Education, 5425 Gullen Mall
Detroit, MI 48202

Michigan State University
Rehabilitation Counseling Prgm
Counseling, Educ Psych and Spec Educ
237 Erickson Hall
East Lansing, MI 48824-1034
http://ed-web3.educ.msu.edu/ord

Western Michigan University
Rehabilitation Counseling Prgm
The Graduate College
3404 Sangren Hall, Mail Stop 5218
Kalamazoo, MI 49008
www.wmich.edu

Minnesota

Minnesota State University - Mankato
Rehabilitation Counseling Prgm
Dept of Speech, Hearing, and Rehabilitation Svcs
College of Allied Health and Nursing
103 Armstrong Hall
Mankato, MN 56001
http://ahn.mnsu.edu/rehabilitation

St Cloud State University
Rehabilitation Counseling Prgm
Dept of Counselor Education and Ed Psych
720 4th Ave S
St Cloud, MN 56301-4498
www.stcloudstate.edu/ceep/rehab

Mississippi

Jackson State University
Rehabilitation Counseling Prgm
PO Box 18829
Jackson, MS 39217
www.jsums.edu

Mississippi State University
Rehabilitation Counseling Prgm
Counseling, Ed Psych and Special Education
Mail Stop 9727
Mississippi State, MS 39762
www.msstate.edu/dept/rehab/Graduate/rehab.html

Missouri

Maryville University
Rehabilitation Counseling Prgm
650 Maryville University Dr
St Louis, MO 63141

Montana

Montana State University Billings
Rehabilitation Counseling Prgm
Dept of Rehabilitation and Human Services
1500 N 30th St
Billings, MT 59101-0298
www.msubillings.edu

New Jersey

Univ of Medicine & Dent of New Jersey
Rehabilitation Counseling Prgm
Dept of Psychiatric Rehabilitation
1776 Raritan Rd
Scotch Plains, NJ 07076
http://shrp.umdnj.edu/programs/graduate.html

New York

University at Buffalo - SUNY
Rehabilitation Counseling Prgm
Dept of Counseling, School, and Educ Psych
409 Baldy Hall
Buffalo, NY 14260-1000

Hofstra University
Rehabilitation Counseling Prgm
119 Hofstra University, 160 Hagedorn
Hempstead, NY 11549-1190
www.hofstra.edu

CUNY Hunter College
Rehabilitation Counseling Prgm
Dept of Educ Found and Counseling Prgms
695 Park Ave
New York, NY 10021

North Carolina

University of North Carolina - Chapel Hill
Rehabilitation Counseling Prgm
CB 7205, 2088 Bondurant Hall
Chapel Hill, NC 27599
www.med.unc.edu

North Carolina A&T State University
Rehabilitation Counseling Prgm
1601 E Market St
Greensboro, NC 27411
www.ncat.edu

East Carolina University
Rehabilitation Counseling Prgm
Dept of Rehabilitation Studies
School of Allied Health Sciences
Greenville, NC 27858-4353
www.ecu.edu/rehb

Winston-Salem State University
Rehabilitation Counseling Prgm
Anderson Center
601 Martin Luther King Jr Dr
Winston-Salem, NC 27110
www.wssu.edu/wssu

Ohio

Ohio University
Rehabilitation Counseling Prgm
201 McCracken Hall
Athens, OH 45701

Bowling Green State University
Rehabilitation Counseling Prgm
School of Intervention Services
Bowling Green, OH 43403-0255
www.bgsu.edu

Wright State University
Rehabilitation Counseling Prgm
M052 Creative Arts Center
Dayton, OH 45435-0001
www.wright.edu

Kent State University
Rehabilitation Counseling Prgm
405 White Hall
Kent, OH 44242
www.kent.edu

Oklahoma

East Central University
Rehabilitation Counseling Prgm
Box C-1
Ada, OK 74820
www.ecok.edu

Langston University
Rehabilitation Counseling Prgm
4205 N Lincoln Blvd
Oklahoma City, OK 73105
www.lunet.edu

Oregon

Western Oregon University
Rehabilitation Counseling Prgm
Education Bldg 220
Monmouth, OR 97361
www.wou.edu/rehab

Portland State University
Rehabilitation Counseling Prgm
PO Box 751
Portland, OR 97207-0751
www.webmail.pdx.edu

Pennsylvania

Edinboro University of Pennsylvania
Rehabilitation Counseling Prgm
322 Butterfield Hall
Edinboro, PA 16444
www.edinboro.edu/cwis/education/counseling/
    rehab_counseling.html

University of Pittsburgh
Rehabilitation Counseling Prgm
5044 Forbes Tower
3600 Forbes at Atwood St
Pittsburgh, PA 15260
www.pitt.edu

University of Scranton
Rehabilitation Counseling Prgm
Dept of Counseling and Human Services
Scranton, PA 18510-4523
http://matrix.scranton.edu

Penn State University
Rehabilitation Counseling Prgm
327 Cedar Bldg
University Park, PA 16802-3110
www.ed.psu.edu/cecprs

Puerto Rico

Pontifical Catholic University of Puerto Rico
Rehabilitation Counseling Prgm
Department of Social Sciences
2250 Las Ameritas Ave, Suite 655
Ponce, PR 00717-9997

University of Puerto Rico
Rehabilitation Counseling Prgm
College of Social Science
PO Box 23345
San Juan, PR 00931-3345

Rhode Island

Salve Regina University
Rehabilitation Counseling Prgm
100 Ochre Point Ave
Newport, RI 02840
www.salve.edu/graduatestudies/programs/rc

South Carolina

University of South Carolina
Rehabilitation Counseling Prgm
School of Medicine
3555 Harden St Ext, Suite B20
Columbia, SC 29208
www.med.sc.edu

South Carolina State University
Rehabilitation Counseling Prgm
300 College St NE
Orangeburg, SC 29117-0001
www.scsu.edu

South Dakota

University of South Dakota
Rehabilitation Counseling Prgm
Dept of Counseling & Human Resource Development
College of Education & Counseling
Box 507, Wenona Hall 311
Brookings, SD 57007-0095

Tennessee

University of Tennessee - Knoxville
Rehabilitation Counseling Prgm
A522 Claxton Complex
Knoxville, TN 37996-3452
web.utk.edu/~edpsych/rehabilitation_counseling

University of Memphis
Rehabilitation Counseling Prgm
Dept of Counseling, Educ Psych and Research
119D Patterson Hall
Memphis, TN 38152
www.memphis.edu

Texas

University of Texas at Austin
Rehabilitation Counseling Prgm
Special Education
1 University Station, D5300
Austin, TX 78712

Univ of Texas Southwestern Med Ctr
Rehabilitation Counseling Prgm
5323 Harry Hines Blvd
Dallas, TX 75390-9088
www.utsouthwestern.edu

University of North Texas
Rehabilitation Counseling Prgm
Dept of Rehab Social Work and Addiction
PO Box 311456
Denton, TX 76203
www.unt.edu

Univ of Texas - Pan American
Rehabilitation Counseling Prgm
1201 W University Dr
Edinburg, TX 78539-2999
www.panam.edu

Texas Tech University
Rehabilitation Counseling Prgm
Rehabilitation Sciences
3601 Fourth St, M/S 6225, Suite 2C-200
Lubbock, TX 79430-6225
www.ttu.edu

Stephen F Austin State University
Rehabilitation Counseling Prgm
Dept of Human Services
PO Box 13019/SFA Station
Nacogdoches, TX 75962-3019
www.sfasu.edu/hs

Utah

Utah State University
Rehabilitation Counseling Prgm
Dept of Special Educ and Rehab
2865 Old Main Hill
Logan, UT 84322-2865
www.rce.usu.edu

Virginia

Virginia Commonwealth University
Rehabilitation Counseling Prgm
Dept of Rehab Counseling
1112 E Clay St, Box 980330
Richmond, VA 23298-0330
views.vcu.edu/sahp/rehab

Washington

Western Washington University
Rehabilitation Counseling Prgm
6912 220th St SW
Suite 105
Mountlake Terrace, WA 98043
www.wwu.edu/rc

West Virginia

West Virginia University
Rehabilitation Counseling Prgm
502 Allen Hall, PO Box 6122
Morgantown, WV 26506-6122
www.wvu.edu

COUNSELING

Wisconsin

University of Wisconsin - Madison
Rehabilitation Counseling Prgm
Rehab Psych and Special Educ
432 N Murray St
Madison, WI 53706
www.wisc.edu

University of Wisconsin - Stout
Rehabilitation Counseling Prgm
Dept of Rehabilitation and Counseling
250F Vocational Rehabilitation
Menomonie, WI 54751
www.uwstout.edu

Rehabilitation Counselor

Programs*	Class Capacity	Begins	Length (months)	Award	Res. Tuition	Non-res. Tuition	Offers:† 1	2	3	4
Iowa										
Univ of Iowa (Iowa City)	15	Jun	23, 48	Cert, MA, PhD			•		•	
Kentucky										
Univ of Kentucky (Lexington)	100	Aug	16	MRC	$16,500	$34,600	•		•	•

*Data are shown only for programs that completed the 2011 AMA Survey of Health Professions Education Programs.

†Key to Offers: 1: Evening or weekend classes; 2: Non-English instruction; 3: Cultural competence instruction; 4: Distance education component.

Dentistry and Related Fields

Includes:
- Dental assistant
- Dental hygienist
- Dental laboratory technician
- Dentist

History

From the early 1940s until 1975, the American Dental Association's (ADA's) Council on Dental Education was the agency recognized as the national accrediting organization for dentistry and dental-related educational programs. In 1975, this accreditation authority was transferred to the Commission on Accreditation of Dental and Dental Auxiliary Educational Programs, an expanded agency established to provide representation of all groups affected by its accrediting activities. In 1979, the name of the Commission was changed to the Commission on Dental Accreditation (CODA). The accreditation standards for educational programs in dental assisting, dental hygiene, and dental laboratory technology have been revised several times over the years to reflect the dental profession's changing needs and educational trends.

Dental Assistant

The dental assistant increases the efficiency of the dental care team by aiding the dentist in the delivery of oral health care. The dental assistant performs a wide range of tasks requiring both interpersonal and technical skills. Duties range from aiding and educating patients to preparing and sterilizing dental instruments and performing administrative work.

History

In 1957, the Council on Dental Education sponsored the first national workshop on dental assisting. Practicing dentists, dental educators, and dental assistants made recommendations for the education and certification of dental assistants. These recommendations were considered in developing the first *Requirements for an Accredited Program in Dental Assisting Education*, which were approved by the ADA House of Delegates in 1960. Prior to 1960, the American Dental Assistants Association (ADAA) approved courses of training for dental assistants, varying in length from 104-clock hours to 2 academic years. Subsequent to the adoption in 1960 of the first accreditation standards, the Council on Dental Education granted provisional approval to those programs approved by the ADAA that were at least 1 academic year in length until site visits could be conducted. Thus, 26 programs appeared on the first list of accredited dental assisting programs, published in 1961.

Career Description

Dental assistants are responsible for:
- Helping patients feel comfortable before, during, and after treatment
- Assisting the dentist during treatment
- Exposing and processing dental radiographs (x-rays) (*Note:* Currently, 31 states require dental assistants to complete additional education and/or examinations to perform this function.)
- Recording the patient's medical history and taking blood pressure and pulse
- Preparing and sterilizing instruments and equipment for the dentist's use
- Providing patients with oral care instructions following such procedures as surgery or placement of a restoration (filling)
- Teaching patients proper brushing and flossing techniques
- Making impressions of patients' teeth for study casts (*Note:* Most states consider this to be an expanded function, requiring additional education and/or examination to perform it.)
- Performing administrative and scheduling tasks, including using a personal computer, communicating by telephone, and maintaining an inventory supply system.

Many states provide a career ladder for dental assistants, allowing them to perform expanded functions, most often with additional education, examinations, and/or credentials. The Dental Assisting National Board (DANB) provides state-specific information on dental assisting requirements and which duties they are allowed to perform; see: *www.danb.org*.

Employment Characteristics

Most of the more than 247,000 active dental assistants are employed by general dentists. In addition, dental specialists employ dental assistants. Most assistants work chairside, although they may also participate in the business aspects of the practice. Besides dental offices, other employment settings available to dental assistants include:
- Schools and clinics (public health dentistry)
- Hospitals (assisting dentists who are treating bedridden patients or in more elaborate dental procedures performed only in hospitals)
- Dental school clinics
- Insurance companies (processing dental insurance claims)
- Vocational schools, technical institutes, community colleges, and universities (teaching others to be dental assistants)

Dental assisting offers both flexibility and stability. Dental assistants have the flexibility to work full or part time. According to DANB's 2010 CDA Salary Survey (*www.danb.org/PDFs/2010SalarySurvey.pdf*), those who are Certified Dental Assistants (CDAs) by DANB work in the dental assisting field for an average of 15.7 years, 8.7 years with the same employer dentist.

Excellent career opportunities exist for nontraditional dental assisting students, seeking career change or job reentry after a period of unemployment, or from a culturally diverse background. Many dental assisting education programs offer more flexible program designs that meet the needs of nontraditional students by offering a variety of educational options, such as part-time or evening hours.

Salary

The salary of a dental assistant varies, depending on the responsibilities associated with the specific position, the individual's training, and the geographic location of employment. The average wage for a full-time DANB-certified dental assistant, in all practice settings, is $18.50 an hour, while non-certified dental assistants employed in general dentistry offices earn, on average, $16.46 an hour (DANB's 2010 CDA Salary Survey, *www.danb.org/PDFs/ 2010SalarySurvey.pdf*).

The May 2011 data from the US Bureau of Labor Statistics show that wages at the 10th percentile are $23,080, the 50th percentile (median) at $34,140, and the 90th percentile at $47,720 (*www.bls.gov/oes/current/oes319091.htm*). For more information, refer to *www.ama-assn.org/go/hpsalary*.

In addition to salary, dental assistants may receive benefit packages from their employers, including health and disability insurance coverage, dues for membership in professional organizations, an allowance for uniforms, profit sharing plans, and paid vacations.

Employment Outlook

Most areas of the country are currently reporting shortages of dental assistants. Owing to the success of preventive dentistry in reducing the incidence of oral disease, senior citizens—a growing population—will retain their teeth longer and will be even more aware of the importance of regular dental care. Employment is expected to grow 31% from 2010 to 2020, which is much faster than the average for all occupations. (*www.bls.gov/oco/ocos163.htm*).

Educational Programs

Length. Nine to 11 months.
   Prerequisites. High school diploma or equivalent.

Certification

Dental assistants can earn one of two national certifications through the Dental Assisting National Board (DANB): the Certified Dental Assistant (CDA) and the Certified Orthodontic Assistant (COA).

To become a CDA, a dental assistant must meet eligibility prerequisites (graduation from a Commission Dental Accreditation (CODA)-accredited program or two years of dental assisting experience) and pass the CDA exam. The exam is composed of three component exams: Radiation Health and Safety (RHS), Infection Control (ICE), and General Chairside Assisting (GC). The ICE and RHS component exams do not have any eligibility requirements.

Eligible candidates may take all three component exams separately or in one test administration (the full CDA exam). Candidates will earn DANB CDA Certification if they pass all three component exams within a five-year period. Passing all three components of the CDA exam as required qualifies a dental assistant to use the Certified Dental Assistant (CDA) certification mark for a period of 1 year. To become a COA, a dental assistant must meet eligibility prerequisites and then pass the Certified Orthodontic Assistant (COA) exam, which is composed of two component exams: Infection Control (ICE) and Orthodontic Assisting (OA). The ICE component exam does not have any eligibility requirements.

Eligible candidates may take both component exams separately or in one test administration (the full COA exam). Candidates will earn the DANB COA Certification if they pass both component

exams within a five-year period. Passing both components of the COA exam as required qualifies a dental assistant to use the Certified Orthodontic Assistant (COA) certification mark for a period of one year.

Thirty-seven states, plus the District of Columbia, the Veterans Administration, and the US Air Force, currently recognize or require dental assistants to take the CDA exam or one of the CDA component exams. Most states do not have separate requirements for orthodontic assistants. For those that do, the COA exam is required or recognized in Maryland, Massachusetts, and Oregon. State regulations vary, and some states offer registration or licensure in addition to this national certification program. For state-specific information about dental assisting requirements, contact your state's dental board or go to *www.danb.org*.

Recertification

To maintain eligibility to continue to use the CDA or COA certification marks, individuals must meet DANB's Recertification Requirements, which consist of holding current DANB-accepted CPR certification, completing at least 12 hours of continuing dental education annually, and paying an annual renewal fee (currently $55).

Inquiries

Careers/Curriculum
American Dental Association
211 East Chicago Avenue
Chicago, IL 60611-2678
312 440-2390
www.ada.org/careers

American Dental Education Association
1400 K Street NW, Suite 1100
Washington, DC 20005
202 289-7201
www.adea.org

American Dental Assistants Association
35 East Wacker Drive, Suite 1730
Chicago, IL 60601
312 541-1550
www.dentalassistant.org

Certification
Dental Assisting National Board, Inc
444 North Michigan Avenue, Suite 900
Chicago, IL 60611
800 FOR-DANB 367-3262
E-mail: *danbmail@danb.org*
www.danb.org

Program Accreditation
Commission on Dental Accreditation
American Dental Association
211 East Chicago Avenue
Chicago, IL 60611-2678
312 440-4653
www.ada.org

Note: Adapted in part from the Bureau of Labor Statistics, US Department of Labor, *Occupational Outlook Handbook*, Dental Assistants, at *www.bls.gov/oco/ocos163.htm*.

Dental Assistant

Alabama

James H Faulkner State Community College
Dental Assistant Prgm
1900 Hwy 31 S
Bay Minette, AL 36507-2619
http://faulknerstate.edu

Lawson State Community College - Bessemer Campus
Dental Assistant Prgm
1109 9th Ave SW
Bessemer, AL 35022

Calhoun Community College
Dental Assistant Prgm
PO Box 2216
Decatur, AL 35609-2216
www.calhoun.edu

Wallace State Community College
Dental Assistant Prgm
801 Main St NW
PO Box 2000
Hanceville, AL 35077-2000

Fortis College
Dental Assistant Prgm
3590 Pleasant Valley Rd
Mobile, AL 36609

Trenholm State Technical College
Dental Assistant Prgm
1225 Air Base Blvd
Montgomery, AL 36108
www.trenholmtech.cc.al.us

Alaska

University of Alaska Anchorage
Dental Assistant Prgm
3211 Providence Dr, AHS 124
Anchorage, AK 99508-8371
www.uaa.alaska.edu

Arizona

Phoenix College
Dental Assistant Prgm
1202 W Thomas Rd
Phoenix, AZ 85013
www.phoenixcollege.edu/dental

Rio Salado College
Dental Assistant Prgm
2323 W 14th St
Tempe, AZ 85281

Pima Community College
Dental Assistant Prgm
2202 W Anklam Rd
Tucson, AZ 85709
www.pima.edu

Arkansas

Arkansas Northeastern College
Dental Assistant Prgm
I-55 and Hwy 148
PO Box 36
Burdette, AR 72321
www.anc.edu

Pulaski Technical College
Dental Assistant Prgm
3000 W Scenic Dr
North Little Rock, AR 72118-3399
www.pulaskitech.edu

California

College of Alameda
Dental Assistant Prgm
555 Atlantic Ave
Alameda, CA 94501

Heald College - Concord Campus
Dental Assistant Prgm
5130 Commercial Circle
Concord, CA 94520
www.heald.edu

Orange Coast College
Dental Assistant Prgm
2701 Fairview Rd
Costa Mesa, CA 92628-0120

Cypress College
Dental Assistant Prgm
9200 Valley View St
Cypress, CA 90630

College of the Redwoods
Dental Assistant Prgm
7351 Tompkins Hill Rd
Eureka, CA 95501
www.redwoods.edu

Citrus College
Dental Assistant Prgm
1000 W Foothill
Glendora, CA 91741
www.citruscollege.edu

Heald College - Hayward Campus
Dental Assistant Prgm
25500 Industrial Blvd
Hayward, CA 94545
www.heald.edu

College of Marin
Dental Assistant Prgm
835 College Ave
Kentfield, CA 94904
www.marin.edu

Hacienda LaPuente Adult Education
Dental Assistant Prgm
14101 E Nelson Ave
La Puente, CA 91746

Foothill College
Dental Assistant Prgm
12345 El Monte Rd
Los Altos Hills, CA 94022
www.foothill.edu/bio/programs/dentala

Modesto Junior College
Dental Assistant Prgm
435 College Ave
Modesto, CA 95350

Monterey Peninsula College
Dental Assistant Prgm
980 Fremont St
Monterey, CA 93940

Moreno Valley College
Dental Assistant Prgm
16130 Lasselle St
Moreno Valley, CA 92551-2045

Cerritos College
Dental Assistant Prgm
11110 E Alondra Blvd
Norwalk, CA 90650
www.cerritos.edu

Pasadena City College
Dental Assistant Prgm
1570 E Colorado Blvd
Pasadena, CA 91106
www.pasadena.edu

Diablo Valley College
Dental Assistant Prgm
321 Golf Club Rd
Pleasant Hill, CA 94523

Chaffey College
Dental Assistant Prgm
5885 Haven Ave
Rancho Cucamonga, CA 91737-3002
http://http:www.chaffey.edu

Sacramento City College
Dental Assistant Prgm
3835 Freeport Blvd
Sacramento, CA 95822
www.scc.losrios.edu

San Diego Mesa College
Dental Assistant Prgm
7250 Mesa College Dr
San Diego, CA 92111-4999
www.sdmesa.edu

City College of San Francisco
Dental Assistant Prgm
50 Phelan Ave
San Francisco, CA 94112
www.ccsf.edu

San Jose City College
Dental Assistant Prgm
2100 Moorpark Ave
San Jose, CA 95128-2799
www.sjcc.edu

Palomar Community College
Dental Assistant Prgm
1140 W Mission Rd
San Marcos, CA 92069
www.palomar.edu

College of San Mateo
Dental Assistant Prgm
1700 W Hillsdale Blvd
San Mateo, CA 94402-3795
www.collegeofsanmateo.edu/dentalassisting

Contra Costa College
Dental Assistant Prgm
2600 Mission Bell Dr
San Pablo, CA 94806
www.contracosta.cc.ca.us

Santa Rosa Junior College
Dental Assistant Prgm
1501 Mendocino Ave
Santa Rosa, CA 95401-4395
www.santarosa.edu

Heald College - Stockton Campus
Dental Assistant Prgm
1605 E March Lane
Stockton, CA 95210

Colorado

T H Pickens Technical Center
Dental Assistant Prgm
500 Airport Blvd
Aurora, CO 80011
www.pickenstech.org

IntelliTec Medical Institute
Dental Assistant Prgm
2345 N Academy Blvd
Colorado Springs, CO 80909

Pikes Peak Community College
Dental Assistant Prgm
11195 Highway 83
Campus Box R13
Colorado Springs, CO 80921-3602
www.ppcc.edu

Front Range Comm College
Dental Assistant Prgm
4616 S Shields
Fort Collins, CO 80526-8312
www.frontrange.edu

Pueblo Community College
Dental Assistant Prgm
900 W Orman Ave, MT Rm 122B
Pueblo, CO 81004
www.pueblocc.edu

Connecticut

Tunxis Community College
Dental Assistant Prgm
271 Scott Swamp Rd
Farmington, CT 06032-3187
txcc.commnet.edu

A I Prince Technical High School
Dental Assistant Prgm
401 Flatbush Ave
Hartford, CT 06106
www.cttech.org/prince

Lincoln College of New England
Dental Assistant Prgm
2279 Mt Vernon Rd
Southington, CT 06489
www.briarwoodcollege.com/

Windham Regional Vocational Tech School
Dental Assistant Prgm
210 Birch St
Willimantic, CT 06226

Florida

South Florida Community College
Dental Assistant Prgm
600 W College Dr
Avon Park, FL 33825
www.www.southflorida.edu

Manatee Technical Institute
Dental Assistant Prgm
5520 Lakewood Ranch Blvd
Bradenton, FL 34211
www.manateetechnicalinstitute.org

Brevard Community College
Dental Assistant Prgm
1519 Clearlake Rd
Cocoa, FL 32922
www.brevardcc.edu

Atlantic Technical Center
Dental Assistant Prgm
4700 Coconut Creek Parkway
Coconut Creek, FL 33063

Daytona State College, Daytona Beach Campus
Dental Assistant Prgm
1200 W International Speedway Blvd
Daytona Beach, FL 32120
www.daytonastate.edu

Lincoln Technical Institute - Fern Park Campus
Dental Assistant Prgm
7275 Estapona Circle
Fern Park, FL 32730
www.americareschoolofnursing.com

Broward College
Dental Assistant Prgm
3501 SW Davie Rd-Bldg 8
Fort Lauderdale, FL 33314
www.broward.edu

Indian River State College
Dental Assistant Prgm
Dental Assisting Technology and Management
3209 Virginia Ave
Fort Pierce, FL 34981-5599
www.ircc.edu

Sanford-Brown Institute - Ft Lauderdale
Dental Assistant Prgm
1201 West Cypress Creek Rd
Ft Lauderdale , FL 33309

Santa Fe College
Dental Assistant Prgm
3000 NW 83rd St, Bldg W
Gainesville, FL 32606

Florida State College at Jacksonville
Dental Assistant Prgm
4501 Capper Rd
Room A314F
Jacksonville, FL 32218

Sanford Brown Institute - Jacksonville
Dental Assistant Prgm
10255 Fortune Parkway
Suite 501
Jacksonville, FL 32256

Palm Beach State College
Dental Assistant Prgm
4200 Congress Ave
Lake Worth, FL 33461
http://pbcc.edu

Traviss Career Center
Dental Assistant Prgm
3225 Winter Lake Rd
Lakeland, FL 33803

Robert Morgan Educational Center
Dental Assistant Prgm
18180 SW 122nd Ave
Miami, FL 33177

Lorenzo Walker Institute of Technology
Dental Assistant Prgm
3702 Estey Ave
Naples, FL 34104
www.lwit.edu

Northwest Florida State College
Dental Assistant Prgm
100 College Blvd
Niceville, FL 32578
www.owcc.cc.fl.us

College of Central Florida
Dental Assistant Prgm
3001 SW College Rd
PO Box 1388
Ocala, FL 34479
www.gocfcc.com

Concorde Career Institute
Dental Assistant Prgm
3444 McCrory Place
Orlando, FL 32803

Orlando Tech
Dental Assistant Prgm
301 W Amelia St
Orlando, FL 32801
www.orlandotech.ocps.net

Gulf Coast State College
Dental Assistant Prgm
5230 W US Hwy 98
Panama City, FL 32401-1041
www.gulfcoast.edu

Charlotte Technical Center
Dental Assistant Prgm
18300 Toledo Blade Blvd
Port Charlotte, FL 33948-3399
www.ccps.k12.fl.us

Pinellas Technical Education Centers - St Petersburg Campus
Dental Assistant Prgm
901 34th St South
St Petersburg, FL 33711
myptec.org

Tallahassee Community College
Dental Assistant Prgm
444 Appleyard Dr
Tallahassee, FL 32304
www.tcc.fl.edu

Erwin Technical Center
Dental Assistant Prgm
2010 E Hillsborough Ave
Tampa, FL 33610
erwin.edu

Hillsborough Community College
Dental Assistant Prgm
Dale Mabry Campus
PO Box 30030
Tampa, FL 33614
www.hccfl.edu/dm

Georgia

Albany Technical College
Dental Assistant Prgm
1704 S Slappey Blvd
Albany, GA 31701-3514
www.albanytech.edu

Athens Technical College
Dental Assistant Prgm
Allied Health and Nursing
800 US Hwy 29 N
Athens, GA 30601
www.athenstech.edu

Atlanta Technical College
Dental Assistant Prgm
1560 Metropolitan Pkwy SW Rm 2157
Atlanta, GA 30310-4446
www.atlantatech.edu

Augusta Technical College
Dental Assistant Prgm
3200 Augusta Tech Dr
Augusta, GA 30906
www.augustatech.edu

Columbus Technical College
Dental Assistant Prgm
928 Manchester Expressway
Columbus, GA 31904
www.columbustech.edu

Southern Crescent Technical College
Dental Assistant Prgm
501 Varsity Rd
Griffin, GA 30223

Gwinnett Technical College
Dental Assistant Prgm
5150 Sugarloaf Pkwy
Lawrenceville, GA 30043

Lanier Technical College
Dental Assistant Prgm
2990 Landrum Education Dr
Oakwood, GA 30566
www.lanier.tec.ga.us

Georgia Northwestern Technical College
Dental Assistant Prgm
466 Brock Rd
Rockmart, GA 30153
www.coosavalleytech.edu

Savannah Technical College
Dental Assistant Prgm
5717 White Bluff Rd
Savannah, GA 31405-5521
www.savannahtech.edu

Fortis College
Dental Assistant Prgm
2108 Cobb Pkwy
Smyrna, GA 30080
www.medixschool.edu

Ogeechee Technical College
Dental Assistant Prgm
1 Joe Kennedy Blvd
Statesboro, GA 30458-8049
www.ogeecheetech.edu

Wiregrass Georgia Technical College
Dental Assistant Prgm
PO Box 928-4089 Val Tech Rd
Valdosta, GA 31603-0928

Hawaii

Heald College - Honolulu Campus
Dental Assistant Prgm
1500 Kapiolani Blvd
Honolulu, HI 96814

Maui Community College
Dental Assistant Prgm
310 Kaahumana Ave
Kahului, HI 96732

Idaho

Carrington College of Boise
Dental Assistant Prgm
1200 N Liberty St
Boise, ID 83704
www.apolloboise.com

College of Western Idaho
Dental Assistant Prgm
5500 East Opportunity Drive
Nampa, ID 83706

Illinois

John A Logan College
Dental Assistant Prgm
700 Logan College Rd
Carterville, IL 62918

Kaskaskia College
Dental Assistant Prgm
27210 College Rd
Centralia, IL 62801
www.kaskaskia.edu

Elgin Community College
Dental Assistant Prgm
1700 Spartan Dr
Elgin, IL 60123
www.elgin.edu

Lewis & Clark Community College
Dental Assistant Prgm
5800 Godfrey Rd, RiverBend Arena RM 235
Godfrey, IL 62035
www.lc.edu

Illinois Valley Community College
Dental Assistant Prgm
815 N Orlando Smith Ave
Oglesby, IL 61348-9691
www.ivcc.edu

Indiana

Ivy Tech Community College
Dental Assistant Prgm
104 W 53rd St
Anderson, IN 46013
www.ivytech.edu

Columbus Area Career Connection/Ivy Tech St
Dental Assistant Prgm
230 S Marr Rd
Columbus, IN 47201

University of Southern Indiana
Dental Assistant Prgm
8600 University Blvd
Evansville, IN 47712

Indiana Univ - Purdue Univ Ft Wayne
Dental Assistant Prgm
2101 Coliseum Blvd E
Fort Wayne, IN 46805
www.ipfw.edu/denta

Indiana University Northwest
Dental Assistant Prgm
3400 Broadway St
Gary, IN 46408
www.iun.edu

Indiana University
Dental Assistant Prgm
1121 W Michigan St
Indianapolis, IN 46202-5186
www.iusd.iupui.edu

International Business Coll - Indianapolis
Dental Assistant Prgm
7205 Shadeland Station
Indianapolis, IN 46256

Kaplan College
Dental Assistant Prgm
7302 Woodland Dr
Indianapolis, IN 46278

Ivy Tech Community College
Dental Assistant Prgm
700 E Firmin St
Kokomo, IN 46902

Ivy Tech Community College - Lafayette
Dental Assistant Prgm
3101 S Creasy Ln
PO Box 6299
Lafayette, IN 47903-6299

Ivy Tech Community College - South Bend
Dental Assistant Prgm
220 Dean Johnson Blvd
South Bend, IN 46601

Iowa

Des Moines Area Community College
Dental Assistant Prgm
2006 S Ankeny Blvd
Ankeny, IA 50023-3993

Eastern Iowa Community College
Cosponsor: Scott Community College
Dental Assistant Prgm
500 Belmont Rd
Bettendorf, IA 52722-5649
www.eicc.edu

Kirkwood Community College
Dental Assistant Prgm
6301 Kirkwood Blvd SW, PO Box 2068
Cedar Rapids, IA 52406-9973

Iowa Western Community College
Dental Assistant Prgm
2700 College Rd, PO Box 4C
Council Bluffs, IA 51503
www.iwcc.edu

Vatterott College - Des Moines Campus
Dental Assistant Prgm
6100 Thornton Ave, Ste 290
Des Moines, IA 50321
www.vatterott-college.edu

Marshalltown Community College
Dental Assistant Prgm
3700 S Center St
Marshalltown, IA 50158
www.iavalley.edu/mcc/about/programs-degrees/
DentalAssisting.html

Northeast Iowa Community College
Dental Assistant Prgm
10250 Sundown Rd
Peosta, IA 52068
www.nicc.edu

Western Iowa Tech Community College
Dental Assistant Prgm
4647 Stone Ave, PO Box 5199
Sioux City, IA 51102-5199
www.witcc.edu

Hawkeye Community College
Dental Assistant Prgm
1501 E Orange Rd, PO Box 8015
Waterloo, IA 50704
www.hawkeyecollege.edu

Kansas

Flint Hills Technical College
Dental Assistant Prgm
3301 W 18th Ave
Emporia, KS 66801
www.fhtc.edu

Salina Area Technical College
Dental Assistant Prgm
2562 Centennial Rd
Salina, KS 67401
SalinaTech.edu

Wichita Area Technical College
Dental Assistant Prgm
324 N Emporia
Wichita, KS 67202
www.watc.edu

Kentucky

Bluegrass Community and Technical College
Dental Assistant Prgm
164 Opportunity Way
Lexington, KY 40511-1020
www.bluegrass.kctcs.edu

West Kentucky Community & Technical College
Dental Assistant Prgm
4810 Alben Barkley Dr
Paducah, KY 42001
www.westkentucky.kctcs.edu

Maine

Univ of Maine Augusta (Bangor)
Dental Assistant Prgm
Lincoln Hall, 29 Texas Ave
Bangor, ME 04401-4324
www.uma.maine.edu

Maryland

All-State Career - Healthcare Division
Dental Assistant Prgm
2200 Broening Highway
Suite 280
Baltimore, MD 21224

Fortis College - Towson
Dental Assistant Prgm
700 York Rd
Towson, MD 21204
www.medixschool.com

Massachusetts

Kaplan Career Institute - Boston
Dental Assistant Prgm
540 Commonwealth Ave
Boston, MA 02215

Massasoit Community College
Dental Assistant Prgm
900 Randolph St
Canton, MA 02021
www.massasoit.mass.edu

Mount Wachusett Community College
Dental Assistant Prgm
Fitchburg Campus
275 Nichols Rd
Gardner, MA 01420

Northern Essex Community College
Dental Assistant Prgm
45 Franklin St
Lawrence, MA 01841
www.necc.mass.edu/healthprofessions

Middlesex Community College
Dental Assistant Prgm
33 Kearney Square
Lowell, MA 01852

Charles H McCann Technical School
Dental Assistant Prgm
70 Hodges Cross Rd
North Adams, MA 01247

Southeastern Technical Institute
Dental Assistant Prgm
250 Foundry St
South Easton, MA 02375

Springfield Technical Community College
Dental Assistant Prgm
One Armory Sq
PO Box 9000
Springfield, MA 01102
stcc.edu

The Salter School
Dental Assistant Prgm
184 West Boylston St
West Boylston, MA 01583

Quinsigamond Community College
Dental Assistant Prgm
670 W Boylston St
Worcester, MA 01606

Michigan

Washtenaw Community College
Dental Assistant Prgm
4800 E Huron River Dr
Ann Arbor, MI 48105
www.wccnet.edu/health/dental.php

Baker College of Auburn Hills
Dental Assistant Prgm
1500 University Drive
Auburn Hills, MI 48326

Lake Michigan College
Dental Assistant Prgm
2755 E Napier Ave
Benton Harbor, MI 49022
www.lakemichigancollege.edu

Kaplan Career Institute - Dearborn Campus
Dental Assistant Prgm
18440 Ford Rd
Detroit, MI 48228

Wayne County Community College District
Dental Assistant Prgm
8551 Greenfield, Rm 308A
Detroit, MI 48228
www.wcccd.edu

Mott Community College
Dental Assistant Prgm
1401 E Court St
Flint, MI 48503

Grand Rapids Community College
Dental Assistant Prgm
143 Bostwick St NE
Grand Rapids, MI 49503

Baker College of Port Huron
Dental Assistant Prgm
3403 Lapeer Rd
Port Huron, MI 48060

Northwestern Michigan College
Dental Assistant Prgm
1701 E Front St
Traverse City, MI 49686
www.nmc.edu

Delta College
Dental Assistant Prgm
1961 Delta Rd
University Center, MI 48710

Minnesota

Northwest Technical College - Bemidji
Dental Assistant Prgm
905 Grant Ave SE
Bemidji, MN 56601
www.ntcmn.edu

Central Lakes College
Dental Assistant Prgm
501 W College Dr
Brainerd, MN 56401
www.clcmn.edu

Minnesota West Comm & Tech College
Dental Assistant Prgm
1011 First St W
Canby, MN 56220

Herzing University - Lakeland Academy Division
Dental Assistant Prgm
5700 W Broadway Ave
Crystal, MN 55428
http://herzing.edu

Hennepin Technical College
Dental Assistant Prgm
13100 College View Dr
Eden Prairie, MN 55347
www.hennepintech.edu

Hibbing Community College
Dental Assistant Prgm
1515 E 25th St
Hibbing, MN 55747
www.hcc.mnscu.edu

Minneapolis Community & Technical College
Dental Assistant Prgm
1501 Hennepin Ave S
Minneapolis, MN 55403
www.minneapolis.edu

Minnesota State Comm & Tech Coll - Moorhead
Dental Assistant Prgm
1900 28th Ave S
Moorhead, MN 56560-4899
www.minnesota.edu

South Central College - North Mankato Campus
Dental Assistant Prgm
1920 Lee Blvd
North Mankato, MN 56003
www.southcentral.edu

Rochester Community & Technical College
Dental Assistant Prgm
851 30th Ave SE
Rochester, MN 55904
www.rctc.edu

Dakota County Technical College
Dental Assistant Prgm
1300 145th St E
Rosemount, MN 55068
www.dctc.edu

St Cloud Technical and Community College
Dental Assistant Prgm
1540 Northway Dr
St Cloud, MN 56303-1240
www.sctc.edu

Century College
Dental Assistant Prgm
3300 Century Ave N
White Bear Lake, MN 55110

Mississippi

Pearl River Community College
Dental Assistant Prgm
5448 US Hwy 49 S
Hattiesburg, MS 39401
www.prcc/edu

Hinds Community College
Dental Assistant Prgm
1750 Chadwick Dr
Jackson, MS 39204
www.hindscc.edu

Meridian Community College
Dental Assistant Prgm
910 Highway 19 North
Meridian, MS 39305

Missouri

Nichols Career Center
Dental Assistant Prgm
605 Union St
Jefferson City, MO 65101
www.jcps.k12.mo.us

Concorde Career College - Kansas City
Dental Assistant Prgm
3239 Broadway Blvd
Kansas City, MO 64111
http://ww.concorde.edu

Metropolitan Community College - Penn Valley
Dental Assistant Prgm
3201 SW Trafficway
Kansas City, MO 64111-2764
www.mcckc.edu

Ozarks Technical Community College
Dental Assistant Prgm
1001 E Chestnut Expressway
Springfield, MO 65802
www.otc.edu

Missouri College
Dental Assistant Prgm
10121 Manchester Rd
St Louis, MO 63122-1583
www.missouricollege.com

St Louis Community College - Forest Park
Dental Assistant Prgm
5600 Oakland Ave
St Louis, MO 63110-1393
http://stlcc.edu/fp/dentalassisting

Montana

Montana State Univ - Great Falls Coll of Tech
Dental Assistant Prgm
2100 16th Ave S
Great Falls, MT 59405
www.msugf.edu

Salish Kootenai College
Dental Assistant Prgm
Box 70
58138 Hwy 93
Pablo, MT 59855
www.skc.edu

Nebraska

Central Community College
Dental Assistant Prgm
PO Box 1024
Hastings, NE 68902-1024
www.cccneb.edu

Southeast Community College
Dental Assistant Prgm
8800 O St
Lincoln, NE 68520-1299
www.southeast.edu

Mid-Plains Community College
Dental Assistant Prgm
1101 Halligan Dr
North Platte, NE 69101
www.mpcc.edu

Kaplan University - Omaha
Dental Assistant Prgm
5425 North 103rd St
Omaha, NE 68134

Metropolitan Community College
Dental Assistant Prgm
PO Box 3777
Omaha, NE 68103-0777

Vatterott College - Omaha Campus
Dental Assistant Prgm
11818 I St
Omaha, NE 68137
www.vatterott-college.edu

Nevada

College of Southern Nevada
Dental Assistant Prgm
6375 W Charleston Blvd
Las Vegas, NV 89146
www.csn.edu

Truckee Meadows Community College
Dental Assistant Prgm
7000 Dandini Blvd
Reno, NV 89512-3999
www.tmcc.edu

New Hampshire

NHTI, Concord's Community College
Dental Assistant Prgm
31 College Dr
Concord, NH 03301-7412
www.nhti.edu

New Jersey

Camden County College
Dental Assistant Prgm
PO Box 200
Blackwood, NJ 08012
www.camdencc.edu

Cumberland County Technical Education Center
Dental Assistant Prgm
601 Bridgeton Ave
Bridgeton, NJ 08302

Cape May County Technical Institute
Dental Assistant Prgm
188 Crest Haven Rd
Cape May Courthouse, NJ 08210

The Institute for Health Education
Dental Assistant Prgm
600 Pavonia Ave, 1st Floor
Jersey City, NJ 07305

Univ of Medicine & Dent of New Jersey
Dental Assistant Prgm
1776 Raritan Rd
Scotch Plains, NJ 07076
www. umdnj.edu

Fortis Institute
Dental Assistant Prgm
201 Willowbrook Blvd 2nd Floor
Wayne, NJ 07470
http://berdaninstitute.com

Burlington County Institute of Technology
Dental Assistant Prgm
695 Woodlane Rd
Westampton, NJ 08060

New Mexico

Central New Mexico Community College
Dental Assistant Prgm
525 Buena Vista SE
Albuquerque, NM 87106
www.tvi.edu

University of New Mexico - Gallup
Dental Assistant Prgm
200 College Rd
Gallup, NM 87301
www.gallup.unm.edu

Dona Ana Community College
Dental Assistant Prgm
3400 S Espina St
Las Cruces, NM 88007
http://dabcc.nmsu.edu

Luna Community College
Dental Assistant Prgm
366 Luna Drive
Las Vegas, NM 87701

Santa Fe Community College
Dental Assistant Prgm
CertDental Assisting, AAS in Dental Health
6401 Richards Ave, Room 421B
Santa Fe, NM 87509
www.sfccnm.edu/dental

New York

SUNY Educational Opportunity Center
Dental Assistant Prgm
465 Washington St
Buffalo, NY 14203

Monroe Community College
Dental Assistant Prgm
1000 E Henrietta Rd
Rochester, NY 14623-5780

North Carolina

Asheville-Buncombe Technical Comm College
Dental Assistant Prgm
340 Victoria Rd
Asheville, NC 28801
www.abtech.edu

University of North Carolina - Chapel Hill
Dental Assistant Prgm
CB 7450
Chapel Hill, NC 27599-7450
www.dent.unc.edu

Central Piedmont Community College
Dental Assistant Prgm
3210 CPCC West Campus Dr
Charlotte, NC 28208
www.cpcc.edu

Wayne Community College
Dental Assistant Prgm
3000 Wayne Memorial Dr
Goldsboro, NC 27533
www.waynecc.edu

Alamance Community College
Dental Assistant Prgm
PO Box 8000
Graham, NC 27253-8000
www.alamance.cc.nc.us

Coastal Carolina Community College
Dental Assistant Prgm
444 Western Blvd
Jacksonville, NC 28546
www.coastalcarolina.edu

Guilford Technical Community College
Dental Assistant Prgm
PO Box 309
601 High Point Rd
Jamestown, NC 27282
www.gtcc.edu

Western Piedmont Community College
Dental Assistant Prgm
1001 Burkemont Ave
Morganton, NC 28655

Miller-Motte College - Raleigh
Dental Assistant Prgm
3901 Capital Blvd
Suite 151
Raleigh, NC 27604

Wake Technical Community College
Dental Assistant Prgm
9101 Fayetteville Rd
Raleigh, NC 27603-5696
www.waketech.edu

Rowan-Cabarrus Community College
Dental Assistant Prgm
PO Box 1595
1333 Jake Alexander Blvd
Salisbury, NC 28145-1595
www.rowancabarrus.edu

Central Carolina Community College
Dental Assistant Prgm
900 S Vance St
Suite 220-B
Sanford, NC 27330

Montgomery Community College
Dental Assistant Prgm
1011 Page St
Troy, NC 27371

Wilkes Community College
Dental Assistant Prgm
PO Box 120
Wilkesboro, NC 28697-0120
www.wilkescc.edu

Martin Commuity College
Dental Assistant Prgm
1161 Kehukee Park Rd
Williamston, NC 27892-9988
www.martincc.edu

Cape Fear Community College
Dental Assistant Prgm
411 N Front St
Wilmington, NC 28401-3993
http://cfcc.edu

Miller-Motte College
Dental Assistant Prgm
5000 Market St
Wilmington, NC 28405

Forsyth Technical Community College
Dental Assistant Prgm
2100 Silas Creek Pkwy
Winston-Salem, NC 27103

North Dakota

North Dakota State College of Science
Dental Assistant Prgm
800 N Sixth St
Wahpeton, ND 58076
ndscs.edu

Ohio

Fortis College
Dental Assistant Prgm
2545 Bailey Rd
Cuyahoga Falls, OH 44221

Miami-Jacobs Career College
Dental Assistant Prgm
875 W Central Ave
Springboro, OH 45066

Eastern Gateway Community College
Dental Assistant Prgm
4000 Sunset Blvd
Steubenville, OH 43952
www.jcc.edu

Choffin Career & Technical Center
Dental Assistant Prgm
200 E Wood St
Youngstown, OH 44503
www.choffincareer.com

Oklahoma

Rose State College
Dental Assistant Prgm
6420 SE 15th St
Midwest City, OK 73110
www.rose.edu

Moore Norman Technology Center
Dental Assistant Prgm
4701 12th Ave NW
Norman, OK 73069
www.mntechnology.com

Francis Tuttle Technology Center
Dental Assistant Prgm
12777 N Rockwell Ave
Oklahoma City, OK 73142-2789

Metro Tech Health Careers Center
Dental Assistant Prgm
1720 Springlake Dr
Oklahoma City, OK 73111

Western Technology Center Western Technology Center
Dental Assistant Prgm
2605 E Main St
Weatherford, OK 73096

Oregon

Linn-Benton Community College
Dental Assistant Prgm
6500 SW Pacific Blvd
Albany, OR 97321
http://linnbenton.edu

Central Oregon Community College
Dental Assistant Prgm
2600 NW College Way
Bend, OR 97701
www.cocc.edu

Lane Community College
Dental Assistant Prgm
4000 E 30th Ave
Eugene, OR 97405

Blue Mountain Community College
Dental Assistant Prgm
2411 NW Carden
PO Box 100
Pendleton, OR 97801
www.bluecc.edu

Concorde Career College - Portland
Dental Assistant Prgm
1425 NE Irving St, Bldg 300
Portland, OR 97232

Portland Community College
Dental Assistant Prgm
PO Box 19000
Portland, OR 97280-0990
www.pcc.edu

Chemeketa Community College
Dental Assistant Prgm
4000 Lancaster Dr NE
PO Box 14007
Salem, OR 97309-7070
www.chemeketa.edu

Pennsylvania

Harcum College
Dental Assistant Prgm
750 Montgomery Ave
Bryn Mawr, PA 19010

Harrisburg Area Community College
Dental Assistant Prgm
One HACC Dr
Harrisburg, PA 17110-2999

Manor College
Dental Assistant Prgm
Expanded Functions Dental Assististing Program
700 Fox Chase Rd
Jenkintown, PA 19046-3399
www.manor.edu/.com
Notes: The program includes Expanded Functions Dental
 Assisting and a part-time 200-hour Expanded
 Functions program for CDAs.

Commonwealth Tech Inst at Hiram G Andrews Ctr
Dental Assistant Prgm
727 Goucher St
Johnstown, PA 15905

YTI Career Institute YTI Career Institute - Lancaster Campus
Dental Assistant Prgm
3050 Hempland Rd
Lancaster, PA 17601

Luzerne County Community College
Dental Assistant Prgm
1333 S Prospect St
Nanticoke, PA 18634-3899
www.luzerne.edu

Bradford School - Pittsburgh
Dental Assistant Prgm
125 West Station Square Dr, Ste 129
Pittsburgh, PA 15219

Westmoreland County Community College
Dental Assistant Prgm
145 Pavilion Ln
Youngwood, PA 15697-1895
www.wccc.edu

Puerto Rico

University of Puerto Rico
Dental Assistant Prgm
Medical Sciences Campus
PO Box 365067
San Juan, PR 00936-5067

Rhode Island

Community College of Rhode Island
Dental Assistant Prgm
1762 Louisquisset Pike
Lincoln, RI 02865
www.ccri.edu

Lincoln Tech Institute
Dental Assistant Prgm
622 George Washington Highway
Lincoln, RI 02865

South Carolina

Aiken Technical College
Dental Assistant Prgm
PO Drawer 696
Aiken, SC 29802

Trident Technical College
Dental Assistant Prgm
PO Box 118067
Charleston, SC 29423-8067
www.tridenttech.edu

Midlands Technical College
Dental Assistant Prgm
Expanded Duty Dental Assisting
PO Box 2408
Columbia, SC 29202
midlandstech.edu

Horry - Georgetown Technical College
Dental Assistant Prgm
2050 Hwy 501 E, Box 261966
Conway, SC 29528-6066
www.hgtc.edu

Florence-Darlington Technical College
Dental Assistant Prgm
PO Box 100548
Florence, SC 29501-0548
www.fdtc.edu

Greenville Technical College
Dental Assistant Prgm
South Pleasantburg Ave
PO Box 5616 - Station B
Greenville, SC 29606-5616

Tri-County Technical College
Dental Assistant Prgm
PO Box 587
Pendleton, SC 29670
www.tctc.edu

York Technical College
Dental Assistant Prgm
Expanded Duty DA Program
452 S Anderson Rd
Rock Hill, SC 29730

Spartanburg Community College
Dental Assistant Prgm
PO Drawer 4386, Highway I-85
Spartanburg, SC 29305-4386
www.sccsc.edu

South Dakota

Lake Area Technical Institute
Dental Assistant Prgm
230 11th St NE
Watertown, SD 57201
http://sweb.lakeareatech.edu/dental/

Tennessee

Chattanooga State Community College
Dental Assistant Prgm
4501 Amnicola Hwy
Chattanooga, TN 37406-1097
www.chattanoogastate.edu/allied_health/
   dental_assisting/

Tennessee Technology Center - Dickson
Dental Assistant Prgm
740 Hwy 46 South
Dickson, TN 37055
www.ttcdickson.edu

Northeast State Community College
Dental Assistant Prgm
1000 W Jason Witten Way
Elizabethton, TN 37643
www.northeaststate.edu

Volunteer State Community College
Dental Assistant Prgm
1480 Nashville Pike
Gallatin, TN 37066

Tennessee Technology Center - Knoxville
Dental Assistant Prgm
1100 Liberty St
Knoxville, TN 37919
www.knoxville.tec.tn.us

Concorde Career College - Memphis
Dental Assistant Prgm
5100 Poplar Ave, Ste 132
Memphis, TN 38137
www.concordecareercolleges.com

Tennessee Technology Center - Memphis
Dental Assistant Prgm
550 Alabama Ave
Memphis, TN 38105-3604
www.ttcmemphis.edu

Tennessee Technology Center - Murfreesboro
Dental Assistant Prgm
1303 Old Fort Pkwy
Murfreesboro, TN 37129
www.ttcmurfreesboro.edu

Kaplan Career Institute
Dental Assistant Prgm
750 Envious Lane
Nashville, TN 37217

Texas

Del Mar College
Dental Assistant Prgm
101 Baldwin Blvd
Corpus Christi, TX 78404-3897
www.delmar.edu/da

Concorde Career College - Dallas
Dental Assistant Prgm
12606 Greenville Ave
Suite 130
Dallas, TX 75243

Sanford-Brown College - Dallas
Dental Assistant Prgm
1250 Mockingbird Lane
Suite 150
Dallas, TX 75247

Grayson County College
Dental Assistant Prgm
6101 Grayson Dr
Box 48
Denison, TX 75020-8299
www.grayson.edu

El Paso Community College
Dental Assistant Prgm
PO Box 20500
El Paso, TX 79998
www.epcc.edu

**Medical Education and Training Campus
   (METC)**
Dental Assistant Prgm
Attn: Standards, Evaluations, and Accreditation
3038 William Hardee Rd, Bldg 895
Fort Sam Houston, TX 78234-2532

Houston Community College
Dental Assistant Prgm
1900 Pressler Dr
Houston, TX 77030
www.hccs.edu

Concorde Career College - San Antonio
Dental Assistant Prgm
4803 NW Loop 410
San Antonio, TX 78229

San Antonio College
Dental Assistant Prgm
1300 San Pedro Ave, NTC 125
San Antonio, TX 78212-4299
www.accd.edu

Texas State Technical College
Dental Assistant Prgm
3801 Campus Dr
Waco, TX 76705
www.waco.tstc.edu

Utah

Davis Applied Technology College
Dental Assistant Prgm
550 East 300 South
Kaysville, UT 84037
www.datc.net

Bridgerland Applied Technology College
Dental Assistant Prgm
1301 West 600 North
Logan, UT 84321
www.bridgerlandatc.org

Ogden-Weber Applied Technology College
Dental Assistant Prgm
200 N Washington Blvd
Ogden, UT 84404-6704

Vermont

Center for Technology - Essex
Dental Assistant Prgm
3 Educational Dr
Essex Junction, VT 05452
www.go-cte.org

Virginia

Germanna Community College
Dental Assistant Prgm
2130 Germanna Highway
Locust Grove, VA 22508

Centura College
Dental Assistant Prgm
7020 North Military Highway
Norfolk, VA 23518

Fortis College - Richmond
Dental Assistant Prgm
2000 Westmoreland St
Suite A
Richmond, VA 23230

J Sargeant Reynolds Community College
Dental Assistant Prgm
PO Box 85622
Richmond, VA 23285-5622
www.jsr.vccs.edu

Washington

Bellingham Technical College
Dental Assistant Prgm
3028 Lindbergh Ave
Bellingham, WA 98225
www.btc.ctc.edu

Lake Washington Institute of Technology
Dental Assistant Prgm
11605 132nd Ave NE
Kirkland, WA 98034-8506
www.lwtc.edu/Academics/Programs_of_Study/
   Dental_Assistant.xml

Clover Park Technical College
Dental Assistant Prgm
4500 Steilacoom Blvd SW
Lakewood, WA 98498-4098
www.cptc.ctc.edu

South Puget Sound Community College
Dental Assistant Prgm
2011 Mottman Rd SW
Olympia, WA 98512-6292
www.spscc.ctc.edu

Renton Technical College
Dental Assistant Prgm
3000 NE Fourth St
Renton, WA 98056

Seattle Vocational Institute
Dental Assistant Prgm
2120 S Jackson St
Seattle, WA 98144

Spokane Community College
Dental Assistant Prgm
N 1810 Greene St MS 2090
Spokane, WA 99207

Bates Technical College
Dental Assistant Prgm
1101 S Yakima Ave
Tacoma, WA 98405
www.bates.ctc.edu

West Virginia

Mercer County Technical Education Center
Dental Assistant Prgm
1397 Stafford Dr
Princeton, WV 24740

Wisconsin

Fox Valley Technical College
Dental Assistant Prgm
1825 N Bluemound Dr
Appleton, WI 54913
www.fvtc.edu

Northeast Wisconsin Technical College
Dental Assistant Prgm
2740 W Mason St, PO Box 19042
Green Bay, WI 54307-9042

Blackhawk Technical College
Dental Assistant Prgm
6004 Prairie Rd
PO Box 5009
Janesville, WI 53547-5009
www.blackhawk.edu

Gateway Technical College
Dental Assistant Prgm
3520 30th Ave
Kenosha, WI 53144-1690
www.gtc.edu

Western Technical College
Dental Assistant Prgm
304 N Sixth St, PO Box C-908
La Crosse, WI 54601
www.westerntc.edu

Dental Hygienist

Dental hygienists provide dental hygiene services as they work with dentists in the delivery of dental care to patients. Hygienists are licensed to use their knowledge and clinical skills to provide dental care to patients and their interpersonal skills to motivate and instruct patients on methods to prevent oral disease and maintain oral health.

History

The first dental hygiene accreditation standards were developed by three groups: the American Dental Hygienists' Association, the National Association of Dental Examiners, and the ADA's Council on Dental Education. The standards were submitted to and approved by the ADA House of Delegates in 1947, 5 years prior to the launching of the dental hygiene accreditation program in 1952. The first list of accredited dental hygiene programs was published in 1953, with 21 programs. That number has grown to approximately 300 today.

Career Description

Although the range of services performed by dental hygienists varies from state to state, patient services rendered by dental hygienists frequently include:

- Performing patient screening procedures, such as assessing oral health conditions, reviewing health and dental history, and taking blood pressure, pulse, and temperature; oral cancer screening; head & neck inspection; and dental charting
- Exposing and developing dental radiographs (x-rays)
- Removing calculus and plaque (hard and soft deposits) from teeth
- Applying preventive materials to teeth (eg, sealants and fluorides)
- Teaching patients appropriate oral hygiene techniques
- Counseling patients regarding proper nutrition and its impact on oral health
- Making impressions of patients' teeth for study casts
- Administration of anesthesia (depending upon state practice act)

Employment Characteristics

Most licensed dental hygienists in the United States are employed by general dentists. Additionally, dental specialists (such as periodontists or pediatric dentists) employ dental hygienists. Most hygienists work one to one with patients in providing dental hygiene services.

Dental hygienists also may be employed to provide dental hygiene care for patients in hospitals, nursing homes, public health clinics, and schools. Depending on the level of education and experience achieved, dental hygienists also can apply their skills and knowledge to other career activities, such as teaching. Research, public health, and business administration are other options. In addition, employment opportunities may be available with companies that market dental-related materials and equipment.

In some states, dental hygienists may also own their own dental hygiene business or practice on an independent contracting basis. These practitioners are not actually employed by dentists but provide dental hygiene services through contractual agreements.

As a career, dental hygiene also offers both stability and flexibility. Many hygienists also have considerable flexibility to undertake a full- or part-time schedule with evening or weekend hours.

Salary

The salary of a dental hygienist varies, depending on the responsibilities associated with the specific position, the geographic location of employment, and the type of practice or other setting in which the hygienist works. May 2011 data from the US Bureau of Labor Statistics (BLS) show that wages at the 10th percentile are $46,020, the 50th percentile (median) at $69,280, and the 90th percentile at $94,850 (*www.bls.gov/oes/current/oes292021.htm*).

In addition, many full-time dental hygienists receive benefit packages from their dentist/employers, which may include health insurance coverage, dues for membership in professional organizations, paid vacations and sick leave, and tuition assistance for continuing education. Most state dental boards require mandatory continuing education for maintenance of the dental hygiene license.

For more information, refer to *www.ama-assn.org/go/hpsalary*.

Employment Outlook

According to BLS projections, employment of dental hygienists is expected to grow 38 percent through 2020, which is much faster than the average for all occupations. This projected growth ranks dental hygienists among the fastest growing occupations, in response to increasing demand for dental care and more use of hygienists.

The demand for dental services will grow because of population growth, older people increasingly retaining more teeth, and a growing emphasis on preventive dental care. To help meet this demand, facilities that provide dental care, particularly dentists' offices, will increasingly employ dental hygienists, often to perform services that have been performed by dentists in the past. Ongoing research indicating a link between oral health and general health also will spur the demand for preventative dental services, which are typically provided by dental hygienists.

Excellent career opportunities exist for nontraditional dental hygiene students, who might meet one or more of the following criteria: over 23 years of age, seeking career change or job reentry after a period of unemployment, or from a culturally diverse background. Some dental hygiene education programs offer more flexible program designs that meet the needs of nontraditional students by offering a variety of educational options, such as part-time or evening hours.

Educational Programs

Length. The majority of community college-based dental hygiene programs offer a two-year associate degree. University-based dental hygiene programs may offer baccalaureate and master's degrees, which generally require at least two or more years of further education.

Prerequisites. Admission requirements vary, depending on the institution. High school-level courses such as health, biology, psychology, chemistry, mathematics, and speech will be beneficial in a dental hygiene career. Many programs prefer individuals who have completed at least one year of college, and some baccalaureate degree programs require applicants to have completed two years of college.

Curriculum. Dental hygiene education programs provide supervised patient care experiences. Programs also include courses in:
- Liberal arts (English, speech, sociology, and psychology)
- Basic sciences (anatomy, physiology, chemistry, biochemistry, immunology, nutrition, pharmacology, microbiology, and general pathology)
- Clinical sciences (dental hygiene; tooth morphology; head, neck, and oral anatomy; oral embryology and histology; oral pathology; radiography; periodontology; pain management; radiology; and dental materials)

After completing a dental hygiene program, dental hygienists can pursue additional training in such areas as education, health administration, basic sciences, and public health.

Licensure

Dental hygienists are licensed by each state to provide dental hygiene care and patient education. Eligibility for state licensure usually includes graduation from a dental hygiene education program accredited by the Commission on Dental Accreditation. In addition to requiring a passing score on the state-authorized licensure examination, which tests candidates' clinical dental hygiene skills as well as their knowledge of dental hygiene and related subjects, almost all states require candidates for licensure to obtain a passing score on the Dental Hygiene National Board Examination (a comprehensive written examination).

Upon receipt of license, a dental hygienist may use RDH, signifying Registered Dental Hygienist, after his/her name.

Inquiries

Careers/Curriculum
American Dental Association
211 East Chicago Avenue
Chicago, IL 60611-2678
312 440-2390
www.ada.org/careers

American Dental Education Association
1400 K Street NW, Suite 1100
Washington, DC 20005
202 289-7201
www.adea.org

American Dental Hygienists' Association
444 North Michigan Avenue, Suite 3400
Chicago, IL 60611
312 440-8900
www.adha.org

Program Accreditation
Commission on Dental Accreditation
American Dental Association
211 E Chicago Avenue
Chicago, IL 60611-2678
312 440-4653
www.ada.org

Note: Adapted in part from the Bureau of Labor Statistics, US Department of Labor, *Occupational Outlook Handbook,* Dental Hygienists, at *www.bls.gov/oco/ocos097.htm*.

Dental Hygienist

Alabama

Fortis Institute - Birmingham Tri-State Business Institute
Dental Hygiene Prgm
100 London Parkway
Suite 150
Birmingham, AL 35211

Wallace State Community College
Dental Hygiene Prgm
PO Box 2000
801 Main St
Hanceville, AL 35077-2000

Alaska

University of Alaska Anchorage
Dental Hygiene Prgm
3211 Providence Dr, AHS 154
Anchorage, AK 99508-8371
www.uaa.alaska.edu/alliedhealth/

University of Alaska - Fairbanks - Community and Technical College
Dental Hygiene Prgm
Tanana Valley Campus
604 Barnette St
Fairbanks, AK 99701

Arizona

Mohave Community College
Dental Hygiene Prgm
3400 Highway 95
Bullhead City, AZ 86442
www.mohave.edu

Northern Arizona University
Dental Hygiene Prgm
Box 15065
Flagstaff, AZ 86011-5065
www.nau.edu/hp/dept/dh/
Prgm Dir: Marge Reveal, Chair
Tel: 928 523-0520   *Fax:* 928 523-6195
E-mail: Marjorie.Reveal@nau.edu

Carrington College - Mesa
Dental Hygiene Prgm
1300 S Country Club Drive
Suite 2
Mesa, AZ 85210

Mesa Community College
Dental Hygiene Prgm
7110 E McKellips Rd
Mesa, AZ 85207
www.maricopa.edu

Fortis College - Phoenix
Dental Hygiene Prgm
555 N 18th St
Suite 110
Phoenix, AZ 85006

Phoenix College
Dental Hygiene Prgm
1202 W Thomas Rd
Phoenix, AZ 85013

Rio Salado College
Dental Hygiene Prgm
2323 W 14th St
Temple, AZ 85281-6950
www.riosalado.maricopa.edu

Pima Community College
Dental Hygiene Prgm
2202 W Anklam Rd
Tucson, AZ 85709
www.pima.edu

Arkansas

University of Arkansas - Fort Smith
Dental Hygiene Prgm
5210 Grand Ave, PO Box 3649
Fort Smith, AR 72913-3649
www.uafortsmith.edu

University of Arkansas for Medical Sciences
Dental Hygiene Prgm
4301 W Markham St, Slot 609
Little Rock, AR 72205
www.uams.edu/chrp/dentalhygiene
Prgm Dir: Susan Long, RDH EdD
Tel: 501 686-5735   *Fax:* 501 686-8519
E-mail: longsusanl@uams.edu

California

West Coast University
Dental Hygiene Prgm
1477 S Manchester Ave
Anaheim, CA 92802

Cabrillo College
Dental Hygiene Prgm
6500 Soquel Dr
Aptos, CA 95003
www.cabrillo.edu

Southwestern College
Dental Hygiene Prgm
900 Otay Lakes Rd
Chula Vista, CA 91910
www.swccd.edu

West Los Angeles College
Dental Hygiene Prgm
9000 Overland Ave
Culver City, CA 90230
www.wlac.edu
Prgm Dir: Carmen Dones, Chair of Allied Health
Tel: 310 287-4464   *Fax:* 310 287-4461
E-mail: donescm@wlac.edu

Cypress College
Dental Hygiene Prgm
9200 Valley View St
Cypress, CA 90630
http://CypressCollege.edu
Prgm Dir: Carol Green, RDH MA
Tel: 714 484-7292   *Fax:* 714 484-7447
E-mail: cgreen@cypresscollege.edu

Fresno City College
Dental Hygiene Prgm
1101 E University Ave
Fresno, CA 93741

Concorde Career College - Garden Grove
Dental Hygiene Prgm
12951 Euclid St
Garden Grove, CA 92840

Chabot College
Dental Hygiene Prgm
25555 Hesperian Blvd
Hayward, CA 94545
http://chabotweb.clpccd.cc.ca.us/

Loma Linda University
Dental Hygiene Prgm
School of Dentistry
11092 Anderson St
Loma Linda, CA 92350

Foothill College
Dental Hygiene Prgm
12345 El Monte Rd
Los Altos Hills, CA 94022
www.foothill.edu/bio/programs/dentalh/

University of Southern California
Dental Hygiene Prgm
University Park MC0641
Los Angeles, CA 90089-6041
www.usc.edu

Riverside Comm Coll - Moreno Valley Campus
Cosponsor: Moreno Valley College
Dental Hygiene Prgm
16130 Lasselle St
Moreno Valley, CA 92551
www.mvc.edu

Cerritos College
Dental Hygiene Prgm
11110 E Alondra Blvd
Norwalk, CA 90650
www.cerritos.edu

Oxnard College
Dental Hygiene Prgm
4000 S Rose Ave
Oxnard, CA 93033-6699
www.oxnardcollege.edu

Pasadena City College
Dental Hygiene Prgm
1570 E Colorado Blvd
Pasadena, CA 91106
www.pasadena.edu

Diablo Valley College
Dental Hygiene Prgm
321 Golf Club Rd
Pleasant Hill, CA 94523
www.dvc.edu

San Joaquin Valley College
Dental Hygiene Prgm
10641 Church St
Rancho Cucamonga, CA 91730

Shasta College
Dental Hygiene Prgm
11555 Old Oregon Trail
PO Box 496006
Redding, CA 96049-6006
www.shastacollege.edu

Sacramento City College
Dental Hygiene Prgm
3835 Freeport Blvd
Sacramento, CA 95822
www.scc.losrios.edu
Notes: Students receive an instrument issue of
   approximately $4,000.

Concorde Career College - San Bernardino
Dental Hygiene Prgm
201 East Airport Drive
San Bernardino, CA 92408

Concorde Career College - San Diego
Dental Hygiene Prgm
4393 Imperial Ave
San Diego, CA 92113-1964

Carrington College California
Dental Hygiene Prgm
6201 San Ignacio Ave
San Jose , CA 95119

Santa Rosa Junior College
Dental Hygiene Prgm
1501 Mendocino Ave
Santa Rosa, CA 95401-4395

University of the Pacific Arthur A Dugoni School of Dentistry
Dental Hygiene Prgm
3061 Pacific Ave
Stockton, CA 95209

Taft College
Dental Hygiene Prgm
29 Emmons Park Dr, Box 1437
Taft, CA 93268
www.taft.cc.ca.us

San Joaquin Valley College - Visalia
Dental Hygiene Prgm
8400 W Mineral King
Visalia, CA 93291
www.sjvc.edu

Colorado

Concorde Career College - Aurora
Dental Hygiene Prgm
111 N Havana St
Aurora, CO 80010

University of Colorado at Denver
Dental Hygiene Prgm
School of Dental Medicine
13065 E 17th Ave, Rm 104
Mail Stop F-848, PO Box 6508
Aurora, CO 80045

Community College of Denver
Dental Hygiene Prgm
Dental Hygiene Program
1062 Akron Way, Bldg 753
Denver, CO 80230
www.ccd.edu/dental

Pueblo Community College
Dental Hygiene Prgm
900 W Orman Ave
Pueblo, CO 81004
www.pueblocc.edu

Colorado Northwestern Community College
Dental Hygiene Prgm
500 Kennedy Dr
Rangley, CO 81648
www.cncc.edu

Connecticut

University of Bridgeport
Dental Hygiene Prgm
Fones School of Dental Hygiene
30 Hazel St
Bridgeport, CT 06601

Tunxis Community College
Dental Hygiene Prgm
271 Scott Swamp Rd
Farmington, CT 06032-3187
http://tunxis.commnet.edu

Lincoln College of New England
Dental Hygiene Prgm
2279 Mount Vernon Rd
Southington, CT 06489

University of New Haven
Dental Hygiene Prgm
300 Orange Ave
West Haven, CT 06516
www.newhaven.edu

Delaware

Delaware Technical Community College - Wilmington
Dental Hygiene Prgm
333 Shipley St
Wilmington, DE 19801
www.dtcc.edu/wilmington/ah

District of Columbia

Howard University
Dental Hygiene Prgm
600 W St NW, Rm 401
Washington, DC 20059
www.howard.edu

Florida

South Florida Community College
Dental Hygiene Prgm
600 W College Dr
Avon Park, FL 33825
www.southflorida.edu

State College of Florida, Manatee-Sarasota - Manatee-Sarasota
Dental Hygiene Prgm
5840 26th St W
Bradenton, FL 34207
www.scf.edu

Brevard Community College
Dental Hygiene Prgm
1519 Clearlake Rd
Cocoa, FL 32922
www.brevardcc.edu

Daytona State College, Daytona Beach Campus
Dental Hygiene Prgm
1155 County Rd 4139
DeLand, FL 32724
www.daytonastate.edu

Broward College
Dental Hygiene Prgm
3501 SW Davie Rd
Fort Lauderdale, FL 33314
www.broward.edu
Prgm Dir: Joyce Abraham, CDA RDH BA
Tel: 954 201-6904   *Fax:* 954 201-6397
E-mail: jabraham@broward.edu

Edison State College
Dental Hygiene Prgm
8099 College Pkwy
Fort Myers, FL 33906-6210
www.edison.edu
Prgm Dir: Karen Molumby, CDA RDH MBA
Tel: 239 985-8322   *Fax:* 239 985-8352
E-mail: kmolumby@edison.edu

Indian River State College
Dental Hygiene Prgm
3209 Virginia Ave
Fort Pierce, FL 34981-5599
www.ircc.edu

Sanford-Brown Institute - Ft Lauderdale
Dental Hygiene Prgm
1201 West Cypress Creek Rd
Ft Lauderdale , FL 33309

Santa Fe College
Dental Hygiene Prgm
3000 NW 83rd St, Bldg W81
Gainesville, FL 32606

Florida State College at Jacksonville
Dental Hygiene Prgm
4501 Capper Rd
Jacksonville, FL 32218
www.fccj.org

Sanford Brown Institute - Jacksonville
Dental Hygiene Prgm
10255 Fortune Pkway
Suite 501
Jacskonville, FL 32256

Palm Beach State College
Dental Hygiene Prgm
4200 Congress Ave
Lake Worth, FL 33461
www.pbcc.edu/dentalhealth.xml

Dade Medical College
Dental Hygiene Prgm
Medical Ctr Campus
950 NW 20th St
Miami, FL 33127

Pasco-Hernando Community College
Dental Hygiene Prgm
10230 Ridge Rd, M-144
New Port Richey, FL 34654-5199
www.pasco-hernandocc.com

Sanford Brown Institute - Orlando
Dental Hygiene Prgm
5959 Lake Ellenor Drive
Orlando, FL 32809

Valencia College
Dental Hygiene Prgm
1800 S Kirkman Rd
Orlando, FL 32811
valenciacc.edu/asdegrees/health/dh.cfm

Gulf Coast State College
Dental Hygiene Prgm
5230 W US Hwy 98
Panama City, FL 32401-1041

Pensacola State College
Dental Hygiene Prgm
5555 Hwy 98 W
Pensacola, FL 32507

St Petersburg College
Dental Hygiene Prgm
PO Box 13489
St Petersburg, FL 33781
www.spjc.edu/hec/dental

Tallahassee Community College
Dental Hygiene Prgm
444 Appleyard Dr
Tallahassee, FL 32304-2895
www.tcc.fl.edu

Hillsborough Community College
Dental Hygiene Prgm
4001 Tampa Bay Blvd
Tampa, FL 33614-2754

Georgia

Darton College
Dental Hygiene Prgm
2400 Gillionville Rd
Albany, GA 31707
www.darton.edu/Programs/AlliedHealth/denthyg.htm

Athens Technical College
Dental Hygiene Prgm
800 US Hwy 29 N
Athens, GA 30601-1500
www.athenstech.edu

Atlanta Technical College
Dental Hygiene Prgm
1560 Metropolitan Parkway SW
Atlanta, GA 30310

Georgia Health Sciences University
Dental Hygiene Prgm
1120 15th St, AD3103
Augusta, GA 30912-0200
www.georgiahealth.edu

Columbus Technical College
Dental Hygiene Prgm
928 Manchester Expressway
Columbus, GA 31904-6572

West Georgia Technical College
Dental Hygiene Prgm
4600 Timber Ridge Dr
Douglasville, GA 30135
www.westcentraltech.edu

Georgia Perimeter College
Dental Hygiene Prgm
2101 Womack Rd
Dunwoody, GA 30338-4497
www.gpc.edu

Central Georgia Technical College
Dental Hygiene Prgm
300 Macon Tech Drive
Macon, GA 31206
http://centralgatech.edu

Clayton State University
Dental Hygiene Prgm
2000 Clayton State Blvd
Suite T-105
Morrow, GA 30260
www.clayton.edu

Lanier Technical College
Dental Hygiene Prgm
2990 Landrum Education Dr
Oakwood, GA 30566
www.laniertech.edu

Georgia Highlands College
Dental Hygiene Prgm
415 E Third Ave
Rome, GA 30161
www.highlands.edu/dental

Armstrong Atlantic State University
Dental Hygiene Prgm
11935 Abercorn St
Savannah, GA 31419-1997

Savannah Technical College
Dental Hygiene Prgm
5717 White Bluff Rd
Savannah, GA 31405

Fortis College
Dental Hygiene Prgm
2108 Cobb Highway
Smyrna, GA 30080

Wiregrass Georgia Technical College
Cosponsor: Valdosta Technical College
Dental Hygiene Prgm
4089 Val Tech Rd, PO Box 928
Valdosta, GA 31603

Southeastern Technical College
Dental Hygiene Prgm
3001 East First St
Vidalia, GA 30474

Middle Georgia Technical College
Dental Hygiene Prgm
80 Cohen Walker Dr
Warner Robins, GA 31088-2729
www.middlegatech.edu

Hawaii

University of Hawaii at Manoa
Dental Hygiene Prgm
2445 Campus Rd, Rm 200-B
Honolulu, HI 96822

University of Hawaii Maui College
Dental Hygiene Prgm
310 W Ka'ahumanu Ave
Kahului, HI 96732

Idaho

Carrington College of Boise
Dental Hygiene Prgm
1200 N Liberty St
Boise, ID 83704
www.apollo.edu

Idaho State University
Dental Hygiene Prgm
Box 8048
Pocatello, ID 83209-8380
www.isu.edu/departments/dentalhy

College of Southern Idaho
Dental Hygiene Prgm
315 Falls Ave
PO Box 1238
Twin Falls, ID 83301

Illinois

Southern Illinois University Carbondale
Dental Hygiene Prgm
School of Allied Health
Mail Code 6615
Carbondale, IL 62901
www.siu.edu/~sah/dh/home.htm

John A Logan College
Dental Hygiene Prgm
700 Logan College Rd
Carterville, IL 62918
www.jalc.edu

Parkland College
Dental Hygiene Prgm
2400 W Bradley Ave
Champaign, IL 61821
www.parkland.edu

Kennedy-King College
Dental Hygiene Prgm
UIC College of Dentistry, Rm 201 S, Mail Code 621
801 S Paulina St
Chicago, IL 60612

Prairie State College
Dental Hygiene Prgm
202 S Halsted St
Chicago Heights, IL 60411
www.prairiestate.edu

Carl Sandburg College
Dental Hygiene Prgm
2400 Tom L Wilson Blvd
209 E Main St
Galesburg, IL 61401

College of DuPage
Dental Hygiene Prgm
425 Fawell Blvd
Glen Ellyn, IL 60137

Lewis & Clark Community College
Dental Hygiene Prgm
5800 Godfrey Rd
Godfrey, IL 62035
www.lc.edu

Lake Land College
Dental Hygiene Prgm
5001 Lake Land Blvd
Mattoon, IL 61938-9366
http://lakeland.cc.il.us

Harper College
Dental Hygiene Prgm
1200 W Algonquin Rd
Palatine, IL 60067

Illinois Central College
Dental Hygiene Prgm
201 SW Adams St
Peoria, IL 61635-0001

Rock Valley College
Dental Hygiene Prgm
4151 Samuelson Rd
Rockford, IL 61109
www.rockvalleycollege.edu

Sanford Brown College - Skokie
Dental Hygiene Prgm
4930 Oakton St
2nd Floor
Skokie, IL 60007

College of Lake County
Dental Hygiene Prgm
33 N Genesee St
Waukegan, IL 60085

Indiana

Ivy Tech Community College - Anderson Campus
Dental Hygiene Prgm
104 West 53rd St
Anderson, IN 46013

University of Southern Indiana
Dental Hygiene Prgm
8600 University Blvd
Evansville, IN 47712
health.usi.edu/acadprog/denthygn/

Indiana Univ - Purdue Univ Ft Wayne
Dental Hygiene Prgm
2101 Coliseum Blvd E
Fort Wayne, IN 46805
www.ipfw.edu/dental/hygiene/default.shtml

Indiana University Northwest
Dental Hygiene Prgm
3400 Broadway St
Gary, IN 46408
www.iun.edu

Indiana University
Dental Hygiene Prgm
School of Dentistry
1121 W Michigan St
Indianapolis, IN 46202-5186

Indiana University South Bend
Dental Hygiene Prgm
1700 Mishawaka Ave
South Bend, IN 46634
www.iusb.edu

Ivy Tech Community College - South Bend
Dental Hygiene Prgm
220 Dean Johnson Blvd
South Bend, IN 46601

Iowa

Des Moines Area Community College
Dental Hygiene Prgm
2006 S Ankeny Blvd
Building 9
Ankeny, IA 50023-3993
http://go.dmacc.edu/programs/dentalhygiene/pages/welcome.aspx

Kirkwood Community College
Dental Hygiene Prgm
6301 Kirkwood Blvd SW, PO Box 2068
Cedar Rapids, IA 52406
www.kirkwoodcollege.com

Iowa Western Community College
Dental Hygiene Prgm
2700 College Rd, PO Box 4C
Council Bluffs, IA 51502-3004
www.iwcc.edu

Iowa Central Community College
Dental Hygiene Prgm
One Triton Circle
Fort Dodge, IA 50501

Hawkeye Community College
Dental Hygiene Prgm
1501 E Orange Rd
PO Box 8015
Waterloo, IA 50704
www.hawkeyecollege.edu

Kansas

Flint Hills Technical College
Dental Hygiene Prgm
3301 W 18th Ave
Emporia, KS 66801

Kaplan Career Institute - Boston
Dental Hygiene Prgm
3136 Dickens Ave
Manhattan, KS 66503

Johnson County Community College
Dental Hygiene Prgm
12345 College Blvd
Overland Park, KS 66210-1299
www.jccc.edu

Wichita State University
Dental Hygiene Prgm
1845 N Fairmount
Wichita, KS 67260-0144
www.wichita.edu/dh

Kentucky

Western Kentucky University
Dental Hygiene Prgm
Academic Complex, Rm 201
Bowling Green, KY 42101

Henderson Community College
Dental Hygiene Prgm
2660 S Green St
Henderson, KY 42420
www.hencc.kctcs.edu

Bluegrass Community and Technical College
Dental Hygiene Prgm
Room 250 Oswald Bldg
Cooper Dr
Lexington, KY 40506
www.bluegrass.kctcs.edu/LCC/DHY

University of Louisville
Dental Hygiene Prgm
School of Dentistry
501 S Preston St
Louisville, KY 40292

Big Sandy Community & Technical College
Dental Hygiene Prgm
1 Bert T Combs Dr
Prestonsburg, KY 41653
www.bigsandy.kctcs.edu

Louisiana

University of Louisiana at Monroe
Dental Hygiene Prgm
700 University Ave
Monroe, LA 71209

Louisiana State University
Dental Hygiene Prgm
School of Dentistry
1100 Florida Ave
New Orleans, LA 70119
www.lsuhsc.edu

Southern Univ at Shreveport
Dental Hygiene Prgm
3050 Martin Luther King Jr Dr
Shreveport, LA 71107
www.susla.edu

Maine

Univ of Maine Augusta (Bangor)
Dental Hygiene Prgm
29 Texas Ave
Bangor, ME 04401-4324
www.uma.maine.edu

University of New England
Dental Hygiene Prgm
Westbrook College Campus
716 Stevens Ave
Portland, ME 04103-2670
www.une.edu

Maryland

Baltimore City Community College
Dental Hygiene Prgm
2901 Liberty Heights Ave
Baltimore, MD 21215
www.bccc.edu

Community College of Baltimore County
Dental Hygiene Prgm
7200 Sollers Point Rd
Baltimore, MD 21222

University of Maryland, Baltimore
Dental Hygiene Prgm
Division of Dental Hygiene
650 W Baltimore St, Rm 1202
Baltimore, MD 21201
www.dental.umaryland.edu

Northern Virginia Community College
Dental Hygiene Prgm
Bethesda, MD 20816

Allegany College of Maryland
Dental Hygiene Prgm
12401 Willowbrook Rd SE
Cumberland, MD 21502-2596

Fortis Institute - Landover
Dental Hygiene Prgm
4351 Garden City Drive
Landover, MD 20785

Massachusetts

Mass College of Pharmacy & Health Sciences
Dental Hygiene Prgm
179 Longwood Ave
Boston, MA 02115-5896
www.mcphs.edu/academics/programs/dental_hygiene/bs
_dental_hygiene/

Bristol Community College
Dental Hygiene Prgm
777 Elsbree St
Fall River, MA 02720
www.bristol.mass.edu

Mount Wachusett Community College
Dental Hygiene Prgm
Dental Hygiene Program
444 Green St
Gardner, MA 01440

Middlesex Community College
Dental Hygiene Prgm
33 Kearney Square
Lowell, MA 01852
www.middlesex.mass.edu

Mt Ida College
Dental Hygiene Prgm
777 Dedham St
Newton Centre, MA 02459

Springfield Technical Community College
Dental Hygiene Prgm
One Armory Square, Ste 1
PO Box 9000
Springfield, MA 01102-9000
www.stcc.edu

Cape Cod Community College
Dental Hygiene Prgm
2240 Iyannough Rd
West Barnstable, MA 02668-1599
www.capecod.edu

Quinsigamond Community College
Dental Hygiene Prgm
670 W Boylston St
Worcester, MA 01606

Michigan

University of Michigan
Dental Hygiene Prgm
1011 N University
Ann Arbor, MI 48109-1078
www.dent.umich.edu/depts/pom/hygiene/

Baker College of Auburn Hills
Dental Hygiene Prgm
1500 University Drive
Auburn Hills, MI 48326

Kellogg Community College
Dental Hygiene Prgm
450 North Ave
Battle Creek, MI 49017
www.kellogg.edu

Ferris State University
Dental Hygiene Prgm
200 Ferris Dr
Big Rapids, MI 49307-2740
www.ferris.edu

Wayne County Community College District
Dental Hygiene Prgm
8551 Greenfield, Rm 310
Detroit, MI 48228
www.wcccd.edu

Mott Community College
Dental Hygiene Prgm
1401 E Court St
Flint, MI 48503
http://mcc.edu

Grand Rapids Community College
Dental Hygiene Prgm
143 Bostwick St NE
Grand Rapids, MI 49503
www.grcc.edu/dental

Kalamazoo Valley Community College
Dental Hygiene Prgm
6767 West O Ave, Box 4070
Kalamazoo, MI 49003-4070
http://kvcc.edu

Lansing Community College
Dental Hygiene Prgm
MC 3100D Health and Human Service Careers
PO Box 40010
Lansing, MI 48901-7210
www.lcc.edu/humanhealth/dental/

Baker College of Port Huron
Dental Hygiene Prgm
3403 Lapeer Rd
Port Huron, MI 48060
www.baker.edu

Delta College
Dental Hygiene Prgm
1961 Delta Rd
University Center, MI 48710
www.delta.edu

Oakland Community College
Dental Hygiene Prgm
7350 Cooley Lake Rd
Waterford, MI 48327
www.oaklandcc.edu

Minnesota

Normandale Community College
Dental Hygiene Prgm
9700 France Ave S
Bloomington, MN 55431
www.normandale.edu

Herzing University
Dental Hygiene Prgm
5700 W Broadway Ave
Crystal, MN 55428
www.herzing.edu

Lake Superior College
Dental Hygiene Prgm
2101 Trinity Rd
Duluth, MN 55811
www.lsc.edu

Argosy University Twin Cities Campus
Dental Hygiene Prgm
1515 Central Parkway
Eagan, MN 55121
www.argosyu.edu

Minnesota State University - Mankato
Dental Hygiene Prgm
3 Morris Hall
Mankato, MN 56001

University of Minnesota
Dental Hygiene Prgm
9-372 Moos Tower
515 Delaware St SE
Minneapolis, MN 55455
www.dentistry.umn.edu

Minnesota State Comm & Tech Coll - Moorhead
Dental Hygiene Prgm
Allied Dental Careers Dept
1900 28th Ave S
Moorhead, MN 56560-4899
www.minnesota.edu

Rochester Community & Technical College
Dental Hygiene Prgm
851 30th Ave SE
Rochester, MN 55904
www.roch.edu

St Cloud Technical and Community College
Dental Hygiene Prgm
1540 Northway Dr
St Cloud, MN 56303-1240
www.sctcc.edu

Century College
Dental Hygiene Prgm
3300 Century Ave N
White Bear Lake, MN 55110
www.century.cc.mn.us/

Mississippi

Northeast Mississippi Community College
Dental Hygiene Prgm
Cunningham Blvd
Booneville, MS 38829

Pearl River Community College
Dental Hygiene Prgm
5448 US Hwy 49 S
Hattiesburg, MS 39401
www.prcc.edu

University of Mississippi Medical Center
Dental Hygiene Prgm
2500 N State St, SHRP
Jackson, MS 39216-4505
http://shrp.umc.edu

Meridian Community College
Dental Hygiene Prgm
910 Hwy 19 N
Meridian, MS 39307
www.meridiancc.edu

Mississippi Delta Community College
Dental Hygiene Prgm
PO Box 668
Highway 3 at Cherry St
Moorhead, MS 38761

Missouri

Missouri College
Dental Hygiene Prgm
1405 S Hanley Rd
Brentwood, MO 63144

Missouri Southern State University
Dental Hygiene Prgm
3950 E Newman
Joplin, MO 64801-1595
www.mssu.edu

Concorde Career College - Kansas City
Dental Hygiene Prgm
3239 Broadway
Kansas City, MO 64111

University of Missouri - Kansas City
Dental Hygiene Prgm
650 E 25th St Rm 415
Kansas City, MO 64108
www.umkc.edu/dentistry

State Fair Community College
Dental Hygiene Prgm
3201 W 16th St
Sedalia, MO 65301
www.sfccmo.edu

Ozarks Technical Community College
Dental Hygiene Prgm
1001 E Chestnut Expressway
Springfield, MO 65802
www.otc.edu

North Central Missouri College
Dental Hygiene Prgm
Hillyard Technical Center
3434 Faraon St
St Joseph, MO 64506

St Louis Community College - Forest Park
Dental Hygiene Prgm
5600 Oakland Ave
4th Floor, Tower A
St Louis, MO 63110-1393
http://stlcc.edu

Montana

Montana State Univ - Great Falls Coll of Tech
Dental Hygiene Prgm
2100 16th Ave S
Great Falls, MT 59405
www.msugf.edu

Nebraska

Central Community College
Dental Hygiene Prgm
PO Box 1024
Hastings, NE 68902-1024
www.cccneb.edu

University of Nebraska - Lincoln
Dental Hygiene Prgm
40th and Holdrege Sts
Lincoln, NE 68583-0740
www.unmc.edu/dentistry

Nevada

College of Southern Nevada
Dental Hygiene Prgm
6375 W Charleston Blvd
W1A
Las Vegas, NV 89146
sites.csn.edu/health/overview-dental.html

Truckee Meadows Community College
Dental Hygiene Prgm
7000 Dandini Blvd, RMDT 417-H
Reno, NV 89512-3999
www.tmcc.edu

New Hampshire

NHTI, Concord's Community College
Dental Hygiene Prgm
31 College Dr
Concord, NH 03301-7412
www.nhti.edu

New Jersey

Camden County College
Dental Hygiene Prgm
PO Box 200
Blackwood, NJ 08012

Middlesex County College
Dental Hygiene Prgm
2600 Woodbridge Ave, PO Box 3050
Edison, NJ 08818-3050

Eastern International College
Dental Hygiene Prgm
3000 JF Kennedy Blvd 3rd floor
Jersey City, NJ 07306

Bergen Community College
Dental Hygiene Prgm
400 Paramus Rd S-337
Paramus, NJ 07652
bergen.edu

Burlington County College
Dental Hygiene Prgm
601 Pemberton-Browns Mills Rd
Pemberton, NJ 08068
www.bcc.edu/pages/1.asp#

Univ of Medicine & Dent of New Jersey
Dental Hygiene Prgm
1776 Raritan Rd
Scotch Plains, NJ 07076
www.umdnj.edu

New Mexico

Pima Medical Institute - Albuquerque
Dental Hygiene Prgm
4400 Cutler Ave NE
Albuquerque, NM 87110

University of New Mexico
Dental Hygiene Prgm
Division of Dental Hygiene
Health Science Center
2320 Tucker NE
Albuquerque, NM 87131-1391
http://hsc.unm.edu/som/dentalhy

San Juan College
Dental Hygiene Prgm
4601 College Blvd
Farmington, NM 87402-4699
www.sanjuancollege.edu/hygiene

Dona Ana Community College
Dental Hygiene Prgm
New Mexico State University
3400 S Espina St
Las Cruces, NM 88003

Eastern New Mexico University - Roswell
Dental Hygiene Prgm
PO Box 6000
52 University Blvd
Roswell, NM 88202-6000

New York

Broome Community College
Dental Hygiene Prgm
PO Box 1017
Binghamton, NY 13902
http://web.sunybroome.edu/healthsciences/den/

Eugenio Maria De Hostos Community College
Dental Hygiene Prgm
500 Grand Concourse
Bronx, NY 10451

New York City College of Technology
Dental Hygiene Prgm
Dental Hygiene Department P201
300 Jay St
Brooklyn, NY 11201-2983
www.citytech.cuny.edu

Farmingdale State College, SUNY
Dental Hygiene Prgm
2350 Broadhollow Rd
Farmingdale, NY 11735
www.farmingdale.edu

Orange County Community College
Dental Hygiene Prgm
115 South St
Middletown, NY 10940
www.sunyorange.edu/dentalhygiene

New York University
Dental Hygiene Prgm
345 E 24th St
New York, NY 10010
www.nyu.edu/dental

Briarcliffe College
Dental Hygiene Prgm
225 West Main St
Patchogue, NY 11772

Monroe Community College
Dental Hygiene Prgm
1000 E Henrietta Rd
Rochester, NY 14623-5780

SUNY at Canton
Cosponsor: Mohawk Valley Community College
Dental Hygiene Prgm
125 Brookley Rd
Rome, NY 13440
www.canton.edu/can/
    can_start.taf?oage=study_school_healthmed

Hudson Valley Community College
Dental Hygiene Prgm
80 Vandenburgh Ave
Troy, NY 12180
www.hvcc.edu

Erie Community College
Dental Hygiene Prgm
6205 Main St
Williamsville, NY 14221-7095
www.ecc.edu
Notes: Sixty students are accepted to clinical courses
each fall at our modern two-year-old facility.
Pre-dental hygiene option available for applicants
who do not meet admission requirements.

North Carolina

Asheville-Buncombe Technical Comm College
Dental Hygiene Prgm
340 Victoria Rd
Asheville, NC 28801
www.abtech.edu

University of North Carolina
Dental Hygiene Prgm
Dental Hygiene Prgms
3220 Old Dental Bldg, CB 7450
Chapel Hill, NC 27599-7450
www.dent.unc.edu

Central Piedmont Community College
Dental Hygiene Prgm
1201 Elizabeth Ave, Kings Dr
Charlotte, NC 28204

Fayetteville Technical Community College
Dental Hygiene Prgm
2201 Hull Rd, PO Box 35236
Fayetteville, NC 28303
www.faytechcc.edu

Wayne Community College
Dental Hygiene Prgm
3000 Wayne Memorial Dr
Goldsboro, NC 27533
www.waynecc.edu

Catawba Valley Community College
Dental Hygiene Prgm
2550 Hwy 70 SE
Hickory, NC 28602
www.cvcc.edu/prog_study/health/dhygiene/

Coastal Carolina Community College
Dental Hygiene Prgm
444 Western Blvd
Jacksonville, NC 28546
http://CoastalCarolina.edu

Guilford Technical Community College
Dental Hygiene Prgm
PO Box 309
Jamestown, NC 27282
www.gtcc.edu

Wake Technical Community College
Dental Hygiene Prgm
2901 Holston Lane
Raleigh, NC 27610
www.waketech.edu

Central Carolina Community College
Dental Hygiene Prgm
900 S Vance St
Suite 220-B
Sanford, NC 27330

Halifax Community College
Dental Hygiene Prgm
PO Drawer 809
Weldon, NC 27890-0809
www.hcc.cc.nc.us

Cape Fear Community College
Dental Hygiene Prgm
411 N Front St
Wilmington, NC 28401-3993

Forsyth Technical Community College
Dental Hygiene Prgm
2100 Silas Creek Pkwy
Winston-Salem, NC 27103-5197

North Dakota

North Dakota State College of Science
Dental Hygiene Prgm
800 N Sixth St
Wahpeton, ND 58076

Ohio

University of Cincinnati
Cosponsor: Raymond Walters College
Dental Hygiene Prgm
9555 Plainfield Rd
Cincinnati, OH 45236

Cuyahoga Community College
Dental Hygiene Prgm
2900 Community College Ave
Cleveland, OH 44115
www.tri-c.edu/programs/healthcareers/dentalhygiene/
    Pages/default.aspx

Columbus State Community College
Dental Hygiene Prgm
550 E Spring St, PO Box 1609
Union Hall 410
Columbus, OH 43216
www.cscc.edu

The Ohio State University
Dental Hygiene Prgm
305 W 12th Ave
PO Box 182357
Columbus, OH 43218-2357
www.dent.osu.edu/dhy

Sinclair Community College
Dental Hygiene Prgm
444 W Third St
Dayton, OH 45402

Lorain County Community College
Dental Hygiene Prgm
1005 N Abbe Rd
Elyria, OH 44035-1691

Lakeland Community College
Dental Hygiene Prgm
7700 Clocktower Dr
Kirtland, OH 44094-5198

Rhodes State College
Dental Hygiene Prgm
4240 Campus Dr
Lima, OH 45804

Stark State College
Dental Hygiene Prgm
6200 Frank Ave NW
North Canton, OH 44720-7299
www.starkstate.edu

Shawnee State University
Dental Hygiene Prgm
940 Second St
Portsmouth, OH 45662
www.shawnee.edu

Owens Community College
Dental Hygiene Prgm
PO Box 10,000
Toledo, OH 43699
www.owens.edu

Youngstown State University
Dental Hygiene Prgm
Dept of Health Professions
One University Plaza
Youngstown, OH 44555
www.ysu.edu

Oklahoma

Rose State College
Dental Hygiene Prgm
6420 SE 15th St
Midwest City, OK 73110
www.rose.edu

Univ of Oklahoma Health Sciences Center
Dental Hygiene Prgm
PO Box 26901
Oklahoma City, OK 73117
dentistry.ouhsc.edu/prospectivestudents_2_2_1.php

Tulsa Community College
Dental Hygiene Prgm
909 S Boston Ave, Rm MP 458
Tulsa, OK 74119-2094
www.tulsacc.edu

Oregon

Lane Community College
Dental Hygiene Prgm
4000 E 30th Ave
Eugene, OR 97405

Mt Hood Community College
Dental Hygiene Prgm
26000 SE Stark St
Gresham, OR 97030
www.mhcc.edu

**Pacific University School of Dental Health
    Science**
Dental Hygiene Prgm
222 SE 8th Ave, Suite 271
Hillsboro, OR 97123

Oregon Institute of Technology
Dental Hygiene Prgm
3201 Campus Dr
Semon Hall #214
Klamath Falls, OR 97601
www.oit.edu

Carrington College Portland
Dental Hygiene Prgm
917 Lloyd Center, First Floor
Portland, OR 97232

Portland Community College
Dental Hygiene Prgm
PO Box 19000
Portland, OR 97219-0990
www.pcc.edu

Pennsylvania

Northampton Community College
Dental Hygiene Prgm
3835 Green Pond Rd
Bethlehem, PA 18020

Montgomery County Community College
Dental Hygiene Prgm
340 DeKalb Pike
Blue Bell, PA 19422-0758
www.mc3.edu

Harcum College
Dental Hygiene Prgm
750 Montgomery Ave
Bryn Mawr, PA 19010
www.harcum.edu

Tri-State Business Institute
Dental Hygiene Prgm
5757 W Ridge Rd
Erie, PA 16506
www.tsbi.edu

Harrisburg Area Community College
Dental Hygiene Prgm
One HACC Dr SM-102
Harrisburg, PA 17110-2999
www.hacc.edu

Manor College
Dental Hygiene Prgm
700 Fox Chase Rd
Jenkintown, PA 19046-3399
www.manor.edu

Luzerne County Community College
Dental Hygiene Prgm
1333 S Prospect St
Nanticoke, PA 18634-3899
www.luzerne.edu

Community College of Philadelphia
Dental Hygiene Prgm
1700 Spring Garden St
Philadelphia, PA 19130
www.ccp.edu

University of Pittsburgh
Dental Hygiene Prgm
3501 Terrace St
B-82 Salk Hall
Pittsburgh, PA 15261
www.dental.pitt.edu/students/dental_hygiene.php

Fortis Institute
Dental Hygiene Prgm
517 Ash St
Scranton, PA 18509

Pennsylvania College of Technology
Dental Hygiene Prgm
One College Ave
Williamsport, PA 17701
www.pct.edu/schools/hs/dental

Westmoreland County Community College
Dental Hygiene Prgm
145 Pavilion Ln
Youngwood, PA 15697-1895
www.wccc.edu

Rhode Island

Community College of Rhode Island
Dental Hygiene Prgm
1762 Louisquisset Pike
Lincoln, RI 02865-4585
www.ccri.edu

South Carolina

Trident Technical College
Dental Hygiene Prgm
PO Box 118067
7000 Rivers Ave
Charleston, SC 29423-8067
www.tridenttech.edu

Horry - Georgetown Technical College
Dental Hygiene Prgm
PO Box 261966
2050 Highway 501 East
Conway, SC 29528-6066
www.hgtc.edu

Florence-Darlington Technical College
Dental Hygiene Prgm
PO Box 100548
Florence, SC 29501-0548

Greenville Technical College
Dental Hygiene Prgm
PO Box 5616
Greenville, SC 29606-5616
www.gvltec.edu

York Technical College
Dental Hygiene Prgm
452 S Anderson Rd
Rock Hill, SC 29730

Midlands Technical College
Dental Hygiene Prgm
PO Box 2408
West Columbia, SC 29202

South Dakota

University of South Dakota
Dental Hygiene Prgm
120 East Hall 414, E Clark St
Vermillion, SD 57069
www.usd.edu/dh

Tennessee

Chattanooga State Community College
Dental Hygiene Prgm
4501 Amnicola Hwy
Chattanooga, TN 37406-1097
www.chattanoogastate.edu

East Tennessee State University
Dental Hygiene Prgm
PO Box 70690
Johnson City, TN 37614-0690
www.etsu.edu/cpah/dental

Hiwassee College
Dental Hygiene Prgm
225 Hiwassee College Dr
Madisonville, TN 37354

Concorde Career College - Memphis
Dental Hygiene Prgm
5100 Poplar Ave
Suite 132
Memphis, TN 38137

University of Tennessee Health Science Ctr
Dental Hygiene Prgm
930 Madison Ave, Ste 600
Memphis, TN 38163
www.utmem.edu/allied/dental_hygiene_home.html

Remington College - Nashville Campus
Dental Hygiene Prgm
441 Donelson Pike
Suite 150
Nashville, TN 37214

Tennessee State University
Dental Hygiene Prgm
3500 John A Merritt Blvd
Nashville, TN 37209-1561

Roane State Community College
Dental Hygiene Prgm
701 Briarcliff Ave
Oak Ridge, TN 37830-8795
www.rscc.cc.tn.us

Texas

Amarillo College
Dental Hygiene Prgm
PO Box 447
Amarillo, TX 79178
www.actx.edu

Austin Community College
Dental Hygiene Prgm
Eastview Campus, Department of Dental Hygiene
3401 Webberville Rd
Austin, TX 78702
www.austincc.edu/health/dhyg

Lamar Institute of Technology
Dental Hygiene Prgm
PO Box 10061
Beaumont, TX 77710
www.lit.edu

Coastal Bend College
Dental Hygiene Prgm
3800 Charco Rd
Beeville, TX 78102
http://coastalbend.edu

Howard College
Dental Hygiene Prgm
1001 Birdwell Ln
Big Spring, TX 79720
www.howardcollege.edu

Blinn College
Dental Hygiene Prgm
PO Box 6030
Bryan, TX 77805-6030
www.blinn.edu

Del Mar College
Dental Hygiene Prgm
101 Baldwin Blvd
Corpus Christi, TX 78404
www.delmar.edu/dh

Baylor College of Dentistry, Texas A&M HSC
Dental Hygiene Prgm
The Texas A & M University System Health Science
  Center
PO Box 660677
Dallas, TX 75266-0677
www.bcd.tamhsc.edu

Concorde Career College - Dallas
Dental Hygiene Prgm
12606 Greenville Ave
Suite 130
Dallas, TX 75243

Sanford-Brown College - Dallas
Dental Hygiene Prgm
1250 West Mockingbird Lane
Suite 150
Dallas, TX 75247

Texas Woman's University
Dental Hygiene Prgm
Box 425796, TWU Station
Denton, TX 76204

El Paso Community College
Dental Hygiene Prgm
PO Box 20500
El Paso, TX 79998
www.epcc.edu

Texas State Technical College - Harlingen
Dental Hygiene Prgm
1902 N Loop 499
Harlingen, TX 78550-3697

**Houston Comm College System - Southeast
  Coll Coleman College for Health Sciences**
Dental Hygiene Prgm
1900 Pressler St
Houston, TX 77030

University of Texas Health Sci Ctr Houston
Dental Hygiene Prgm
6516 M D Anderson Blvd
Suite 1.085
Houston, TX 77030
www.db.uth.tmc.edu/dental_hygiene/

Tarrant County College
Dental Hygiene Prgm
828 Harwood Rd
Hurst, TX 76054
www.tccd.edu/dental

Lone Star College - Kingwood
Dental Hygiene Prgm
20000 Kingwood Dr
Health & Science Building 118A
Kingwood, TX 77339
www.lonestar.edu

Collin College
Dental Hygiene Prgm
2200 W University Dr
McKinney, TX 75070-8001

Northeast Texas Community College
Dental Hygiene Prgm
PO Box 1307
Mt. Pleasant , TX 75456

Concorde Career College - San Antonio
Dental Hygiene Prgm
4803 NW Loop 410
Suite 200
San Antonio, TX 78229

UT Health Science Center - San Antonio
Dental Hygiene Prgm
7703 Floyd Curl Dr MSC 6244
San Antonio, TX 78229-3900

Temple College
Dental Hygiene Prgm
2600 S First St
Temple, TX 76504-7435

Tyler Junior College
Dental Hygiene Prgm
PO Box 9020
Tyler, TX 75711
www.tjc.edu

Wharton County Junior College
Dental Hygiene Prgm
911 Boling Hwy
Wharton, TX 77488
www.wcjc.edu

Midwestern State University
Dental Hygiene Prgm
3410 Taft Blvd
Wichita Falls, TX 76308-2099
www.mwsu.edu

Utah

Weber State University
Dental Hygiene Prgm
3920 University Circle
Ogden, UT 84408-3920
www.weber.edu/dentalhyg

The Utah College of Dental Hygiene
Dental Hygiene Prgm
1176 South 1480 West
Orem, UT 84058

Utah Valley University
Dental Hygiene Prgm
800 W University Pkwy
Orem, UT 84058

Fortis College - Salt Lake City
Dental Hygiene Prgm
3949 South 700 East
Suite 150
Salt Lake City, UT 84107

Dixie State College of Utah
Dental Hygiene Prgm
225 South 700 East
St George, UT 84770

Salt Lake Community College
Dental Hygiene Prgm
3491 Wights Fort Rd
Jordan HTC 115R
West Jordan, UT 84088
www.slcc.edu/dentalhygiene/

Vermont

Vermont Technical College
Dental Hygiene Prgm
301 Lawrence Place
Williston Campus
Williston, VT 05495
www.vtc.edu

Virginia

Old Dominion University
Dental Hygiene Prgm
Gene W Hirschfeld School of Dental Hygiene
2011 Health Science Building, 4608 Hampton Blvd
Norfolk, VA 23529-0499
www.odu.edu/dental

Virginia Commonwealth University
Dental Hygiene Prgm
School of Dentistry
PO Box 980566
Richmond, VA 23298-0566
www.dentistry.vcu.edu

Virginia Western Community College
Dental Hygiene Prgm
3097 Colonial Ave
Roanoke, VA 24015
www.vw.vccs.edu/health/denthome.htm

Thomas Nelson Community College
Dental Hygiene Prgm
4601 Opportunity Way
Williamsburg, VA 23188

Wytheville Community College
Dental Hygiene Prgm
1000 E Main St
Wytheville, VA 24382

Washington

Bellingham Technical College
Dental Hygiene Prgm
3028 Lindbergh Ave
Bellingham, WA 98225

Lake Washington Institute of Technology
Dental Hygiene Prgm
11605 132nd Ave NE
Kirkland, WA 98034
www.lwtchost.ctc.edu/programs2/dental

Pierce College
Dental Hygiene Prgm
9401 Farwest Dr SW
Lakewood, WA 98498-1999

Columbia Basin College
Dental Hygiene Prgm
2600 N 20th Ave
MS T-1
Pasco, WA 99301
www.columbiabasin.edu

Pima Medical Institute - Seattle
Dental Hygiene Prgm
9709 3rd Ave NE
Suite 400
Seattle, WA 98115

Shoreline Community College
Dental Hygiene Prgm
16101 Greenwood Ave N 2500 Bldg
Shoreline, WA 98133
http://success.shore.ctc.edu/dental/

Eastern Washington University
Dental Hygiene Prgm
310 N Riverpoint Blvd Box E
Spokane, WA 99202

Clark College
Dental Hygiene Prgm
1933 Fort Vancouver Way
Vancouver, WA 98663

Yakima Valley Community College
Dental Hygiene Prgm
PO Box 22520
Yakima, WA 98907-2520
www.yvcc.edu

West Virginia

Bridgemont Community and Technical College
Dental Hygiene Prgm
Department of Dental Hygiene
619 2nd Ave
Fayetteville, WV 25840

West Virginia University
Dental Hygiene Prgm
Health Science Ctr N, PO Box 9425
Morgantown, WV 26506-9425
www.hsc.wvu.edu/sod/departments/Hygiene/

Southern West Virginia Comm & Tech College
Dental Hygiene Prgm
Dempsey Branch Rd
PO Box 2900
Mount Gay, WV 25637
www.southernwv.edu

West Liberty State College
Dental Hygiene Prgm
PO Box 295
CSC 121
West Liberty, WV 26074-0295
www.westliberty.edu

Wisconsin

Fox Valley Technical College
Dental Hygiene Prgm
1825 Bluemound Dr
Appleton, WI 54914
www.fvtc.edu

Chippewa Valley Technical College Dental Dept.
Dental Hygiene Prgm
620 West Clairemont Ave
Eau Claire, WI 54701

Northeast Wisconsin Technical College
Dental Hygiene Prgm
2740 W Mason St, PO Box 19042
Green Bay, WI 54307-9042
www.nwtc.edu

Western Technical College Western Technical College
Dental Hygiene Prgm
1300 Badger St
Health Science Center
La Crosse, WI 54602-0908

Madison Area Technical College
Dental Hygiene Prgm
211 N Carroll St
Madison, WI 53703
www.matcmadison.edu

Milwaukee Area Technical College
Dental Hygiene Prgm
700 W State St
Milwaukee, WI 53233

Waukesha County Technical College
Dental Hygiene Prgm
800 Main St
Pewaukee, WI 53072
www.wctc.edu

Northcentral Technical College
Dental Hygiene Prgm
1000 Campus Dr
Wausau, WI 54401
www.ntc.edu

Wyoming

Laramie County Community College
Dental Hygiene Prgm
1400 E College Dr
Cheyenne, WY 82007-3299
www.lccc.cc.wy.us

Sheridan College
Dental Hygiene Prgm
3059 Coffeen Ave
Sheridan, WY 82801
www.sheridan.edu

Dental Hygienist

Programs*	Class Capacity	Begins	Length (months)	Award	Res. Tuition	Non-res. Tuition		Offers:† 1	2	3	4
Arizona											
Northern Arizona Univ (Flagstaff)	30	Aug	30	BS	$7,212	$17,711	per year	•		•	•
Arkansas											
Univ of Arkansas for Medical Sciences (Little Rock)	32	Aug	19	AS, BS	$8,575	$19,635				•	
California											
Cypress College	20	Aug	18	Cert, AS	$1,080	$6,240				•	
West Los Angeles College (Culver City)	25	Sep	21	Dipl, AS	$1,586	$13,420	per year			•	•
Florida											
Broward College (Fort Lauderdale)	16	Aug	12	AS	$3,253	$11,347				•	
Edison State College (Fort Myers)	18	Aug	18	AS	$3,955	$14,670	per year			•	

*Data are shown only for programs that completed the 2011 AMA Survey of Health Professions Education Programs.

†Key to Offers: 1: Evening or weekend classes; 2: Non-English instruction; 3: Cultural competence instruction; 4: Distance education component.

Dental Laboratory Technician

Dental laboratory technicians make dental prostheses—replacements for natural teeth, including dentures and crowns. The hallmarks of the qualified dental laboratory technician are skill in using small hand instruments, accuracy, artistic ability, and attention to detail to create practical and esthetically pleasing replacements.

History

The first educational standards for the education of dental laboratory technicians, adopted by the ADA House of Delegates in 1946, were rescinded and revised in 1957. Between 1946 and 1957, four programs for training dental laboratory technicians were developed, and the establishment of new programs remained static through 1965. From 1966 to 1979, the number of accredited dental laboratory technology programs increased from 4 to 59. Since that time, the number has decreased to approximately 20.

Career Description

Dental laboratory technicians seldom interact directly with patients; rather, they work with dentists by following detailed written instructions to make dental prostheses, which are replacements for natural teeth that enable people who have lost some or all of their teeth to eat, chew, talk, and smile in a manner similar to the way they did before. The dental technician uses impressions (molds) of the patient's teeth or oral soft tissues to create full dentures, removable partial dentures or fixed bridges, crowns, and orthodontic appliances and splints.

Dental technicians use sophisticated instruments and equipment and work with a variety of materials for replacing damaged or missing tooth structure, including waxes, plastics, precious and nonprecious alloys, stainless steel, and porcelain.

Employment Characteristics

Most of the more than 46,000 active dental laboratory technicians in the United States today work in commercial dental laboratories, which on average employ between three to five technicians. In addition, some dentists employ dental technicians in their private dental offices. Other employment opportunities for dental technicians include dental schools, hospitals, the military, and companies that manufacture dental prosthetic materials. Dental laboratory technician education programs also offer teaching positions for qualified technicians.

Salary

The starting salary of a dental technician varies depending on the responsibilities associated with the specific position and the geographic location of employment. May 2011 data from the US Bureau of Labor Statistics (BLS) show that wages at the 10th percentile were $21,070, the 50th percentile (median) at $35,590, and the 90th percentile at $59,360 (*www.bls.gov/oes/current/ oes519081.htm*).

In addition to salary, many dental technicians receive benefit packages from their employers, which may include health and disability insurance coverage, reimbursement for continuing education programs, and paid vacations and holidays. Experienced technicians may become self-employed by opening their own dental laboratories, leading to greater financial rewards.

For more information, refer to *www.ama-assn.org/go/hpsalary*.

Employment Outlook

The BLS projects that employment of dental laboratory technicians is expected to experience little or no change from 2010-2020. Baby boomers are more likely to retain their teeth than previous generation, so growth has been taking place at a steady rate.

Excellent career opportunities exist for nontraditional dental technology students, who might be seeking career change or job reentry after a period of unemployment, or from a culturally diverse background.

Educational Programs

Length. Most dental laboratory technicians receive their education and training through a two-year program at a community college, vocational school, technical college, or dental school, for which they may receive a certificate or an associate degree.

Prerequisites. High school diploma or its equivalent, although the Commission strongly encourages formal college-level education. High school students interested in becoming dental laboratory technicians should take courses in mathematics and science. Courses in metal and wood shop, art, drafting, and computers are recommended. Courses in management and business may help those wishing to operate their own laboratories.

Certification

Dental laboratory technicians can become certified by passing an examination, administered by the National Board for Certification in Dental Laboratory Technology, which evaluates their technical skills and knowledge. Passing this examination qualifies a dental technician to use the designation Certified Dental Technician (CDT). A CDT specializes in one or more of five areas: complete dentures, partial dentures, crowns and bridges, ceramics, and orthodontics.

Dental technicians are eligible to take the examination if they have completed a dental laboratory technology program accredited by the Commission on Dental Accreditation and have two years of professional experience or have completed five years of work experience as dental technicians, or have graduated from a nonaccredited program and have three years of professional experience and passed a comprehensive examination.

Inquiries

Careers/Curriculum
American Dental Association
211 East Chicago Avenue
Chicago, IL 60611-2678
312 440-2390
www.ada.org/careers

American Dental Education Association
1400 K Street NW, Suite 1100
Washington, DC 20005
202 289-7201
www.adea.org

Laboratory Conference Section Board of the American Dental
    Trade Association
4222 King Street W
Alexandria, VA 22302
703 379-7755

National Association of Dental Laboratories
325 John Knox Road, L103
Tallahassee, FL 32303
800 950-1150
www.nadl.org

Certification
National Board for Certification in Dental Laboratory Technology
325 John Knox Road, L103
Tallahassee, FL 32303
800 684-5310
www.nbccert.org

Program Accreditation
Commission on Dental Accreditation
American Dental Association
211 East Chicago Avenue
Chicago, IL 60611-2678
(312) 440-4653
www.ada.org

Note: Adapted in part from the Bureau of Labor Statistics, US
Department of Labor, *Occupational Outlook Handbook*, Medical,
Dental, and Ophthalmic Laboratory Technicians, at
www.bls.gov/oco/ocos238.htm.

Dental Laboratory Technician

Arizona

Pima Community College
Dental Lab Technician Prgm
2202 W Anklam Rd, HRP 220
Tucson, AZ 85709-0080

California

Los Angeles City College
Dental Lab Technician Prgm
855 N Vermont Ave
Los Angeles, CA 90029
www.lacitycollege.edu

Pasadena City College
Dental Lab Technician Prgm
1570 E Colorado Blvd R505
Pasadena, CA 91106
www.pasadena.edu

Florida

McFatter Technical Center
Dental Lab Technician Prgm
6500 Nova Dr
Davie, FL 33317
http://mcfattertech.com

Indian River State College
Dental Lab Technician Prgm
3209 Virginia Ave
Fort Pierce, FL 34981-5599
www.ircc.edu

Georgia

Atlanta Technical College
Dental Lab Technician Prgm
1560 Metropolitan Pkwy SW
Atlanta, GA 30310-4446
www.atlantatech.org

Indiana

Indiana Univ - Purdue Univ Ft Wayne
Dental Lab Technician Prgm
2101 Coliseum Blvd E
Fort Wayne, IN 46805
www.ipfw.edu/dlt

Iowa

Kirkwood Community College
Dental Lab Technician Prgm
6301 Kirkwood Blvd SW, PO Box 2068
Cedar Rapids, IA 52406-9973
www.kirkwood.edu

Kentucky

Bluegrass Community and Technical College
Dental Lab Technician Prgm
470 Cooper Dr, 330 Oswald Bldg
Lexington, KY 40506-0235
www.bluegrass.kctcs.edu/ahDLT/

Louisiana

Louisiana State University
Dental Lab Technician Prgm
School of Dentistry
1100 Florida Ave
Box 222
New Orleans, LA 70119
www.lsusd.lsuhsc.edu

Massachusetts

Middlesex Community College
Dental Lab Technician Prgm
33 Kearney Square
Lowell, MA 01852

New York

New York City College of Technology
Dental Lab Technician Prgm
300 Jay St
Brooklyn, NY 11201-2983
www.citytech.cuny.edu

Erie Community College
Dental Lab Technician Prgm
4041 Southwestern Blvd
Orchard Park, NY 14127-2199
www.ecc.edu

North Carolina

Durham Technical Community College
Dental Lab Technician Prgm
1637 Lawson St
Durham, NC 27703
www.durhamtech.edu

Oregon

Portland Community College
Dental Lab Technician Prgm
PO Box 19000
Portland, OR 97280-0990

Texas

**Medical Education and Training Campus
    (METC)**
Dental Lab Technician Prgm
Attn: Standards, Evaluations, and Accreditation
3038 William Hardee Rd, Building 895
Ft. Sam Houston, TX 78234-2532

San Antonio College
Dental Lab Technician Prgm
1300 San Pedro Ave
NAHC 134
San Antonio, TX 78212-2499
www.uthscsa.edu/sah/dlt.html

Virginia

J Sargeant Reynolds Community College
Dental Lab Technician Prgm
PO Box 85622
700 East Jackson St
Richmond, VA 23285-5622
www.reynolds.edu

Washington

Bates Technical College
Dental Lab Technician Prgm
1101 S Yakima Ave
Tacoma, WA 98405
www.bates.ctc.edu

Dentist

Career Description

Dentists diagnose, prevent, and treat problems with teeth or mouth tissue. They remove decay, fill cavities, examine x-rays, place protective plastic sealants on children's teeth, straighten teeth, and repair fractured teeth. They also perform corrective surgery on gums and supporting bones to treat gum diseases. Dentists extract teeth and make models and measurements for dentures to replace missing teeth. They provide instruction on diet, brushing, flossing, the use of fluorides, and other aspects of dental care. They also administer anesthetics and write prescriptions for antibiotics and other medications.

Dentists use a variety of equipment, including x-ray machines; drills; and instruments such as mouth mirrors, probes, forceps, brushes, and scalpels. They wear masks, gloves, and safety glasses to protect themselves and their patients from infectious diseases.

Dentists in private practice oversee a variety of administrative tasks, including bookkeeping and buying equipment and supplies. They may employ and supervise dental hygienists, dental assistants, dental laboratory technicians, and receptionists.

More than 80 percent of dentists are general practitioners, handling a variety of dental needs. Other dentists practice in any of nine specialty areas.

- *Orthodontists*, the largest group of specialists, straighten teeth by applying pressure to the teeth with braces or retainers.
- *Oral and maxillofacial surgeons*, the next largest group, operate on the mouth and jaws.
- *Pediatric dentists* focus on dentistry for children
- *Periodontists* treat gums and bone supporting the teeth
- *Prosthodontists* replace missing teeth with permanent fixtures, such as crowns and bridges, or with removable fixtures such as dentures
- *Endodontists* perform root canal therapy
- *Public health dentists* promote good dental health and prevention of dental diseases within the community
- *Oral pathologists* study oral diseases
- *Oral and maxillofacial radiologists* diagnose diseases in the head and neck through the use of imaging technologies

Teaching, dental research and dental industry comprise additional rewarding career options for both general practitioners and dental specialists. Dentists also work in public health agencies, hospitals, the military and other settings.

Employment Characteristics

Most dentists work four or five days a week. Some work evenings and weekends to meet their patients' needs. Most full-time dentists work between 35 and 40 hours a week, but others work more. Initially, dentists may work more hours as they establish their practice. Experienced dentists often work fewer hours. Many continue in part-time practice well beyond the usual retirement age.

Most dentists are solo practitioners, meaning that they own their own businesses and work alone or with a small staff. Some dentists have partners, and a few work for other dentists as associate dentists.

Salary

Dentists' average income places them in the highest five percent of US family income. May 2011 data from the US Bureau of Labor Statistics (BLS) show that wages at the 50th percentile (median) were $142,740 (*www.bls.gov/oes/current/oes291021.htm*).

For more information, refer to *www.ama-assn.org/go/hpsalary*.

Employment Outlook

The BLS projects that employment of dentists will grow by 21 percent through 2020, which is faster than the average for all occupations. The demand for dental services is expected to continue to increase. The overall US population is growing, and the elderly segment of the population is growing even faster; these phenomena will increase the demand for dental care. Many members of the baby-boom generation will need complicated dental work. In addition, elderly people are more likely to retain their teeth than were their predecessors, so they will require much more care than in the past. The younger generation will continue to need preventive checkups despite an overall increase in the dental health of the public over the last few decades. Recently, some private insurance providers have increased their dental coverage. If this trend continues, people with new or expanded dental insurance will be more likely to visit a dentist than in the past. Also, although they are currently a small proportion of dental expenditures, cosmetic dental services, such as providing teeth-whitening treatments, will become increasingly popular. This trend is expected to continue as new technologies allow these procedures to take less time and be much less invasive.

Employment of dentists, however, is not expected to keep pace with the increased demand for dental services. Productivity increases from new technology, as well as the tendency to assign more tasks to dental hygienists and assistants, will allow dentists to perform more work than they have in the past. As their practices expand, dentists are likely to hire more hygienists and dental assistants to handle routine services.

Dentists will increasingly provide care and instruction aimed at preventing the loss of teeth, rather than simply providing treatments such as fillings. Improvements in dental technology also will allow dentists to offer more effective and less painful treatment to their patients. For example, National Institute of Dental and Craniofacial Research (NIDCR) clinical and basic research that may revolutionize the practice of dentistry includes:

- Postnatal stem cell research aimed at tissue regeneration
- Salivary research, which is expected to yield new diagnostic tests
- Gene transfer therapy that may induce the salivary glands to produce hormones, antibodies, or other agents to prevent or treat oral and systemic disease
- Stem cells, possibly derived from the patient's own deciduous teeth, used to repair bone defects
- Small "labs-on-a-chip" placed intraorally to analyze hundreds of different components in oral fluids as early indicators of oral and systemic disease
- Restorative procedures and new dental materials to retain teeth

Need for Minority Dentists

There is a critical need in many underserved communities where minority and disadvantaged people are not getting the dental care they need. Recent data shows that minority dentists treat a very high number of minority patients.

More underrepresented minority dentists (African American, Hispanic and American Indian) are necessary to eliminate the barriers to oral care. This need is expected to increase, in light of US Census projections that minority populations will make up more than 50 percent of the US population by 2050.

Educational Programs

Award, Length. Dental schools award the degree of Doctor of Dental Surgery (DDS) or Doctor of Dental Medicine (DMD); programs are four years.

Prerequisites. Those interested in a career in dentistry are encouraged to obtain broad exposure to science and math while in high school and to enroll in college preparatory classes in biology, algebra, and chemistry. In addition, it is recommended to continue taking natural science courses in college such as general biology, organic and inorganic chemistry, and physics. Majoring in science is not a must, but completion of pre-dental science requirements is necessary. A college undergraduate degree is recommended in preparation for dental school. Most dental students have completed four years of college.

Other good ways to learn more about the field and prepare for a career in dentistry:

- Ask to volunteer or job shadow at your family dentist's office, orthodontist's office and pediatric dentist's office
- Talk with admission officers about financial aid resources and dental school requirements
- Join the American Student Dental Association (ASDA)
- Take the Dental Admissions Test (DAT) a year before entering dental school

Curriculum. The four years of study leading to the DDS or DMD degree are divided into two components. Years one and two encompass:

- Classroom and laboratory instruction in basic health sciences (including anatomy, biochemistry, histology, microbiology, pharmacology, and physiology), with an emphasis on dental aspects

- Basic principles of oral diagnosis and treatment; students may practice on manikins and models, and may begin treating patients later in the second year

Years three and four cover the following:

- Treatment of patients under the supervision of licensed dental faculty. Procedures cover the broad scope of general dentistry and include opportunities to work in a variety of settings, e.g., community clinics, hospitals, and outpatient clinics
- Practice management courses, including instruction in effective communication skills, the use of allied dental personnel, and business management

Licensure, Certification, Registration

All states require dentists to be licensed to practice. In most states, a candidate must graduate from a US dental school accredited by the ADA Commission on Dental Accreditation and pass written and practical examinations to qualify for licensure. Requirements include two to four years of postgraduate education and, in some cases, the completion of a special state examination.

Inquiries

Education, Careers, Resources
American Dental Association
211 East Chicago Avenue
Chicago, IL 60611-2678
312 440-2500
www.ada.org/student

Program Accreditation
American Dental Association
Commission on Dental Accreditation (CODA)
211 East Chicago Avenue
Chicago, IL 60611-2678
312 440-2500
www.ada.org/prof/ed/accred/commission

Note: Adapted in part from the Bureau of Labor Statistics, US Department of Labor, *Occupational Outlook Handbook*, Dentists, at *www.bls.gov/oco/ocos072.htm*.

Dentist

Alabama

University of Alabama
Dentistry Prgm
School of Dentistry
1530 3rd Ave South, SDB 406
Birmingham, AL 35294-0007
www.dental.uab.edu

Arizona

Midwestern University - Glendale Campus
Dentistry Prgm
College of Dental Medicine
19555 N 59th Ave
Glendale, AZ 85308

AT Still University of Health Sciences
Dentistry Prgm
Arizona School of Dentistry & Oral Health
5850 East Still Circle
Mesa, AZ 85206
www.atsu.edu/asdoh

California

Loma Linda University
Dentistry Prgm
School of Dentistry
11092 Anderson St
Loma Linda, CA 92350

University of California - Los Angeles
Dentistry Prgm
School of Dentistry
10833 Le Conte Ave -CHS 53-038
Los Angeles, CA 90095-1668
www.dent.ucla.edu

University of Southern California
Dentistry Prgm
925 W 34th St
Suite 203
Los Angeles, CA 90089-0641
www.usc.edu/hsc/dental

Western Univ of Health Sciences
Dentistry Prgm
College of Dental Medicine
309 E Second St
Pomona, CA 91766-1854

University of California - San Francisco
Dentistry Prgm
School of Dentistry
513 Parnassus Ave, S630
San Francisco, CA 94143-0430
www.ucsf.edu

University of the Pacific
Dentistry Prgm
Arthur A Dugoni School of Dentistry
2155 Webster St
San Francisco, CA 94115
www.dental.pacific.edu

Colorado

University of Colorado Denver - Anschutz MC
Dentistry Prgm
Mail Stop F831
13065 E 17th Ave - Room 302
Aurora, CO 80045
www.unmc.edu/dentistry

Connecticut

University of Connecticut
Dentistry Prgm
School of Dental Medicine, Office of the Dean
263 Farmington Ave
Farmington, CT 06030
sdm.uchc.edu

District of Columbia

Howard University
Dentistry Prgm
College of Dentistry
600 W St, NW
Washington, DC 20059-0001
www.howard.edu

Florida

Lake Erie Coll of Osteopathic Medicine
Dentistry Prgm
5000 Lakewood Ranch Blvd
Bradenton, FL 34211

Nova Southeastern University
Dentistry Prgm
College of Dental Medicine
3200 S University Drive
Ft. Lauderdale, FL 33328
dental.nova.edu

University of Florida
Dentistry Prgm
1395 Center Drive, Rm D4-6
PO Box 100405
Gainesville, FL 32610-0405
dental.ufl.edu

Georgia

Georgia Health Sciences University
Dentistry Prgm
College of Dental Medicine
1120 15th St, GC-5202A
Augusta, GA 30912-0200
www.mcg.edu/SOD

Illinois

Southern Illinois University Edwardsville
Dentistry Prgm
School of Dental Medicine
2800 College Ave, Bldg 273
Alton, IL 62002
www.siue.edu/sdm/

University of Illinois at Chicago
Dentistry Prgm
College of Dentistry (M/C 621)
801 South Paulina St, Rm 102
Chicago, IL 60612-7211
www.dentistry.uic.edu

Midwestern University
Dentistry Prgm
555 31st St
Downers Grove, IL 60515

Indiana

Indiana University
Dentistry Prgm
1121 West Michigan St
Room DS104
Indianapolis, IN 46202-5186
www.iusd.iupui.edu

Iowa

University of Iowa
Dentistry Prgm
801 Newton Rd
N308 Dental Science Building
Iowa City, IA 52242-1010
www.dentistry.uiowa.edu

Kentucky

University of Kentucky
Dentistry Prgm
800 Rose St
D-136 Chandler Medical Ctr
Lexington, KY 40536-0297
www.mc.uky.edu/Dentistry

University of Louisville
Dentistry Prgm
School of Dentistry, Office of the Dean
501 S Preston - Room 227
Louisville, KY 40202
www.dental.louisville.edu/dental

Louisiana

Louisiana State University
Dentistry Prgm
Box 141
8000 GSRI Rd
New Orleans, LA 70119-2799
www.lsusd.lsuhsc.edu

Maryland

University of Maryland, Baltimore
Dentistry Prgm
School of Dentistry
650 W Baltimore St, Room 6404
Ste 6402
Baltimore, MD 21201
www.dental.umaryland.edu

Massachusetts

Boston University
Dentistry Prgm
100 E Newton St, Suite G317
Boston, MA 02118
www.dentalshcool.bu.edu

Harvard Medical School
Dentistry Prgm
188 Longwood Ave
Boston, MA 02115
www.hsdm.med.harvard.edu

Tufts University
Dentistry Prgm
School of Dental Medicine
One Kneeland St - 15th floor
Boston, MA 02111
www.tufts.edu/dental

Michigan

University of Michigan
Dentistry Prgm
School of Dentistry
1011 N University Ave, 1234
Ann Arbor, MI 48109-1078
www.dent.umich.edu

University of Detroit Mercy
Dentistry Prgm
School of Dentistry
2700 Martin Luther King Jr Blvd
MB 98
Detroit, MI 48208-2576
www.udmercy.edu/dental

Minnesota

University of Minnesota
Dentistry Prgm
School of Dentistry
15-238 Moos Tower, 515 Delaware St SE
Minneapolis, MN 55455
www.dentistry.umn.edu

Mississippi

University of Mississippi Medical Center
Dentistry Prgm
School of Dentistry
2500 N State St
Jackson, MS 39216-4505

Missouri

University of Missouri - Kansas City
Dentistry Prgm
650 E 25th St
Kansas City, MO 64108
www.umkc.edu/dentistry

Nebraska

University of Nebraska Medical Center
Dentistry Prgm
College of Dentistry
40th and Holdrege Sts, Box 830740
Lincoln, NE 68583-0740

Creighton University
Dentistry Prgm
School of Dentistry
2500 California Plaza
Omaha, NE 68178-0240
cudental.creighton.edu

Nevada

University of Nevada - Las Vegas
Dentistry Prgm
School of Dental Medicine, Office of the Dean
1001 Shadow Lane, MS 7410
Las Vegas, NV 89106-4124
dentalschool.unlv.edu

New Jersey

Univ of Medicine & Dent of New Jersey
Dentistry Prgm
New Jersey Dental School
110 Bergen St, Rm B815
Newark, NJ 07103-2425
www.umdnj.edu

New York

University at Buffalo - SUNY
Dentistry Prgm
School of Dental Medicine
325 Squire Hall
3435 Main Street
Buffalo, NY 14214-8006
www.sdm.buffalo.edu

Columbia University
Dentistry Prgm
College of Dental Medicine
630 W 168th St, PH7 East - 122, Box 20
New York, NY 10032
cpmcnet.columbia.edu/dept/dental

New York University
Dentistry Prgm
Office of the Dean, 10th Floor
345 East 24th St
New York, NY 10010
www.nyu.edu/dental

State University at Stony Brook
Dentistry Prgm
School of Dental Medicine
160 Rockland Hall - Sullivan Hall
Stony Brook, NY 11794-8700
www.hsc.stonybrook.edu/dental

North Carolina

University of North Carolina Hospitals
Dentistry Prgm
1090 Old Dental Building
CB 7450
Chapell Hill, NC 27599-7450

East Carolina University
Dentistry Prgm
Lakeside Annex 7, Mail Stop 701
Greenville, NC 27832-4354

Ohio

Case Western Reserve University
Dentistry Prgm
10900 Euclid Ave
Cleveland, OH 44106-4905
dental.case.edu

The Ohio State University
Dentistry Prgm
College of Dentistry; Office of the Dean
305 W 12th Ave
PO Box 182357
Columbus, OH 43210-1267
www.dent.ohio-state.edu

Oklahoma

University of Oklahoma Health Sciences Center
Dentistry Prgm
College of Dentistry
1201 N Stonewall Ave
Oklahoma City, OK 73117
dentistry.ouhsc.edu

Oregon

Oregon Health & Science University
Dentistry Prgm
School of Dentistry
611 SW Campus Dr
Portland, OR 97239
www.ohsu.edu/sod/admissions

Pennsylvania

Temple University
Dentistry Prgm
Maurice H Kornberg School of Dentistry
3223 North Broad St
Philadelphia, PA 19140
www.temple.edu/dentistry

Univ of Penn School of Dental Medicine
Dentistry Prgm
School of Dental Medicine
Robert Schattner Center, 240 South 40th St
Philadelphia, PA 19104-6030
www.dental.upenn.edu

University of Pittsburgh
Dentistry Prgm
School of Dental Medicine
3501 Terrace St, 440 Salk Hall
Pittsburgh, PA 15261
www.dental.pitt.edu

Puerto Rico

University of Puerto Rico
Dentistry Prgm
Medical Sciences Campus
PO Box 365067 - Main Bldg Office #A103B
San Juan, PR 00936-5067
www.dental.rcm.upr.edu

South Carolina

Medical University of South Carolina
Dentistry Prgm
171 Ashley Ave; MSC 507, Basic Science Bldg Rm 447
PO Box 250507
Charleston, SC 29425
www.gradstudies.musc.edu/dentistry/dental.html

Tennessee

University of Tennessee Health Science Ctr
Dentistry Prgm
875 Union Ave
Memphis, TN 38163
www.utmem.edu/dentistry

Meharry Medical College
Dentistry Prgm
School of Dentistry
1005 DB Todd Jr Blvd
Nashville, TN 37208
www.dentistry.mmc.edu

Texas

Baylor College of Dentistry, Texas A&M HSC
Dentistry Prgm
3302 Gaston Ave
Dallas, TX 75246

University of Texas Health Sci Ctr Houston
Dentistry Prgm
School of Dentistry at Houston
6516 MD Anderson Blvd #147
Houston, TX 77030
www.db.uth.tmc.edu

UT Health Science Center - San Antonio
Dentistry Prgm
San Antonio Dental School
7703 Floyd Curl Drive, MC 7906
San Antonio, TX 78229-3900
www.dental.uthscsa.edu

Utah

Roseman University of Health Sciences
Dentistry Prgm
Dean, South Jordan Campus, College of Dental Medicine
10920 S Riverfront Parkway
South Jordan, UT 84095

Virginia

Virginia Commonwealth Univ/Health System
Dentistry Prgm
Office of the Vice President for Health Sciences
1012 East Marshall St, PO Box 980549
Richmond, VA 23298-0549
www.dentistry.vcu.edu

Washington

University of Washington
Dentistry Prgm
School of Dentistry, Box 356365
1959 NE Pacific St, D322 Health Sc Bldg
Seattle, WA 98195
www.dental.washington.edu

West Virginia

West Virginia University
Dentistry Prgm
School of Dentistry
1150 HSC North, PO Box 9400
Morgantown, WV 26506-9400
www.hsc.wvu.edu/sod

Wisconsin

Marquette University
Dentistry Prgm
1801 W Wisconsin Ave
PO Box 1881
Milwaukee, WI 53201
www.dental.mu.edu

Dietetics

Includes:
- Dietitian/nutritionist
- Dietetic technician

History

Important dates in the history of dietetics and the American Dietetics Association (ADA):

1917—The American Dietetics Association is founded

1928—A list of hospitals with approved courses for student dietitians is published

1974—Essentials were published for dietetic technician programs for food service management and nutrition care support personnel

1974—The ADA is first recognized by the US Department of Health, Education, and Welfare, now the US Department of Education (ED) as the accrediting agency for dietetic internships and coordinated undergraduate programs. The ED now recognizes the Commission on Accreditation for Dietetics Education (CADE) as an accrediting agency for coordinated and didactic graduate and undergraduate programs, post-baccalaureate dietetic internships, and associate degree technician programs.

1994—The ADA bylaws are amended to demonstrate the administrative autonomy of the body charged with accreditation, the CADE.

Dietitian/Nutritionist

Career Description

Dietetics is the science of applying food and nutrition to health. Registered Dietitians are nutritionists who integrate and apply the principles derived from the sciences of food, nutrition, biochemistry, physiology, food management, and behavior to achieve and maintain the health status of the public they serve.

Employment Characteristics

Clinical registered dietitians are a vital part of the medical team in hospitals, nursing homes, health maintenance organizations, and other health care facilities. As a key member of the health care team, the clinical RD provides medical nutrition therapy and the use of specific nutrition services to treat chronic conditions, illnesses, or injuries. Opportunities for advancement are available by choosing a particular area of nutrition practice, such as diabetes, heart disease, or pediatrics, or by expanding into hospital administration.

Community registered dietitians work in public and home health agencies, day care centers, health and recreation clubs, and in government-funded programs that feed and counsel families, the elderly, pregnant women, children, and individuals with special needs. Wherever proper nutrition can help improve quality of life, community RDs reach out to the public to teach, monitor, and advise.

Educator registered dietitians work in colleges, universities, and medical centers, teaching future physicians, nurses, dietitians, and dietetic technicians the science of foods and nutrition.

Research registered dietitians work in government agencies, food and pharmaceutical companies, and major universities and medical centers. They conduct or direct experiments to answer critical nutrition questions, find alternative foods, and form dietary recommendations for the public.

Consultant registered dietitians work under contract with health care or food companies or in their own business. In private practice, they perform nutrition screening and assessment of their own clients and those referred to them by physicians. They counsel on weight loss, cholesterol reduction, and a variety of other diet-related concerns. Those under contract with health care facilities consult with food service or restaurant managers, food vendors or distributors, athletes, nursing home residents, or company employees.

Management registered dietitians work in health care institutions, schools, cafeterias, and restaurants, playing a key role where food is served. They are responsible for personnel management, menu planning, budgeting, and purchasing.

Business registered dietitians work in food- and nutrition-related industries, in such areas as communications, consumer affairs, product development, sales, marketing, advertising, and public relations.

Salary

According to the American Dietetic Association (ADA) 2011 Dietetics Compensation and Benefits Survey, among registered dietitians employed full time in dietetics in their primary position for less than five years, half earn between $54,470 to 66,560 per year. Salary levels may vary with location, scope of responsibility, and supply of job applicants. Salary also increases as experience increases; many RDs, particularly those in management and business earn incomes averaging $72,580 per year.

May 2011 data from the US Bureau of Labor Statistics (BLS) show that wages at the 10th percentile are $34,300, the 50th percentile (median) at $54,470, and the 90th percentile at $76,400 (*www.bls.gov/oes/current/oes291031.htm*). Median annual wages in the industries employing the largest numbers of dietitians and nutritionists in May 2009 (from largest to smallest) were:

General medical and surgical hospitals	$55,240
Nursing care facilities	$56,220
Local government	$50,230
Outpatient care centers	$57,350
Special food services	$54,000

For more information, refer to *www.ama-assn.org/go/hpsalary*.

Employment Outlook

The BLS projects that employment of dietitians and nutritionists is expected to increase nine percent from 2008 through 2018, about as fast as the average for all occupations. Job growth will result from an increasing emphasis on disease prevention through improved dietary habits. A growing and aging population will boost demand for nutritional counseling and treatment in hospitals, residential care facilities, schools, prisons, community health programs, and home health care agencies. Public interest in nutrition and increased emphasis on health education and prudent lifestyles also will spur demand, especially in food service management.

Educational Programs

Length. The professional component is a minimum of two years at the baccalaureate or graduate degree level. Post-baccalaureate dietetic internship programs vary from six months to two years, depending on study design and integration in a graduate program. Following completion of academic and supervised practice requirements, individuals are eligible to take a national certification examination for registered dietitians. Most states also regulate dietitians and nutritionists. National certification as a RD will meet state requirements.

Prerequisites. Variable for programs at the baccalaureate and graduate degree levels, depending on the degree offered and institutional requirements. Applicants to post-baccalaureate dietetic internship programs must have completed a baccalaureate degree from a US regionally accredited college or university or equivalent foreign degree and Commission on Accreditation for Dietetics Education (CADE)-approved didactic coursework.

Curriculum. Didactic curriculum requirements focus on food and nutrition sciences and management, supported by the physical and biological as well as behavioral and social sciences, in addition to business, economics, and communication. The supervised practice curriculum provides experiences to develop the skills and competence to practice dietetics.

Program Types

Coordinated Program in Dietetics (CP)
- An academic program in a regionally accredited college or university granting a baccalaureate or graduate degree
- Includes didactic instruction and a minimum of 900 to 1,200 hours of supervised practice experiences, which may be planned concurrently with or following the didactic component
- Graduates are eligible to write the registration examination for dietitians

Didactic Program in Dietetics (DPD)
- An academic program in a regionally accredited college or university granting a baccalaureate or graduate degree
- Graduates can apply for a dietetic internship program leading to eligibility to write the registration examination for dietitians

Dietetic Internship (DI)
- A supervised practice program sponsored by a health care facility, college or university, federal or state agency, business, or corporation
- Minimum of 900 to 1,200 hours of supervised practice experiences
- Entry requires completion of CADE-approved Didactic Program in Dietetics and at least a baccalaureate degree from a US regionally accredited college or university or foreign equivalent
- May be full-time or part-time and vary from six months to two years
- Graduates are eligible to write the registration examination for dietitians

Inquiries

Careers

Inquiries regarding careers in dietetics and nutrition should be addressed to:
Accreditation and Education Programs
American Dietetic Association
120 South Riverside Plaza, Suite 2000
Chicago, IL 60606-6995
312 899-0040, Ext 5400
E-mail: *education@eatright.org*

Certification/Registration

Inquiries regarding dietitian registration should be addressed to:
Commission on Dietetic Registration
120 South Riverside Plaza, Suite 2000
Chicago, IL 60606-6995
312 899-0040, Ext 5500
E-mail: *cdr@eatright.org*

Program Accreditation

Accreditation Council for Education in Nutrition and Dietetics
American Dietetic Association
120 S Riverside Plaza, Suite 2000
Chicago, IL 60606-6995
312 899-0040, Ext 5400
E-mail: *education@eatright.org*

Accredited Programs

A list of accredited programs with selected information is available on the ADA web site at: *www.eatright.org/ACEND/*

Note: Adapted in part from the Bureau of Labor Statistics, US Department of Labor, *Occupational Outlook Handbook,* Dietitians and Nutritionists, at *www.bls.gov/oco/ocos077.htm.*

Dietitian/Nutritionist

Alabama

Auburn University
Dietetics-Didactic Prgm
Nutrition and Food Science
328 Spidle Hall
Auburn, AL 36849-5605
www.humsci.auburn.edu

Samford University
Dietetics-Didactic Prgm
Family and Consumer Educ
800 Lakeshore Dr
Birmingham, AL 35229-2239
www.samford.edu

University of Alabama at Birmingham
Dietetic Internship Prgm
Dept of Nutrition Sciences
Webb Bldg Rm 212
1675 University Blvd
Birmingham, AL 35294
www.uab.edu/nutrition

Oakwood College
Dietetic Internship Prgm
Family and Consumer Science
7000 Adventist Blvd
Huntsville, AL 35896
www.oakwood.edu

University of Montevallo
Dietetics-Didactic Prgm
Family and Consumer Sciences
Station 6385 Bloch Hall
Montevallo, AL 35115-6000
www.montevallo.edu

Alabama State Department of Education
Dietetic Internship Prgm
Child Nutrition Programs
5163 Gordon Persons Building
PO Box 302101
Montgomery, AL 36130-2101
www.alsde.edu

Alabama A&M University
Dietetics-Didactic Prgm
Nutrition and Hospitality Mgmt
Div of Family & Consumer Serv PO Box 639
Normal, AL 35762-0639
www.aamu.edu

University of Alabama
Dietetics-Coordinated Prgm
Human Nutrition and Hosp Mgmt
PO Box 870158, 206 Doster Hall
Tuscaloosa, AL 35487-0158
www.ches.ua.edu

University of Alabama
Dietetics-Didactic Prgm
Human Nutrition and Hosp Mgmt
PO Box 870158
Tuscaloosa, AL 35487-0158
www.ches.ua.edu

Tuskegee University
Dietetics-Didactic Prgm
Food and Nutrition Sciences
204 Campbell Hall
Tuskegee, AL 36088
www.tuskegee.edu

Alaska

University of Alaska Anchorage
Dietetic Internship Prgm
3211 Providence Dr
108 Cuddy Center
Anchorage, AK 99508
www.uaa.alaska.edu

University of Alaska Anchorage
Dietetics-Didactic Prgm
Division of Culinary Arts and Hospitality
3211 Providence Drive
Anchorage, AK 99508-4645

Arizona

Arizona State University at the Polytechnic Campus
Dietetics-Didactic Prgm
Department of Nutrition
7001 E Williams Field Rd
Mesa, AZ 85212
www.east.asu.edu/ecollege/nutrition

Arizona State University at the Polytechnic Campus
Dietetic Internship Prgm
Department of Nutrition
7001 E Williams Field Rd, Bldg 20
Mesa, AZ 85212
www.east.asu.edu/ecollege/nutrition

Maricopa County Dept of Public Health
Dietetic Internship Prgm
Office of Nutrition Services
4041 North Central, Suite 700 C
Phoenix, AZ 85012

Paradise Valley Unified School District
Dietetic Internship Prgm
20621 N 32nd St
Phoenix, AZ 85050
www.pvusd.k12.az.us

Southwestern DI Consortium (PhD)
Dietetic Internship Prgm
Phoenix Indian Medical Center
Phoenix, AZ 85016

Carondelet St Mary's Hospital
Dietetic Internship Prgm
Morrisons Custom Mgmt Co
1601 W St Mary's Rd
Tucson, AZ 85745
www.azdpac.org/programinfo.cfm?PID=100020

University of Arizona
Dietetics-Didactic Prgm
Dept of Nutritional Sciences
PO Box 210038, Shantz 309
Tucson, AZ 85721-0038
www.ag.arizona.edu/NSC/nschome.htm

University of Arizona
Dietetic Internship Prgm
University Medical Center Support Services
1501 N Campbell Ave
PO Box 245088
Tucson, AZ 85724-5088
www.arizona.edu

Arkansas

Henderson State University
Dietetics-Didactic Prgm
Dept of Family and Consumer Sciences
PO Box 7504
Arkadelphia, AR 71999-0001
www.hsu.edu

Ouachita Baptist University
Dietetics-Didactic Prgm
Dept of Biology
PO Box 3769
Arkadelphia, AR 71998-0001
www.obu.edu/biology/program_in_dietetics.htm

University of Central Arkansas
Dietetics-Didactic Prgm
Family and Consumer Sciences
McAlister Hall 100
Conway, AR 72035
www.uca.edu/divisions/academic/chas/diet.html

University of Central Arkansas
Dietetic Internship Prgm
Family and Consumer Sciences
McAlister Hall 100
Conway, AR 72035
www.uca.edu/divisions/academic/chas/diet.html

University of Arkansas
Dietetics-Didactic Prgm
Human Environmental Sciences
118 HOEC
Fayetteville, AR 72701
www.uark.edu/depts/hesweb

University of Arkansas for Medical Sciences
Dietetic Internship Prgm
Veterans Affairs Med Ctr
4301 W Markham St, Slot 627
Little Rock, AR 72205-7199
www.uams.edu/chrp/dietnutrition/

University of Arkansas at Pine Bluff
Dietetics-Didactic Prgm
1200 North University Drive
Mail Slot 4971
Pine Bluff, AR 71601
www.uapb.edu

Harding University
Dietetics-Didactic Prgm
Family and Consumer Sciences
900 E Center Ave, Box 12233
Searcy, AR 72149-0001

Arkansas State University
Dietetics-Coordinated Prgm
College of Nursing and Health Professions
Nutritional Science
PO Box 910
State University, AR 72467-0910
www.astate.edu/conhp

California

Clinica Sierra Vista
Dietetic Internship Prgm
1430 Truxtun Ave, Ste 120
Bakersfield, CA 93301-3834

University of California - Berkeley
Dietetics-Didactic Prgm
Dept of Nutritional Sciences and Toxicology
119 Morgan Hall
Berkeley, CA 94720-3104
http://nutrition.berkeley.edu

California State University - Chico
Dietetics-Didactic Prgm
Dept of Biological Sciences
Tehama Hall 124
Chico, CA 95929-0002

California State University - Chico
Dietetic Internship Prgm
Nutrition and Food Sciences
Dept of Biological Sciences
Chico, CA 95929-0002
www.csuchico.edu/biol/nfsc

University of California - Davis
Dietetics-Didactic Prgm
Dept of Nutrition
One Shields Ave
Davis, CA 95616-8669
www.ucdavis.edu

California State University - Fresno
Dietetics-Didactic Prgm
Dept of Ecology Food Science and Nutrition
5300 N Campus Dr MS FF17
Fresno, CA 93740-8019
http://cast.csufresno.edu/fsn

California State University - Fresno
Dietetic Internship Prgm
Dept of Ecology Food Science and Nutrition
5300 N Campus Dr MS FF17
Fresno, CA 93740-8019
http://cast.csufresno.edu/fsn

Public Health Foundation Enterprises
Dietetic Internship Prgm
WIC Program
12781 Schabarum Ave
Irwindale, CA 91706-6802
www.phfewic.org

Loma Linda University
Dietetics-Coordinated Prgm
School of Public Health, Nutrition Dept
Nichol Hall, Rm 1102
Loma Linda, CA 92350
www.llu.edu/llu/nutrition

California State University - Long Beach
Dietetic Internship Prgm
Family and Consumer Sciences
1250 Bellflower Blvd
Long Beach, CA 90840-0501
www.csulb.edu/~gcfrank

California State University - Long Beach
Dietetics-Didactic Prgm
Family and Consumer Sciences
1250 Bellflower Blvd
Long Beach, CA 90840-0501
www.csulb.edu

California State University - Los Angeles
Dietetics-Didactic Prgm
Health and Nutritional Sciences
5151 State University Dr
Los Angeles, CA 90032-8162
www.calstatelal.edu/dept/hnut_sci/dept_pro.htm

California State University - Los Angeles
Dietetics-Coordinated Prgm
Kinesiology and Nutritional Science
5151 State University Dr
Los Angeles, CA 90032-8172
www.calstatela.edu/dept/hnut_sci/dept_pro.htm

Center for Child Development/Disabilities/UAP
Cosponsor: Children's Hosp of Los Angeles
Dietetic Internship Prgm
Child Development and Developmental Disorders
Mailstop 53, PO Box 54700
Los Angeles, CA 90054-0700

Los Angeles County+USC Healthcare Network
Dietetic Internship Prgm
Morrison Management Specialists
1200 N State St, Rm 1506
Los Angeles, CA 90033-4525

VA Greater Los Angeles Healthcare System
Dietetic Internship Prgm
Nutrition and Food Dept 120
11301 Wilshire Blvd
Los Angeles, CA 90073

Pepperdine University
Dietetics-Didactic Prgm
RAC108C, Nutritional Sciences
24255 Pacific Coast Hwy
Malibu, CA 90263-4325
www.pepperdine.edu

Napa State Hospital
Dietetic Internship Prgm
2100 Napa Vallejo Hwy
Napa, CA 94558-6293

California State University - Northridge
Dietetic Internship Prgm
Family Environmental Sciences
18111 Nordhoff St
Northridge, CA 91330-8308
www.csundi.com

California State University - Northridge
Dietetics-Didactic Prgm
Family Environmental Sciences
18111 Nordhoff St
Northridge, CA 91330-8308
www.csun.edu

Patton State Hospital
Dietetic Internship Prgm
3102 E Highland Ave
Patton, CA 92369

California State Polytechnic University
Dietetics-Didactic Prgm
Foods and Nutrition Dept
3801 W Temple Ave
Pomona, CA 91768-2557
www.csupomona.edu

California State Polytechnic University
Dietetic Internship Prgm
Foods and Nutri/Home Economics
3801 W Temple Ave
Pomona, CA 91768-2557
www.csupomona.edu/~kcaldwellfreeman

Porterville Development Center
Dietetic Internship Prgm
PO Box 2000
Porterville, CA 93258-2000

Central Valley WIC Dietetic Internship
Dietetic Internship Prgm
1560 E Manning Ave
Reedley, CA 93654

California State University - Sacramento
Dietetics-Didactic Prgm
Human Environmental Sciences
6000 J St
Sacramento, CA 95819-6053
www.csus.edu

California State University - Sacramento
Dietetic Internship Prgm
6000 J St
Sacramento, CA 95819-6053
www.cce.csus.edu/programs/di/

UC Davis Medical Center
Dietetic Internship Prgm
2315 Stockton Blvd
Sacramento, CA 95817

California State University - San Bernardino
Dietetics-Didactic Prgm
Health Science and Human Ecology
5500 University Pkwy
San Bernardino, CA 92407-2318
http://health.csusb.edu/dchen

Point Loma Nazarene University (PhD)
Dietetics-Didactic Prgm
3900 Lomaland Dr
San Diego, CA 92106

San Diego State University
Dietetics-Didactic Prgm
Exercise and Nutritional Sciences
5500 Campanile Dr
San Diego, CA 92182-7251
www.sdsu.edu

San Diego State University
Dietetic Internship Prgm
WIC Dietetic Internship
5500 Campanile Dr
San Diego, CA 92111
www.rohan.sdsu.edu

VA San Diego Healthcare System
Dietetic Internship Prgm
Dietetics and Clinical Nutrition Serv 120
3350 La Jolla Village Dr
San Diego, CA 92161-0002

San Francisco State University
Dietetic Internship Prgm
Cons and Fam Studies
1600 Holloway Ave
San Francisco, CA 94132
www.sfsu.edu

San Francisco State University
Dietetics-Didactic Prgm
Cons and Fam Studies
1600 Holloway Ave
San Francisco, CA 94132-1722
www.sfsu.edu

University of California - San Francisco
Dietetic Internship Prgm
Medical Center, Box 0212 Rm M-294
Dept of Nutrition & Dietetics
San Francisco, CA 94143-0212
www.ucsf.edu

San Jose State University
Dietetics-Didactic Prgm
Nutrition and Food Science
San Jose, CA 95192-0058

San Jose State University
Dietetic Internship Prgm
Nutrition Food and Science
One Washington Square
San Jose, CA 95192-0058

California Polytechnic State University
Dietetic Internship Prgm
Food Science and Nutrition
San Luis Obispo, CA 93407

California Polytechnic State University
Dietetics-Didactic Prgm
Food Science and Nutrition
San Luis Obispo, CA 93407
www.calpoly.edu

Olive View/UCLA Medical Center
Dietetic Internship Prgm
Dept of Food and Nutrition
14445 Olive View Dr, Rm 1C112
Sylmar, CA 91342-1438

Colorado

Penrose Hospital
Dietetic Internship Prgm
Nutrition Services
PO Box 7021
Colorado Springs, CO 80933-7021

University of Colorado at Colorado Springs
Dietetics-Didactic Prgm
1420 Austin Bluffs Parkway
Colorado Springs, CO 80933

Johnson & Wales University
Dietetics-Didactic Prgm
7150 Montview Blvd
Denver, CO 80220

Metropolitan State College of Denver
Dietetics-Didactic Prgm
Department of Health Professions
Campus Box 33, PO Box 173362
Denver, CO 80217-3362
www.mscd.edu

Colorado State University
Dietetics-Didactic Prgm
Department of Food Science and Human Nutrition
Gifford Building, Room 234
Fort Collins, CO 80523-1571
www.fshn.cahs.colostate.edu

Colorado State University
Dietetics-Coordinated Prgm
Food Sci and Human Nutrition
Gifford Bldg 205
Fort Collins, CO 80523-1571
www.fshn.cahs.colostate.edu

University of Northern Colorado
Dietetic Internship Prgm
Community Health and Nutrition
CHN Box 93-501 20th St
Greeley, CO 80639
www.unco.edu/dietetic

University of Northern Colorado
Dietetics-Didactic Prgm
Community Health and Nutrition
CHN, Box 93-501 20th St
Greeley, CO 80639
www.univnorthco.edu

Tri-County Health Department
Dietetic Internship Prgm
Nutrition Services
4857 S Broadway
Greenwood Village, CO 80111

Connecticut

Danbury Hospital
Dietetic Internship Prgm
24 Hospital Ave
Danbury, CT 06810-6077
www.danburyhospital.org

Yale-New Haven Hospital
Dietetic Internship Prgm
Food and Nutrition
20 York St GBB
New Haven, CT 06504
www.ynhh.org/general/training.html#diet

University of Connecticut
Dietetic Internship Prgm
School of Allied Health
358 Mansfield Rd, Unit 2101
Storrs, CT 06269-2101
www.alliedhealth.uconn.edu

University of Connecticut
Dietetics-Coordinated Prgm
School of Allied Health
358 Mansfield Rd, Unit 2101
Storrs, CT 06269-2101
www.alliedhealth.uconn.edu

University of Connecticut
Dietetics-Didactic Prgm
Nutritional Sciences U-4017
3624 Horsebarn Rd Extension
Storrs, CT 06269
www.canr.uconn.edu/nusci

Saint Joseph College
Dietetic Internship Prgm
Department of Nutrition
1678 Asylum Ave
West Hartford, CT 06117-2700
www.sjc.edu/dietetics

Saint Joseph College
Dietetics-Didactic Prgm
Nutrition and Family Studies
1678 Asylum Ave
West Hartford, CT 06117-2700
www.sjc.edu

University of New Haven
Dietetics-Didactic Prgm
College of Arts and Sciences
300 Orange Ave
West Haven, CT 06516-1916
www.newhaven.edu

Delaware

Delaware State University
Dietetics-Didactic Prgm
Dept of Family and Consumer Sciences
1200 N Dupont Hwy
Dover, DE 19901-2277
www.desu.edu

University of Delaware-Christiana Care Health
Dietetics-Didactic Prgm
Dept of Nutrition and Dietetics
234A Alison Hall
Newark, DE 19716-3301
www.udel.edu

University of Delaware-Christiana Care Health
Dietetic Internship Prgm
Nutrition and Dietetics
315 Alison Hall
Newark, DE 19716
www.udel.edu

District of Columbia

Howard University
Dietetics-Coordinated Prgm
Nutritional Sciences
6th and Bryant Sts NW, Annex I
Washington, DC 20059
www.howard.edu

University of the District of Columbia
Dietetics-Didactic Prgm
Biological and Environmental Sciences
Bldg 44 Rm 200-2, 4200 Connecticut Ave NW
Washington, DC 20008-1173

Florida

Bay Pines VA Medical Center
Dietetic Internship Prgm
Bay Pines, FL 33744

University of Florida
Dietetics-Didactic Prgm
Food Sci and Human Nutrition
PO Box 110370
Gainesville, FL 32611-0370
www.ufl.edu

University of Florida
Dietetic Internship Prgm
Food Sci and Human Nutrition
359 FSB, PO Box 110370
Gainesville, FL 32611
http://fshn.ifas.ufl.edu

St Luke's Hosp/Mayo Clinic Jacksonville
Dietetic Internship Prgm
4500 San Pablo Rd
Jacksonville, FL 32224

University of North Florida
Dietetic Internship Prgm
Dept of Health Science
4567 St Johns Bluff Rd S
J Brooks Brown Hall, Bldg 39
Jacksonville, FL 32224-2646
www.unf.edu/coh

University of North Florida
Dietetics-Didactic Prgm
College of Health
4567 St Johns Bluff Rd S
Jacksonville, FL 32224-2645
www.unf.edu

Florida International University
Dietetics-Coordinated Prgm
Dept of Dietetics and Nutrition
11200 SW 8th St
Miami, FL 33199
www.fiu.edu

Florida International University
Dietetics-Didactic Prgm
Dietetics and Nutrition
11200 SW 8th St
Miami, FL 33199
http://w3.fiu.edu

Pasco County Health Department
Dietetic Internship Prgm
Nutrition Div
10841 Little Rd
New Port Richey, FL 34654-2533
www.doh.state.fl.us/chdpasco/default.html

Sarasota District Schools
Dietetic Internship Prgm
Food and Nutrition Services
101 Old Venice Rd
Osprey, FL 34229-9023
www.sarasota.k12.fl.us/~fns

Keiser University
Dietetics-Coordinated Prgm
Dietetics and Nutrition
1640 SW 145th Ave
Pembroke Pines, FL 33027
www.keiseruniversity.edu/dietetics-and-nutrition-bs.php

Sarasota Memorial Hospital
Dietetic Internship Prgm
Food and Nutrition Services
1700 S Tamiami Trail
Sarasota, FL 34239-3555
www.smh.com

Florida Department of Education
Dietetic Internship Prgm
325 W Gaines St, Rm 1032
Tallahassee, FL 32399-0400

Florida State University
Dietetic Internship Prgm
Nutrition Food and Exercise Sciences
400 Sandels Bldg
Tallahassee, FL 32306-1493
www.fsu.edu

Florida State University
Dietetics-Didactic Prgm
Nutrition Food and Exercise Sciences
436 Sandels Bldg
Tallahassee, FL 32306-1493
www.fsu.edu

James A Haley Veteran's Hospital
Dietetic Internship Prgm
13000 N Bruce B Downs Blvd
Tampa, FL 33612-4745

Georgia

University of Georgia
Dietetic Internship Prgm
Dept of Foods and Nutrition
Dawson Hall
Athens, GA 30602
www.fcs.uga.edu

University of Georgia
Dietetics-Didactic Prgm
Dept of Foods and Nutrition
Dawson Hall
Athens, GA 30602

Div of Pub Hlth/Georgia Dept of Hum Res
Dietetic Internship Prgm
Office of Nutrition
Two Peachtree St NW, Suite 11-254
Atlanta, GA 30303-3142
http://health.state.ga.us/

Emory University Hospital
Dietetic Internship Prgm
Food and Nutrition Services
1364 Clifton Rd NE, Rm FG06
Atlanta, GA 30322
http://medshare.emory.org/EHC/FNSWeb.nsf

Georgia State University
Dietetics-Didactic Prgm
Dept of Nutrition and Dietetics
MSC2A0880, 33 Gilmer St SE, Unit 2
Atlanta, GA 30303-3083
www.gsu.edu

Georgia State University
Dietetic Internship Prgm
Dept of Nutrition and Dietetics
University Plaza
Atlanta, GA 30303-3083
www.gsu.edu

Georgia State University
Dietetics-Coordinated Prgm
Division of Nutrition
PO Box 3995
Atlanta, GA 30302-3995

Morrison Chartwells
Dietetic Internship Prgm
Distance Education Dietetic Internship
5801 Peachtree Dunwoody Rd NE
Atlanta, GA 30342
www.rdinternship.com

Augusta Area Dietetic Internship
Cosponsor: Morrison Health Care Foodservice
Dietetic Internship Prgm
University Hospital
1350 Walton Way
Augusta, GA 30901-2629
www.universityhealth.org

Fort Valley State University
Dietetics-Didactic Prgm
Family and Consumer Sciences
1005 State University Dr, PO Box 4622 FVSU
Fort Valley, GA 31030

Life University
Dietetics-Didactic Prgm
Dept of Nutrition
1269 Barclay Circle
Marietta, GA 30060-2903

Life University
Dietetic Internship Prgm
1269 Barclay Circle SE
110 Annex B
Marietta, GA 30060-2903

Southern Regional Medical Center
Dietetic Internship Prgm
11 Upper Riverdale Rd SW
Riverdale, GA 30274-2600
www.southernregional.org

Georgia Southern University
Dietetics-Didactic Prgm
Family and Consumer Sciences
Box 8034
Statesboro, GA 30460
www.georgiasouthern.edu

Hawaii

University of Hawaii at Manoa
Dietetics-Didactic Prgm
Food Sci and Human Nutrition
Ag Sciences III, 1955 East West Rd, Rm 3141
Honolulu, HI 96822-2218
www.hawaii.edu/dietetics

Idaho

University of Idaho
Dietetics-Coordinated Prgm
Family and Consumer Science
College of Agriculture
Moscow, ID 83844-3183
www.uidaho.edu/fcs

Idaho State University
Dietetics-Didactic Prgm
Health and Nutrition Science
Campus Box 8109, 1291 East Terry, MLK Way
Pocatello, ID 83209-8109
www.isu.edu

Idaho State University
Dietetic Internship Prgm
Health and Nutrition Sciences
Campus Box 8109
Pocatello, ID 83209-8109
www.isu.edu

Illinois

Olivet Nazarene University
Dietetics-Didactic Prgm
Family and Consumer Sciences
One University Dr
Bourbonnais, IL 60914
http://web.olivet.edu/facs

Southern Illinois University Carbondale
Dietetics-Didactic Prgm
Animal Sci Food and Nutrition
Mailcode 4317
875 S Normal Ave
Carbondale, IL 62901-4317

Southern Illinois University Carbondale
Dietetic Internship Prgm
Food and Nutrition
Mail Code 4317
Carbondale, IL 62901-4317
www.siu.edu/cwis

Eastern Illinois University
Dietetics-Didactic Prgm
Family and Consumer Sci, Klehm Hall 109-B
600 Lincoln Ave, Klehm Hall 1433
Charleston, IL 61920-3099
www.eiu.edu/~famsci

Eastern Illinois University
Dietetic Internship Prgm
Family and Consumer Sciences
600 Lincoln Ave, Klehm Hall 1433
Charleston, IL 61920-3099
www.eiu.edu/~dietetic

Rush University Medical Center
Dietetic Internship Prgm
1653 W Congress Pkwy
425 Triangle Office Bldg
Chicago, IL 60612-3864
www.rushu.rush.edu/health/dept.html

University of Illinois at Chicago
Dietetics-Didactic Prgm
Chicago, IL 60612

University of Illinois at Chicago
Dietetics-Coordinated Prgm
Human Nutrition and Dietetics
1919 W Taylor St, M/C 517
Chicago, IL 60612-7256

Northern Illinois University
Dietetic Internship Prgm
Family Consumer and Nutri Sciences
DeKalb, IL 60115-2854
www.fcns.niu.edu

Northern Illinois University
Dietetics-Didactic Prgm
Family Consumer and Nutri Sciences
DeKalb, IL 60115-2854
www.niu.edu

Ingalls Memorial Hospital
Dietetic Internship Prgm
One Ingalls Dr
Harvey, IL 60426
www.ingalls.org

Edward Hines Jr. VA Hospital
Dietetic Internship Prgm
Nutrition and Food Service (120D)
PO Box 5000
Hines, IL 60141
www.hines.med.va.gov/

Benedictine University
Dietetics-Didactic Prgm
Dept of Nutrition
5700 College Rd
Lisle, IL 60532-0900
www.ben.edu/nutrition

Benedictine University
Dietetic Internship Prgm
Dept of Nutrition
5700 College Rd Birck-329
Lisle, IL 60532-0900
www.ben.edu

Western Illinois University
Dietetics-Didactic Prgm
Family and Consumer Sciences
Macomb, IL 61455
www.wiu.edu/users/mifcs

Loyola University of Chicago
Dietetic Internship Prgm
2160 S First Ave
2873 Maguire Center
Maywood, IL 60153
www.luc.edu

Illinois State University
Dietetic Internship Prgm
Dept of Family and Consumer Sciences
Campus Box 5060
Normal, IL 61790-5060
www.cast.ilstu.edu/isudi

Illinois State University
Dietetics-Didactic Prgm
Family and Consumer Sciences
Campus Box 5060
Normal, IL 61790-5060
www.cast.ilstu.edu/fcs

Bradley University
Dietetics-Didactic Prgm
Family and Consumer Sciences
1501 W Bradley Ave
Peoria, IL 61625-0015
www.bradley.edu

Bradley University
Dietetic Internship Prgm
Department of Family and Consumer Sciences
Bradley Hall 21
1501 West Bradley Ave
Peoria, IL 61625-0001
www.bradley.edu/academic/departments/fcs/programs/
internship/

OSF Saint Francis Medical Center
Dietetic Internship Prgm
530 NE Glen Oak Ave
Peoria, IL 61637-0001
www.osfsaintfrancis.org

Dominican University
Dietetics-Coordinated Prgm
7900 W Division
River Forest, IL 60305

Dominican University
Dietetics-Didactic Prgm
Dept of Nutrition Sciences
7900 W Division St
River Forest, IL 60305-1066
www.dom.edu

Univ of Illinois at Urbana-Champaign
Dietetic Internship Prgm
Dept of Food Science and Human Nutrition
443 Bevier Hall, 905 S Goodwin Ave
Urbana, IL 61801
www.aces.uiuc.edu/~dietetic

Univ of Illinois at Urbana-Champaign
Dietetics-Didactic Prgm
Food Sci and Human Nutri, 345 Bevier Hall
905 S Goodwin Ave
Urbana, IL 61801-3852
www.fshn.uiuc.edu/Dietetics

Indiana

Indiana University - Bloomington
Dietetics-Didactic Prgm
Applied Health Science
HPER 116
1025 E 7th St
Bloomington, IN 47405-7109

University of Southern Indiana
Dietetics-Didactic Prgm
College of Nursing and Health Professions HP 2088
Food and Nutrition Department
8600 University Boulevard
Evansville, IN 47712-3596
http://health.usi.edu/acadprog/fdnutr/default.asp

Indiana University
Dietetic Internship Prgm
Nutrition/Diet Prgm, Sch of Allied Hlth
Ball Residence, Rm 114
1226 W Michigan St
Indianapolis, IN 46202-5180

Ball State University
Dietetic Internship Prgm
Family and Consumer Sciences
150 Applied Technology Bldg
Muncie, IN 47306
www.bsu.edu

Ball State University
Dietetics-Didactic Prgm
Family and Consumer Sciences
Muncie, IN 47306-0250
www.bsu.edu

Indiana State University
Dietetics-Coordinated Prgm
Family and Consumer Sciences
Terre Haute, IN 47809

Purdue University
Dietetics-Coordinated Prgm
Dept of Foods and Nutrition
700 W State St
West Lafayette, IN 47907-2059
www.cfs.purdue.edu

Purdue University
Dietetics-Didactic Prgm
Dept of Foods and Nutrition
1264 Stone Hall
West Lafayette, IN 47907-1264
www.purdue.edu

Iowa

Iowa State University
Dietetic Internship Prgm
Food Sci and Human Nutrition
220 MacKay Hall
Ames, IA 50011
www.dietetics.iastate.edu

Iowa State University
Dietetics-Didactic Prgm
Food Sci and Human Nutrition
220 MacKay Hall
Ames, IA 50011-1120
www.dietetics.iastate.edu

University of Iowa Hospitals & Clinics
Dietetic Internship Prgm
200 Hawkins Dr, W146GH
Iowa City, IA 52242-1051
www.uihealthcare.com/

Kansas

University of Kansas Medical Center
Dietetic Internship Prgm
Dept of Dietetics and Nutrition
3901 Rainbow Blvd
Kansas City, KS 66160-7250
www2.kumc.edu/sah/dn/

Kansas State University
Dietetics-Coordinated Prgm
Hotel Rest Inst Mgmt and Diet
Justin Hall 104
Manhattan, KS 66506-1404
www.ksu.edu/humec/hrimd

Kansas State University
Dietetics-Didactic Prgm
Hotel Rest Inst Mgmt and Diet
Justin Hall 104
Manhattan, KS 66506-1404
www.ksu.edu/humec/hrimd

Kentucky

Western Kentucky University
Dietetics-Didactic Prgm
Consumer and Family Sci, Acad Complex 302F
One Big Red Way
Bowling Green, KY 42101-3576
www.wku.edu/dietetics

Univ of Kentucky Hospital
Dietetic Internship Prgm
Nutrition Services
H507 UKCMC, 800 Rose St
Lexington, KY 40536-0293
www.hes.eku.edu

University of Kentucky
Dietetic Internship Prgm
Human Environmental Sciences
204 Funkhouser Bldg
Lexington, KY 40506-0054
www.uky.edu

University of Kentucky
Dietetics-Coordinated Prgm
Nutrition and Food Science
210C Erikson Hall
Lexington, KY 40506-0050
www.uky.edu

University of Kentucky
Dietetics-Didactic Prgm
Nutrition and Food Science
204 Funkhouser Bldg
Lexington, KY 40506-0050
www.uky.edu

Murray State University
Dietetics-Didactic Prgm
Food Serv Systems Management
200 N Oakley, Applied Sciences Bldg
Murray, KY 42071-3345
www.murraystate.edu

Murray State University
Dietetic Internship Prgm
Nutrition Dietetics and Food Management
200 N Oakley, Applied Sciences Bldg
Murray, KY 42071-3345
www.murraystate.edu

Eastern Kentucky University
Dietetic Internship Prgm
Human Environmental Sciences
102 Burrier Bldg, 521 Lancaster Ave
Richmond, KY 40475-3107
www.fcs.eku.edu

Eastern Kentucky University
Dietetics-Didactic Prgm
Human Environmental Sciences
102 Burrier Bldg
Richmond, KY 40475
www.fcs.eku.edu

Louisiana

Louisiana State University
Dietetics-Didactic Prgm
School of Human Ecology
Baton Rouge, LA 70803-4300
http://sun.huec.lsu.edu

Southern Univ and A&M College
Dietetics-Didactic Prgm
Agriculture and Home Econ
PO Box 11342
Baton Rouge, LA 70813-1342
www.subr.edu

Southern Univ and A&M College
Dietetic Internship Prgm
PO Box 11342
Baton Rouge, LA 70813-1342
www.subr.edu

North Oaks Medical Center
Dietetic Internship Prgm
Nutritional Services
PO Box 2668
Hammond, LA 70404-2668
www.northoaks.org

University of Louisiana at Lafayette
Dietetic Internship Prgm
School of Human Resources
PO Box 40399, McKinley St
Lafayette, LA 70504-0399
www.louisiana.edu

University of Louisiana at Lafayette
Dietetics-Didactic Prgm
Coll of Applied Life Sciences
Sch of Human Res, Box 40399, McKinley St
Lafayette, LA 70504-0399
www.sustainablelouisiana/humr.org

McNeese State University
Dietetics-Didactic Prgm
PO Box 92820
Lake Charles, LA 70609

McNeese State University
Dietetic Internship Prgm
PO Box 92820 MSU
Lake Charles, LA 70609-2820

Tulane University
Dietetic Internship Prgm
Pub Hlth and Comm Hlth Sciences
1440 Canal St, Suite 2317
New Orleans, LA 70112-2699

Louisiana Tech University
Dietetics-Didactic Prgm
College of Human Ecology
PO Box 3167
Ruston, LA 71272
www.latech.edu/ans/human-ecology/index.shtml

Louisiana Tech University
Dietetic Internship Prgm
College of Human Ecology
PO Box 3167
Ruston, LA 71272
www.latech.edu/ans/human-ecology/index.shtml

Nicholls State University
Dietetics-Didactic Prgm
Family and Consumer Sciences
Box 2014
Thibodaux, LA 70310

Maine

University of Maine - Orono
Dietetic Internship Prgm
Food Sci and Human Nutrition
5735 Hitchner Hall, Rm 113
Orono, ME 04469-5749
www.umaine.edu

University of Maine - Orono
Dietetics-Didactic Prgm
Food Sci and Human Nutrition
5735 Hitchner Hall
Orono, ME 04469-5735
www.fsn.umaine.edu

Maryland

Johns Hopkins Bayview Medical Center
Dietetics-Coordinated Prgm
4940 Eastern Ave
Baltimore, MD 21224

Johns Hopkins Bayview Medical Center
Dietetic Internship Prgm
Clinical Nutrition Dept
4940 Eastern Ave
Baltimore, MD 21224-2735
www.jhbmc.jhu.edu/nutri

Morgan State University
Dietetics-Didactic Prgm
Dept of Family and Consumer Sci, Jenkins Bldg, Rm
   403-A
1700 E Cold Spring Ln
Baltimore, MD 21251
www.morgan.edu

University of Maryland Medical System
Dietetic Internship Prgm
Food and Nutrition Services
22 S Greene St
Baltimore, MD 21201-1595

National Institutes of Health
Dietetic Internship Prgm
Nutrition Dept, Clinical Ctr, Bldg 10 Rm B1S-234
10 Center Dr MSC 1078
Bethesda, MD 20892-1078
www.cc.nih.gov/nutr

Univ of Maryland at College Park
Dietetic Internship Prgm
Dept of Nutrition and Food Science
0112 Skinner Bldg
College Park, MD 20742
www.nfsc.umd.edu

Univ of Maryland at College Park
Dietetics-Didactic Prgm
Dept of Nutrition and Food Science
College Park, MD 20742-7521
www.nfsc.umd.edu

Sodexho Health Care Services, Mid Atlantic
Dietetic Internship Prgm
10500 Little Patuxent Pkwy, Ste 620
Columbia, MD 21044
www.dieteticintern.com/

University of Maryland Eastern Shore
Dietetics-Didactic Prgm
Dept of Human Ecology
Princess Anne, MD 21853-1299
www.umes.edu/ecology/ap4.htm

University of Maryland Eastern Shore
Dietetic Internship Prgm
Dept of Human Ecology
Princess Anne, MD 21853-1299
www.umes.edu/ecology/ap4.htm

Massachusetts

University of Massachusetts - Amherst
Dietetics-Didactic Prgm
Dept of Nutrition Box 31420
213 Chenoweth Laboratory, 100 Holdsworth Way
Amherst, MA 01003-9282
www.umass.edu

Beth Israel Deaconess Medical Center
Dietetic Internship Prgm
330 Brookline Ave
Boston, MA 02215-5491
www.bidmc.harvard.edu/dietetic

Boston University
Dietetic Internship Prgm
Graduate Nutrition Div
635 Commonwealth Ave
Boston, MA 02215-1605
www.bu.edu/sargent

Boston University /Sargent College
Dietetics-Didactic Prgm
635 Commonwealth Ave
Boston, MA 02215-1605
www.bu.edu/sargent

Brigham & Women's Hospital
Dietetic Internship Prgm
75 Francis St
Boston, MA 02115-6195
www.brighamandwomens.org/

Frances Stern Nutrition Center
Dietetic Internship Prgm
New England Medical Center, Tufts University
750 Washington St, Box 783
Boston, MA 02111-1533
www.tufts.edu/nutrition/program/dietetic_internship

Massachusetts General Hospital
Dietetic Internship Prgm
Dept of Dietetics
Boston, MA 02114
www.massgeneral.org

Simmons College
Dietetics-Didactic Prgm
Dept of Nutrition
300 The Fenway
Boston, MA 02115-5898
www.simmons.edu

Simmons College
Dietetic Internship Prgm
Dept of Nutrition
300 The Fenway
Boston, MA 02115
www.simmons.edu

Mount Auburn Hospital
Dietetic Internship Prgm
330 Mount Auburn St
Cambridge, MA 02138
www.mountauburnhospital.org/

Framingham State University
Dietetics-Coordinated Prgm
Family and Consumer Sciences
100 State St
Framingham, MA 01701-9101
www.framingham.edu

Framingham State University
Dietetics-Didactic Prgm
Family and Consumer Sciences
100 State St
Framingham, MA 01701-9101
www.framingham.edu

University of Massachusetts - Amherst
Dietetic Internship Prgm
Academic Programs
100 Venture Way, Suite 201
Hadley, MA 01035
www.umass.edu/contined

Sodexho Health Care Services
Dietetic Internship Prgm
Southcoast Hospitals Group
101 Page St
New Bedford, MA 02740-3464
www.southcoast.org/jobs/interns-dietary.html

Sodexho Health Care Services
Dietetic Internship Prgm
101 Page St
Waltham, MA 02451
www.dieteticintern.com

Michigan

University of Michigan
Dietetics-Didactic Prgm
School of Public Health
Human Nutrition Prgm
1420 Washington Heights M6150
Ann Arbor, MI 48109-2029

University of Michigan
Dietetic Internship Prgm
School of Public Health
1420 Washington Heights M6150
Ann Arbor, MI 48109-2029

University of Michigan Hospitals & Health Ctr
Dietetic Internship Prgm
UH2C227/0056
1500 E Medical Ctr Dr
Ann Arbor, MI 48109-0056
www.med.umich.edu/pfans/internship

Andrews University
Dietetic Internship Prgm
Dept of Nutrition
Berrien Springs, MI 49104-0210
www.andrews.edu

Andrews University
Dietetics-Didactic Prgm
Dept of Nutrition
Berrien Springs, MI 49104-0210
www.andrews.edu.

Harper University Hospital
Dietetic Internship Prgm
Dept of Nutrition and Food Svcs
3901 Beaubien Ave
Detroit, MI 48201-2018
www.harperhospital.org/harper/diet/intro

Henry Ford Hospital
Dietetic Internship Prgm
Dept of Food and Nutrition Services
2799 W Grand Blvd
Detroit, MI 48202-2689

DIETETICS

Wayne State University
Dietetics-Coordinated Prgm
Nutrition and Food Science
3009 Science Hall
Detroit, MI 48202
www.wayne.edu

Michigan State University
Dietetics-Didactic Prgm
Food Science and Human Nutrition
210 Trout FSHN Bldg
East Lansing, MI 48824-1224
www.msu.edu/unit/fshn

Michigan State University
Dietetic Internship Prgm
Dept of Food Science and Human Nutrition
2100 Anthony Hall
East Lansing, MI 48824-1225
www.msu.edu/unit/fshn/grad/intern.html

Hurley Medical Center
Dietetic Internship Prgm
Nutrition Service Dept
One Hurley Plaza
Flint, MI 48503-5993

Western Michigan University
Dietetics-Didactic Prgm
Family and Consumer Sciences
3024 Kohrman Hall
Kalamazoo, MI 49008
www.wmich.edu

Western Michigan University
Dietetic Internship Prgm
Family and Consumer Sciences
3025 Kohrman Hall
Kalamazoo, MI 49008-5067
www.wmich.edu

Madonna University
Dietetics-Didactic Prgm
Dept of Biological and Health Sciences
36600 Schoolcraft Rd
Livonia, MI 48150-1173
www.madonna.edu

Central Michigan University
Dietetics-Didactic Prgm
Human Environmental Studies
205 Wightman Hall
Mount Pleasant, MI 48859
http://nutrition.cmich.edu

Central Michigan University
Dietetic Internship Prgm
Human Environmental Studies
205 Wightman Hall
Mount Pleasant, MI 48859-3652
http://nutrition.cmich.edu

Eastern Michigan University
Dietetics-Coordinated Prgm
206 Roosevelt Hall
Ypsilanti, MI 48197
www.emich.edu

Minnesota

Minnesota State University - Mankato
Dietetics-Didactic Prgm
Family Consumer Sciences Department
102 Wiecking Center
Mankato, MN 56001
www.mnsu.edu

University of Minnesota
Dietetics-Coordinated Prgm
Division of Epidemiology and Community Health
West Bank Office Building, Suite 300
1300 South Second Street
Minneapolis, MN 55454
www.sph.umn.edu/programs/phn/curriculum/
    coordinated.asp

University of Minnesota Med Ctr - Fairview
Dietetic Internship Prgm
2450 Riverside Ave
Minneapolis, MN 55454
www.fairview-university.fairview.org/

Veterans Affairs Medical Center
Dietetic Internship Prgm
Nutrition and Food Service
One Veterans Dr
Minneapolis, MN 55417
www.va.gov/nfs

Concordia College - Moorhead
Dietetics-Didactic Prgm
Family and Nutrition Sciences
Moorhead, MN 56562
www.cord.edu

Concordia College - Moorhead
Dietetic Internship Prgm
Dept of Family and Nutrition Sciences
901 S 8th St
Moorhead, MN 56562
www.cord.edu

St Mary's Hospital
Cosponsor: Mayo Medical Center
Dietetic Internship Prgm
1216 2nd St SW
Rochester, MN 55902-1906
www.mayo.edu

College of St Benedict/St John's University
Dietetics-Didactic Prgm
Nutrition Dept
37 S College Ave
St Joseph, MN 56374-2099
www.csbsju.edu/nutrition

Saint Catherine University - St Paul
Dietetics-Didactic Prgm
Family Consumer and Nutri Sci, MC 4182
2004 Randolph Ave
St Paul, MN 55105-1750
www.stkate.edu

University of Minnesota - St Paul
Dietetics-Didactic Prgm
225 Food Science and Nutrition
1334 Eckles Ave
St Paul, MN 55108-6099
www1.umn.edu/twincities/index.php

University of Minnesota - St Paul
Dietetic Internship Prgm
225 Food Science and Nutrition
1334 Eckles Ave
St Paul, MN 55108-6099
http://fscn.che.umn.edu/index.html

Mississippi

Alcorn State University
Dietetics-Didactic Prgm
Family and Consumer Sciences
1000 ASU Dr #839
Alcorn State, MS 39096-7500
www.alcorn.edu/HumanSciences

Delta State University
Dietetics-Coordinated Prgm
Div of Family and Consumer Sciences
PO Box 3273
Cleveland, MS 38733
www.deltastate.edu/pages/1.asp

University of Southern Mississippi
Dietetic Internship Prgm
Family and Consumer Sciences
PO Box 5172
Hattiesburg, MS 39406-5035
www.usm.edu/nfs/

University of Southern Mississippi
Dietetics-Didactic Prgm
Family and Consumer Science
118 College Dr #5172
Hattiesburg, MS 39406
www.usm.edu/nfs

Mississippi State University
Dietetic Internship Prgm
School of Human Sciences Box 9745
128 Lloyd Ricks
Mississippi State, MS 39762-9745
www.msstate.edu

Mississippi State University
Dietetics-Didactic Prgm
School of Human Sciences
PO Box 9805, 107 Herzer, Stone Blvd
Mississippi State, MS 39762-9745
www.msstate.edu

University of Mississippi
Dietetics-Coordinated Prgm
Department of Nutrition and Hospitality Management
222 Lenoir Hall
University, MS 38677
www.olemiss.edu/depts/fcs/Food_and_Nutrition/

University of Mississippi
Dietetics-Didactic Prgm
Family and Consumer Sciences
110 Meek Hall, PO Box 1848
University, MS 38677-1848

Missouri

Southeast Missouri State University
Dietetic Internship Prgm
Dept of Human Enviromental Studies
One University Plaza
Cape Girardeau, MO 63701-4799
www5.semo.edu/dietetic_internship

Southeast Missouri State University
Dietetics-Didactic Prgm
Dept of Human Environmental Studies
One University Plaza MS 5750
Cape Girardeau, MO 63701-4799
www.semo.edu

University of Missouri
Dietetics-Coordinated Prgm
106 McKee
Columbia, MO 65211-0001
www.missouri.edu/~nutsci

Missouri Dept of Health & Senior Service
Dietetic Internship Prgm
PO Box 570
Jefferson City, MO 65102-0570

ARAMARK Healthcare Kansas City
Dietetic Internship Prgm
St Joseph Health System
1000 Carondelet Dr
Kansas City, MO 64114-4802
www.aramark.com

DIETETICS

Northwest Missouri State University
Dietetics-Didactic Prgm
Coll of Educ and Human Services
Family and Consumer Sciences, Rm 309 Admin Bldg
Maryville, MO 64468-6001
www.nwmissouri.edu

College of the Ozarks
Dietetics-Didactic Prgm
Dietetics and Nutrition Educ
PO Box 17
Point Lookout, MO 65726-0017
www.cofo.edu

Cox College of Nursing and Health Sciences
Dietetic Internship Prgm
Springfield, MO 65802

Missouri State University
Dietetics-Didactic Prgm
Dept of Biomedical Sciences
901 S National Ave
Springfield, MO 65804
www.missouristate.edu

DVA Medical Center
Dietetic Internship Prgm
Jefferson Barracks Div-Nutri and Food Serv 120/JB
One Jefferson Barracks Dr
St Louis, MO 63125
www.va.gov/nfs/StLouisVA

Fontbonne University
Dietetics-Didactic Prgm
Human Environmental Sciences
6800 Wydown Blvd
St Louis, MO 63105-3098

Saint Louis University Doisy College of Health Sciences
Dietetic Internship Prgm
Dept of Nutri and Diet, Rm 3076
3437 Caroline St
St Louis, MO 63104-1111
www.slu.edu/colleges/AH

Saint Louis University Doisy College of Health Sciences
Dietetics-Didactic Prgm
Dept of Nutri and Diet, Rm 3076
3437 Caroline St
St Louis, MO 63104-1111
www.slu.edu/x2270.xml

University of Central Missouri
Dietetics-Didactic Prgm
Dept of Health and Human Performance
Morrow 100
Warrensburg, MO 64093
www.cmsu.edu/dietetics

Montana

Montana State University
Dietetic Internship Prgm
Montana Dietetic Internship
205B Herrick Hall
PO Box 173540
Bozeman, MT 59717-3540
www.montana.edu/ehhd/hhd/facultyandstaff/
    ckaiser.htm

Montana State University
Dietetics-Didactic Prgm
Health and Human Development
101 MH H&PE Complex
Bozeman, MT 59717
www.montana.edu/wwwhhd

Nebraska

University of Nebraska - Lincoln
Dietetics-Didactic Prgm
Nutrition Science and Dietetics
104H Ruth Leverton Hall
Lincoln, NE 68583-0806
www.unl.edu

University of Nebraska - Lincoln
Dietetic Internship Prgm
Nutrition Science and Dietetics
120 Ruth Leverton Hall
Lincoln, NE 68583-0806
http://cehs.unl.edu/nhs/internships/dieteticintern.shtml

University of Nebraska Medical Center
Dietetic Internship Prgm
981200 Nebraska Medical Center
Omaha, NE 68198-1200
www.unmc.edu/alliedhealth/mne

Nevada

University of Nevada - Las Vegas
Dietetic Internship Prgm
4505 Maryland Pkwy
Las Vegas, NV 89154

University of Nevada - Las Vegas
Dietetics-Didactic Prgm
Box 453026
4505 S Maryland Pkwy
Las Vegas, NV 89154-3026

University of Nevada - Reno
Dietetics-Didactic Prgm
Dept of Nutrition
SFB Mail Stop 142
Reno, NV 89557
www.unr.edu

University of Nevada - Reno
Dietetic Internship Prgm
Dept of Nutrition
Mail Stop 142
Reno, NV 89557-0132
www.cabnr.unr.edu/nutrition

New Hampshire

University of New Hampshire
Dietetic Internship Prgm
Nutrition Assessment and Counseling Services
Kendall Hall
Durham, NH 03824
www.dieteticinternship.unh.edu

University of New Hampshire
Dietetics-Didactic Prgm
Animal and Nutri Sci Human Nutrition Ctr
Kendall Hall
129 Main St
Durham, NH 03824
www.anscandnutr.unh.edu

Keene State College
Dietetics-Didactic Prgm
Health Sciences/Nutrition
Joslin House MS 2903
229 Main St
Keene, NH 03435-2903
www.keene.edu/programs/hlsc

Keene State College
Dietetic Internship Prgm
229 Main St, M2903
Keene, NH 03431
www.keene.edu/academics/dietetics

New Jersey

College of St Elizabeth
Dietetic Internship Prgm
Dept of Foods and Nutrition
Henderson Hall, 2 Convent Rd
Morristown, NJ 07960-6989
www.cse.edu

College of St Elizabeth
Dietetics-Didactic Prgm
Dept of Foods and Nutrition
2 Convent Rd
153 Henderson Hall
Morristown, NJ 07960-6989
www.cse.edu

Rutgers University
Dietetics-Didactic Prgm
Nutrition Sci, 229B Davison Hall
26 Nichol Ave
New Brunswick, NJ 08901-2882
www.rutgers.edu

Univ of Medicine & Dent of New Jersey
Dietetics-Coordinated Prgm
School of Health Related Profs Primary Care Dept
1776 Raritan Rd
Scotch Plains, NJ 07076
http://shrp.umdnj.edu/programs/dietetic

Univ of Medicine & Dent of New Jersey
Dietetic Internship Prgm
School of Health Related Professions
1776 Raritan Rd
Scotch Plains, NJ 07076
http://shrp.umdnj.edu/programs/dietetic

Montclair State University
Dietetics-Didactic Prgm
Dept of Human Ecology
111 Finley
University Hall
Upper Montclair, NJ 07043
www.montclair.edu

Montclair State University
Dietetic Internship Prgm
Dept of Home Ecology
University Hall
Upper Montclair, NJ 07043

South Jersey Healthcare Regional Med Center
Dietetic Internship Prgm
1505 W Sherman Ave
Vineland, NJ 08360

New Mexico

University of New Mexico
Dietetic Internship Prgm
Individual Family and Community Education
Nutrition MSC05 3040
Albuquerque, NM 87131-1231
www.unm.edu

University of New Mexico
Dietetics-Didactic Prgm
Individual Family and Community Education
Nutrition MSC05 3040
Albuquerque, NM 87131-1231
www.unm.edu

New Mexico State University
Dietetics-Didactic Prgm
Dept of Family and Consumer Sciences
Box 30003, MSC 3470
Las Cruces, NM 88003-8003
www.nmsu.edu/~famcon

New York

CUNY Herbert H Lehman College
Dietetic Internship Prgm
Dept of Health Services
250 Bedford Park Blvd W
Bronx, NY 10468-1589
www.lehman.cuny.edu/deannss/healthsci/di/info.html

CUNY Herbert H Lehman College
Dietetics-Didactic Prgm
Dept of Health Serv Dietetics Food and Nutrition
Bedford Park Blvd W
Bronx, NY 10468-1589
www.lehman.cuny.edu

James J Peters VA Medical Center
Dietetic Internship Prgm
Nutrition and Food Program (120)
130 W Kingsbridge Rd
Bronx, NY 10468-3904
www.va.gov/visns/visn03/diethome.asp

CUNY Brooklyn College
Dietetic Internship Prgm
Dept of Health and Nutrition Sciences
2900 Bedford Ave
Brooklyn, NY 11210-2889
http://academic.brooklyn.cuny.edu/hns

CUNY Brooklyn College
Dietetics-Didactic Prgm
Dept of Health and Nutrition Sciences
2900 Bedford Ave
Brooklyn, NY 11210-2889
http://academic.brooklyn.cuny.edu/hns

Long Island University - C W Post Campus
Dietetics-Didactic Prgm
Dept of Nutrition, Life Science Bldg
720 Northern Blvd
Brookville, NY 11548
www.liu.edu/nutrit

Long Island University - C W Post Campus
Dietetic Internship Prgm
Dept of Nutrition
720 Northern Blvd
Brookville, NY 11548
www.cwpost.liu.edu/nutrit

Buffalo State, SUNY
Dietetics-Coordinated Prgm
Dietetics and Nutrition Dept, Caudell Hall 207
1300 Elmwood Ave
Caudell Hall 207
Buffalo, NY 14222-1095
www.buffalostate.edu

Buffalo State, SUNY
Dietetics-Didactic Prgm
Dietetics and Nutrition Dept
1300 Elmwood Ave
Caudell Hall 207
Buffalo, NY 14222-1095
www.buffalostate.edu

D'Youville College
Dietetics-Coordinated Prgm
320 Porter Ave
Buffalo, NY 14201-1084
www.dyc.edu

University at Buffalo - SUNY
Dietetic Internship Prgm
15 Farber Hall
3435 Main St
Buffalo, NY 14214
www.phhp.buffalo.edu/ens/nutrition/ntr-internship.html

Sodexho Health Care Services
Cosponsor: NY Metropolitan Dietetic Internship
Dietetic Internship Prgm
90 Merrick Ave, Ste 210
East Meadow, NY 11554
http://dieteticintern.com/NYmetro/

CUNY Queens College
Dietetic Internship Prgm
Family Nutri and Exercise Sciences
65-30 Kissena Blvd
Flushing, NY 11367-1597
www.qc.edu/FNES/dietintern.html

CUNY Queens College
Dietetics-Didactic Prgm
Dept of Family, Nutri and Exercise Sciences
65-30 Kissena Blvd
Flushing, NY 11367-1597
www.qc.edu

Cornell University
Dietetics-Didactic Prgm
Div of Nutritional Sciences
373 MVR Hall
Ithaca, NY 14853-4401
www.nutrition.cornell.edu/dns7_dietetic.html

Cornell University
Dietetic Internship Prgm
Division of Nutritional Sciences
225 Savage Hall
Ithaca, NY 14853-4401
www.nutrition.cornell.edu/dns7_dieteticintern.html

North Shore-Long Island Jewish Hlth System
Dietetic Internship Prgm
300 Community Dr
Manhasset, NY 11030

Columbia University Teachers College
Dietetic Internship Prgm
Dept of Health and Behavior Studies
525 W 120th St, Box 137
New York, NY 10027-6625
www.tc.columbia.edu/hbs/nutrition

CUNY Hunter College
Dietetic Internship Prgm
School of Health Sciences
425 E 25th St, Box 896
New York, NY 10010-2590
www.hunter.cuny.edu/schoolhp/phn/dietetic_internship

CUNY Hunter College
Dietetics-Didactic Prgm
Brookdale Hlth Science Ctr
425 E 25th St
New York, NY 10010-2590

New York University
Dietetics-Didactic Prgm
Nutrition and Food Studies
35 W 4th St, 10th Fl, Rm 1077
New York, NY 10012-1172
www.nyu.edu/education/nutrition

New York University
Dietetic Internship Prgm
Nutrition and Food Studies
35 W 4th St, 10th Fl
New York, NY 10011-1172
www.nyu.edu/education/nutrition

New York-Presbyterian Hospital
Dietetic Internship Prgm
525 E 68th St AN-833
Box 92
New York, NY 10021-4873
www.nyp.org/nutrition

New York Institute of Technology
Dietetics-Didactic Prgm
Clinical Nutrition Dept
NYCOM II, Rm 334
Old Westbury, NY 11568-8000
www.nyit.edu

SUNY College at Oneonta
Dietetic Internship Prgm
Dept of Human Ecology
39 Denison Hall
Oneonta, NY 13820
www.oneonta.edu/academics/dieteticinternship

SUNY College at Oneonta
Dietetics-Didactic Prgm
Dept of Human Ecology
104C Human Ecology
Oneonta, NY 13820-4015
www.oneonta.edu/academics/huec/dietetics4.asp

SUNY College at Plattsburgh
Dietetics-Didactic Prgm
Nutrition and Food Studies
101 Broad St
Plattsburgh, NY 12901-2681
www.plattsburgh.edu

Rochester Institute of Technology
Dietetics-Didactic Prgm
Hospitality and Service Management
14 Lomb Memorial Dr
Rochester, NY 14623-5604
www.rit.edu

Stony Brook University
Dietetic Internship Prgm
Department of Family Medicine
Health Sciences Center Level 4, Rm 050
Stony Brook, NY 11794-8461
www.hsc.stonybrook.edu/SOM/fammed/intern_program

Syracuse University
Dietetic Internship Prgm
Nutrition and Foodservice Mgmt
034 Slocum Hall
Syracuse, NY 13244-1250
www.hshp.syr.edu/schools/nhm/academics/grad/mams/
    dietetic

Syracuse University
Dietetics-Didactic Prgm
Nutrition and Foodservice Mgmt
034 Slocum Hall
Syracuse, NY 13244-1250

The Sage Colleges
Dietetics-Didactic Prgm
Div of Health and Rehab Sciences, Ackerman Hall
45 Ferry St
Ackerman Hall
Troy, NY 12180-4115
www.sage.edu

The Sage Colleges
Dietetic Internship Prgm
45 Ferry St
Troy, NY 12180-4115
www.sage.edu

North Carolina

Appalachian State University
Dietetics-Didactic Prgm
Family and Consumer Sciences
Boone, NC 28608-2630
www.appstate.edu

Appalachian State University
Dietetic Internship Prgm
Family and Consumer Sciences
PO Box 32056
Boone, NC 28608-2056
www.appstate.edu

University of North Carolina - Chapel Hill
Dietetics-Coordinated Prgm
McGavran-Greenberg Hall
Dept of Nutrition CB 7461
Chapel Hill, NC 27599-7461
www.sph.unc.edu/nutr

University of North Carolina - Chapel Hill
Dietetics-Didactic Prgm
McGavran-Greenburg Hall
Dept of Nutrition CB 7461
Chapel Hill, NC 27599-7461
www.sph.unc.edu/nutr

Western Carolina University
Dietetic Internship Prgm
Nutrition/Sciences
Dept of Health Sciences
Cullowhee, NC 28723
www.wcu.edu

Western Carolina University
Dietetics-Didactic Prgm
Dept of Health Sciences
Cullowhee, NC 28723
www.wcu.edu

North Carolina Central University
Dietetics-Didactic Prgm
Dept of Human Sciences
PO Box 19615
Durham, NC 27707-0099
www.nccu.edu

North Carolina Central University
Dietetic Internship Prgm
Dept of Human Sciences
PO Box 19615
Durham, NC 27707-0099
www.nccu.edu

North Carolina A&T State University
Dietetics-Didactic Prgm
Dept of Human Environment and Families
102 Benbow Hall, 1601 E Market St
Greensboro, NC 27411-1064
www.ag.ncat.edu/academics/fcs/dietetics/index.htm

University of North Carolina - Greensboro
Dietetics-Didactic Prgm
Nutrition and Foodservice Systems
PO Box 26170
Greensboro, NC 27402-6170
www.uncg.edu/nutrition

University of North Carolina - Greensboro
Dietetic Internship Prgm
Dept of Nutrition and Food Service Systems
1000 Spring Garden St
318 Stone Bldg
Greensboro, NC 27402-6170
www.uncg.edu/nutrition

East Carolina University
Dietetics-Didactic Prgm
School of Human Environmental Sciences
Nutrition & Hospitality Mgmt
Greenville, NC 27858-4353
www.ecu.edu

East Carolina University
Dietetic Internship Prgm
School of Human Environmental Sciences
Nutrition & Hospitality Mgmt
155 Rivers Bldg
Greenville, NC 27858-4353
www.ecu.edu

Lenoir - Rhyne University
Dietetic Internship Prgm
Solmaz Institute
PO Box 7155
Hickory, NC 28603-7155
www.lr.edu

Meredith College
Dietetics-Didactic Prgm
Human Environmental Sciences
3800 Hillsborough St
Raleigh, NC 27607-5298

Meredith College
Dietetic Internship Prgm
Human Environmental Sciences
3800 Hillsborough St
Raleigh, NC 27607-5298
www.meredith.edu

North Dakota

North Dakota State University
Dietetics-Coordinated Prgm
Dept of Health, Nutrition, and Exercise Science
PO Box 5057
EML Hall 351
Fargo, ND 58105-5057
www.ndsu.nodak.edu

North Dakota State University
Dietetics-Didactic Prgm
Dept of Health, Nutrition, and Exercise Science
PO Box 5057
EML Hall 351
Fargo, ND 58105
www.ndsu.nodak.edu

University of North Dakota
Dietetics-Coordinated Prgm
Nutrition and Dietetics
PO Box 8237
Grand Forks, ND 58202-8237
www.und.edu

Ohio

The University of Akron
Dietetics-Coordinated Prgm
Home Econ and Family Ecology
215 Schrank Hall S
Akron, OH 44325-6103
www.uakron.edu/fcs

The University of Akron
Dietetics-Didactic Prgm
School of Family and Consumer Sciences
215 Schrank Hall S
Akron, OH 44325-6103
www3.uakron.edu/fcs

Ashland University
Dietetics-Didactic Prgm
Department of Family and Consumer Sciences
401 College Ave
Ashland, OH 44805-3799
www.ashland.edu

Ohio University
Dietetics-Didactic Prgm
Human and Consumer Sciences
Grover Center W324
Athens, OH 45701-2979
www.ohiou.edu

Bluffton College
Dietetics-Didactic Prgm
Family and Consumer Sciences
1 University Dr, Box 1346
Bluffton, OH 45817-1196
www.bluffton.edu/fcs

Bowling Green State University
Dietetic Internship Prgm
Family and Consumer Sciences
Bowling Green, OH 43403-0254
www.bgsu.edu

Bowling Green State University
Dietetics-Didactic Prgm
Family and Consumer Sciences
206 Johnston Hall
Bowling Green, OH 43403-0254
www.bgsu.edu/colleges/edhd/FCS

Christ Hospital
Dietetic Internship Prgm
Food and Nutrition Services
2139 Auburn Ave
Cincinnati, OH 45219-2906
www.health-alliance.com Html

Good Samaritan Hospital
Dietetic Internship Prgm
Nutrition Dept
375 Dixmyth Ave
Cincinnati, OH 45220-2489

University of Cincinnati
Dietetics-Didactic Prgm
Dept of Health Sciences
363C Hastings & William French Bldg, Box 670394
Cincinnati, OH 45267-0394
www.cahs.uc.edu

University of Cincinnati
Dietetics-Coordinated Prgm
PO Box 210063
Cincinnati, OH 45267

Case Western Reserve University
Dietetic Internship Prgm
Dept of Nutrition, School of Medicine
10900 Euclid Ave
Cleveland, OH 44106-1712

Case Western Reserve University
Dietetics-Didactic Prgm
Dept of Nutrition
10900 Euclid Ave
Cleveland, OH 44106-4906
www.case.edu

Cleveland Clinic Foundation
Dietetic Internship Prgm
Nutrition Therapy M17
9500 Euclid Ave
Cleveland, OH 44195
www.clevelandclinic.org/education/diet

Louis Stokes Cleveland VA Med Ctr
Dietetic Internship Prgm
10701 East Blvd
Cleveland, OH 44106-1702
www.cwru.edu/med/nutrition/clevamc.html

MetroHealth Medical Center
Dietetic Internship Prgm
2500 MetroHealth Dr
Cleveland, OH 44109-1998
www.metrohealth.org/

University Hospitals Case Medical Center
Dietetic Internship Prgm
11100 Euclid Ave
Lakeside 5021
Cleveland, OH 44106-5000
www.cwru.edu/med/nutrition/uhocle.html

Mt Carmel College of Nursing
Dietetic Internship Prgm
127 S Davis Ave
Columbus, OH 43222-1504
www.mccn.edu

The Ohio State University
Dietetic Internship Prgm
Dept of Human Nutrition and Food Managemnt
325 Campbell Hall, 1787 Neil Ave
Columbus, OH 43210-1220
http://hec.osu.edu/hn

The Ohio State University
Dietetics-Didactic Prgm
Dept of Human Nutrition and Food Management
1787 Neil Ave
Columbus, OH 43210-1220
http://hec.osu.edu/hn

The Ohio State University
Dietetics-Coordinated Prgm
Sch of Allied Medical Profs
1583 Perry St
Columbus, OH 43210-1234
www.osu.edu

The Ohio State University
Dietetic Internship Prgm
School of Allied Medical Profs
Med Dietetics, 1583 Perry St
Columbus, OH 43210-1234
www.osu.edu

Miami Valley Hospital
Dietetic Internship Prgm
One Wyoming St
Dayton, OH 45409-2793
www.miamivalleyhospital.com

University of Dayton
Dietetics-Didactic Prgm
Health and Sports Science
300 College Park Ave
Dayton, OH 45469-1210
www.udayton.edu

Kent State University
Dietetics-Didactic Prgm
Family and Consumer Studies
Nixson Hall, Nutrition & Dietetics
Kent, OH 44242
www.dept.kent.edu/f&cs

Kent State University
Dietetic Internship Prgm
100 Nixson Hall
Kent, OH 44242
www.kent.edu

Miami University
Dietetics-Didactic Prgm
Phys Ed Hlth and Sports Studies
100A Phillips Hall
Oxford, OH 45056
www.miami.muohio.edu

Youngstown State University
Dietetics-Didactic Prgm
Human Ecology Dept
One University Plaza
Youngstown, OH 44555-0001
www.ysu.edu

Youngstown State University
Dietetics-Coordinated Prgm
One University Plaza
Youngstown, OH 44555-0001
www.ysu.edu

Oklahoma

University of Central Oklahoma
Dietetic Internship Prgm
Human Environmental Sciences
100 N University Dr
Edmond, OK 73034
www.educ.ucok.edu

University of Central Oklahoma
Dietetics-Didactic Prgm
College of Education
Human Environmental Sciences
Edmond, OK 73034
www.ucok.edu

Langston University
Dietetics-Didactic Prgm
Dept of Home Ecology
302 Jones Hall
PO Box 1500
Langston, OK 73050
www.lunet.edu

Univ of Oklahoma Health Sciences Center
Dietetics-Coordinated Prgm
Dept of Nutritional Sciences
801 NE 13th, PO Box 26901
Oklahoma City, OK 73190
www.ouhsc.edu

Univ of Oklahoma Health Sciences Center
Dietetic Internship Prgm
College of Allied Hlth, Dept of Nutri Sci
PO Box 26901 CHB
Oklahoma City, OK 73190
www.ah.ouhsc.edu/main

Univ of Oklahoma Health Sciences Center
Dietetics-Didactic Prgm
College of Allied Health
Nutritional Sci, PO Box 26901
Oklahoma City, OK 73190
www.ah.ouhsc.edu/main

Oklahoma State University
Dietetic Internship Prgm
Dept of Nutritional Sciences
HES 301
Stillwater, OK 74078-6337
http://ches.okstate.edu/nsci/

Oklahoma State University
Dietetics-Didactic Prgm
Nutritional Sciences Dept
301 HES
Stillwater, OK 74078-6141
http://ches.okstate.edu/nsci/

Northeastern State University
Dietetics-Didactic Prgm
Coll of Business and Technology
600 N Grand, 210A PA Bldg
Tahlequah, OK 74464-2399
http://arapaho.nsuok.edu/~fcs

Oregon

Oregon State University
Dietetics-Didactic Prgm
Nutrition and Food Mgmt
212 Milam Hall
Corvallis, OR 97331-5103
www.oregonstate.edu

Oregon State University
Dietetic Internship Prgm
School of Biological and Population Health Sci
Dept of Nutrition and Exercise Sciences
200 Milam Hall
Corvallis, OR 97331
www.hhs.oregonstate.edu/nes/dietetics/
    dietetic-internship-osudi

Oregon Health & Science University
Dietetic Internship Prgm
EJH-10-FM 10
3181 SW Sam Jackson Park Rd
Portland, OR 97201-3098
www.ohsu.edu/dietetic

Mid Willamette Valley Dietetic Internship
Dietetic Internship Prgm
1955 Dallas Hwy NW, Ste 1200
Salem, OR 97304
www.capitalmanor.com/internship.htm

Pennsylvania

Cedar Crest College
Dietetics-Didactic Prgm
100 College Dr
Allentown, PA 18104-6196
www.cedarcrest.edu/Redesign/homepage5/index.htm

Cedar Crest College
Dietetic Internship Prgm
Dietetic Internship
100 College Drive
Allentown, PA 18104-6196
www.cedarcrest.edu/ca/academics/nutrition/
    dietetic_internship.shtm

Sodexho Health Care Services
Dietetic Internship Prgm
6081 Hamilton Blvd
PO Box 3501
Allentown, PA 18106-0501
www.woodco.com

Geisinger Medical Center
Dietetic Internship Prgm
100 N Academy Ave
Danville, PA 17822-0115
www.geisinger.org

Messiah College
Dietetics-Didactic Prgm
Dept of Natural Sciences
One College Ave
Box 3030
Grantham, PA 17027
www.messiah.edu

Seton Hill University
Dietetics-Coordinated Prgm
Family and Consumer Sciences
Seton Hill Dr
Greensburg, PA 15601-1599
www.setonhill.edu

Immaculata University
Dietetics-Didactic Prgm
Fashion Foods and Nutrition
Box 722
Immaculata, PA 19345-0722
www.immaculata.edu

Immaculata University
Dietetic Internship Prgm
Nutrition Educ
Box 500, Graduate Div
Immaculata, PA 19345-0901
www.immaculata.edu

Indiana University of Pennsylvania
Dietetics-Didactic Prgm
Dept of Food and Nutrition
911 South Dr
Ackerman Hall 14
Indiana, PA 15705-1087
www.hhs.iup.edu/fn

Indiana University of Pennsylvania
Dietetic Internship Prgm
Dept of Food and Nutrition
Ackerman Hall 14
911 South Dr
Indiana, PA 15705-1087
www.hhs.iup.edu/fn

Mansfield University
Dietetics-Didactic Prgm
203C Elliott Hall
Dept of Health Sciences
Mansfield, PA 16933
www.mnsfld.edu/~health/index.htm

ARAMARK Healthcare
Dietetic Internship Prgm
c/o Joan Reedon
1101 Market St, 19th Floor
Philadelphia, PA 19107-2934
www.aramark.com/Careers/DieteticInternships

Drexel University College of Medicine
Dietetics-Didactic Prgm
Nutrition and Food Sciences
3141 Chestnut St
Philadelphia, PA 19104-2875
www.drexel.edu

La Salle University
Dietetics-Didactic Prgm
1900 W Olney Ave
Philadelphia, PA 19141-1199
www.lasalle.edu

La Salle University
Dietetics-Coordinated Prgm
1900 W Olney Ave
Philadelphia, PA 19141-1199
www.lasalle.edu

Adagio Health
Dietetic Internship Prgm
960 Penn Ave, Ste 600
Pittsburgh, PA 15222-1417
www.adagiohealth.org

University of Pittsburgh
Dietetics-Didactic Prgm
Health and Rehab Science
4048 Forbes Tower
Pittsburgh, PA 15260-1802
www.pitt.edu

University of Pittsburgh
Dietetics-Coordinated Prgm
Health and Rehab Sciences
4048 Forbes Tower
Pittsburgh, PA 15260-1802
www.shrs.pitt.edu/cdn

Marywood University
Dietetics-Didactic Prgm
Dept of Nutrition and Dietetics
2300 Adams Ave
Scranton, PA 18509-1514
www.marywood.edu/departments/nutr_diet/home.html

Marywood University
Dietetic Internship Prgm
Dept of Nutrition and Dietetics
2300 Adams Ave
Scranton, PA 18509-1514
www.marywood.edu/departments/nutr_diet/home.html

Marywood University
Dietetics-Coordinated Prgm
Dept of Nutrition and Dietetics
2300 Adams Ave
Scranton, PA 18509-1598
www.marywood.edu/departments/nutr_diet/home.html

Penn State University
Dietetic Internship Prgm
Nutrition Dept Coll of Hlth and Human Dev
5126 Henderson Bldg
University Park, PA 16802
http://nutrition.hhdev.psu.edu/internship/index.html

Penn State University
Dietetics-Didactic Prgm
Nutrition Dept
Coll of Hlth & Human Development
S-126 Henderson Bldg
University Park, PA 16802-6500
http://nutrition.hhdev.psu.edu/internship/index.html

Sodexho Health Care Services
Dietetic Internship Prgm
Fuld Campus
Rte 532 & General Sullivan Rd
PO Box 602-0601
Washington Cross, PA 18977
www.dieteticintern.com/NJ-Phila

West Chester University
Dietetics-Didactic Prgm
H302 Department of Health
Sturzebecker Health Sciences Center
West Chester, PA 19383
www.wcupa.edu

Puerto Rico

Universidad Del Turabo
Dietetics-Coordinated Prgm
Gurabo, PR 00778

Puerto Rico Department of Health
Dietetic Internship Prgm
PO Box 70184
San Juan, PR 00936

University of Puerto Rico
Dietetic Internship Prgm
College of Health Related Professions
Med Sci Campus, PO Box 365067
San Juan, PR 00936-5067
http://cprsweb.rcm.upr.edu

University of Puerto Rico
Dietetics-Didactic Prgm
Box 23347 UPR Station
Rio Piedras Campus
San Juan, PR 00931-3347

VA Caribbean Healthcare System
Dietetic Internship Prgm
10 Calle Casia
San Juan, PR 00921

Rhode Island

University of Rhode Island
Dietetics-Didactic Prgm
Food Science and Nutrition
110 Ranger Hall
Kingston, RI 02881-0804
www.uri.edu/cels/fsn

University of Rhode Island
Dietetic Internship Prgm
Food Science and Nutrition
106 Ranger Hall
Kingston, RI 02881
www.uri.edu/cels/fsn

Johnson & Wales University
Dietetics-Didactic Prgm
College of Culinary Arts
One Washington Square
Providence, RI 02905
www.jwu.edu

South Carolina

Medical University of South Carolina
Dietetic Internship Prgm
96 Jonathan Lucas St, Ste 219K
PO Box 250327
Charleston, SC 29425
www.musc.edu/dieteticinternship

Clemson University
Dietetics-Didactic Prgm
Dept of Food Science
223 Poole, Agricultural Center
Box 340316
Clemson, SC 29634-0371
www.clemson.edu/foodscience

SC Dept of Health & Environmental Control
Dietetic Internship Prgm
Mills Complex
PO Box 101106
Columbia, SC 29211-0106
www.scdhec.gov

South Carolina State University
Dietetics-Didactic Prgm
Staley Hall PO Box 7657
300 College Ave
Orangeburg, SC 29117-0001

Winthrop University
Dietetics-Didactic Prgm
Dept of Human Nutrition
302 Life Sciences Bldg
Rock Hill, SC 29733
www.winthrop.edu/nutrition

Winthrop University
Dietetic Internship Prgm
Dept of Human Nutrition
302 Life Sciences Bldg
Rock Hill, SC 29733
www.winthrop.edu/nutrition/dietetic.htm

South Dakota

South Dakota State University
Dietetics-Didactic Prgm
Family and Consumer Sciences
PO Box 2275A
Brookings, SD 57007-0497
www3.sdstate.edu

University of South Dakota
Dietetic Internship Prgm
School of Medicine
1400 W 22nd St
Sioux Falls, SD 57105
www.usd.edu/cd/dieteticinternship

Tennessee

University of Tennessee - Chattanooga
Dietetics-Didactic Prgm
Dept of Human Ecology, #4204
615 McCallie Ave
Chattanooga, TN 37403
www.utc.edu

Tennessee Technological University
Dietetics-Didactic Prgm
School of Home Economics
Box 5035
Cookeville, TN 38505
www.tntech.edu

Carson-Newman College
Dietetics-Didactic Prgm
PO Box 71881
2130 Branner Ave
Jefferson City, TN 37760-7001
www.cn.edu

East Tennessee State University
Dietetic Internship Prgm
Applied Human Sciences-STAT
PO Box 70671
Johnson City, TN 37614-0671
www.etsu.edu/scitech/ahsc/ahsc.htm

East Tennessee State University
Dietetics-Didactic Prgm
Applied Human Sciences
PO Box 70671
Johnson City, TN 37614-0671
www.etsu.edu

University of Tennessee - Knoxville
Dietetics-Didactic Prgm
Dept of Nutrition
1215 W Cumberland Ave
229 Jessie Harris Bldg
Knoxville, TN 37996-1920

University of Tennessee - Knoxville
Dietetic Internship Prgm
Human Ecology, Dept of Nutrition
1215 Cumberland Ave, Rm 229
Knoxville, TN 37996-1920
http://nutrition.utk.edu

University of Tennessee - Martin
Dietetics-Didactic Prgm
Dept of Family and Consumer Sci
340 Gooch Hall
Martin, TN 38238-5045
www.utm.edu

University of Tennessee - Martin
Dietetic Internship Prgm
Human Environmental Sciences
340 Gooch Hall
Martin, TN 38238-5045
www.utm.edu

Memphis VA Medical Center
Dietetic Internship Prgm
Nutrition and Food Services (120)
1030 Jefferson Ave
Building 1 CW267D
Memphis, TN 38104
www.dieteticinternship.va.gov

University of Memphis
Dietetics-Didactic Prgm
Consumer Science and Education
Fieldhouse 1611
Memphis, TN 38152
http://hss.memphis.edu

University of Memphis
Dietetic Internship Prgm
Dept of Health and Sport Science
161A Fieldhouse
Memphis, TN 38152
www.memphis.edu

Middle Tennessee State University
Dietetics-Didactic Prgm
Dept of Human Sciences
PO Box 86
Murfreesboro, TN 37132
www.mtsu.edu

National HealthCare LP
Dietetic Internship Prgm
PO Box 1398
Murfreesboro, TN 37133-1398
www.nhccare.com/di.htm

Lipscomb University
Dietetic Internship Prgm
3901 Granny White Pike
Nashville, TN 37204-3951
www.lipscomb.edu

Lipscomb University
Dietetics-Didactic Prgm
Family and Consumer Sciences
3901 Granny White Pike
Nashville, TN 37204-3951
www.lipscomb.edu

Tennessee State University
Dietetics-Didactic Prgm
Family Consumer Sciences PO Box 9538
3500 John A Merritt Blvd
Nashville, TN 37209-1561
www.tnstate.edu/sacs

Vanderbilt University Medical Center
Dietetic Internship Prgm
B-802TVC
1301 22nd Ave S
Nashville, TN 37232-5510
www.mc.vanderbilt.edu/alliedhealth

Texas

Abilene Christian University
Dietetics-Didactic Prgm
Family and Consumer Sciences
ACU Box 28155
Abilene, TX 79699
www.acu.edu

Texas WIC
Dietetic Internship Prgm
Bureau of Nutrition Services
1100 W 49th St
Austin, TX 78756
www.dshs.state.tx.us/

University of Texas at Austin
Dietetics-Coordinated Prgm
Dept of Human Ecology
1 University Station, A2700
Austin, TX 78712-1097
www.he.utexas.edu

University of Texas at Austin
Dietetics-Didactic Prgm
Dept of Human Ecology
1 University Station, A2700
Austin, TX 78712
www.utexas.edu/depts/he

Lamar University
Dietetics-Didactic Prgm
Family and Consumer Sciences
PO Box 10035
Beaumont, TX 77710-0035
www.lamar.edu

Lamar University
Dietetic Internship Prgm
Family and Consumer Sciences
PO Box 10035
Beaumont, TX 77710-0035
www.lamar.edu

Texas A&M University
Dietetic Internship Prgm
Dept of Animal Science
2253 TAMU
College Station, TX 77843-2253
http://nfs.tamu.edu

Texas A&M University
Dietetics-Didactic Prgm
Human Nutrition Section
2253 TAMU
College Station, TX 77843-2471
http://nfs.tamu.edu

Baylor University Med Center
Dietetic Internship Prgm
3500 Gaston Ave
Dallas, TX 75246-2045
www.baylorhealth.com/locations/bumc/

Presbyterian Hospital of Dallas
Dietetic Internship Prgm
8200 Walnut Hill Ln
Dallas, TX 75231-4402
www.phscare.org/phd/dietetics

Univ of Texas Southwestern Med Ctr
Dietetics-Coordinated Prgm
Dept of Clinical Nutrition
5323 Harry Hines Blvd
Dallas, TX 75390-8877
www.utsouthwestern.edu/clinnut

Texas Woman's University
Dietetic Internship Prgm
Nutrition and Food Sciences
PO Box 425888
Denton, TX 76204-5888
www.twu.edu/hs/nfs/intern.htm Htm

Texas Woman's University
Dietetics-Didactic Prgm
Nutrition and Food Sciences
304 Administration Dr, Clock Tower
Denton, TX 76201
www.twu.edu/hs/nfs

Univ of Texas - Pan American
Dietetics-Coordinated Prgm
Health and Human Services
1201 W University Dr
Edinburg, TX 78539-2909
www.panam.edu

US Military Dietetic Internship Consortium
Dietetic Internship Prgm
Nutrition Care Div
3851 Roger Brooke Dr
Fort Sam Houston, TX 78234-6200
www.amsc.amedd.army.mil/training.asp

Texas Christian University
Dietetics-Coordinated Prgm
Dept of Nutrition and Dietetics
TCU Box 298600
Fort Worth, TX 76129
www.tcu.edu

Texas Christian University
Dietetics-Didactic Prgm
Dept of Nutrition and Dietetics
TCU Box 298600
Fort Worth, TX 76129
www.tcu.edu

Michael E DeBakey VA Medical Center
Dietetic Internship Prgm
2002 Holcombe Blvd
Houston, TX 77030-4298
www.va.gov/nfs/HoustonVAMC

Texas Southern University
Dietetics-Didactic Prgm
Human Svcs and Consumer Sci
3100 Cleburne Ave
Houston, TX 77004-4575
www.tsu.edu

Texas Woman's University
Dietetic Internship Prgm
1130 John Freeman Blvd
Houston, TX 77030-2897
www.twu.edu/hs/nfs/hintern.htm

University of Houston
Dietetic Internship Prgm
Human Development and Consumer Sci
4800 Calhoun Rd
Houston, TX 77204-6020
www.hhp.uh.edu/internship

University of Houston
Dietetics-Didactic Prgm
Human Development and Consumer Sci
4800 Calhoun Rd
Houston, TX 77204-6861
http://hhp.uh.edu/nutrition

University of Texas Health Sci Ctr Houston
Dietetic Internship Prgm
Sch of Public Hlth, E619 RAS Bldg
1200 Herman Pressler St
Houston, TX 77030
www.sph.uth.tmc.edu

Sam Houston State University
Dietetics-Didactic Prgm
Food Science and Nutrition
SHSU Box 2177
1700 Sam Houston Ave
Huntsville, TX 77341-2177
www.shsu.edu/~hec_www

Sam Houston State University
Dietetic Internship Prgm
PO Box 2177
1700 Sam Houston Ave
Huntsville, TX 77341-2177
www.shsu.edu/~hec_www

Texas A&M University - Kingsville
Dietetics-Didactic Prgm
Dept of Human Sciences
MSC 168, 700 University Blvd
Kingsville, TX 78363
www.tamu.edu

Texas A&M University - Kingsville
Dietetic Internship Prgm
Dept of Human Sciences
MSC 168, 700 University Blvd
Kingsville, TX 78363-8202
www.tamu.edu

US Military Dietetic Internship Consortium
Dietetic Internship Prgm
Wilford Hall Medical Center
959 MDTS/MTN, 2200 Bergquist Dr, Suite 1
Lackland AFB, TX 78236-5300

UT Health Science Center - San Antonio
Dietetics-Coordinated Prgm
1937 East Bustamante St
Laredo, TX 78041-5416
www.uthscsa.edu/sah/index.asp

Texas Tech University
Dietetic Internship Prgm
Dept of Educ, Nutr, Rest, and Hotel Mgmt
PO Box 41162, 15th and Akron St
Lubbock, TX 79409-1162
www.hs.ttu.edu/intern

Texas Tech University
Dietetics-Didactic Prgm
Educ Nutri and Rest Hotel Mgmt
PO Box 41162, 15th and Akron St
Lubbock, TX 79409-1162
www.hs.ttu.edu

Stephen F Austin State University
Dietetics-Didactic Prgm
Dept of Human Sciences
SFA Station, PO Box 13014
Nacogdoches, TX 75962-3014
www.sfasu.edu

Stephen F Austin State University
Dietetic Internship Prgm
Dept of Human Sciences
SFA Station, PO Box 13014
Nacogdoches, TX 75962-3014
www.sfasu.edu/di

Prairie View A&M University
Dietetics-Didactic Prgm
Dept of Human Sciences
PO Box 4329
Prairie View, TX 77446-4329
www.pvamu.edu

Prairie View A&M University
Dietetic Internship Prgm
Box 4329
Prairie View, TX 77446
www.pvamu.edu

Baptist Health System
Dietetic Internship Prgm
Food and Nutrition Services
111 Dallas St
San Antonio, TX 78205-1201
www.baptisthealthsystem.com

The University of the Incarnate Word
Dietetics-Didactic Prgm
4301 Broadway St
San Antonio, TX 78209-6318
www.uiw.edu

The University of the Incarnate Word
Dietetic Internship Prgm
4301 Broadway Box 311
San Antonio, TX 78209
www.uiw.edu

Texas State University - San Marcos
Dietetic Internship Prgm
Family and Consumer Sciences
601 University Dr
San Marcos, TX 78666-4616
www.txstate.edu

Texas State University - San Marcos
Dietetics-Didactic Prgm
Family and Consumer Sciences
601 University Dr
San Marcos, TX 78666-4616
www.txstate.edu

Baylor University
Dietetics-Didactic Prgm
Family and Consumer Sciences
BU Box 97346
Waco, TX 76798-7346

Utah

Utah State University
Dietetics-Didactic Prgm
8700 Old Main Hill
Logan, UT 84322-8700
www.usu.edu/~dietetic

Utah State University
Dietetics-Coordinated Prgm
Nutrition and Food Science
Logan, UT 84322-8700
www.usu.edu/~dietetic

Brigham Young University
Dietetic Internship Prgm
Food Science and Nutrition
S219 ESC, PO Box 24620
Provo, UT 84602-4620
http://ndfs.byu.edu

Brigham Young University
Dietetics-Didactic Prgm
Food Science and Nutrition
S219 ESC, PO Box 24620
Provo, UT 84602-4620
http://ndfs.byu.edu

University of Utah
Dietetics-Coordinated Prgm
Div of Foods and Nutrition
250 South 1850 East #214
Salt Lake City, UT 84112
www.health.utah.edu/nutr/

Utah State University - Salt Lake
Dietetic Internship Prgm
5250 S Commerce Dr Ste 300
Salt Lake City, UT 84107
http://extension.usu.edu/intern intern

Vermont

University of Vermont
Dietetics-Coordinated Prgm
349 Waterman Bldg
Burlington, VT 05405

University of Vermont
Dietetics-Didactic Prgm
Dept of Nutritional Sciences
Terrill Hall
Burlington, VT 05405
http://nutrition.uvm.edu

Virginia

Virginia Polytechnic Inst & State Univ
Dietetics-Didactic Prgm
Human Nutrition Foods and Exercise
College of Agriculture and Life Sciences
Blacksburg, VA 24061-0430
www.hnfe.vt.edu

Virginia Polytechnic Inst & State Univ
Dietetic Internship Prgm
338 Wallace Hall
Blacksburg, VA 24061-0430
www.hnfe.vt.edu

University of Virginia Health System
Dietetic Internship Prgm
Box 800673
Charlottesville, VA 22908
http://hsc.virginia.edu/internet/dietetics

James Madison University
Dietetics-Didactic Prgm
Dept of Health Sciences MSC 4301
HHS 3140
Harrisonburg, VA 22807
www.jmu.edu

Norfolk State University
Dietetics-Didactic Prgm
700 Park Ave
Norfolk, VA 23504

Virginia State University
Dietetic Internship Prgm
PO Box 9211
Petersburg, VA 23806
www.vsu.edu

Virginia State University
Dietetics-Didactic Prgm
Dept of Human Ecology, Box 9211
Petersburg, VA 23806-0001
www.vsu.edu

DIETETICS

177

Radford University
Dietetics-Didactic Prgm
Dept of Health Services
PO Box 6962
Radford, VA 24142-5826
www.radford.edu/~fdsn-web

Virginia Commonwealth Univ/Health System
Dietetic Internship Prgm
PO Box 980294
Richmond, VA 23298-0294
http://views.vcu.edu/dietetic

Virginia Department of Health
Dietetic Internship Prgm
Div of WIC and Community Nutrition Services
109 Governor St, 9th Fl
Richmond, VA 23219

Washington

Central Washington University
Dietetics-Didactic Prgm
Family and Consumer Sciences
400 E University Way
Ellensburg, WA 98926-7565
www.cwu.edu

Central Washington University
Dietetic Internship Prgm
Family and Consumer Sciences
400 E University Way
Ellensburg, WA 98929-7565
www.cwu.edu/~fandcs/internship.html

Bastyr University
Dietetics-Didactic Prgm
14500 Juanita Dr NE
Kenmore, WA 98028-4966
www.bastyr.edu

Bastyr University
Dietetic Internship Prgm
Nutrition Program
14500 Juanita Dr NE
Kenmore, WA 98028-4966

Washington State University
Dietetics-Didactic Prgm
Food Sci and Human Nutrition
FSHN 120, PO Box 646376
Pullman, WA 99164-6376
http://fshn.wsu.edu

Washington State University
Dietetics-Coordinated Prgm
106 FSHN Bldg
PO Box 646376
Pullman, WA 99164-6376
http://fshn.wsu.edu

Sea Mar Community Health Center
Dietetic Internship Prgm
8915 14th Ave S
Seattle, WA 98108-4807
www.seamar.org www.seamar.org

Seattle Pacific University
Dietetics-Didactic Prgm
Family and Consumer Sciences
3307 3rd Ave W
Ste 211
Seattle, WA 98119-1997
www.spu.edu/depts/fcs

Washington State University - Spokane
Dietetics-Coordinated Prgm
310 N Riverpoint Blvd Box M
Spokane, WA 99210
www.wsu.edu

West Virginia

Marshall University
Dietetics-Didactic Prgm
One John Marshall Dr
Huntington, WV 25755-9521
www.marshall.edu

Marshall University
Dietetic Internship Prgm
Corbly Hall 203 Family and Consumer Sci
One John Marshall Dr
Huntington, WV 25755-9521
www.marshall.edu

West Virginia University
Dietetics-Didactic Prgm
Coll of Agriculture and Forestry
PO Box 6108
Morgantown, WV 26506-6124
www.caf.wvu.edu

West Virginia University
Dietetic Internship Prgm
Coll of Agriculture and Forestry
PO Box 6108
Morgantown, WV 26506-6124
www.caf.wvu.edu

West Virginia University Hospitals
Dietetic Internship Prgm
Dept of Nutrition and Environmental Serv
Medical Center Dr, PO Box 8016
Morgantown, WV 26506-8016
www.hsc.wvu.edu/di

Wisconsin

University of Wisconsin - Green Bay
Dietetics-Didactic Prgm
Human Biology Dept LS 423
2420 Nicolet Dr
Green Bay, WI 54311-7001
www.uwgb.edu/humbio/program/Majors.htm

University of Wisconsin - Green Bay
Dietetic Internship Prgm
2420 Nicolet Dr
Human Biology Dept ES 301
Green Bay, WI 54311-7001
www.uwgb.edu/humbio/dietetics/Index.htm

Viterbo University
Dietetics-Coordinated Prgm
Nutrition and Dietetics Dept
900 Viterbo Dr
La Crosse, WI 54601-4797
www.viterbo.edu

Viterbo University
Dietetic Internship Prgm
Nutrition and Dietetics Dept
900 Viterbo Dr
La Crosse, WI 54601-4797
www.viterbo.edu

University of Wisconsin - Madison
Dietetics-Didactic Prgm
Dept of Nutritional Sciences
1415 Linden Dr
Madison, WI 53706-1571
http://nutrisci.wisc.edu

University of Wisconsin Hospital and Clinics
Dietetic Internship Prgm
Food and Nutrition Services F4/120
600 Highland Ave
Madison, WI 53792-1510
www.uwhealth.org

University of Wisconsin - Stout
Dietetic Internship Prgm
Dept of Food and Nutrition
222 Home Economics Bldg
415 10th Ave
Menomonie, WI 54751
www.uwstout.edu/programs/msfns/intern

University of Wisconsin - Stout
Dietetics-Didactic Prgm
College of Human Development
415 E 10th Ave
Menomonie, WI 54751-0790
www.uwstout.edu/programs/bsd

Mount Mary College
Dietetic Internship Prgm
Graduate Program in Dietetics
2900 N Menomonee River Pkwy
Milwaukee, WI 53222-4597
www.mtmary.edu/dietetics.htm

Mount Mary College
Dietetics-Coordinated Prgm
Dept of Dietetics
2900 N Menomonee River Pkwy
Milwaukee, WI 53222-4597
www.mtmary.edu

University of Wisconsin - Stevens Point
Dietetics-Didactic Prgm
Health Promotion and Human Development
202 CPS
Stevens Point, WI 54481
www.uwsp.edu

Wyoming

University of Wyoming
Dietetics-Didactic Prgm
Dept of Family and Consumer Sciences
1000 E University Ave
Laramie, WY 82071-3354
www.uwyo.edu/family

Dietetic Technician

Career Description
Dietetic technicians assist in shaping the public's food choices and provide nutrition assessment and counseling to persons with illnesses or injuries. Technicians work under the supervision of the registered dietitian. They often screen patients to identify nutrition problems, provide uncomplicated patient education and counseling to individuals and groups, develop menus and recipes, supervise food service personnel, purchase food, and monitor inventory and food quality.

Employment Characteristics
As an integral part of the nutrition care team, dietetic technicians work with registered dietitians in a number of different settings, such as hospitals, public health nutrition programs, and long-term care facilities. Technicians also work in child nutrition and school lunch programs, community wellness centers, health clubs, nutrition programs for the elderly, food companies, restaurants, and food service management.

Salary
According to the American Dietetic Association (ADA) 2011 Dietetics Compensation and Benefits Survey, half of all registered dietetic technicians employed full-time in their primary position for less than five years earn annual incomes of between $26,060 to 44,630. Salary levels may vary based on location, scope of responsibility, and supply of DTRs.

For more information, refer to *www.ama-assn.org/go/hpsalary*.

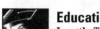

Educational Programs
Length. Two years (associate degree), combining classroom and supervised practical experience, at a US regionally accredited college or university. After completing this program, individuals are eligible to take the registration examination for dietetic technicians. Those who pass the exam become Dietetic Technicians, Registered, and can use the initials "DTR" after their names.

Prerequisites. Applicants must have a high school diploma or equivalency and must meet institutional entrance requirements.

Curriculum. Didactic instruction and a minimum of 450 hours of supervised practice experiences make up the curriculum. Food, nutrition, and management courses are emphasized, supported by the sciences, especially biology, anatomy, and chemistry. Mathematics, English, sociology, psychology, communications, and business courses are also important.

Inquiries

Careers
Inquiries regarding careers in dietetics and nutrition should be addressed to:
Accreditation and Education Programs
American Dietetic Association
120 South Riverside Plaza, Suite 2000
Chicago, IL 60606-6995
312 899-0040, Ext 5400
E-mail: *education@eatright.org*

Certification/Registration
Inquiries regarding dietetic technician registration should be addressed to:
Commission on Dietetic Registration
120 South Riverside Plaza, Suite 2000
Chicago, IL 60606-6995
312 899-0040, Ext 5500
E-mail: *cdr@eatright.org*

Program Accreditation
Accreditation Council for Education in Nutrition and Dietetics
American Dietetic Association
120 South Riverside Plaza, Suite 2000
Chicago, IL 60606-6995
312 899-0040, Ext 5400
E-mail: *education@eatright.org*

Accredited Programs
A list of accredited programs with selected information is available on the ADA web site at: *http://www.eatright.org/ACEND/*

Dietetic Technician

Arizona

Chandler-Gilbert Community College
Dietetic Technician-AD Prgm
2626 East Pecos Rd
Chandler, AZ 85225
cgcmail.maricopa.edu

Central Arizona College
Dietetic Technician-AD Prgm
8470 N Overfield Rd
Coolidge, AZ 85228-9030
www.centralaz.edu

Paradise Valley Community College
Dietetic Technician-AD Prgm
18401 N 32nd St
Phoenix, AZ 85032
www.pvc.maricopa.edu

Arkansas

Black River Technical College
Dietetic Technician-AD Prgm
PO Box 468
Pocahontas, AR 72455
www.blackrivertech.org

California

Orange Coast College
Dietetic Technician-AD Prgm
2701 Fairview Rd
Costa Mesa, CA 92628-0120

Los Angeles City College
Dietetic Technician-AD Prgm
Family and Consumer Studies
855 N Vermont Ave
Los Angeles, CA 90029-3590
www.lacc.cc.ca.us

Merritt College
Dietetic Technician-AD Prgm
12500 Campus Dr
Oakland, CA 94619-3107

Chaffey College
Dietetic Technician-AD Prgm
Food Service Management
5885 Haven Ave
Rancho Cucamonga, CA 91737-3002
www.chaffey.edu

Santa Rosa Junior College
Dietetic Technician-AD Prgm
Dietetic Technician Program
Consumer and Family Studies Department
1501 Mendocino Ave
Santa Rosa, CA 95401-4395
www.santarosa.edu/instruction/

Connecticut

Gateway Community College
Dietetic Technician-AD Prgm
88 Bassett Rd
New Haven, CT 06473
www.gwctc.commnet.edu

Lincoln College of New England
Dietetic Technician-AD Prgm
2279 Mount Vernon Rd
Southington, CT 06489-1007
www.lincolncollegene.edu

Florida

Florida State College at Jacksonville
Dietetic Technician-AD Prgm
North Campus, 4501 Capper Rd
Jacksonville, FL 32218-4436
www.fccj.org

Hillsborough Community College
Dietetic Technician-AD Prgm
Dietetic Technician Program
PO Box 30030
Tampa, FL 33630-3030
www.hccfl.edu

Illinois

Parkland College
Dietetic Technician-AD Prgm
2400 West Bradley Ave
Champaign, IL 61821-1899
www.parkland.edu

Harper College
Dietetic Technician-AD Prgm
1200 W Algonquin Rd
Palatine, IL 60067-7398
www.harpercollege.edu

Louisiana

Delgado Community College
Dietetic Technician-AD Prgm
615 City Park Ave
New Orleans, LA 70119
www.dcc.edu

Maine

Southern Maine Community College
Dietetic Technician-AD Prgm
2 Fort Rd
South Portland, ME 04106
www.smccme.edu

Maryland

Baltimore City Community College
Dietetic Technician-AD Prgm
Dept of Allied Health
2901 Liberty Heights Ave
Baltimore, MD 21215-7893
www.bccc.state.md.us

Massachusetts

Laboure College
Dietetic Technician-AD Prgm
2120 Dorchester Ave
Boston, MA 02124-5698
www.Laboure.edu

Michigan

Wayne County Community College District
Dietetic Technician-AD Prgm
Northwest Campus
8551 Greenfield Rd
Detroit, MI 48226
wcccd.edu

Minnesota

Normandale Community College
Dietetic Technician-AD Prgm
9700 France Ave S
Bloomington, MN 55431-4309
www.normandale.mnscu.edu

Missouri

St Louis Community College - Florissant Valley
Dietetic Technician-AD Prgm
3400 Pershall Rd
St Louis, MO 63135-1499
www.stlcc.edu

Montana

Montana State Univ - Great Falls Coll of Tech
Dietetic Technician-AD Prgm
2100 16th Ave South
Great Falls, MT 59405

Nebraska

Southeast Community College
Dietetic Technician-AD Prgm
8800 O St
Lincoln, NE 68520-1227
www.southeast.edu

Nevada

Truckee Meadows Community College
Dietetic Technician-AD Prgm
7000 Dandini Blvd, RDMT 334J
Reno, NV 89512-3999
www.tmcc.edu

New Hampshire

University of New Hampshire
Dietetic Technician-AD Prgm
Thompson School of Applied Sci
6A Putnam Hall
Durham, NH 03824
www.unh.edu

New Jersey

Camden County College
Dietetic Technician-AD Prgm
PO Box 200
College Dr
Blackwood, NJ 08012-0200
www.camdencc.edu

Middlesex County College
Dietetic Technician-AD Prgm
2600 Woodbridge Ave, PO Box 3050
Edison, NJ 08818-3050
www.middlesex.cc.nj.us

New York

LaGuardia Community College
Dietetic Technician-AD Prgm
City University of New York
31-10 Thomson Ave, Rm E300
Long Island City, NY 11101-3071
www.lagcc.cuny.edu

SUNY at Morrisville
Dietetic Technician-AD Prgm
Bailey Annex
Morrisville, NY 13408

Suffolk County Community College - Eastern Campus
Dietetic Technician-AD Prgm
121 Speonk-Riverhead Rd
Riverhead, NY 11901-3499
www.sunysuffolk.edu

Westchester Community College
Dietetic Technician-AD Prgm
75 Grasslands Rd
Student Center Building, Rm 215
Valhalla, NY 10595-1698
www.sunywcc.edu

Erie Community College - North Campus
Dietetic Technician-AD Prgm
6205 Main St
Williamsville, NY 14221-7095
www.ecc.edu

Trocaire College
Dietetic Technician-AD Prgm
6681 Transit Rd
Williamsville, NY 14221
www.trocaire.edu

North Carolina

Gaston College - Lincolnton
Dietetic Technician-AD Prgm
PO Box 600
Lincolnton, NC 28093
www.gaston.edu

Ohio

Cincinnati State Tech & Comm College
Dietetic Technician-AD Prgm
Health Technologies Div
3520 Central Pkwy
Cincinnati, OH 45223-2690
www.cincinnatistate.edu

Cuyahoga Community College
Dietetic Technician-AD Prgm
2900 Community College Ave
Cleveland, OH 44115-3196
www.tri-c.edu

Columbus State Community College
Dietetic Technician-AD Prgm
550 E Spring St, PO Box 1609
Columbus, OH 43216-1609
www.cscc.edu

Sinclair Community College
Dietetic Technician-AD Prgm
444 W Third St
Dayton, OH 45402-1460
www.sinclair.edu

Owens Community College
Dietetic Technician-AD Prgm
PO Box 10000
Oregon Rd
Toledo, OH 43699-1947
www.owens.edu

Youngstown State University
Dietetic Technician-AD Prgm
Dept of Human Ecology
One University Plaza
Youngstown, OH 44555-3344
www.ysu.edu

Oklahoma

Oklahoma State University
Dietetic Technician-AD Prgm
900 North Portland Ave
Oklahoma City, OK 73107-6120

Pennsylvania

Community College of Allegheny County
Dietetic Technician-AD Prgm
808 Ridge Ave
Pittsburgh, PA 15212-6097
www.ccac.edu

Penn State University
Dietetic Technician-AD Prgm
Coll of Health and Human Development
Hotel Rest & Recreation Mgmt
201 Mateer Bldg
University Park, PA 16802-1307
www.worldcampus.psu.edu

Tennessee

Southwest Tennessee Community College
Dietetic Technician-AD Prgm
PO Box 780
Union A-106
Memphis, TN 38101-0780
www.southwest.tn.edu

Texas

Tarrant County College - Southeast Campus
Dietetic Technician-AD Prgm
2100 Southeast Pkwy
Arlington, TX 76018
www.tccd.edu/campus/default.asp?menu=3

Wisconsin

Milwaukee Area Technical College
Dietetic Technician-AD Prgm
1200 S 71st St
West Allis, WI 53214-3110
www.matc.edu

DIETETICS

Expressive/Creative Arts Therapies

Includes:
- Art therapist
- Dance/movement therapist
- Music therapist

Art Therapist

History

Art therapy emerged as a distinct profession in the 1940s when hospitals and rehabilitation facilities increasingly began to include art therapy programs along with traditional "talk" therapies, underscoring the recognition that art making enhanced recovery, health and wellness. Since that time, the profession of art therapy has grown into an effective and important method of assessment and treatment with children, adults, families, and groups in a variety of settings, with art therapy having gained attention within the fields of psychiatry, medicine, psychology, counseling, education, and arts. Today, there are approximately 30 approved master's degree programs in art therapy across the United States.

The American Art Therapy Association, the official member organization for art therapy professionals and students, was founded in 1969 to develop and promote educational, professional and ethical standards for the field of art therapy. The AATA sponsors annual conferences, approves educational programs, and publishes *Art Therapy: Journal of the American Art Therapy Association*, the quarterly *American Art Therapy Association Newsletter*, the Monthly Update, books, and monographs.

Career Description

Art therapy is a mental health profession that uses the creative process of art making to improve and enhance the physical, mental, and emotional well being of individuals of all ages. It is based on the belief that the creative process of artistic self-expression helps people resolve conflicts and problems, develop interpersonal skills, manage behavior, reduce stress, increase self-esteem and self-awareness, and achieve insight. Art therapy integrates the fields of human development, visual art (drawing, painting, sculpture, and other art forms), and the creative process with models of counseling and psychotherapy. Art therapy programs and art therapists are found in a variety of settings, including hospitals and clinics, social service and community agencies, wellness centers, educational institutions, veterans' health facilities, and private practices. Art therapy is used with children, adolescents, adults, older adults, groups, and families to assess and treat the following:
- Anxiety, depression, and other mental and emotional conditions
- Substance abuse and other addictions
- Family and relationship issues
- Abuse and domestic violence
- Social and emotional difficulties related to disability and illness
- Trauma and loss
- Physical, cognitive, and neurological conditions
- Psychosocial difficulties related to chronic illnesses

Art therapists use drawing, painting, and other art processes to assess and treat clients with emotional, cognitive, physical, and/or developmental needs and disorders. Using their skills in evaluation and psychotherapy, they choose materials and interventions appropriate to their clients' needs and design sessions to achieve therapeutic goals and objectives. Art therapists also maintain appropriate charts, records, and periodic reports on client progress as required by agency guidelines and professional standards; participate in professional staff meetings and conferences; and provide information and consultation regarding the client's clinical progress. They also may function as supervisors, administrators, consultants, and expert witnesses. With the growing acceptance of complementary therapies and recent research findings on art therapy with medical populations, art therapy is increasingly being applied in practice for a variety of patient groups. For example, art therapists work with cancer, burn, pain, post-surgery, HIV-positive, asthma, and substance abuse patients, and with pediatric, geriatric, and other medical populations. In hospitals, art therapists may be part of psychiatric departments, child life programs, arts in hospital programs, or creative arts therapies or activity therapies departments.

An understanding of the application of various art media and art processes to treatment is central to the practice of art therapy. In general, an art therapist must be sensitive to a variety of human needs and possess emotional stability, patience, interpersonal skills, and a capacity for insight into psychological processes. An art therapist also must be an attentive listener and keen observer and be able to develop a rapport with people. Flexibility and a sense of humor are important in adapting to work with people with a wide range of mental health and health care needs and in a variety of settings. Many art therapists also hold credentials in mental health counseling or marriage and family therapy because of their training and experience.

Employment Characteristics

Art therapists work in many different health care environments, including:
- Hospitals and clinics (medical and psychiatric)
- Outpatient mental health agencies and day treatment facilities
- Residential treatment centers
- Domestic violence shelters and treatment settings
- Community agencies that serve individuals with disabilities
- Correctional facilities
- Elder care facilities
- Art studios
- Private practice
- Schools, colleges, and universities

An art therapist may work as part of a team that includes physicians, psychologists, nurses, mental health counselors, marriage and family therapists, rehabilitation counselors, social workers, and/or teachers. Together, they determine each client's therapeutic goals and objectives and implement a treatment plan. Other art therapists work independently and maintain private practices with children, adolescents, adults, groups, and/or families.

Salary

Earnings for art therapists vary depending on type of practice, job responsibilities, and practice location. The average entry-level income (2009 data) is approximately $39,000; median income is between $30,000 and $50,000; and top earning potential between $80,000 and $149,000. Art therapists who possess doctoral degrees and/or licensure or who qualify in their state to conduct a private practice can earn an average of $85 to $150 plus per hour as independent practitioners.

For more information, refer to *www.ama-assn.org/go/hpsalary*.

Educational Programs

Length. Art therapy master's degree programs are a minimum of two years and must include at least 24 graduate credit hours in the art therapy core curriculum. All AATA-approved educational programs include professional and mental health counseling competencies so that graduates can meet credential requirements for both art therapy board certification and counseling licensure.

Prerequisites. Applicants to master's degree programs must hold a baccalaureate degree from an accredited U.S. institution or have equivalent academic preparation from an institution outside the United States. In addition, prospective students must submit a portfolio of original artwork and must document 15 semester hours in studio art and 12 semester hours in psychology.

Curriculum. Educational requirements include
- Theories of art therapy, counseling, and psychotherapy
- Psychopathology
- Ethics and standards of practice
- Assessment and evaluation
- Individual, group, and family techniques
- Human and creative development
- Multicultural issues

- Research methods
- Practicum experiences in clinical, community, and/or other settings

Registration and Certification

The Art Therapy Credentials Board (ATCB) offers three levels of credentials:
- Registered Art Therapist (ATR), requiring specific graduate-level education in art therapy and documentation of supervised postgraduate clinical experience
- Board Certified Art Therapist (ATR-BC), which requires the successful completion of the national examination and demonstration of comprehensive knowledge of the theories and clinical skills used in art therapy
- An advanced supervisory credential (ATCS) for professional art therapists who have acquired specific training and skills in supervision and to ensure that supervisees receive the best training available.

Inquiries

Education, Program Approval, Careers, Resources
American Art Therapy Association (AATA), Inc
225 North Fairfax Street
Alexandria, VA 22314
703 548-5861
E-mail: *info@americanarttherapyassociation.org*
www.americanarttherapyassociation.org

Registration/Certification
Art Therapy Credentials Board (ATCB), Inc
3 Terrace Way
Greensboro, NC 27403-3660
877 213-2822 Toll-free
336 482-2856
E-mail: *atcb@nbcc.org*
www.atcb.org

Art Therapist

California

Notre Dame de Namur University
Art Therapy Prgm
1500 Ralston Ave
Belmont, CA 94002
www.ndnu.edu

Phillips Graduate Institute
Art Therapy Prgm
5445 Balboa Blvd
Encino, CA 91316-1509
www.pgi.edu

Loyola Marymount University
Art Therapy Prgm
Grad Dept of Marital and Family Therapy
1 LMU Dr
Los Angeles, CA 90045-2659
www.lmu.edu/mft

Colorado

Naropa University
Art Therapy Prgm
2130 Arapahoe Ave
Boulder, CO 80302
www.naropa.edu

Connecticut

Albertus Magnus College
Art Therapy Prgm
700 Prospect St
New Haven, CT 06511
www.albertus.edu

District of Columbia

George Washington University
Art Therapy Prgm
2129 G St NW, Bldg L, Rear
Washington, DC 20052
www.gwu.edu/~artx

Florida

Florida State University
Art Therapy Prgm
028 William Johnston Building
Tallahassee, FL 32306-1232
www.fsu.edu/~are

Illinois

Adler School of Professional Psychology
Art Therapy Prgm
65 E Wacker Pl, Ste 2100
Chicago, IL 60601-7298
www.adler.edu

School of the Art Institute of Chicago
Art Therapy Prgm
Dept of Art Therapy
37 S Wabash
Chicago, IL 60603-3103
www.saic.edu

Southern Illinois University Edwardsville
Art Therapy Prgm
Dept of Art and Design
Box 1764
Edwardsville, IL 62026-1764
www.siue.edu/artsandsciences/art/arttherapy/

Kansas

Emporia State University
Art Therapy Prgm
1200 Commercial St, Campus Box 4036
Emporia, KS 66801
www.emporia.edu/physpe/arttherapy/athp.html
Prgm Dir: Gaelynn Wolf Bordonaro, PhD ATR-BC
Tel: 620 341-5809
E-mail: gwolf@emporia.edu

Kentucky

University of Louisville
Art Therapy Prgm
Coll of Education and Human Dev Expressive Therapies
Louisville, KY 40292
louisville.edu/education/departments/ecpy/exp-therapy

Massachusetts

Lesley University
Art Therapy Prgm
Expressive Therapies
29 Everett St
Cambridge, MA 02138
www.lesley.edu

Springfield College
Art Therapy Prgm
Visual & Performing Arts
263 Alden St
Springfield, MA 01109-3797
www.springfieldcollege.edu
Prgm Dir: Simone Alter-Muri, Professor of Art
Therapy/Counseling and Art Education
Tel: 413 748-3752   *Fax:* 413 748-3580
E-mail: simone_alter-muri@springfieldcollege.edu

Michigan

Wayne State University
Art Therapy Prgm
163 Community Arts Bldg
Detroit, MI 48202
www.wayne.edu

New Jersey

Caldwell College
Art Therapy Prgm
9 Ryerson Ave
Caldwell, NJ 07006
www.caldwell.edu

New Mexico

Southwestern College
Art Therapy Prgm
Art Therapy/Counseling
PO Box 4788
Santa Fe, NM 87502-4788
www.swc.edu

New York

Pratt Institute
Art Therapy Prgm
200 Willoughby Ave
East 3
Brooklyn, NY 11205
www.pratt.edu

Long Island University - C W Post Campus
Art Therapy Prgm
720 Northern Blvd
Brookville, NY 11548
www.liu.edu

Hofstra University
Art Therapy Prgm
124 Hofstra University
Hempstead, NY 11549-1240
www.hofstra.edu

College of New Rochelle
Art Therapy Prgm
29 Castle Pl
Chapel Hall G 15
New Rochelle, NY 10805
www.cnr.edu

New York University
Art Therapy Prgm
34 Stuyvesant St
New York, NY 10003
www.nyu.edu

School of Visual Arts
Art Therapy Prgm
209 E 23rd St
New York, NY 10010
www.sva.edu

Nazareth College of Rochester
Art Therapy Prgm
Dr Ellen Horovitz
4245 East Ave
Rochester, NY 14618-3790
www.naz.edu/health-and-human-services/
creative-arts-therapy
Prgm Dir: Ellen G Horovitz, PhD ATR-BC LCAT RYT
Tel: 585 389-2535   *Fax:* 585 586-2452
E-mail: ehorovi4@naz.edu

Ohio

Ursuline College
Art Therapy Prgm
2550 Lander Rd
Pepper Pike, OH 44124
www.ursuline.edu
Prgm Dir: Gail Rule-Hoffman, MEd ATR-BC LPC-S
LICDC
Tel: 440 646-8139   *Fax:* 440 684-6135
E-mail: grulehoffman@ursuline.edu

Oregon

Marylhurst University
Art Therapy Prgm
Dept of Graduate Studies in Art Therapy Counseling
17600 Pacific Hwy, PO Box 261
Marylhurst, OR 97036
www.marylhurst.edu
Prgm Dir: Christine Turner, ATR-BC LPC NCC ACS
Tel: 503 699-6244   *Fax:* 503 534-4062
E-mail: cturner@marylhurst.edu

Pennsylvania

Seton Hill University
Art Therapy Prgm
PO Box 467F, Seton Hill Dr
Greensburg, PA 15601
www.setonhill.edu

Drexel University College of Medicine
Art Therapy Prgm
Hahnemann Creative Arts in Therapy Program
245 N 15th St
Philadelphia, PA 19102-1192
www.drexel.edu/cnhp/creativearts/

Marywood University
Art Therapy Prgm
Art Dept
2300 Adams Ave
Scranton, PA 18509

Quebec, Canada

Concordia University
Art Therapy Prgm
1455 de Maisonneuve Blvd W
Montreal, QC H3G 1M8

Virginia

Eastern Virginia Medical School
Art Therapy Prgm
PO Box 1980
Norfolk, VA 23501
www.evms.edu/hlthprof/art-therapy.html

Washington

Antioch University - Seattle
Art Therapy Prgm
2326 Sixth Ave
Seattle, WA 98121-1814
www.antiochsea.edu

Wisconsin

Mount Mary College
Art Therapy Prgm
2900 N Menomonee River Pkwy
Milwaukee, WI 53222-4545
www.mtmary.edu

Programs*	Class Capacity	Begins	Length (months)	Award	Res. Tuition	Non-res. Tuition	Offers:† 1	2	3	4
Kansas										
Emporia State Univ	20	Aug Jan	2	MS, MS MHC	$6,200	$16,300			•	
Massachusetts										
Springfield College	25	Sep	18	MS			•		•	
New York										
Nazareth College of Rochester	25	Sep May	24	Dipl, MS, MCAT	$21,300	$21,300	•		•	•
Ohio										
Ursuline College (Pepper Pike)	20	Aug Jan May	24	Dipl, MA	$18,000		•		•	
Oregon										
Marylhurst Univ	20	Sep	21	Cert, MA			•		•	

*Data are shown only for programs that completed the 2011 AMA Survey of Health Professions Education Programs.

†Key to Offers: 1: Evening or weekend classes; 2: Non-English instruction; 3: Cultural competence instruction; 4: Distance education component.

EXPRESSIVE/CREATIVE ARTS THERAPIES

Dance/Movement Therapist

Emerging as a distinct profession in the 1940s, dance/movement therapy, a creative arts therapy, is rooted in the expressive nature of dance itself. Dance is the most fundamental of the arts, involving a direct expression and experience of oneself through the body. It is a basic form of authentic communication, and as such it is an especially effective medium for therapy. Based in the belief that the body, mind, and spirit are interconnected, dance/movement therapy is defined by the American Dance Therapy Association (ADTA) as "The psychotherapeutic use of movement as a process that furthers the emotional, cognitive, social, and physical integration of the individual."

Career Description
Dance/movement therapists work with individuals of all ages, groups, and families in a wide variety of settings. They focus on helping their clients improve self-esteem and body image, develop effective communication skills and relationships, expand their movement vocabulary, and gain insight into patterns of behavior, as well as create new options for coping with problems. Dance/movement therapy can be a powerful tool for treatment of trauma and other mental and medical health problems, stress management, and the prevention of physical and mental health problems. Movement is the primary medium that dance/movement therapists use for observation, assessment, research, therapeutic interaction, and interventions.

Employment Characteristics
Dance/movement therapists work in settings that include psychiatric and rehabilitation facilities, schools, nursing homes, drug treatment centers, counseling centers, medical facilities, crisis centers, and wellness and alternative health care centers. Dance/movement therapy is used with people of all ages, races, and ethnic backgrounds in individual, couples, family, and group therapy formats.

There are approximately 1,300 dance/movement therapists in 46 states and 41 foreign countries.

Educational Programs
Length. Professional training for US dance/movement therapists is on the graduate level. Graduates receive a master's degree in dance/movement therapy or related degree title. Graduates from an ADTA-approved dance/movement therapy program are eligible for the R-DMT (Registered Dance/Movement Therapist) credential upon completion of graduate studies. Approved programs have met the basic educational standards of the ADTA, which include that the program's parent institution is accredited by its regional accreditation association.

Prerequisites. Extensive dance experience and a liberal arts background with coursework in psychology are required. For specific prerequisites, contact each graduate program.

Certification/Registration
The Dance/Movement Therapy Certification Board distinguishes between dance/movement therapists prepared to work in professional settings within a team under supervision and board-certified individuals who are prepared for the responsibilities of working independently in private practice, teaching, or providing supervision.

- *R-DMT: Registered Dance/Movement Therapist*—Therapists with this title have a master's degree and are fully qualified to work in a professional treatment system.
- *BC-DMT: Board Certified Dance/Movement Therapist*— Therapists with this title have met additional certification requirements and are fully qualified to teach, provide supervision, and engage in private practice.

Inquiries
American Dance Therapy Association
Dance/Movement Therapy Certification Board, Inc.
10632 Little Patuxent Parkway, Suite 108
Columbia, MD 21044-3263
410 997-4040
www.adta.org

Dance/Movement Therapist

Colorado

Naropa University
Dance/Movement Therapy Prgm
2130 Arapahoe Ave
Boulder, CO 80302
www.naropa.edu

Illinois

Columbia College
Dance/Movement Therapy Prgm
600 S Michigan Ave
Chicago, IL 60605-9988
www.colum.graddance.edu

Massachusetts

Lesley University
Dance/Movement Therapy Prgm
29 Everett St
Cambridge, MA 02138

New York

Pratt Institute
Dance/Movement Therapy Prgm
East 3, 200 Willoughby Ave
Brooklyn, NY 11205
www.pratt.edu/ad/ather

Music Therapist

Career Description
Music therapists use music within a therapeutic relationship to address physical, emotional, cognitive, and social needs of individuals of all ages, improving quality of life for persons who are well and meeting the needs of children and adults with disabilities or illnesses. After assessing the strengths and needs of each client, qualified music therapists develop a treatment plan with goals and objectives and then provide the indicated treatment. Music therapists structure the use of both instrumental and vocal music strategies to facilitate changes that are non-musical in nature. They may improvise or compose music with clients, accompany and conduct group music experiences, provide instrument instruction, direct music and movement interventions, or structure music listening opportunities. Music therapists provide services for children and adults with psychiatric disorders, developmental disabilities, speech and hearing impairments, physical disabilities, and neurological impairments, among others. Music therapy interventions can be designed to promote wellness, manage stress, improve physical functioning, alleviate pain, enhance memory and cognitive functioning, improve communication, and provide unique opportunities for interaction. Depending upon the needs of the clients involved, music therapy sessions are offered on an individual or group basis. Music therapists are usually members of an interdisciplinary team of health care professionals who work collaboratively to address clients treatment needs.

Personal Qualifications
Music therapists should have a genuine interest in people and a desire to help others empower themselves. The essence of music therapy practice involves establishing caring and professional relationships with people of all ages and abilities. Empathy, patience, tact, a sense of humor, imagination, creativity, and an understanding of oneself are important characteristics for professionals in this field. People thinking about music therapy as a career must be accomplished musicians. They must be versatile and able to adjust to changing circumstances. Music therapists must express themselves well in speech and in writing. In addition, they must be able to work well with other health care providers.

Employment Characteristics
Music therapists are employed in many different settings, including general and psychiatric hospitals, mental health agencies, physical rehabilitation centers, nursing homes, public and private schools, substance abuse programs, forensic facilities, hospice programs, and day care facilities. Typically, full-time therapists work a standard 40-hour workweek. Some therapists prefer part-time work and choose to develop contracts with specific agencies, providing music therapy services for an hourly or contractual fee. In addition, a growing number of clinicians are choosing to start private practices in music therapy to benefit from opportunities provided through self-employment.

Salary
According to the American Music Therapy Association (AMTA), the overall average salary for full-time music therapists was $48,066 in 2011. Individual salaries can vary by population served, work setting, geographic location, years of experience, and level of graduate education completed. The income range reported in 2011 included salaries up to $188,000.
For more information, refer to *www.ama-assn.org/go/hpsalary*.

Future Outlook
As an increasing number of consumers seek noninvasive, alternative and complementary therapies as treatment options, the need for music therapists continues to rise. The profession is currently experiencing an increase in requests for music therapy services with individuals diagnosed with autism as well as in early intervention programs and special education settings, in addition to an increased need for music therapy services with individuals diagnosed with Alzheimer disease in skilled facilities and community-based treatment programs. Other employment areas demonstrating growth include mental health settings, medical facilities, and self-employment/private practice opportunities.

Educational Programs
Length. Those who wish to become music therapists must earn a bachelor degree or higher in music therapy from one of over 70 AMTA-approved colleges and universities. NASM accreditation is a criterion for AMTA approval. Entry-level study requires academic coursework and 1,200 hours of clinical training, including a supervised internship.
Prerequisites. For entry into undergraduate programs, a high school diploma is required, along with demonstration of musicianship. Candidates for the master degree must hold a baccalaureate degree or equivalent in music therapy (see ertification below) or be working concurrently toward fulfilling degree equivalency requirements.
Curriculum. The curriculum is designed to impart entry-level competencies in three main areas: musical foundations, clinical foundations, and music therapy foundations and principles. Graduate programs in music therapy examine, with greater breadth and depth, issues relevant to the clinical, professional, and academic preparation of music therapists, usually in combination with established methods of research inquiry.

Certification
At the completion of academic and clinical training, students are eligible to take the national examination administered by the Certification Board for Music Therapists (CBMT), an independent, nonprofit certifying agency fully accredited by the National Commission for Certifying Agencies. After successful completion of the CBMT examination, graduates are issued the credential necessary for professional practice, Music Therapist-Board Certified (MT-BC). To demonstrate continued competence and to maintain this credential, music therapists are required to complete 100 hours of continuing music therapy education, or to retake and pass the CBMT examination within every five-year recertification cycle. *Note:* Those therapists on the

National Registry with the CMT (Certified Music Therapist) or RMT (Registered Music Therapist) credentials are qualified to practice under these certifications until 2020.

Inquiries

Education and Careers
American Music Therapy Association (AMTA)
8455 Colesville Road, Suite 1000
Silver Spring, MD 20910
301 589-3300
E-mail: *info@musictherapy.org*
www.musictherapy.org

Certification
Certification Board for Music Therapists (CBMT)
506 East Lancaster Avenue, Suite 102
Downingtown, PA 19335
800 765-2268 or 610 269-8900
E-mail: *info@cbmt.org*
www.cbmt.org

Program Accreditation
National Association of Schools of Music (NASM)
11250 Roger Bacon Drive, Suite 21
Reston, VA 20190
703 437-0700
E-mail: *info@arts-accredit.org*
http://nasm.arts-accredit.org

Music Therapist

Alabama

Auburn University
Music Therapy Prgm
Auburn, AL 36849-5420
auburn.edu/music

Samford University
Music Therapy Prgm
800 Lakeshore Dr
Birmingham, AL 35229
www.samford.edu/arts/music

University of Alabama at Birmingham
Music Therapy Prgm
Birmingham, AL 35294
www.music.uab.edu

University of North Alabama
Music Therapy Prgm
Florence, AL 35632-0001
www.una.edu/music

Univ of Alabama at Birmingham - Huntsville
Music Therapy Prgm
Roberts Hall 102
Huntsville, AL 35899
www.uah.edu/music

Jacksonville State University
Music Therapy Prgm
700 Pelham Rd North
Jacksonville, AL 36265
music.jsu.edu

Judson College
Music Therapy Prgm
302 Bibb St
Marion, AL 36756
www.judson.edu

University of Mobile
Music Therapy Prgm
5735 College Parkway
Mobile, AL 36613-2842
www.umobile.edu

University of South Alabama
Music Therapy Prgm
307 N University Blvd
Mobile, AL 36688-0002
www.southalabama.edu/music

University of Montevallo
Music Therapy Prgm
Montevallo, AL 35115
www.montevallo.edu/music

Alabama State University
Music Therapy Prgm
915 South Jackson St
Montgomery, AL 36104
www.alasu.edu

Huntingdon College
Music Therapy Prgm
1500 East Fairview Ave
Montgomery, AL 36106-2148
www.huntingdon.edu

Troy University
Music Therapy Prgm
114 Smith Hall
Troy, AL 36082
www.troy.edu

Stillman College
Music Therapy Prgm
PO Box 1430
Tuscaloosa, AL 35403
www.stillman.edu

University of Alabama
Music Therapy Prgm
School of Music
PO Box 870366
Tuscaloosa, AL 35487-0366
www.musictherapy.ua.edu

Alaska

University of Alaska Anchorage
Music Therapy Prgm
3211 Providence Dr
Anchorage, AK 99508
www.uaa.alaska.edu/music

University of Alaska - Fairbanks
Music Therapy Prgm
Fairbanks, AK 99775-5660

Arizona

Arizona State University
Music Therapy Prgm
School of Music
PO Box 870405
Tempe, AZ 85287-0405
www.asu.edu

University of Arizona
Music Therapy Prgm
Tucson, AZ 85721
www.music.arizona.edu

Arkansas

Ouachita Baptist University
Music Therapy Prgm
410 Ouachita St
Arkadelphia, AR 71998-0001
www.obu.edu

Hendrix College
Music Therapy Prgm
1600 Washington Ave
Conway, AR 72032
www.hendrix.edu

University of Central Arkansas
Music Therapy Prgm
201 Donaghey Ave
Conway, AR 72035-0001
uca.edu/cfac/music

University of Arkansas
Music Therapy Prgm
Fayetteville, AR 72701
music.uark.edu

University of Arkansas - Fort Smith
Music Therapy Prgm
5210 Grand Ave
Fort Smith, AR 72913
www.uafortsmith.edu

University of Arkansas at Little Rock
Music Therapy Prgm
2801 S University Ave
Little Rock, AR 72204
ualr.edu/music

Southern Arkansas University
Music Therapy Prgm
Magnolia, AR 71754-8000
www.saumag.edu

U of Arkansas at Monticello Coll of Tech
Music Therapy Prgm
PO Box 3607
Monticello, AR 71656
www.uamont.edu

University of Arkansas at Pine Bluff
Music Therapy Prgm
1200 North University Drive
Pine Bluff, AR 71611
www.uapb.edu

Arkansas State University
Music Therapy Prgm
State University, AR 72467
www.clt.astate.edu/finearts/music

California

Pacific Union College
Music Therapy Prgm
One Angwin Ave
Angwin, CA 94508-9797
www.puc.edu/academics/departments/music/home

Azusa Pacific University
Music Therapy Prgm
901 E Alosta Ave
Azusa, CA 91702

California State University - Dominguez Hills
Music Therapy Prgm
1000 East Victoria St
Carson, CA 90747
cah.csudh.edu/dnp/music/index.asp

California State University - Chico
Music Therapy Prgm
400 W First St
Chico, CA 95929-0805
www.csuchico.edu/mus

California State University - Fresno
Music Therapy Prgm
2380 E Keats Ave
Fresno, CA 93740-8024
www.csufresno.edu/music

California State University - East Bay
Music Therapy Prgm
Hayward, CA 94542
www.class.csueastbay.edu/music

Biola University
Music Therapy Prgm
13800 Biola Ave
La Mirada, CA 90639
www.biola.edu/music

California State University - Long Beach
Music Therapy Prgm
1250 Bellflower Blvd
Long Beach, CA 90840-7101
www.csulb.edu/~music

Loyola Marymount University
Music Therapy Prgm
One LMU Drive
Los Angeles, CA 90045-2659
cfa.lmu.edu/programs/music.htm

University of Southern California
Music Therapy Prgm
University Park
Los Angeles, CA 90089-0851
www.usc.edu/music

California State University - Northridge
Music Therapy Prgm
18111 Nordhoff St
Northridge, CA 91330
www.csun.edu

Chapman University
Music Therapy Prgm
School of Music
One University Dr
Orange, CA 92866
www1.chapman.edu/music/

California State University - San Bernardino
Music Therapy Prgm
5500 University Parkway
San Bernardino, CA 92407
music.csusb.edu

Point Loma Nazarene University
Music Therapy Prgm
3900 Lomaland Drive
San Diego, CA 92106-2899
www.pointloma.edu/music

San Francisco State University
Music Therapy Prgm
1600 Holloway Ave
San Francisco, CA 94132
musicdance.sfsu.edu

San Jose State University
Music Therapy Prgm
One Washington Square
San Jose, CA 95192-0095
www.sjsu.edu/depts/music

California Polytechnic State University
Music Therapy Prgm
One Grand Ave
San Luis Obispo, CA 93407-0326
www.music.calpoly.edu

University of the Pacific
Music Therapy Prgm
Conservatory of Music
3601 Pacific Ave
Stockton, CA 95211
http://web.pacific.edu/x1458.xml

California State University - Stanislaus
Music Therapy Prgm
One University Circle
Turlock, CA 95382
www.csustan.edu/music

Colorado

Adams State College
Music Therapy Prgm
208 Edgemont Blvd
Alamosa, CO 81102
www.music.adams.edu

University of Colorado at Boulder
Music Therapy Prgm
Boulder, CO 80309-0301
www.colorado.edu/music

Metropolitan State College of Denver
Music Therapy Prgm
Denver, CO 80217-3362
music.mscd.edu

Fort Lewis College
Music Therapy Prgm
1000 Rim Drive
Durango, CO 81301
www.fortlewis.edu

Colorado State University
Music Therapy Prgm
School of the Arts
Department of Music, Theatre and Dance
Fort Collins, CO 80523-1178
www.colostate.edu

Colorado Mesa University
Music Therapy Prgm
1100 North Ave
Grand Junction, CO 81501
www.coloradomesa.edu

Colorado Christian University
Music Therapy Prgm
8787 West Alameda Ave
Lakewood, CO 80226
www.ccu.edu

Colorado State University - Pueblo
Music Therapy Prgm
2200 Bonforte Blvd
Pueblo, CO 81001-4901
chass.colostate-pueblo.edu/music

Connecticut

Western Connecticut State University
Music Therapy Prgm
Danbury, CT 06810
www.wcsu.edu/music

Central Connecticut State University
Music Therapy Prgm
1615 Stanley St
New Britain, CT 06050
www.ccsu.edu

Yale University School of Medicine
Music Therapy Prgm
New Haven, CT 06520-8246
www.music.yale.edu

University of Connecticut
Music Therapy Prgm
Storrs, CT 06269-1012
www.music.uconn.edu

The Hartt School
Music Therapy Prgm
West Hartford, CT 06117
www.hartford.edu/hartt/community

Delaware

University of Delaware-Christiana Care Health
Music Therapy Prgm
Newark, DE 19716
www.music.udel.edu

District of Columbia

George Washington University
Music Therapy Prgm
Washington, DC 20052
www.gwu.edu/~music

Howard University
Music Therapy Prgm
College of Arts and Sciences, Music Dept
6th and Fairmont St NW
Washington, DC 20059

Florida

Florida Atlantic University
Music Therapy Prgm
Boca Raton, FL 33431
www.fau.edu/music

The Players School of Music
Music Therapy Prgm
923 McMullen Booth Rd
Clearwater, FL 33759
www.playerschool.com

University of Miami
Music Therapy Prgm
Frost School of Music
PO Box 248165
Coral Gables, FL 33124

Stetson University
Music Therapy Prgm
Deland, FL 32723
www.stetson.edu/music

University of Florida
Music Therapy Prgm
Gainesville, FL 32611-7900
www.arts.ufl.edu/music

University of North Florida
Music Therapy Prgm
1 University of North Florida Drive
Jacksonville, FL 32224-2645
www.unf.edu/coas/music

EXPRESSIVE/CREATIVE ARTS THERAPIES

Florida International University
Music Therapy Prgm
11200 Southwest 8th St
Miami, FL 33199
music.fiu.edu

New World Symphony
Music Therapy Prgm
500 17th St
Miami Beach, FL 33139
www.nws.edu

University of Central Florida
Music Therapy Prgm
4000 Central Florida Blvd
Orlando, FL 32816-1354
www.music.ucf.edu

University of West Florida
Music Therapy Prgm
11000 University Parkway
Pensacola, FL 32514-5751
www.uwf.edu/music

Florida State University
Music Therapy Prgm
College of Music
Tallahassee, FL 32306-1180

University of South Florida
Music Therapy Prgm
Tampa, FL 33620
music.arts.usf.edu

University of Tampa
Music Therapy Prgm
Department of Music
Tampa, FL 33606
www.ut.edu

Palm Beach Atlantic University
Music Therapy Prgm
West Palm Beach, FL 33416-4708
www.pba.edu

Rollins College
Music Therapy Prgm
Winter Park, FL 32789
www.rollins.edu/music

Georgia

University of Georgia
Music Therapy Prgm
School of Music
Fine Arts Bldg
Athens, GA 30602-3153

Georgia State University
Music Therapy Prgm
Atlanta, GA 30302-4097
www.music.gsu.edu

University of West Georgia
Music Therapy Prgm
1601 Maple St
Carrollton, GA 30118-2210
www.westga.edu/~musicdpt

Columbus State University
Music Therapy Prgm
4225 University Ave
Columbus, GA 31907-5645
music.colstate.edu

Kennesaw State University
Music Therapy Prgm
1000 Chastain Rd
Kennesaw, GA 30144
www.kennesaw.edu/music

Georgia College & State University
Music Therapy Prgm
C BX 067
Milledgeville, GA 31061
http://musictherapy.gcsu.edu

Georgia Southern University
Music Therapy Prgm
Statesboro, GA 30460-8052
class.georgiasouthern.edu/music

Valdosta State University
Music Therapy Prgm
Valdosta, GA 31698
www.valdosta.edu/music

Hawaii

University of Hawaii at Manoa
Music Therapy Prgm
Honolulu, HI 96822
www.hawaii.edu/uhmmusic

Idaho

Boise State University
Music Therapy Prgm
1910 University Dr
Boise, ID 83725-1560
www.boisestate.edu/music

University of Idaho
Music Therapy Prgm
Moscow, ID 83844-4015
music.uidaho.edu

Northwest Nazarene University
Music Therapy Prgm
623 Holly St
Nampa, ID 83686
www.nnu.edu/music

Idaho State University
Music Therapy Prgm
921 S 8th Ave
Pocatello, ID 83209
www.isu.edu/music

Illinois

Illinois Wesleyan University
Music Therapy Prgm
Bloomington, IL 61702-2900
www.iwu.edu/music

Olivet Nazarene University
Music Therapy Prgm
One University Dr
Bourbonnais, IL 60914
music.olivet.edu

Southern Illinois University Carbondale
Music Therapy Prgm
Carbondale, IL 62901
www.siu.edu/~music

Eastern Illinois University
Music Therapy Prgm
600 Lincoln Ave
Charleston, IL 61920
www.eiu.edu/~music

DePaul University
Music Therapy Prgm
804 W Belden Ave
Chicago, IL 60614
music.depaul.edu

Northeastern Illinois University
Music Therapy Prgm
5500 North Saint Louis Ave
Chicago, IL 60625-4699
www.neiu.edu/~music

Millikin University
Music Therapy Prgm
1184 West Main St
Decatur, IL 62522
www.millikin.edu/music

Northern Illinois University
Music Therapy Prgm
1425 West Lincoln Highway
DeKalb, IL 60115-2828
www.niu.edu/music

Southern Illinois University Edwardsville
Music Therapy Prgm
Edwardsville, IL 62026
www.siue.edu/MUSIC

Northwestern University
Music Therapy Prgm
711 Elgin Rd
Evanston, IL 60208-1200
www.music.northwestern.edu

Western Illinois University
Music Therapy Prgm
Music Dept
Macomb, IL 61455
www.wiu.edu

Illinois State University
Music Therapy Prgm
5660 School of Music
Normal, IL 61790-5660

Univ of Illinois at Urbana-Champaign
Music Therapy Prgm
1114 West Nevada St
Urbana, IL 61801
www.music.uiuc.edu

Indiana

Indiana University
Music Therapy Prgm
1201 East Third St
Bloomington, IN 47405
www.music.indiana.edu

University of Evansville
Music Therapy Prgm
Dept of Music
1800 Lincoln Ave
Evansville, IN 47722
http://music.evansville.edu

Indiana Univ - Purdue Univ Ft Wayne
Music Therapy Prgm
2101 Coliseum Blvd E
Fort Wayne, IN 46805-1499
www.ipfw.edu/academics/programs/undergraduate/m/
    music-therapy/

DePauw University
Music Therapy Prgm
605 South College St
Greencastle, IN 46135
www.depauw.edu/music

Indiana Univ-Purdue Univ-Indianapolis
Music Therapy Prgm
Department of Music and Arts Technology
535 W Michigan St, IT 379
Indianapolis, IN 46202
www.music.iupui.edu

University of Indianapolis
Music Therapy Prgm
1400 East Hanna Ave
Indianapolis, IN 46227
music.uindy.edu

Ball State University
Music Therapy Prgm
Muncie, IN 47306-0410
www.bsu.edu/music

St Mary of the Woods College
Music Therapy Prgm
Dept of Performing and Visual Arts
St Mary of the Woods, IN 47876
www.smwc.edu

Indiana State University
Music Therapy Prgm
Terre Haute, IN 47809
www.indstate.edu/music

Valparaiso University
Music Therapy Prgm
Valparaiso, IN 46383-6493
www.valpo.edu/music

Iowa

Iowa State University
Music Therapy Prgm
Ames, IA 50011
www.music.iastate.edu

University of Northern Iowa
Music Therapy Prgm
Cedar Falls, IA 50614-0246
www.uni.edu/music

University of Iowa
Music Therapy Prgm
School of Music
Voxman Music Bldg
Iowa City, IA 52242
www.uiowa.edu

Wartburg College
Music Therapy Prgm
Music Department, 100 Wartburg Blvd
Waverly, IA 50677

Kansas

Fort Hays State University
Music Therapy Prgm
600 Park St
Hays, KS 67601-4099
www.fhsu.edu/music

University of Kansas
Music Therapy Prgm
Art, Music Ed and Music Therapy
311 Bailey Hall
Lawrence, KS 66045
www.ku.edu

Kansas State University
Music Therapy Prgm
Manhattan, KS 66506-4702
www.k-state.edu/music

Pittsburg State University
Music Therapy Prgm
1701 South Broadway
Pittsburg, KS 66762-7511
www.pittstate.edu/music

Washburn University
Music Therapy Prgm
Topeka, KS 66621
www.washburn.edu/music

Kentucky

Western Kentucky University
Music Therapy Prgm
1906 College Heights Blvd
Bowling Green, KY 42101-1029
www.wku.edu/music

Northern Kentucky University
Music Therapy Prgm
Nunn Drive
Highland Heights, KY 41099
music.nku.edu

University of Kentucky
Music Therapy Prgm
Lexington, KY 40506-0022
www.uky.edu/finearts/music

University of Louisville
Music Therapy Prgm
School of Music
Louisville, KY 40292
www.louisville.edu/music/therapy

Murray State University
Music Therapy Prgm
Murray, KY 42071-0009
www.murraystate.edu/chfa/music

Eastern Kentucky University
Music Therapy Prgm
Richmond, KY 40475
www.music.eku.edu

Louisiana

Louisiana State University
Music Therapy Prgm
Baton Rouge, LA 70803
www.music.lsu.edu

Southeastern Louisiana University
Music Therapy Prgm
Hammond, LA 70402
www.selu.edu/music

University of Louisiana at Lafayette
Music Therapy Prgm
Lafayette, LA 70504-1207
music.louisiana.edu

University of Louisiana at Monroe
Music Therapy Prgm
Monroe, LA 71209-0250
www.ulm.edu/music

Northwestern State University
Music Therapy Prgm
Northwestern State University of Louisiana
140 Central Ave
Natchitoches, LA 71497
www.nsula.edu/capa/music

Loyola University New Orleans
Music Therapy Prgm
College of Music
6363 St Charles Ave
New Orleans, LA 70118
www.loyno.edu

University of New Orleans
Music Therapy Prgm
Lakefront
New Orleans, LA 70148
www.music.uno.edu

Maine

University of Southern Maine
Music Therapy Prgm
37 College Ave
Gorham, ME 04038
www.usm.maine.edu/music

Maryland

Univ of Maryland at College Park
Music Therapy Prgm
College Park, MD 20742-1211
www.music.umd.edu

Montgomery College
Music Therapy Prgm
51 Mannakee St
Rockville, MD 20850
www.montgomerycollege.edu/departments/musicrv

Salisbury University
Music Therapy Prgm
1101 Camden Ave
Salisbury, MD 21801-6860
www.salisbury.edu/musicdept

Towson University
Music Therapy Prgm
8000 York Rd
Towson, MD 21252-0001
www.towson.edu/music

Massachusetts

University of Massachusetts - Amherst
Music Therapy Prgm
Amherst, MA 01003
www.umass.edu/music

Berklee College of Music
Music Therapy Prgm
Chair, Music Therapy Dept
1140 Boylston St
Boston, MA 02215-3693
www.berklee.edu

Lesley University
Music Therapy Prgm
Expressive Therapics Division
29 Everett St
Cambridge, MA 02138
www.lesley.edu

University of Massachusetts - Lowell
Music Therapy Prgm
Lowell, MA 01854
www.uml.edu/dept/music

Anna Maria College
Music Therapy Prgm
Dept of Music, Box 45
Paxton, MA 01612-1198
www.annamaria.edu

Salem State University
Music Therapy Prgm
352 Lafayette St
Salem, MA 01970
www.salemstate.edu/music

Westfield State College
Music Therapy Prgm
577 Western Ave
Westfield, MA 01086-1630
www.wsc.ma.edu/music

Michigan

Albion College
Music Therapy Prgm
611 E Porter St
Albion, MI 49224
www.albion.edu/music

Grand Valley State University
Music Therapy Prgm
1 Campus Drive
Allendale, MI 49401-9403
www.gvsu.edu/music

University of Michigan
Music Therapy Prgm
Ann Arbor, MI 48109-2085
www.music.umich.edu

Andrews University
Music Therapy Prgm
100 Old US 31
Berrien Springs, MI 49104
www.andrews.edu/music

Wayne State University
Music Therapy Prgm
1321 Old Main
Detroit, MI 48202
music.wayne.edu

Michigan State University
Music Therapy Prgm
School of Music
East Lansing, MI 48824-1043
www.music.msu.edu

Calvin College
Music Therapy Prgm
3201 Burton St, Southeast
Grand Rapids, MI 49546
www.calvin.edu/music

Western Michigan University
Music Therapy Prgm
School of Music
1903 W Michigan Ave
Kalamazoo, MI 49008-3834
www.wmich.edu/musictherapy

Northern Michigan University
Music Therapy Prgm
1401 Presque Isle Ave
Marquette, MI 49855-5365
www.nmu.edu/music

Central Michigan University
Music Therapy Prgm
Mount Pleasant, MI 48859
www.music.cmich.edu

Saginaw Valley State University
Music Therapy Prgm
7400 Bay Rd
University City, MI 48710
www.svsu.edu/abs/music

Eastern Michigan University
Music Therapy Prgm
Dept of Music and Dance
N101 Alexander Bldg
Ypsilanti, MI 48197
www.emich.edu/music/html/music_therapy.html

Minnesota

Bemidji State University
Music Therapy Prgm
1500 Birchmont Drive, Northeast
Bemidji, MN 56601-2699
www.bemidjistate.edu/academics/departments/music

University of Minnesota - Duluth
Music Therapy Prgm
1201 Ordean Court
Duluth, MN 55812
www.d.umn.edu/music

Augsburg College
Music Therapy Prgm
2211 Riverside Ave
Minneapolis, MN 55454
www.augsburg.edu

University of Minnesota
Music Therapy Prgm
School of Music
2106 4th St S
Minneapolis, MN 55455

St Cloud State University
Music Therapy Prgm
720 Fourth Ave South
Saint Cloud, MN 56301-4498
www.stcloudstate.edu/music

College of St Benedict/St John's University
Music Therapy Prgm
37 S College Ave
Saint Joseph, MN 56374
www.csbsju.edu/music

Winona State University
Music Therapy Prgm
Winona, MN 55987-5838
www.winona.edu/music

Mississippi

Mississippi University for Women
Music Therapy Prgm
Department of Music and Theatre W-70
1100 College St
Columbus, MS 39701

William Carey University
Music Therapy Prgm
498 Tuscan Ave
Hattiesburg, MS 39401
www.wmcarey.edu

University of Mississippi
Music Therapy Prgm
University, MS 38677
www.olemiss.edu/depts/music

Missouri

Southwest Baptist University
Music Therapy Prgm
1600 University Ave
Bolivar, MO 65613-2496
www.sbuniv.edu/music

Southeast Missouri State University
Music Therapy Prgm
One University Plaza
Cape Girardeau, MO 63701
www.semo.edu/music

University of Missouri
Music Therapy Prgm
Columbia, MO 65211
music.missouri.edu

University of Missouri - Kansas City
Music Therapy Prgm
Conservatory of Music, 316 Grant Hall
4949 Cherry
Kansas City, MO 64110-2229

Truman State University
Music Therapy Prgm
100 East Normal St
Kirksville, MO 63501
music.truman.edu

Northwest Missouri State University
Music Therapy Prgm
800 University Dr
Maryville, MO 64468
www.nwmissouri.edu/dept/music

Missouri Western State University
Music Therapy Prgm
4525 Downs Dr
Saint Joseph, MO 64507-2294
www.missouriwestern.edu/music

Drury University
Music Therapy Prgm
900 N Benton Ave
Springfield, MO 65802

Maryville University
Music Therapy Prgm
650 Maryville University Dr
St Louis, MO 63141
www.maryville.edu

University of Central Missouri
Music Therapy Prgm
Warrensburg, MO 64093
www.ucmo.edu/music

Montana

Montana State University Billings
Music Therapy Prgm
Billings, MT 59101-0298
www.msubillings.edu/cas/music

Montana State University
Music Therapy Prgm
Bozeman, MT 59717-3420
www.montana.edu/music

Nebraska

University of Nebraska - Kearney
Music Therapy Prgm
2506 12th Ave
Kearney, NE 68849-3220
www.unk.edu/acad/music/

Nebraska Wesleyan University
Music Therapy Prgm
5000 St Paul Ave
Lincoln, NE 68504-2794
www.music.nebrwesleyan.edu

University of Nebraska - Lincoln
Music Therapy Prgm
Lincoln, NE 68588-0100
www.unl.edu/music

University of Nebraska - Omaha
Music Therapy Prgm
Omaha, NE 68182-0245
www.music.unomaha.edu

Nevada

University of Nevada - Las Vegas
Music Therapy Prgm
4505 Maryland Pkwy
Las Vegas, NV 89154-5025
music.unlv.edu

University of Nevada - Reno
Music Therapy Prgm
Reno, NV 89557-0049
www.unr.edu/cla/music

New Hampshire

University of New Hampshire
Music Therapy Prgm
Durham, NH 03824
www.unh.edu/music

Keene State College
Music Therapy Prgm
229 Main St
Keene, NH 03435-2402
music.keene.edu

New Jersey

The College of New Jersey
Music Therapy Prgm
Ewing, NJ 08628-0718
www.tcnj.edu/~music

Montclair State University
Music Therapy Prgm
Montclair, NJ 07043
www.montclair.edu/music

Montclair State University
Music Therapy Prgm
Music Dept
Upper Montclair, NJ 07043
www.montclair.edu/music

New Mexico

University of New Mexico
Music Therapy Prgm
Albuquerque, NM 87131-1411
music.unm.edu

New Mexico State University
Music Therapy Prgm
Las Cruces, NM 88003
www.nmsu.edu/~music

New York

Binghamton University
Music Therapy Prgm
State University of New York
Vestal Parkway East
Binghamton, NY 13902-6000
www2.binghamton.edu/music

SUNY Fredonia
Music Therapy Prgm
School of Music
Mason Hall
Fredonia, NY 14063
www.fredonia.edu/som/musTherapy.asp

Ithaca College
Music Therapy Prgm
Ithaca, NY 14850
www.ithaca.edu/music

SUNY at New Paltz
Music Therapy Prgm
Music Dept
1 Hawk Dr
New Paltz, NY 12561

New York University
Music Therapy Prgm
35 W 4th St
New York, NY 10012
www.nyu.edu

Nazareth College of Rochester
Music Therapy Prgm
4245 East Ave
Rochester, NY 14618
www.naz.edu

Roberts Wesleyan College
Music Therapy Prgm
2301 Westside Drive
Rochester, NY 14624
www.roberts.edu/music

North Carolina

Appalachian State University
Music Therapy Prgm
Hayes School of Music
813 River St
Boone, NC 28608
www.music.appstate.edu

Queens University of Charlotte
Music Therapy Prgm
Music Dept
1900 Selwyn Ave
Charlotte, NC 28274
www.queens.edu

North Carolina A&T State University
Music Therapy Prgm
1601 East Market St
Greensboro, NC 27411
www.ncat.edu/~music

East Carolina University
Music Therapy Prgm
212 A J Fletcher Music Center
Greenville, NC 27858
www.ecu.edu

Meredith College
Music Therapy Prgm
3800 Hillsborough St
Raleigh, NC 27607-5298
www.meredith.edu/music

North Dakota

University of North Dakota
Music Therapy Prgm
3350 Campus Rd, Stop 7125
HFA Building, Rm 110
Grand Forks, ND 58202
www.undmusic.org

Minot State University
Music Therapy Prgm
500 University Ave W
Minot, ND 58707
minotstateu.edu/music

Ohio

The University of Akron
Music Therapy Prgm
Akron, OH 44325-1002
www.uakron.edu/music

Ohio University
Music Therapy Prgm
School of Music
440 Music Bldg
Athens, OH 45701
www.ohio.edu

Baldwin-Wallace College
Music Therapy Prgm
Cleveland Consortium
275 Eastland Rd
Berea, OH 44017
www.bw.edu

Bowling Green State University
Music Therapy Prgm
Bowling Green, OH 43403-0290
www.bgsu.edu/music

Xavier University
Music Therapy Prgm
3800 Victory Pkwy
Cincinnati, OH 45207
www.xu.edu/music

Case Western Reserve University
Music Therapy Prgm
10900 Euclid Ave
Cleveland, OH 44106-7105
www.music.case.edu

Cleveland State University
Music Therapy Prgm
Cleveland, OH 44115-2403
www.csuohio.edu/music

Capital University
Music Therapy Prgm
One College and Main
Columbus, OH 43209-2394
music.capital.edu

University of Dayton
Music Therapy Prgm
Music Dept
300 College Park Ave
Dayton, OH 45469-0290
www.udayton.edu

Kent State University
Music Therapy Prgm
Kent, OH 44242-0001
dept.kent.edu/music

University of Toledo
Music Therapy Prgm
Toledo, OH 43606-3390
www.utoledo.edu/as/music

College of Wooster
Cosponsor: Cleveland Music Therapy Consortium
Music Therapy Prgm
Dept of Music
Wooster, OH 44691
www.wooster.edu

Oklahoma

University of Oklahoma
Music Therapy Prgm
Norman, OK 73019-2071
www.music.ou.edu

Oklahoma Christian University
Music Therapy Prgm
Oklahoma City, OK 73136-1100
www.oc.edu/music

Oklahoma State University
Music Therapy Prgm
Stillwater, OK 74078-4077
music.okstate.edu

Northeastern State University
Music Therapy Prgm
605 N Grand Ave
Tahlequah, OK 74464
www.nsumusic.com

Southwestern Oklahoma State University
Music Therapy Prgm
Music Therapy Division
100 Campus Dr
Weatherford, OK 73096
www.swosu.edu/music/therapy
Prgm Dir: ChihChen Sophia Lee, PhD MT-BC
Tel: 580 774-3218   *Fax:* 580 774-3714
E-mail: sophia.lee@swosu.edu

EXPRESSIVE/CREATIVE ARTS THERAPIES

Ontario, Canada

University of Windsor
Music Therapy Prgm
School of Music
Windsor, ON N9B 3P4
www.uwindsor.ca/music

Oregon

University of Oregon
Music Therapy Prgm
Eugene, OR 97403-1225
music.uoregon.edu

Marylhurst University
Music Therapy Prgm
17600 Pacific Hwy (Hwy 43)
Marylhurst, OR 97036-0261
www.marylhurst.edu

Linfield College
Music Therapy Prgm
McMinnville, OR 97128
www.linfield.edu/music

Portland State University
Music Therapy Prgm
Portland, OR 97207-0751
www.pdx.edu/music

Pennsylvania

Bloomsburg University
Music Therapy Prgm
400 E Second St
Bloomsburg, PA 17815
www.bloomu.edu/academic/mus

Elizabethtown College
Music Therapy Prgm
Dept of Fine and Performing Arts
One Alpha Dr
Elizabethtown, PA 17022-2298
www.etown.edu

Messiah College
Music Therapy Prgm
One College Ave
Grantham, PA 17027
www.messiah.edu/music

Immaculata University
Music Therapy Prgm
Dept of Music
Box 703
Immaculata, PA 19345
www.immaculata.edu

Indiana University of Pennsylvania
Music Therapy Prgm
422 S Eleventh St
Indiana, PA 15705
www.arts.iup.edu/music

Mansfield University
Music Therapy Prgm
Dept of Music
Mansfield, PA 16933

Drexel University College of Medicine
Music Therapy Prgm
245 N 15th St, MS 905
Philadelphia, PA 19102-1192

Temple University
Music Therapy Prgm
Boyer College of Music and Dance 012-00
Philadelphia, PA 19122
www.temple.edu/musictherapy

Duquesne University
Music Therapy Prgm
Mary Pappert School of Music
600 Forbes Ave
Pittsburgh, PA 15282
www.duq.edu

Marywood University
Music Therapy Prgm
2300 Adams Ave
Scranton, PA 18509
www.marywood.edu

Susquehanna Health / Williamsport Hospital
Music Therapy Prgm
Susquehanna University
514 University Ave
Selinsgrove, PA 17870
www.susqu.edu/music

Slippery Rock University of Pennsylvania
Music Therapy Prgm
Dept of Music
Slippery Rock, PA 16057

Penn State University
Music Therapy Prgm
University Park, PA 16802
www.music.psu.edu

Rhode Island

University of Rhode Island
Music Therapy Prgm
Kingston, RI 02881-0820
www.uri.edu/artsci/mus

Rhode Island College
Music Therapy Prgm
600 Mount Pleasant Ave
Providence, RI 02908-1991
www.ric.edu/mtd/music

South Carolina

Charleston Southern University
Music Therapy Prgm
9200 University Blvd, PO Box 118087
Charleston, SC 29423-8087
www.csuniv.edu

College of Charleston
Music Therapy Prgm
66 George St
Charleston, SC 29424-0001

University of South Carolina
Music Therapy Prgm
Columbia, SC 29208
www.music.sc.edu

South Dakota

University of South Dakota
Music Therapy Prgm
414 E Clark St
Vermillion, SD 57069
www.usd.edu/cfa/Music

Tennessee

University of Tennessee - Chattanooga
Music Therapy Prgm
615 McCallie Ave
Chattanooga, TN 37403
www.utc.edu/music

Austin Peay State University
Music Therapy Prgm
Clarksville, TN 37044
www.apsu.edu/music

Tennessee Technological University
Music Therapy Prgm
Dept of Music and Art
Box 5045
Cookeville, TN 38505

Union University
Music Therapy Prgm
1050 Union University Drive
Jackson, TN 38305-3697
www.uu.edu/academics/coas/music

East Tennessee State University
Music Therapy Prgm
Johnson City, TN 37614
www.etsu.edu/music

University of Tennessee - Knoxville
Music Therapy Prgm
Knoxville, TN 37996-2600
www.music.utk.edu

University of Memphis
Music Therapy Prgm
3775 Central Ave
Memphis, TN 38152

Middle Tennessee State University
Music Therapy Prgm
1301 East Main St
Murfreesboro, TN 37132
www.mtsumusic.com

Belmont University
Music Therapy Prgm
1900 Belmont Blvd
Nashville, TN 37212-3757
www.belmont.edu/music

Lipscomb University
Music Therapy Prgm
One University Park Drive
Nashville, TN 37204-3951
music.lipscomb.edu

Tennessee State University
Music Therapy Prgm
3500 John A Merritt Blvd
Nashville, TN 37209-1561
www.tnstate.edu/music

Texas

Abilene Christian University
Music Therapy Prgm
Abilene, TX 79699-8274
www.acu.edu/music

University of Texas at Arlington
Music Therapy Prgm
Arlington, TX 76019
www.uta.edu/music

University of Texas at Austin
Music Therapy Prgm
One University Station, E3100
Austin, TX 78712-0435
www.music.utexas.edu

West Texas A&M University
Music Therapy Prgm
Dept of Music
WTAMU Box 60879
Canyon, TX 79016-0001

Texas A&M University - Commerce
Music Therapy Prgm
Commerce, TX 75428
www7.tamu-commerce.edu/music

Del Mar College
Music Therapy Prgm
101 Baldwin Blvd
Corpus Christi, TX 78404-3897
www.delmar.edu/music

Southern Methodist University
Music Therapy Prgm
Meadows School of the Arts
Div of Music Therapy
Dallas, TX 75275
www.smu.edu

Texas Woman's University
Music Therapy Prgm
PO Box 425768
TWU Station
Denton, TX 76204
www.twu.edu

University of North Texas
Music Therapy Prgm
Denton, TX 76203-5017
www.music.unt.edu

University of Texas at El Paso
Music Therapy Prgm
El Paso, TX 79968-0552
www.utep.edu/music

Texas Christian University
Music Therapy Prgm
Fort Worth, TX 76129
www.music.tcu.edu

Texas Wesleyan University
Music Therapy Prgm
1201 Wesleyan St
Fort Worth, TX 76105
www. web3.txwes.edu/music/music/index.htm

University of Houston
Music Therapy Prgm
Houston, TX 77204-4017
www.music.uh.edu

Sam Houston State University
Music Therapy Prgm
School of Music, Box 2208, SHSU
Huntsville, TX 77341

Texas Tech University
Music Therapy Prgm
Lubbock, TX 79409-2033
www.depts.ttu.edu/music

Stephen F Austin State University
Music Therapy Prgm
Nacogdoches, TX 75962-3043
www.music.sfasu.edu

Angelo State University
Music Therapy Prgm
San Angelo, TX 76909
www.angelo.edu/dept/artmusic

The University of the Incarnate Word
Music Therapy Prgm
4301 Broadway Ave
PO Box 340
San Antonio, TX 78209
www.uiw.edu
Prgm Dir: Janice Dvorkin, DPsy ACMT
Tel: 210 829-3856   *Fax:* 210 829-3880
E-mail: dvorkin@uiwtx.edu

Texas State University - San Marcos
Music Therapy Prgm
San Marcos, TX 78666-4616
www.music.txstate.edu

Tarleton State University
Music Therapy Prgm
Stephenville, TX 76402
www.tarleton.edu/~music

Utah

Utah State University
Music Therapy Prgm
4015 Old Main Hill, Department of Music
Logan, UT 84322
www.usu.edu

Brigham Young University
Music Therapy Prgm
Provo, UT 84602-6410
music.byu.edu

University of Utah
Music Therapy Prgm
1375 East Presidents Circle
Salt Lake City, UT 84112
www.music.utah.edu

Virginia

Virginia Polytechnic Inst & State Univ
Music Therapy Prgm
Blacksburg, VA 24061
www.music.vt.edu

George Mason University
Music Therapy Prgm
4400 University Dr
Fairfax, VA 22030-4444
music.gmu.edu

Longwood University
Music Therapy Prgm
Farmville, VA 23909
www.longwood.edu/music

James Madison University
Music Therapy Prgm
800 S Main St
Harrisonburg, VA 22801
www.jmu.edu/music

Radford University
Music Therapy Prgm
Dept of Music
Radford, VA 24142
www.radford.edu

Shenandoah University
Music Therapy Prgm
1460 University Dr
Winchester, VA 22601-5195
www.su.edu

Washington

Western Washington University
Music Therapy Prgm
Bellingham, WA 98225-9107
www.wwu.edu/music

Central Washington University
Music Therapy Prgm
400 East University Way
Ellensburg, WA 98926-7458
www.cwu.edu/~music

Washington State University
Music Therapy Prgm
Pullman, WA 99164-5300
www.libarts.wsu.edu/music

University of Washington
Music Therapy Prgm
Seattle, WA 98195-3450
www.music.washington.edu

Pacific Lutheran University
Music Therapy Prgm
Tacoma, WA 98447
www.plu.edu/~music/

University of Puget Sound
Music Therapy Prgm
Tacoma, WA 98416-1076
www.ups.edu/music

West Virginia

Marshall University
Music Therapy Prgm
One John Marshall Dr
Huntington, WV 25755
www.marshall.edu/cofa/music

Wisconsin

University of Wisconsin - Eau Claire
Music Therapy Prgm
Dept of Public Health Professions
College of Nursing and Health Sciences
Eau Claire, WI 54702-4004
www.uwec.edu/ph/mt/index.htm

Carthage College
Music Therapy Prgm
2001 Alford Park Drive
Kenosha, WI 53140-1994
www.carthage.edu/departments/music

University of Wisconsin - La Crosse
Music Therapy Prgm
La Crosse, WI 54601
www.uwlax.edu/music

University of Wisconsin - Madison
Music Therapy Prgm
455 N Park St
Madison, WI 53706
www.music.wisc.edu

Alverno College
Music Therapy Prgm
3401 S 39th St, PO Box 3439222
Milwaukee, WI 53234-3922
www.alverno.edu

University of Wisconsin - Oshkosh
Music Therapy Prgm
800 Algoma Blvd
Oshkosh, WI 54901
www.uwosh.edu

University of Wisconsin - River Falls
Music Therapy Prgm
River Falls, WI 54022-5001
www.uwrf.edu/music

University of Wisconsin - Stevens Point
Music Therapy Prgm
2100 Main St
Stevens Point, WI 54481
www.uwsp.edu/music

University of Wisconsin - Superior
Music Therapy Prgm
Belknap and Catlin
Superior, WI 54880-4500
www.uwsuper.edu/music

University of Wisconsin - Whitewater
Music Therapy Prgm
800 W Main St
Whitewater, WI 53190
www.academics.uww.edu/cac/music

Wyoming

University of Wyoming
Music Therapy Prgm
1000 East University Ave
Laramie, WY 82071-3037
www.uwyo.edu/music

EXPRESSIVE/CREATIVE ARTS THERAPIES

Northwest College
Music Therapy Prgm
231 Sixth St
Powell, WY 82716
www.northwestmusic.org

Health Information and Communication

Includes:
- Cancer registrar
- Health care manager
- Health information administrator
- Health information technician
- Medical coder
- Medical librarian
- Medical transcriptionist

Cancer Registrar

Cancer registrars are data management experts who report cancer statistics for various health care agencies. Registrars work closely with physicians, administrators, researchers, and health care planners to provide support for cancer program development, ensure compliance of reporting standards, and serve as a valuable resource for cancer information with the ultimate goal of preventing and controlling cancer. The cancer registrar is involved in managing and analyzing clinical cancer information for the purpose of education, research, and outcome measurement.

Career Description

Cancer registrars possess the clinical and technical knowledge and skills necessary to maintain components of the disease-related data collection systems consistent with medical, administrative, ethical, and legal and accreditation requirements of the health care delivery system. The cancer registrar's primary responsibility is to ensure that timely, accurate, and complete data are incorporated and maintained on all types of cancer diagnosed and/or treated within an institution or other defined population. Information is entered into the database manually and through database linkage and computer interfaces.

Cancer registrars bridge the information gap by capturing a complete summary of the patient's disease from diagnosis through their lifetime. The information is not limited to the episodic information contained in the health care facility record. The summary or abstract is an ongoing account of the cancer patient's history, diagnosis, treatment, and current status and includes information from sources outside of the health care facility.

In addition to managing and reporting cancer data, registrars serve in multiple other professional activities. Cancer registrars participate in cancer program, institution, and community benefit activities as part of the active leadership structure. Registrars provide benchmarking services, monitor quality of care and clinical practice guidelines, assess patterns of care and referrals, and monitor adverse outcomes including mortality and co-morbidity. Cancer registrars can provide consultative services on many issues including registry management and program standards.

Employment Characteristics

Employment opportunities for cancer registrars are found in health care facilities, cancer research organizations, clinical trials, federal and state public health agencies, pharmaceutical companies, computer vendors, and consulting firms. Registrars' expertise is in demand in almost any organization with a focus on cancer or cancer data.

Salary

According to the National Cancer Registrars Association (NCRA), entry-level salaries average between $39,506 and $55,134. ("NCRA Frontline Workers in Cancer Data Management: Workforce Analysis Study of the Cancer Registry Field," September 2005.) For more information, refer to *www.ama-assn.org/go/hpsalary*.

Educational Programs

Length. Beginning in 2010, the requirement to sit for certification is a minimum of an associate's degree in Cancer Information Management or an associate, baccalaureate or masters degree in a recognized allied health field plus 1,950 hours of experience in the cancer registry field. Detailed information is available at *www.ctrexam.org/eligibility*.

Prerequisites. Applicants for the associate degree program for Cancer Information Management and other accepted allied health degrees should have a high school diploma or equivalent, medical terminology, and anatomy and physiology.

Curriculum. The preprofessional curriculum should include appropriate general education credits predicated on the requirements of the academic institution. The professional curriculum requires:

- Cancer Registry Structure and Management
  - Introduction to Cancer Registries
  - Legal and Ethical Issues and Standards
  - Registry Organization; Types of Registries
  - Cancer Registry Management
  - National Standard Setters
- Cancer Registry Operations
  - Case Ascertainment
  - Disease Registry Files
  - Principles of Abstracting and Data Set Identification
  - Registry Standards and Networking
  - Registry Standards for Approved Cancer Programs
- Cancer Disease, Coding and Staging
  - Cancer and Its Natural Disease Course
  - Coding Systems (ICD-O-3)
  - Coding Diagnosis
  - Evaluating Extent of Disease
  - American Joint Committee on Cancer
  - Summary Staging
  - Collaborative Staging
- Oncology Treatment and Coding
  - Surgery
  - Surgical Coding
  - Radiation Coding
  - Chemotherapy

- ○ Chemotherapy Coding
- ○ Immunotherapy
- ○ Immunotherapy Coding
- ○ Hormonal Treatment
- ○ Hormonal Therapy Coding
- ○ Alternative, Palliative and Experimental Treatments
- ○ Other Treatment Coding
- ○ Clinical Trials
- ○ Coding and Monitoring
- Abstracting Methods
  - ○ Components of the Medical Record
  - ○ Structure and Content of Source Documents
  - ○ Abstracting Principles
  - ○ Abstracting Medical Records
- Outcomes and Data Quality and Utilization
  - ○ Policies and Procedures
  - ○ Cancer Patient Methodology
  - ○ Statistics and Epidemiology
  - ○ Database Management

Certification

The National Cancer Registers Association's Council on Certification administers a semi-annual examination for those eligible to become Certified Tumor Registrars (CTR). Candidates must meet eligibility requirements that include a combination of experience in the cancer registry field and the appropriate education. Persons who have successfully completed the certification exam have demonstrated that they have met or exceeded the standard level of experience and technical knowledge required for effective cancer data management. To maintain certification, the NCRA's current continuing education requirement's of 20 hours every years must be met. Detailed information is available at: *www.ctrexam.org/eligibility.*

Inquiries

Careers, Program Accreditation
National Cancer Registrars Association
1340 Braddock Place, Suite 203
Alexandria, VA 22314
703 299-6640
703 299-6620 Fax
E-mail: *info@ncra-usa.org*
www.ncra-usa.org

Certification
National Cancer Registers Association, Council on Certification
1340 Braddock Place, Suite 203
Alexandria, VA 22314
703 299-6640
E-mail: *ctrexam@ncra-usa.org*
www.ctrexam.org

Cancer Registrar

California

Santa Barbara City College
Cancer Registrar Prgm
721 Cliff Dr
Santa Barbara, CA 93109
www.sbcc.edu

Georgia

Ogeechee Technical College
Cancer Registrar Prgm
One Joe Kennedy Blvd
Statesboro, GA 30458
www.ogeecheetech.edu

Illinois

American Health Information Management Assoc
Cancer Registrar Prgm
233 N Michigan Ave, Ste 2150
Chicago, IL 60601
campus.ahima.org/campus/course_info/CRM/crm_intro.html

Iowa

Scott Community College
Cancer Registrar Prgm
Bettendorf, IA 52722
www.eic.edu/highschool/programs/career/health_careers/cim.html

North Carolina

Davidson County Community College
Cancer Registrar Prgm
PO Box 1287
Lexington, NC 27293
www.davidsonccc.edu

Ohio

Owens Community College
Cancer Registrar Prgm
PO Box 10,000
Toledo, OH 43699
www.owens.edu/cim

Texas

San Jacinto College South
Cancer Registrar Prgm
5800 Uvalde Rd
Houston, TX 77049
www.sjcd.cc.tx.us

Health Care Manager

The health care management profession includes individuals with specialized training either at the undergraduate and/or graduate levels in the traditional management disciplines, but taught in a health care context, combined with coursework in policy and public health.

Health care managers, also known as health services managers, health administrators, or health care executives, direct the operation of hospitals, health systems and other types of organizations. They are responsible for facilities, services, programs, staff, budgets, relations with other organizations, and other management aspects, depending on the type and size of the organization.

Career Description

Health care managers work in a variety of settings, including hospital and health systems management, medical groups, pharmaceutical and biotechnology companies, care management organizations, health information technology firms, supply chain companies, government/policy organizations, investment banks, health insurers, and health care management consulting firms. Some graduates may also work with large corporations directing their health and other benefits programs.

Employment Characteristics

According to the Bureau of Labor and Statistics, employment in the field of health care management is expected to grow 16 percent through 2018. The health care industry will continue to expand and diversify, requiring managers to help ensure smooth business operations.

Salary

Salaries vary depending on the employer and geographic location. Data from the US Bureau of Labor Statistics (BLS) for May 2011 show that wages at the 10th percentile are $52,730, the 50th percentile (median) at $86,400, and the 90th percentile at $147,890 (*www.bls.gov/oes/current/oes119111.htm*).

According to the American College of Healthcare Executives (ACHE), each management level in the acute care sector has its own responsibilities, qualifications, salary range, and typical work hours.

Entry-level salaries may average between $40,000 and $60,000—but can be higher. With some experience, salaries typically are $65,000 to $110,000. Salaries for upper-level positions depend on the size of the organization. For smaller hospitals, this might be $130,000, although publications such as Modern Healthcare periodically list salaries for health care managers in larger organizations that can be substantially higher. For the largest organizations this may be a factor of three to ten (or more) times higher than this level. To find out what to expect as an entry-level manager, mid-level manager, and senior-level executive, visit ACHE's website at *www.ache.org/CARSVCS/ CareerFAQ/intro.cfm*.

Educational Programs

Medical and health services managers must be familiar with management principles and practices. A master's degree in health services administration, long-term care administration, health sciences, public health,

public administration, or business administration is the standard credential for most generalist positions in this field. However, a bachelor's degree is adequate for some entry-level positions in smaller facilities, at the departmental level within health care organizations, and in health information management.

Length. Baccalaureate degree programs are four years; master's programs are generally two years.

Prerequisites. Applicants for the four-year baccalaureate degree program should have a high school diploma or equivalent. A four-year baccalaureate degree—BS or BA—which is the primary prerequisite for admission to a graduate program, can be earned in any field of study ranging from health care management and business to biology, sociology, policy, public health, government, social work, or allied health professions. Some coursework in economics and statistics is helpful, but not generally a requirement. In the past, most students chose the traditional route of a master's degree in health administration or public health. Today, however, students are investigating other options, including degrees in business with course concentration in health services management. Some schools offer a joint degree—a master's degree in both business administration and public health, for example, or in both health care management and law.

Sometimes physicians, nurses, or other practicing health professionals decide to earn this credential to become more involved in leadership roles. In certain cases, students will complete the master's degree prior to going to medical, nursing or other academic programs.

Lists and descriptions of programs granting degrees in health care management/health administration are available at *www.aupha.org/DirectoryOfPrograms/*.

Curriculum. The pre-professional curriculum should include appropriate general education credit predicated on the requirements of the academic institution. The professional curriculum can include coursework in health care policy and law, marketing, organizational behavior, health care financing, human resources, health information management, and other health care management topics. Academic programs may also include a supervised internship, residency, or fellowship. For specifics on curriculum, refer to *www.aupha.org/DirectoryOfPrograms/*.

Inquiries

Careers

For information about career opportunities in health care management and professional credentialing, contact:

American College of Healthcare Executives
One N. Franklin St., Suite 1700
Chicago, IL 60606
(312) 424-2800
www.ache.org

For information about career opportunities in medical group practices and ambulatory care management, contact:
Medical Group Management Association
104 Inverness Terrace East
Englewood, CO 80112
(301) 799-1111
www.mgma.org

Education

For information about undergraduate and graduate academic programs in this field, and a list of certified undergraduate programs, contact:

Association of University Programs in Health Administration
2000 North 14th St., Suite 780
Arlington, VA 22201
(703) 894-0940
www.aupha.org

Program Accreditation

For a list of accredited graduate programs in medical and health services administration, contact:

Commission on Accreditation of Healthcare Management
  Education
2111 Wilson Blvd., Suite 700
Arlington, VA 22201
(703) 351-5010
www.cahme.org

Note: Adapted in part from the Bureau of Labor Statistics, US Department of Labor, *Occupational Outlook Handbook,* Medical and Health Services Managers, at *www.bls.gov/oco/ocos014.htm*.

Health Information Administrator

Definition of Health Information Management

The health information management profession includes managers, technicians, and specialists expert in systems and processes for health information management, including:

- Planning: Formulating strategic, functional, and user requirements for health information
- Engineering: Designing information flow, data models, and definitions
- Administration: Managing data collection and storage, information retrieval, and release
- Application: Analyzing, interpreting, classifying, and coding data and facilitating information use by others
- Policy: Establishing and implementing security, confidentiality, retention, integrity, and access standards

Career Description

Graduates of baccalaureate degree educational programs in health information management are known as health information administrators and apply their training and expertise in both science and management to develop, implement, and/or administer health care data collection and reporting systems to assure the integrity and availability of the information resources needed to support authorized users and decision-makers. Health information managers have expertise in developing and managing effective processes and systems to assure the integrity of health care data and to preserve the complete, accurate, and legal source of patient data (patient medical records). Health information managers use their expertise to develop and manage effective processes and systems to preserve patient privacy, confidentiality, and the security of health information maintained in paper or computerized systems. Common job titles held by health information administrators in today's job market are related to line, staff, and/or technical positions such as director, assistant director, manager, privacy officer, compliance officer, claims analyst, clinical information analyst, HIM educator, and so forth. It is anticipated that job titles will change (eg, health information engineer, clinical information coordinator, data administrator, information security officer) as health care enterprises expand their reliance on information systems and technology. Health information administrators have, and will continue to assume, roles that directly contribute to the development of computer-based patient record systems and a national health information infrastructure.

The tasks or functions performed by health information administrators are numerous and are continually changing within the work environment. Although the job title and work setting will dictate the actual tasks performed by the health information administrator, in general this individual performs tasks related to the management of health information and the systems used to collect, store, process, retrieve, analyze, disseminate, and communicate that information, regardless of the physical medium in which information is maintained. In addition, health information administrators assess the uses of information and identify what information is available and where there are inconsistencies, gaps, and duplications in health data sources. They are capable of planning and designing and maintaining systems and serving as pivotal team members in the development of computer-based patient record systems and other enterprise-wide information systems. Their

responsibilities also include serving as brokers of information services. Among the information services provided are a design and requirements definition for clinical and administrative systems development, data administration, data quality management, data security management, decision support design and data analyses, and management of information-intensive areas such as clinical quality/performance assessment and utilization and case management.

Employment Characteristics

Presently, opportunities for practice are found in numerous settings such as acute care general hospitals, managed care organizations, consulting firms, claims and reimbursement organizations, accounting firms, home health care agencies, long-term care facilities, corrections facilities, drug companies, behavioral health care organizations, insurance companies, state and federal health care agencies, public health care computing industries and health care vendors. Practice opportunities are unlimited.

Salary

According to the American Health Information Management Association (AHIMA), entry-level salaries average between $40,000 and $75,000. For more information, refer to *www.ama-assn.org/go/ hpsalary* and *http://www.hicareers.com/Toolbox/salarystudy.aspx.*

Educational Programs

Length. Baccalaureate degree programs are 4 years. Post-baccalaureate and other certificate programs are generally 1 year.

Prerequisites. Applicants for the 4-year baccalaureate degree program should have a high school diploma or equivalent. Applicants for the 1-year post-baccalaureate certificate program should have a baccalaureate degree that includes coursework in science and statistics, as specified.

Curriculum. The pre-professional curriculum should include appropriate general education credit predicated on the requirements of the academic institution. The professional curriculum requires:

- Biomedical sciences (anatomy, physiology, language of medicine, pharmacology, and disease processes)
- Information technology (microcomputer applications, programming, system architectures and operating systems, introduction to database concepts, and data communications)
- Health care delivery systems
- Legal aspects of health care and ethical issues
- Organization and management (managerial principles, human resources management and development, financial management for health care, organizational behavior, and interpersonal skills)
- Quantitative methods and research methodologies (introductory and advanced health care statistics/epidemiology, research methods in health care)
- Health care information requirements and standards
- Health care information systems (computer applications in health care, systems analysis and design)

- Health data content and structures, classification, nomenclature and reimbursement systems, clinical quality assessment, and performance improvement
- Biomedical and health services research support
- Health information services management
- A capstone experience/practicum/project

 Inquiries

Careers
www.HICareers.com

Professional Credentialing
American Health Information Management Association
233 N Michigan Avenue, Suite 2150
Chicago, IL 60601-5800
312 233-1100
www.ahima.org

Program Accreditation
Commission on Accreditation for Health Informatics and
Information Management Education (CAHIIM)
233 N Michigan Avenue, Suite 2150
Chicago, IL 60601-5800
312 233-1100
312 233-1429 Fax
www.cahiim.org

Health Information Technician

Definition of Health Information Management

The health information management profession includes managers, technicians, and specialists expert in systems and processes for health information management, including:

- Planning: Formulating strategic, functional, and user requirements for health information
- Engineering: Designing information flow, data models, and definitions
- Administration: Managing data collection and storage, information retrieval, and release
- Application: Analyzing, interpreting, classifying, and coding data and facilitating information use by others
- Policy: Establishing and implementing security, confidentiality, retention, integrity, and access standards

Career Description

Graduates of associate degree programs are known as health information technicians and conduct health data collection, monitoring, maintenance, and reporting activities in accordance with established data quality principles, legal and regulatory standards, and professional best practice guidelines. These functions encompass, among other areas, monitoring electronic and paper-based documentation and processing and using health data for billing and reporting purposes through use of various electronic systems. Common job titles held by health information technicians in today's job market include reimbursement specialist, information access and disclosure specialist, coder, medical record technician, clinical documentation specialist, Electronic Medical Records Technician, data quality coordinator, supervisor, etc. It is anticipated that job titles will change as health care enterprises expand their reliance on information systems and technology. Health information technicians have, and will continue to assume, roles that support efforts toward the development and implementation of computer-based patient record systems and a national health information infrastructure.

The tasks or functions performed by health information technicians are numerous and continually changing within the work environment. The job title and work setting will dictate the actual tasks performed by the health information technician. However, in general, these individuals perform tasks related to the use, analysis, validation, presentation, data abstracting, analysis, coding, release of information, data privacy and security, retrieval, quality measurement, and control of health care data regardless of the physical medium in which information is maintained. Their task responsibilities may also include supervising personnel.

Employment Characteristics

Presently, opportunities for practice are found in numerous settings such as acute care general hospitals, managed care organizations, physician office practices, home health care agencies, long-term care facilities, correctional facilities, behavioral health care organizations, insurance companies, ambulatory settings, and state and federal health care agencies, and public health departments and health care vendors. Practice opportunities are unlimited.

Salary

According to AHIMA, entry-level salaries average between $30,000 and $50,000. For more information, refer to *www.ama-assn.org/go/hpsalary* and *http://www.hicareers.com/Toolbox/salarystudy.aspx.*

Educational Programs

Length. Programs are generally 2 years, offering an associate degree.

Prerequisites. High school diploma or equivalent.

Curriculum. In addition to general education courses, the professional component of the technician program requires:

- Biomedical sciences (anatomy, physiology, language of medicine, disease processes, and pharmacology)
- Information technology (microcomputer applications and computers in health care)
- Health data content and structure
- Health care delivery systems, organization and supervision, health care statistics, and data literacy
- Clinical quality assessment and performance improvement
- Clinical classification systems
- Reimbursement methodologies
- Legal and ethical issues
- Supervised professional practice experiences in health information departments of health care facilities and agencies

Inquiries

Careers
www.HICarreers.com

Professional Credentialing
American Health Information Management Association
233 N Michigan Avenue, Suite 2150
Chicago, IL 60601-5800
312 233-1100
www.ahima.org

Program Accreditation
Commission on Accreditation for Health Informatics and Information Management Education (CAHIIM)
233 N Michigan Avenue, Suite 2150
Chicago, IL 60601-5800
312 233-1100
312 233-1429 Fax
www.cahiim.org

Medical Coder

Each time a patient receives medical care, the physician or other health professional must document the services that are provided. Since each of these encounters is unique, the medical coder assigns alpha-numeric codes that are specific to the patient's symptoms and diagnosis and identify each procedure and other service performed. This series of codes provides the insurance carrier with a detailed account of the encounter and ensures that providers are correctly compensated for their services. These codes are also important for making critical clinical decisions and for statistical research and health planning analysis.

Career opportunities include:

- Inpatient hospital coder
- Outpatient coder
- Coding abstracting analyst
- Insurance claim analyst
- Insurance fraud investigator
- Managed care organization coder
- Procedural coder
- Physician's office/clinic coder

Career Description

The medical coder must be detail-oriented and exhibit a high degree of accuracy and a working knowledge of medical terminology, anatomy, and physiology. In addition to the responsibilities described above, the medical coder must maintain current knowledge of medical coding rules and regulations pertaining especially to medical coding compliance and reimbursement and must integrate changes into the medical practice. The medical coder has an ongoing responsibility to educate health professionals regarding updates in coding rules and guidelines and to teach them how to provide accurate and detailed documentation of each patient encounter.

Employment Characteristics

The medical coder is integral to the health information management team and may work in physician offices, hospital inpatient and outpatient facilities, ambulatory surgical centers, home health care facilities, long-term care facilities, and behavioral health care organizations as well as for insurance and drug companies. Other professional opportunities include training medical coders, auditing and teaching for consulting firms, and fraud and abuse investigation for state and federal healthcare agencies. With the use of electronic medical records, many medical coders also can work from remote locations or home offices.

Salary

A 2010 survey by the American Academy of Professional Coders (AAPC) found that the annual average salary for certified medical coders is $45,404, versus $38,290 for non-certified coders. Salary varies based on educational credentials, certification status, experience, position responsibilities, and geographic location, from approximately $37,000 to $69,000. For more salary detail, refer to *http://news.aapc.com/index.php/category/medical-coding-salary-surveys/*.

Education

To prepare for a career as a medical coder, an individual may choose from several pathways, including on-the-job training with certified professional coders (CPCs), online training, book-based self-study programs, or instructor-led classroom training at a community college or trade school.

Certification

Several organizations offer certification for medical coders; nationally recognized organizations include the AAPC and American Health Information Management Association (AHIMA). Certification exams are proctored and take up to six hours to complete. Online exams are recognized by other certification organizations.

Continuing education is imperative for medical coders to stay current in a rapidly changing industry. A medical coder certified with the AAPC, for example, must complete 32 continuing education units (CEUs) every two years to maintain certification. CEUs may be earned by attending workshops, local chapter meetings, and state and national conferences as well as by presenting at conferences, reading articles and then taking a quiz in the Coding Edge, and participating in qualifying Webinars.

Inquiries

Careers, Program Accreditation, Certification
American Academy of Professional Coders (AAPC)
2480 South 3850 West, Suite B
Salt Lake City, UT 84120
800 626-CODE (2633)
www.aapc.com

American Health Information Management Association (AHIMA)
233 North Michigan Avenue, Suite 2150
Chicago, IL 60601-5800
312 233-1100
E-mail: *info@ahima.org*
www.ahima.org/careers

Medical librarians are information professionals who specialize in health resources and provide medical information for physicians, allied health professionals, patients, consumers, students, and corporations. Using materials ranging from traditional print sources to electronic databases, medical librarians devise and use innovative strategies to assess and deliver information to their clients. Physicians often call upon medical librarians to provide life-saving information for patient care.

Career Description

Medical librarians help improve the quality of patient care by helping health care professionals stay abreast of new developments and treatments. Additionally, they find relevant health information for patients and consumers, serve as educators for students pursuing health care degrees, and provide training in the location and use of medical resources. Increasingly medical librarians use technology to design Web sites and distance education programs and to construct digital libraries. Others work for Internet companies and electronic publishers that index and organize information for the Web. Medical librarians also participate as members of research teams on university campuses and serve health care corporations, such as insurance and pharmaceutical companies, by providing information necessary for developing new products and services.

In administrative roles, medical librarians serve as directors, chief information officers, and deans or associate deans of information technology departments. Librarians ensure their informational mission is accomplished by providing leadership and strategic planning for their institutions, managing multimillion dollar budgets, pursuing grant funding, and developing marketing and public relations plans for their libraries.

Medical librarians work closely with support staff in the library to accomplish day-to-day tasks. Known as medical library assistants, these support staff provide critical operations support in all areas of the library, including circulation, serials management, acquisitions, interlibrary loan, cataloging, billing, and reference services. Some states have associations and special interest groups that support the educational needs of library support staff. Such organizations include the New York State Library Assistants' Association (NYSLAA) and the Metropolitan New York Library Council's Library Assistants, Support Staff and Associates special interest group. NYSLAA sponsors a Certificate of Achievement Program that recognizes library assistants for their contributions to libraries and the library profession.

Employment Characteristics

Medical librarians and medical library assistants are employed anywhere health information is needed, including hospitals, academic medical centers, clinics, colleges, universities, professional schools, consumer health libraries, research centers, foundations, biotechnology centers, insurance companies, medical equipment manufacturers, pharmaceutical companies, publishers, and federal state and local government agencies.

Salary

Salaries vary according to the type and location of the institution, level of responsibility and technical skill, and length of employment. According to the Medical Library Association (MLA), the average starting salary for entry-level medical librarians was $43,400 in 2008. The overall average salary for experienced medical librarians was $65,796. Library directors can earn over $150,000 per year.

For more information, refer to *www.ama-assn.org/go/hpsalary*.

Educational Programs

Length. Programs are one to two years and result in a master's degree.

Prerequisites. Medical librarians must have a master of library and information science degree from an American Library Association-accredited school. An undergraduate degree in any field is necessary for admission to a master's program. Undergraduate courses in biology, medical sciences, medical terminology, computer science, education, and management are helpful. Medical librarians may also apply for membership in the Academy of Health Information Professionals, a credentialing program for medical librarians sponsored by the Medical Library Association.

Curriculum. Programs leading to a master of library and information science degree include a wide variety of courses. All students take core courses in research, information resources, cataloging, and management and choose between tracks for public, school, academic, or special libraries. Upon choosing a track, the student and academic advisor select courses that reflect the student's career goals. Those wishing to focus on systems and technology will take a variety of technology courses in addition to the core and specialty track courses. Medical librarianship falls within the special library curriculum in many schools of library and information science. Medical library curriculum courses include resources for consumer health information, resources and services for health sciences information, medical informatics, and resources and services for special populations.

Inquiries

Careers/Credentialing

Medical Library Association
65 East Wacker Place, Suite 1900
Chicago, IL 60601-7246
312 419-9094
E-mail: *mlapd2@mlahq.org*
www.mlanet.org/career

Library Assistants

New York State Library Assistants' Association
www.nyslaa.org
Metropolitan New York Library Council
Library Assistants, Support Staff and Associates
Vergie Savage-Branch
Cornell University Medical College Library
1300 York Avenue
New York, NY 10021
(212) 746-6091
www.metro.org/SIGs/lassa.html

HEALTH INFORMATION AND COMMUNICATION

Program Accreditation
American Library Association, Committee on Accreditation/Office
   for Accreditation
Karen O'Brien, Director
50 East Huron
Chicago, IL 60611
(312) 280-2434
E-mail: *kobrien@ala.org*

Medical Librarian

Alabama

University of Alabama
Medical Librarian Prgm
School of Library and Information Studies
Box 870252
515 Gorgas Library, Capstone Dr
Tuscaloosa, AL 35487-0252
www.slis.ua.edu

Alberta, Canada

University of Alberta
Medical Librarian Prgm
School for Library and information Studies
3-20 Rutherford S
Edmonton, AB T6G 2J4

Arizona

University of Arizona
Medical Librarian Prgm
School of Information Resources and Library Science
1515 E First St
Tucson, AZ 85719
www.sir.arizona.edu

British Columbia, Canada

University of British Columbia
Medical Librarian Prgm
School of Library, Archival and Information Studies
Suite 301, 6190 Agronomy Rd
Vancouver, BC V6T 1Z3
www.slais.ubc.ca

California

University of California - Los Angeles
Medical Librarian Prgm
Graduate School of Education and Information
Studies Bldg
Box 351520
Los Angeles, CA 90095-1520

San Jose State University
Medical Librarian Prgm
School of Library and Information Science
One Washington Square
San Jose, CA 95192-0029

Connecticut

Southern Connecticut State University
Medical Librarian Prgm
Information and Library Sciences
501 Crescent St
New Haven, CT 06515
www.southernct.edu/departments/ils

District of Columbia

Catholic University of America
Medical Librarian Prgm
School of Library and Information Science
620 Michigan Ave NE
Washington, DC 20064

Florida

Florida State University
Medical Librarian Prgm
School of Information Studies
Shores Bldg
Tallahassee, FL 32306-2100
www.lis.fsu.edu

University of South Florida
Medical Librarian Prgm
School of Library and Information Sciences
4202 E Fowler Ave
CIS 1040
Tampa, FL 33620
www.cas.usf.edu/lis

Hawaii

University of Hawaii at Manoa
Medical Librarian Prgm
Library and Information Science Program
2550 McCarthy Mall
Honolulu, HI 96822
www.hawaii.edu/slis

Illinois

Univ of Illinois at Urbana-Champaign
Medical Librarian Prgm
Graduate School of Library and Information Science
501 E Daniel St
Champaign, IL 61820-6211

Dominican University
Medical Librarian Prgm
Graduate School of Library and Information Science
7900 W Division St
River Forest, IL 60305
www.gslis.dom.edu

Indiana

Indiana University - Indianapolis
Medical Librarian Prgm
School of Library and Information Science at
   Indianapolis
755 W Michigan St
Indianapolis, IN 46202
http://slis.iupui.edu

Iowa

University of Iowa
Medical Librarian Prgm
School of Library and Information Science
3087 Main Library
Iowa City, IA 52242-1420
www.uiowa.edu/~libsci

Kansas

Emporia State University
Medical Librarian Prgm
School of Library and Information Management
1200 Commerical, Campus Box 4025
Emporia, KS 66801
www.slim.emporia.edu

Kentucky

University of Kentucky
Medical Librarian Prgm
School of Library and Information Science
502 King Library
Lexington, KY 40506-0039
www.uky.edu/cis/slis

Louisiana

Louisiana State University
Medical Librarian Prgm
School of Library and Information Science
267 Coates Hall
Baton Rouge, LA 70803
http://slis.lsu.edu

Maryland

University of Maryland, Baltimore
Medical Librarian Prgm
College of Information Studies
4105 Hornbake Bldg
College Park, MD 20742
www.clis.umd.edu

Massachusetts

Simmons College
Medical Librarian Prgm
Graduate School of Library and Information Science
300 The Fenway
Boston, MA 02115
www.simmons.edu/gslis

Michigan

University of Michigan
Medical Librarian Prgm
School of Information
550 E University Ave, 304 W Hall Bldg
Ann Arbor, MI 48109-1092
www.si.umich.edu

Wayne State University
Medical Librarian Prgm
Library and Information Science Program
106 Kresge Library
Detroit, MI 48202
www.lisp.wayne.edu

Mississippi

University of Southern Mississippi
Medical Librarian Prgm
School of Library and Information Science
118 College Dr #5146
Hattiesburg, MS 39406-0001
www.usm.edu/slis

Missouri

University of Missouri
Medical Librarian Prgm
Information Science and Learning Technologies
303 Townsend Hall
Columbia, MO 65211
www.sislt.missouri.edu

New Jersey

Rutgers University
Medical Librarian Prgm
Dept of Library and Information Science
4 Huntington St
New Brunswick, NJ 08901-1071
www.scils.rutgers.edu

New York

University at Albany/State U of New York
Medical Librarian Prgm
School of Inform Science and Policy Draper 113
135 Western Ave
Albany, NY 12222
www.albany.edu/sisp

Long Island University - C W Post Campus
Medical Librarian Prgm
Palmer School of Library and Information Science
720 Northern Blvd
Brookville, NY 11548
www.liu.edu/palmer

University at Buffalo - SUNY
Medical Librarian Prgm
Library and Information Studies
534 Baldy Hall
Buffalo, NY 14260
www.informatics.buffalo.edu/lis

CUNY Queens College
Medical Librarian Prgm
Graduate School of Library and Information Studies
65-30 Kissena Blvd
Flushing, NY 11367-1597
www.qc.edu/gslis

St John's University
Medical Librarian Prgm
Division of Library and Information Science
8000 Utopia Pkwy
Jamaica, NY 11439
www.stjohns.edu/libraryscience

Pratt Institute
Medical Librarian Prgm
School of Information and Library Science
144 W 14th St, 6th Fl
New York, NY 10011
www.pratt.edu/sils

Syracuse University
Medical Librarian Prgm
School of Information Studies
4-206 Center for Science and Technology
Syracuse, NY 13244
www.ist.syr.edu

North Carolina

University of North Carolina - Chapel Hill
Medical Librarian Prgm
School of Information and Library Science
100 Manning Hall, CB 3360
Chapel Hill, NC 27599-3360
www.ils.unc.edu

North Carolina Central University
Medical Librarian Prgm
School of Library and Information Sciences
1800 Fayetteville St
Durham, NC 27707
www.nccu.edu

University of North Carolina - Greensboro
Medical Librarian Prgm
Dept of Library and Information Studies
349 Curry Bldg
Greensboro, NC 27401-6170
www.uncg.edu

Nova Scotia, Canada

Dalhousie University
Medical Librarian Prgm
School of Library and Information Studies
3rd Fl, Killiam Library
Halifax, NS B3H 3J5
www.mgmt.dal.ca/slis

Ohio

Kent State University
Medical Librarian Prgm
School of Library and Information Sciences
PO Box 5190
Kent, OH 44242-0001
www.slis.kent.edu

Oklahoma

University of Oklahoma
Medical Librarian Prgm
School of Library and Information Studies
401 W Brooks, Rm 120
Norman, OK 73019-6032
www.ou.edu/cas/slis

Ontario, Canada

University of Western Ontario
Medical Librarian Prgm
Graduate Programs in Library and Information Science
255 Middlesex College
London, ON N6A 5B7
www.fims.uwo.ca

University of Toronto
Medical Librarian Prgm
Master of Information Studies
Faculty of Information Studies
140 St George St
Toronto, ON M5S 3G6
www.fis.utoronto.ca

Pennsylvania

Clarion University of Pennsylvania
Medical Librarian Prgm
Department of Library Science
210 Carlson Library Bldg
840 Wood St
Clarion, PA 16214
www.clarion.edu/libsci

Drexel University College of Medicine
Medical Librarian Prgm
College of Information Science and Technology
3141 Chestnut St
Philadelphia, PA 19104-2875
www.cis.drexel.edu

University of Pittsburgh
Medical Librarian Prgm
Department of Library and Information Science
135 N Bellefield Ave
Pittsburgh, PA 15260
www.sis.pitt.edu

Puerto Rico

University of Puerto Rico
Medical Librarian Prgm
Information Science and Technologies
PO Box 210906
San Juan, PR 00031-1906
www.upr.edu/home1600.html

Quebec, Canada

McGill University
Medical Librarian Prgm
Graduate School of Library and Information Studies
3459 McTavish St, MS 57-F
Montreal, QC H3A 1Y1
www.gslis.mcgill.ca

University de Montreal
Medical Librarian Prgm
Ecole de bibiotheconomie et des sciences de
    l'information
CP 6128, Succursale Centre-ville
Montreal, QC H3C 3J7
www.ebsi.umontreal.ca

Rhode Island

University of Rhode Island
Medical Librarian Prgm
Graduate School of Library and Information Studies
Rodman Hall
94 W Alumni Ave
Kingston, RI 02881
www.uri.edu/artsci/lsc

South Carolina

University of South Carolina
Medical Librarian Prgm
School of Library and Information Science
Davis College
Columbia, SC 29208
www.libsci.sc.edu

Tennessee

University of Tennessee - Knoxville
Medical Librarian Prgm
School of Information Sciences
451 Communications Bldg
1345 Circle Park Dr
Knoxville, TN 37996-0341
www.sis.utk.edu

Texas

University of Texas at Austin
Medical Librarian Prgm
School of Information
1 University Station D7000
Austin, TX 78712-0390
www.ischool.utexas.edu

HEALTH INFORMATION AND COMMUNICATION

Texas Woman's University
Medical Librarian Prgm
School of Library and Information Studies
PO Box 425438
Denton, TX 76204-5438
www.twu.edu/cope/slis

University of North Texas
Medical Librarian Prgm
School of Library and Information Sciences
PO Box 311068
Denton, TX 76203-1068
www.unt.edu/slis

Washington

University of Washington
Medical Librarian Prgm
Information School
370 Mary Gates Hall
Box 352840
Seattle, WA 98195-2840
www.ischool.washington.edu

Wisconsin

University of Wisconsin - Madison
Medical Librarian Prgm
Library and Information Studies
600 N Park St
Rm 4217, H C White Hall
Madison, WI 53706

University of Wisconsin - Milwaukee
Medical Librarian Prgm
School of Information Studies
PO Box 413
Milwaukee, WI 53201
www.sois.uwm.edu

Medical Transcriptionist

Medical transcriptionists are specialists in medical language and health care documentation who interpret and transcribe dictation by physicians and other health professionals regarding patient assessment, workup, therapeutic procedures, clinical course, diagnosis, prognosis, and so on, editing dictated material for grammar and clarity as necessary and appropriate.

Career Description

In the broadest sense, medical transcription is the act of translating from oral to written form (on paper or electronically) the record of a person's encounter with a health care professional. Medical transcriptionists (MTs) are specialists in medical language and health care documentation. They interpret and transcribe dictation by physicians and other health care professionals regarding patient assessment, workup, therapeutic procedures, clinical course, diagnosis, prognosis, etc, editing dictated material for grammar and clarity as necessary and appropriate.

Physicians and other health care providers employ state-of-the-art electronic technology to dictate and transmit highly technical and confidential information about their patients. These medical professionals rely on skilled medical transcriptionists to transform spoken words into comprehensive records that accurately communicate medical information.

Speech recognition systems also may be used as an intermediary to translate the medical professional's dictation into rough draft. The medical transcriptionist is on the frontline to implement risk management by further refining the draft into a finished document. This requires listening to dictation while reading the draft created via speech recognition technology and editing the text on a computer screen. This editing may range from minimal to extensive, depending on the capabilities of the speech recognition software and the dictating habits of the originator, and may include correction of content as well as punctuation, grammar, and style.

Secretarial keyboarding and *technical language editing/transcription* should not be confused. The primary skills necessary for performance of quality medical transcription are extensive medical knowledge and understanding, sound judgment, deductive reasoning, and the ability to detect medical inconsistencies in dictation. For example, a diagnosis inconsistent with the patient's history and symptoms may be mistakenly dictated. As a foremost partner in risk management, the medical transcriptionist questions, seeks clarification, verifies the information, and enters the correct information into the report.

Employment Characteristics

Medical transcriptionists use their talents in a variety of health care settings where dictation for the purpose of health care documentation requires transcription; these include:

- Physician's offices
- Public and private hospitals
- Teaching hospitals
- Medical schools
- Medical transcription businesses
- Clinics
- Laboratories
- Pathology and radiology departments
- Insurance companies
- Medical libraries
- Government medical facilities
- Rehabilitation centers
- Legal offices
- Research centers
- Veterinary medical facilities
- Associations representing the health care industry

In addition, many MTs work from their homes as independent contractors, subcontractors, or home-based employees.

Medical transcriptionists work with physicians and surgeons in multiple specialties, as well as with pharmacists, therapists, technicians, nurses, dietitians, social workers, psychologists, and other medical personnel. All of these health care providers rely on information that is received, accurately documented, and disseminated by the medical transcriptionist.

Qualified medical transcriptionists who wish to expand their professional responsibilities may become quality assurance specialists, editors, or supervisors. Experienced medical transcriptionists may become teachers, working in schools and colleges to educate future medical transcription professionals as managers, department heads, or owners of medical transcription businesses.

Salary

Medical transcriptionists may be paid in any of a variety of ways, but chiefly by the hour, by production, or by a combination of hourly pay plus incentive pay for production.

Data from the US Bureau of Labor Statistics (BLS) for May 2009 show that wages at the 10th percentile were $22,010, the 50th percentile (median) at $33,480, and the 90th percentile at $46,680 (*www.bls.gov/oes/current/oes319094.htm*).

For more information, refer to *www.ama-assn.org/go/hpsalary*.

Employment Outlook

BLS data project that employment of medical transcriptionists will grow by 6 percent through 2020, slower than average for all occupations. Demand for medical transcription services will continue to be spurred by a growing and aging population. Older age groups receive proportionally greater numbers of medical tests, treatments, and procedures that require documentation. A high level of demand for transcription services also will be sustained by the continued need for electronic documentation that can be shared easily among providers, third-party payers, regulators, consumers, and health information systems. Growing numbers of medical transcriptionists will be needed to amend patients' records, edit documents from speech recognition systems, and identify discrepancies in medical reports.

Contracting out transcription work overseas and advancements in speech recognition technology are not expected to significantly reduce the need for well-trained medical transcriptionists. Outsourcing transcription work abroad—to countries such as India, Pakistan, Philippines, Barbados, and Canada—has grown more popular as transmitting confidential health information over the Internet has become more secure; however, the demand for overseas transcription services is expected only to supplement the demand for well-trained domestic medical transcriptionists. In addition, reports transcribed by overseas medical transcription services usually require editing for accuracy by domestic medical transcriptionists before they meet US quality standards.

Speech recognition technology allows physicians and other health professionals to dictate medical reports to a computer, which immediately creates an electronic document. In spite of the advances in this technology, the software has been slow to grasp and analyze the human voice, the English language, and the medical vernacular with all its diversity. As a result, there will continue to be a need for skilled medical transcriptionists to identify and appropriately edit the inevitable errors created by speech recognition systems and to create a final document.

Educational Programs

In general, MT courses take nine to 18 months to complete. Prospective students should look for schools that emphasize excellence in medical transcription rather than those focusing on the ideas of working at home or completing a program rapidly. Accordingly, the Association for Healthcare Documentation Integrity (AHDI) recently established an education program approval process to evaluate medical transcription programs. A joint committee, the Approval Committee for Certificate Programs, (ACCP) was established by AHDI and the American Health Information Management Association (AHIMA) for certifying and approving medical transcription education programs, with the first school approved in 2005. Approved programs satisfy all requirements AHDI has established and have demonstrated a meritorious record of job placement for their graduates. These programs are highly regarded by MT employers who seek out these graduates because of their job readiness. For a list of these programs, see *www.ahdionline.org/scriptcontent/ mtapproved.cfm*.

When evaluating an educational program, a potential student should ask about the amount of authentic physician dictation which is used for practice and then make appropriate use of every opportunity to practice. If the dictation is not available, even the best student is unlikely to succeed. "Authentic dictation" is actually dictated by real clinicians under real circumstances; regardless how hard anyone tries to duplicate authenticity, there is something about reading that gives it a rhythm and flow that you will not encounter in real life.

In addition, one should ask whether there are real transcriptionists (preferably CMTs) teaching the transcription practice portion of the program or mentoring students through transcription practice. Real MTs bring on-the-job experience to academic studies and to transcription practice. Also, it's recommended to interview the instructors and directors of the programs to get a personal sense of rapport (or lack thereof).

Certification and Registration

The AHDI issues two credentials and one designation:
- Registered Medical Transcriptionist (RMT)—The AHDI offers a voluntary credentialing exam to individuals who wish to become RMTs. This exam is applicable for recent graduates of medical transcription education programs, single-specialty transcriptionists, or MTs with fewer than two years' experience in acute care. This exam is considered a level 1 exam. Individuals interested in this exam may not hold a CMT credential.
- Certified Medical Transcriptionist (CMT)—The AHDI offers a voluntary certification exam to individuals who wish to become CMTs. Individuals interested in this exam should have two years of acute care (or equivalent) transcription experience. This exam is considered a level 2 "expert" exam.

- Fellow of AAMT (FAAMT)—This designation signifies those who have achieved a balance of successful activities in the profession that goes beyond regular transcription practice.

No educational program can offer "certification." Although a program may provide its graduates with a certificate of completion, this is not the same as either the RMT or the CMT credentials, which are achieved only through successful completion of examinations administered by Prometric for the AHDI in electronic testing centers throughout the world. The AHDI believes that the CMT credential should be the eventual goal for every working medical transcriptionist.

Inquiries

Careers, Program Accreditation
Association for Healthcare Documentation Integrity
4230 Kiernan Avenue, Suite 130
Modesto, CA 95356
800 982-2182 or 209 527-9620
E-mail: *ahdi@ahdionline.org*
www.ahdionline.org

For careers information, see *www.ahdionline.org/scriptcontent/ Downloads/AboutMT.pdf*

American Health Information Management Association (AHIMA)
233 North Michigan Avenue, Suite 2150
Chicago, IL 60601-5800
312 233-1100
E-mail: *info@ahima.org*
www.ahima.org/careers

Certification
Association for Healthcare Documentation Integrity
4230 Kiernan Avenue, Suite 130
Modesto, CA 95356
800 982-2182 or 209 527-9620
E-mail: *ahdi@ahdionline.org*
www.ahdionline.org

Note: Adapted in part from the Bureau of Labor Statistics, US Department of Labor, *Occupational Outlook Handbook*, Medical Transcriptionists, at *www.bls.gov/oco/ocos271.htm*.

Medical Transcriptionist

British Columbia, Canada

CanScribe Career Centre
Medical Transcriptionist Prgm
223 3121 Hill Rd
Lake Country, BC V4V 1G1
www.canscribe.com

Florida

Seminole State College
Medical Transcriptionist Prgm
850 South SR 434
Altamonte Spring, FL 32714
www.scc-fl.edu/medicaltran

Sheridan Technical Center
Medical Transcriptionist Prgm
5400 Sheridan St
Hollywood, FL 33201
www.sheridantechnical.com/medtranscription

Winter Park Tech
Medical Transcriptionist Prgm
901 W Webster Ave
Winter Park, FL 32789
www.wpt.ocps.net/

Illinois

Richland Community College
Medical Transcriptionist Prgm
One College Park
Decatur, IL 62521
www.richland.edu/programs/ot/medtrans

Nebraska

Metropolitan Community College
Medical Transcriptionist Prgm
PO Box 3777
Omaha, NE 68103
www.mccneb.edu

New York

A&H Training
Medical Transcriptionist Prgm
4 British American Blvd
Latham, NY 12110
www.ahtraining.com

North Carolina

TRS Institute
Medical Transcriptionist Prgm
628 Green Valley Rd
Suite 300
Greenboro, NC 27408
www.trsinstitute.com

Guilford Technical Community College
Medical Transcriptionist Prgm
PO Box 309
Jamestown, NC 27282
www.gtcc.edu/distance/degreeonline/index.aspx

Ohio

Medical Transcription Education Center, Inc.
Medical Transcriptionist Prgm
3634 West Market St
Suite 103
Fairlawn, OH 44333
www.mtecinc.com

South Carolina

Trident Technical College
Medical Transcriptionist Prgm
7000 Rivers Ave
North Charleston, SC 29406
www.tridenttech.edu/ce_22423.htm

Tennessee

Columbia State Community College
Medical Transcriptionist Prgm
1665 Hampshire Pike
Columbia, TN 38401
www.columbiastate.edu/
    ecd-online-medical-transcription

Roane State Community College
Medical Transcriptionist Prgm
276 Patton Lane
Harriman, TN 37748
www.roanestate.edu/keyword.asp?keyword=MDT

Texas

Med-Line School of Medical Transcription
Medical Transcriptionist Prgm
12006 Annette Rd
Angleton, TX 77515
www.medlineschool.com

Central Texas College
Medical Transcriptionist Prgm
PO Box 1800
Killeen, TX 76549
www.ctcd.edu

Utah

Career Step
Medical Transcriptionist Prgm
1220 N Main St
Suite 6
Springville, UT 84663
www.careerstep.com

Washington

Everett Community College
Medical Transcriptionist Prgm
2000 Tower St
Everett, WA 98201
www.everettcc.edu/medtrans

Wisconsin

Lakeshore Technical College
Medical Transcriptionist Prgm
1290 North Ave
Cleveland, WI 53015
www.goltoltc.com

HEALTH INFORMATION AND COMMUNICATION

Laboratory Science

Includes:
- Blood bank technology-specialist
- Clinical assistant
- Clinical laboratory scientist/medical technologist
- Clinical laboratory technician/medical laboratory technician
- Cytogenetic technologist
- Cytotechnologist
- Diagnostic molecular scientist
- Histotechnician
- Histotechnologist
- Pathologists' assistant
- Phlebotomist

Blood Bank Technology-Specialist

Specialists in blood bank technology (SBBs) perform both routine and specialized tests in blood donor centers, transfusion services, reference laboratories, and research facilities. SBBs use methodology that conforms to the Standards for Blood Centers and Transfusion Services of the American Association of Blood Banks (AABB).

Career Description
Specialists in blood bank technology demonstrate a superior level of technical proficiency and problem-solving ability in such areas as:

- Testing for blood group antigens, compatibility, and antibody identification
- Investigating abnormalities such as hemolytic diseases of the newborn, hemolytic anemias, and adverse reactions to transfusion
- Supporting physicians in transfusion therapy for patients with coagulopathies (diseases affecting blood clotting) or candidates for organ and cellular transplantation/therapy
- Performing blood collection and processing, including selecting donors, collecting blood, typing blood, molecular testing, and performing viral marker testing to ensure the safety of the patient.

Accordingly, supervision, management, and/or teaching make up a considerable part of the responsibilities of the specialist in blood bank technology educational program.

Employment Characteristics
Specialists in blood bank technology work in many types of facilities, including community blood centers, private hospital blood banks, university-affiliated blood banks, transfusion services, and independent laboratories. They also may be part of a university faculty. Specialists may have some weekend and night duty, including emergency calls. Qualified specialists may advance to supervisory or administrative positions or move into teaching or research activities. The criteria for advancement in this field are experience, technical expertise, and completion of advanced education courses.

Salary
According to the 2010 Wage and Vacancy Survey conducted by the American Society for Clinical Pathology (ASCP), the median average hourly rate for staff SBBs is $28.62 per hour or $59,530 annually. Supervisory SBBs earn a median average wage of $34.20 per hour or $71,136 annually. The survey results were published in the March 2011 issue of *LabMedicine*, available at *http://labmed.ascpjournals.org/content/42/3/141*.

For more information, refer to *www.ama-assn.org/go/hpsalary*.

Educational Programs
Length. Most educational programs are approximately 12 months. Some programs offer a master's degree and are approximately 24 months.

Prerequisites. Applicants must be certified in medical technology by the Board of Certification and possess a baccalaureate degree from a regionally accredited college or university. If applicants are not certified in medical technology by the Board of Certification, they must possess both a baccalaureate degree from a regionally accredited college or university with a major in any of the biological or physical sciences and have work experience in a blood bank.

Curriculum. Each specific educational program defines its own criteria for measurement of student achievement, and the sequence of instruction is at the discretion of the medical director and the program director and/or educational coordinator of the program. The clinical material available in the educational program provides the student with a full range of experiences. The educational design and environment are conducive to the development of competence in all technical areas of the modern blood bank. The didactic experience covers all theoretical concepts of blood bank immunohematology and transfusion medicine.

Inquiries

Careers/Curriculum
American Association of Blood Banks (AABB)
8101 Glenbrook Road
Bethesda, MD 20814-2749
301 215-6482
www.aabb.org

Certification/Registration
Board of Certification
PO Box 12277
Chicago, IL 60612-0277
312 738-1336
E-mail: *boc@ascp.org*

Program Accreditation

Commission on Accreditation of Allied Health Education Programs (CAAHEP)

1361 Park Street, Clearwater, FL 33756

727 210-2350

727 210-2354 Fax

E-mail: *mail@caahep.org*

www.caahep.org

in collaboration with:

Committee on Accreditation of SBB Schools

American Association of Blood Banks (AABB)

8101 Glenbrook Road

Bethesda, MD 20814-2749

301 215-6482 Education Department

E-mail: *education@aabb.org*

www.aabb.org

Specialist in Blood Bank Technology

Arizona

Blood Systems Laboratories
Specialist in BB Tech Prgm
2424 W Erie
Tempe, AZ 85282

California

American Red Cross Blood Services - Southern California Region
Specialist in BB Tech Prgm
100 Red Cross Way
Pomona, CA 91768

Florida

Transfusion Med Acad Ctr FL Blood Svcs
Specialist in BB Tech Prgm
10100 Dr Martin Luther King Jr St North
St Petersburg, FL 33716-3806
www.fbsblood.org
Prgm Dir: Marjorie Doty, MT(ASCP)SBB
Tel: 727 568-5433, Ext   *Fax:* 727 568-1177
E-mail: mdoty@fbsblood.org

Illinois

Rush University
Specialist in BB Tech Prgm
Department of Clinical Laboratory Sciences
600 S Paulina St, Suite 1021B-AAC
Chicago, IL 60612-3833
www.rush.edu
Notes: Program is offered online. Graduate credit is earned.

Indiana

Indiana Blood Center
Specialist in BB Tech Prgm
3450 N Meridian St
Indianapolis, IN 46208
www.indianablood.org

Louisiana

Medical Center of Louisiana
Specialist in BB Tech Prgm
Blood Bank Department
Medical Center of LA, Blood Bank
2021 Perdido Street
New Orleans, LA 70112
www.mclno.org

Maryland

Johns Hopkins Hospital
Specialist in BB Tech Prgm
Carnegie Bldg #656
600 N Wolfe St
Baltimore, MD 21287-6667
www.jhmi.edu
Prgm Dir: Lorraine Blagg, Education & Development Coordinator
Tel: 410 502-9584   *Fax:* 410 955-0618
E-mail: lblagg1@jhmi.edu

NIH Clinical Center Department of Transfusion
Specialist in BB Tech Prgm
Department of Transfusion Medicine, Bldg 10
10 Center Dr MSC 1184, Rm 1C 711
NIH/CC/DTM Bldg 10
Bethesda, MD 20892-1184
www.clinicalcenter.nih.gov

Walter Reed National Military Med Ctr
Cosponsor: Armed Services Blood Bank Fellowship
Specialist in BB Tech Prgm
8901 Wisconsin Ave
Building 9, BSMT, Room 0712
Bethesda, MD 20889-5600
www.militaryblood.dod.mil/fellow
Prgm Dir: William Turcan, MT(ASCP)SBB
Tel: 301 295-8605
E-mail: william.turcan@med.navy.mil

Ohio

University of Cincinnati Medical Center
Cosponsor: Hoxworth Blood Center
Specialist in BB Tech Prgm
3130 Highland Ave, PO Box 670055
Transfusion and Transplantation Sciences
Cincinnati, OH 45267-0055
www.grad.uc.edu and www.hoxworth.org
Prgm Dir: Ronald A Sacher, MD
Tel: 513 558-1203   *Fax:* 513 558-1279
E-mail: ronald.sacher@uc.edu

American Red Cross Blood Services - Central Ohio Region
Specialist in BB Tech Prgm
995 E Broad
Immunohematology Reference Laboratory
Columbus, OH 43205
Prgm Dir: Joanne Kosanke, MT(ASCP)SBB
Tel: 614 253-2740, Ext   *Fax:* 614 253-2487
E-mail: joanne.kosanke@redcross.org
Notes: The program is for part-time students.

Community Blood Center/Community Tissue Svc
Specialist in BB Tech Prgm
349 S Main St
Dayton, OH 45402-2715
www.cbccts.org

Texas

Univ of Texas Southwestern Med Ctr
Specialist in BB Tech Prgm
5323 Harry Hines Blvd
Dallas, TX 75390-8878
www.utsouthwestern.edu/mls

University of Texas Medical Branch
Specialist in BB Tech Prgm
301 University Blvd
SHP-CLS-SBB program
Pathology/Blood Bank
Galveston, TX 77555-1140
http://http:www.utmb.edu/sbb
Prgm Dir: Janet Vincent, Education Coordinator
Tel: 409 772-9476   *Fax:* 409 772-9470
E-mail: jvincent@utmb.edu

Gulf Coast School of Blood Bank Technology
Specialist in BB Tech Prgm
1400 La Concha Ln
Houston, TX 77054-1802
www.giveblood.org
Prgm Dir: Clare Wong, MT(ASCP)SBB SLS
Tel: 713 791-6201   *Fax:* 713 791-6610
E-mail: cwong@giveblood.org

UT Health Science Center - San Antonio
Cosponsor: University Hospital Health System
Specialist in BB Tech Prgm
Dept of Clinical Laboratory Sci, 6246
7703 Floyd Curl Dr
San Antonio, TX 78229-3900
www.uthscsa.edu

Wisconsin

BloodCenter of Wisconsin
Specialist in BB Tech Prgm
638 N 18th St
PO Box 2178
Milwaukee, WI 53233
www.bcw.edu/bins/site/templates/bloodcenter_default.asp?area_2=public%2Feducation%2Fsbb+progr

Specialist in Blood Bank Technology

Programs*	Class Capacity	Begins	Length (months)	Award	Res. Tuition	Non-res. Tuition	Offers:† 1 2 3 4
Florida							
Transfusion Med Acad Ctr FL Blood Svcs (St Petersburg)	6	Mar	12	Cert	$3,000	$3,000	•
Maryland							
Johns Hopkins Hospital (Baltimore)	3	Sep	52	Cert			
Walter Reed National Military Med Ctr (Bethesda)	8	Jul	18	Cert, SBB, MSHS			
Ohio							
American Red Cross Blood Services - Central Ohio Region (Columbus)	2	Jan	18		$3,000	$3,000 per year	
Univ of Cincinnati Medical Center	2	Sep	15	Dipl, Cert, MS	$12,000	$21,000	
Texas							
Gulf Coast School of Blood Bank Technology (Houston)	6	May	12	Cert			•
Univ of Texas Medical Branch (Galveston)	25	Mar	12	Cert	$3,000	per year	•

*Data are shown only for programs that completed the 2011 AMA Survey of Health Professions Education Programs.

†Key to Offers: 1: Evening or weekend classes; 2: Non-English instruction; 3: Cultural competence instruction; 4: Distance education component.

Clinical Assistant

Laboratory tests play an important role in the detection, diagnosis, and treatment of diseases. Clinical assistants are formally prepared multiskilled health care providers with a laboratory focus. Clinical assistants are trained to work under the supervision of an appropriately qualified person in chemistry, donor room collection screening, component processing, hematology, immunology, microbiology, phlebotomy, and/or urinalysis.

Career Description

Clinical assistants follow standard operating procedures to collect specimens; prepare blood and body fluid specimens for analysis according to standard operating procedures; prepare/reconstitute reagents, standards, and controls according to standard operating procedure; perform appropriate tests at the clinical assistant level; perform and record vital sign measurements; and follow established quality control protocols. Clinical assistants follow infection control and safety practices and use information systems necessary to accomplish job functions.

Employment Characteristics

Many clinical assistants are employed in hospital laboratories. Others are employed in physicians' private laboratories and clinics; by the armed forces; or by city, state, and federal health agencies.

Salary

Salaries vary depending on the employer and geographic location. According to the 2010 Wage and Vacancy Survey conducted by the American Society for Clinical Pathology (ASCP), staff-level laboratory assistants earn a median average wage of $13.52 per hour and $28,122 annually. For supervisors, the median average pay rate was $19.50 per hour or $40,560 annually. The survey results were published in the March 2011 issue of *LabMedicine*, available at *http://labmed.ascpjournals.org/ content/42/3/141*.

For more information, refer to *www.ama-assn.org/go/hpsalary*.

Educational Programs

Length. Approved programs culminate in a postsecondary certificate.

Prerequisites. High school diploma or equivalent. The applicant must also meet the admission requirements of the sponsoring institution.

Curriculum. Clinical assistant programs are conducted in junior or community colleges, hospitals, medical laboratories, proprietary schools, and other equivalent postsecondary educational institutions.

Inquiries

Careers/Curriculum

American Medical Technologists
10700 West Higgins Road, Suite 150
Rosemont, IL 60018
(847) 823-5169
E-mail: *mail@amt1.com*
www.amt1.com

American Society for Clinical Laboratory Science
6701 Democracy Boulevard, Suite 300
Bethesda, MD 20817
(301) 657-2768
E-mail: *ascls@ascls.org*
www.ascls.org

American Society for Clinical Pathology
33 West Monroe, Suite 1600
Chicago, IL 60603
(312) 541-4999
E-mail: *info@ascp.org*
www.ascp.org

Certification/Registration

American Society for Clinical Pathology
Board of Certification
PO Box 12270
Chicago, IL 60612
(312) 738-1336, Ext 1341
E-mail: *boc@ascp.org*
www.ascp.org

American Association of Bioanalysts
Board of Registry
906 Olive Street, Suite 1200
St. Louis, MO 63101-1434
www.aab.org

American Medical Technologists
10700 West Higgins Road, Suite 150
Rosemont, IL 60018
(847) 823-5169
E-mail: *mail@amt1.com*
www.amt1.com

Program Accreditation

Dianne M Cearlock, PhD, Chief Executive Officer
National Accrediting Agency for Clinical Laboratory Sciences
5600 North River Road, Suite 720
Rosemont, IL 60018
(773) 714-8880
E-mail: *dcearlock@naacls.org*
www.naacls.org

Clinical Assistant

Iowa

Indian Hills Community College
Clinical Assisting Prgm
Ottumwa, IA 52501

Massachusetts

Springfield Technical Community College
Clinical Assisting Prgm
Clinical Laboratory Assistant Program
2 Armory Square
Springfield, MA 01102
http://STCC.edu

Michigan

Northern Michigan University
Clinical Assisting Prgm
Clinical Sciences Department
3515 West Science, 1401 Presque Isle Ave
Marquette, MI 49855-5301
www.nmu.edu/cls/cls.htm

Oregon

Clackamas Community College
Clinical Assisting Prgm
19600 South Molalla Ave
Oregon City, OR 97045-7998
www.clackamas.cc.or.us

Pennsylvania

Community College of Allegheny County
Clinical Assisting Prgm
1750 N Clairton Rd, Route 885
West Mifflin, PA 15122

Washington

Edmonds Community College
Clinical Assisting Prgm
20000 68th Ave W
Lynwood, WA 98036
www.edcc.edu

Clinical Laboratory Scientist/Medical Technologist

Laboratory tests play an important role in the detection, diagnosis, and treatment of many diseases. Clinical laboratory scientists/medical technologists perform these tests in conjunction with pathologists (physicians who diagnose the causes and nature of disease) and other physicians or scientists who specialize in clinical chemistry, microbiology, or the other biological sciences. Clinical laboratory scientists/medical technologists develop data on the blood, tissues, and fluids of the human body by using a variety of precise methodologies and technologies.

Career Description

In addition to possessing the skills of clinical laboratory technicians/medical laboratory technicians, clinical laboratory scientists/medical technologists perform complex analyses, fine-line discrimination, and error correction. They are able to recognize the interdependency of tests and have knowledge of physiological conditions affecting test results so that they can confirm these results and develop data that may be used by a physician in determining the presence, extent, and, as far as possible, cause of a disease.

Clinical laboratory scientists/medical technologists assume responsibility and are held accountable for accurate results. They establish and monitor quality assurance and quality improvement programs and design or modify procedures as necessary. Tests and procedures performed or supervised by clinical laboratory scientists/medical technologists in the clinical laboratory focus on major areas of hematology, microbiology, immunohematology, immunology, clinical chemistry, and urinalysis.

Employment Characteristics

Most clinical laboratory scientists/medical technologists are employed in hospital laboratories. Others are employed in physicians' private laboratories and clinics; by the armed forces; by city, state, and federal health agencies; in industrial medical laboratories; in pharmaceutical houses; in numerous public and private research programs dedicated to the study of specific diseases; and as faculty of accredited programs preparing medical laboratory personnel. While many graduates are employed in the clinical laboratory setting, career options are abundant, with opportunities in all areas of health care. As a clinical laboratory scientist/medical technologist, one may decide to specialize in:

- Biomedical research and development
- Andrology and assisted reproductive technology laboratories
- Organ transplantation
- Genetic testing
- Infection control
- Health information management
- Health care industry
- Consultative and entrepreneurial opportunities
- Forensic testing
- Immunohematology (Specialist in Blood Banking or SBB)
- Specialist certification in chemistry, hematology, immunology, or microbiology

Salary

Salaries vary depending on the employer and geographic location. Data from the US Bureau of Labor Statistics (BLS) for May 2011 show that wages at the 10th percentile are $39,550, the 50th percentile (median) at $57,010, and the 90th percentile at $78,160 (*www.bls.gov/oes/current/oes292011.htm*).

According to the 2010 Wage and Vacancy Survey conducted by the American Society for Clinical Pathology (ASCP), full-time, certified clinical laboratory scientists/medical technologists at the staff level earn a national median average wage of $26.16 per hour or $54,412 annually. Supervisors earned a median average wage of $31.68 per hour or $65,478 per year. The survey results were published in the March 2011 issue of *LabMedicine*, available at *http://labmed.ascpjournals.org/content/42/3/141*.

For more information, refer to *www.ama-assn.org/go/hpsalary*.

Employment Outlook

According to the BLS, employment of clinical laboratory workers (both clinical laboratory technologists and technicians) is expected to grow by 14 percent between 2008 and 2018, faster than the average for all occupations. The volume of laboratory tests continues to increase with both population growth and the development of new types of tests.

Educational Programs

Length. Programs are at least one year of professional/clinical education in conjunction with either a baccalaureate or a master's degree.

Prerequisites. College courses and number of required credits are those necessary to ensure admission of a student who is prepared for the clinical educational program. Content areas should include general chemistry, general biological sciences, organic and/or biochemistry, microbiology, immunology, and mathematics. Survey courses do not qualify as fulfillment of chemistry and biological science prerequisites, and remedial mathematics courses will not satisfy the mathematics requirement.

College/university programs that integrate preprofessional and professional coursework are structured with professional courses in the junior and senior years or at the graduate level.

Curriculum. There must be a structured laboratory program, including instruction pertaining to theory and practice in hematology, clinical chemistry, microbiology, immunology, and immunohematology. The program must culminate in a baccalaureate degree for those students not already possessing the degree but may also culminate in a master's degree.

Inquiries

Careers/Curriculum
American Medical Technologists
10700 West Higgins Road, Suite 150
Rosemont, IL 60018
847 823-5169
E-mail: *mail@amt1.com*
www.amt1.com

American Society for Clinical Laboratory Science
6701 Democracy Blvd., Suite 300
Bethesda, MD 20817
301 657-2768
E-mail: *ascls@ascls.org*
www.ascls.org

American Society for Clinical Pathology
33 West Monroe, Suite 1600
Chicago, IL 60603
312 541-4999
E-mail: *info@ascp.org*
www.ascp.org

Certification/Registration
American Society for Clinical Pathology
Board of Certification
PO Box 12270
Chicago, IL 60612
312 738-1336, Ext 1341
www.ascp.org

American Association of Bioanalysts
Board of Registry
906 Olive Street, Suite 1200
St Louis, MO 63101-1434
www.aab.org

American Medical Technologists
10700 West Higgins Road, Suite 150
Rosemont, IL 60018
847 823-5169
E-mail: *mail@amt1.com*
www.amt1.com

Program Accreditation
Dianne M Cearlock, PhD
Chief Executive Officer (CEO)
National Accrediting Agency for Clinical Laboratory Sciences
5600 North River Road, Suite 720
Rosemont, IL 60018
773 714-8880
E-mail: *dcearlock@naacls.org*
www.naacls.org

Note: Adapted in part from the Bureau of Labor Statistics, US Department of Labor, *Occupational Outlook Handbook,* Clinical Laboratory Technologists and Technicians, at *www.bls.gov/oco/ocos096.htm.*

Clinical Laboratory Scientist/Medical Technologist

Alabama

University of Alabama at Birmingham
Clin Lab Scientist/Med Technologist Prgm
1530 3rd Ave S
SHPB 434
Birmingham, AL 35294-1212
http://main.uab.edu/Shrp/default.aspx?pid=78012

Auburn University at Montgomery
Clin Lab Scientist/Med Technologist Prgm
Division of Clinical Laboratory Science
PO Box 244023
Montgomery, AL 36124-3146
www.aum.edu/cls

Baptist Medical Center South
Clin Lab Scientist/Med Technologist Prgm
2105 E South Blvd
PO Box 11010
BMCS Laboratory
Montgomery, AL 36111-0100
baptistfirst.org

Tuskegee University
Clin Lab Scientist/Med Technologist Prgm
School of Nursing and Allied Health
Basil O'Connor Hall
Tuskegee, AL 36088
www.Tuskegee.edu

Alaska

University of Alaska Anchorage
Clin Lab Scientist/Med Technologist Prgm
3211 Providence Dr
AHS 172, University of Alaska Anchorage
Anchorage, AK 99508-4614
http://alliedhealth.uaa.alaska.edu

Arizona

DeVry University - Phoenix
Clin Lab Scientist/Med Technologist Prgm
2149 W Dunlap Ave
Phoenix, AZ 85021
www.devry.edu/programs/clinical_laboratory_science/

Arizona State University
Clin Lab Scientist/Med Technologist Prgm
School of Life Sciences
PO Box 874501
Tempe, AZ 85287-4501
http://sols.asu.edu/cls/

Arkansas

Baptist Health Schools Little Rock
Clin Lab Scientist/Med Technologist Prgm
11900 Colonel Glenn Rd, Ste 1000
Little Rock, AR 72210
www.bhslr.edu

University of Arkansas for Medical Sciences
Clin Lab Scientist/Med Technologist Prgm
4301 W Markham St, Slot 597
Little Rock, AR 72205
www.uams.edu/chrp/medtech/

Arkansas State University
Clin Lab Scientist/Med Technologist Prgm
PO Box 910
State University, AR 72467
www2.astate.edu/a/conhp/cls/index.dot

California

California State University - Dominguez Hills
Clin Lab Scientist/Med Technologist Prgm
1000 E Victoria Blvd
College of Professional Studies, WHA 330
Carson, CA 90747-9960
www.csudh.edu/cps/hhs/dhs/cs/

Arrowhead Regional Medical Center
Clin Lab Scientist/Med Technologist Prgm
400 N Pepper Ave
Clinical Laboratory
Colton, CA 92324

Loma Linda University
Clin Lab Scientist/Med Technologist Prgm
School of Allied Health Professions, Dept of CLS
Nichol Hall, Rm A918
Loma Linda, CA 92350
www.llu.edu/llu/sahp/clinlab/mthome.html

Univ of California Irvine Med Ctr
Clin Lab Scientist/Med Technologist Prgm
101 City Dr S, Rte 38
Orange, CA 92868
www.ucihs.uci.edu/com/pathology/medtechprog.html

Eisenhower Memorial Hospital
Clin Lab Scientist/Med Technologist Prgm
39000 Bob Hope Dr
Kiewit Bldg, Suite 402
Rancho Mirage, CA 92270

Univ of California Davis Health System
Clin Lab Scientist/Med Technologist Prgm
Specialty Testing Center
3740 Business Dr
Sacramento, CA 95820
www.ucdmc.ucdavis.edu/pathology/
    education/cls_training_program/

Univ of California San Diego Med Ctr
Clin Lab Scientist/Med Technologist Prgm
UCSD Clinical Laboratory Science Training Program
200 West Arbor Drive
San Diego, CA 92103-8320

San Francisco State University
Clin Lab Scientist/Med Technologist Prgm
Ctr for Biomedical Laboratory Sci 211
1600 Holloway Ave SCI 202
San Francisco, CA 94132
http://chhsweb.sfsu.edu/cls

San Jose State University
Clin Lab Scientist/Med Technologist Prgm
One Washington Square
San Jose, CA 95192-0100
www.sjsu.edu/cls

Santa Barbara Cottage Hospital
Clin Lab Scientist/Med Technologist Prgm
Pueblo at Bath Sts
PO Box 689
Santa Barbara, CA 93102
www.cottagehealthsystem.org

Colorado

Penrose Hospital
Clin Lab Scientist/Med Technologist Prgm
2222 N Nevada Ave
Colorado Springs, CO 80907-7021
www.penrosestfrancis.org

Metropolitan State College of Denver
Clin Lab Scientist/Med Technologist Prgm
1719 E 19th Ave 5CS
Denver, CO 80218
www.MedLabEd.org

Parkview Medical Center
Clin Lab Scientist/Med Technologist Prgm
Parkview Laboratory, 400 W 16th St
Pueblo, CO 81003
www.parkviewmc.com/pmc.nsf/view/
    schoolofmedicaltech

Connecticut

University of Bridgeport
Clin Lab Scientist/Med Technologist Prgm
Medical Technology
169 University Ave
Bridgeport, CT 06604
www.bridgeport.edu

Danbury Hospital
Clin Lab Scientist/Med Technologist Prgm
School of Medical Technology
24 Hospital Ave
Danbury, CT 06810
www.danburyhospital.org/body.cfm?id=610

Hartford Hospital
Clin Lab Scientist/Med Technologist Prgm
School of Allied Health
560 Hudson St
Hartford, CT 06106
www.harthosp.org

University of Hartford
Clin Lab Scientist/Med Technologist Prgm
Dana Hall, Rm 429
200 Bloomfield Ave
West Hartford, CT 06117-1599
www.hartford.edu

Delaware

University of Delaware-Christiana Care Health
Clin Lab Scientist/Med Technologist Prgm
Dept of Medical Technology
305 Willard Hall Education Building
Newark, DE 19716
www.udel.edu/medtech

District of Columbia

George Washington University
Clin Lab Scientist/Med Technologist Prgm
2300 I St NW, Ste 503
Washington, DC 20037
www.gwumc.edu/healthsci/programs/cls/

Howard University
Clin Lab Scientist/Med Technologist Prgm
6th & Bryant Sts NW
Coll of Phar, Nursing & Allied Hlth Sciences
Dept of Clinical Laboratory Science, Annex 1
Washington, DC 20059
www.howard.edu

Washington Hospital Center
Clin Lab Scientist/Med Technologist Prgm
110 Irving St NW
Department of Pathology and Laboratory Medicine
Washington, DC 20010
www.whcenter.org/departments/pathology

Florida

Santa Fe College
Clin Lab Scientist/Med Technologist Prgm
14180 NW 119th Terrace
Alachua, FL 32615
www.sfcollege.edu/centers/perry/
    index.php?section=clinical_lab_sciences

Florida Gulf Coast University
Clin Lab Scientist/Med Technologist Prgm
10501 FGCU Blvd South
College of Health Professions
Fort Myers, FL 33965-6565
www.fgcu.edu/chp/hs

St Vincent's Medical Center
Clin Lab Scientist/Med Technologist Prgm
1 Shircliff Way
Jacksonville, FL 32204
www.jaxhealth.com/medicalscience

University of North Florida
Clin Lab Scientist/Med Technologist Prgm
Medical Laboratory Science Program
1 UNF Drive
Jacksonville, FL 32224

University of Central Florida
Clin Lab Scientist/Med Technologist Prgm
4000 Central Florida Blvd, HPA II 335A
Orlando, FL 32816-2360
www.biomed.ucf.edu

University of West Florida
Clin Lab Scientist/Med Technologist Prgm
11000 University Pkwy
Pensacola, FL 32514-5751
http://uwf.edu/clinicallabsciences

Bayfront Medical Center
Clin Lab Scientist/Med Technologist Prgm
701 Sixth St S
St Petersburg, FL 33701
www.bayfront.org

Tampa General Hospital
Clin Lab Scientist/Med Technologist Prgm
PO Box 1289
1 Tampa General Cirlcle
Tampa, FL 33606
www.tgh.org/medicaltechnology.htm

Georgia

Emory University System of Health Care
Clin Lab Scientist/Med Technologist Prgm
1364 Clifton Rd, NE, Suite 175
Atlanta, GA 30322
www.emoryhealthcare.org/medtech

Georgia Health Sciences University
Clin Lab Scientist/Med Technologist Prgm
EC-3422
987 St Sebastian Way
Augusta, GA 30912-0500
www.mcg.edu/sah/brt/cls/index.html

Armstrong Atlantic State University
Clin Lab Scientist/Med Technologist Prgm
11935 Abercorn St
Savannah, GA 31419-1997
www.medtech.armstrong.edu

Thomas University
Clin Lab Scientist/Med Technologist Prgm
1501 Millpond Rd
Thomasville, GA 31792
www.thomasu.edu/cls.htm

Hawaii

University of Hawaii at Manoa
Clin Lab Scientist/Med Technologist Prgm
1960 East-West Rd, Bio C206
Honolulu, HI 96822
www.hawaii.edu/medtech/Medtech.html

Idaho

Idaho State University
Clin Lab Scientist/Med Technologist Prgm
Dept of Biological Sciences
741 S Seventh, Box 8007
Pocatello, ID 83209
http://isu.edu/cls

Illinois

Loyola University of Chicago
Clin Lab Scientist/Med Technologist Prgm
School of Continuing and Professional Studies
820 North Michigan Ave - Lewis Towers Suite 401
Chicago, IL 60611
www.luc.edu/scps/clinicallabscience_curriculum.html

Rush University
Clin Lab Scientist/Med Technologist Prgm
600 S Paulina, Ste 1019 AAC
Department of Clinical Laboratory Sciences
Chicago, IL 60612-3833
www.rushu.rush.edu

Northern Illinois University
Clin Lab Scientist/Med Technologist Prgm
Clinical Laboratory Sciences
Dusable 163
DeKalb, IL 60115-2825
www.niu.edu/ahcd/undergrad/clinical_lab.shtml

NorthShore University Health System
Cosponsor: Evanston Hospital
Clin Lab Scientist/Med Technologist Prgm
2650 Ridge Ave, Room 1905C
Department of Pathology and Laboratory Medicine
Evanston, IL 60201
www.NorthShore.org/academicprograms

Edward Hines Jr. VA Hospital
Clin Lab Scientist/Med Technologist Prgm
5000 South 5th Ave
PO Box 5000/113/School
Hines, IL 60141-3030
www.hines.med.va.gov/edu/mt.htm

Illinois State University
Clin Lab Scientist/Med Technologist Prgm
5220 Health Sciences
Normal, IL 61790-5220
www.healthsciences.ilstu.edu/clinical_lab_science/

OSF Saint Francis Medical Center
Clin Lab Scientist/Med Technologist Prgm
530 NE Glen Oak Ave
School of CLS/HT
Peoria, IL 61637
www.osfhealthcare.org

St John's Hospital
Clin Lab Scientist/Med Technologist Prgm
800 E Carpenter St
Springfield, IL 62769
www.st-johns.org

University of Illinois at Springfield
Clin Lab Scientist/Med Technologist Prgm
One University Plaza
MS HSB 314
Springfield, IL 62703
www.uis.edu/clinicallabscience

Indiana

St Francis Hospital & Health Centers
Clin Lab Scientist/Med Technologist Prgm
1600 Albany St
Beech Grove, IN 46107
www.stfrancishospitals.org

Parkview Hospital
Clin Lab Scientist/Med Technologist Prgm
328 Ley Rd
Fort Wayne, IN 46825
http://lab.parkview.com/default.aspx

St Margaret Mercy Healthcare Centers
Clin Lab Scientist/Med Technologist Prgm
5454 Hohman Ave
Hammond, IN 46320
www.ssfhs.org

Indiana University
Clin Lab Scientist/Med Technologist Prgm
Clarian Pathology Laboratory Building, Room 6027F
350 W 11th St
Indianapolis, IN 46202
www.pathology.iupui.edu/CLS

Indiana University Health
Clin Lab Scientist/Med Technologist Prgm
350 W 11th St
CPL-6002 E
Indianapolis, IN 46202
www.clarian.org/portal/patients/education?clarian
ContentID=/education/new_allied_health/train

St Joseph Medical Center
Clin Lab Scientist/Med Technologist Prgm
1907 W Sycamore St
Kokomo, IN 46901

Ball Memorial Hospital/PA Labs,Inc.
Cosponsor: PA Labs Inc
Clin Lab Scientist/Med Technologist Prgm
2401 W University Ave
Muncie, IN 47303
www.palab.com

Good Samaritan Hospital
Clin Lab Scientist/Med Technologist Prgm
520 S Seventh St
Vincennes, IN 47591
www.gshvin.org

Iowa

St Luke's Hospital
Clin Lab Scientist/Med Technologist Prgm
1026 A Ave NE
Cedar Rapids, IA 52402
www.stlukescr.org

Mercy Medical Center - Des Moines
Clin Lab Scientist/Med Technologist Prgm
1111 6th Ave
Des Moines, IA 50314
www.mercydesmoines.org/school_clin_lab_sci/

Mercy Medical Center - Sioux City
Clin Lab Scientist/Med Technologist Prgm
801 5th St
Sioux City, IA 51101
www.mercysiouxcity.com/services/clinical/

St. Luke's College/St. Luke's Regl Med Ctr
Clin Lab Scientist/Med Technologist Prgm
2720 Stone Park Blvd
Sioux City, IA 51104
www.stlukescollege.edu

Allen College
Clin Lab Scientist/Med Technologist Prgm
Clinical Laboratory Science Program
1825 Logan Ave
Waterloo, IA 50703
www.allencollege.edu

Kansas

University of Kansas Medical Center
Clin Lab Scientist/Med Technologist Prgm
3901 Rainbow Blvd, MS 4048
G014 Eaton Molecular Pathology
Kansas City, KS 66160
www.cls.kumc.edu

Wichita State University
Clin Lab Scientist/Med Technologist Prgm
1845 Fairmount St
Campus Box 43
Wichita, KS 67260-0043
http://webs.wichita.edu/?u=chp_mt&p=/index

Kentucky

St Elizabeth Medical Center
Clin Lab Scientist/Med Technologist Prgm
One Medical Village Dr
Edgewood, KY 41017
www.stelizabeth.com/services/our_services/training/
medtechschool/index.asp

University of Kentucky
Clin Lab Scientist/Med Technologist Prgm
Division of Clinical and Reproductive Sciences
900 S Limestone
Room 126G Wethington Building
Lexington, KY 40536-0200
www.mc.uky.edu/CLS/Undergraduate/3+1Option.htm

Bellarmine University
Clin Lab Scientist/Med Technologist Prgm
Lansing Sch of Nursing & Hlth Sci, 108 Pasteur Hall
2001 Newburg Rd
Louisville, KY 40205-0671
www.bellarmine.edu/lansing/cls/

Owensboro Medical Health System
Clin Lab Scientist/Med Technologist Prgm
PO Box 20007
Laboratory
Owensboro, KY 42304-0007
www.omhs.org

Eastern Kentucky University
Clin Lab Scientist/Med Technologist Prgm
Dizney 220
521 Lancaster Ave
Richmond, KY 40475-3102
www.eku.edu/cls

Louisiana

Rapides Regional Medical Center
Clin Lab Scientist/Med Technologist Prgm
211 Fourth St, PO Box 30101
Alexandria, LA 71301
www.rapidesregional.com

Our Lady of the Lake College
Clin Lab Scientist/Med Technologist Prgm
7443 Picardy Ave
Baton Rouge, LA 70808
www.ololcollege-edu.org/content/
admissions-academic-programs-Clinical-
Laboratory-Sciences

Lake Charles Memorial Hospital
Clin Lab Scientist/Med Technologist Prgm
1701 Oak Park Blvd
Lake Charles, LA 70601
www.LCMH.com

McNeese State University
Clin Lab Scientist/Med Technologist Prgm
4205 Ryan St
Box 92000
Lake Charles, LA 70609-2000
http://faculty.mcneese.edu/jbushnel/clswebpagef06.htm

University of Louisiana at Monroe
Clin Lab Scientist/Med Technologist Prgm
700 University Ave
Monroe, LA 71209-0700

Louisiana State Univ Health Sciences Center
Clin Lab Scientist/Med Technologist Prgm
1900 Gravier St, 10C5
LSU Health Sciences Center, Department of Clinical
Laborator
New Orleans, LA 70112
www.lsuhsc.edu

LSU Health Science Center Shreveport
Clin Lab Scientist/Med Technologist Prgm
PO Box 33932
1501 Kings Hwy
Shreveport, LA 71103
www.sh.lsuhsc.edu/ah

Overton Brooks VA Medical Center
Clin Lab Scientist/Med Technologist Prgm
510 E Stoner Ave
Shreveport, LA 71101-4295

Maine

Eastern Maine Medical Center
Clin Lab Scientist/Med Technologist Prgm
489 State St
Bangor, ME 04401
www.medtech.emmc.org

Maryland

Morgan State University
Clin Lab Scientist/Med Technologist Prgm
Cold Spring Ln & Hillen Rd
1700 E Cold Spring Ln
Baltimore, MD 21215
www.morgan.edu/medical technolgy

University of Maryland, Baltimore
Clin Lab Scientist/Med Technologist Prgm
Clin Lab Scientist/Med & Research Technology Prgm
100 Penn St, AHB Room 435
Baltimore, MD 21201-1082
http://medschool.umaryland.edu/dmrt

Walter Reed National Military Med Ctr
Clin Lab Scientist/Med Technologist Prgm
Department of Pathology
8901 Wisconsin Ave
Bethesda, MD 20889-5600
www.wramc.amedd.army.mil/patients/healthcare/
pathology/pages/labofficers.aspx

Salisbury University
Clin Lab Scientist/Med Technologist Prgm
1101 Camden Ave
312B Devilbiss Hall
Salisbury, MD 21801
www.salisbury.edu/healthsci/MEDTECH/

Stevenson University
Clin Lab Scientist/Med Technologist Prgm
1525 Greenspring Valley Rd
Stevenson, MD 21153
www.stevenson.edu

Massachusetts

University of Massachusetts - Lowell
Clin Lab Scientist/Med Technologist Prgm
Department of Clinical Laboratory and Nutritional
    Sciences
3 Solomont Way Suite 4/Weed Hall
Lowell, MA 01854
www.uml.edu/SHE/CLNS

University of Massachusetts - Dartmouth
Clin Lab Scientist/Med Technologist Prgm
Dept of Med Lab Science
285 Old Westport Rd
North Dartmouth, MA 02747-2300
www.umassd.edu/cas/medlabscience/welcome.cfm

Berkshire Medical Center
Clin Lab Scientist/Med Technologist Prgm
725 North St
School of Medical Technology
Pittsfield, MA 01201
www.berkshirehealthsystems.com

Michigan

Andrews University
Clin Lab Scientist/Med Technologist Prgm
Department of Clinical and Laboratory Sciences
Halenz Hall 327
Berrien Springs, MI 49104-0400
www.andrews.edu/CAS/CLS

Ferris State University
Clin Lab Scientist/Med Technologist Prgm
VFS210A
200 Ferris Dr
Big Rapids, MI 49307-2740
www.ferris.edu/cls

DMC University Laboratories
Clin Lab Scientist/Med Technologist Prgm
4201 St Antoine
DMC University Laboratories
Detroit, MI 48201
www.dmc.org/univlab

Wayne State University
Clin Lab Scientist/Med Technologist Prgm
Room 329 Mortuary Science Building
5439 Woodward Ave
Detroit, MI 48202
http:cphs.wayne.edu/cls/index.php

Michigan State University
Clin Lab Scientist/Med Technologist Prgm
322 N Kedzie Hall
Biomedical Laboratory Diagnostics Program
East Lansing, MI 48824
www.bld.msu.edu

Hurley Medical Center
Clin Lab Scientist/Med Technologist Prgm
One Hurley Plaza
Flint, MI 48503
http://hurleymc.com/?id=63&sid=1

Grand Valley State University
Clin Lab Scientist/Med Technologist Prgm
301 Michigan St NE, Ste 200
Cook-DeVos Center for Health Sciences
Grand Rapids, MI 49503-3314
www.gvsu.edu/cls/

St John Health
Clin Lab Scientist/Med Technologist Prgm
19251 Mack Ave, Ste 101
Grosse Pointe Woods, MI 48236
www.stjohn.org/labcareers

Madonna University
Clin Lab Scientist/Med Technologist Prgm
Medical Technology Program
Livonia, MI 48150
www.Madonna.edu

Northern Michigan University
Clin Lab Scientist/Med Technologist Prgm
1401 Presque Isle Ave
3513 West Science
Marquette, MI 49855
www.nmu.edu/cls/cls.htm

Beaumont Hospital - Royal Oak
Clin Lab Scientist/Med Technologist Prgm
3601 W 13 Mile Rd
Department of Clinical Pathology, RI 105
Royal Oak, MI 48073-6769
www.beaumonthospitals.com/alliedhealth

Saginaw Valley State University
Clin Lab Scientist/Med Technologist Prgm
7400 Bay Rd
University Center, MI 48710
www.svsu.edu/acadprog/departments/
    medical-laboratory-science.html

Eastern Michigan University
Clin Lab Scientist/Med Technologist Prgm
316 Marshall Building
Ypsilanti, MI 48197
www.emich.edu/hs/CLSindex.html

Minnesota

Argosy University Twin Cities Campus
Clin Lab Scientist/Med Technologist Prgm
1515 Central Parkway
Eagan, MN 55121
www.argosyu.edu

Fairview Health Services
Clin Lab Scientist/Med Technologist Prgm
2450 Riverside Ave F180-56
Minneapolis, MN 55454
www.fairview.org/cls

Hennepin County Medical Center
Clin Lab Scientist/Med Technologist Prgm
701 Park Ave, Clin Lab P4
Clinical Laboratories
Minneapolis, MN 55415
www.hcmc.org/a_z/EducationPrograms/CLS.htm

University of Minnesota
Clin Lab Scientist/Med Technologist Prgm
420 Delaware St SE, MMC 711
Minneapolis, MN 55455
www.cls.umn.edu

Mayo Clinic
Clin Lab Scientist/Med Technologist Prgm
200 1st St, SW
Rochester, MN 55905
www.mayo.edu/mshs/lab-science-rch.html

St Cloud State University
Clin Lab Scientist/Med Technologist Prgm
162 Wick Science Building
720 Fourth Ave South
St Cloud, MN 56301-4498
www.stcloudstate.edu/healthsciences/MedLabScience

Winona State University
Clin Lab Scientist/Med Technologist Prgm
22224 East Burns Valley Rd
Winona, MN 55987
www.winona.edu

Mississippi

University of Southern Mississippi
Clin Lab Scientist/Med Technologist Prgm
118 College Dr, #5134
Hattiesburg, MS 39406-0001
www.usm.edu/medtech

Mississippi Baptist Medical Center
Clin Lab Scientist/Med Technologist Prgm
1225 N State St
Jackson, MS 39202
www.mbhs.org

University of Mississippi Medical Center
Clin Lab Scientist/Med Technologist Prgm
2500 N State St
Jackson, MS 39216
http://shrp.umc.edu/CLS/index.html

North Mississippi Medical Center
Clin Lab Scientist/Med Technologist Prgm
830 S Gloster
North Mississippi Medical Center
Tupelo, MS 38801
www.nmhs.net/medtech

Missouri

Southeast Missouri Hospital Coll of Nursing
Clin Lab Scientist/Med Technologist Prgm
2001 William St
Cape Girardeau, MO 63703
www.southeastmissourihospital.com/college

St John's Regional Medical Center
Clin Lab Scientist/Med Technologist Prgm
2727 McClelland Blvd
Joplin, MO 64804-1695
www.stj.com

Saint Luke's Hospital
Clin Lab Scientist/Med Technologist Prgm
4401 Wornall Rd
Department of Pathology
Kansas City, MO 64111
www.saintlukeshealthsystem.org/slhs/Services/
    Medical_and_Health_Education/
    Program_in_Clinical

North Kansas City Hospital
Clin Lab Scientist/Med Technologist Prgm
2800 Clay Edwards Dr
North Kansas City, MO 64116-3220
www.nkch.org/lab

Cox Medical Centers
Clin Lab Scientist/Med Technologist Prgm
3801 S National Ave
Springfield, MO 65807
www.coxhealth.com

Saint Louis University
Clin Lab Scientist/Med Technologist Prgm
3437 Caroline St Rm 3102
Dept of Clinical Laboratory Science
St Louis, MO 63104-1111
www.slu.edu/x2361.xml

St John's Mercy Medical Center
Clin Lab Scientist/Med Technologist Prgm
615 S New Ballas Rd
School of Clinical Laboratory Science
St Louis, MO 63141
www.stjohnsmercy.org/sjmmc/departmentservices/scls

Mercy Hospital Springfield - St. Louis
Clin Lab Scientist/Med Technologist Prgm
School of Clinical Laboratory Science
615 South New Ballas Rd
St. Louis, MO 63141-8277
www.stjohnsmercy.org/sjmmc/departmentservices/scls

Montana

Montana State University
Clin Lab Scientist/Med Technologist Prgm
109 Lewis Hall
Bozeman, MT 59717-3520
www.montana.edu/wwwmb

Nebraska

Nebraska Methodist Hospital
Clin Lab Scientist/Med Technologist Prgm
Pathology Center
8303 Dodge St
Omaha, NE 68114
www.unmc.edu/alliedhealth/cls

University of Nebraska Medical Center
Clin Lab Scientist/Med Technologist Prgm
984010 Nebraska Medical Center
Omaha, NE 68198-4010
http://unmc.edu/alliedhealth/cls

Nevada

University of Nevada - Las Vegas
Clin Lab Scientist/Med Technologist Prgm
4505 Maryland Pkwy
Mail Box 453021
Las Vegas, NV 89154-3021
http://alliedhealth.unlv.edu/cls/

New Hampshire

University of New Hampshire
Clin Lab Scientist/Med Technologist Prgm
210 Kendall Hall
129 Main St
Durham, NH 03824
www.mls.unh.edu

New Jersey

Monmouth Medical Center
Clin Lab Scientist/Med Technologist Prgm
300 2nd Ave
Long Branch, NJ 07740

Atlantic Health - Morristown Memorial Hosp
Clin Lab Scientist/Med Technologist Prgm
100 Madison Ave
Laboratory- Box 17
Morristown, NJ 07962
www.atlantichealth.org/Atlantic/
   For+Professionals+%26+Med+Ed/

Jersey Shore University Medical Center
Clin Lab Scientist/Med Technologist Prgm
Florence M Cook School of Medical Laboratory Science
1945 Corlies Ave
Mehandru Pavilion 3
Neptune, NJ 07753
www.jerseyshoreuniversitymedicalcenter.com/
   index.cfm/HealthProf/ClinicalLab/index.cfm

Univ of Medicine & Dent of New Jersey
Clin Lab Scientist/Med Technologist Prgm
School of Health Related Professions
65 Bergen St
Newark, NJ 07107-3006
http://shrp.umdnj.edu/programs/cls/medic.htm

The Valley Hospital
Clin Lab Scientist/Med Technologist Prgm
223 N Van Dien Ave
Ridgewood, NJ 07450

New Mexico

University of New Mexico
Clin Lab Scientist/Med Technologist Prgm
MSC09 5250
1 University of New Mexico
Albuquerque, NM 87131-0001
http://hsc.unm.edu/som/pathology/medlab/

New York

Albany Medical College
Clin Lab Scientist/Med Technologist Prgm
106 New Scotland Ave
Health Science Department
Albany, NY 12208
www.acphs.edu/BSBTCLSgrid.php

New York Methodist Hospital
Clin Lab Scientist/Med Technologist Prgm
1401 Kings Highway, 2nd Floor
Center for Allied Health Education
Brooklyn, NY 11229
www.nymahe.org

Long Island University - C W Post Campus
Clin Lab Scientist/Med Technologist Prgm
720 Northern Blvd
Life Science Building, Rm 349
CW Post Campus
Brookville, NY 11548
www.cwpost.liu.edu/cwis/cwp/health/biomed/

University at Buffalo - SUNY
Clin Lab Scientist/Med Technologist Prgm
26 Cary Hall
3435 Main St
Buffalo, NY 14214-3005
www.smbs.buffalo.edu/cls/

St John's University
Clin Lab Scientist/Med Technologist Prgm
Dr Andrew J Bartilucci Center
175-05 Horace Harding Expwy
Fresh Meadows, NY 11365
www.stjohns.edu

Woman's Christian Association Hospital
Clin Lab Scientist/Med Technologist Prgm
PO Box 840
207 Foote Ave
Jamestown, NY 14702-0840
www.wcahospital.org/mtschool

Marist College
Clin Lab Scientist/Med Technologist Prgm
Dept of Medical Laboratory Sciences, DN 228
Donnelly Hall, Rm 109
3399 North Rd
Poughkeepsie, NY 12601-1387
http://Marist.edu

Rochester General Hospital
Clin Lab Scientist/Med Technologist Prgm
1425 Portland Ave
Rochester, NY 14621
www.rochestergeneral.org

CUNY College of Staten Island
Clin Lab Scientist/Med Technologist Prgm
2800 Victory Blvd
Building 6S, Room 143
Staten Island, NY 10314
www.csi.cuny.edu

Stony Brook University
Clin Lab Scientist/Med Technologist Prgm
Sch of Hlth Tech and Management
Department of Clinical Laboratory Sciences
Stony Brook, NY 11794-8205
www.hsc.stonybrook.edu/shtm/

SUNY Upstate Medical University
Clin Lab Scientist/Med Technologist Prgm
750 E Adams St
Dept of Clinical Laboratory Science
Rm 2156 Weiskotten Hall
Syracuse, NY 13210
www.upstate.edu/chp/mt/

North Carolina

University of North Carolina
Clin Lab Scientist/Med Technologist Prgm
4100 Bondurant Hall, CB # 7145
Division of Clinical Laboratory Science
Chapel Hill, NC 27599-7145
www.unc.edu/ahs/clinical

Carolinas College of Health Sciences
Clin Lab Scientist/Med Technologist Prgm
PO Box 32861
1200 Blythe Blvd
Charlotte, NC 28203
www.carolinascollege.edu

East Carolina University
Clin Lab Scientist/Med Technologist Prgm
Department of Clinical Laboratory Science
Mail Stop 674
Health Sciences Building, 3410
Greenville, NC 27858-4353
www.edu.edu/clsc

Wake Forest University Baptist Medical Center
Clin Lab Scientist/Med Technologist Prgm
Medical Center Blvd
Department of Pathology
Winston-Salem, NC 27157
www1.wfubmc.edu/pathology/medtech

Winston-Salem State University
Clin Lab Scientist/Med Technologist Prgm
CLS Dept FL Atkins Ste 401
601 Martin Luther King Jr Dr
Winston-Salem, NC 27110
www.wssu.edu/wssu

North Dakota

Sanford Medical Center/Sanford Health
Clin Lab Scientist/Med Technologist Prgm
801 Broadway North
PO Box MC
Fargo, ND 58122-0040
www.meritcare.com/jobs/students/lab/index.aspx

University of North Dakota
Clin Lab Scientist/Med Technologist Prgm
SMHS, Dept of Pathology/CLS Program
501 North Columbia Rd Stop 9037
Grand Forks, ND 58202-9037
http://pathology.med.und.nodak.edu/cls/

Ohio

Ohio Northern University
Clin Lab Scientist/Med Technologist Prgm
525 S Main St
Ada, OH 45810
www.onu.edu/wcocls

Akron Children's Hospital
Cosponsor: Akron General Med Center and Summa
   Health System
Clin Lab Scientist/Med Technologist Prgm
One Perkins Square
Akron, OH 44308-1062
www.akronchildrens.org/cms/site/8a472fd91240f270/
   index.html

Bowling Green State University
Clin Lab Scientist/Med Technologist Prgm
504 Life Science Bldg
Bowling Green, OH 43403
www.bgsu.edu/departments/pah/medt/

University of Cincinnati
Clin Lab Scientist/Med Technologist Prgm
3202 Eden Ave
371 French East, ML 0394
Cincinnati, OH 45267-0394
www.cahs.uc.edu/departments/MedicalT.cfm

Cleveland Clinic Foundation
Clin Lab Scientist/Med Technologist Prgm
9500 Euclid Ave
CL-45
Cleveland, OH 44195-5131
www.clevelandclinic.org/mtschool

The Ohio State University
Clin Lab Scientist/Med Technologist Prgm
453 W 10th Ave
Medical Technology Div, 535 Atwell Hall
Columbus, OH 43210
www.amp.osu.edu/mt/

Wright State University
Clin Lab Scientist/Med Technologist Prgm
235 Biological Sciences Building
3640 Colonel Glenn Hwy
Dayton, OH 45435
www.wright.edu/biology/programs/cls

Southwest General Health Center
Clin Lab Scientist/Med Technologist Prgm
18697 E Bagley Rd
Middleburg Heights, OH 44130
www.swgeneral.com

St Vincent Mercy Medical Center
Clin Lab Scientist/Med Technologist Prgm
2222 Cherry St
Toledo, OH 43608
www.ehealthconnection.com/regions/toledo/

University of Toledo
Clin Lab Scientist/Med Technologist Prgm
Department of Biological Sciences, MS#601
2801 W Bancroft St
Toledo, OH 43606
www.utoledo.edu/nsm/bio/undergrad/medtech_html

Oklahoma

Valley View Regional Hospital
Clin Lab Scientist/Med Technologist Prgm
430 N Monta Vista
c/o Laboratory
Ada, OK 74820
www.valeyviewregional.com/medicalservices/laboratory

Comanche County Memorial Hospital
Clin Lab Scientist/Med Technologist Prgm
PO Box 129
3401 West Gore Blvd
Lawton, OK 73505
www.sites.google.com/site/ccmhmtschool

Northeastern State University
Clin Lab Scientist/Med Technologist Prgm
Department of Health Professions, Coll of Sci and Hlth
   Profe
2400 West Shawnee, Rm 145
Muskogee, OK 74401
http://nsuok.edu

Saint Francis Hospital
Clin Lab Scientist/Med Technologist Prgm
6161 S Yale Ave
Tulsa, OK 74136
www.saintfrancislab.com

Oregon

Oregon Health & Science University
Cosponsor: Oregon Insitute of Technology
Clin Lab Scientist/Med Technologist Prgm
3181 SW Sam Jackson Park Rd MTGH
Portland, OR 97239-3098
www.oit.edu/portland/cls

Pennsylvania

Altoona Regional Health System
Clin Lab Scientist/Med Technologist Prgm
620 Howard Ave
Altoona, PA 16601-4899
www.altoonaregional.org/medtech/

Neumann University
Clin Lab Scientist/Med Technologist Prgm
One Neumann Dr
Aston, PA 19014
www.neumann.edu

Pocono Medical Center Laboratory
Clin Lab Scientist/Med Technologist Prgm
Medical Technology Clinical Internship
206 East Brown St
East Stroudsburg, PA 18301
www.poconohealthsystem.org

Saint Vincent Health Center
Clin Lab Scientist/Med Technologist Prgm
232 W 25th St
Erie, PA 16544-0002
www.saintvincenthealth.com/medicalprofessionals/
   medical_technology.htm

Conemaugh Valley Memorial Hospital
Clin Lab Scientist/Med Technologist Prgm
1086 Franklin St
Johnstown, PA 15905-4398
www.conemaugh.org

Lancaster Gen Coll of Nursing & Hlth Sciences
Clin Lab Scientist/Med Technologist Prgm
410 N Lime St
Lancaster, PA 17602
www.lancastergeneralcollege.edu

Pennsylvania Hospital
Clin Lab Scientist/Med Technologist Prgm
800 Spruce St
Room 756 Preston Building
Philadelphia, PA 19107
www.uphs.upenn.edu/pahedu/med_tech

St Christopher's Hospital for Children
Clin Lab Scientist/Med Technologist Prgm
Dept of Pathology and Laboratory Medicine
E Erie Ave at N Front St
3601 A St
Philadelphia, PA 19134
www.stchristophershospital.com/CWSContent/
   stchristophershospital/ourServices/medicalServices/

Thomas Jefferson University
Clin Lab Scientist/Med Technologist Prgm
130 S 9th St, Ste 1924
Philadelphia, PA 19107
www.jefferson.edu/jchp/ls

Reading Hospital & Medical Center
Clin Lab Scientist/Med Technologist Prgm
PO Box 16052
Reading, PA 19612-6052
www.readinghospital.org/oth/Page.asp?PageID=
   OTH000418

Robert Packer Hospital
Cosponsor: Guthrie Health Systems
Clin Lab Scientist/Med Technologist Prgm
One Guthrie Square
Sayre, PA 18840
www.guthrie.org/medtech

Mount Nittany Medical Center
Clin Lab Scientist/Med Technologist Prgm
1800 E Park Ave
Clinical Laboratory Science School
State College, PA 16803
www.mountnittany.org

Williamsport Hosp & Medical Center
Clin Lab Scientist/Med Technologist Prgm
777 Rural Ave
c/o Williamsport Hospital Lab
Williamsport, PA 17701
www.susquehannahealth.org

York Hospital/WellSpan Health
Clin Lab Scientist/Med Technologist Prgm
1001 S George St
Allied Health - CLS Program
York, PA 17405-7198
www.wellspan.org/EducationResearch/
   AlliedHealthEducation_YHLabScience.htm

Puerto Rico

Pontifical Catholic University of Puerto Rico
Clin Lab Scientist/Med Technologist Prgm
2250 Las Americas Ave, Ste 588
Ponce, PR 00717-9997
www.pucpr.edu

Inter American University of Puerto Rico
Clin Lab Scientist/Med Technologist Prgm
Call Box 5100
San German, PR 00683-9801
www.sg.inter.edu

Inter American University of Puerto Rico
Clin Lab Scientist/Med Technologist Prgm
PO Box 191293
Francisco Sein State Rd 1
San Juan, PR 00919-1293
www.metro.inter.edu

University of Puerto Rico
Clin Lab Scientist/Med Technologist Prgm
Med Sciences Campus - School of Health Professions
PO Box 365067
San Juan, PR 00927
http://cprsweb.rcm.upr.edu/tecnologiamedica.asp

Qatar

Qatar University
Clin Lab Scientist/Med Technologist Prgm
PO 2713
Doha, Qatar, QA
www.qu.edu.qa/artssciences/health/programs/
biomedical/index.php

Rhode Island

Our Lady of Fatima Hospital
Clin Lab Scientist/Med Technologist Prgm
200 High Service Ave
North Providence, RI 02904
www.saintjosephri.com

Rhode Island Hospital
Clin Lab Scientist/Med Technologist Prgm
593 Eddy St
PO Building, Rm 034
Providence, RI 02903

South Carolina

Palmetto Health Baptist
Clin Lab Scientist/Med Technologist Prgm
Taylor at Marion Sts
Columbia, SC 29220
www.palmettohealth.org/body.cfm?id=246

McLeod Regional Medical Center
Clin Lab Scientist/Med Technologist Prgm
PO Box 100551
Medical Park West Suite 350
305 E Cheves St
Florence, SC 29506
www.peedeeahec.net

Lexington Medical Center
Clin Lab Scientist/Med Technologist Prgm
2720 Sunset Blvd
West Columbia, SC 29169
www.lexmed.com/medical_services/
School_of_Medical_Tech.htm

South Dakota

South Dakota State University
Clin Lab Scientist/Med Technologist Prgm
121 Shepard Hall
SAV 131, Box 2202
Brookings, SD 57007-0896
www.sdstate.edu

Sanford USD Medical Center
Clin Lab Scientist/Med Technologist Prgm
1305 W 18th St
Sanford USD Medical Center, Lab
Sioux Falls, SD 57117-5039
www.sanfordhealth.org/clsmtprogram

Tennessee

Austin Peay State University
Clin Lab Scientist/Med Technologist Prgm
PO Box 4668
Allied Health Sciences
Clarksville, TN 37044
www.apsu.edu/medtech

Lincoln Memorial University
Clin Lab Scientist/Med Technologist Prgm
6965 Cumberland Gap Pkwy
Harrogate, TN 37752
www.lmunet.edu/academics/programs/medical.html

University of Tennessee Medical Center
Clin Lab Scientist/Med Technologist Prgm
1924 Alcoa Hwy SW
Knoxville, TN 37920
www.utmedicalcenter.org/health_professionals/
educational_services/medical_technology_program

Baptist College of Health Sciences
Clin Lab Scientist/Med Technologist Prgm
1003 Monroe Ave
Memphis, TN 38104
www.bchs.edu

University of Tennessee Health Science Ctr
Clin Lab Scientist/Med Technologist Prgm
930 Madison Ave, Suite 664
Memphis, TN 38163
www.utmem.edu/allied/mthome.html

Vanderbilt University Medical Center
Clin Lab Scientist/Med Technologist Prgm
4605D The Vanderbilt Clinic
1301 Medical Center Dr
Nashville, TN 37232-5310
www.mc.vanderbilt.edu/medtech/

Texas

Austin State Hospital
Clin Lab Scientist/Med Technologist Prgm
4110 Guadalupe St
Austin, TX 78751-4296
www.dshs.state.tx.us/mhhospitals/AustinSH/
ResMedTech.shtm

CHRISTUS Hospital - St Elizabeth
Clin Lab Scientist/Med Technologist Prgm
2830 Calder St, PO Box 5405
Beaumont, TX 77726-5405
www.christusste.org

Texas A&M University - Corpus Christi
Clin Lab Scientist/Med Technologist Prgm
College of Science and Technology
6300 Ocean Dr
Corpus Christi, TX 78412
http://lsci.tamucc.edu/bims/Main/CLS

Univ of Texas Southwestern Med Ctr
Clin Lab Scientist/Med Technologist Prgm
5323 Harry Hines Blvd
Dallas, TX 75390-8878
www.utsouthwestern.edu/mls

Univ of Texas - Pan American
Clin Lab Scientist/Med Technologist Prgm
1201 W University Dr
Edinburg, TX 78539
http://portal.utpa.edu/utpa_main/daa_home/hshs_home
/clinlab_home

University of Texas at El Paso
Clin Lab Scientist/Med Technologist Prgm
1101 N Campbell, Rm 718
El Paso, TX 79902
http://academics.utep.edu/Default.aspx?alias=
academics.utep.edu/cls

Tarleton State University
Clin Lab Scientist/Med Technologist Prgm
1501 Enderly Place
Fort Worth, TX 76104
www.tarleton.edu/~clinlab

University of Texas Medical Branch
Clin Lab Scientist/Med Technologist Prgm
School of Allied Hlth Sciences
301 University Blvd
Galveston, TX 77555-1140
www.sahs.utmb.edu/cls/

Texas Southern University
Clin Lab Scientist/Med Technologist Prgm
3100 Cleburne Ave
Houston, TX 77004
www.tsu.edu

The Methodist Hospital
Clin Lab Scientist/Med Technologist Prgm
6565 Fannin, B154
Houston, TX 77030
www.methodisthealth.com

Univ of Texas M D Anderson Cancer Ctr
Clin Lab Scientist/Med Technologist Prgm
1515 Holcombe Blvd Unit 002
Houston, TX 77030
www.mdanderson.org/healthsciences

Texas Tech Univ Health Sciences Center
Clin Lab Scientist/Med Technologist Prgm
School of Allied Health Sciences
3601 4th St MS 8261
Lubbock, TX 79430
www.ttuhsc.edu/pages/alh

UT Health Science Center - San Antonio
Clin Lab Scientist/Med Technologist Prgm
7703 Floyd Curl Dr
Dept of Clinical Laboratory Sciences - MC 6246
San Antonio, TX 78229-3900
www.uthscsa.edu/sah/cls/cls.html

Texas State University - San Marcos
Clin Lab Scientist/Med Technologist Prgm
601 University Dr
San Marcos, TX 78666-4616
www.health.txstate.edu/cls

Scott & White Hospital
Clin Lab Scientist/Med Technologist Prgm
2401 S 31st St
Temple, TX 76508
http://cls.sw.org

United Regional Health Care Systems
Clin Lab Scientist/Med Technologist Prgm
1600 Eleventh St
Wichita Falls, TX 76301

Utah

Weber State University
Clin Lab Scientist/Med Technologist Prgm
3905 University Circle
Ogden, UT 84408-3905
www.weber.edu/cls

Brigham Young University
Clin Lab Scientist/Med Technologist Prgm
379 WIDB
Provo, UT 84602
http://mmbio.byu.edu/home/Academic_Programs/

University of Utah Health Science Center
Clin Lab Scientist/Med Technologist Prgm
Dept of Pathology
30 North 1900 East
Salt Lake City, UT 84132
http://path.utah.edu/mls

Dixie State College of Utah
Clin Lab Scientist/Med Technologist Prgm
Medical Labortory Science Program
225 S 700 East
St. George, UT 84770

Vermont

University of Vermont
Clin Lab Scientist/Med Technologist Prgm
Medical Laboratory and Radiation Sciences
302 Rowell Hall
106 Carrigan Drive
Burlington, VT 05405
www.uvm.edu/~mlrs/?Page=programs/
mls_program.html&SM=programs_menu.html

Virginia

Inova Fairfax Hospital
Clin Lab Scientist/Med Technologist Prgm
3300 Gallows Rd
Falls Church, VA 22042

Augusta Medical Center
Clin Lab Scientist/Med Technologist Prgm
PO Box 1000
78 Medical Center Dr
Fishersville, VA 22939
www.augustamed.com/cls

Rockingham Memorial Hospital
Clin Lab Scientist/Med Technologist Prgm
235 Cantrell Ave
Harrisonburg, VA 22801
www.rmhonline.com

Norfolk State University
Clin Lab Scientist/Med Technologist Prgm
700 Park Ave
Norfolk, VA 23504
www.nsu.edu

Old Dominion University
Clin Lab Scientist/Med Technologist Prgm
School of Med Laboratory and Radiation Sciences
2118 Health Sciences Bldg
Norfolk, VA 23529
http://hs.odu.edu/medlab/academics/medtech/

Virginia Commonwealth University
Cosponsor: VCU Medical Center
Clin Lab Scientist/Med Technologist Prgm
PO Box 980583, Medical Center Campus
301 College St
Richmond, VA 23298-0583
www.sahp.vcu.edu/cls

Carilion Medical Center / Jefferson College of Health Sciences
Clin Lab Scientist/Med Technologist Prgm
Carilion Roanoke Community Hospital
101 Elm Ave SW
Roanoke, VA 24013

Washington

University of Washington
Clin Lab Scientist/Med Technologist Prgm
School of Medicine
Dept of Laboratory Medicine, Box 357110
Seattle, WA 98195-7110
http://depts.washington.edu/labweb/Education/
MedTech/

Providence Sacred Heart Medical Center
Clin Lab Scientist/Med Technologist Prgm
101 W Eighth Ave
Spokane, WA 99220-2555
www.shmclab.org

Heritage University
Clin Lab Scientist/Med Technologist Prgm
3240 Fort Rd
Toppenish, WA 98948
www.heritage.edu

West Virginia

Marshall University
Clin Lab Scientist/Med Technologist Prgm
One John Marshall Dr
Huntington, WV 25755
www.marshall.edu/clinical

West Virginia University
Clin Lab Scientist/Med Technologist Prgm
2163E Health Sciences Ctr N, PO Box 9211
Morgantown, WV 26506-9211
www.hsc.wvu.edu/som/medtech

West Liberty State College
Clin Lab Scientist/Med Technologist Prgm
Dept of Health Sciences
325C Main Hall
CSC 140
West Liberty, WV 26074
www.westliberty.edu

Wisconsin

Affinity Health System - St Elizabeth Hosp
Clin Lab Scientist/Med Technologist Prgm
1506 S Oneida St
Appleton, WI 54915
www.affinityhealth.org

Sacred Heart Hospital
Clin Lab Scientist/Med Technologist Prgm
900 W Clairemont Ave
Eau Claire, WI 54701
www.sacredhearteauclaire.org/OurServices/Laboratory/

University of Wisconsin - Madison
Clin Lab Scientist/Med Technologist Prgm
1300 University Ave
6173 MSC
Madison, WI 53706
www.clsmedtech.wisc.edu

Saint Joseph's Hospital / Marshfield Clinic
Clin Lab Scientist/Med Technologist Prgm
Marshfield Laboratories
1000 N Oak Ave
Marshfield, WI 54449
www.marshfieldlabs.org/marshfieldlabs/
default.aspx?page=laboratorycareer

Clement J Zablocki VA Medical Center
Clin Lab Scientist/Med Technologist Prgm
5000 W National Ave
Milwaukee, WI 53295

Marquette University
Clin Lab Scientist/Med Technologist Prgm
PO Box 1881
Milwaukee, WI 53201-1881
www.marquette.edu/chs/clls/

University of Wisconsin - Milwaukee
Clin Lab Scientist/Med Technologist Prgm
Department of Health Sciences
PO Box 413
Enderis Hall - 411
Milwaukee, WI 53201
www4.uwm.edu/chs/academics/undergraduate/
healthsciences/

University of Wisconsin - Stevens Point
Clin Lab Scientist/Med Technologist Prgm
D127 Science Bldg
UW-Stevens Point College of Professional Studies
Stevens Point, WI 54481
www.uwsp.edu/hlthsci

Aspirus Wausau Hospital
Clin Lab Scientist/Med Technologist Prgm
333 Pine Ridge Blvd
Wausau, WI 54401
www.aspirus.org/ourServices/index.cfm?catID=
1&subCatID=11&pageID=123

Clinical Laboratory Technician/Medical Laboratory Technician

Laboratory tests play an important role in the detection, diagnosis, and treatment of many diseases and in the promotion of health. Clinical laboratory technicians/medical laboratory technicians perform these tests under the supervision or direction of pathologists (physicians who diagnose the causes and nature of disease) and other physicians, clinical laboratory scientists/medical technologists, or other scientists who specialize in clinical chemistry, microbiology, or the other biological sciences. Clinical laboratory technicians/medical laboratory technicians develop data on the blood, tissues, and fluids of the human body by using a variety of precise methodologies and technologies.

Career Description

Clinical laboratory technicians/medical laboratory technicians typically hold an associate degree and perform all the routine tests in an up-to-date medical laboratory and can demonstrate discrimination between closely similar items and correction of errors by the use of preset strategies. The technician has knowledge of specific techniques and instruments and is able to recognize factors that directly affect procedures and results. The technician also monitors quality assurance procedures.

Employment Characteristics

Most clinical laboratory technicians/medical laboratory technicians work in hospital, clinic, or physician office laboratories.

Salary

Salaries vary, depending upon the employer and geographic location. Data from the US Bureau of Labor Statistics (BLS) for May 2011 show that wages at the 10th percentile are $24,580, the 50th percentile (median) at $36,950, and the 90th percentile at $57,330 (*www.bls.gov/oes/current/oes292012.htm*).

According to the 2010 Wage and Vacancy Survey conducted by the American Society for Clinical Pathology (ASCP), the average median hourly wage is $19.78 per hour or $40,768 per year for staff-level clinical laboratory technicians/medical laboratory technicians employees, while supervisors earned a median average wage of $23.72 per hour or $49,338 yearly. The survey results were published in the March 2011 issue of *LabMedicine*; available at *http://labmed.ascpjournals.org/content/42/3/141*.

For more information, refer to *www.ama-assn.org/go/hpsalary*.

Educational Programs

Length. The period of education is usually two academic years and typically culminates in an associate degree.

Prerequisites. High school diploma or equivalent. The applicant also must meet the admission requirements of the sponsoring educational institution.

Curriculum. Associate degree programs are conducted in junior or community colleges, in two-year divisions of universities and colleges, or in other recognized institutions granting associate degrees. Courses are taught on campus and usually in affiliated hospitals. Classroom and laboratory classes focus on general knowledge and basic skills; understanding principles and master procedures of laboratory testing; and basic laboratory mathemat-

ics, computer technology, communication skills, and interpersonal relationships and responsibilities. The clinical courses include application of basic principles commonly used in the diagnostic laboratory. Clinical instruction includes procedures in hematology, microbiology, immunohematology, immunology, clinical chemistry, and urinalysis.

Inquiries

Careers/Curriculum
American Medical Technologists
10700 West Higgins Road, Suite 150
Rosemont, IL 60018
847 823-5169
E-mail: *mail@amt1.com*
www.amt1.com

American Society for Clinical Laboratory Science
6701 Democracy Blvd., Suite 300
Bethesda, MD 20817
301 657-2768
E-mail: *ascls@ascls.org*
www.ascls.org

American Society for Clinical Pathology
33 West Monroe, Suite 1600
Chicago, IL 60603
312 541-4999
E-mail: *info@ascp.org*
www.ascp.org

Certification/Registration
American Society for Clinical Pathology
Board of Certification
PO Box 12270
Chicago, IL 60612
312 738-1336, Ext 1341
E-mail: *boc@ascp.org*
www.ascp.org

American Association of Bioanalysts
Board of Registry
906 Olive Street, Suite 1200
St. Louis, MO 63101-1434
www.aab.org

American Medical Technologists
10700 West Higgins Road, Suite 150
Rosemont, IL 60018
847 823-5169
E-mail: *mail@amt1.com*
www.amt1.com

Program Accreditation
Dianne M Cearlock, PhD, Chief Executive Officer
National Accrediting Agency for Clinical Laboratory Sciences
5600 North River Road, Suite 720
Rosemont, IL 60018
773 714-8880
E-mail: *dcearlock@naacls.org*
www.naacls.org

Clinical Laboratory Technician/Medical Laboratory Technician

Alabama

Jefferson State Community College
Clin Lab Technician/Med Lab Technician Prgm
2601 Carson Rd
Birmingham, AL 35215
www.jeffstateonline.com

Calhoun Community College
Clin Lab Technician/Med Lab Technician Prgm
PO Box 2216
Decatur, AL 35609-2216

Gadsden State Community College
Clin Lab Technician/Med Lab Technician Prgm
PO Box 227 Gadsden State Community College
1001 George Wallace Dr
Bevill Hall
Gadsden, AL 35902-0227
www.gadsdenstate.edu

Wallace State Community College
Clin Lab Technician/Med Lab Technician Prgm
801 Main St NW
PO Box 2000
Hanceville, AL 35077-2000
www.wallacestate.edu

Alaska

University of Alaska Anchorage
Clin Lab Technician/Med Lab Technician Prgm
AHS 172
3211 Providence Dr
Anchorage, AK 99508-4614
www.uaa.alaska.edu/ctc/alliedhealth/
    medlab/labtech.cfm

Arizona

Brookline College - Phoenix
Clin Lab Technician/Med Lab Technician Prgm
2445 W Dunlap Ave, Suite 100
Phoenix, AZ 85021
http://brooklinecollege.edu

Phoenix College
Clin Lab Technician/Med Lab Technician Prgm
1202 W Thomas Rd
Phoenix, AZ 85013
www.phoenixcollege.edu/he/mlt

Pima Community College
Clin Lab Technician/Med Lab Technician Prgm
2202 W Anklam Rd
Tucson, AZ 85709
www.pima.edu

Arkansas

Arkansas State University - Beebe
Clin Lab Technician/Med Lab Technician Prgm
PO Box 1000
Beebe, AR 72012
www.asub.edu

South Arkansas Community College
Clin Lab Technician/Med Lab Technician Prgm
PO Box 7010
El Dorado, AR 71731-7070
www.southark.edu

North Arkansas College
Clin Lab Technician/Med Lab Technician Prgm
1515 Pioneer Dr
Harrison, AR 72601-5599
www.northark.edu

Phillips Community College/U of Arkansas
Clin Lab Technician/Med Lab Technician Prgm
PO Box 785
1000 Campus Drive
Helena-West Helena, AR 72342
www.pccua.edu

National Park Community College
Clin Lab Technician/Med Lab Technician Prgm
101 College Dr
Hot Springs, AR 71913-9174
www.npcc.edu

Arkansas State University
Clin Lab Technician/Med Lab Technician Prgm
PO Box 910
State University, AR 72467
www2.astate.edu/a/conhp/cls/index.dot

California

Southwestern College
Clin Lab Technician/Med Lab Technician Prgm
900 Otay Lakes Rd
Chula Vista, CA 91910
www.swccd.edu

De Anza College
Clin Lab Technician/Med Lab Technician Prgm
21250 Stevens Creek Blvd
Cupertino, CA 95014
www.deanza.edu

Folsom Lake College
Clin Lab Technician/Med Lab Technician Prgm
10 College Parkway
Folsom, CA 95630
www.flc.losrios.edu

Diablo Valley College
Clin Lab Technician/Med Lab Technician Prgm
321 Golf Club Rd
Pleasant Hill, CA 94523

Kaiser Permanente School of Allied Health Sci
Clin Lab Technician/Med Lab Technician Prgm
938 Marina South
Richmond, CA 94804

Hartnell Community College
Clin Lab Technician/Med Lab Technician Prgm
156 Homestead Ave
Salinas, CA 93901-1697
www.hartnell.edu

Naval School of Health Sciences, San Diego
Clin Lab Technician/Med Lab Technician Prgm
34101 Farenholt Ave
San Diego, CA 92134-5291
www.navy.med.mil/nshs-sd/
Notes: Note: Program for military personnel only

Institute of Medical Education
Clin Lab Technician/Med Lab Technician Prgm
130 Park Center Plaza
San Jose, CA 95113
www.imededu.com

College of the Canyons
Clin Lab Technician/Med Lab Technician Prgm
26455 Rockwell Canyon Rd
Santa Clarita, CA 91355
www.canyons.edu/MLT

Colorado

Arapahoe Community College
Clin Lab Technician/Med Lab Technician Prgm
5900 S Santa Fe Dr
PO Box 9002
Littleton, CO 80160-9002
www.arapahoe.edu

Delaware

**Delaware Technical Community College -
    Owens Campus**
Clin Lab Technician/Med Lab Technician Prgm
PO Box 610
Rte 18 Seashore Highway
Georgetown, DE 19947
www.dtcc.edu/owens/medlab

Florida

Brevard Community College
Clin Lab Technician/Med Lab Technician Prgm
1519 Clearlake Rd
Cocoa, FL 32922
www.brevardcc.edu

Keiser University
Clin Lab Technician/Med Lab Technician Prgm
1500 NW 49th St
Fort Lauderdale, FL 33309
www.keiseruniversity.edu

MedVance Institute - Fort Lauderdale
Clin Lab Technician/Med Lab Technician Prgm
4850 West Oakland Park Blvd, Suite 200
Fort Lauderdale, FL 33313

Southwest Florida College - Fort Myers
Clin Lab Technician/Med Lab Technician Prgm
1685 Medical Lane
Fort Myers, FL 33907
www.swfc.edu

Indian River State College
Clin Lab Technician/Med Lab Technician Prgm
3209 Virginia Ave
Fort Pierce, FL 34981
www.irsc.edu

Florida State College at Jacksonville
Clin Lab Technician/Med Lab Technician Prgm
North Campus, 4501 Capper Rd
Jacksonville, FL 32218
http://catalog.fccj.edu/preview_program.php?catoid=
    1&poid=59&bc=1

Dade Medical College
Clin Lab Technician/Med Lab Technician Prgm
Medical Center Campus
950 NW 20th St
Miami, FL 33127
www.mdc.edu/medical/AHT/MLT/default.asp

MedVance Institute - West Palm Beach
Clin Lab Technician/Med Lab Technician Prgm
1630 South Congress Ave, Suite 300
Palm Springs, FL 33461

St Petersburg College
Clin Lab Technician/Med Lab Technician Prgm
PO Box 13489
St Petersburg, FL 33733
www.spcollege.edu/hec/medlab

Southwest Florida College - Tampa
Clin Lab Technician/Med Lab Technician Prgm
3910 Riga Blvd
Tampa, FL 33619
www.swfc.edu

Georgia

Darton College
Clin Lab Technician/Med Lab Technician Prgm
2400 Gillionville Rd
Albany, GA 31707
www.darton.edu/programs/AlliedHealth/mlt/

College of Coastal Georgia
Clin Lab Technician/Med Lab Technician Prgm
3700 Altama Ave
Brunswick, GA 31520
www.ccga.edu

Chattahoochee Technical College
Clin Lab Technician/Med Lab Technician Prgm
1645 Bluffs Parkway
Canton, GA 30114

North Georgia Technical College
Clin Lab Technician/Med Lab Technician Prgm
Hwy 197 N, PO Box 65
1500 Hwy 197 N
Clarkesville, GA 30523
www.northgatech.edu

Georgia Piedmont Technical College
Clin Lab Technician/Med Lab Technician Prgm
495 N Indian Creek Dr
Clarkston, GA 30021-2397
www.dekalbtech.edu

Dalton State College
Clin Lab Technician/Med Lab Technician Prgm
650 College Dr
Dalton, GA 30728
www.daltonstate.edu/technicaldivision/mlt

Central Georgia Technical College
Clin Lab Technician/Med Lab Technician Prgm
3300 Macon Tech Dr
Macon, GA 31206
www.centralgatech.edu/catalog/section6/ah/ML03.htm

Miller-Motte Technical College - Macon
Clin Lab Technician/Med Lab Technician Prgm
(McCann School of Business & Technology MLT
    Consortium)
175 Tom Hill Senior Rd
Macon, GA 31210

Lanier Technical College
Clin Lab Technician/Med Lab Technician Prgm
2990 Landrum Education Dr
Oakwood, GA 30566
laniertech.edu

Southwest Georgia Technical College
Clin Lab Technician/Med Lab Technician Prgm
15689 US Hwy 19 N
Thomasville, GA 31792
www.swgtc.net

Wiregrass Georgia Technical College
Clin Lab Technician/Med Lab Technician Prgm
4089 Val Tech Rd
Valdosta, GA 31602-0929
www.valdostatech.org/site/academics/degree/
    med_lab.asp

Southeastern Technical College
Clin Lab Technician/Med Lab Technician Prgm
3001 E First St
Vidalia, GA 30474
www.southeasterntech.edu

West Georgia Technical College
Clin Lab Technician/Med Lab Technician Prgm
178 Murphy Campus Blvd
Waco, GA 30182
www.westcentraltech.edu

Okefenokee Technical College
Clin Lab Technician/Med Lab Technician Prgm
1701 Carswell Ave
Waycross, GA 31503
www.okefenokeetech.edu

Hawaii

Kapiolani Community College
Clin Lab Technician/Med Lab Technician Prgm
4303 Diamond Head Rd
Health Sciences/MLT Program
Honolulu, HI 96816
www.kcc.hawaii.edu/object/mlt.html

Illinois

Southwestern Illinois College
Clin Lab Technician/Med Lab Technician Prgm
2500 Carlyle Rd
Belleville, IL 62221-5899
www.swic.edu

Sanford-Brown College - Collinsville
Clin Lab Technician/Med Lab Technician Prgm
1101 Eastport Plaza Drive
Collinsville, IL 62234
www.sanfordbrown.edu

Oakton Community College
Clin Lab Technician/Med Lab Technician Prgm
1600 E Golf Rd
Division 1
Des Plaines, IL 60016
www.oakton.edu/acad/dept/mlt/

Illinois Central College
Clin Lab Technician/Med Lab Technician Prgm
Thomas K Thomas Bldg
201 SW Adams St
One College Drive
East Peoria, IL 61635-0001
www.icc.edu

Elgin Community College
Clin Lab Technician/Med Lab Technician Prgm
1700 Spartan Dr
Elgin, IL 60123-7193
www.elgin.edu

Southern Illinois Collegiate Common Market
Clin Lab Technician/Med Lab Technician Prgm
3213 S Park Ave
Herrin, IL 62948
http://siccm.com

Kankakee Community College
Clin Lab Technician/Med Lab Technician Prgm
100 College Dr
Kankakee, IL 60901
www.kcc.edu

Blessing Hospital
Clin Lab Technician/Med Lab Technician Prgm
Broadway at 11th St
Quincy, IL 62301
www.blessinghealthsystem.com

Indiana

Medtech College-Fort Wayne
Clin Lab Technician/Med Lab Technician Prgm
7230 Engle Rd, Suite 200
Ft. Wayne, IN 46804
www.medtechcollege.edu

MedTech College-Greenwood
Clin Lab Technician/Med Lab Technician Prgm
1500 American Way
Greenwood, IN 46143
www.medtechcollege.edu

Harrison College
Clin Lab Technician/Med Lab Technician Prgm
8150 Brookville Rd
Indianapolis, IN 46239
www.harrison.edu

MedTech College-Indianapolis
Clin Lab Technician/Med Lab Technician Prgm
6612 E 75th St
Indianapolis, IN 46250
www.medtechcollege.edu

**Ivy Tech Community College - Southern
    Indiana**
Clin Lab Technician/Med Lab Technician Prgm
8204 Hwy 311
Sellersburg, IN 47172
www.ivytech.edu/sellersburg

Ivy Tech Community College - South Bend
Clin Lab Technician/Med Lab Technician Prgm
220 Dean Johnson Blvd
South Bend, IN 46601-3415
www.ivytech.edu/schools/health/
    medical-laboratory-tech/index.html

Ivy Tech Community College
Clin Lab Technician/Med Lab Technician Prgm
8000 Education Dr
Terre Haute, IN 47802-4898
www.ivytech.edu/terrehaute

Iowa

Des Moines Area Community College
Clin Lab Technician/Med Lab Technician Prgm
2006 S Ankeny Blvd, Bldg 9
Ankeny, IA 50023
http://go.dmacc.edu/programs/medlabtech/pages/
    welcome.aspx

Iowa Central Community College
Clin Lab Technician/Med Lab Technician Prgm
330 Ave M
One Triton Circle
Fort Dodge, IA 50501
www.iccc.cc.ia.us/health/files/labtech.htm

Indian Hills Community College
Clin Lab Technician/Med Lab Technician Prgm
655 Indian Hills Drive, Bldg 21
Ottumwa, IA 52501

Hawkeye Community College
Clin Lab Technician/Med Lab Technician Prgm
1501 E Orange Rd, PO Box 8015
Waterloo, IA 50704
www.hawkeyecollege.edu

Kansas

Barton County Community College
Clin Lab Technician/Med Lab Technician Prgm
245 NE 30th Rd
Great Bend, KS 67530-9283
www.bartonccc.edu/mlt/home

Seward County Community College
Clin Lab Technician/Med Lab Technician Prgm
PO Box 1137
520 N Washington
Liberal, KS 67901
www.sccc.edu

Kentucky

Henderson Community College /MCC Consortium
Clin Lab Technician/Med Lab Technician Prgm
Henderson Community College
2660 S Green St
Henderson, KY 42420
www.henderson.kctcs.edu

Jefferson Community and Technical College
Clin Lab Technician/Med Lab Technician Prgm
109 E Broadway
Louisville, KY 40202
www.jefferson.kctcs.edu/academics/Programs_of_Study/
CLT

HCC/MCC Consortium
Cosponsor: Madisonville Community College
Clin Lab Technician/Med Lab Technician Prgm
2000 College Drive Health Campus
750 N Laffoon St
Madisonville, KY 42431
www.madisonville.kctcs.edu

West Kentucky Community & Technical College
Clin Lab Technician/Med Lab Technician Prgm
4810 Alben Barkley Drive
PO Box 7380
Paducah, KY 42002
www.westkentucky.kctcs.edu

Southeast Kentucky Comm & Tech College
Clin Lab Technician/Med Lab Technician Prgm
3300 US Highway 25E S
Pineville, KY 40977

Eastern Kentucky University
Clin Lab Technician/Med Lab Technician Prgm
Dizney 220
521 Lancaster Ave
Richmond, KY 40475-3102

Somerset Community College
Clin Lab Technician/Med Lab Technician Prgm
808 Monticello St
Somerset, KY 42501
www.somerset.kctcs.edu

Louisiana

Louisiana State University - Alexandria
Clin Lab Technician/Med Lab Technician Prgm
8100 Hwy 71 S
LSUA Dept of Allied Health
Alexandria, LA 71302-9121
www.lsua.edu

Fortis College
Clin Lab Technician/Med Lab Technician Prgm
9255 Interline Ave
Baton Rouge, LA 70809
www.medvance.edu

Acadiana Technical College - Lafayette Campus
Clin Lab Technician/Med Lab Technician Prgm
1101 Bertrand Ave
Lafayette, LA 70506
www.greateracadianaregion.net/lafayette/index.htm

Delgado Community College
Clin Lab Technician/Med Lab Technician Prgm
615 City Park Ave
New Orleans, LA 70119
www.dcc.edu

Southern Univ at Shreveport
Clin Lab Technician/Med Lab Technician Prgm
3050 Martin Luther King Jr Dr
Shreveport, LA 71107
www.susla.edu

Maine

University of Maine at Presque Isle
Cosponsor: University of Maine at Augusta
Clin Lab Technician/Med Lab Technician Prgm
181 Main St
Presque Isle, ME 04769
www.umpi.edu/campus-directory/
medical-laboratory-technology

Maryland

Anne Arundel Community College
Clin Lab Technician/Med Lab Technician Prgm
101 College Parkway
Arnold, MD 21012

Community College of Baltimore County
Clin Lab Technician/Med Lab Technician Prgm
7201 Rossville Blvd
Baltimore, MD 21237
http://ccbcmd.edu/allied_health/MLT.html

Allegany College of Maryland
Clin Lab Technician/Med Lab Technician Prgm
12401 Willowbrook Rd SE
Cumberland, MD 21502-2596
www.allegany.edu

College of Southern Maryland
Clin Lab Technician/Med Lab Technician Prgm
8730 Mitchell Rd PO Box 910
La Plata, MD 20646-0910

Massachusetts

Bunker Hill Community College
Clin Lab Technician/Med Lab Technician Prgm
250 New Rutherford Ave
Charlestown, MA 02129

Bristol Community College
Clin Lab Technician/Med Lab Technician Prgm
777 Elsbree St
Fall River, MA 02720
www.bristolcc.edu

Mount Wachusett Community College
Clin Lab Technician/Med Lab Technician Prgm
242 Green St
Heywood Hospital - Laboratory
Gardner, MA 01440
www.mwcc.edu/programs/cls/faq.html

Quincy College
Clin Lab Technician/Med Lab Technician Prgm
24 Saville Ave
Quincy, MA 02169

Springfield Technical Community College
Clin Lab Technician/Med Lab Technician Prgm
2 Armory Square
PO Box 9000
Springfield, MA 01102
http://STCC.edu

Michigan

Baker College of Owosso
Clin Lab Technician/Med Lab Technician Prgm
4500 Enterprise Dr
Allen Park, MI 48101
www.baker.edu

Kellogg Community College
Clin Lab Technician/Med Lab Technician Prgm
450 North Ave
Battle Creek, MI 49017
www.kellogg.edu/alliedhealth/mlt/mltmain.html

Ferris State University
Clin Lab Technician/Med Lab Technician Prgm
VFS210A
200 Ferris Dr
Big Rapids, MI 49307-2740
www.ferris.edu/cls

Baker College of Jackson
Clin Lab Technician/Med Lab Technician Prgm
2800 Springport Rd
Jackson, MI 49202
www.baker.edu

Northern Michigan University
Clin Lab Technician/Med Lab Technician Prgm
3513 West Science Bldg
Marquette, MI 49855
www.nmu.edu/cls/cls.htm

Baker College of Owosso
Clin Lab Technician/Med Lab Technician Prgm
1020 S Washington St
Owosso, MI 48867
www.baker.edu

Baker College of Port Huron
Clin Lab Technician/Med Lab Technician Prgm
3403 Lapeer Rd
Port Huron, MI 48060
www.baker.edu

Macomb Community College
Clin Lab Technician/Med Lab Technician Prgm
14500 E Twelve Mile Rd
Warren, MI 48088
www.macomb.edu

Minnesota

Alexandria Technical College
Clin Lab Technician/Med Lab Technician Prgm
1601 Jefferson St
Alexandria, MN 56308
http://web.alextech.edu

North Hennepin Community College
Clin Lab Technician/Med Lab Technician Prgm
7411 85th Ave N
North Hennepin Community College MLT Program
SC126C
Brooklyn Park, MN 55445
www.nhcc.edu/What_Can_I_Study/
Programs_and_Majors/Medical_Lab_Technology/
index.cfm

Lake Superior College
Clin Lab Technician/Med Lab Technician Prgm
2101 Trinity Rd
Duluth, MN 55811
www.lsc.edu

Argosy University Twin Cities Campus
Clin Lab Technician/Med Lab Technician Prgm
1515 Central Parkway
Eagan, MN 55121
www.argosyu.edu

South Central College
Clin Lab Technician/Med Lab Technician Prgm
1225 3rd St SW
Faribault, MN 55021
http://southcentral.edu

Minnesota State Community and Technical Coll
Clin Lab Technician/Med Lab Technician Prgm
1414 College Way
Fergus Falls, MN 56537
www.minnesota.edu

Hibbing Community College
Clin Lab Technician/Med Lab Technician Prgm
1515 E 25th St
Hibbing, MN 55746
www.hibbing.edu

Rasmussen College - Lake Elmo
Clin Lab Technician/Med Lab Technician Prgm
8565 Eagle Point Circle
Lake Elmo, MN 55042
www.rasmussen.edu/locations/minnesota/twin-cities/
    lake-elmo-woodbury/

Rasmussen College - Mankato
Clin Lab Technician/Med Lab Technician Prgm
130 Saint Andrews Drive
Mankato, MN 56001
www.rasmussen.edu/locations/minnesota/mankato/

Rasmussen College - Moorhead
Clin Lab Technician/Med Lab Technician Prgm
1250 29th Ave South
Moorhead, MN 56560
www.rasmussen.edu/locations/minnesota/moorhead/

Saint Paul College
Clin Lab Technician/Med Lab Technician Prgm
235 Marshall Ave
St Paul, MN 55102-1807
www.saintpaul.edu

Rasmussen College - St. Cloud
Clin Lab Technician/Med Lab Technician Prgm
226 Park Ave South
St. Cloud, MN 56301
www.rasmussen.edu/locations/minnesota/st-cloud/

Minnesota West Comm & Tech College
Clin Lab Technician/Med Lab Technician Prgm
1450 Collegeway Dr
Worthington, MN 56187

Mississippi

Northeast Mississippi Community College
Clin Lab Technician/Med Lab Technician Prgm
101 Cunningham Blvd
Booneville, MS 38829
www.nemcc.edu

Mississippi Gulf Coast Community College
Clin Lab Technician/Med Lab Technician Prgm
2300 Hwy 90, PO Box 100
Gautier, MS 39553
www.mgccc.edu

Miller-Motte Technical College - Gulfport
Clin Lab Technician/Med Lab Technician Prgm
(McCann School of Business & Technology MLT
    Consortium)
12121 Highway 49 North
Gulfport, MS 39503

Pearl River Community College
Clin Lab Technician/Med Lab Technician Prgm
5448 US Hwy 49 S
Hattiesburg, MS 39401
www.prcc.edu

Hinds Community College
Clin Lab Technician/Med Lab Technician Prgm
Nursing/Allied Hlth Ctr
1750 Chadwick Dr
Jackson, MS 39204-3402
www.hindscc.edu/HealthRelatedProfessions/MLT

Meridian Community College
Clin Lab Technician/Med Lab Technician Prgm
910 Hwy 19 N
Meridian, MS 39307
www.meridiancc.edu/mlt

Mississippi Delta Community College
Clin Lab Technician/Med Lab Technician Prgm
PO Box 668
Moorhead, MS 38761
www.msdelta.edu/healthsciences/mlt/medlabindex.html

Copiah-Lincoln Community College
Clin Lab Technician/Med Lab Technician Prgm
PO Box 457
Wesson, MS 39191-0457
www.colin.edu/careertech/MedicalLab

Missouri

National American University
Clin Lab Technician/Med Lab Technician Prgm
7490 NW 87th St
Kansas City, MO 64153
www.national.edu

Moberly Area Community College
Clin Lab Technician/Med Lab Technician Prgm
Advanced Technology 2900 Doreli Lane
Mexico, MO 65265
www.macc.edu/~mlt/

Three Rivers Community College
Clin Lab Technician/Med Lab Technician Prgm
2080 Three Rivers Blvd
Poplar Bluff, MO 63901
www.trcc.edu

Ozarks Technical Community College
Clin Lab Technician/Med Lab Technician Prgm
1001 E Chestnut Expressway
Springfield, MO 65802

St Louis Community College - Forest Park
Clin Lab Technician/Med Lab Technician Prgm
5600 Oakland Ave
St Louis, MO 63110
www.stlcc.edu/Programs/
    Clinical_Laboratory_Technology

Nebraska

Central Community College
Clin Lab Technician/Med Lab Technician Prgm
PO Box 1024
E Hwy 6
550 South Technical Blvd
Hastings, NE 68902-1024
http://cccneb.edu

Southeast Community College
Clin Lab Technician/Med Lab Technician Prgm
8800 O St
Lincoln, NE 68520
www.southeast.edu

Mid-Plains Community College
Clin Lab Technician/Med Lab Technician Prgm
North Campus
1101 Halligan Dr
North Platte, NE 69101
www.medlabtek.net

Nevada

College of Southern Nevada
Clin Lab Technician/Med Lab Technician Prgm
6375 W Charleston Blvd
Las Vegas, NV 89146
www.csn.edu/health.asp

New Hampshire

River Valley Community College
Clin Lab Technician/Med Lab Technician Prgm
1 College Drive
Claremont, NH 03743-9707
www.rivervalley.edu/clt.html

New Jersey

Camden County College
Clin Lab Technician/Med Lab Technician Prgm
PO Box 200
College Dr
Blackwood, NJ 08012
www.camdencc.edu

Middlesex County College
Clin Lab Technician/Med Lab Technician Prgm
2600 Woodbridge Ave
LH221
Edison, NJ 08818-3050
www.middlesexcc.edu/academi/med

Brookdale Community College /Meridian Health
Clin Lab Technician/Med Lab Technician Prgm
765 Newman Springs Rd
Lincroft, NJ 07738-1543
www.brookdalecc.edu

Mercer County Community College
Clin Lab Technician/Med Lab Technician Prgm
PO Box B
1200 Old Trenton Rd
Trenton, NJ 08690
www.mccc.edu

New Mexico

Central New Mexico Community College
Clin Lab Technician/Med Lab Technician Prgm
525 Buena Vista SE
Albuquerque, NM 87106
www.cnm.edu

San Juan College
Clin Lab Technician/Med Lab Technician Prgm
4601 College Blvd
Farmington, NM 87402
www.sanjuancollege.edu/mlt

University of New Mexico - Gallup
Clin Lab Technician/Med Lab Technician Prgm
200 College Rd
Gallup, NM 87301
www.unm.edu

New York

Broome Community College
Clin Lab Technician/Med Lab Technician Prgm
PO Box 1017
Binghamton, NY 13902
www.sunybroome.edu

Farmingdale State College, SUNY
Clin Lab Technician/Med Lab Technician Prgm
2350 Broadhollow Rd
Gleeson 344
Farmingdale, NY 11735
www.farmingdale.edu/quicklinks/
    IFS_Medical_Laboratory_Tech.html

Nassau Community College
Clin Lab Technician/Med Lab Technician Prgm
One Education Dr
AHS Department
Garden City, NY 11530
www.ncc.edu/Academics/AcademicDepartments/ 120
AlliedHealthSciences/MedicalLabTech/

Orange County Community College
Clin Lab Technician/Med Lab Technician Prgm
115 South St
Middletown, NY 10940
www.sunyorange.edu

Dutchess Community College
Clin Lab Technician/Med Lab Technician Prgm
53 Pendell Rd
Poughkeepsie, NY 12601
www.sunydutchess.edu/academics/departments/
AlliedHealthandBiologicalSciences/AlliedHealthand

Erie Community College - North Campus
Clin Lab Technician/Med Lab Technician Prgm
6205 Main St
Williamsville, NY 14221
www.ecc.edu

North Carolina

Asheville-Buncombe Technical Comm College
Clin Lab Technician/Med Lab Technician Prgm
340 Victoria Rd
Rhododendron Building
Asheville, NC 28801
www.abtech.edu

Central Piedmont Community College
Clin Lab Technician/Med Lab Technician Prgm
PO Box 35009
Health Sciences Division, Central Piedmont Community
College
Charlotte, NC 28235-5009
www.cpcc.edu/health_sciences/
medical-laboratory-technology

College of The Albemarle
Clin Lab Technician/Med Lab Technician Prgm
PO Box 2327
Elizabeth City, NC 27906-2327
www.albemarle.edu

Alamance Community College
Clin Lab Technician/Med Lab Technician Prgm
PO Box 8000
1247 Jimmie Kerr Rd
Graham, NC 27253-8000
www.alamancecc.edu

Coastal Carolina Community College
Clin Lab Technician/Med Lab Technician Prgm
444 Western Blvd
Jacksonville, NC 28546-6816
www.coastalcarolina.edu

Davidson County Community College
Clin Lab Technician/Med Lab Technician Prgm
PO Box 1287
297 DCCC Rd Thomasville NC 27360
Lexington, NC 27293-1287
www.davidsonccc.edu

Stanly Community College
Clin Lab Technician/Med Lab Technician Prgm
102 Stanly Parkway
Locust, NC 28097
www.stanly.edu

Western Piedmont Community College
Clin Lab Technician/Med Lab Technician Prgm
1001 Burkemont Ave
Morganton, NC 28655-0680
www.wpcc.edu

Sandhills Community College
Clin Lab Technician/Med Lab Technician Prgm
3395 Airport Rd
Pinehurst, NC 28374
www.sandhills.edu/degrees-programs/health-sciences/
medical-laboratory-technology.html

Wake Technical Community College
Clin Lab Technician/Med Lab Technician Prgm
9101 Fayetteville Rd
Wake Tech Health Sciences Campus, 2901 Holston Lane
Raleigh, NC 27610
www.waketech.edu

Southwestern Community College
Clin Lab Technician/Med Lab Technician Prgm
447 College Dr
Sylva, NC 28779
www.southwesternccc.edu/mlt

Davidson County Community College
Clin Lab Technician/Med Lab Technician Prgm
297 DCCC Rd
PO Box 1287 Lexington NC 27293-1287
Thomasville, NC 27360
www.davidsonccc.edu/academics/
ht-medical-lab-tech.htm

Beaufort County Community College
Clin Lab Technician/Med Lab Technician Prgm
PO Box 1069
Highway 264 E
BCCC
Washington, NC 27889
www.beaufort.cc.nc.us/progrm/Allied%20Health/MLT/
mlt.htm

Halifax Community College
Clin Lab Technician/Med Lab Technician Prgm
PO Box 809
100 College Drive
Weldon, NC 27890
www.halifaxcc.edu

Southeastern Community College
Clin Lab Technician/Med Lab Technician Prgm
PO Box 151
Whiteville, NC 28472
www.sccnc.edu

North Dakota

Turtle Mountain Community College
Clin Lab Technician/Med Lab Technician Prgm
PO Box 340
Belcourt, ND 58316
www.tm.edu

Bismarck State College
Clin Lab Technician/Med Lab Technician Prgm
1500 Edwards Ave
PO Box 5587
Bismarck, ND 58506-5587
www.bismarckstate.edu

Rasmussen College - Bismarck
Clin Lab Technician/Med Lab Technician Prgm
1701 E Century Ave
Bismarck, ND 58503
www.rasmussen.edu/locations/north-dakota/bismarck/

Ohio

Akron Institute of Herzing College
Clin Lab Technician/Med Lab Technician Prgm
1600 South Arlington St, Suite 100
Akron, OH 44306

Cincinnati State Tech & Comm College
Clin Lab Technician/Med Lab Technician Prgm
3520 Central Pkwy
Health and Public Safety Division
Cincinnati, OH 45223
www.cincinnatistate.edu

Cuyahoga Community College
Clin Lab Technician/Med Lab Technician Prgm
Metro Campus Health Careers and Science Bldg, 126I
2900 Community College Ave
Cleveland, OH 44115-3196
www.tri-c.edu/programs/healthcareers/medicallab/
Pages/default.aspx

Columbus State Community College
Clin Lab Technician/Med Lab Technician Prgm
550 E Spring St
Union Hall 315
Columbus, OH 43216-1609
www.cscc.edu/mlt

Lorain County Community College
Clin Lab Technician/Med Lab Technician Prgm
1005 N Abbe Rd
HS210A
Elyria, OH 44035
www.lorainccc.edu/Academic+Programs/
Associates+Degree+and+Certificate+Programs/
clinical+labor

Lakeland Community College
Clin Lab Technician/Med Lab Technician Prgm
7700 Clocktower Dr
Lakeland Community College
Kirtland, OH 44094-5198
www.lakelandcc.edu/academic/sh/mlt/index.asp

Washington State Community College
Clin Lab Technician/Med Lab Technician Prgm
710 Colegate Dr
Marietta, OH 45750
www.wscc.edu/academics/health/
medicallaboratorytechnology.asp

Marion Technical College
Clin Lab Technician/Med Lab Technician Prgm
1467 Mt Vernon Ave
Marion, OH 43302
www.mtc.edu

Stark State College
Clin Lab Technician/Med Lab Technician Prgm
6200 Frank Ave NW
North Canton, OH 44720
www.starkstate.edu/academics/health/medlabtech.htm

Edison Community College
Clin Lab Technician/Med Lab Technician Prgm
1973 Edison Drive
Piqua, OH 45356
www.edisonohio.edu

Shawnee State University
Clin Lab Technician/Med Lab Technician Prgm
940 Second St
Portsmouth, OH 45662
www.shawnee.edu/acad/hs/mlt/index.html

Clark State Community College
Clin Lab Technician/Med Lab Technician Prgm
570 E Leffel Ln
Springfield, OH 45501-0570
www.clarkstate.edu/programdetails.php?Program=74

Eastern Gateway Community College
Clin Lab Technician/Med Lab Technician Prgm
4000 Sunset Blvd
Steubenville, OH 43952
www.egcc.edu

Youngstown State University
Clin Lab Technician/Med Lab Technician Prgm
Dept of Health Professions
One University Plaza
Youngstown, OH 44555
http://bchhs.ysu.edu/healthprofessions/medtech/
histotech.htm

Zane State College
Clin Lab Technician/Med Lab Technician Prgm
1555 Newark Rd
Zanesville, OH 43701
www.zanestate.edu

Oklahoma

Northeastern Oklahoma A&M College
Clin Lab Technician/Med Lab Technician Prgm
Second and I Sts NE
200 I St NE
Miami, OK 74354
www.neo.edu

Rose State College
Clin Lab Technician/Med Lab Technician Prgm
6420 SE 15th St
Midwest City, OK 73110
www.rose.edu

Platt College
Clin Lab Technician/Med Lab Technician Prgm
Platt College MLT Consortium
201 N Eastern
Moore, OK 73160

Platt College
Clin Lab Technician/Med Lab Technician Prgm
Platt College MLT Consortium
2727 W Memorial Rd
Oklahoma City, OK 73134

Seminole State College
Clin Lab Technician/Med Lab Technician Prgm
PO Box 351
2701 Boren Blvd
Seminole, OK 74818-0351
http://sscok.edu

Platt College
Clin Lab Technician/Med Lab Technician Prgm
Platt College MLT Consortium
3801 S Sheridan
Tulsa, OK 74145

Tulsa Community College
Clin Lab Technician/Med Lab Technician Prgm
10300 E 81st S
Tulsa, OK 74133
www.tulsacc.edu

Eastern Oklahoma State College
Clin Lab Technician/Med Lab Technician Prgm
1301 West Main St
Wilburton, OK 74578
www.eosc.edu

Oregon

Portland Community College
Clin Lab Technician/Med Lab Technician Prgm
PO Box 19000
CA JH-201
705 N Killingsworth St
Portland, OR 97217
www.pcc.edu/programs/medical-lab/

Pennsylvania

McCann School of Business and Technology - Allentown
Clin Lab Technician/Med Lab Technician Prgm
(McCann School of Business & Technology MLT
Consortium)
220 N Irving St
Allentown, PA 18109

Montgomery County Community College
Clin Lab Technician/Med Lab Technician Prgm
340 DeKalb Pike
PO Box 400
Science Center 340
Blue Bell, PA 19422
www.mc3.edu/Media/Website%20Resources/pdf/
academics/health/mlt-info-pack.pdf

Harcum College
Clin Lab Technician/Med Lab Technician Prgm
750 Montgomery Ave
Bryn Mawr, PA 19010
www.harcum.edu

McCann School of Business and Technology - Carlisle
Clin Lab Technician/Med Lab Technician Prgm
(McCann School of Business & Technology MLT
Consortium)
346 York Rd
Carlisle, PA 17013

Mount Aloysius College
Clin Lab Technician/Med Lab Technician Prgm
7373 Admiral Peary Highway
Cresson, PA 16630

McCann School of Business and Technology - Dickson City
Clin Lab Technician/Med Lab Technician Prgm
(McCann School of Business & Technology MLT
Consortium)
2227 Scranton Carbondale Highway
Dickson City, PA 18519

Fortis Institute-Erie
Clin Lab Technician/Med Lab Technician Prgm
5757 West 26th St
Erie, PA 16505

Harrisburg Area Community College
Clin Lab Technician/Med Lab Technician Prgm
1 HACC Drive, SM 114E
Harrisburg, PA 17110-2999
www.hacc.edu/HealthCareers/ProgramsOffered/
MedicalLaboratoryTech/index.cfm

McCann School of Business and Technology - Hazleton
Clin Lab Technician/Med Lab Technician Prgm
(McCann School of Business & Technology MLT
Consortium)
370 Maplewood Drive Humboldt Industrial Park
Hazle Township, PA 18202

Penn State University - Hazleton
Clin Lab Technician/Med Lab Technician Prgm
76 University Dr
Hazleton, PA 18202
www.hn.psu.edu/Academics/MLTassoc.htm?cn21

Mercyhurst University
Clin Lab Technician/Med Lab Technician Prgm
16 W Division St
North East, PA 16428

Community College of Philadelphia
Clin Lab Technician/Med Lab Technician Prgm
1700 Spring Garden St
CLT Program
Philadelphia, PA 19130
www.ccp.edu/academicprograms

McCann School of Business and Technology - Pottsville
Clin Lab Technician/Med Lab Technician Prgm
(McCann School of Business & Technology MLT
Consortium)
2650 Woodglen Rd
Pottsville, PA 17901

Reading Area Community College
Clin Lab Technician/Med Lab Technician Prgm
Ten S Second St, PO Box 1706
Reading, PA 19603

Laurel Technical Institute
Clin Lab Technician/Med Lab Technician Prgm
200 Stering Ave
Sharon, PA 16146

McCann School of Business and Technology - Sunbury
Clin Lab Technician/Med Lab Technician Prgm
(McCann School of Business & Technology MLT
Consortium)
1147 North Fourth St
Sunbury, PA 17801

Laurel Business Institute
Clin Lab Technician/Med Lab Technician Prgm
11 E Penn St, PO Box 877
Uniontown, PA 15401
www.laurel.edu

Community College of Allegheny County
Clin Lab Technician/Med Lab Technician Prgm
1750 Clairton Rd, Rte 885
West Mifflin, PA 15122
www.ccac.edu

Rhode Island

Community College of Rhode Island
Clin Lab Technician/Med Lab Technician Prgm
1762 Louisquisset Pike
Allied Health Department
Lincoln, RI 02865
www.ccri.edu/alliedhealth/clinicallab

South Carolina

Trident Technical College
Clin Lab Technician/Med Lab Technician Prgm
PO Box 118067
7000 Rivers Ave
Charleston, SC 29423-8067
www.tridenttech.edu/3740.htm

Midlands Technical College
Clin Lab Technician/Med Lab Technician Prgm
PO Box 2408
Columbia, SC 29202
www.midlandstech.edu/medlab/

Florence-Darlington Technical College
Clin Lab Technician/Med Lab Technician Prgm
PO Box 100548
Florence, SC 29501-0548
www.fdtc.edu

Greenville Technical College
Clin Lab Technician/Med Lab Technician Prgm
PO Box 5616, Station B
MS 4021
Greenville, SC 29606
www.gvltec.edu/display.aspx?id=898

Tri-County Technical College
Clin Lab Technician/Med Lab Technician Prgm
PO Box 587
7900 Hwy 76
Pendleton, SC 29670-0587
www.tctc.edu

York Technical College
Clin Lab Technician/Med Lab Technician Prgm
452 S Anderson Rd
Rock Hill, SC 29730
www.yorktech.com

Spartanburg Community College
Clin Lab Technician/Med Lab Technician Prgm
PO Drawer 4386
Bus I-85 and New Cut Rd
Spartanburg, SC 29305
www.sccsc.edu/HHS/MedLab

South Dakota

Mitchell Technical Institute
Clin Lab Technician/Med Lab Technician Prgm
821 N Capital
Mitchell, SD 57301
www.mitchelltech.edu

Lake Area Technical Institute
Clin Lab Technician/Med Lab Technician Prgm
230 11th St NE
Watertown, SD 57201
lakeareatech.edu

Tennessee

Fortis Institute
Clin Lab Technician/Med Lab Technician Prgm
1025 Highway 111
Cookeville, TN 38501
www.medvance.org

Volunteer State Community College
Clin Lab Technician/Med Lab Technician Prgm
1480 Nashville Pike
Gallatin, TN 37066
www.volstate.edu/medlabtech

Jackson State Community College
Clin Lab Technician/Med Lab Technician Prgm
Allied Health Department
2046 N Parkway
Jackson, TN 38301-3797
www.jscc.edu/academics/departments/allied-health/
    medical-laboratory-technician.html

Northeast State Community College
Clin Lab Technician/Med Lab Technician Prgm
300 West Main St
Kingsport, TN 37660
www.northeaststate.edu

Southwest Tennessee Community College
Clin Lab Technician/Med Lab Technician Prgm
PO Box 780
761 Linden Ave
Memphis, TN 38126
www.southwest.tn.edu

Fortis Institute
Clin Lab Technician/Med Lab Technician Prgm
3354 Perimeter Hill Drive
Nashville, TN 37211
www.medvance.edu

Texas

Amarillo College
Clin Lab Technician/Med Lab Technician Prgm
PO Box 447
Amarillo, TX 79178
www.actx.edu/medical_lab and www.actx.edu/mltonline

Austin Community College
Clin Lab Technician/Med Lab Technician Prgm
Eastview Campus
3401 Webberville Rd
Austin, TX 78702
www.austincc.edu/health/mlt/

Univ TX at Brownsville/TX Southmost Coll
Clin Lab Technician/Med Lab Technician Prgm
80 Ft Brown
Brownsville, TX 78520
http://blue.utb.edu/medlabtech/

Del Mar College
Clin Lab Technician/Med Lab Technician Prgm
101 Baldwin
Corpus Christi, TX 78404
www.delmar.edu/mlt

Navarro College
Clin Lab Technician/Med Lab Technician Prgm
3200 W 7th Ave
Corsicana, TX 75110-4899
www.navarrocollege.edu

El Centro College
Clin Lab Technician/Med Lab Technician Prgm
801 Main St
Dallas, TX 75202-3604
www.elcentrocollege.edu/MedicalLabTech

Platt College
Clin Lab Technician/Med Lab Technician Prgm
Platt College MLT Consortium
2974 LBJ Freeway
Dallas, TX 75234

Grayson County College
Clin Lab Technician/Med Lab Technician Prgm
6101 Grayson Dr
Denison, TX 75020
www.grayson.edu

El Paso Community College
Clin Lab Technician/Med Lab Technician Prgm
PO Box 20500
El Paso, TX 79998
www.epcc.edu

Medical Education and Training Campus (METC)
Clin Lab Technician/Med Lab Technician Prgm
Academy of Health Sciences
3151 Scott Rd
Fort Sam Houston, TX 78234-6137
www.dcss.cs.amedd.army.mil/

Tarleton State University
Clin Lab Technician/Med Lab Technician Prgm
1501 Enderly Place
Fort Worth, TX 76104
www.tarleton.edu

Houston Community College
Clin Lab Technician/Med Lab Technician Prgm
1900 Pressler Dr
Houston, TX 77030
www.coleman.hccs.edu

Sanford-Brown College - Houston
Clin Lab Technician/Med Lab Technician Prgm
9999 Richmond Ave
Houston, TX 77042

Central Texas College
Clin Lab Technician/Med Lab Technician Prgm
6200 W Central TX Expressway, PO Box 1800
Killeen, TX 76540
www.ctcd.edu

Laredo Community College
Clin Lab Technician/Med Lab Technician Prgm
West End Washington St
Laredo, TX 78040
www.laredo.edu

Northeast Texas Community College
Clin Lab Technician/Med Lab Technician Prgm
PO Box 1307
Mount Pleasant, TX 75456
www2.ntcc.edu/Academics/MedicalLabTechnician/

Lamar State College - Orange
Clin Lab Technician/Med Lab Technician Prgm
410 Front St
Orange, TX 77630
www.lsco.edu

San Jacinto College Central
Clin Lab Technician/Med Lab Technician Prgm
8060 Spencer Hwy, PO Box 2007
Pasadena, TX 77505
www.sjcd.edu

St Philip's College
Clin Lab Technician/Med Lab Technician Prgm
1801 Martin Luther King Dr
San Antonio, TX 78203-2098
www.accd.edu/spc/acad/ahd/mlab/mlabprogram.aspx

882d Training Group, 382 Training Squadron
Clin Lab Technician/Med Lab Technician Prgm
382nd Training Squadron/XYAC
917 Missile Rd, Suite 3
Sheppard AFB, TX 76311-2263

Tyler Junior College
Clin Lab Technician/Med Lab Technician Prgm
PO Box 9020
Tyler, TX 75711-9020
www.tjc.edu/medlab/home.asp

Victoria College
Clin Lab Technician/Med Lab Technician Prgm
2200 E Red River
Victoria, TX 77901
www.victoriacollege.edu/medicallaboratorytechnology

McLennan Community College
Clin Lab Technician/Med Lab Technician Prgm
1400 College Dr
Waco, TX 76708
www.mclennan.edu

882d Training Group, 382 Training Squadron
Clin Lab Technician/Med Lab Technician Prgm
939 Missile Rd
Sheppard AFB
Wichita Falls, TX 76311-2245

Utah

Weber State University
Clin Lab Technician/Med Lab Technician Prgm
3905 University Cirlce
Ogden, UT 84408-3905
http://weber.edu/cls

Virginia

Centra Health Systems of Lynchburg
Clin Lab Technician/Med Lab Technician Prgm
3300 Rivermont Ave
Lynchburg, VA 24503

J Sargeant Reynolds Community College
Clin Lab Technician/Med Lab Technician Prgm
PO Box 85622
Richmond, VA 23285-5622
www.jsr.vccs.edu/curriculum/programs/
    marketingprograms/Medical_Laboratory_Tec

Northern Virginia Community College
Clin Lab Technician/Med Lab Technician Prgm
6699 Springfield Center Drive
Springfield, VA 22150
www.nvcc.edu

Wytheville Community College
Clin Lab Technician/Med Lab Technician Prgm
1000 E Main St
Wytheville, VA 24382
www.wcc.vccs.edu/academics/programs/medlab.php

Washington

Clover Park Technical College
Clin Lab Technician/Med Lab Technician Prgm
4500 Steilacoom Blvd SW
Lakewood, WA 98499-4098
www.cptc.edu

Shoreline Community College
Clin Lab Technician/Med Lab Technician Prgm
16101 Greenwood Ave N
MLT Program, Health Occupations Division
Seattle, WA 98133
www.shoreline.edu/shoreline.medlablocal.html

Wenatchee Valley College
Clin Lab Technician/Med Lab Technician Prgm
1201 S Miller St
Central Washington Hospital
Wenatchee, WA 98801
www.wvc.edu/directory/departments/medlabtech

West Virginia

Bluefield Regional Medical Center
Cosponsor: New River Technical and Community College
Clin Lab Technician/Med Lab Technician Prgm
BRMC 500 Cherry St
Bluefield, WV 24701-3306
www.brmcwv.org

Fairmont State Univ
Cosponsor: Pierpont Community & Technical College
Clin Lab Technician/Med Lab Technician Prgm
1201 Locust Ave
211 Education Building
Fairmont, WV 26554
www.pierpont.edu/academics/ctc_mlt/default.asp

Marshall University
Clin Lab Technician/Med Lab Technician Prgm
Clinical Lab Science Dept
One John Marshall Dr
Huntington, WV 25755
www.marshall.edu/cohp
Notes: The program is a 2+2 career ladder program with
all students completing the MLT/CLT curriculum.
Students may take the required courses for the
CLS/MT curriculum on a part-time basis.

Southern West Virginia Comm & Tech College
Clin Lab Technician/Med Lab Technician Prgm
Logan Campus, PO Box 2900
Dempsey Branch Rd
Mount Gay, WV 25637
http://southernwv.edu

Wisconsin

Herzing University
Clin Lab Technician/Med Lab Technician Prgm
555 S Executive Drive
Brookfield, WI 53005
www.herzing.edu

Chippewa Valley Technical College
Clin Lab Technician/Med Lab Technician Prgm
620 W Clairemont Ave
Eau Claire, WI 54701
www.cvtc.edu/Programs/DeptPages/CLT/
MLTHomePage.html

Southwest Wisconsin Technical College
Clin Lab Technician/Med Lab Technician Prgm
1800 Bronson Blvd
Fennimore, WI 53809
www.swtc.edu

Moraine Park Technical College
Clin Lab Technician/Med Lab Technician Prgm
235 N National Ave
PO Box 1940
Fond du Lac, WI 54936-1940
www.morainepark.edu

Northeast Wisconsin Technical College
Clin Lab Technician/Med Lab Technician Prgm
2740 W Mason St, PO Box 19042
Green Bay, WI 54307-9042
www.nwtc.edu

Rasmussen College - Green Bay
Clin Lab Technician/Med Lab Technician Prgm
904 South Taylor St
Green Bay, WI 54303
www.rasmussen.edu

Western Technical College
Clin Lab Technician/Med Lab Technician Prgm
PO Box C-908
400 7th St North
La Crosse, WI 54601
www.westerntc.edu/ClassInformation/
ProgramInformation.aspx?PROGRAM_NBR=105131

Madison Area Technical College
Clin Lab Technician/Med Lab Technician Prgm
3550 Anderson St
Madison, WI 53704-2599
http://programs.matcmadison.edu/programs/
clinical-laboratory-technician

Milwaukee Area Technical College
Clin Lab Technician/Med Lab Technician Prgm
700 W State St
Milwaukee, WI 53233-1443
http://matc.edu/student/offerings/cllab.html

Blackhawk Technical College
Clin Lab Technician/Med Lab Technician Prgm
210 Fourth Ave
Monroe, WI 53566
www.blackhawk.edu

Northcentral Technical College
Clin Lab Technician/Med Lab Technician Prgm
1000 W Campus Drive
Wausau, WI 54401-1899
www.ntc.edu

Wyoming

Casper College
Clin Lab Technician/Med Lab Technician Prgm
125 College Drive
Casper, WY 82601
www.caspercollege.edu

Cytogenetic Technologist

Laboratory tests play an important role in the detection, diagnosis, and treatment of diseases. Cytogenetic technologists study the morphology of chromosomes and their relationship to disease. Cytogenetic analysis provides important data for the diagnosis, prognosis, and treatment of genetic disorders and malignant diseases.

Career Description

Cytogenetic technologists evaluate the correct methodof collection, transport, and handling of various specimen types for cytogenetic analysis; identify culture techniques based on tissue type and reason for referral; and perform chromosomal staining, microscopic analysis, and karyotyping (organizing chromosomes according to a standardized ideogram). In addition to practicing good general laboratory skills, quality assurance principles, and safety protocols, cytogenetic technologists understand the legal implications of their work environment and exhibit appropriate ethical and professional health care standards while demonstrating professional conduct, stress management, and interpersonal and communication skills with patients, peers, other health care personnel, and the public.

Employment Characteristics

Cytogenetic technologists are employed in hospital laboratories, private medical laboratories, and research facilities. They may also serve as faculty in cytogenetic education programs.

Salary

Salaries vary depending upon the employer and geographic location.

For more information, refer to *www.ama-assn.org/go/hpsalary*.

Educational Programs

Length. Programs are at least one year. Cytogenetic technologists attend a baccalaureate or postbaccalaureate program that includes professional and clinical education. Certification is desired by most employers.

Prerequisites. College courses and a number of required credits necessary to ensure admission of a student who is prepared for the clinical education program. College and university programs that integrate preprofessional and professional coursework are structured with professional courses in the junior and senior years or at the graduate level.

Curriculum. Cytogenetic technology programs are conducted in colleges and universities, hospitals, private medical laboratories, and other equivalent postsecondary educational institutions. The areas of study that must be included in either the professional program or as prerequisites are biology, chemistry, biochemistry or cellular biology, genetics, cytogenetics, hematology, microbiology, immunology, laboratory information systems, laboratory safety, and quality control.

Inquiries

Careers/Curriculum

American Medical Technologists
10700 West Higgins Road, Suite 150
Rosemont, IL 60018
847 823-5169
E-mail: *mail@amt1.com*
www.amt1.com

American Society for Clinical Laboratory Science
6701 Democracy Blvd., Suite 300
Bethesda, MD 20817
301 657-2768
E-mail: *ascls@ascls.org*
www.ascls.org

American Society for Clinical Pathology
33 West Monroe, Suite 1600
Chicago, IL 60603
312 541-4999
E-mail: *info@ascp.org*
www.ascp.org

Association of Genetic Technologists
Executive Office
PO Box 15945-288
Lenexa, KS 66285
913 541-9077

Certification/Registration

American Society for Clinical Pathology
Board of Certification
PO Box 12270
Chicago, IL 60612
312 738-1336, Ext 1341
E-mail: *boc@ascp.org*
www.ascp.org

American Association of Bioanalysts
Board of Registry
906 Olive Street, Suite 1200
St. Louis, MO 63101-1434
www.aab.org

American Medical Technologists
10700 West Higgins Road, Suite 150
Rosemont, IL 60018
847 823-5169
E-mail: *mail@amt1.com*
www.amt1.com

Program Accreditation

Dianne M Cearlock, PhD, Chief Executive Officer
National Accrediting Agency for Clinical Laboratory Sciences
5600 North River Rd, Suite 720
Rosemont, IL 60018
773 714-8880
E-mail: *dcearlock@naacls.org*
www.naacls.org

Cytogenetic Technologist

California

Cedars Sinai Medical Center
Cytogenetic Technology Prgm
Stephen Spielberg Building, 8723 Alden Drive
SSB-143
Los Angeles, CA 90048

Quest Diagnostics Nichols Institute
Cytogenetic Technology Prgm
33608 Ortega Highway
San Juan Capistrano, CA 92690

Connecticut

University of Connecticut
Cytogenetic Technology Prgm
School of Allied Health, 222 Koons Halls
358 Mansfield Rd, Unit 2101
Storrs, CT 06269
www. allied health.uconn.edu

Georgia

Kennesaw State University
Cytogenetic Technology Prgm
1000 Chastain Rd
Bldg 12
Kennesaw, GA 30144-5591
http://science.kennesaw.edu/biophys/cytogene

Michigan

Northern Michigan University
Cytogenetic Technology Prgm
3711 West Science
Dept of Clinical Lab Science
Marquette, MI 49855-5346
www.nmu.edu

Minnesota

Mayo Clinic
Cytogenetic Technology Prgm
522 Hilton Bldg
200 First St SW
Rochester, MN 55905
www.mayo.edu/mshs/cytogen-career.html

Texas

Univ of Texas M D Anderson Cancer Ctr
Cytogenetic Technology PrgmUnit 146, 1515 Holcombe
    Blvd
The School of Health Professions - Unit 2
Houston, TX 77030-4095
www.mdanderson.org/healthsciences

UT Health Science Center - San Antonio
Cytogenetic Technology Prgm
Dept of Clin Lab Sci
7703 Floyd Curl Dr
San Antonio, TX 78229-3900
www.uthscsa.edu/sah/cls/cls.html

Cytotechnologist

Cytology is the study of the structure and the function of cells. Cytotechnologists are specially trained technologists who work with pathologists to evaluate cellular material from virtually all body sites primarily utilizing the microscope. Paramount to cytotechnologists is the microscopic recognition of normal and abnormal cytologic changes, including, but not limited to, malignant neoplasms, precancerous lesions, infectious agents, and inflammatory processes in gynecologic, non-gynecologic, and fine needle aspiration specimens. Cytotechnologists possess the technical skills for a wide variety of cytologic laboratory specimen preparations and a basic knowledge of contemporary procedures and technologies.

History

In the pioneer days of clinical pathology, it was the rare pathologist who did not have an assistant. These first technical "assistants," some of whom were trained by George N Papanicolaou, MD, famed American anatomist and cytologist, were always the product of an apprentice-type training. As their number, and the number of apprentice programs grew, there was a need to certify that the apprentices had mastered the knowledge of cytology. The Board of Registry of the American Society for Clinical Pathology (ASCP) offered the examination for what was then called the cytology technician for the first time in 1957.

In 1962, the Cytology Committee of the ASCP and the ASCP Board of Schools developed the *Essentials of an Acceptable School of Cytotechnology*, which were adopted by the House of Delegates of the American Medical Association (AMA). Until 1975, representatives of the ASCP served on the Cytotechnology Programs Review Committee of the National Accrediting Agency for Clinical Laboratory Sciences (NAACLS), which replaced the ASCP Board of Schools in 1974. In 1975, the American Society of Cytology (ASC) was recognized as the organization that would collaborate with the AMA Council on Medical Education (CME) in the accreditation of cytotechnology programs. The ASC formed the Cytotechnology Programs Review Committee (CPRC) to assume the responsibilities formerly handled by NACCLS. The Standards (Essentials) and Guidelines for an Accredited Educational Program for the Cytotechnologist were revised and adopted in 1967, 1977, 1983, 1992, and 1998.

The Commission on Accreditation of Allied Health Education Programs (CAAHEP) was incorporated as a non-profit organization on July 1, 1994, and assumed from the AMA Committee on Allied Health Education and Accreditation (CAHEA) the role as the leading accrediting agency for the majority of allied heath fields. The AMA continued to be CAAHEP's primary sponsor through a three-year transition period ending on December 31, 1996. Currently, the AMA is one of CAAHEP's approximately 70 member organizations.

While CAAHEP is the ultimate accrediting body, the day-to-day work of accreditation is the responsibility of CAAHEP's Committees on Accreditation (CoAs), one for each of the CAAHEP-accredited professions. These committees are composed of professionals from the individual disciplines. The Cytotechnology Programs Review Committee is the CoA for the profession of cytotechnology.

Career Description

Cell specimens may be obtained from various body sites, such as the female reproductive tract, the lung, or any body cavity shedding cells. Using special techniques, slides are first prepared from these specimens. Cytotechnologists then examine the slides microscopically, mark cellular changes that are most representative of a disease process, provide an initial interpretation, and submit to a pathologist for final evaluation. Cytotechnologists can make the final diagnosis for specimens of the female reproductive tract if it is negative for any abnormalities. Using the findings of cytotechnologists, the pathologist is then able, in many instances, to diagnose cancer and other diseases long before they can be detected by other methods. In recent years, fine needles have been used to aspirate lesions, often deeply seated in the body, thus greatly enhancing the ability to diagnose tumors located in otherwise inaccessible sites. Frequently, cytotechnologists will assist with fine needle aspirations (FNA) by providing an assessment of cellular adequacy and in processing the specimens.

Employment Characteristics

Most cytotechnologists work in hospitals or in commercial laboratories. With experience, cytotechnologists may also work in private industry or in supervisory, research, and teaching capacities. In addition, cytotechnologists who are board certified may take the Molecular Biology certification examination of the American Society for Clinical Pathology (ASCP), leading to another professional development and practice opportunity.

Salary

Employment opportunities and salaries vary depending on geographic location, experience, and ability.

According to the 2010 Wage and Vacancy Survey conducted by the American Society for Clinical Pathology (ASCP), staff-level cytotechnologists earn a median average salary of $29.44 per hour or $61,235 per year; supervisors earn a median average rate of $34.26 per hour or $71,261 annually. The survey results were published in the March 2011 issue of *LabMedicine*, available at *http://labmed.ascpjournals.org/content/42/3/141*.

For more information, refer to *www.ama-assn.org/go/hpsalary*.

Educational Programs

Length. The length of the program depends significantly on its organizational structure. In general, after completion of the prerequisite course work, at least one calendar year of structured professional instruction in cytotechnology is necessary to achieve program objectives and to establish entry-level competencies.

Prerequisites. Applicants should be well grounded in the biological sciences and in basic chemistry. This entails that students have a minimum of 28 semester hours of biological sciences and chemistry upon completion of a cytotechnology program, and three semester hours of mathematics and/or statistics. In addition, applicants are also required to have a baccalaureate degree in order to qualify for the national certification exam.

Curriculum. The curriculum includes the principles of cytopreparation of cell samples, cytologic evaluation of cell samples from all body sites, introduction to principles of management, research, and education as they apply to the cytology laboratory, and cytology as applied in clinical medicine. Also, as molecular diagnostics becomes increasingly important in the field of pathology, programs are incorporating instruction in immunohistochemistry, cytogenetics, in situ hybridization, polymerase chain reaction, and flow cytometry. Upon completion of a cytotechnology program, graduates will possess the technical skills to evaluate a wide variety of cytologic preparations and have a basic knowledge of contemporary procedures and technologies used in cytopathology.

Inquiries

Careers/Curriculum
American Society of Cytopathology
100 West 10th Street, Suite 605
Wilmington, DE 19801
302 543-6583
E-mail: *asc@cytopathology.org*
www.cytopathology.org

American Society for Cytotechnology
1500 Sunday Drive, Suite 102
Raleigh, NC 27607
919 861-5571 or (800 948-3947
E-mail: *info@asct.com*
www.asct.com

Certification/Registration
American Society for Clinical Pathology
Board of Certification
PO Box 12270
Chicago, IL 60612
312 738-1336
www.ascp.org

Program Accreditation
Commission on Accreditation of Allied Health Education Programs
  (CAAHEP)
1361 Park Street, Clearwater, FL 33756
727 210-2350
727 210-2354 Fax
E-mail: *mail@caahep.org*
www.caahep.org

in collaboration with:
Cytotechnology Programs Review Committee
American Society of Cytopathology
100 West 10th Street, Suite 605
Wilmington, DE 19801
302 543-6583
E-mail: *dmacintyre@cytopathology.org*

Cytotechnologist

Alabama

University of Alabama at Birmingham
Cytotechnology Prgm
Sch of Health Professions
1705 University Blvd
RMSB 440
Birmingham, AL 35294-1212
www.uab.edu/msct
Prgm Dir: Vivian Pijuan-Thompson, PhD CT(ASCP)
Tel: 205 934-3378   *Fax:* 205 975-7302
E-mail: pijuan@uab.edu

Auburn University at Montgomery
Cytotechnology Prgm
204B Moore Hall
PO Box 244023 School of Sciences
Montgomery, AL 36124-4023
www.aum.edu/cls

Arkansas

University of Arkansas for Medical Sciences
Cytotechnology Prgm
College of Health Related Professions
4301 W Markham St, # 517
Little Rock, AR 72205-9985
www.uams.edu/chrp/cytotechnology/

California

Loma Linda University
Cytotechnology Prgm
Dept of Clinical Laboratory Science
Anderson/Barton Rd, NH A918
School of Allied Health Professions, Dept of Clin Lab Sci
Loma Linda, CA 92350
www.llu.edu/llu/sahp/clinlab/cthome.html

Greater LA Cytotechnology Training Consortium
Cytotechnology Prgm
Department of Pathology
UCLA Medical Center, A7-147
10833 Le Conte Ave
Los Angeles, CA 90095-1732
www.Pathology.ucla.edu

Indiana

Indiana University School of Medicine
Cytotechnology Prgm
350 West 11th St, Room 6002J
Indianapolis, IN 46202
http://medicine.iu.edu/hpp/

Kansas

University of Kansas Medical Center
Cytotechnology Prgm
3901 Rainbow Blvd, Mail Stop 4048
Mail Stop 4048
Kansas City, KS 66160-7281
www.kumc.edu

Michigan

DMC University Laboratories
Cytotechnology Prgm
4707 St Antoine Blvd
Old Hutzel Hospital-Cytopathology Department
Detroit, MI 48201
www.dmc.org
Prgm Dir: Joy Raymond, SCT(ASCP)CM
Tel: 313 745-0928   *Fax:* 313 745-7158
E-mail: jraymond@dmc.org

Minnesota

Mayo School of Health Sciences
Cytotechnology Prgm
200 First St SW
Rochester, MN 55905
www.mayo.edu/education
Notes: Program inactive in 2009-2010 to adapt curriculum to changing needs in the profession, and reactivated in 2010-2011.

Mississippi

University of Mississippi Medical Center
Cytotechnology Prgm
School of Health Related Professions
2500 N State St
Jackson, MS 39216
www.umc.edu
Prgm Dir: Zelma Cason, MS SCT(ASCP)
Tel: 601 984-6358   *Fax:* 601 815-1717
E-mail: zcason@umc.edu

Missouri

Saint Louis University
Cytotechnology Prgm
Cytotechnology Program Doisy College of Health Sciences
3437 Caroline St
St Louis, MO 63104-1111
www.slu.edu
Prgm Dir: Linda Hoechst, MA SCT(ASCP)(IAC)
Tel: 314 977-8685   *Fax:* 314 977-8503
E-mail: lhoechs1@slu.edu

Nebraska

University of Nebraska Medical Center
Cytotechnology Prgm
984142 Nebraska Medical Center
Omaha, NE 68198-4142
www.unmc.edu

New Jersey

Thomas Edison State College
Cytotechnology Prgm
1776 Raritan Rd
Scotch Plains, NJ 07076
www.umdnj.edu

Univ of Medicine & Dent of New Jersey
Cytotechnology Prgm
School of Health Related Professions
1776 Raritan Rd
Scotch Plains, NJ 07076-2997
www.umdnj.edu

New York

Albany College of Pharmacy and Health Science
Cytotechnology Prgm
106 New Scotland Ave
Albany, NY 12208-3492
www.acp.edu

Memorial Sloan-Kettering Cancer Ctr
Cytotechnology Prgm
1275 York Ave, C596
New York, NY 10021
www.mskcc.org
Prgm Dir: Maria A Friedlander, MPA CT(ASCP)CMIAC
Tel: 212 639-5900 *Fax:* 212 639-6318
E-mail: angelesm@mskcc.org

North Carolina

Central Piedmont Community College
Cytotechnology Prgm
Health Sciences Division
PO Box 35009
Charlotte, NC 28235
www.cpcc.edu

North Dakota

University of North Dakota
Cytotechnology Prgm
School of Medicine & Health Sciences Room 3124
501 N Columbia Rd, Stop 9037
Grand Forks, ND 58202-9037
www.und.nodak.edu

Pennsylvania

Thomas Jefferson University
Cytotechnology Prgm
Cytotechnology/Cell Sciences Prgm
Jefferson School of Hlth Prof, Dept of Bioscience Tech
Edison Bldg, Ste 1924, 130 S Ninth St, Rm 1924
Philadelphia, PA 19107-5233
www.jefferson.edu/jchp/ls
Prgm Dir: Shirley E Greening, MS JD CT(ASCP) CFIAC
Tel: 215 503-7844 *Fax:* 215 503-2189
E-mail: shirley.greening@jefferson.edu

Univ Health Center of Pittsburgh
Cytotechnology Prgm
Anisa I Kanbour School of Cytopathology
300 Halket St Magee Womens Hospital
Pittsburgh, PA 15213-3180
path.upmc.edu
Prgm Dir: Judith Modery
Tel: 412 641-4664 *Fax:* 412 641-5258
E-mail: jmodery@magee.edu

Puerto Rico

University of Puerto Rico
Cytotechnology Prgm
College of Allied Health Professions
PO Box 365067 Ofc 701
San Juan, PR 00936-5067
www.rcm.upr.edu

Rhode Island

University of Rhode Island
Cytotechnology Prgm
Office of Special Programs
Room 302E, 80 Washington St
Feinstein Providence Campus
Providence, RI 02903
www.uri.edu/cels/cmb

Tennessee

University of Tennessee Health Science Ctr
Cytotechnology Prgm
Coll of Allied Hlth Sciences
930 Madison Ave, Suite 674
Dept of Clinical Laboratory Sciences
Memphis, TN 38163
www.uthsc.edu/allied/cytohome.html
Prgm Dir: Barbara D Benstein, PhD SCT(ASCP)
Tel: 901 448-6304 *Fax:* 901 448-7545
E-mail: bdubrayb@uthsc.edu

Texas

Medical Education and Training Campus (METC)
Cytotechnology Prgm
Building 2841
Room 2303, 3851 Scott Rd
Department of Clinical Support Services
Fort Sam Houston, TX 78234-6137
www.bamc.amedd.army.mil

Univ of Texas M D Anderson Cancer Ctr
Cytotechnology Prgm
School of Health Professions
1515 Holcombe Blvd, Unit 2
Houston, TX 77030-4009
www.mdanderson.org/healthsciences

Utah

University of Utah Health Science Center
Cytotechnology Prgm
ARUP Laboratory
500 Chipeta Way
Salt Lake City, UT 84108
www.utah.edu

Vermont

Fletcher Allen Health Care
Cytotechnology Prgm
111 Colchester Ave
Burlington, VT 05401
www.fletcherallen.org/cytoschool
Prgm Dir: Sandra Giroux, MS SCT(ASCP) CFIAC
Tel: 802 847-5133 *Fax:* 802 847-3632
E-mail: Sandra.Giroux@vtmednet.org

Virginia

Old Dominion University
Cytotechnology Prgm
2118 Technology Building
Hampton Blvd
Norfolk, VA 23529
www.odu.edu/cyto

West Virginia

Cabell Huntington Hospital
Cytotechnology Prgm
1340 Hal Greer Blvd
Huntington, WV 25701
www.cabellhuntington.org

Wisconsin

Wisconsin State Laboratory of Hygiene
Cytotechnology Prgm
465 Henry Mall
Madison, WI 53706
www.slh.wisc.edu/cytology/index.php

Marshfield Clinic
Cosponsor: St. Joseph's Hospital
Cytotechnology Prgm
1000 N Oak Ave
Marshfield, WI 54449-5795
www.marshfieldlabs.org/marshfieldlabs/
default.aspx?page=laboratorycareer

University of Wisconsin - Milwaukee
Cytotechnology Prgm
College of Health Sciences
2400 East Hartford Ave
PO Box 413 Enderis Hall 463
Milwaukee, WI 53201
www4.uwm.edu/chs/academics/undergraduate/
healthsciences/cytotechnology

Cytotechnologist

Programs*	Class Capacity	Begins	Length (months)	Award	Res. Tuition	Non-res. Tuition		Offers:† 1	2	3	4
Alabama											
Univ of Alabama at Birmingham	12	Aug	16	Cert, MS	$23,356	$53,418	per year				•
Michigan											
DMC Univ Laboratories (Detroit)	5	Sep	12	Cert							
Mississippi											
Univ of Mississippi Medical Center (Jackson)	24	Jun	12	BS	$5,439	$13,894	per year				
Missouri											
Saint Louis Univ (St Louis)	12	Jun	12	Cert, BSCT, Post Bacc	$37,420	$37,420	total tuition				
New York											
Memorial Sloan-Kettering Cancer Ctr (New York)	4	Aug	12	Cert, CT	$8,000	$8,000	per year				
Pennsylvania											
Thomas Jefferson Univ (Philadelphia)	24	Sep	12	BS MS	$33,776	$33,776	total tuition			•	
Univ Health Center of Pittsburgh	8	Jul	12	Cert	$7,000	$7,000	per year				
Tennessee											
Univ of Tennessee Health Science Ctr (Memphis)	6	Aug	21	MS	$1,122	$26,544	per year				
Vermont											
Fletcher Allen Health Care (Burlington)	6	Sep	12	Cert, BS	$7,000	$7,000	per year				

*Data are shown only for programs that completed the 2011 AMA Survey of Health Professions Education Programs.

†Key to Offers: 1: Evening or weekend classes; 2: Non-English instruction; 3: Cultural competence instruction; 4: Distance education component.

Diagnostic Molecular Scientist

The diagnostic molecular scientist performs diagnostic assay or testing using a variety of manual techniques and precision instruments. The results of these tests are used to detect and diagnose disease and other abnormalities. The main responsibilities of the diagnostic molecular scientist are all aspects of genetic testing, including DNA and RNA isolation, amplification and detection, infectious disease testing, and viral load analysis.

Career Description

Diagnostic molecular scientists provide service in the molecular diagnosis of acquired, inherited, and infectious diseases. This includes researching, evaluating, implementing, and monitoring methods of collection, transport, and handling of various specimen types for molecular analysis; researching and developing principles, practices, and applications of molecular-based testing for laboratory utilization and clinical decisions for client outcomes; and performing appropriate techniques utilizing instrumentation and information management systems for molecular analysis and correlating results with acquired, inherited, and infectious diseases. Finally, diagnostic molecular scientists apply the principles of management and supervision when they function as section supervisors and of educational methodology when they teach students.

Employment Characteristics

Most diagnostic molecular scientists work in hospital laboratories.

Educational Programs

Length. Programs for the diagnostic molecular scientist usually lead to a master's degree.

Prerequisites. College level courses as required by the sponsoring institution.

Curriculum. The curriculum includes both didactic instruction and practical demonstration in the areas of organic and/or biochemistry, genetics, cell biology, microbiology, immunology, diagnostic molecular biology, principles and methodologies for all major areas commonly practiced by a modern diagnostic molecular laboratory, and clinical significance of laboratory procedures in diagnosis and treatment. It also includes principles and practices of:

- Laboratory administration, supervision, safety, and problem solving
- Quality management
- Computer science (including acquisition and evaluation of laboratory information systems)
- Professional conduct

Inquiries

Careers/Curriculum

American Medical Technologists
10700 West Higgins Road, Suite 150
Rosemont, IL 60018
847 823-5169
E-mail: *mail@amt1.com*
www.amt1.com

American Society for Clinical Laboratory Science
6701 Democracy Blvd., Suite 300
Bethesda, MD 20817
301 657-2768
E-mail: *ascls@ascls.org*
www.ascls.org

American Society for Clinical Pathology
33 West Monroe, Suite 1600
Chicago, IL 60603
312 541-4999
E-mail: *info@ascp.org*
www.ascp.org

Certification/Registration

American Society for Clinical Pathology
Board of Certification
PO Box 12270
Chicago, IL 60612
312 738-1336, Ext 1341
www.ascp.org

American Association of Bioanalysts
Board of Registry
906 Olive Street, Suite 1200
St. Louis, MO 63101-1434
www.aab.org

Program Accreditation

Dianne M Cearlock, PhD
Chief Executive Officer (CEO)
National Accrediting Agency for Clinical Laboratory Sciences
5600 River Rd, Suite 720
Rosemont, IL 60018
773 714-8880
E-mail: *dcearlock@naacls.org*
www.naacls.org

Diagnostic Molecular Scientist

Connecticut

University of Connecticut
Diagnostic Molecular Scientist Prgm
Molecular Diagnostics Program
358 Mansfield Rd, Room 222, Koons Hall, Unit 2101
Storrs, CT 06269
www.alliedhealth.uconn.edu

Kansas

University of Kansas Medical Center
Diagnostic Molecular Scientist Prgm
G014 Eaton
3901 Rainbow Blvd, MS 4048
Kansas City, KS 66160
www.cls.kumc.edu

Michigan

Michigan State University
Diagnostic Molecular Scientist Prgm
Biomedical Laboratory Diagnostics Program
322 N Kedzie Hall
East Lansing, MI 48824-1031
www.bld/msu/edu

Northern Michigan University
Diagnostic Molecular Scientist Prgm
1401 Presque Isle Ave
3513 W Science Bldg
Marquette, MI 49855-5346
www.nmu.edu

New York

SUNY Upstate Medical University
Diagnostic Molecular Scientist Prgm
750 E Adams St
2156 Weiskotten Hall
Syracuse, NY 13210
www.upstate.edu/chp/mb

North Carolina

University of North Carolina - Chapel Hill
Diagnostic Molecular Scientist Prgm
Division of Clinical Laboratory Sciences
CB 7145, Bondurant Hall, Suite 4100
Chapel Hill, NC 27599-7145
www.med.unc.edu/ahs/clinical/mds

Texas

Univ of Texas M D Anderson Cancer Ctr
Diagnostic Molecular Scientist Prgm
Program in Molecular Genetic Technology
1515 Holcombe Blvd, Unit 146
Houston, TX 77030
www.mdanderson.org/healthsciences

Texas Tech Univ Health Sciences Center
Diagnostic Molecular Scientist Prgm
Dept of Laboratory Sciences & Primary Care
3601 Fourth St, 2-B-181, MS 6281
Lubbock, TX 79430
www.ttuhsc.edu

Histotechnician

Physicians (usually pathologists) and other scientists specializing in biological sciences or related clinical areas such as chemistry work in partnership with medical laboratory workers to analyze blood, tissues, and fluids from humans (and sometimes animals), using a variety of precision instruments. The results of these tests are used to detect and diagnose disease and other abnormalities.

The main responsibility of the histotechnician in the clinical laboratory is preparing sections of body tissue for examination by a pathologist. This includes the preparation of tissue specimens of human and animal origin for diagnostic, research, or teaching purposes. Tissue sections prepared by the histotechnician for a variety of disease entities enable the pathologist to diagnose body dysfunction and malignancy.

Career Description

Histotechnicians process sections of body tissue by fixation, dehydration, embedding, sectioning, decalcification, microincineration, mounting, and routine and special staining. They identify tissue structures, cell components, and their staining characteristics and relate them to physiological functions; and institute proper procedures to maintain accuracy and precision.

Employment Characteristics

Most histotechnicians work in hospital or reference laboratories.

Salary

According to the 2010 Wage and Vacancy Survey conducted by the American Society for Clinical Pathology (ASCP), histotechnicians earn an average median wage of $22.68 per hour or $47,174 annually; supervisors earn a median average wage of $29.48 per hour or $61,318 per year. The survey results were published in the March 2011 issue of *LabMedicine*, available at *http:// labmed.ascpjournals.org/ content/42/3/141*.

For more information, refer to *www.ama-assn.org/go/hpsalary*.

Educational Programs

Length. Programs for the histotechnician are 12 months, unless the curriculum is an integral part of a college program.

Prerequisites. High school diploma or equivalent to enter a college-based program. For admission into hospital-based programs, credentials ranging from a high school diploma to an associate degree may be required. Each program will have its own prerequisites for the amount of education required, including specific biology, chemistry, and math courses that are required before acceptance into the program.

Curriculum. The curriculum includes both didactic instruction and practical demonstration in the areas of:

- Medical ethics
- Medical terminology
- Chemistry
- Laboratory mathematics
- Computer technology
- Organic and/or biochemistry
- Immunology
- Anatomy
- Histology
- Histochemistry
- Quality control
- Instrumentation
- Microscopy
- Processing techniques
- Laboratory safety
- Preparation of museum specimens
- Record procedures

It is recommended that the curriculum be an integral part of a junior or community college program culminating in an associate degree and that the course of study include chemistry, biology, and mathematics.

Inquiries

Careers/Curriculum

American Society for Clinical Pathology
33 West Monroe, Suite 1600
Chicago, IL 60603
312 541-4999
E-mail: *info@ascp.org*
www.ascp.org

National Society for Histotechnology
10320 Little Patuxent Parkway, Suite 804
Columbia, MD 21044
443 535-4060
E-mail: *histo@nsh.org*
www.nsh.org

Certification/Registration

American Society for Clinical Pathology
Board of Certification
33 West Monroe, Suite 1600
Chicago, IL 60603
800 267-2727, option 2
312 738-1336, Ext 1341
E-mail: *boc@ascp.org*
www.ascp.org

Program Accreditation

Dianne M Cearlock, PhD, Chief Executive Officer
National Accrediting Agency for Clinical Laboratory Sciences
5600 North River Road, Suite 720
Rosemont, IL 60018
847 939-3597 or 773 714-8880
E-mail: *info@naacls.org*
www.naacls.org

Histotechnician

Arizona

Phoenix College
Histotechnician Prgm
1202 W Thomas Rd
Phoenix, AZ 85013

Arkansas

Baptist Health Schools Little Rock
Histotechnician Prgm
11900 Colonel Glenn Rd, Ste 1000
Little Rock, AR 72206
www.bhslr.edu

California

TPMG Regional Laboratory
Histotechnician Prgm
1725 Eastshore Hwy
Berkeley, CA 94710

Mt San Antonio College
Histotechnician Prgm
1100 N Grand Ave
Walnut, CA 91789-1399
www.mtsac.edu

Connecticut

Goodwin College
Histotechnician Prgm
745 Burnside Ave
403 Main St
1 Riverside Drive
East Hartford, CT 06118
www.goodwincollege.org

Delaware

Delaware Technical Community College
Cosponsor: Christiana Care Health Services
Histotechnician Prgm
333 N Shipley St
WSE 308M
Wilmington, DE 19801
www.dtcc.edu/wilmington/ah/htt.html

Florida

Florida State College at Jacksonville
Histotechnician Prgm
North Campus, 4501 Capper Rd
Jacksonville, FL 32218
http://catalog.fccj.edu/
    preview_program.php?catoid=1&poid=58&bc=1

Lakeland Regional Medical Center
Histotechnician Prgm
1324 Lakeland Hills Blvd
Lakeland, FL 33805

Dade Medical College
Histotechnician Prgm
950 NW 20 St #2239
Miami, FL 33127-4693
www.mdc.edu/medical/AHT/Histotechnology/default.asp

Keiser University
Histotechnician Prgm
5600 Lake Underhill Rd
Orlando, FL 32807
www.keiseruniversity.edu

Keiser University
Histotechnician Prgm
12520 Pines Blvd
Pembroke Pines, FL 33027

Georgia

Darton College
Histotechnician Prgm
2400 Gillionville Rd
Albany, GA 31707
www.darton.edu/programs/AlliedHealth/certificates/
Hist-Cert.php

Illinois

Elgin Community College
Histotechnician Prgm
1700 Spartan Drive
Elgin, IL 60123
www.elgin.edu/hst2

OSF Saint Francis Medical Center
Histotechnician Prgm
School of CLS/HT
530 NE Glen Oak Ave
Peoria, IL 61637-0001
www.osfsaintfrancis.org

Indiana

Indiana University
Histotechnician Prgm
350 West 11th St
Room 4084
Indianapolis, IN 46202
http://medicine.iu.edu/histo

Maryland

Harford Community College
Histotechnician Prgm
401 Thomas Run Rd
Bel Air, MD 21015
www.harford.edu

Michigan

DMC University Laboratories
Histotechnician Prgm
4707 St Antoine Blvd
Detroit, MI 48201
www.dmcul.org/univlab/histology.html

Lansing Community College
Histotechnician Prgm
Ingham Intermediate School District
611 Hagadorn Rd
Mason, MI 48854-9592
www.lcc.edu/science/

Beaumont Hospital - Royal Oak
Histotechnician Prgm
Department of Anatomic Pathology
3601 W 13 Mile Rd
Royal Oak, MI 48073-6769
www.beaumonthospitals.com/alliedhealth

Minnesota

North Hennepin Community College
Histotechnician Prgm
7411 85th Ave North
Brooklyn Park, MN 55445

Argosy University Twin Cities Campus
Histotechnician Prgm
1515 Central Parkway
Eagan, MN 55121
www.argosyu.edu

Mayo Clinic
Histotechnician Prgm
200 1st St SW, Hilton 1082
Rochester, MN 55905
www.mayo.edu/mshs/histology-career.html

New York

State University of New York at Cobleskill
Histotechnician Prgm
111 Schenectady Ave
Cobleskill, NY 12043
www.Cobleskill.edu/academics/lasschool/nas/
    histoprog.asp

North Carolina

Davidson County Community College
Histotechnician Prgm
PO Box 1287
Lexington, NC 27293
www.davidsonccc.edu/academics/
    hwp-histotechnology.htm

North Dakota

University of North Dakota
Histotechnician Prgm
School of Medicine & Health Sciences, Dept of Pathology
Stop Box 9037
501 N Columbia Rd
Grand Forks, ND 58203-9037
http://pathology.med.und.nodak.edu/histotech/

Ohio

Columbus State Community College
Histotechnician Prgm
550 E Spring St
CSCC - 519 Union Hall
Columbus, OH 43215
www.cscc.edu/histology

Lakeland Community College
Histotechnician Prgm
7700 Clocktower Drive
Kirtland, OH 44094

Youngstown State University
Histotechnician Prgm
Dept of Health Professions
One University Plaza
Youngstown, OH 44555
http://bchhs.ysu.edu/healthprofessions/medtech/
    histotech.htm

Pennsylvania

Harcum College
Histotechnician Prgm
750 Montgomery Ave
Bryn Mawr, PA 19010

Conemaugh Valley Memorial Hospital
Histotechnician Prgm
1086 Franklin St
Johnstown, PA 15905-4305
www.conemaugh.org

University of Pittsburgh
Histotechnician Prgm
Magee-Womens Hospital of UPMC
300 Halket St
Pittsburgh, PA 15213
www.path.upmc.edu/histotechnology/Index.htm

Rhode Island

Community College of Rhode Island
Histotechnician Prgm
1762 Louisquisset Pike
Allied Health Department
Lincoln, RI 02865
www.ccri.edu/alliedhealth/histotechnician

Texas

**Medical Education and Training Campus
(METC)**
Histotechnician Prgm
Histotechnician Program
3085 Wilson Way
Fort Sam Houston, TX 78234-6402
www.metc.mil

Tarleton State University
Histotechnician Prgm
1501 Enderly Place
Fort Worth, TX 76104
www.tarleton.edu/~clinlab

Houston Community College
Histotechnician Prgm
1900 Pressler Dr
Houston, TX 77030
www.Coleman.hccs.edu

Univ of Texas M D Anderson Cancer Ctr
Histotechnician Prgm
1515 Holcombe Blvd, Box 206
Unit 2
Houston, TX 77030
www.mdanderson.org/healthsciences

St Philip's College
Histotechnician Prgm
1801 Martin Luther King Dr
San Antonio, TX 78203
www.accd.edu/spc/acad/ahd/hist/hlabprogram.aspx

UT Health Science Center - San Antonio
Histotechnician Prgm
7703 Floyd Curl Dr
Dept of Pathology
San Antonio, TX 78229
http://pathology.uthscsa.edu/strl/histology/
    services-training.shtml

Virginia

Old Dominion University
Histotechnician Prgm
School of Medical Lab & Radiation Sci
2118 Health Sci Bldg ODU
Norfolk, VA 23529
http://hs.odu.edu/medlab/academics/histo

Washington

Clover Park Technical College
Histotechnician Prgm
5400 Steilacoom Blvd
Lakewood, WA 98499
www.cptc.edu

Wisconsin

Saint Joseph's Hospital / Marshfield Clinic
Histotechnician Prgm
611 St Joseph Ave
1000 N Oak
Marshfield, WI 54449-1898
www.marshfieldlaboratories.org/career.asp

Histotechnologist

Physicians (usually pathologists) and other scientists specializing in biological sciences or related clinical areas such as chemistry work in partnership with medical laboratory workers to analyze blood, tissues, and fluids from humans (and sometimes animals), using a variety of precision instruments. The results of these tests are used to detect and diagnose disease and other abnormalities.

The main responsibility of the histotechnologist in the clinical laboratory is preparing sections of body tissue for examination by a pathologist. This includes the preparation of tissue specimens of human and animal origin for diagnostic, research, or teaching purposes. Tissue sections prepared by the histotechnologist for a variety of disease entities enable the pathologist to diagnose body dysfunction and malignancy.

Career Description

Histotechnologists process sections of body tissue by fixation, dehydration, embedding, sectioning, decalcification, microincineration, mounting, and routine and special staining. In addition, histotechnologists perform the more complex procedures for processing and staining tissues, including troubleshooting and problem solving routine and special stains, immunohistochemistry, and muscle enzyme histochemistry. They identify tissue structures, cell components, and their staining characteristics and relate them to physiological functions; implement and test new techniques and procedures; make judgments concerning the results of quality control measures; and institute proper procedures to maintain accuracy and precision. Histotechnologists apply the principles of management and supervision when they function as section supervisors and of educational methodology when they teach students.

Employment Characteristics

Most histotechnologists work in hospital, reference, or research laboratories.

Salary

According to the 2010 Wage and Vacancy Survey conducted by the American Society for Clinical Pathology (ASCP), available at *http://labmed.ascpjournals.org/content/42/3/141*, histotechnologists at the staff level earn a median average wage of $26 per hour or $54,080 annually; for those at the supervisory level, these figures are $32.10 and $66,768, respectively.

For more information, refer to *www.ama-assn.org/go/hpsalary*.

Educational Programs

Length, Award. Programs based in colleges/universities are four years and lead to a baccalaureate degree; those based in hospitals require a baccalaureate degree for admission, and culminate with a certificate.

Prerequisites. A high school diploma or equivalent is required for entrance into a college/university-based program. A baccalaureate degree with courses in biology, chemistry and math is required for entrance into a hospital-based program.

Curriculum. The curriculum includes both didactic instruction and practical demonstration in the areas of

- Medical ethics
- Medical terminology
- Chemistry
- Laboratory mathematics
- Computer technology
- Organic and/or biochemistry
- Immunohistochemistry/Immunofluorescence
- Electron microscopy
- Management
- Anatomy
- Histology
- Histochemistry
- Quality Control
- Instrumentation
- Microscopy
- Processing techniques
- Preparation of museum specimens
- Record and administration procedures
- Muscle enzyme histochemistry
- In situ hybridization
- Laboratory safety
- Management principles
- Education methodology
- Cost analysis
- Research techniques
- Federal, state, and accrediting agencies rules and regulations

The baccalaureate-level program includes coursework designed to provide supervisors and teachers with advanced capabilities.

Inquiries

Careers/Curriculum

American Society for Clinical Pathology
33 West Monroe, Suite 1600
Chicago, IL 60603
312 541-4999
E-mail: *info@ascp.org*
www.ascp.org

National Society for Histotechnology
10320 Little Patuxent Parkway, Suite 804
Columbia, MD 21044
443 535-4060
E-mail: *histo@nsh.org*
www.nsh.org

Certification/Registration

American Society for Clinical Pathology
Board of Certification
33 West Monroe, Suite 1600
Chicago, IL 60603
800 267-2727, option 2
312 738-1336, Ext 1341
E-mail: *boc@ascp.org*
www.ascp.org

Program Accreditation
Dianne M Cearlock, PhD, Chief Executive Officer
National Accrediting Agency for Clinical Laboratory Sciences
5600 North River Road, Suite 720
Rosemont, IL 60018
847 939-3597 or 773 714-8880
E-mail: *info@naacls.org*
www.naacls.org

Histotechnologist

Florida

Barry University
Histotechnology Prgm
11300 NE Second Ave
Miami Shores, FL 33161-6695
www.barry.edu/histo

Michigan

Beaumont Hospital - Royal Oak
Histotechnology Prgm
Anatomic Pathology/Beaumont Hospital
3601 W 13 Mile Rd
Royal Oak, MI 48073-6769
www.beaumonthospitals.com/alliedhealth

Pennsylvania

Drexel University College of Medicine
Histotechnology Prgm
245 N 15th St
Philadelphia, PA 19102
www.drexelmed.edu

South Carolina

Medical University of South Carolina Medical Center
Histotechnology Prgm
165 Ashley Ave
MSC 908
Charleston, SC 29425-0908
www.musc.edu/histoprogram

Tennessee

University of Tennessee Health Science Ctr
Histotechnology Prgm
930 Madison Ave, Suite 664
Memphis, TN 38163
www.utmem.edu/allied/cytohome.html

Texas

Univ of Texas M D Anderson Cancer Ctr
Histotechnology Prgm
1515 Holcombe Blvd
Unit 0002
Houston, TX 77030
www.mdanderson.org/healthsciences

West Virginia

West Virginia University
Histotechnology Prgm
Health Science Center
PO Box 9211
Morgantown, WV 26506

Anatomic pathologists are physicians who examine tissue specimens from patients and perform autopsies to diagnose the disease processes involved. Pathologists' assistants participate in autopsies and in the examination, dissection, and processing of tissue specimens. They function as physician extenders.

Career Description

The following services are provided under the direct supervision of a licensed and board-certified pathologist and should include, but not be limited to the following:

Surgical pathology. Assisting in the preparation and performance of surgical specimen dissection by ensuring appropriate specimen accessioning, obtaining pertinent clinical information and studies, describing gross anatomic features, dissecting surgical specimens, preparing and submitting tissue for histologic processing, obtaining and submitting specimens for additional analytic procedures (immunostaining, flow cytometry, image analysis, bacterial and viral cultures, toxicology, etc), and assisting in photographing gross and microscopic specimens.

Autopsy pathology. Assisting in the performance of postmortem examination by ascertaining proper legal authorization; obtaining and reviewing the patient's chart and other pertinent clinical data and studies; notifying involved personnel of all special procedures and techniques required; coordinating special requests for specimens; notifying involved clinicians and appropriate authorities and individuals; assisting in the postmortem examination; selecting and preparing tissue for histologic processing and special studies; obtaining specimens for biological and toxicologic analysis; assisting in photographing gross and microscopic specimens and photomicrography; and participating in the completion of the autopsy report.

Additional duties. Assuming duties as may be assigned relative to teaching, administrative, supervisory, and budgetary functions in anatomic pathology.

Employment Characteristics

Pathologists' assistants are employed in a variety of settings, including community and regional hospitals, university medical centers, private pathology laboratories, and medical examiners/ coroners' offices.

Salary

Salaries vary with geographic location and type of employing institution. According to the 2010 Wage and Vacancy Survey conducted by the American Society for Clinical Pathology (ASCP), staff-level pathologists' assistants earn a median average wage of $35.00 per hour or $72,800 annually; supervisors earn a median average rate of $37.80 per hour or $77,376 annually. The survey results were published in the March 2011 issue of *LabMedicine*, available at *http://labmed.ascpjournals.org/content/42/3/141*.

For more information, refer to *www.ama-assn.org/go/hpsalary*.

Educational Programs

Length. Minimum of 22 months.
Degree. Most programs are at the master's level.
Prerequisites. Variable among programs and dependent on the degree offered. Baccalaureate programs require a minimum of 60 hours of acceptable credits, with variable specific requirements.

Curriculum. The curriculum includes both didactic and practical training to provide a sound background in the basic medical sciences and the necessary skills to work in an anatomic pathology laboratory. Coursework includes anatomy, physiology, and medical terminology, as well as general, systemic, pediatric, and forensic pathology. Clinical training includes autopsy pathology, surgical pathology, forensic pathology, and medical photography.

Inquiries

Careers/Curriculum
American Association of Pathologists' Assistants
2345 Rice Street, Suite 220
St Paul, MN 55113
800 532-AAPA or 651 697-9264
E-mail: *msok@associationdevlopment.org* or *executivedirector@pathassist.org*
www.pathassist.org

American Society for Clinical Pathology
33 West Monroe, Suite 1600
Chicago, IL 60603
312 541-4999
E-mail: *info@ascp.org*
www.ascp.org

Certification/Registration
American Society for Clinical Pathology
Board of Certification
PO Box 12270
Chicago, IL 60612
312 738-1336, Ext 1341
www.ascp.org

Program Accreditation
Dianne M Cearlock, PhD
Chief Executive Officer (CEO)
National Accrediting Agency for Clinical Laboratory Sciences
5600 North River Rd, Suite 720
Rosemont, IL 60018
773 714-8880
E-mail: *dcearlock@naacls.org*
www.naacls.org

Pathologists' Assistant

Alberta, Canada

University of Calgary
Pathologists' Assistant Prgm
Diagnostic & Scientific Centre, Rm C411, 9, 3535
    Research Rd
Calgary, AB T2N 4Z6
www.pathology.ucalgary.ca

Connecticut

Quinnipiac University
Pathologists' Assistant Prgm
275 Mount Carmel Ave
Hamden, CT 06518
www.quinnipiac.edu

Illinois

Rosalind Franklin University of Medicine
Pathologists' Assistant Prgm
3333 Green Bay Rd
Pathologists' Assistant Department
North Chicago, IL 60064
www.rosalindfranklin.edu/dnn/chp/home/CHP/
    PathologistsAssistant/tabid/1459/Default.aspx

Indiana

Indiana University
Pathologists' Assistant Prgm
350 W 11th St, Rm 4029A
Clarian Pathology Laboratory
Indianapolis, IN 46202
www.pathology.iupui.edu/grad

Maryland

University of Maryland, Baltimore
Pathologists' Assistant Prgm
Dept of Pathology 22 South Greene St
MSTF, Room 700B
10 South Pine St
Baltimore, MD 21201
http://medschool.umaryland.edu/pathology/pa.asp

Michigan

Wayne State University
Cosponsor: Eugene Applebaum College of Pharmacy &
    Health Sci
Pathologists' Assistant Prgm
Department of Fundamental & Appl Sci, Mort Sci
5439 Woodward Ave
Detroit, MI 48202
www.mortsci.wayne.edu

North Carolina

Duke University Medical Center
Pathologists' Assistant Prgm
Box 3712 DUMC
Department of Pathology
Durham, NC 27710
http://pathology.mc.duke.edu/website/
    WebForm.aspx?id=AP_PathAssistMain

Ontario, Canada

University of Western Ontario
Pathologists' Assistant Prgm
Dental Sciences Building Room 4044
1151 Richmond St, North
London, ON
www.uwo.ca/pathol/gradprogram.html

Pennsylvania

Drexel University College of Medicine
Pathologists' Assistant Prgm
Office of Professional Studies in the Health Sciences
Mail Stop 344, Room 4807
245 N 15th St
Philadelphia, PA 19102
www.drexelmed.edu/Home/AcademicPrograms/
    ProfessionalStudiesintheHealthSciences/Programs/
    Maste

West Virginia

West Virginia University
Pathologists' Assistant Prgm
2146H Health Sciences North
Dept of Pathology, Box 9203
Morgantown, WV 26506
www.hsc.wvu.edu/som/pa/

Laboratory tests play an important role in the detection, diagnosis, and treatment of diseases. Phlebotomists collect blood specimens for many of these tests. Phlebotomists practice safe blood collection and handling techniques that protect patients from injury, safeguard themselves from accidents, and produce high-quality specimens while demonstrating compassion for the patient.

Career Description

Phlebotomists collect, transport, handle, and process blood specimens for analysis; identify and select equipment, supplies, and additives used in blood collection; and understand factors that affect specimen collection procedures and test results. Recognizing the importance of specimen collection in the overall patient care system, phlebotomists adhere to infection control and safety policies and procedures. They monitor quality control within predetermined limits while demonstrating professional conduct, stress management, and communication skills with patients, peers, and other health care personnel as well as with the public.

Employment Characteristics

Many phlebotomists are employed in hospital laboratories. Others are employed in physicians' private laboratories and clinics; by the armed forces; by city, state, and federal health agencies; in industrial medical laboratories; in pharmaceutical houses; in numerous public and private research programs; and as faculty of approved programs preparing medical laboratory personnel.

Salary

Salaries vary depending on the employer and geographic location. According to the 2010 Wage and Vacancy Survey conducted by the American Society for Clinical Pathology (ASCP), staff phlebotomists earn a median average wage of $13.50 per hour or $28,080 per year; average pay for supervisors is $20.08 per hour or $41,766 annually. The survey results were published in the March 2010 issue of *LabMedicine*, available at *http://labmed.ascpjournals.org/content/42/3/141*.

For more information, refer to *www.ama-assn.org/go/hpsalary*.

Educational Programs

Length. Approved programs contain at least 100 hours of clinical practicum and culminate in a post-secondary certificate.

Prerequisites. High school diploma or equivalent. The applicant must also meet the admission requirements of the sponsoring institution.

Curriculum. Phlebotomy programs are conducted in junior or community colleges, hospitals, medical laboratories, proprietary schools, and other equivalent postsecondary educational institutions. The curriculum includes didactic instruction and 100 hours of applied experiences, performance of a minimum of 100 successful unaided collections, and instruction in a variety of collection techniques, including vacuum collection devices, syringe, and capillary/skin-puncture methods.

Inquiries

Careers/Curriculum

American Medical Technologists
10700 West Higgins Road, Suite 150
Rosemont, IL 60018
847 823-5169
E-mail: *mail@amt1.com*
www.amt1.com

American Society for Clinical Laboratory Science
6701 Democracy Boulevard, Suite 300
Bethesda, MD 20817
301 657-2768
E-mail: *ascls@ascls.org*
www.ascls.org

American Society for Clinical Pathology
33 West Monroe, Suite 1600
Chicago, IL 60603
312 541-4999
E-mail: *info@ascp.org*
www.ascp.org

National Phlebotomy Association
1901 Brightseat Road
Landover, MD 20785
301 386-4200
E-mail: *naltphle@aol.com*
www.nationalphlebotomy.org

Certification/Registration

American Society for Clinical Pathology
Board of Certification
PO Box 12270
Chicago, IL 60612
312 738-1336, Ext 1341
E-mail: *boc@ascp.org*
www.ascp.org

American Association of Bioanalysts
Board of Registry
906 Olive Street, Suite 1200
St. Louis, MO 63101-1434
www.aab.org

American Medical Technologists
10700 West Higgins Road, Suite 150
Rosemont, IL 60018
847 823-5169
E-mail: *mail@amt1.com*
www.amt1.com

Program Accreditation

Dianne M Cearlock, PhD, Chief Executive Officer
National Accrediting Agency for Clinical Laboratory Sciences
5600 North River Road, Suite 720
Rosemont, IL 60018
(773) 714-8880
E-mail: *dcearlock@naacls.org*
www.naacls.org

Phlebotomist

Arizona

Arizona Medical Training Institute
Phlebotomy Prgm
1530 North Country Club, Suite 11
Mesa, AZ 85201
www.azmti.com

Arkansas

South Arkansas Community College
Phlebotomy Prgm
300 South West Ave
El Dorado, AR 71730

Phillips Community College/U of Arkansas
Phlebotomy Prgm
1000 Campus Dr, PO Box 785
Helena-West Helena, AR 72342
www.pccua.edu

Southeast Arkansas College
Phlebotomy Prgm
1900 Hazel St
Pine Bluff, AR 71603
www.seark.edu

California

California Institute of Medical Science, Inc
Phlebotomy Prgm
1901 E Shields, Suite B-118
Fresno, CA 93726

Colorado

Front Range Comm College
Phlebotomy Prgm
800 South Taft
Loveland, CO 80537
www.frontrange.edu

Florida

Florida Hospital
Phlebotomy Prgm
601 E Rollins St
Orlando, FL 32803
www.floridahospital.com

Georgia

Dalton State College
Phlebotomy Prgm
650 College Dr
Dalton, GA 30720-3778
www.daltonstate.edu

Hawaii

Kapiolani Community College /University of Hawaii - Kapiolani
Phlebotomy Prgm
4303 Diamond Head Rd
Health Sciences Dept, Kauila 121
Honolulu, HI 96816

Illinois

Moraine Valley Community College
Phlebotomy Prgm
Career Programs B-150
9000 W College Parkway
Palos Hills, IL 60465
www.morainevalley.edu/HealthSciences/Phlebotomy/
   phlebotomy.htm

South Suburban College
Phlebotomy Prgm
15800 S State St
South Holland, IL 60473
www.southsuburbancollege.edu

College of Lake County
Phlebotomy Prgm
33 N Genesee St
#S307
Waukegan, IL 60085
www.clcillinois.edu/programs/mlt/

Indiana

In Training Inc College of Adult Education
Phlebotomy Prgm
182 Deanna Drive
Lowell, IN 46356
www.intrainingcollege.com

Ivy Tech Community College
Phlebotomy Prgm
220 Dean Johnson Blvd
South Bend, IN 46601
www.ivytech.edu/schools/health/index.html

Iowa

St. Luke's College/St. Luke's Regl Med Ctr
Phlebotomy Prgm
2720 Stone Park Blvd
Sioux City, IA 51104

Louisiana

Rapides Regional Medical Center
Phlebotomy Prgm
211 Fourth St
Box 30101
Alexandria, LA 71301-8421
www.rapidesregional.com

Bossier Parish Community College
Phlebotomy Prgm
3220 East Texas St
Bossier City, LA 71111
www.bpcc.edu

L E Fletcher Technical Community College
Phlebotomy Prgm
310 St Charles St
PO Box 5033
Houma, LA 70361
www.ftcc.edu

Delgado Community College
Phlebotomy Prgm
615 City Park Ave
New Orleans, LA 70119
www.dcc.edu

Southern Univ at Shreveport
Phlebotomy Prgm
3050 Martin Luther King Jr Dr
Shreveport, LA 71107
www.susla.edu

Maryland

Kaplan College - Hagerstown
Phlebotomy Prgm
18618 Crestwood Dr
Hagerstown, MD 21742
www.kc-hagerstown.com

Michigan

Baker College of Auburn Hills
Phlebotomy Prgm
1500 University Drive
Auburn Hills, MI 48326-2642

Mid Michigan Community College
Phlebotomy Prgm
703 N McEwan
Clare, MI 48617
www.midmich.cc.mi.us

DMC University Laboratories
Phlebotomy Prgm
4707 St Antoine Blvd
Detroit, MI 48201

Medright Incorporated
Phlebotomy Prgm
427 Allen Rd
Ferndale, MI 48220
www.medright.org

Baker College of Owosso
Phlebotomy Prgm
1020 S Washington St
Owosso, MI 48867
www.baker.edu

Minnesota

Hennepin County Medical Center
Phlebotomy Prgm
Clinical Laboratories, P4
701 Park Ave
Minneapolis, MN 55415

Minneapolis Community & Technical College
Phlebotomy Prgm
1501 Hennepin Ave
Minneapolis, MN 55403

Saint Catherine University - Minneapolis
Phlebotomy Prgm
601 25th Ave S
Minneapolis, MN 55454
www.stkate.edu/academic/phlebotomy

Mayo Clinic
Phlebotomy Prgm
200 First St SW
Rochester, MN 55905

Mississippi

University of Southern Mississippi
Phlebotomy Prgm
118 College Drive, PO Box 5134
Hattiesburg, MS 39406

Missouri

Saint Luke's Hospital
Phlebotomy Prgm
4401 Wornall Rd
Kansas City, MO 64111
www.saintlukeshealthsystem.org

Nevada

University of Nevada - Las Vegas
Phlebotomy Prgm
4505 Maryland Parkway
Las Vegas, NV 89154-3021

New Jersey

Univ of Medicine & Dent of New Jersey
Phlebotomy Prgm
65 Bergen St
Bergen Bldg GB-159
PO Box 1709
Newark, NJ 07101-1709
http://shrp.umdnj.edu/programs/cls/phlebotomy.htm

New York

Trocaire College
Phlebotomy Prgm
360 Choate Ave
Buffalo, NY 14220
www.trocaire.edu

Nicholas H Noyes Memorial Hospital
Phlebotomy Prgm
111 Clara Barton St
Dansville, NY 14437
www.noyes-health.org

Orange County Community College
Phlebotomy Prgm
115 South St
Middletown, NY 10940
www.sunyorange.edu

Rochester General Hospital
Phlebotomy Prgm
1425 Portland Ave
Rochester, NY 14621
www.rochestergeneral.org

North Carolina

Asheville-Buncombe Technical Comm College
Phlebotomy Prgm
340 Victoria Rd
Rhododendron Building
Asheville, NC 28801
www.abtech.edu

Carolinas College of Health Sciences
Phlebotomy Prgm
PO Box 32861
1200 Blythe Blvd
Charlotte, NC 28203
www.carolinascollege.edu

Fayetteville Technical Community College
Phlebotomy Prgm
2201 Hull Rd, PO Box 35236
Fayetteville, NC 28303
www.faytechcc.edu

Wake Technical Community College
Phlebotomy Prgm
9101 Fayetteville Rd
Wake Tech Health Sciences Campus, 2901 Holston Lane
Raleigh, NC 27610
http://waketech.edu

Nash Community College
Phlebotomy Prgm
522 N Old Carriage Rd, PO Box 7480
Rocky Mount, NC 27804
www.nashcc.edu

Brunswick Community College
Phlebotomy Prgm
PO Box 30
50 College Rd
Supply, NC 28462
http://brunswickcc.edu

Southwestern Community College
Phlebotomy Prgm
447 College Dr
Sylva, NC 28779
www.southwesterncc.edu/acadprog/pbt.htm

Halifax Community College
Phlebotomy Prgm
PO Drawer 809
Hwy 158
100 College Drive
Weldon, NC 27890
www.halifaxcc.edu

Rockingham Community College
Phlebotomy Prgm
PO Box 38
Wentworth, NC 27375-0038
www.rockinghamcc.edu

Southeastern Community College
Phlebotomy Prgm
PO Box 151
Whiteville, NC 28472
www.sccnc.edu

Cape Fear Community College
Phlebotomy Prgm
411 N Front St
Wilmington, NC 28401-3993
www.cfcc.edu

North Dakota

Turtle Mountain Community College
Phlebotomy Prgm
PO Box 340
Belcourt, ND 58316

Bismarck State College
Phlebotomy Prgm
PO Box 5587
1500 Edwards Ave
Bismarck, ND 58506-5587
www.bismarckstate.edu

NDSU/Sanford Health Consortium
Phlebotomy Prgm
737 Broadway
Fargo, ND 58122
www.meritcare.com

Ohio

Collins Career Center
Phlebotomy Prgm
11627 State Route 243
Chesapeake, OH 45619
www.collins-cc.k12.oh.us

Cuyahoga Community College
Phlebotomy Prgm
Metropolitan Campus MHCS 126
2900 Community College Ave
Cleveland, OH 44115-3196
www.tri-c.edu/programs/healthcareers/medicallab/
Pages/CertificateLaboratoryPhlebotomy.aspx

Columbus State Community College
Phlebotomy Prgm
550 E Spring St
Union 519 Columbus State Community College
Columbus, OH 43215
www.cscc.edu/phlebotomy

Lorain County Community College
Phlebotomy Prgm
1005 N Abbe Rd
HS210A
Elyria, OH 44035
www.lorainccc.edu/Academic+Programs/
Associates+Degree+and+Certificate+Programs/
p.htm

Edison Community College
Phlebotomy Prgm
1973 Edison Dr
Piqua, OH 45356
www.edisonohio.edu

Trumbull Memorial Hospital
Phlebotomy Prgm
1350 E Market St
Warren, OH 44482-1269

Zane State College
Phlebotomy Prgm
1555 Newark Rd
Zanesville, OH 43701
www.zanestate.edu

Oklahoma

Seminole State College
Phlebotomy Prgm
2701 Boren Blvd
Seminole, OK 74818

Tulsa Community College
Phlebotomy Prgm
10300 E 81st S
Tulsa, OK 74133
www.tulsacc.edu

Pennsylvania

Montgomery County Community College
Phlebotomy Prgm
340 DeKalb Pike
PO Box 400
Science Center 340
Blue Bell, PA 19468
www.mc3.edu/academics/divisions/health-sciences/mlt

Community College of Beaver County
Phlebotomy Prgm
1 Campus Dr
Monaca, PA 15061
www.ccbc.edu

Community College of Philadelphia
Phlebotomy Prgm
1700 Spring Garden St
Philadelphia, PA 19130
www.ccp.edu/academic

Tennessee

Southwest Tennessee Community College
Phlebotomy Prgm
PO Box 780
761 Linden Ave
Memphis, TN 38126
www.southwest.tn.edu

Texas

Austin Community College
Phlebotomy Prgm
Eastview Campus
3401 Webberville Rd
Austin, TX 78712
www.austincc.edu/health/phb

Weatherford College
Phlebotomy Prgm
225 College Park Dr
Weatherford, TX 76086

Wisconsin

Milwaukee Area Technical College
Phlebotomy Prgm
Health Occupations Division
700 W State St
Milwaukee, WI 53233-1443
http://matc.edu/student/offerings/phleb.html

Mid-State Technical College
Phlebotomy Prgm
933 Michigan Ave
Stevens Point, WI 54481-3141
www.mstc.edu/phlebotomytechnician/index.htm

Northcentral Technical College
Phlebotomy Prgm
1000 W Campus Drive
Wausau, WI 54401
www.ntc.edu

Medical Imaging and Radiation Therapy

Includes:
- Diagnostic medical sonographer
- Magnetic resonance technologist
- Medical dosimetrist
- Nuclear medicine technologist
- Radiation therapist
- Radiographer
- Radiologist assistant

Post-Primary Specialties in Radiologic Technology

Practitioners of the following post-primary specialties in radiologic technology are eligible for certification by the American Registry of Radiologic Technologists. Candidates for certification must be certified in radiography, radiation therapy, or nuclear medicine and document specific clinical competencies to be eligible for the certification examination.
- Bone densitometry
- Breast sonography
- Cardiac-interventional radiography
- Computed tomography
- Magnetic resonance imaging (both a primary and post-primary track)
- Mammography
- Quality management
- Vascular sonography
- Vascular-interventional radiography
- Sonography (both a primary and post-primary track)

Diagnostic Medical Sonographer

The diagnostic medical sonographer provides patient services using medical ultrasound (high-frequency sound waves that produce images of internal structures). Working under the supervision of a physician responsible for the use and interpretation of ultrasound procedures, the sonographer gathers sonographic data which physician uses to diagnose a variety of conditions and diseases.

History

In 1972, the American Society of Ultrasound Technical Specialists (ASUTS) appointed a committee to explore the mechanism of accreditation of educational programs for the ultrasound technical specialist through the AMA Council on Medical Education (CME). In 1974, the occupation of diagnostic medical sonography received recognition by the AMA.

From 1974 to 1979, the Standards (Essentials) of an Accredited Educational Program for the Diagnostic Medical Sonographer were developed. Because of the multidisciplinary nature of diagnostic ultrasound, many interested medical and allied health organizations collaborated in drafting the Standards. Educational programs were first accredited in January 1982. In 1995, the Commission on Accreditation of Allied Health Education Programs (CAAHEP) took over the oversight of program accreditation from the AMA. The Standards were most recently revised in 2007.

Career Description

The sonographer provides patients with diagnostic services in a variety of medical settings that assist the physician in the interpretation of ultrasound procedures. These duties include
- Obtaining, reviewing, and integrating pertinent patient history and supporting clinical data to facilitate optimum diagnostic results
- Performing appropriate procedures and recording anatomical, pathological, and/or physiological data for interpretation by a physician
- Recording and processing sonographic data and other pertinent observations made during the procedure for presentation to the interpreting physician
- Exercising discretion and judgment in the performance of sonographic services
- Providing patient education related to medical ultrasound
- Promoting principles of good health

According to the US Bureau of Labor Statistics, sonographers may specialize in the fields noted below. Formal training in diagnostic medical sonography is offered through hospital-based programs, two-year associate degree programs, and/or four-year baccalaureate degree programs. Diagnostic medical sonography programs are accredited by the Commission on Accreditation of Allied Health Education Programs (CAAHEP) and include general, cardiac and/or vascular learning concentrations in their curriculum.
- Obstetric and gynecologic sonographers specialize in the imaging of the female reproductive system. Included in the discipline is one of the more well-known uses of sonography: examining the fetus of a pregnant woman to track the baby's growth and health.
- *Abdominal sonographers* inspect a patient's abdominal cavity to help diagnose and treat conditions primarily involving the gallbladder, bile ducts, kidneys, liver, pancreas, spleen, and male reproductive system. Abdominal sonographers also are prepared to scan superficial parts of the body, such as the thyroid, scrotum, and breast as well as some portions of the chest, although studies of the heart using sonography usually are done by echocardiographers.
- *Neurosonographers* focus on the nervous system, including the brain and spine. In neonatal care, neurosonographers study and diagnose neurological and nervous system disorders in premature infants. They also may scan blood vessels to check for abnormalities indicating a stroke in infants diagnosed with sickle-cell anemia. Like other sonographers, neurosonographers operate transducers to perform the sonogram, but use frequencies and beam shapes different from those used by obstetric and abdominal sonographers.
- *Breast sonographers* use sonography to study diseases of the breasts. Sonography aids mammography in the differentiation of breast lesions, which may identify a lesion as benign or suspi-

cious for malignancy. Breast sonographers use high-frequency transducers, made exclusively to study breast tissue.

- *Vascular sonographers* specialize in evaluating disease of the vascular system. Through use of Doppler and imaging, they can assess vessels for plaque, thrombus, and/or post-treatment evaluations.
- *Cardiac sonographers* use diagnostic medical sonography to evaluate the fetal, pediatric and adult heart. Cardiac sonography is used to evaluate heart chamber size and function as well as the presence of congenital and acquired heart disease.

Employment Characteristics

Diagnostic medical sonographers may be employed in hospitals, clinics, private offices, or industry. Most full-time sonographers work about 40 hours a week and may provide on-call support which constitutes being on call and readily available to report to work within the response time established by the medical facilities.

Salary

Data from the US Bureau of Labor Statistics from May 2011 show that wages at the 10th percentile are $44,950, the 50th percentile (median) at $65,210, and the 90th percentile at $90,640 (*www.bls.gov/oes/current/oes292032.htm*).

For more information, refer to www.ama-assn.org/go/hpsalary.

Employment Outlook

The demand for sonographers, including suitably qualified educators, researchers, and administrators, continues to exceed the supply; BLS data show that employment is expected to increase by about 44 percent through 2020—faster than the average for all occupations. The supply and demand ratio affects salaries, depending on experience and responsibilities.

Educational Programs

Length. Accredited programs are between one and four years (certificate, associate, and baccalaureate level), depending on program design, objectives, and the degree or certificate awarded.

Prerequisites. Applicants to a one-year program must possess qualifications in a clinically related allied health profession. Applicants to two-year programs must be high school graduates (or equivalent) with an educational background in basic science, general physics, and algebra. All applicants must demonstrate satisfactory completion of the following courses at college level: general physics, biological science, algebra, and communication skills.

Skills potential and practicing sonographers should exhibit include social perceptiveness, strong hand-eye coordination, learning strategies, critical thinking skills, instructional skills, active listening, active learning, reading comprehension, and written/oral expression.

Curriculum. Curricula of accredited programs include physical sciences, applied biological sciences, patient care, clinical medicine, applications of ultrasound, instrumentation, related diagnostic procedures, and image evaluation. A plan for well-structured, competency-based clinical education is an essential part of the curriculum of all sonography programs.

Certification and Licensure

Some states are now passing laws requiring licensure for diagnostic medical sonographers. Most of these states accept certification by a nationally registered

organization as a component of the licensure process. Two states that have established licensing requirements are Oregon and New Mexico. Organizations such as the American Registry for Diagnostic Medical Sonography (ARDMS), the American Registry of Radiologic Technologists (ARRT), and Cardiovascular Credentialing International (CCI) certify the competency of sonographers through certification. Because certification provides an independent, objective measure of an individual's professional standing, many employers prefer to hire registered sonographers. Certification with ARDMS requires passing a sonography principles and instrumentation examination, in addition to passing an exam in a specialty such as obstetric and gynecologic sonography, abdominal sonography, neurosonography, breast sonography, fetal echocardiography, pediatric echocardiography, adult echocardiography, and vascular echocardiography. Registration by ARRT requires passing an examination in general sonography, vascular sonography, or breast sonography. CCI certification involves passing a combined basic cardiovascular science exam and specialty exam such as the Registered Cardiac Sonographer or Registered Congenital Cardiac Sonographer registry exams.

To keep their certification current, sonographers must complete continuing education to stay abreast of technological advances related to the occupation. Intersocietal Accreditation Commission (IAC) is requiring that accredited labs must have a process in place to ensure that echocardiographer sonographers be credentialed by 2014 and vascular sonographers by 2017.

Inquiries

Careers/Curriculum
Society of Diagnostic Medical Sonography
2745 Dallas Parkway, Suite 350
Plano, TX 75093-4706
214 473-8057
E-mail: *info@sdms.org*
www.sdms.org

Society for Vascular Ultrasound
4601 Presidents Drive, Suite 260
Lanham, MD 20706-4831
301 459-7550 or 800 SVU-VEIN 800 788-8346)
www.svunet.org

American Society of Echocardiography
2100 Gateway Centre Blvd Suite 310
Morrisville , NC 27560
919 861-5574
www.asecho.org

Certification
American Registry for Diagnostic Medical Sonography
51 Monroe Street, Plaza East Ore
Rockville, MD 20852
301 738-8401
www.ardms.org

American Registry of Radiologic Technologists
1255 Northland Drive
St Paul, MN 55120-1155
651 687-0048
www.arrt.org

Cardiovascular Credentialing International
1500 Sunday Drive, Suite 102
Raleigh, NC 27607
800 326-0268
www.cci-online.org

Program Accreditation

Commission on Accreditation of Allied Health Education Programs (CAAHEP) in collaboration with:

Joint Review Committee on Education in Diagnostic Medical Sonography

6021 University Boulevard, Suite 500
Ellicott City, MD 21043
443 973-3251
866 738-3444 Fax
E-mail: *mail@jrcdms.org*

Note: Adapted in part from the Bureau of Labor Statistics, US Department of Labor, *Occupational Outlook Handbook*, Diagnostic Medical Sonographers, at *www.bls.gov/oco/ ocos273.htm*.

Diagnostic Medical Sonographer

Alabama

Virginia College - Birmingham
Diagnostic Med Sonography (General/Vascular) Prgm
488 Palisades Blvd
Birmingham, AL 35209

Wallace State Community College
Diagnostic Med Sonography (General) Prgm
PO Box 2000, 801 Main St NW
Hanceville, AL 35077-2000
www.wallacestate.edu
Prgm Dir: Janet E Money, RDMS CNMT
Tel: 256 352-8318   *Fax:* 256 352-8320
E-mail: janet.money@wallacestate.edu

Trenholm State Technical College
Diagnostic Med Sonography (General) Prgm
1225 Air Base Blvd P O Box 10048
Montgomery, AL 36108

Lurleen B Wallace Community College
Diagnostic Med Sonography (General) Prgm
1706 North Main St PO Box 910
Opp, AL 36467

Institute of Ultrasound Diagnostics
Diagnostic Med Sonography (General) Prgm
31214 Coleman Lane, Suite A
Spanish Fort, AL 36527
www.iudmed.com

Arizona

GateWay Community College
Diagnostic Med Sonography (General) Prgm
108 N 40th St Health Sciences Division
Phoenix, AZ 85034
www.gatewaycc.edu
Prgm Dir: Bryan Dodd,
Tel: 602 286-8486   *Fax:* 602 288-8480
E-mail: dodd@gatewaycc.edu

Arkansas

University of Arkansas - Fort Smith
Diagnostic Med Sonography (General) Prgm
5210 Grand Ave, PO Box 3649
College of Health Sciences
Fort Smith, AR 72913
www.uaforthsmith.edu

University of Arkansas for Medical Sciences
Diagnostic Med Sonography (General) Prgm
4301 W Markham St, Mail Slot 563-B
Little Rock, AR 72205
www.uams.edu

Arkansas State University
Diagnostic Med Sonography (General) Prgm
PO Box 910
106 N Caraway Rd
State University, AR 72467
www.astate.edu

California

Platt College Los Angeles, LLC
Diagnostic Med Sonography (General) Prgm
1000 South Fremont Ave Suite A9 West
Alhambra, CA 91803

Orange Coast College
Diagnostic Med Sonography (General) Prgm
2701 Fairview Rd
Costa Mesa, CA 92626
www.orangecoastcollege.edu

Cypress College
Diagnostic Med Sonography (General) Prgm
9200 Valley View
Health Science Division
Cypress, CA 90630
www.cypresscollege.edu

Community Regional Medical Center
Diagnostic Med Sonography (General/Cardiac) Prgm
2823 Fresno St
Fresno, CA 93721

Loma Linda University
Diagnostic Med Sonography (General) Prgm
Sch of Allied Hlth Profs
11234 Anderson St
Loma Linda, CA 92354
www.llu.edu

Foothill College
Diagnostic Med Sonography (General) Prgm
12345 El Monte Rd
Los Altos Hills, CA 94022-4599
www.foothill.edu
Prgm Dir: Kathleen Austin, BS RDMS RT
Tel: 650 949-7304   *Fax:* 650 949-7686
E-mail: austinkathleen@fhda.edu

Charles Drew University of Medicine and Sci
Diagnostic Med Sonography (General) Prgm
1731 E 120th St
Los Angeles, CA 90059

Merced College
Diagnostic Med Sonography (General/Cardiac) Prgm
3600 M St
Merced, CA 95348-2806
www.mccd.edu

Kaiser Permanente School of Allied Health Sci
Diagnostic Med Sonography (General) Prgm
938 Marina Way S
Richmond, CA 94553
www.kpsahs.org

Univ of California San Diego Med Ctr
Diagnostic Med Sonography (General) Prgm
200 W Arbor Dr
San Diego, CA 92103-8759
www.radtech.ucsd.edu

Santa Barbara City College
Diagnostic Med Sonography (General) Prgm
721 Cliff Dr
Santa Barbara, CA 93109-2394

Colorado

University of Colorado Denver - Anschutz MC
Diagnostic Med Sonography (General) Prgm
U of Colorado Hospital, Dept of Ultrasound F-720
1635 Aurora Court
Aurora, CO 80045
www.medschool.ucdenver.edu/radiology

Connecticut

St Francis Hospital & Medical Center
Cosponsor: The Hofman Heart Institute of Connecticut
Diagnostic Med Sonography (Cardiac) Prgm
114 Woodland St
Hartford, CT 06105
www.stfranciscare.org

Yale-New Haven Hospital
Diagnostic Med Sonography (General/Cardiac) Prgm
20 York St SP 2-122
New Haven, CT 06504

Delaware

Delaware Technical Community College
Cosponsor: Christiana Care Health System
Diagnostic Med Sonography (Gen/Card/Vascular) Prgm
Riverside Medical Arts Complex, Suite 101
700 W Lea Blvd
Wilmington, DE 19802
www.dtcc.edu
Prgm Dir: Lily O Lee, BS RDMS RVT
Tel: 302 765-4588   *Fax:* 302 765-4599
E-mail: lillee@christianacare.org

District of Columbia

George Washington University
Diagnostic Med Sonography (Gen/Card/Vascular) Prgm
900 23rd St NW, #6180
Washington, DC 20037
www.gwumc.edu/healthsci/

Florida

Broward College
Diagnostic Med Sonography (General/Cardiac) Prgm
North Campus Bldg 41
1000 Coconut Creek Blvd
Coconut Creek, FL 33066
www.broward.edu
Prgm Dir: Karen Hoban, MS RDMS RDCS RVT RT(R)
Tel: 954 201-2089   *Fax:* 954 201-2348
E-mail: khoban@broward.edu

Keiser University
Diagnostic Med Sonography (General) Prgm
1800 Business Park Blvd
Daytona Beach, FL 32114
www.keiseruniversity.edu

Institute of Allied Medical Professions
Diagnostic Med Sonography (General/Cardiac) Prgm
5150 Linton Blvd Suite 340
Delray Beach, FL 33484

Keiser University
Diagnostic Med Sonography (General) Prgm
1500 NW 49th St
Fort Lauderdale, FL 33309
www.keiseruniversity.edu

Nova Southeastern University
Diagnostic Med Sonography (Vascular) Prgm
3200 S University Dr
College of Allied Health and Nursing
Fort Lauderdale, FL 33328
www.nova.edu/sonography

Sanford-Brown Institute - Ft Lauderdale
Diagnostic Med Sonography (General) Prgm
1201 West Cypress Creek Rd
Fort Lauderdale, FL 33309

Santa Fe College
Diagnostic Med Sonography (General) Prgm
3000 NW 83rd St
Gainesville, FL 32606

St Vincent's Medical Center
Diagnostic Med Sonography (General/Vascular) Prgm
1 Shircliff Way
Jacksonville, FL 32204
www.jaxhealth.com
Prgm Dir: Chemene Wilson, MHSc RT(R) RDMS RVT
Tel: 904 308-8272   *Fax:* 904 308-5109
E-mail: cwils002@stvincentshealth.com

Keiser University
Diagnostic Med Sonography (General) Prgm
900 S Babcock St
Melbourne, FL 32901

Dade Medical College
Diagnostic Med Sonography (General/Cardiac) Prgm
Medical Center Campus
950 NW 20th St
Miami, FL 33127-4693
www.mdc.edu

Central Florida Institute
Diagnostic Med Sonography (General) Prgm
6000 Cinderlande Parkway
Orlando, FL 32810

Florida Hospital College of Health Sciences
Diagnostic Med Sonography (Gen/Card/Vascular) Prgm
671 Winyah Drive
Orlando, FL 32803

Valencia College
Diagnostic Med Sonography (General) Prgm
PO Box 3028
1800 S Kirkman Rd, MP 4-14
Orlando, FL 32811
www.valenciacc.edu/Sonography

Palm Beach State College
Diagnostic Med Sonography (General) Prgm
3160 PGA Blvd
Palm Beach Gardens, FL 33410
www.pbcc.edu

Central Florida Institute
Diagnostic Med Sonography (General) Prgm
30522 US Highway 19 North
Palm Harbor, FL 34684

Hillsborough Community College
Diagnostic Med Sonography (General) Prgm
PO Box 30030
Tampa, FL 33630-3030
www.hccfl.edu/depts/healthsci/sonography

Polk State College
Diagnostic Med Sonography (General) Prgm
999 Ave H, NE
Winter Haven, FL 33881-4299

Georgia

Athens Technical College
Diagnostic Med Sonography (General) Prgm
800 US Hwy 29 N
Athens, GA 30601

Grady Health System
Diagnostic Med Sonography (General) Prgm
PO Box 26095
80 Jesse Hill Jr Dr SE
Atlanta, GA 30303-3050
www.gradyhealth.org/imaging
Prgm Dir: Judy K Billings, BSRT RT(R) RDMS
Tel: 404 616-5032   *Fax:* 404 616-3512
E-mail: jbillings@gmh.edu

Sanford-Brown Institute
Diagnostic Med Sonography (General) Prgm
1140 Hammond Dr, Ste A 1150
Atlanta, GA 30328
www.sb-atlanta.com

Georgia Health Sciences University
Diagnostic Med Sonography (General) Prgm
School of Allied Health
987 Sebastian Way
Augusta, GA 30912
www.mcg.edu

Georgia Northwestern Technical College
Diagnostic Med Sonography (Gen/Card/Vascular) Prgm
General, Vascular, and Echocardiography concentrations
1 Maurice Culberson Dr
Rome, GA 30161
www.gntc.edu

Ogeechee Technical College
Diagnostic Med Sonography (General/Cardiac) Prgm
1 Joe Kennedy Blvd
Statesboro, GA 30458
www.ogeecheetech.edu

Idaho

Boise State University
Diagnostic Med Sonography (General) Prgm
Radiologic Sciences Department
1910 University Dr MS #1845
Boise, ID 83725-1845
hs.boisestate.edu/radsci/sonography/
Prgm Dir: Joie Burns, MS RT(R)(S) RDMS RVT
Tel: 208 426-1382   *Fax:* 208 426-4459
E-mail: jburns@boisestate.edu

Illinois

Southern Illinois University Carbondale
Diagnostic Med Sonography (General) Prgm
1365 Douglas Dr, Mailcode 6615
College of Applied Sciences & Arts
Carbondale, IL 62901
www.siu.edu

John A Logan College
Diagnostic Med Sonography (Cardiac) Prgm
700 Logan College Rd
Carterville, IL 62918
www.jalc.edu

Northwestern Memorial Hospital
Diagnostic Med Sonography (General) Prgm
541 N Fairbanks Court, Suite 950
Chicago, IL 60611
www.nmh.org
Notes: A BS degree may be earned by enrolling in one of
three academic affiliates and completing three years
of BS prerequisites at that institution, and then being
accepted into the DMS program at Northwestern
Memorial for 18 months of training.

Rush University
Diagnostic Med Sonography (Vascular) Prgm
600 S Paulina, Ste 440
Suite 1019A
Chicago, IL 60612
www.rushu.rush.edu

College of DuPage
Diagnostic Med Sonography (General/Vascular) Prgm
425 Fawell Blvd
Glen Ellyn, IL 60137
www.cod.edu

Harper College
Diagnostic Med Sonography (General/Cardiac) Prgm
1200 W Algonquin Rd
Division of Health Careers and Public Safety
Palatine, IL 60067-7398
www.HarperCollege.edu

Triton College
Diagnostic Med Sonography (General) Prgm
2000 N Fifth Ave
River Grove, IL 60171
www.triton.edu

Indiana

St Anthony Medical Center
Diagnostic Med Sonography (Cardiac) Prgm
Saint Anthony School of Echocardiography
1201 S Main St
Crown Point, IN 46307

University of Southern Indiana
Diagnostic Med Sonography (Gen/Card/Vascular) Prgm
800 University Blvd
Evansville, IN 47712

Iowa

Mercy College of Health Sciences
Diagnostic Med Sonography (General/Cardiac) Prgm
928 Sixth Ave
Des Moines, IA 50309-1239
www.mchs.edu

University of Iowa Hospitals & Clinics
Diagnostic Med Sonography (Gen/Card/Vascular) Prgm
C-723 Radiology
200 Hawkins Dr
Iowa City, IA 52242-1077
www.medicine.uiowa.edu/RadSci/medical_sonography

Kansas

University of Kansas Medical Center
Diagnostic Med Sonography (Gen/Card/Vascular) Prgm
2105 Bell Memorial Hospital
3901 Rainbow Rd MS 4032
Kansas City, KS 66160
www.kumc.edu

Washburn University
Diagnostic Med Sonography (Gen/Card/Vascular) Prgm
1700 SW College Ave
Dept of Allied Health Benton Hall Room 106
Topeka, KS 66621
www.washburn.edu

Kentucky

Bowling Green Technical College
Diagnostic Med Sonography (General) Prgm
1845 Loop Dr
Bowling Green, KY 42101-3601
www.kctcs.edu

Hazard Community & Technical College
Diagnostic Med Sonography (General/Vascular) Prgm
One Community College Drive
Hazard, KY 41701

Jefferson Community and Technical College
Diagnostic Med Sonography (General/Vascular) Prgm
800 W Chestnut St
Louisville, KY 40203

Morehead State University
Diagnostic Med Sonography (General) Prgm
150 University Blvd, Center for Health, Education, &
   Researc
Morehead, KY 40351-1689
www.moreheadstate.edu

**West Kentucky Community & Technical
   College**
Diagnostic Med Sonography (General) Prgm
4810 Alben Barkley Dr, PO Box 7380
Paducah, KY 42002
www.westkentucky.kctcs.edu
Prgm Dir: Alice Robertson, BS RT(R) RDMS
Tel: 270 534-3487, Ext   *Fax:* 270 534-3498
E-mail: alice.robertson@kctcs.edu

St Catharine College
Diagnostic Med Sonography (Gen/Card/Vascular) Prgm
2735 Bardstown Rd
St Catharine, KY 40061
www.sccky.edu

Louisiana

Louisiana State University at Eunice
Diagnostic Med Sonography (General) Prgm
PO Box 1129
Eunice, LA 70535
www.lsue.edu

Delgado Community College
Diagnostic Med Sonography (General) Prgm
615 City Park Ave
New Orleans, LA 70119
www.dcc.edu
Prgm Dir: John Geshner, BA RDMS RDCS
Tel: 504 671-1340   *Fax:* 504 568-5494
E-mail: jgeshn@dcc.edu

Maine

Kennebec Valley Community College
Diagnostic Med Sonography (General) Prgm
92 Western Ave
Fairfield, ME 4937

Maryland

Johns Hopkins Hospital
Diagnostic Med Sonography (General) Prgm
Radiology Admin B-179
600 N Wolfe St, Blalock B-179
Baltimore, MD 21287
www.jhmi.edu

University of Maryland Baltimore County
Cosponsor: UMBC Training Centers, LLC
Diagnostic Med Sonography (Gen/Card/Vascular) Prgm
1450 S Rolling Rd
Baltimore, MD 21227
www.umbctrainingcenters.com
Prgm Dir: Lyna El-Khoury Rumbarger, BS RDCS
Tel: 443 543-5423   *Fax:* 443 543-5410
E-mail: lrumbarger@umbctraining.com

Sanford-Brown Institute - Landover
Diagnostic Med Sonography (General) Prgm
8401 Corporate Dr Suite 500
Landover, MD 20785

Montgomery College
Diagnostic Med Sonography (Gen/Card/Vascular) Prgm
7977 Georgia Ave
Silver Spring, MD 20910
http://montgomerycollege.edu/dms

Massachusetts

Middlesex Community College
Diagnostic Med Sonography (General) Prgm
Springs Rd
Bldg 6
Bedford, MA 01730
www.Middlesex.mass.edu

Bunker Hill Community College
Diagnostic Med Sonography (General/Cardiac) Prgm
250 New Rutherford Ave
Boston, MA 02129-2991
www.bhcc.edu

Springfield Technical Community College
Diagnostic Med Sonography (General) Prgm
One Armory Square
PO Box 9000 - Suite 1
Springfield, MA 01102-9000
www.stcc.edu
Prgm Dir: David J Sloan, BA RDMS RVT
Tel: 413 755-4915   *Fax:* 413 755-4764
E-mail: djsloan@stcc.edu

Michigan

Baker College of Auburn Hills
Diagnostic Med Sonography (Gen/Card/Vascular) Prgm
1500 University Drive
Auburn Hills, MI 48326

Ferris State University
Diagnostic Med Sonography (General) Prgm
200 Ferris Drive
Big Rapids, MI 49307

Henry Ford Hospital
Diagnostic Med Sonography (General) Prgm
2799 W Grand Blvd
Rm WC 370, Clinical Bldg
Detroit, MI 48202
www.henryfordhealth.org

Grand Valley State University
Diagnostic Med Sonography (Gen/Card/Vascular) Prgm
301 Michigan St NW Suite 200
Grand Rapids, MI 49503

Jackson Community College
Diagnostic Med Sonography (Gen/Card/Vascular) Prgm
2111 Emmons Rd
Jackson, MI 49201
www.jccmi.edu

Baker College of Owosso
Diagnostic Med Sonography (General) Prgm
1020 S Washington St
Owosso, MI 48867

Oakland Community College - Southfield
Diagnostic Med Sonography (General) Prgm
22322 Rutland Dr
Southfield, MI 48075
www.oaklandcc.edu

Providence Hospital
Cosponsor: Madonna University
Diagnostic Med Sonography (General/Vascular) Prgm
16001 W Nine Mile Rd
Southfield, MI 48075
http://stjohn.org/alliedhealth/sonography
Prgm Dir: Janette Wybo, BAS RDMS RVT RDCS
Tel: 248 849-5385   *Fax:* 248 849-5395
E-mail: janette.wybo@stjohn.org

Delta College
Diagnostic Med Sonography (General) Prgm
1961 Delta Rd
F-216
University Center, MI 48710
www.delta.edu/health/sonography.aspx
Prgm Dir: Kim Boldt, BS RDMS RVT RDCS
Tel: 989 686-9361   *Fax:* 989 667-2230
E-mail: kboldt@delta.edu

Minnesota

Argosy University Twin Cities Campus
Diagnostic Med Sonography (General/Cardiac) Prgm
General and Echocardiography concentrations
1515 Central Parkway
Eagan, MN 55121
www.argosyu.edu

Saint Catherine University - Minneapolis
Diagnostic Med Sonography (General) Prgm
601 25th Ave S
Minneapolis, MN 55454
www.stkate.edu

Mayo School of Health Sciences
Diagnostic Med Sonography (Gen/Card/Vascular) Prgm
200 First St SW
Rochester, MN 55905
www.mayo.edu/mshs/echo-echo.html

St Cloud Technical and Community College
Diagnostic Med Sonography (General) Prgm
1540 Northway Dr
St Cloud, MN 56303
www.sctc.edu

Mississippi

Hinds Community College
Diagnostic Med Sonography (General) Prgm
1750 Chadwick Dr
Jackson, MS 39204
www.hindscc.edu

Itawamba Community College
Diagnostic Med Sonography (General) Prgm
2176 S Eason Blvd
Tupelo, MS 38804
www.iccms.edu

Missouri

University of Missouri
Diagnostic Med Sonography (General/Vascular) Prgm
409 Lewis Hall
Columbia, MO 65211
www.missouri.edu
Prgm Dir: Moses Hdeib, MD RDMS RDCS RVT
Tel: 573 884-2994   *Fax:* 573 884-8067
E-mail: hdeibm@health.missouri.edu

Sanford-Brown College - Fenton
Diagnostic Med Sonography (General) Prgm
1345 Smizer Mill Rd
Fenton, MO 63026

Saint Luke's Hospital
Diagnostic Med Sonography (General) Prgm
ATTN: Diagnostic Medical Sonography 624 Westport Rd
Kansas City, MO 64111

Rolla Technical Center
Diagnostic Med Sonography (General/Vascular) Prgm
500 Forum Drive
Rolla, MO 65401

Cox Medical Centers
Diagnostic Med Sonography (Gen/Card/Vascular) Prgm
3801 S National Ave
Springfield, MO 65807
www.coxhealth.com

St Louis Community College - Forest Park
Diagnostic Med Sonography (Gen/Card/Vascular) Prgm
5600 Oakland Ave
St Louis, MO 63110
www.stlcc.edu

Hillyard Technical Center
Diagnostic Med Sonography (General/Vascular) Prgm
3434 Faraon St
St. Joseph, MO 64506

Nebraska

BryanLGH College of Health Sciences
Diagnostic Med Sonography (General) Prgm
5035 Everett St
Lincoln, NE 68506
www.bryanlghcollege.org

Nebraska Methodist College
Diagnostic Med Sonography (Gen/Card/Vascular) Prgm
8501 W Dodge Rd
Omaha, NE 68114

University of Nebraska Medical Center
Diagnostic Med Sonography (General) Prgm
Division of Radiation Sciences Technology Educ
984545 Nebraska Medical Center
Omaha, NE 68198-4545
www.unmc.edu/alliedhealth/dms
Prgm Dir: Kim Michael, MA RT(R) RDMS RVT
Tel: 402 559-1189   *Fax:* 402 559-4667
E-mail: kkmichael@unmc.edu

Nevada

College of Southern Nevada
Diagnostic Med Sonography (Gen/Card/Vascular) Prgm
6375 W Charleston Blvd, W3K
Las Vegas, NV 89146
www.csn.edu

New Hampshire

NHTI, Concord's Community College
Diagnostic Med Sonography (General) Prgm
31 College Dr
Concord, NH 03301-7412
www.ccsnh.edu

New Jersey

Sanford-Brown Institute
Diagnostic Med Sonography (General) Prgm
675 US 1 Plaza Gill Ln, 2nd Fl
Iselin, NJ 08830
www.sb-nj.com

Bergen Community College
Diagnostic Med Sonography (General/Cardiac) Prgm
400 Paramus Rd
Paramus, NJ 07652-1595
www.bergen.edu

JFK Medical Center - Muhlenberg Schools
Diagnostic Med Sonography (General) Prgm
Park Ave and Randolph Rd
Harold B and Dorothy A Snyder Schools
Plainfield, NJ 07061

Univ of Medicine & Dent of New Jersey
Diagnostic Med Sonography (General) Prgm
School of Health Related Professions
1776 Raritan Rd, Room 507
Scotch Plains, NJ 07076
www.umdnj.edu

Gloucester County College
Diagnostic Med Sonography (General) Prgm
1400 Tanyard Rd
Sewell, NJ 08080
www.gccnj.edu

New Mexico

Central New Mexico Community College
Diagnostic Med Sonography (General) Prgm
525 Buena Vista SE
Albuquerque, NM 87106
www.cnm.edu

Dona Ana Community College
Diagnostic Med Sonography (General) Prgm
MSC3DA PO Box 30001
3400 S Espina St
Las Cruces, NM 88003-8001
http://dacc.nmsu.edu/hps/sonography

New York

Long Island University - Brooklyn Campus
Diagnostic Med Sonography (Vascular) Prgm
1 University Plaza (M-101)
School of Continuing Studies
Brooklyn, NY 11201-5372
www.liu.edu

New York Methodist Hospital
Diagnostic Med Sonography (General) Prgm
1401 Kings Highway
Brooklyn, NY 11229

SUNY Downstate Medical Center
Diagnostic Med Sonography (General/Cardiac) Prgm
College of Health Related Professions
450 Clarkson Ave, Box 1192
Brooklyn, NY 11203
www.downstate.edu/chrp

Sanford-Brown Institute - Garden City
Diagnostic Med Sonography (General) Prgm
711 Stewart Ave Suite 200
Garden City, NY 11530

New York University
Diagnostic Med Sonography (General/Cardiac) Prgm
726 Broadway Room 652
New York, NY 10003-6688
www.scps.nyu.edu/degcert/
   degree_info.jsp?stDegType=AS

Sanford-Brown Institute
Diagnostic Med Sonography (General) Prgm
120 East 16th St 4th Floor
New York, NY 10003

Western Suffolk BOCES
Diagnostic Med Sonography (Gen/Card/Vascular) Prgm
School of Sonography
152 Laurel Hill Rd
Northport, NY 11768
www.wsboces.org

Rochester Institute of Technology
Diagnostic Med Sonography (General) Prgm
153 Lomb Memorial Drive
Rochester, NY 14623
www.rit.edu

Hudson Valley Community College
Diagnostic Med Sonography (General/Cardiac) Prgm
80 Vandenburgh Ave
Troy, NY 12180
www.hvcc.edu

Sanford-Brown Institute - White Plains
Diagnostic Med Sonography (General) Prgm
333 Westchester Ave
White Plains, NY 10604

North Carolina

Asheville-Buncombe Technical Comm College
Diagnostic Med Sonography (General/Vascular) Prgm
340 Victoria Rd
Asheville, NC 28801
www.abtech.edu

Pitt Community College
Diagnostic Med Sonography (General/Cardiac) Prgm
PO Drawer 7007
Greenville, NC 27835-7007
www.pittcc.edu

Caldwell Comm College & Tech Institute
Diagnostic Med Sonography (General/Cardiac) Prgm
2855 Hickory Blvd
Hudson, NC 28638
www.cccti.edu
Prgm Dir: Kimberlee B Watts, MS RDMS
Tel: 828 726-2322   *Fax:* 828 726-2489
E-mail: kwatts@cccti.edu

South Piedmont Community College
Diagnostic Med Sonography (General) Prgm
4209 Old Charlotte Highway
Monroe, NC 28110

Johnston Community College
Diagnostic Med Sonography (Gen/Card/Vascular) Prgm
PO Box 2350
245 College Rd
Smithfield, NC 27577
www.johnstoncc.edu

Southwestern Community College
Diagnostic Med Sonography (General) Prgm
447 College Dr
Sylva, NC 28779
www.southwesterncc.edu

Cape Fear Community College
Diagnostic Med Sonography (General) Prgm
411 N Front St
Wilmington, NC 28401
www.cfcc.edu

Forsyth Technical Community College
Diagnostic Med Sonography (General) Prgm
2100 Silas Creek Pkwy
Bob Green Hall
Winston-Salem, NC 27103
www.forsythtech.edu

Ohio

Mercy Medical Center
Diagnostic Med Sonography (General) Prgm
1320 Mercy Dr NW
Canton, OH 44708
www.cantonmercy.com

Collins Career Center - Chesapeake
Diagnostic Med Sonography (General/Vascular) Prgm
11627 State Rte 243
Chesapeake, OH 45619

Cincinnati State Tech & Comm College
Diagnostic Med Sonography (Gen/Card/Vascular) Prgm
3250 Central Pkwy
Cincinnati, OH 45223
www.cincinnatistate.edu

Lorain County Community College
Diagnostic Med Sonography (General) Prgm
1005 N Abbe Rd
Elyria, OH 44035
www.lorainccc.edu

Kettering College of Medical Arts
Diagnostic Med Sonography (Gen/Card/Vascular) Prgm
3737 Southern Blvd
Kettering, OH 45429
kcma.edu

Sanford-Brown College
Diagnostic Med Sonography (General) Prgm
17535 Rosbough Dr
Suite 150
Middleburg Heights, OH 44130
www.sbcleveland.com

Central Ohio Technical College
Diagnostic Med Sonography (Gen/Card/Vascular) Prgm
1179 University Dr
Newark, OH 43055-1767
www.cotc.edu

Cuyahoga Community College
Diagnostic Med Sonography (Gen/Card/Vascular) Prgm
11000 Pleasant Valley Rd
Parma, OH 44130
www.tri-c.edu

University of Rio Grande
Cosponsor: Rio Grande Community College
Diagnostic Med Sonography (General) Prgm
PO Box 500
218 N College Ave
Rio Grande, OH 45674-0500
www.rio.edu

Owens Community College
Diagnostic Med Sonography (General) Prgm
30334 Oregon Rd
PO Box 10000
Toledo, OH 43699-1947
www.owens.edu

Oklahoma

Moore Norman Technology Center
Diagnostic Med Sonography (General) Prgm
4701 12th Ave NW
Norman, OK 73069
www.mntechnology.com

Oklahoma State University
Diagnostic Med Sonography (Cardiac) Prgm
900 N Portland Ave
Oklahoma City, OK 73107

Univ of Oklahoma Health Sciences Center
Diagnostic Med Sonography (General/Cardiac) Prgm
Dept Medical Imaging & Radiation Sciences, Suite 3021
College of Allied Health, 1200 N Stonewall
Oklahoma City, OK 73117-1215
www.ah.ouhsc.edu/mirs/academic_programs.asp
Prgm Dir: Kari Boyce, PhD RDMS RDCS
Tel: 405 271-6477   Fax: 405 271-1424
E-mail: kari-boyce@ouhsc.edu

Pennsylvania

Northampton Community College
Diagnostic Med Sonography (General) Prgm
3835 Green Pond Rd
Bethlehem, PA 18020
www.northampton.edu

Mount Aloysius College
Diagnostic Med Sonography (General) Prgm
7373 Admiral Peary Highway
Cresson, PA 16630

Misericordia University
Diagnostic Med Sonography (General) Prgm
301 Lake St
McAuley-Walsh Room 310
Dallas, PA 18612
www.misericordia.edu

Great Lakes Institute of Technology
Diagnostic Med Sonography (General) Prgm
5100 Peach St
Erie, PA 16509

Harrisburg Area Community College
Diagnostic Med Sonography (General) Prgm
1 HACC Dr
Harrisburg, PA 17110-2999
www.hacc.edu

Lancaster Gen Coll of Nursing & Hlth Sciences
Diagnostic Med Sonography (General) Prgm
410 N Lime St
Lancaster, PA 17602
www.lancastergeneralcollege.edu

Community College of Allegheny County
Diagnostic Med Sonography (General/Cardiac) Prgm
595 Beatty Rd
Boyce Campus
Monroeville, PA 15146
www.ccac.edu

Thomas Jefferson University
Diagnostic Med Sonography (Gen/Card/Vascular) Prgm
Radiologic Sciences
130 S Ninth St, Ste 1011
Philadelphia, PA 19107
www.jefferson.edu/jchp/di/

Sanford-Brown Institute - Pittsburgh
Diagnostic Med Sonography (General) Prgm
421 Seventh Ave
Pittsburgh, PA 15219

Lackawanna College
Diagnostic Med Sonography (General/Vascular) Prgm
501 Vine St
Scranton, PA 18509
www.lackawanna.edu

South Hills School of Business & Technology
Diagnostic Med Sonography (Gen/Card/Vascular) Prgm
480 Waupelani Drive
State College, PA 16801

Crozer-Keystone Medical Center
Diagnostic Med Sonography (General) Prgm
North Campus Rm 214A
One Medical Center Blvd
Upland, PA 19013
www.crozer.org

Wilkes-Barre General Hospital
Cosponsor: Wyoming Valley Health Care System
Diagnostic Med Sonography (General) Prgm
575 N River St
Wilkes-Barre, PA 18764
www.wvhcs.org

Rhode Island

Community College of Rhode Island
Diagnostic Med Sonography (Gen/Card/Vascular) Prgm
1762 Louisquisset Pike
Lincoln, RI 02865

Rhode Island Hospital
Diagnostic Med Sonography (General) Prgm
4 Davol Square, Building A, Box 162
Providence, RI 02903
www.lifespan.org/diagimag

South Carolina

Greenville Technical College
Diagnostic Med Sonography (General) Prgm
PO Box 5616
Greenville, SC 29606-5616
www.gvltec.edu

Horry - Georgetown Technical College
Diagnostic Med Sonography (General) Prgm
Grand Strand Campus 743 Hemlock Ave
Myrtle Beach, SC 29577

South Dakota

Southeast Technical Institute
Diagnostic Med Sonography (General) Prgm
2320 N Career Ave
Sioux Falls, SD 57107
www.southeasttech.com

Tennessee

Chattanooga State Community College
Diagnostic Med Sonography (Gen/Card/Vascular) Prgm
CBIH 124
4501 Amnicola Highway
Chattanooga, TN 37406
www.chattanoogastate.edu
Prgm Dir: Jody Hancock, MAEd RDMS RVT RT(R)
Tel: 423 697-3341   Fax: 423 697-3324
E-mail: jody.hancock@chattanoogastate.edu

Volunteer State Community College
Diagnostic Med Sonography (General) Prgm
1480 Nashville Pike
Gallatin, TN 37066-3188
www.volstate.edu

Baptist College of Health Sciences
Diagnostic Med Sonography (General/Vascular) Prgm
1003 Monroe Ave
Memphis, TN 38104
www.bchs.edu

Methodist Le Bonheur Healthcare
Diagnostic Med Sonography (General) Prgm
Dept of Radiology
1265 Union Ave
Memphis, TN 38104
www.methodisthealth.org

Vanderbilt University Medical Center
Diagnostic Med Sonography (General) Prgm
1161 21st Ave S
MCN-CCC1121
Nashville, TN 37232-2675
www.vanderbilt.edu

Texas

Austin Community College
Diagnostic Med Sonography (Gen/Card/Vascular) Prgm
3401 Webberville Rd
Building 9000
Austin, TX 78702
www.austincc.edu/health/sono
Prgm Dir: Regina Swearengin, BS RDMS
Tel: 512 223-5944   *Fax:* 512 223-5895
E-mail: ginas@austincc.edu

Lamar Institute of Technology
Diagnostic Med Sonography (General) Prgm
PO Box 10061
855 E Lavaca
Beaumont, TX 77710
www.lit.edu

Univ TX at Brownsville/TX Southmost Coll
Diagnostic Med Sonography (General) Prgm
80 Ft Brown
Brownsville, TX 78620
www.utb.edu

Del Mar College
Diagnostic Med Sonography (General/Cardiac) Prgm
101 Baldwin Blvd
Corpus Christi, TX 78404
www.delmar.edu

Lone Star College-CyFair
Diagnostic Med Sonography (General/Vascular) Prgm
9191 Barker-Cypress Rd
Cypress, TX 77433
www.nhmccd.edu

El Centro College
Diagnostic Med Sonography (General) Prgm
Main and Lamar Sts
Dallas, TX 75202
www.elcentrocollege.edu/sonography

Sanford-Brown College - Dallas
Diagnostic Med Sonography (General) Prgm
1250 W Mockingbird Ln
Suite 150
Dallas, TX 75247
http://sbdallas.com

El Paso Community College
Diagnostic Med Sonography (General) Prgm
PO Box 20500
El Paso, TX 79998
www.epcc.edu
Prgm Dir: Nora M Balderas, BS RT(R) RDMS
Tel: 915 831-3722, Ext   *Fax:* 915 831-4114
E-mail: norab@epcc.edu

Harris County Hosp Dist/Ben Taub Gen Hosp
Diagnostic Med Sonography (General) Prgm
9250 Kirby Suite 1800
Houston, TX 77054

Houston Community College
Diagnostic Med Sonography (General) Prgm
1900 Pressler Dr
Houston, TX 77030
www.hccs.edu

Sanford-Brown College - Houston
Diagnostic Med Sonography (General) Prgm
10500 Forum Place Dr #200
Houston, TX 77036
www.sbhouston.com

Angelina College
Diagnostic Med Sonography (General) Prgm
PO Box 1768 3500 South First St
Lufkin, TX 75902

Midland College
Diagnostic Med Sonography (General) Prgm
3600 N Garfield
Midland, TX 79705
www.midland.edu

Temple College
Diagnostic Med Sonography (General) Prgm
2600 S First St
Temple, TX 76504

Tyler Junior College
Diagnostic Med Sonography (General) Prgm
PO Box 9020
Tyler, TX 75711
www.tjc.edu

Weatherford College
Diagnostic Med Sonography (General/Vascular) Prgm
225 College Park Drive
Weatherford, TX 76086

Virginia

Southside Regional Medical Center
Diagnostic Med Sonography (General) Prgm
SRMC Professional Schools 737 South Sycamore St
Petersburg, VA 23803

Northern Virginia Community College
Diagnostic Med Sonography (General) Prgm
6699 Springfield Center Drive
Springfield, VA 22150

Tidewater Community College
Diagnostic Med Sonography (General) Prgm
1700 College Crescent
Virginia Beach, VA 23453
www.tcc.edu/healthprofessions/

Washington

Bellevue College
Diagnostic Med Sonography (General/Cardiac) Prgm
3000 Landerholm Circle SE, Rm B243
Bellevue, WA 98007-6484
www.bellevuecollege.edu

Seattle University
Diagnostic Med Sonography (Gen/Card/Vascular) Prgm
Diagnostic Ultrasound Dept
901 12th Ave, PO Box 222000
Seattle, WA 98122-4360
www.seattleu.edu

Spokane Community College
Diagnostic Med Sonography (General) Prgm
1810 N Greene St, MS 1090
Spokane, WA 99217
www.scc.spokane.edu/?dms

Tacoma Community College
Diagnostic Med Sonography (General) Prgm
6501 S 19th St Building 19
Tacoma, WA 98466

West Virginia

Mountain State University
Diagnostic Med Sonography (General) Prgm
PO Box 9003
410 Neville St
Beckley, WV 25801
www.mountainstate.edu

West Virginia University Hospitals
Diagnostic Med Sonography (General) Prgm
PO Box 8062
Medical Center Dr
Morgantown, WV 26506
www.wvuhradtech.com
Prgm Dir: Mandy Kooser,
Tel: 304 598-4187, Ext   *Fax:* 304 598-4072
E-mail: kooserm@wvuhealthcare.com

Wisconsin

Chippewa Valley Technical College
Diagnostic Med Sonography (General) Prgm
620 W Clairemont Ave
Eau Claire, WI 54701
www.cvtc.edu

Northeast Wisconsin Technical College
Diagnostic Med Sonography (General) Prgm
2740 W Mason St
PO Box 19042
Green Bay, WI 54307-9042
www.nwtc.edu

Blackhawk Technical College
Diagnostic Med Sonography (General/Vascular) Prgm
6004 Prairie Rd PO Box 5009
Janesville, WI 53547

University of Wisconsin Hospital and Clinics
Diagnostic Med Sonography (General/Cardiac) Prgm
School of Diagnostic Medical Sonography
610 N Whitney Way, Suite 440
Madison, WI 53705
www.uwhealth.org/ultrasoundschool
Prgm Dir: Bridgett Willey, MS RDMS RDCS RVT RT(R)
Tel: 608 263-7635   *Fax:* 608 263-9208
E-mail: Bwilley@uwhealth.org
Notes: For the certificate option, students pay $1,000 per
   semester (Total $6,000 for the 24 months). For the
   degree option, students pay by the credit hour.

Aurora St Luke's Medical Center
Diagnostic Med Sonography (General/Vascular) Prgm
180 W Grange Ave
Milwaukee, WI 53207
www.aurorahealthcare.org

Columbia St Mary's Hospitals
Diagnostic Med Sonography (General/Vascular) Prgm
2121 E Newport Ave
Milwaukee, WI 53211
www.ccon.edu

Wheaton Franciscan Healthcare - St Francis
Diagnostic Med Sonography (General) Prgm
3237 S 16th St
Milwaukee, WI 53215
www.wfhealthcare.org

Wyoming

Laramie County Community College
Diagnostic Med Sonography (General) Prgm
1400 East College Drive
Cheyenne, WY 82007

Diagnostic Medical Sonographer

Programs*	Class Capacity	Begins	Length (months)	Award	Res. Tuition	Non-res. Tuition		Offers:† 1	2	3	4
Alabama											
Wallace State Community College (Hanceville)	25	Aug	18	Dipl, AAS	$7,350	$14,700	per year			•	
Arizona											
GateWay Community College (Phoenix)	32	Aug	21	Dipl, Cert, AAS	$4,180		per year				
California											
Foothill College (Los Altos Hills)	30	Sep	18	AS	$1,278	$6,412				•	•
Delaware											
Delaware Technical Community College (Wilmington)	12	May	24	AAS	$4,000	$10,000	per year			•	
Florida											
Broward College (Coconut Creek)	15	Jan	24	AAS	$3,709	$9,767	per year			•	
St Vincent's Medical Center (Jacksonville)	6	Jul	18	Cert	$1,750	$1,750	per year			•	
Georgia											
Grady Health System (Atlanta)	10	Sep Mar	18	Cert	$8,700	$8,700	per year			•	
Idaho											
Boise State Univ	7	Aug	12	BS	$5,566	$15,966	per year				•
Kentucky											
West Kentucky Community & Technical College (Paducah)	12	Aug	18	Cert, AAS	$10,000	$33,000					•
Louisiana											
Delgado Community College (New Orleans)	12	Aug	16	Cert							
Maryland											
Univ of Maryland Baltimore County	44	Jul	14	Cert	$18,995	$18,995	per year			•	
Massachusetts											
Springfield Technical Community College	10	Sep	24	AS	$5,000	$12,000	per year			•	
Michigan											
Delta College (Univ Center)	14	Oct	18, 24	Dipl, Cert, AAS	$4,368	$6,760				•	
Providence Hospital (Southfield)	5	May	18	Cert	$3,000	$3,000	per year				
Missouri											
Univ of Missouri (Columbia)	19	Jun	24	BHS, MHS						•	•
Nebraska											
Univ of Nebraska Medical Center (Omaha)	8	Aug	12	BS	$9,371	$27,800				•	
North Carolina											
Caldwell Comm College & Tech Institute (Hudson)	35	Aug	21	AAS	$2,500	$9,500	per year			•	
Oklahoma											
Univ of Oklahoma Health Sciences Center (Oklahoma City)	32	Jun	48	BS	$4,234	$16,282				•	•
Tennessee											
Chattanooga State Community College	25	Aug	12	Cert	$5,100	$19,550				•	•
Texas											
Austin Community College	30	Summer	22, 28	AAS	$5,566	$15,690				•	•
El Paso Community College	10	Jul	22, 24	AAS						•	
West Virginia											
West Virginia Univ Hospitals (Morgantown)	3	Jul	18	Cert	$2,000	$2,000					
Wisconsin											
Univ of Wisconsin Hospital and Clinics (Madison)	16	Sep	24	Cert, BS						•	

*Data are shown only for programs that completed the 2011 AMA Survey of Health Professions Education Programs.

†Key to Offers: 1: Evening or weekend classes; 2: Non-English instruction; 3: Cultural competence instruction; 4: Distance education component.

Magnetic Resonance Technologist

Magnetic resonance technologists use radiowaves, magnetic fields, and computerized equipment to produce images of body tissues, organs, and vessels. MR technologists provide quality patient care while producing images of anatomy that permit accurate diagnoses. MR technologists critical-thinking skills to adapt procedural requirements to each patient and specific area of study.

Career Description

Magnetic resonance technologists apply knowledge of anatomy, physiology, positioning, and MR protocols in the performance of their responsibilities. They must be able to communicate effectively. The MR technologist must show competence and compassion in meeting the special needs of each patient.

Employment Characteristics

Magnetic resonance technologists are employed in health care facilities including hospitals, specialized imaging centers, urgent care clinics, and physician offices. Career advancement opportunities are available to qualified individuals as educators or as imaging department administrators. Several states require licensure as a condition of practice.

Salary

Salaries and benefits are generally competitive with other health professions and vary according to experience and employment location. Data from the 2010 Wage and Salary Survey of the American Society of Radiologic Technologists (ASRT) indicate that the average salary for practitioners with less than 2 years of experience is $50,350; the overall average is $65,099.

For more information, refer to *www.ama-assn.org/go/hpsalary*.

Educational Programs

Length. Program length varies, depending on program design, objectives, prerequisite requirements, and the degree or certificate awarded.

Curriculum. Many programs, though not all, require radiographer certification as a prerequisite. The competency-based curriculum of an accredited program includes extensive components of professional and structured clinical courses. Contact a particular program for information on specific courses and prerequisites. A Multiorganizational Curriculum is used. This curriculum is a project of the ASRT, Association of Educators in Imaging and Radiologic Sciences (AEIRS), and the Section for Magnetic Resonance Technologists (SMRT) of the International Society for Magnetic Resonance in Medicine (ISMRM).

Inquiries

Careers/Curriculum

American Society of Radiologic Technologists (ASRT)
15000 Central Avenue SE
Albuquerque, NM 87123
505 298-4500
E-mail: *customerinfo@asrt.org*
www.asrt.org

Association of Education in Imaging and Radiologic Sciences (AEIRS)
PO Box 90204
Albuquerque, NM 87199-0204
505 823-4740
E-mail: *office@aeirs.org*
www.aeirs.org

Section for Magnetic Resonance Technologists (SMRT)
2030 Addison Street, 7th Floor
Berkeley, CA 94704
510 841-1899
E-mail: *infoeismrm.org*
www.ismrm.org/smrt/

Certification/Registration

American Registry of Radiologic Technologists
1255 Northland Drive
St Paul, MN 55120
651 687-0048
www.arrt.org

Program Accreditation

Joint Review Committee on Education in Radiologic Technology
20 North Wacker Drive, Suite 2850
Chicago, IL 60606-3182
312 704-5300
E-mail: *mail@jrcert.org*
www.jrcert.org

MEDICAL IMAGING & RADIATION THERAPY

Magnetic Resonance Technologist

Arkansas

Arkansas State University
Magnetic Resonance Technologist Prgm
State University, AR 72467

Nebraska

University of Nebraska Medical Center
Magnetic Resonance Technologist Prgm
Omaha, NE 68198

Pennsylvania

Thomas Jefferson University
Magnetic Resonance Technologist Prgm
130 S 9th St, Ste 1005
Philadelphia, PA 19107
www.jefferson.edu

Rhode Island

Rhode Island Hospital
Magnetic Resonance Technologist Prgm
Providence, RI 02903

West Virginia

West Virginia University Hospitals
Cosponsor: Center for Advanced Imaging at WVU
Magnetic Resonance Technologist Prgm
Medical Center Drive Box 8062
Morgantown, WV 26506
www.wvuhradtech.com

Medical Dosimetrist

Medical dosimetrists, in collaboration with radiation oncologists and medical physicists, generate radiation dose distributions and dose calculations to design radiation treatment plans that will deliver a prescribed dose of radiation to a defined anatomic area.

Career Description

Medical dosimetrists apply knowledge of anatomy and physiology, oncologic pathology, radiation biology, radiation oncology techniques, treatment planning and dosimetry procedures, and computer computation in the performance of their duties. The medical dosimetrist is responsible for designing a radiation oncologist (physician)-prescribed course of treatment, considering dose-limiting structures and the need for special casts and immobilization devices. They must be able to communicate effectively.

Medical Physics

A related field to medical dosimetry is medical physics, an applied branch of physics that uses the concepts and methods of physics in diagnosis and treatment of human disease. It is allied with medical electronics, bioengineering, and health physics. Professionals in this field ensure radiation safety and helping to develop improved imaging techniques (eg, mammography CT, MR, and ultrasound). They also contribute to development of therapeutic techniques (eg, prostate implants, stereotactic radiosurgery), collaborate with radiation oncologists to design treatment plans, and monitor equipment and procedures to ensure that cancer patients receive the prescribed dose of radiation to the correct location. (Source: American Association of Physicists in Medicine; available at *www.aapm.org/publicgeneral/default.asp*)

Employment Characteristics

Medical dosimetrists are employed in health care facilities, including hospitals, cancer centers, and private offices. They are also employed in settings where their responsibilities focus on education, management, research, and sales.

Salary

Salaries and benefits vary with experience and employment location but are competitive with other health specialties. Data from the 2010 Wage and Salary Survey of the American Society of Radiologic Technologists

(ASRT) indicate that the average salary for practitioners with less than two years of experience is $54,528; the overall average is $95,279.

For more information, refer to *www.ama-assn.org/go/hpsalary*.

Educational Programs

Length. Program length varies, depending on program design, objectives, and the degree or certificate awarded.

Curriculum. Most programs require prerequisite work in radiation therapy or radiation physics. The competency-based curriculum of an accredited program includes extensive components of professional and structured clinical courses. Interested individuals should contact a particular program for information on specific courses and prerequisites.

Inquiries

Careers/Curriculum
American Association of Medical Dosimetrists
c/o Credentialing Services
One Physics Ellipse
College Park, MD 20740
301 209-3320
E-mail: *aamd@aapm.org*
www.medicaldosimetry.org

Certification/Registration
Medical Dosimetrist Certification Board
15000 Commerce Parkway, Suite C
Mount Laurel, NJ 08054
866 813-MDCB (6322)
E-mail: *info@mdcb.org*
www.mdcb.org

Program Accreditation
Joint Review Committee on Education in Radiologic Technology
20 North Wacker Drive, Suite 2850
Chicago, IL 60606-3182
312 704-5300
E-mail: *mail@jrcert.org*
www.jrcert.org

Medical Dosimetrist

Arkansas

University of Arkansas for Medical Sciences College of Medicine
Medical Dosimetry Prgm
4301 W Markham St
Little Rock, AR 72205

California

Loma Linda University
Medical Dosimetry Prgm
Loma Linda, CA 92350

Illinois

Southern Illinois University Carbondale
Medical Dosimetry Prgm
MC 6615
Carbondale, IL 62901
www.siuc.edu

Indiana

Indiana University
Medical Dosimetry Prgm
Indianapolis, IN 46202

Maryland

University of Maryland Medical System
Medical Dosimetry Prgm
Baltimore, MD 21201-1595

New York

Roswell Park Cancer Institute
Medical Dosimetry Prgm
Elm St
Buffalo, NY 14263

North Carolina

University of North Carolina Hospitals
Medical Dosimetry Prgm
101 Manning Dr
Chapel Hill, NC 27514-7512
www.med.unc.edu/radone

Pitt Community College
Medical Dosimetry Prgm
PO Drawer 7007
Greenville, NC 27835-7007

Ohio

Cleveland Clinic Foundation
Medical Dosimetry Prgm
Cleveland, OH 44195

Oklahoma

**University of Oklahoma Health Sciences
Center**
Medical Dosimetry Prgm
Oklahoma City, OK 73117

Pennsylvania

Thomas Jefferson University
Medical Dosimetry Prgm
Jefferson College of Health Professions
130 S 9th St, Suite 1520
Philadelphia, PA 19107

Texas

Univ of Texas M D Anderson Cancer Ctr
Medical Dosimetry Prgm
1515 Holcombe Blvd, Unit 190
Houston, TX 77030
www.mdanderson.org

UT Health Science Center - San Antonio
Medical Dosimetry Prgm
San Antonio, TX 78229

Washington

Bellevue College
Medical Dosimetry Prgm
3000 Landerholm Circle SE
Bellevue, WA 98007-6484

Wisconsin

University of Wisconsin - La Crosse
Medical Dosimetry Prgm
1725 State St 4094 HSC
La Crosse, WI 54601
www.uwlax.edu/md

MEDICAL IMAGING & RADIATION THERAPY

Nuclear medicine is the medical specialty that utilizes the properties of radioactive nuclides to make diagnostic evaluations of the anatomic and physiologic conditions of the body and to provide therapy with unsealed radioactive sources. The nuclear medicine technologist is an allied health professional who, under the direction of an authorized user, is committed to applying the art and skill of diagnostic evaluation and therapeutics through the safe and effective use of radiopharmaceuticals and pharmaceuticals.

History

The Joint Review Committee on Educational Programs in Nuclear Medicine Technology (JRCNMT), the agency that accredits nuclear medicine technology educational programs, was formed in 1970.

The first *Essentials of an Accredited Educational Program for the Nuclear Medicine Technologist* was adopted by the collaborating organizations in 1969. The *Essentials* were substantially revised in 1976, 1984, 1991, 1997, and 2003. A new edition, *Accreditation Standards for Nuclear Medicine Technologist Education*, went into effect in 2011. This document outlines the requirements for an educational program to receive accreditation.

Career Description

Nuclear medicine technologists obtain adequate knowledge of a patient's medical history to understand the illness or condition and evaluate the appropriateness of the pending diagnostic or therapeutic procedure; instruct patients before and during procedures; evaluate whether patient preparation is satisfactory before beginning a procedure; and recognize emergency patient conditions and initiate life-saving first aid when necessary.

They apply knowledge of radiation physics and safety regulations to limit radiation exposure; prepare and administer radiopharmaceuticals; use radiation detection devices that measure the quantity and distribution of radionuclides deposited in the patient; and apply quality control techniques as part of a quality assurance program covering all procedures and products in the laboratory.

Administrative functions of a nuclear medicine technologist may include supervising nuclear medicine technologists, students, and other health care personnel; participating in procuring supplies and equipment; documenting laboratory operations; and participating in departmental inspections conducted by various licensing, regulatory and accrediting agencies.

Employment Characteristics

Opportunities in nuclear medicine technology may be found in major medical centers, smaller hospitals, and independent imaging centers. Opportunities also are available for obtaining positions in clinical research, education, and administration.

Salary

Salaries vary depending on the employer and geographic location. Data from the 2007 Wage and Salary Survey of the American Society of Radiologic Technologists (ASRT) indicate that the average salary for practitioners with less than 2 years of experience is $56,400, the overall average

is $69,083, and the average salary of the top 5% of earners is $95,906.

Data from the US Bureau of Labor Statistics from May 2011 show that wages at the 10th percentile are $49,640, the 50th percentile (median) at $69,450, and the 90th percentile at $92,960 (*www.bls.gov/oes/current/oes292033.htm*).

For more information, refer to *www.ama-assn.org/go/hpsalary*.

Educational Programs

Length. The professional portion of programs ranges from one to two years. Institutions offering accredited programs may provide an integrated educational sequence leading to an associate or baccalaureate degree over a period of two or four years.

Prerequisites. Applicants for admission must have graduated from high school or the equivalent and have acquired postsecondary competencies in human anatomy and physiology, general physics, college algebra, medical terminology, oral and written communications, humanities, social science, and chemistry.

Curriculum. The curriculum includes:

- Patient care
- Cross-sectional anatomy
- Statistics
- Nuclear medicine and radiation physics
- Radiation biology
- Radiation safety and protection
- Radionuclide chemistry and radiopharmacy
- Nuclear instrumentation
- Positron emission tomography (PET)
- Computed tomography (CT)
- Medical ethics and law
- Healthcare administration
- Health sciences research methods
- Medical informatics
- Pharmacology
- Computer applications for nuclear medicine
- Diagnostic nuclear medicine procedures
- Immunology
- Radionuclide therapy
- Quality control and quality assurance

Inquiries

Careers/Curriculum
American Society of Radiologic Technologists
15000 Central Avenue SE
Albuquerque, NM 87123
www.asrt.org

Society of Nuclear Medicine—Technologist Section
1850 Samuel Morse Drive
Reston, VA 22090-5316
703 708-9000
www.snm.org

Certification/Registration

Nuclear Medicine Technology Certification Board
3558 Habersham at Northlake, Building I
Tucker, GA 30084
404 315-1739
www.nmtcb.org

American Registry of Radiologic Technologists
1255 Northland Drive
Mendota Heights, MN 55120
651 687-0048
www.arrt.org

Program Accreditation

Joint Review Committee on Educational Programs in Nuclear
    Medicine Technology (JRCNMT)
2000 West Danforth Road, Suite 130, #203
Edmond, OK 73003
405 285-0546
E-mail: *jrcnmt@coxinet.net*
www.jrcnmt.org

Note: Adapted in part from the Bureau of Labor Statistics, US Department of Labor, Occupational *Outlook Handbook*, 2010-2011 Edition, Nuclear Medicine Technologists, on the Internet at *www.bls.gov/oco/ocos104.htm*.

Nuclear Medicine Technologist

Alabama

University of Alabama at Birmingham
Nuclear Medicine Technology Prgm
SHPB 441
1530 Third Ave S
Birmingham, AL 35294
www.uab.edu/NMTProgram

Arizona

GateWay Community College
Nuclear Medicine Technology Prgm
108 N 40th St
Phoenix, AZ 85034
www.gatewaycc.edu/Programs/NuclearMedicine/
Prgm Dir: Jeanne Dial,
Tel: 602 286-8512   *Fax:* 602 286-8480
E-mail: dial@gatewaycc.edu

Arkansas

Baptist Health Schools Little Rock
Nuclear Medicine Technology Prgm
11900 Colonel Glenn Rd, Ste 1000
Little Rock, AR 72210
bhslr.edu
Prgm Dir: Sharon Ward, MA CNMT RT(N) ASCP(N)
Tel: 501 202-7447   *Fax:* 501 202-7712
E-mail: sharon.ward@baptist-health.org

University of Arkansas for Medical Sciences
Nuclear Medicine Technology Prgm
4301 W Markham St #714
Little Rock, AR 72205
www.uams.edu/chrp/nuclearmedicine

California

VA Palo Alto Health Care System
Nuclear Medicine Technology Prgm
3801 Miranda Ave
Nuclear Medicine (115
Palo Alto, CA 94304
www.palo-alto.med.va.gov/nucmed

Kaiser Permanente School of Allied Health Sci
Nuclear Medicine Technology Prgm
938 Marina Way S
Richmond, CA 94804
www.kpsahs.org

Harbor UCLA Medical Center
Nuclear Medicine Technology Prgm
1000 W Carson St, Box 23
Torrance, CA 90509
www.humc.edu

Connecticut

Gateway Community College
Nuclear Medicine Technology Prgm
88 Bassett Rd
North Haven, CT 06473
www.gwctc.commnet.edu/academics.aspx?id=425

Lincoln College of New England
Nuclear Medicine Technology Prgm
2279 Mount Vernon Rd
Southington, CT 06489
www.lincolncollegene.edu/programs/
    associates-degree-college/
    nuclear-medicine-technology-degre

Delaware

Delaware Technical Community College
Nuclear Medicine Technology Prgm
700 W Lea Blvd, Ste 101
Wilmington, DE 19805
www.dtcc.edu/wilmington/ah
Prgm Dir: Tammy Holdren, BS CNMT RT(N)(CT)
Tel: 302 765-4590, Ext   *Fax:* 302 765-4599
E-mail: tholdren@christianacare.org

Florida

Institute of Allied Medical Professions
Nuclear Medicine Technology Prgm
5150 Linton Blvd, Ste 340
Delray Beach, FL 33484
www.iamp.edu

Santa Fe College
Nuclear Medicine Technology Prgm
3000 NW 83rd St
Health Sciences, W-Bldg
Gainesville, FL 32606
dept.sfcollege.edu/health/nucmed
Prgm Dir: Brian Goring, BS CNMT
Tel: 352 395-5672   *Fax:* 352 395-5711
E-mail: brian.goring@sfcollege.edu

St Vincent's Medical Center
Nuclear Medicine Technology Prgm
Medical Sciences Education Department
One Shircliff Way
Jacksonville, FL 32204
www.jaxhealth.com
Notes: CT-certified students are able to complete the
    program in 12 months at a tuition of $4,500.

Jackson Memorial Hospital
Nuclear Medicine Technology Prgm
1611 NW 12th Ave, C-250
Miami, FL 33136
www.jhsmiami.org/body.cfm?id=10708

Florida Hospital College of Health Sciences
Nuclear Medicine Technology Prgm
671 Winyah Dr
Orlando, FL 32803
www.fhchs.edu
Prgm Dir: Joseph Hawkins, MSEd CNMT
Tel: 407 303-9380
E-mail: joe_hawkins@fhchs.edu

Hillsborough Community College
Nuclear Medicine Technology Prgm
Dale Mabry Campus
PO Box 30030
Tampa, FL 33630
www.hccfl.edu
Prgm Dir: Larry Gibson, RT(N) CNMT
Tel: 813 253-7418   *Fax:* 813 253-7491
E-mail: lgibson@hccfl.edu

Georgia

Georgia Health Sciences University
Nuclear Medicine Technology Prgm
Department of Biomedical and Radiological
    Technologies
987 St Sebastian Way
EC2422
Augusta, GA 30912
www.mcg.edu/sah/brt/nmt/

Armstrong Atlantic State University
Nuclear Medicine Technology Prgm
11935 Abercorn St
Savannah, GA 31419
www.radsci.armstrong.edu

Illinois

Northwestern Memorial Hospital
Nuclear Medicine Technology Prgm
School of Nuclear Medicine Technology
541 North Fairbanks Ct, Suite 950
Chicago, IL 60611
www.nmh.org/clinicalschools
Prgm Dir: Lisa Riehle, MS CNMT RT (N)
Tel: 312 926-4461   *Fax:* 312 926-1741
E-mail: lriehle@nmh.org

College of DuPage
Nuclear Medicine Technology Prgm
425 N Fawell Blvd
Glen Ellyn, IL 60137
www.cod.edu

Triton College
Nuclear Medicine Technology Prgm
2000 N Fifth Ave
River Grove, IL 60171
www.triton.edu

Indiana

Indiana University
Nuclear Medicine Technology Prgm
School of Medicine
541 Clinical Dr CL-120
Indianapolis, IN 46202
www.indyrad.iupui.edu/radweb

Iowa

Mercy College of Health Sciences
Nuclear Medicine Technology Prgm
928 6th Ave
Des Moines, IA 50309
www.mchs.edu/acad_nuc_med.cfm

University of Iowa Hospitals & Clinics
Nuclear Medicine Technology Prgm
Dept of Radiology
200 Hawkins Dr, 2800 JPP
Iowa City, IA 52242
www.healthcare.uiowa.edu/radsci/nuclear_medicine/
index.html
Prgm Dir: Anthony Knight, MBA CNMT RT(N)
Tel: 319 356-2954   *Fax:* 319 384-6389
E-mail: anthony-knight@uiowa.edu

Allen College
Nuclear Medicine Technology Prgm
1825 Logan Ave
Waterloo, IA 50703
www.allencollege.edu
Prgm Dir: Jared Seliger,
Tel: 319 226-2081   *Fax:* 319 226-2051
E-mail: seligejd@ihs.org

Kansas

University of Kansas Medical Center
Nuclear Medicine Technology Prgm
3901 Rainbow Blvd
2172 KU Hospital Mail Stop 4032
Kansas City, KS 66160
www.alliedhealth.kumc.edu
Prgm Dir: Tina Crain, MS CNMT RT(R)(N)(QM)
Tel: 913 588-6858   *Fax:* 913 588-8393
E-mail: tcrain@kumc.edu

Kentucky

Bluegrass Community and Technical College
Nuclear Medicine Technology Prgm
330A Oswald Building
470 Cooper Drive
Lexington, KY 40506
www.bluegrass.kctcs.edu/Academics/
Programs_of_Study/
Nuclear_Medicine_and_Molecular_Imaging
Prgm Dir: Charles Coulston, MSEd RT(R)(N) CNMT
Tel: 859 246-6241   *Fax:* 859 246-4671
E-mail: charles.coulston@kctcs.edu

Jefferson Community and Technical College
Nuclear Medicine Technology Prgm
Allied Health Div
109 E Broadway
Louisville, KY 40202

Louisiana

Delgado Community College
Nuclear Medicine Technology Prgm
615 City Park Ave
New Orleans, LA 70119
www.dcc.edu
Prgm Dir: Steve Trichell, BS RT(N)
Tel: 504 671-6232   *Fax:* 504 483-4609
E-mail: strich@dcc.edu

Maine

Central Maine Medical Center
Nuclear Medicine Technology Prgm
70 Middle St
Lewiston, ME 04240
www.cmmccollege.edu
Prgm Dir: Heather Poulin, MS CNMT RTNM
Tel: 207 795-5956   *Fax:* 207 755-5816
E-mail: PoulinHe@cmhc.org

Maryland

Johns Hopkins Hospital
Nuclear Medicine Technology Prgm
600 N Wolfe St
Radiology Admin Blalock B-179
Baltimore, MD 21287
www.jhmi.edu
Prgm Dir: Mary McCormick, PhD CNMT
Tel: 410 528-8299   *Fax:* 410 528-8308
E-mail: mmorga25@jhmi.edu

Prince George's Community College
Nuclear Medicine Technology Prgm
301 Largo Rd
Lanham Hall - 326
Largo, MD 20774
www.pgcc.edu
Prgm Dir: Nancy Meman, BS CNMT RT(N)
Tel: 301 341-3026   *Fax:* 301 386-7528
E-mail: nmeman@pgcc.edu

Massachusetts

Mass College of Pharmacy & Health Sciences
Nuclear Medicine Technology Prgm
179 Longwood Ave, G414
Boston, MA 02115
www.mcphs.edu/academics/programs/
radiologic_sciences/pb_nuc_med_tech/

Salem State University
Nuclear Medicine Technology Prgm
352 Lafayette St
Salem, MA 01970
www.salemstate.edu/biology

Springfield Technical Community College
Nuclear Medicine Technology Prgm
One Armory Sq
Springfield, MA 01102
www.stcc.edu
Prgm Dir: Richard Serino, MEd CNMT
Tel: 413 755-4871   *Fax:* 413 755-4764
E-mail: rserino@stcc.edu

Regis College
Nuclear Medicine Technology Prgm
235 Wellsley St
Weston, MA 02493
www.bidmc.harvard.edu/nmt

UMass Memorial Medical Center
Cosponsor: Worcester State University
Nuclear Medicine Technology Prgm
55 Lake Ave N
Nuclear Medicine
Worcester, MA 01655
www.umassmed.edu/nuclear_med/NMT
Prgm Dir: Leo Nalivaika, MBA CNMT
Tel: 774 442-4253   *Fax:* 774 443-4472
E-mail: leo.nalivaika@umassmemorial.org

Michigan

Ferris State University
Nuclear Medicine Technology Prgm
200 Ferris Dr, VFS 405A
Big Rapids, MI 49307

Beaumont Hospital - Royal Oak
Nuclear Medicine Technology Prgm
3601 W 13 Mile Rd
Royal Oak, MI 48073
Prgm Dir: Mary Premo, BA CNMT RT(N)
Tel: 248 898-4125   *Fax:* 248 898-0487
E-mail: mpremo@beaumont.edu

Macomb Community College
Nuclear Medicine Technology Prgm
14500 E 12 Mile Rd
Warren, MI 48088
www.macomb.edu
Prgm Dir: Sharon Lafferty, MSA CNMT
Tel: 586 286-2191   *Fax:* 586 226-4779
E-mail: laffertys@macomb.edu

Minnesota

Mayo School of Health Sciences
Nuclear Medicine Technology Prgm
Sch of Hlth Sciences
200 First St SW
Rochester, MN 55905
mayo.edu/mshs

Saint Mary's University of Minnesota
Cosponsor: North Shore University
Nuclear Medicine Technology Prgm
700 Terrace Hts #10
Winona, MN 55987

Mississippi

University of Mississippi Medical Center
Nuclear Medicine Technology Prgm
2500 N State St
Jackson, MS 39216
Prgm Dir: Sherry West, Asst Professor MS ARRT(R)(N)
CNMT
Tel: 601 984-2555   *Fax:* 601 984-4986
E-mail: sjwest@umc.edu

Missouri

University of Missouri
Nuclear Medicine Technology Prgm
605 Lewis Hall
Columbia, MO 65211
www.umshp.org/shpsite/shp_home.htm

Research Medical Center
Nuclear Medicine Technology Prgm
2316 E Meyer Blvd
Kansas City, MO 64132
www.researchmedicalcenter.com
Prgm Dir: Charlotte Haupt, MA BS CNMT
Tel: 816 276-4068   *Fax:* 816 276-3138
E-mail: Charlotte.Haupt@hcamidwest.com

Saint Louis University
Nuclear Medicine Technology Prgm
Doisy College of Health Sciences
3437 Caroline St
St Louis, MO 63104
www.slu.edu/x12892.xml
Prgm Dir: William Hubble, MA CNMT RT (R)(N)(CT) FSNMTS
Tel: 314 577-8526, Ext   *Fax:* 314 577-8503
E-mail: hubblewl@slu.edu

Nebraska

University of Nebraska Medical Center
Nuclear Medicine Technology Prgm
984545 Nebraska Medical Center
Omaha, NE 68198
www.unmc.edu/alliedhealth/rste
Prgm Dir: Marcia Hess Smith, BS CNMT
Tel: 402 559-7224   *Fax:* 402 559-4667
E-mail: mhesssmith@unmc.edu

Nevada

University of Nevada - Las Vegas
Nuclear Medicine Technology Prgm
Department of Health Physics and Diagnostic Sciences
4505 S Maryland Pkwy, Box 453037
Las Vegas, NV 89154
www.unlv.edu

New Jersey

JFK Medical Center - Muhlenberg Schools
Nuclear Medicine Technology Prgm
Park Ave and Randolph Rd
Plainfield, NJ 07061
www.muhlenbergschools.org
Prgm Dir: Maunesh Soni, MS MHA CNMT
Tel: 908 668-2770   *Fax:* 908 226-4640
E-mail: msoni@solarishs.org

Univ of Medicine & Dent of New Jersey
Nuclear Medicine Technology Prgm
School of Health Related Professions
1776 Raritan Rd, Rm 540
Scotch Plains, NJ 07076
shrp.umdnj.edu/admissions/brochures_pdf/ 12066_nuclear.pdf
Prgm Dir: Michael Teters, MS RT(N) DABR
Tel: 908 889-2449   *Fax:* 908 889-2487
E-mail: tetersms@umdnj.edu

Gloucester County College
Nuclear Medicine Technology Prgm
1400 Tanyard Rd
Sewell, NJ 08080
gccnj.edu
Prgm Dir: Laura Sharkey, MS Ed BS CNMT
Tel: 856 415-2196   *Fax:* 856 464-8463
E-mail: lsharkey@gccnj.edu

New York

Bronx Community College
Nuclear Medicine Technology Prgm
2155 University Ave
Bronx, NY 10453
www.bcc.cuny.edu

University at Buffalo - SUNY
Nuclear Medicine Technology Prgm
105 Parker Hall, 3435 Main St
Buffalo, NY 14214
www.nucmed.buffalo.edu
Prgm Dir: Elpida Crawford, MS CNMT
Tel: 716 838-5889, Ext   *Fax:* 716 838-4918
E-mail: esc@buffalo.edu

Molloy College
Nuclear Medicine Technology Prgm
1000 Hempstead Ave
PO Box 5002
Rockville Centre, NY 11571

North Carolina

University of North Carolina Hospitals
Nuclear Medicine Technology Prgm
101 Manning Dr
Radiology Administration
Chapel Hill, NC 27514
www.unchealthcare.org/site/nuclear_medicine

Caldwell Comm College & Tech Institute
Nuclear Medicine Technology Prgm
2855 Hickory Blvd
Hudson, NC 28638
www.cccti.edu
Prgm Dir: Jimmy Council, RT(N) CNMT MBA
Tel: 828 726-2370   *Fax:* 828 726-2489
E-mail: jcouncil@cccti.edu

Forsyth Technical Community College
Nuclear Medicine Technology Prgm
2100 Silas Creek Pkwy
Winston-Salem, NC 27103

Ohio

University of Cincinnati
Nuclear Medicine Technology Prgm
3202 Eden Ave
PO Box 670394
Cincinnati, OH 45267
www.cahs.uc.edu/departments/AMIT.cfm

Wexner Medical Center at Ohio State Univ
Nuclear Medicine Technology Prgm
203 Doan Hall
410 W 10th Ave
Columbus, OH 43210
radiology.osu.edu/10995.cfm
Prgm Dir: Stacey Copley, BS CNMT RT(N)
Tel: 614 293-3131   *Fax:* 614 293-2529
E-mail: stacey.copley@osumc.edu
Notes: Application deadline is April 1 for each academic year.

The University of Findlay
Nuclear Medicine Technology Prgm
Nuclear Medicine Institute
1000 N Main St
Findlay, OH 45840
www.findlay.edu/academics/colleges/cohp/ academicprograms/undergraduate/NMIP

Cuyahoga Community College
Nuclear Medicine Technology Prgm
11000 Pleasant Valley Rd
Parma, OH 44130
www.tri-c.edu/programs/healthcareers/nuclearmedicine

Kent State University - Salem Campus
Nuclear Medicine Technology Prgm
2491 State Route 45 South
Salem, OH 44460
www.salem.kent.edu/academics/salem/ris.cfm
Prgm Dir: Janet Berger, BGS CNMT
Tel: 330 337-4261   *Fax:* 330 337-4255
E-mail: jlong1@kent.edu

Oklahoma

Univ of Oklahoma Health Sciences Center
Nuclear Medicine Technology Prgm
1200 N Stonewall
AHB 3021
Oklahoma City, OK 73117
www.ah.ouhsc.edu/main/Programs/ showprograms2.asp?pgID=3&pID=11
Prgm Dir: Vesper Grantham, MEd CNMT RT(N)
Tel: 405 271-6477, Ext   *Fax:* 405 271-1424
E-mail: vesper-grantham@ouhsc.edu

Pennsylvania

Cedar Crest College
Nuclear Medicine Technology Prgm
100 College Dr
Allentown, PA 18104
www.cedarcrest.edu

Misericordia University
Nuclear Medicine Technology Prgm
301 Lake St
Dallas, PA 18612
www.misericordia.edu/ misericordia_pg.cfm?page_id=988&subcat_id=108

Lancaster Gen Coll of Nursing & Hlth Sciences
Nuclear Medicine Technology Prgm
410 N Lime St
Lancaster, PA 17602
www.LancasterGeneralCollege.edu

Robert Morris University
Nuclear Medicine Technology Prgm
6001 University Blvd
Moon Township, PA 15108

Jameson Health System
Nuclear Medicine Technology Prgm
South Campus
1000 S Mercer St
New Castle, PA 16101
Prgm Dir: Shannon Kacenga, AS RT(R)(N)
Tel: 724 658-9001   *Fax:* 724 656-4165
E-mail: skacenga@jamesonhealth.org

Thomas Jefferson University
Nuclear Medicine Technology Prgm
Jefferson College of Health Professions
130 S Ninth St, Suite 1014
Philadelphia, PA 19107
www.jefferson.edu

Community College of Allegheny County
Nuclear Medicine Technology Prgm
808 Ridge Ave
Pittsburgh, PA 15212
www.ccac.edu
Prgm Dir: Carl Mazzetti, BS CNMT
Tel: 412 237-2751   *Fax:* 412 237-6579
E-mail: cmazzett@ccac.edu

Puerto Rico

University of Puerto Rico Medical Science Campus
Nuclear Medicine Technology Prgm
PO Box 365067
San Juan, PR 00936
http://eps.rcm.upr/medicinanuclear.asp
Prgm Dir: Miriam Espada, MPH CNMT
Tel: 787 758-2525, Ext   *Fax:* 787 754-3256
E-mail: miriam.espada@upr.edu

MEDICAL IMAGING & RADIATION THERAPY

Rhode Island

Rhode Island Hospital
Nuclear Medicine Technology Prgm
3 Davol Square, Bldg A, Box 162
Providence, RI 02903
www.rihsdi.org
Prgm Dir: Lisa Tetreault, BS RT(N) CNMT
Tel: 401 528-8531, Ext   *Fax:* 401 457-0219
E-mail: ltetreault1@lifespan.org

South Carolina

Midlands Technical College
Nuclear Medicine Technology Prgm
PO Box 2408
Columbia, SC 29202
www.midlandstech.edu/nucmed/

South Dakota

Southeast Technical Institute
Nuclear Medicine Technology Prgm
2320 N Career Ave
Sioux Falls, SD 57107
Prgm Dir: Doug Warner, MEd CNMT
Tel: 605 367-7625   *Fax:* 605 367-5724
E-mail: douglas.warner@southeasttech.edu

Tennessee

Chattanooga State Community College
Nuclear Medicine Technology Prgm
4501 Amnicola Hwy
Chattanooga, TN 37406
www.chattanoogastate.edu/allied_health/
    nuclear_medicine

South College
Nuclear Medicine Technology Prgm
3904 Lonas Dr
Knoxville, TN 37909
www.southcollegetn.edu

Baptist College of Health Sciences
Nuclear Medicine Technology Prgm
1003 Monroe Ave
Memphis, TN 38104
Prgm Dir: Kathy Hunt, MS CNMT
Tel: 901 572-2642   *Fax:* 901 572-2750
E-mail: Kathy.hunt@bchs.edu

Methodist University Hospital
Nuclear Medicine Technology Prgm
1265 Union Ave
Memphis, TN 38104
methodisthealth.org

Vanderbilt University Medical Center
Nuclear Medicine Technology Prgm
1161 21st Ave South
CCC-1124 MCN
Nashville, TN 37232
www.mc.vanderbilt.edu/radiology
Prgm Dir: James Patton, PhD
Tel: 615 322-0508   *Fax:* 615 322-3764
E-mail: jim.patton@vanderbilt.edu

Texas

Amarillo College
Nuclear Medicine Technology Prgm
PO Box 447
Amarillo, TX 79178
www.actx.edu/nuclear_med

Del Mar College
Nuclear Medicine Technology Prgm
101 Baldwin Blvd
Corpus Christi, TX 78404
www.delmar.edu/nmt/

Baylor University Med Center
Nuclear Medicine Technology Prgm
4500 Crutcher St
Suite 220
Dallas, TX 75246
www.baylorhealth.edu/RAHS

Galveston College
Nuclear Medicine Technology Prgm
4015 Ave Q
Galveston, TX 77550
www.gc.edu

Houston Community College
Nuclear Medicine Technology Prgm
1900 Pressler Dr
Houston, TX 77030
coleman.hccs.edu/nuclearmedicinetechnology

The University of the Incarnate Word
Nuclear Medicine Technology Prgm
4301 Broadway St
CPO-300
San Antonio, TX 78209

Utah

University of Utah Health Science Center
Nuclear Medicine Technology Prgm
50 N Medical Drive
Salt Lake City, UT 84132
medicine.utah.edu/radiology/technologist

Vermont

University of Vermont
Nuclear Medicine Technology Prgm
106 Carrigan Drive
302 Rowell Bldg
Burlington, VT 05405
www.uvm.edu/mlrs

Virginia

Old Dominion University
Nuclear Medicine Technology Prgm
2118 Health Technology Building
Norfolk, VA 23529
http://hs.odu.edu/medlab/academics/nmed/
Prgm Dir: Scott Sechrist, EdD CNMT ARRT(N)
Tel: 757 683-3589   *Fax:* 757 683-5028
E-mail: ssechris@odu.edu

Virginia Commonwealth University
Nuclear Medicine Technology Prgm
701 W Grace St
Box 843057
Richmond, VA 23284
www.sahp.vcu.edu/radsci

Washington

Bellevue College
Nuclear Medicine Technology Prgm
3000 Landerholm Circle SE
Radiation and Imaging Sciences, B243
Bellevue, WA 98007
www.bellevuecollege.edu/nucmed
Prgm Dir: Jennifer Prekeges, MS CNMT
Tel: 425 564-2475   *Fax:* 425 564-4193
E-mail: jennifer.prekeges@bellevuecollege.edu

West Virginia

**Kanawha Valley Community & Technical
    College**
Nuclear Medicine Technology Prgm
PO Box 1000
Cole Complex
Institute, WV 25112
www.kvctc.edu
Prgm Dir: Mark Rucker, MS CNMT
Tel: 304 204-4077   *Fax:* 304 204-4078
E-mail: mrucker@kvctc.edu

West Virginia University Hospitals
Nuclear Medicine Technology Prgm
One Medical Ctr Dr, PO Box 8062
Morgantown, WV 26506
www.wvuhradtech.com
Prgm Dir: Tiffany Davis, MA RT (R)(N) CNMT
Tel: 304 598-4000, Ext   *Fax:* 304 598-4348
E-mail: davistif@wvuhealthcare.com

Wheeling Jesuit University
Nuclear Medicine Technology Prgm
316 Washington Ave
Wheeling, WV 26003
www.wju.edu
Prgm Dir: Robert George, PhD CNMT RT(N)
Tel: 304 243-2387   *Fax:* 304 243-2608
E-mail: rfgeorge@wju.edu
Notes: The program continues to work toward a fifth year
    optional clinical rotation in Computed Tomography.

Wisconsin

Saint Joseph's Hospital
Cosponsor: Marshfield Clinic
Nuclear Medicine Technology Prgm
611 St Joseph Ave
Marshfield, WI 54449
www.stjosephs-marshfield.org/nuclearmedicine
Prgm Dir: Carlyn Johnson, BS CNMT
Tel: 715 387-7787   *Fax:* 715 387-7775
E-mail: carlyn.johnson@ministryhealth.org

Aurora St Luke's Medical Center
Nuclear Medicine Technology Prgm
2900 W Oklahoma Ave
Milwaukee, WI 53201
www.aurorahealthcare.org

Froedtert Hospital
Nuclear Medicine Technology Prgm
9200 W Wisconsin Ave
Milwaukee, WI 53226
www.fmlh.edu
Prgm Dir: Frank Steffel, BS CNMT
Tel: 414 805-2071   *Fax:* 414 771-3460
E-mail: fsteffel@fmlh.edu

Nuclear Medicine Technologist

Programs*	Class Capacity	Begins	Length (months)	Award	Res. Tuition	Non-res. Tuition		Offers:† 1	2	3	4
Arizona											
GateWay Community College (Phoenix)	50	Aug	21, 18	AAS	$4,500	$19,700	per year			•	
Arkansas											
Baptist Health Schools Little Rock	9	Jul	12	Cert	$6,740	$6,740	per year			•	
Delaware											
Delaware Technical Community College (Wilmington)	8	May	24	AAS	$3,708	$9,270	per year	•		•	•
Florida											
Florida Hospital College of Health Sciences (Orlando)	29	Aug	33	BS	$10,080	$10,080	per year			•	
Hillsborough Community College (Tampa)	20	Aug	24	AS	$3,785	$13,838	per year			•	
Santa Fe College (Gainesville)	22	Aug	22	Dipl, Cert, AS	$7,677	$28,306	per year			•	
Illinois											
Northwestern Memorial Hospital (Chicago)	12	Sep	12, 48	Cert, BS (3+1)	$6,500	$6,500	per year			•	
Iowa											
Allen College (Waterloo)	8	Aug	12	Cert, BS	$16,000	$16,000	per year			•	•
Univ of Iowa Hospitals & Clinics (Iowa City)	11	Aug	12	Cert, BS	$9,848	$32,626	per year			•	
Kansas											
Univ of Kansas Medical Center (Kansas City)	6	Sep	12	Cert	$4,500	$4,500	per year			•	
Kentucky											
Bluegrass Community and Technical College (Lexington)	8	Aug	22	AS	$3,300	$11,200				•	
Louisiana											
Delgado Community College (New Orleans)	8	Aug	12		$3,281	$8,447	per year			•	
Maine											
Central Maine Medical Center (Lewiston)	11	Sep Mar (odd yrs)	24	AS	$6,300	$6,300	per year			•	
Maryland											
Johns Hopkins Hospital (Baltimore)	15	Jun	18	Cert	$10,000	$10,000	per year			•	
Prince George's Community College (Largo)	13	Jan	18	Cert, AAS	$2,500	$4,400					
Massachusetts											
Springfield Technical Community College	18	Sep	24	Dipl, AS	$4,500	$12,000					•
UMass Memorial Medical Center (Worcester)	8	Jun	12, 48	Cert, BS	$9,000	$16,000	per year			•	
Michigan											
Beaumont Hospital - Royal Oak	10	Sep	14	Cert	$4,500	$4,500				•	
Macomb Community College (Warren)	18	Aug	21	AAS	$2,400	$4,000	per year			•	
Mississippi											
Univ of Mississippi Medical Center (Jackson)	10	Jun	12	Cert						•	
Missouri											
Research Medical Center (Kansas City)	6	Sep	12	Cert	$3,950	$3,950	per year			•	
Saint Louis Univ (St Louis)	12	Sep	12, 49	BS	$33,470	$33,470	total tuition			•	
Nebraska											
Univ of Nebraska Medical Center (Omaha)	8	Aug	12	BS	$11,453	$33,976				•	
New Jersey											
Gloucester County College (Sewell)	24	Sep	21	AAS	$4,500	$7,000				•	
JFK Medical Center - Muhlenberg Schools (Plainfield)	14	Jan	12	Cert, AS	$27,000					•	
Univ of Medicine & Dent of New Jersey (Scotch Plains)	15	Sep	15	Dipl, Cert, BS	$14,855	$15,665	per year			•	
New York											
Univ at Buffalo - SUNY	15	Aug	18	BS	$7,136	$15,546	per year			•	
North Carolina											
Caldwell Comm College & Tech Institute (Hudson)	15	Aug	21	AAS	$2,712	$11,928	per year				
Ohio											
Kent State Univ - Salem Campus	10	Aug	17	BRIT	$11,380	$25,850	per year				
Wexner Medical Center at Ohio State Univ (Columbus)	10	last week of June	12	Cert	$6,000	$6,000	per year			•	
Oklahoma											
Univ of Oklahoma Health Sciences Center (Oklahoma City)	11	Jun	48	BS	$6,475	$18,525	per year			•	•
Pennsylvania											
Community College of Allegheny County (Pittsburgh)	30	Sep	24	AS	$3,500	$10,500		•			•
Jameson Health System (New Castle)	2	Jul	12	Cert	$4,500	$4,500	per year				
Puerto Rico											
Univ of Puerto Rico Medical Science Campus (San Juan)	7	Aug	12	BS	$2,700		per year		•	•	
Rhode Island											
Rhode Island Hospital (Providence)	10	Jan	16	Cert	$8,000	$8,000				•	
South Dakota											
Southeast Technical Institute (Sioux Falls)	36	Aug	24	Assoc	$10,772	$10,772	per year			•	
Tennessee											
Baptist College of Health Sciences (Memphis)	23	Sep	18	BHS	$8,600	$8,600				•	
Vanderbilt Univ Medical Center (Nashville)	8	Aug	12	Cert, BS							

*Data are shown only for programs that completed the 2011 AMA Survey of Health Professions Education Programs.

†Key to Offers: 1: Evening or weekend classes; 2: Non-English instruction; 3: Cultural competence instruction; 4: Distance education component.

MEDICAL IMAGING & RADIATION THERAPY

Nuclear Medicine Technologist

Programs*	Class Capacity	Begins	Length (months)	Award	Res. Tuition	Non-res. Tuition		Offers:† 1	2	3	4
Virginia											
Old Dominion Univ (Norfolk)	12	Aug	22	BSNMT	$10,104	$28,158				•	
Washington											
Bellevue College	8	Sep	18	Assoc	$4,037	$9,443	per year			•	•
West Virginia											
Kanawha Valley Community & Technical College (Institute)	16	May	24	Assoc	$2,956	$8,638				•	
West Virginia Univ Hospitals (Morgantown)	4	Jul	12	Cert	$2,000	$2,000	per year				
Wheeling Jesuit Univ	18	Aug	48	BS	$23,000	$23,000	per year		•	•	•
Wisconsin											
Froedtert Hospital (Milwaukee)	6	Sep	12	BS	$6,000	$6,000				•	
Saint Joseph's Hospital (Marshfield)	6	Aug	12	Cert	$4,800	$4,800					

*Data are shown only for programs that completed the 2011 AMA Survey of Health Professions Education Programs.

†Key to Offers: 1: Evening or weekend classes; 2: Non-English instruction; 3: Cultural competence instruction; 4: Distance education component.

Radiation Therapist

Radiation therapists deliver prescribed doses of radiation to patients for therapeutic purposes. In fulfilling this primary responsibility, radiation therapists provide appropriate patient care; apply problem-solving and critical thinking skills in administering treatment protocols, tumor localization, and dosimetry; and maintain patient records. Radiation therapists are responsible for applying the principles of radiation protection for patients, themselves, and others.

Career Description

Radiation therapists apply knowledge of anatomy and physiology, oncologic pathology, radiation biology, radiation oncology techniques, treatment planning procedures, and dosimetry in the performance of their duties. They must also communicate effectively.

The radiation therapist accepts responsibility for administering a radiation oncologist (physician)-prescribed course of radiation therapy, providing patient care, and maintaining treatment records. Radiation therapists also assess treatment delivery and changes in daily patient physiologic and psychologic conditions. Additional responsibilities may include tumor localization, dosimetry, patient follow-up, and patient education. Radiation therapists must display competence and compassion in meeting the special needs of the oncology patient.

Employment Characteristics

Radiation therapists are employed in health care facilities, including hospitals, cancer centers and private offices. They are also employed in settings where their responsibilities focus on education, management, research, and sales. Thirty five states require licensure as a condition of practice.

Salary

Salaries and benefits vary with experience and employment location. Data from the 2010 Wage and Salary Survey of the American Society of Radiologic Technologists (ASRT) indicate that the average salary for practitioners with less than 2 years of experience is $57,427, the overall average is $79,124.

Data from the US Bureau of Labor Statistics from May 2011 show that wages at the 10th percentile are $51,210, the 50th percentile (median) at $76,630, and the 90th percentile at $112,540 (*www.bls.gov/oes/current/oes291124.htm*).

For more information, refer to *www.ama-assn.org/go/hpsalary*.

Employment Outlook

Employment of radiation therapists is projected to grow by 20% between 2010 and 2020, which is much faster than the average for all occupations. The growing elderly population is expected to cause an increase in the number of people needing treatment. In addition, as radiation therapy becomes safer and more effective, it will be prescribed more often, leading to an increased demand for therapists. Growth is likely to be rapid across all practice settings, including hospitals, physicians' offices, and outpatient centers.

Educational Programs

Length. Program length varies, depending on program design, objectives, prerequisite requirements, and the degree or certificate awarded. A typical program is two years in length.

Curriculum. The competency-based curriculum of an accredited program includes extensive components of professional and structured clinical courses. Contact a particular program for information on specific courses and prerequisites.

Inquiries

Careers/Curriculum
American Society of Radiologic Technologists
15000 Central Avenue SE
Albuquerque, NM 87123
(505) 298-4500
E-mail: *customerinfo@asrt.org*
www.asrt.org

Certification/Registration
American Registry of Radiologic Technologists
1255 Northland Drive
St Paul, MN 55120
(651) 687-0048
www.arrt.org

Program Accreditation
Joint Review Committee on Education in Radiologic Technology
20 North Wacker Drive, Suite 2850
Chicago, IL 60606-3182
(312) 704-5300
E-mail: *mail@jrcert.org*
www.jrcert.org

Note: Adapted in part from the Bureau of Labor Statistics, US Department of Labor, *Occupational Outlook Handbook, 2010-2011 Edition*, Radiation Therapists, at *www.bls.gov/oco/ocos299.htm*.

Radiation Therapist

Alabama

University of South Alabama
Radiation Therapy Prgm
Department of Radiologic Sciences
5721 USA Drive North, HAHN 3015
Mobile, AL 36688-0002

Arizona

GateWay Community College
Radiation Therapy Prgm
108 N 40th St
Phoenix, AZ 85034

Arkansas

Central Arkansas Radiation Therapy Inst
Radiation Therapy Prgm
PO Box 55050
Little Rock, AR 72215
www.carti.com
Prgm Dir: Debra G Tomlinson, MA RT(R)(T)
Tel: 501 603-8866   *Fax:* 501 614-9880
E-mail: dtomlinson@carti.com

Arkansas State University
Radiation Therapy Prgm
PO Box 910
State University, AR 72467
www.clt.astate.edu/RadSci/RSTherapyhome.htm

California

City of Hope
Radiation Therapy Prgm
1500 E Duarte Rd
Duarte, CA 91010-0269
www.cityofhope.org

Loma Linda University
Radiation Therapy Prgm
Nichol Hall Rm A829
Loma Linda, CA 92350
www.llu.edu/llu/sahp/radtech/radiologistassistant.html

California State University - Long Beach
Radiation Therapy Prgm
1250 Bellflower Blvd
Long Beach, CA 90840-4902

Kaiser Permanente School of Allied Health Sci
Cosponsor: Kaiser Med Ctr - Richmond
Radiation Therapy Prgm
938 Marina Way S
Richmond, CA 94804
www.kpsahs.org

City College of San Francisco
Radiation Therapy Prgm
50 Phelan Ave, Box S91
San Francisco, CA 94112
www.ccsf.edu

Connecticut

Hartford Hospital
Radiation Therapy Prgm
80 Seymour St
Hartford, CT 06115-5037
harthosp.org
Prgm Dir: Nora Uricchio, MEd RT(R)(T)
Tel: 860 972-3956   *Fax:* 860 972-6461
E-mail: nuricch@harthosp.org

Gateway Community College
Radiation Therapy Prgm
88 Bassett Rd
North Haven, CT 06473
www.gwcc.commnet.edu

District of Columbia

Howard University
Radiation Therapy Prgm
515 1/2 W St NW
Washington, DC 20059
www.howard.edu

Florida

21st Century Oncology Inc School of Rad Tech
Radiation Therapy Prgm
Cape Coral Office
1419 SE 8th Terrace
Cape Coral, FL 33990
www.rtsx.com

Institute of Allied Medical Professions
Cosponsor: Cambridge Institute
Radiation Therapy Prgm
5150 Linton Blvd - Suite 340
Delray Beach, FL 33484
www.cambridgehealth.edu

Hillsborough Community College
Radiation Therapy Prgm
PO Box 30030
Tampa, FL 33614
www.hccfl.edu

Georgia

Grady Health System
Radiation Therapy Prgm
80 Jesse Hill Jr Dr SE, PO Box 26095
Atlanta, GA 30303-3050
http://gradyhealthsystem.org/Imaging/index.asp

Institute of Allied Medical Professions
Radiation Therapy Prgm
5673 Peachtree Dunwoody Rd
Suite 450
Atlanta, GA 30342
www.iampga.com

Georgia Health Sciences University
Radiation Therapy Prgm
Health Sciences Building
987 St Sebastian Way, EC-2420
Augusta, GA 30912
www.mcg.edu/sah/brt/radtherapy/

Georgia Northwestern Technical College
Radiation Therapy Prgm
One Maurice Culberson Dr
Rome, GA 30161
www.coosavalleytech.edu

Armstrong Atlantic State University
Radiation Therapy Prgm
11935 Abercorn St
Savannah, GA 31419-1997

Illinois

Southern Illinois University Carbondale
Radiation Therapy Prgm
MC 6615, School of Allied Health
College of Applied Sciences and Arts
Carbondale, IL 62901
www.siuc.edu

Northwestern Memorial Hospital
Radiation Therapy Prgm
251 E Huron St
Galter Pavilion LC-178
Chicago, IL 60611
www.nmh.org/nm/clinical+schools

Swedish American Hospital
Radiation Therapy Prgm
1401 E State St
Rockford, IL 61104

Indiana

Ivy Tech Community College - Bloomington
Radiation Therapy Prgm
200 Daniels Way
Bloomington, IN 47404

Indiana University Northwest
Radiation Therapy Prgm
3400 Broadway St
Gary, IN 46408-1197
www.iun.edu

Indiana University
Radiation Therapy Prgm
School of Medicine-Dept of Radiation Oncology
535 Barnhill Dr, RT 041
Indianapolis, IN 46202
www.iupui.edu

Iowa

University of Iowa Hospitals & Clinics
Radiation Therapy Prgm
200 Hawkins Dr, LL West Addition PFP
Iowa City, IA 52242-1009
Prgm Dir: Mindi J TenNapel, MBA MS RT(R)(T)
Tel: 319 356-8286   *Fax:* 319 356-1530
E-mail: mindi-tennapel@uiowa.edu

Kentucky

St Catharine College
Radiation Therapy Prgm
2735 Bardstown Rd
St Catharine, KY 40061

Louisiana

Delgado Community College
Radiation Therapy Prgm
615 City Park Ave
New Orleans, LA 70119
www.dcc.edu

Maine

Southern Maine Community College
Radiation Therapy Prgm
Two Fort Rd
South Portland, ME 04106
www.smccme.edu

Maryland

Community College of Baltimore County
Radiation Therapy Prgm
7201 Rossville Blvd
Baltimore, MD 21237-9987

Massachusetts

Laboure College
Radiation Therapy Prgm
2120 Dorchester Ave
Boston, MA 02124-5698
www.laboure.edu
Prgm Dir: Pauline E Clancy, MS RT(T)
Tel: 617 296-8300, Ext   *Fax:* 617 296-7947
E-mail: pauline_clancy@laboure.edu

Mass College of Pharmacy & Health Sciences
Radiation Therapy Prgm
179 Longwood Ave
Boston, MA 02115-5896
www.mcphs.edu/academics/programs/
    radiologic_sciences/bs_rad_therapy

Suffolk University
Radiation Therapy Prgm
Physics Department
41 Temple St
Boston, MA 02114

UMass Memorial Medical Center
Radiation Therapy Prgm
Radiation Oncology Department
55 Lake Ave North
Worcester, MA 01655
Prgm Dir: Patricia E Webster, MS RT(T)
Tel: 774 442-5551   *Fax:* 774 442-5006
E-mail: Patricia.Webster@umassmemorial.org

Michigan

Wayne State University
Radiation Therapy Prgm
Eugene Applebaum College of Pharmacy and Health
    Sciences
259 Mack Ave
Detroit, MI 48201
www.bulletins.wayne.edu/ubk-output/med2.html
Prgm Dir: Adam F Kempa, MEd RT(T)
Tel: 313 577-1137   *Fax:* 313 577-0908
E-mail: aa1156@wayne.edu

University of Michigan - Flint
Radiation Therapy Prgm
2102 William S White Bldg
303 E Kearsley St
Flint, MI 48502-1950
www.umflint.edu/PubHealth/radiationtherapy/index.htm
Prgm Dir: Julie A Hollenbeck, BS RT(T)
Tel: 810 424-5368   *Fax:* 810 762-3003
E-mail: hollenbj@umflint.edu

Grand Valley State University
Radiation Therapy Prgm
301 Michigan St NE, Ste 200
Grand Rapids, MI 49503
www.gvsu.edu

Baker College of Jackson
Radiation Therapy Prgm
2800 Springport Rd
Jackson, MI 49202

**Beaumont Hospital - Royal Oak William
    Beaumont Hospital School of Rad Therapy**
Radiation Therapy Prgm
3601 W 13 Mile Rd
Dept of Radiation Oncology
Royal Oak, MI 48073-6769
www.beaumonthospitals.com/
    allied-health-school-of-radiation-therapy

Minnesota

Argosy University Twin Cities Campus
Radiation Therapy Prgm
1515 Central Parkway
Eagan, MN 55121

University of Minnesota Med Ctr - Fairview
Radiation Therapy Prgm
420 Delaware St SE
MMC Box 400
Minneapolis, MN 55455
www.fairview.org/
Prgm Dir: Patricia M Fountinelle, MS RT(R)(T) CMD
Tel: 612 273-5107   *Fax:* 612 273-3589
E-mail: pfounti1@fairview.org

Mayo School of Health Sciences
Cosponsor: College of Medicine, Mayo Clinic
Radiation Therapy Prgm
200 First St SW
Rochester, MN 55905
www.mayo.edu/mshs

Missouri

Saint Louis University
Radiation Therapy Prgm
3437 Caroline St
St Louis, MO 63104
www.slu.edu

Nebraska

University of Nebraska Medical Center
Radiation Therapy Prgm
984545 Nebraska Medical Center
Omaha, NE 68198-4545
www.unmc.edu/alliedhealth/rste
Prgm Dir: Lisa Bartenhagen, MS RT(R)(T)
Tel: 402 559-4236   *Fax:* 402 559-4667
E-mail: labarten@unmc.edu

New Hampshire

NHTI, Concord's Community College
Radiation Therapy Prgm
31 College Dr
Concord, NH 03301
www.nhctc.edu

New Jersey

Cooper University Hospital
Radiation Therapy Prgm
One Cooper Plaza
Camden, NJ 08103
www.cooperhealth.edu

St Barnabas Medical Center
Radiation Therapy Prgm
94 Old Short Hills Rd
Livingston, NJ 07039
www.sbhcs.com

Bergen Community College
Radiation Therapy Prgm
400 Paramus Rd
Paramus, NJ 07652

New York

New York Methodist Hospital
Radiation Therapy Prgm
1401 Kings Highway, 2nd Floor
Brooklyn, NY 11229
www.nymahe.org

Erie Community College - City Campus
Radiation Therapy Prgm
121 Ellicott St
Buffalo, NY 14203
www.ecc.edu

Nassau Community College
Radiation Therapy Prgm
One Education Dr
Garden City, NY 11530
www.ncc.edu
Prgm Dir: Catherine Smyth, MA RT(T)
Tel: 516 572-7491   *Fax:* 516 572-9750
E-mail: catherine.smyth@ncc.edu

Memorial Sloan-Kettering Cancer Ctr
Radiation Therapy Prgm
School of Radiation Therapy
1275 York Ave, Box 22
New York, NY 10065
www.mskcc.org/schoolofradiationtherapy

SUNY Upstate Medical University
Radiation Therapy Prgm
750 E Adams St
Syracuse, NY 13210
www.upstate.edu
Prgm Dir: Joan O'Brien, MSEd RT(T)
Tel: 315 464-8448   *Fax:* 315 464-6940
E-mail: obrienj@upstate.edu

North Carolina

University of North Carolina Hospitals
Radiation Therapy Prgm
101 Manning Drive
Chapel Hill, NC 27514-7512
www.med.unc.edu/radonc

Pitt Community College
Radiation Therapy Prgm
PO Drawer 7007
Greenville, NC 27835-7007
www.pittcc.edu/academics/programs/health-sciences/
    radiation-therapy-diploma/

Forsyth Technical Community College
Radiation Therapy Prgm
2100 Silas Creek Pkwy
Winston-Salem, NC 27104
www.forsythtech.edu
Prgm Dir: Christina R Gibson, MPH RT(R)(T)
Tel: 336 734-7184   *Fax:* 336 734-7444
E-mail: cgibson@forsythtech.edu

Ohio

University of Cincinnati
Radiation Therapy Prgm
234 Goodman Ave, ML 757
Cincinnati, OH 45219

The Ohio State University
Radiation Therapy Prgm
Radiologic Sciences and Therapy
106 Atwell Hall
453 W 10th Ave
Columbus, OH 43210
www.amp.osu.edu/rd

Kent State University - Salem Campus
Radiation Therapy Prgm
2491 State Route 45 South
Salem, OH 44460

Oklahoma

Univ of Oklahoma Health Sciences Center
Radiation Therapy Prgm
PO Box 26901 Rm 451
Oklahoma City, OK 73190
www.ah.ouhsc.edu

Oregon

Oregon Health & Science University
Radiation Therapy Prgm
3181 SW Sam Jackson Park Rd, GH 124
Portland, OR 97239-3098
euston.ohsu.edu/radiation_therapy

Pennsylvania

Gwynedd-Mercy College
Radiation Therapy Prgm
1325 Sumneytown Pike
PO Box 901
Gwynedd Valley, PA 19437-0901
www.gmc.edu

Thomas Jefferson University
Radiation Therapy Prgm
130 S Ninth St, Ste 1012
Philadelphia, PA 19107

Community College of Allegheny County
Radiation Therapy Prgm
808 Ridge Ave, M607
Pittsburgh, PA 15212-6097
www.ccac.edu

Tennessee

Chattanooga State Community College
Radiation Therapy Prgm
4501 Amnicola Hwy
Chattanooga, TN 37406

Baptist College of Health Sciences
Radiation Therapy Prgm
1003 Monroe Ave
Memphis, TN 38104
www.bchs.edu

Vanderbilt University Medical Center
Radiation Therapy Prgm
Center for Radiation Oncology
The Vanderbilt Clinic B 902
Nashville, TN 37232-5671
www.mc.vanderbilt.edu/alliedhealth/radiation

Texas

Amarillo College
Radiation Therapy Prgm
PO Box 447
Amarillo, TX 79105-9973
www.actx.edu/radiation
Prgm Dir: Tony Tackitt, MEd RT(T)
Tel: 806 354-6063   *Fax:* 806 354-6076
E-mail: tmtackitt@actx.edu

Univ of Texas Southwestern Med Ctr
Radiation Therapy Prgm
5323 Harry Hines Blvd, MC-9082
Dallas, TX 75390-9082
www.utsouthwestern.edu

Galveston College
Radiation Therapy Prgm
4015 Ave Q
Galveston, TX 77550-2782
www.gc.edu

Univ of Texas M D Anderson Cancer Ctr
Radiation Therapy Prgm
1515 Holcombe Blvd, PO Unit 190
Houston, TX 77030-4009
www.mdanderson.org/healthsciences

Texas State University - San Marcos
Radiation Therapy Prgm
601 University Dr
San Marcos, TX 78666
www.txstate.edu

Vermont

University of Vermont
Radiation Therapy Prgm
Burlington, VT 05405

Virginia

University of Virginia Health System
Cosponsor: University of Virginia Medical Center
Radiation Therapy Prgm
PO Box 800383
Charlottesville, VA 22908-0383
www.healthsystem.virginia.edu/radonc

Virginia Commonwealth University
Radiation Therapy Prgm
701 W Grace St, Ste 2100
Box 843057
Richmond, VA 23284-3057
www.sahp.vcu.edu/radsci
Prgm Dir: Melanie Dempsey, MS Ed RT(R)(T) CMD
Tel: 804 828-9104   *Fax:* 804 828-5778
E-mail: mcdempsey@vcu.edu

Virginia Western Community College
Radiation Therapy Prgm
PO Box 14007
Roanoke, VA 24038

Washington

Bellevue College
Radiation Therapy Prgm
3000 Landerholm Circle SE, Rm B242
Bellevue, WA 98007-6484
www.bellevuecollege.edu
Prgm Dir: Julius Armstrong, MBA RT(T)
Tel: 425 564-5079   *Fax:* 425 564-4193
E-mail: julius.armstrong@bellevuecollege.edu

West Virginia

West Virginia University Hospitals
Radiation Therapy Prgm
PO Box 8150, Medical Ctr Dr
Morgantown, WV 26506-8150
www.wvuhradtech.com

Wisconsin

University of Wisconsin - La Crosse
Radiation Therapy Prgm
1725 State St, 4094 HSC
La Crosse, WI 54601

Radiation Therapist

Programs*	Class Capacity	Begins	Length (months)	Award	Res. Tuition	Non-res. Tuition		Offers:† 1	2	3	4
Arkansas											
Central Arkansas Radiation Therapy Inst (Little Rock)	15	Aug	12	Cert, BS	$3,000	$3,000	per year			•	
Connecticut											
Hartford Hospital	16	Sep	24, 16	Cert	$5,000	$5,000				•	
Iowa											
Univ of Iowa Hospitals & Clinics (Iowa City)	7	Aug	12	Cert, BS	$7,000	$12,000	per year			•	
Massachusetts											
Laboure College (Boston)	20	Sep	24	AS	$26,000	$26,000	per year			•	•
UMass Memorial Medical Center (Worcester)	7	Sep	15	Cert	$4,500	$4,500	per year			•	
Michigan											
Univ of Michigan - Flint	10	Jun	22	BS	$9,000	$18,000				•	
Wayne State Univ (Detroit)	28	Sep	48	BS(RT)	$12,095	$25,945				•	
Minnesota											
Univ of Minnesota Med Ctr - Fairview (Minneapolis)	15	Sep	12, 16	Cert						•	
Nebraska											
Univ of Nebraska Medical Center (Omaha)	21	Aug	12	Dipl, BS	$8,747	$25,946	per year			•	
New York											
Nassau Community College (Garden City)	47	Sep	24	AAS	$4,825	$9,650				•	
SUNY Upstate Medical Univ (Syracuse)	18	Aug	20	Bacc	$7,905	$21,480	per year			•	
North Carolina											
Forsyth Technical Community College (Winston-Salem)	22	Aug	24, 12	AAS	$2,400	$9,500				•	
Texas											
Amarillo College	10	Jun	24	AAS	$4,132	$9,201	per year			•	•
Virginia											
Virginia Commonwealth Univ (Richmond)	15	Aug	33	BS						•	
Washington											
Bellevue College	25	Sep	24	AA	$4,500	$5,000				•	

*Data are shown only for programs that completed the 2011 AMA Survey of Health Professions Education Programs.

†Key to Offers: 1: Evening or weekend classes; 2: Non-English instruction; 3: Cultural competence instruction; 4: Distance education component.

MEDICAL IMAGING & RADIATION THERAPY

Radiographer

Radiographers use radiation-producing equipment to image tissues, organs, bones, and vessels of the body, as prescribed by physicians, to assist in the diagnosis of disease or injury. Radiographers provide patient care services and are responsible for limiting radiation exposure to patients, themselves, and others. Radiographers use critical-thinking skills to modify technical parameters in order to create diagnostic images based on variable patient conditions.

Career Description

Radiographers apply knowledge of anatomy, physiology, positioning, radiographic technique, and radiation biology and protection in the performance of their responsibilities. They must be able to communicate effectively. Additional duties may include evaluating radiologic equipment, conducting a radiographic quality assurance program, providing patient education, and managing a medical imaging department. The radiographer must display competence and compassion in meeting the special needs of each patient. Career advancement opportunities are available to qualified individuals as educators or as imaging department administrators.

Employment Characteristics

Radiographers are employed in health care facilities—including hospitals, specialized imaging centers, urgent care clinics, and private physician offices and as educators or imaging department administrators. Thirty-nine states require licensure as a condition of practice.

Salary

Salaries and benefits vary according to experience and employment location. Data from the 2010 Wage and Salary Survey of the American Society of Radiologic Technologists (ASRT) indicate that the average salary for practitioners with less than two years of experience is $44,439; the overall average is $53,953.

For more information, refer to *www.ama-assn.org/go/hpsalary*.

Educational Programs

Length. Program length varies, depending on program design, objectives, prerequisite requirements, and the degree or certificate awarded. A typical program is two years in length.

Curriculum. The competency-based curriculum of an accredited program includes extensive components of professional and structured clinical courses. Contact a particular program for information on specific courses and prerequisites.

Inquiries

Careers/Curriculum
American Society of Radiologic Technologists
15000 Central Avenue SE
Albuquerque, NM 87123
(505) 298-4500
E-mail: *customerinfo@asrt.org*
www.asrt.org

Certification/Registration
American Registry of Radiologic Technologists
1255 Northland Drive
St Paul, MN 55120
(651) 687-0048
www.arrt.org

Program Accreditation
Joint Review Committee on Education in Radiologic Technology
20 North Wacker Drive, Suite 2850
Chicago, IL 60606-3182
(312) 704-5300
E-mail: *mail@jrcert.org*
www.jrcert.org

Radiographer

Alabama

Jefferson State Community College
Radiography Prgm
4600 Valleydale Rd
Birmingham, AL 35242
www.jeffstateonline.com

Wallace Community College
Radiography Prgm
1141 Wallace Dr
Dothan, AL 36303
www.wallace.edu

Gadsden State Community College
Radiography Prgm
PO Box 227
Gadsden, AL 35902-0227
http://gadsdenstate.edu
Prgm Dir: Deborah Gay Utz, MEd RT(R)
Tel: 256 549-8468   *Fax:* 256 549-8458
E-mail: gutz@gadsdenstate.edu

Wallace State Community College
Radiography Prgm
PO Box 2000
Hanceville, AL 35077-2000
www.wallacestate.edu

Crestwood Medical Center
Radiography Prgm
One Hospital Dr SE
Huntsville, AL 35801

Huntsville Hospital
Radiography Prgm
101 Sivley Rd
Huntsville, AL 35801
http://huntsvillehospital.org

University of South Alabama
Radiography Prgm
1504 Springhill Ave, Ste 2515
Mobile, AL 36604-3273
www.usouthal.edu/alliedhealth/radiologicsciences

Trenholm State Technical College
Radiography Prgm
1225 Air Base Blvd
PO Box 10048
Montgomery, AL 36108
www.trenholmstate.edu

Southern Union State Community College
Radiography Prgm
1701 Lafayette Pkwy
Opelika, AL 36801
http://suscc.edu

DCH Regional Medical Center
Radiography Prgm
809 University Blvd E
Tuscaloosa, AL 35401
www.dchsystem.com
Prgm Dir: Deborah G Shell, MEd RT(R)
Tel: 205 759-6009   *Fax:* 205 759-7844
E-mail: dshell@dchsystem.com

Arizona

Central Arizona College
Radiography Prgm
273 E Old West Hwy
Apache Junction, AZ 85248-6092

Pima Medical Institute - Mesa
Radiography Prgm
957 S Dobson Rd
Mesa, AZ 85202

Carrington College - Westside
Radiography Prgm
2701 West Bethany Home Rd
Phoenix, AZ 85017
www.carrington.edu

GateWay Community College
Radiography Prgm
108 N 40th St
Phoenix, AZ 85034
www.gatewaycc.edu

Yavapai County Health Department
Radiography Prgm
1100 East Sheldon St
Prescott, AZ 86301
www.yc.edu/radiology

Pima Community College
Radiography Prgm
2202 W Anklam Rd, HRP 220
Tucson, AZ 85709-0080
www.pima.edu

Pima Medical Institute - Tucson
Radiography Prgm
3350 E Grant Rd
Tucson, AZ 85716

Arizona Western College
Radiography Prgm
PO Box 929
Yuma, AZ 85366-0929
www.azwestern.edu

Arkansas

South Arkansas Community College
Radiography Prgm
311 S West Ave
PO Box 7010
El Dorado, AR 71731-7010
www.southark.edu
Prgm Dir: Deborah M Edney, MBA RT(R)
Tel: 870 875-7226   *Fax:* 870 864-7140
E-mail: dedney@southark.edu

University of Arkansas for Medical Sciences
Radiography Prgm
AHEC-Northwest
2907 E Joyce St
Fayetteville, AR 72703

University of Arkansas - Fort Smith
Radiography Prgm
5201 Grand Ave
PO Box 3649
Fort Smith, AR 72913-3649
www.uafortsmith.edu

North Arkansas College
Radiography Prgm
1515 Pioneer Dr
Harrison, AR 72601
www.northark.edu

National Park Community College
Radiography Prgm
101 College Dr
Hot Springs, AR 71913-9174
www.npcc.edu

Baptist Health Schools Little Rock
Radiography Prgm
School of Radiography
11900 Colonel Glenn Rd, Suite 1000
Little Rock, AR 72210-2820
bhslr.org

Saint Vincent Health System
Radiography Prgm
Two St Vincent Circle
Little Rock, AR 72205-5499
www.stvincenthealth.com

University of Arkansas for Medical Sciences
Radiography Prgm
4301 West Markham, #563
Little Rock, AR 72205
www.uams.edu/chrp/imaging

Southeast Arkansas College
Radiography Prgm
1900 Hazel St
Pine Bluff, AR 71603

Arkansas State University
Radiography Prgm
PO Box 910
State University, AR 72467
www.clt.astate.edu/RadSci/
Prgm Dir: Raymond F Winters, MS RT(R)(CT)
Tel: 870 972-3073, Ext   *Fax:* 870 972-3485
E-mail: rwinters@astate.edu

University of Arkansas for Medical Sciences
Radiography Prgm
300 E Sixth St
Texarkana, AR 71854
www.uams.edu/chrp/rad-tech

California

Cabrillo College
Radiography Prgm
6500 Soquel Dr
Aptos, CA 95003
www.cabrillo.edu

Bakersfield College
Radiography Prgm
Radiologic Technology Program
1801 Panorama Dr
Bakersfield, CA 93305
www.bakersfieldcollege.edu/alliedhealth
Prgm Dir: Nancy J Perkins, MA Ed RT(R)(M) CRT
Tel: 661 395-4284   *Fax:* 661 395-4295
E-mail: nperkins@bakersfieldcollege.edu

Mills-Peninsula Health Services
Radiography Prgm
1501 Trousdale Dr
Burlingame, CA 94010
www.mills-peninsula.org

Pima Medical Institute
Radiography Prgm
780 Bay Blvd, Ste 101
Chula Vista, CA 91910
www.pmi.edu/locations/chulavista.asp

Arrowhead Regional Medical Center
Radiography Prgm
400 N Pepper Ave
Colton, CA 92324-1819

Gurnick Academy of Medical Arts
Radiography Prgm
1401 Willow Pass Rd suite 450
Concord, CA 94520
www.gurnick.edu

Orange Coast College
Radiography Prgm
2701 Fairview Rd, PO Box 5005
Costa Mesa, CA 92628-5005
www.occ.cccd.edu

Cypress College
Radiography Prgm
9200 Valley View St
Cypress, CA 90630-5897
http://CypressCollege.edu

Fresno City College
Radiography Prgm
1101 E University Ave
Fresno, CA 93741
www.FresnoCityCollege.edu
Prgm Dir: Joseph J Shultz, MEd RT(R)
Tel: 559 244-2618   *Fax:* 559 244-2626
E-mail: Joseph.Shultz@FresnoCityCollege.edu

Antelope Valley College
Radiography Prgm
3041 W Ave K, Admin Bldg
Lancaster, CA 93534
www.avc.edu

Loma Linda University
Radiography Prgm
School of Allied Health Professions
Nichol Hall Room A829
Loma Linda, CA 92350
www.llu.edu/llu/sahp

Foothill College
Radiography Prgm
12345 El Monte Rd
Los Altos Hills, CA 94022-4599
www.foothill.edu
Prgm Dir: Bonny M Wheeler, MA RT(R)(M)
Tel: 650 949-7563   *Fax:* 650 949-7686
E-mail: WheelerBonny@foothill.edu

Charles Drew University of Medicine and Sci
Radiography Prgm
1731 E 120th St
Los Angeles, CA 90059

East Los Angeles Education and Career Center
Radiography Prgm
2100 Marengo St
Los Angeles, CA 90033

Los Angeles City College
Radiography Prgm
855 N Vermont Ave
Los Angeles, CA 90029
www.lacitycollege.edu
Prgm Dir: John G Radtke, MA RT(R)(N) (CNMT)
Tel: 323 953-4000, Ext   *Fax:* 323 953-4013
E-mail: JGR5150@yahoo.com

Yuba Community College
Radiography Prgm
2088 N Beale Rd
Marysville, CA 95901
www.yccd.edu/radtech

Merced College
Radiography Prgm
3600 M St
Merced, CA 95348-2898
www.mccd.edu/alliedhealth/radtechhp.htm

Moorpark College
Radiography Prgm
7075 Campus Rd
Moorpark, CA 93021
www.moorparkcollege.net
Prgm Dir: Guadalupe Aldana, MS RT(R)
Tel: 805 378-1400, Ext   *Fax:* 805 378-1548
E-mail: laldana@vcccd.edu

Kaplan College - North Hollywood Campus
Radiography Prgm
North Hollywood, CA 91606

California State University - Northridge
Radiography Prgm
18111 Nordhoff St
Northridge, CA 91330-8285
www.csun.edu/~vchsc02t/
Prgm Dir: Anita M Slechta, MS RT(R)(M) FASRT
Tel: 818 677-2475 *Fax:* 818 677-2045
E-mail: anita.slechta@csun.edu

Merritt College
Radiography Prgm
12500 Campus Dr
Oakland, CA 94619
http://merritt.peralta.edu

Pasadena City College
Radiography Prgm
1570 E Colorado Blvd
Pasadena, CA 91106-2003
www.pasadena.edu

Chaffey College
Radiography Prgm
5885 Haven Ave
Rancho Cucamonga, CA 91737
www.chaffey.edu/radtec

Canada College
Radiography Prgm
4200 Farm Hill Blvd
Redwood City, CA 94061
www.canadacollege.edu/radtech/

Kaiser Permanente School of Allied Health Sci
Cosponsor: Richmond Medical Center
Radiography Prgm
938 Marina Way S
Richmond, CA 94804
www.kpsahs.org

San Diego Mesa College
Radiography Prgm
7250 Mesa College Dr
San Diego, CA 92111
www.sdmesa.edu/radiologic-tech

City College of San Francisco
Radiography Prgm
50 Phelan Ave, Box S69
San Francisco, CA 94112
www.ccsf.edu/dmi

Santa Barbara City College
Radiography Prgm
721 Cliff Dr
Santa Barbara, CA 93109-2394
www.sbcc.edu/radiology

Santa Rosa Junior College
Radiography Prgm
1501 Mendocino Ave
Santa Rosa, CA 95401-4395
http://online.santarosa.edu/presentation/page/?29017

San Joaquin General Hospital
Radiography Prgm
PO Box 1020
Stockton, CA 95201
www.sjgeneralhospital.com/

El Camino College
Radiography Prgm
16007 S Crenshaw Blvd
Torrance, CA 90506
www.elcamino.cc.ca.us/

Harbor UCLA Medical Center
Cosponsor: LA County Department of Health Service
Radiography Prgm
1000 W Carson St, Box 27
PO Box 2910
Torrance, CA 90509-2910
www.harbor-ucla-radiology.org
Prgm Dir: Tuyen T Bui, MSHS BSRT(R)(ARRT)
Tel: 310 222-2825, Ext *Fax:* 310 782-3870
E-mail: tubui@dhs.lacounty.gov

Mt San Antonio College
Radiography Prgm
1100 N Grand Ave
Walnut, CA 91789-1399
www.mtsac.edu

Colorado

Red Rocks Community College
Radiography Prgm
5420 Miller St
Arvada, CO 80002
www.rrcc.edu/medicalimaging/

Concorde Career College - Aurora
Radiography Prgm
111 N Havana St
Aurora, CO 80010
www.concorde.edu

Memorial Hospital
Cosponsor: Memorial Health System
Radiography Prgm
1400 E Boulder
175 S Union, Suite 240
Colorado Springs, CO 80909
memorialhealthsystem.com
Prgm Dir: Elaine R Ivan, MA RT(R)(M)
Tel: 719 365-8291 *Fax:* 719 365-5374
E-mail: elaine.ivan@memorialhealthsystem.com

Centura Health-St Anthony Hospitals
Radiography Prgm
1601 Lowell Blvd
Denver, CO 80204-1597
www.centura.org

Community College of Denver - Lowry Campus
Radiography Prgm
1070 Alton Way, Bldg 849
Denver, CO 80230
www.ccd.edu/radiography
Prgm Dir: Catherine B Masters, MEd RT(R)
Tel: 303 365-8391 *Fax:* 303 365-8396
E-mail: catherine.masters@ccd.edu

Pima Medical Institute - Denver
Radiography Prgm
7475 Dakin St, Ste 100
Denver, CO 80221
www.pmi.edu

Colorado Mesa University
Radiography Prgm
1100 North Ave
Grand Junction, CO 81501
www.mesastate.edu

Connecticut

St Vincent's College
Radiography Prgm
2800 Main St
Bridgeport, CT 06606
www.stvincentscollege.edu

Danbury Hospital /Western Connecticut Health Network
Radiography Prgm
24 Hospital Ave
Danbury, CT 06810
www.danburyhospital.org

Quinnipiac University
Radiography Prgm
275 Mount Carmel Ave
Hamden, CT 06518-1908
www.quinnipiac.edu

Capital Community College
Radiography Prgm
950 Main St
Hartford, CT 06103-1207
www.ccc.commnet.edu

Hartford Hospital
Radiography Prgm
560 Hudson St
ERD Room 837
Hartford, CT 06106
www.harthosp.org/alliedhealth/radiography
Prgm Dir: Pamela M Cooke, MEd RT(R)(M)
Tel: 860 972-3955 *Fax:* 860 972-3955
E-mail: pcooke@harthosp.org

Middlesex Community College
Radiography Prgm
100 Training Hill Rd
Middletown, CT 06457

Gateway Community College
Radiography Prgm
88 Bassett Rd
North Haven, CT 06473

Stamford Hospital
Radiography Prgm
Shelburne Rd W Broad St, Box 9317
Stamford, CT 06904-9317
www.stamhealth.org

Naugatuck Valley Community College
Radiography Prgm
750 Chase Pkwy
Waterbury, CT 06708
www.nvcc.commnet.edu

University of Hartford
Radiography Prgm
200 Bloomfield Ave
West Hartford, CT 06117

Windham Community Memorial Hospital
Radiography Prgm
112 Mansfield Ave
Willimantic, CT 06226
www.wcmh.org
Prgm Dir: Carrie L Vincenzo, MHS RRA RT(R)
Tel: 860 456-6195 *Fax:* 860 456-6823
E-mail: cvincenzo@wcmh.org

Delaware

Delaware Technical Community College - Jack F. Owens Campus
Radiography Prgm
PO Box 610, Seashore Hwy
Georgetown, DE 19947
www.dtcc.edu

Delaware Technical Community College - Wilmington Campus
Radiography Prgm
333 Shipley St
Wilmington, DE 19802

District of Columbia

Washington Hospital Center
Radiography Prgm
110 Irving St NW
Washington, DC 20010

Florida

South Florida Community College
Radiography Prgm
600 W College Dr
Avon Park, FL 33825
www.southflorida.edu

West Boca Medical Center
Radiography Prgm
21644 State Rd 7
Boca Raton, FL 33428

Bethesda Memorial Hospital
Radiography Prgm
2815 S Seacrest Blvd
Boynton Beach, FL 33435
www.bethesdaweb.com/Imaging/Radiography Program

State College of Florida, Manatee-Sarasota
Radiography Prgm
5840 26th St W
Bradenton, FL 34207
www.scf.edu/radiography
Prgm Dir: Patrick W Patterson, MS RT(R)(N) CNMT
Tel: 941 752-5245 *Fax:* 941 727-6471
E-mail: patterp@scf.edu

Brevard Community College
Radiography Prgm
1519 Clearlake Rd
Cocoa, FL 32922
www.brevardcc.edu
Prgm Dir: Susan A Sheehan, MS RT(R)(M) (QM)
Tel: 321 433-7591 *Fax:* 321 433-7599
E-mail: sheehans@brevardcc.edu

Halifax Health Medical Center
Radiography Prgm
303 N Clyde Morris Blvd
Daytona Beach, FL 32114
www.halifaxhealth.org/formedicalprofessionals/
  radiography_program.aspx
Prgm Dir: Darcie J Nethery, PhD RT(R)
Tel: 386 254-4075, Ext *Fax:* 386 425-4231
E-mail: darcie.nethery@halifax.org

Keiser University
Radiography Prgm
1800 Business Park Blvd
Daytona Beach, FL 32114
www.keiseruniversity.edu

Institute of Allied Medical Professions - Delray Beach
Cosponsor: Cambridge Institute
Radiography Prgm
Delray Beach, FL 33484

Keiser University
Radiography Prgm
1500 NW 49th St
Fort Lauderdale, FL 33309
www.keiseruniversity.edu

MedVance Institute - Ft Lauderdale Campus/KIMC Investments
Radiography Prgm
4850 W Oakland Park Blvd, Suite 200
Fort Lauderdale, FL 33313
www.medvance.edu

Edison State College
Radiography Prgm
PO Box 60210
8099 College Pkwy SW
Fort Myers, FL 33906-6210
www.edison.edu

Indian River State College
Radiography Prgm
3209 Virginia Ave
Fort Pierce, FL 34982

Santa Fe College
Radiography Prgm
3000 NW 83rd St
Gainesville, FL 32602-6200
http://inst.sfcc.edu/~health/xray/

Dade Medical College - Hollywood Campus
Radiography Prgm
Hollywood, FL

Keiser University, Jacksonville Campus
Radiography Prgm
6430 Southpoint Parkway
Suite 100
Jacksonville, FL 32218
www.keiseruniversity.edu

Mayo Clinic Jacksonville
Cosponsor: Mayo Clinic Florida
Radiography Prgm
4500 San Pablo Rd
Jacksonville, FL 32224
www.mayo.edu/mshs
Notes: We are associated with a junior college that
  provides our students with an associate degree. The
  Mayo program provides a certificate.

Shands Jacksonville Medical Center
Radiography Prgm
School of Radiologic Technology
655 W Eighth St
Jacksonville, FL 32209
jax.shands.org/education/radtech

St Vincent's Medical Center
Radiography Prgm
1 Shircliff Way
Jacksonville, FL 32204
www.jaxhealth.com
Prgm Dir: Karen F Nevins, MSHA RT(R)(QM)
Tel: 904 308-8552 *Fax:* 904 308-5109
E-mail: knevins@jaxhealth.com

Keiser University
Radiography Prgm
2400 Interstate Dr
Lakeland, FL 33805

Lakeland Regional Medical Center
Radiography Prgm
1324 Lakeland Hills Blvd, PO Box 95448
Lakeland, FL 33805
lrmc.com

Keiser University
Radiography Prgm
900 S Babcock St
Melbourne, FL 32901
www.keiseruniversity.edu

Dade Medical College
Radiography Prgm
3721-1 NW 7th St
Miami, FL 33126
www.mdc.edu

Jackson Memorial Hospital
Cosponsor: Univ of Miami
Radiography Prgm
1611 NW 12th Ave
Miami, FL 33136-1094

Keiser University - Kendall Campus
Radiography Prgm
Miami, FL 33127

MedVance Institute
Radiography Prgm
Miami/KIMC Investments, Inc
9035 Sunset Dr, Suite 200
Miami, FL 33173

Miami Dade Comm Coll/Jackson Mem Hosp
Radiography Prgm
950 NW 20th St
Miami, FL 33127-4693
www.mdc.edu

Professional Training Centers
Radiography Prgm
13926 SW 47th St
Miami, FL 33175
www.ptcmatt.com

Marion County School of Radiologic Tech
Cosponsor: Marion County School System
Radiography Prgm
1014 SW Seventh Rd
Ocala, FL 34471
www.mcctae.com
Prgm Dir: Timothy Richardson, MA RT(R)
Tel: 352 671-7222 *Fax:* 352 671-7216
E-mail: Timothy.Richardson@marion.k12.fl.us

Florida Hospital College of Health Sciences
Radiography Prgm
671 Winyah Dr
Orlando, FL 32803

Valencia College
Radiography Prgm
PO Box 3028
Orlando, FL 32802
valenciacc.edu/asdegrees/as.asp

Palm Beach State College
Radiography Prgm
3160 PGA Blvd
Palm Beach Gardens, FL 33418-2893
www.pbcc.edu/x1284.xml

MedVance Institute - West Palm Beach Campus
Radiography Prgm
1630 S Congress Ave
Palm Springs, FL 33461

Gulf Coast State College
Radiography Prgm
School of Radiography
5230 W US Hwy 98
Panama City, FL 32401-1041
www.gulfcoast.edu

Pensacola State College - Warrington Campus
Radiography Prgm
Pensacola Junior College
5555 W Hwy 98
Pensacola, FL 32507-1097
pjc.edu

Keiser University - Sarasota
Radiography Prgm
6151 Lake Osprey Dr
Sarasota, FL 34240
www.keiseruniversity.edu

St Petersburg College
Radiography Prgm
PO Box 13489
St. Petersburg, FL 33733

Everest Univ - Brandon Campus
Radiography Prgm
3924 Coconut Palm Dr
Tampa, FL 33619

Hillsborough Community College
Radiography Prgm
PO Box 30030
Tampa, FL 33630-3030
www.hccfl.edu

Polk State College
Radiography Prgm
999 Ave H NE
Winter Haven, FL 33881-4299
www.polk.edu

Georgia

Chattahoochee Technical College North Metro
Radiography Prgm
5198 Ross Rd
Acworth, GA 30102

Albany Technical College
Radiography Prgm
1704 S Slappey Blvd
Albany, GA 31701

Athens Technical College
Radiography Prgm
800 US Hwy 29 N
Athens, GA 30601-1500
www.athenstech.edu

Emory University
Radiography Prgm
PO Box 25901
Atlanta, GA 30322

Grady Health System
Radiography Prgm
80 Jesse Hill Jr Dr SE
PO Box 26095
Atlanta, GA 30303-3050
www.gradyhealth.org/imaging
Prgm Dir: Cheryl Pressly, MS RT(R)
Tel: 404 616-3611   *Fax:* 404 616-3512
E-mail: cpressly@gmh.edu

University Hospital
Radiography Prgm
1350 Walton Way
Augusta, GA 30901-3599
www.universityhealth.org
Prgm Dir: Patricia S Graham, MBA RT(R)
Tel: 706 774-8646   *Fax:* 706 774-5079
E-mail: pgraham@uh.org

College of Coastal Georgia
Radiography Prgm
1 College Drive
Brunswick, GA 31520-3644
Prgm Dir: Bonnie M Tobias, MSA RT(R)(M(QM)
Tel: 912 279-5864   *Fax:* 912 262-3283
E-mail: BTobias@ccga.edu

Columbus Technical College
Radiography Prgm
928 Manchester Expressway
Columbus, GA 31904-6572
www.columbustech.edu

Dalton State College
Radiography Prgm
650 College Dr
Dalton, GA 30720
www.daltonstate.edu

DeKalb Medical Center
Radiography Prgm
2701 N Decatur Rd
Decatur, GA 30033
www.dekalbmedical.org

West Georgia Technical College - Douglasville
Radiography Prgm
4600 Timber Ridge Dr
Douglasville, GA 30135
www.westcentraltech.edu

Oconee Fall Line Technical College
Radiography Prgm
560 Pinehill Rd
Dublin, GA 31021
www.heartofgatech.edu

West Georgia Technical College - LaGrange
Radiography Prgm
303 Fort Dr
LaGrange, GA 30240
www.westgatech.edu

Gwinnett Technical College
Radiography Prgm
5150 Sugarloaf Pkwy
Lawrenceville, GA 30043
gwinnetttech.edu
Prgm Dir: James A Sass, MEd RT(R)(M)(QM) CIIP
Tel: 678 226-6326   *Fax:* 770 685-1338
E-mail: jsass@gwinnetttech.edu

Moultrie Technical College
Radiography Prgm
800 Veterans Pkwy N
Moultrie, GA 31788
www.moultrietech.edu

Lanier Technical College
Radiography Prgm
2990 Landrum Education Dr
Oakwood, GA 30566
www.laniertech.edu

Georgia Northwestern Technical College
Radiography Prgm
1 Maurice Culberson Dr
Rome, GA 30161

Armstrong Atlantic State University
Radiography Prgm
11935 Abercorn St
Savannah, GA 31419
www.radsci.armstrong.edu
Prgm Dir: Elwin R Tilson, EdD RT(R)(M)(CT)(QM)
    FAEIRS
Tel: 912 344-2939   *Fax:* 912 344-3469
E-mail: elwin.tilson@armstrong.edu

Ogeechee Technical College
Radiography Prgm
One Joe Kennedy Blvd
Statesboro, GA 30458
www.ogeecheetech.edu
Prgm Dir: Janice F Martin, MA RT(R)
Tel: 912 871-1647   *Fax:* 866 425-7011
E-mail: jmartin@ogeecheetech.edu

Southeastern Technical College
Radiography Prgm
3001 E First St
Vidalia, GA 30474

Middle Georgia Technical College
Radiography Prgm
80 Cohen Walker Dr
Warner Robins, GA 31088
www.middlegatech.edu

Okefenokee Technical College
Radiography Prgm
1701 Carswell Ave
Waycross, GA 31503
www.okefenokeetech.edu

Hawaii

Kapiolani Community College
Radiography Prgm
4303 Diamond Head Rd
Honolulu, HI 96816
http://programs.kcc.hawaii.edu
Prgm Dir: Jodi Ann Nakaoka, MEd RT(R)(M)
Tel: 808 734-9251   *Fax:* 808 734-9126
E-mail: jnakaoka@hawaii.edu

Idaho

Boise State University
Radiography Prgm
College of Health Sciences
1910 University Dr
Boise, ID 83725-1845
http://radsci.boisestate.edu

North Idaho College
Radiography Prgm
1000 W Garden Ave
Coeur d'Alene, ID 83814
www.nic.edu

College of Southern Idaho
Radiography Prgm
315 Falls Ave
Twin Falls, ID 83303-1238
www.csi.edu/radiologic_technology/

Illinois

Southwestern Illinois College
Radiography Prgm
2500 Carlyle Rd
Belleville, IL 62221-9989
www.southwestern.cc.il.us/

Northwestern College
Radiography Prgm
7725 S Harlem
Bridgeview, IL 60455

Kaskaskia College
Radiography Prgm
27210 College Rd
Centralia, IL 62801
www.kaskaskia.edu

Parkland College
Radiography Prgm
2400 W Bradley Ave
Champaign, IL 61821-1899
www.parkland.edu

Malcolm X College
Radiography Prgm
1900 W Van Buren St
Chicago, IL 60612
malcolmx.ccc.edu/Academic_Programs/Radiography.asp

Northwestern Memorial Hospital
Radiography Prgm
Chicago, IL 60611

Wright College
Radiography Prgm
4300 N Narragansett Ave
Chicago, IL 60634
wright.ccc.edu
Prgm Dir: Dennis M King, MHS RT(R)
Tel: 773 481-8880   *Fax:* 773 481-8892
E-mail: dking@ccc.edu

Danville Area Community College
Radiography Prgm
2000 E Main St
Danville, IL 61832
www.dacc.edu

Sauk Valley Community College
Radiography Prgm
173 Illinois Rte 2
Dixon, IL 61021-9112
www.svcc.edu
Prgm Dir: Dianna H Brevitt, MAT RT(R)(CT)
Tel: 815 835-6362   *Fax:* 815 288-5651
E-mail: brevitd@svcc.edu

Elgin Community College
Radiography Prgm
1700 Spartan Dr
Elgin, IL 60123

St Francis Hospital
Cosponsor: Resurrection Health Care
Radiography Prgm
355 Ridge Ave
Evanston, IL 60202

College of DuPage
Radiography Prgm
425 N Fawell Blvd
Glen Ellyn, IL 60137-6599
http://cod.edu

College of Lake County
Radiography Prgm
19351 W Washington St
Grayslake, IL 60030-1198
www.clcillinois.edu

Rend Lake College
Radiography Prgm
468 N Ken Gray Pkwy
Ina, IL 62846

McDonough District Hospital
Radiography Prgm
525 E Grant St
Macomb, IL 61455
Prgm Dir: Vincent E Staub, MS RT(R)
Tel: 309 833-4101, Ext   *Fax:* 309 836-1551
E-mail: vestaub@mdh.org

Kishwaukee College
Radiography Prgm
21193 Malta Rd
Malta, IL 60150-9699
www.kishwaukeecollege.edu
Prgm Dir: Carol Guschl, MSEd RT(R)(QM)
Tel: 815 825-2086, Ext   *Fax:* 815 825-2072
E-mail: guschl@kishwaukeecollege.edu

Heartland Community College
Radiography Prgm
1500 W Raab Road
Normal, IL 61761

Olney Central College
Radiography Prgm
305 N West St
Olney, IL 62450
www.iecc.edu

Harper College
Radiography Prgm
Palatine, IL 60067

Moraine Valley Community College
Radiography Prgm
9000 W College Parkway
Palos Hills, IL 60465
www.morainevalley.edu
Prgm Dir: Michael A Gatto, MS RT(R)
Tel: 708 974-5316   *Fax:* 708 974-8316
E-mail: gatto@morainevalley.edu

Illinois Central College
Radiography Prgm
Thomas K Thomas Bldg
201 SW Adams St
Peoria, IL 61635-0001
www.icc.edu

OSF Saint Francis Medical Center
Radiography Prgm
530 NE Glen Oak Ave
Peoria, IL 61637
www.osfsaintfrancis.org

Blessing Hospital
Radiography Prgm
1005 Broadway PO Box 7005
Quincy, IL 62305-7005
www.blessinghealthsystem.org

Triton College
Radiography Prgm
2000 N Fifth Ave
River Grove, IL 60171
www.triton.edu

Trinity College of Nursing & Health Sciences
Radiography Prgm
2122 25th Ave
Rock Island, IL 61201-5317
www.trinityqc.com/homepage_col.cfm?id=1835

Rockford Memorial Hospital
Radiography Prgm
2400 N Rockton Ave
Rockford, IL 61103
www.rhsnet.org
Prgm Dir: Patricia Griesman, MS RT(R)
Tel: 815 971-5480   *Fax:* 815 971-9465
E-mail: pgriesman@rhsnet.org

Swedish American Hospital
Radiography Prgm
1250 E State St
Rockford, IL 61104-2315

Lincoln Land Community College
Radiography Prgm
5250 Shepherd Rd
PO Box 19256
Springfield, IL 62794-9256
www.llcc.edu

Indiana

Columbus Regional Hospital
Radiography Prgm
2400 E 17th St
Columbus, IN 47201
www.crh.org

University of Southern Indiana
Radiography Prgm
8600 University Blvd
Evansville, IN 47712

Indiana Univ - Purdue Univ Ft Wayne
Cosponsor: Parkview Hospital and St. Joseph Hospital
Radiography Prgm
2101 East Coliseum Blvd
Fort Wayne, IN 46805

University of Saint Francis
Radiography Prgm
2701 Spring St
Fort Wayne, IN 46808
www.sf.edu

Indiana University Northwest
Radiography Prgm
3400 Broadway St
Gary, IN 46408-1197
www.iun.edu

Hancock Regional Hospital
Radiography Prgm
801 N State St
Greenfield, IN 46140
www.hancockregional.org

Community Health Network
Radiography Prgm
1500 N Ritter Ave
Indianapolis, IN 46219

Indiana University
Radiography Prgm
541 Clinical Dr 120
Indianapolis, IN 46202-5111
http://ww2.indyrad.iupui.edu/RadWeb/

Ivy Tech Community College
Radiography Prgm
9301 E 59th St
Indianapolis, IN 46216
www.ivytech.edu/indianapolis

St Vincent Health/St Joseph Hospital
Radiography Prgm
2001 W 86th St
Indianapolis, IN 46260
www.stvincent.org/education/radiography
Prgm Dir: Mark E Adkins, MS Ed RT(R)(QM)
Tel: 317 338-3879
E-mail: meadkins@stvincent.org

Indiana University - Kokomo
Radiography Prgm
2300 S Washington St
Kokomo, IN 46902
www.iuk.edu/~koalhe/

King's Daughters' Hospital & Health Services
Radiography Prgm
One King's Daughters' Drive
PO Box 447
Madison, IN 47250
www.kdhhs.org

Ivy Tech Community College - Marion
Radiography Prgm
1015 E 3rd St
Marion, IN 46952
www.ivytech.edu/marion

Ball State University
Radiography Prgm
2000 W University Ave
Muncie, IN 47306
www.bsu.edu/physiology-health/radiography
Prgm Dir: Donna L Long, MSM RT(R)(M)(QM)
Tel: 317 962-3284   *Fax:* 317 962-2102
E-mail: dlong2@iuhealth.org

Reid Hospital & Health Care Services
Radiography Prgm
1100 Reid Parkway
Richmond, IN 47374
www.reidhospital.org
Prgm Dir: Roger A Preston, MSRS RT(R)
Tel: 765 983-3167   *Fax:* 765 983-3260
E-mail: roger.preston@reidhospital.org

Indiana University South Bend
Radiography Prgm
1700 Mishawaka Ave, PO Box 7111
South Bend, IN 46634
www.iusb.edu

Ivy Tech Community College
Radiography Prgm
8000 S Education Dr
Terre Haute, IN 47802

Good Samaritan Hospital
Radiography Prgm
520 S Seventh St
Vincennes, IN 47591
Prgm Dir: Marsha L Cox, MSRS RT(R)(M)
Tel: 812 885-8011   *Fax:* 812 885-3445
E-mail: mcox@gshvin.org

MEDICAL IMAGING & RADIATION THERAPY

Iowa

Scott Community College
Radiography Prgm
500 Belmont Rd
Bettendorf, IA 52722-5649

**St Luke's Hospital dba Mercy/St. Luke's
 School of Radiologic Tech**
Cosponsor: Mercy Medical Center
Radiography Prgm
PO Box 3026
1026 A Ave NE
Cedar Rapids, IA 52406-3026
www.isrt.org/ResourceCenter/mstl.aspx
Prgm Dir: Dana D Schmitz, MEd RT(R)
Tel: 319 369-7077   *Fax:* 319 368-5721
E-mail: schmitdd@crstlukes.com

Jennie Edmundson Memorial Hospital
Radiography Prgm
933 E Pierce St
Council Bluffs, IA 51503
Prgm Dir: Mary Kathleen Rollins, MHA RT(R)(M)
Tel: 712 396-6746   *Fax:* 712 396-6227
E-mail: kate.rollins@nmhs.org

**Iowa Methodist Med Ctr/Iowa Hlth - Des
 Moines**
Radiography Prgm
1200 Pleasant St
Des Moines, IA 50309-1453
www.iowahealth.org/radtech

Mercy College of Health Sciences
Radiography Prgm
928 Sixth Ave
Des Moines, IA 50309
www.mchs.edu

Iowa Central Community College
Radiography Prgm
330 Ave M
Fort Dodge, IA 50501
www.iowacentral.com

University of Iowa Hospitals & Clinics
Radiography Prgm
Radiology, C-723 GH
200 Hawkins Dr
Iowa City, IA 52242-1077
www.medicine.uiowa.edu/RadSci
Prgm Dir: Kathy Martensen, MA RT(R)
Tel: 319 356-4332   *Fax:* 319 384-9574
E-mail: kathy-martensen@uiowa.edu

Mercy Medical Center - North Iowa
Radiography Prgm
1000 Fourth St SW
Mason City, IA 50401

Indian Hills Community College
Radiography Prgm
655 Indian Hills Drive Bldg 21
Ottumwa, IA 52501
www.ihcc.cc.ia.us

Northeast Iowa Community College
Radiography Prgm
Peosta Campus
10250 Sundown Rd
Peosta, IA 52068
www.nicc.edu

St. Luke's College/St. Luke's Regl Med Ctr
Radiography Prgm
2720 Stone Park Blvd
Sioux City, IA 51104
www.stlukescollege.edu

Allen College
Radiography Prgm
1825 Logan Ave
Waterloo, IA 50703
www.allencollege.edu

Covenant Medical Center
Radiography Prgm
3421 W 9th St
Waterloo, IA 50702
covhealth.com/radiology_school.asp
Prgm Dir: Danette M Shook, MA Ed RT(R)(M)(MR)
Tel: 319 272-7419   *Fax:* 319 272-7105
E-mail: Danette.Shook@wfhc.org

Kansas

Fort Hays State University
Radiography Prgm
600 Park St
Hays, KS 67601-4099

Hutchinson Community College
Radiography Prgm
815 N Walnut
Hutchinson, KS 67501
www.hutchcc.edu

Labette Community College
Radiography Prgm
200 S 14th St
Parsons, KS 67357
www.labette.edu

Washburn University
Radiography Prgm
1700 SW College Ave
Topeka, KS 66621
www.washburn.edu

Newman University
Radiography Prgm
3100 McCormick Ave
Wichita, KS 67213
http://newmanu.edu

Kentucky

Bowling Green Technical College
Radiography Prgm
1845 Loop Dr
Bowling Green, KY 42101
www.bowlinggreen.kctcs.edu
Prgm Dir: Lori A Slaughter, MA Ed RT(R)(M)
Tel: 270 901-1081   *Fax:* 270 901-1139
E-mail: lori.slaughter@kctcs.edu

Elizabethtown Community & Technical College
Radiography Prgm
620 College St Rd
Elizabethtown, KY 42701
www.elizabethtown.kctcs.edu

Hazard Community & Technical College
Cosponsor: Southeast Kentucky Community and
 Technical College
Radiography Prgm
One Community College Dr
Hazard, KY 41701
www.hazard.kctcs.edu

Northern Kentucky University
Radiography Prgm
227 Albright Health Ctr
Highland Heights, KY 41099-2104
www.nku.edu/~nursing/radtechhome.html

Bluegrass Community and Technical College
Radiography Prgm
470 Cooper Dr
Lexington, KY 40502-0235
www.bluegrass.kctcs.edu/ah/rad/

Spencerian College - Lexington
Radiography Prgm
1575 Winchester Rd
Lexington, KY 40505
www.spencerian.edu

St Joseph Health System
Radiography Prgm
One St Joseph Dr
Lexington, KY 40504
www.saintjosephhealthcare.org/radiology

Jefferson Community and Technical College
Radiography Prgm
109 E Broadway St
Louisville, KY 40202

Spencerian College
Radiography Prgm
4627 Dixie Hwy
Louisville, KY 40216

Madisonville Community College
Radiography Prgm
750 N Laffoon St
Health Campus
Madisonville, KY 42431
www.madisonville.kctcs.edu
Prgm Dir: Tonia R Gibson, MS RT(R)
Tel: 270 824-1739   *Fax:* 270 824-1879
E-mail: tonia.gibson@kctcs.edu

Morehead State University
Radiography Prgm
Center For Health Education and Research
CHER 210
Morehead, KY 40351
www.morehead-st.edu
Prgm Dir: Barbara L Dehner, MSRS RT (R)(M)(CT)
 FAERS
Tel: 606 783-2651   *Fax:* 606 783-5051
E-mail: b.dehner@moreheadstate.edu

Owensboro Community & Technical College
Radiography Prgm
4800 New Hartford Rd
Owensboro, KY 42303
www.octc.kctcs.edu

**West Kentucky Community & Technical
 College**
Radiography Prgm
4810 Alben Barkley Dr, PO Box 7380
PO Box 7380
Paducah, KY 42002-7408
www.westkentucky.kctcs.edu

Southeast Kentucky Comm & Tech College
Radiography Prgm
3300 US Highway 25E S
Pineville, KY 40977
www.secc.kctcs.edu/AcademicAffairs/AlliedHealth/Radi
 ographyP/

Somerset Community College
Radiography Prgm
808 Monticello St
Somerset, KY 42501

St Catharine College
Radiography Prgm
2735 Bardstown Rd
St Catharine, KY 40061
www.sccky.edu

Louisiana

Louisiana State University - Alexandria
Radiography Prgm
8100 Hwy 71 S
Alexandria, LA 71302

Baton Rouge General Medical Center
Radiography Prgm
3616 North Blvd
Baton Rouge, LA 70806
www.brgeneral.org/sort

Fortis College
Radiography Prgm
Baton Rouge, KIMC Investments, Inc
9255 Interline Ave
Baton Rouge, LA 70809
www.medvance.org

Our Lady of the Lake College
Radiography Prgm
7434 Perkins Rd
Baton Rouge, LA 70808
www.ololcollege.edu
Prgm Dir: Shelly M Pendergrass, BSRT RT(R)
Tel: 225 768-1763   *Fax:* 225 768-0819
E-mail: spenderg@ololcollege.edu

Louisiana State University at Eunice
Radiography Prgm
PO Box 1129
Eunice, LA 70535
www.lsue.edu/radtech

North Oaks Medical Center
Radiography Prgm
PO Box 2668
42367 Deluxe Plaza, Suite 27
Hammond, LA 70404
www.northoaks.org
Prgm Dir: Marsha J Talbert, MS RT(R)
Tel: 985 345-9805   *Fax:* 985 345-9894
E-mail: talbertm@northoaks.org

Lafayette General Medical Center
Radiography Prgm
1214 Coolidge Ave
PO Box 52009 OCS
Lafayette, LA 70505
www.lgmc.com
Prgm Dir: Charlotte S Powell, MS RS LRT
Tel: 337 289-8457   *Fax:* 337 289-8660
E-mail: cpowell@lgmc.com

McNeese State University
Radiography Prgm
Box 92000
Lake Charles, LA 70609
www.mcneese.edu/radtech
Prgm Dir: Gregory L Bradley, MEd RT(R)
Tel: 337 475-5657   *Fax:* 337 475-5664
E-mail: gbradley@mcneese.edu

Career Technical College
Radiography Prgm
2319 Louisville Ave
Monroe, LA 71201
www.careertc.com

University of Louisiana at Monroe
Radiography Prgm
700 University Ave
NURS 321-E
Monroe, LA 71209-0450
www.ulm.edu/radtech

Delgado Community College
Radiography Prgm
615 City Park Ave
New Orleans, LA 70119-4399
www.dcc.edu/ahealth/rad

Our Lady of Holy Cross College
Radiography Prgm
1516 Jefferson Hwy
New Orleans, LA 70121
www.olhcc.edu
Prgm Dir: Chimene Pitre, MS RT(R)(CT)
Tel: 504 842-9208   *Fax:* 504 842-2459
E-mail: cpitre@ochsner.org

Northwestern State University
Radiography Prgm
College of Nursing and Allied Health, Radiologic
    Sciences Pr
1800 Line Ave
Shreveport, LA 71101-4653
http://radiologicsciences.nsula.edu

Southern Univ at Shreveport
Radiography Prgm
610 Texas St, #331
Shreveport, LA 71101
www.susla.edu

Maine

Eastern Maine Community College
Radiography Prgm
354 Hogan Rd
Bangor, ME 04401
www.emcc.edu
Prgm Dir: Susan Roeder, MEd RT(R)(N)
Tel: 207 974-4659   *Fax:* 207 974-4608
E-mail: sroeder@emcc.edu

Kennebec Valley Community College
Radiography Prgm
92 Western Ave
Fairfield, ME 04937
www.kvcc.me.edu

**Central Maine Medical Center College of
    Nursing & Health Professions**
Radiography Prgm
70 Middle St
Lewiston, ME 04240-0305
www.cmmccollege.edu
Prgm Dir: Judith Ripley, MS RT(R)
Tel: 207 795-5974   *Fax:* 207 344-0641
E-mail: ripleyj@cmhc.org
Notes: Hospital-based program affiliated with Central
    Maine Community College in Auburn, ME for an
    associate degree.

Southern Maine Community College
Radiography Prgm
Two Fort Rd
South Portland, ME 04106
www.smmcme.edu

Maryland

Anne Arundel Community College
Radiography Prgm
101 College Pkwy
Arnold, MD 21012-1895

Fortis Institute
Radiography Prgm
6901 Security Blvd, Ste 21
Baltimore, MD 21244

Greater Baltimore Medical Center
Radiography Prgm
6701 N Charles St
Baltimore, MD 21204
GBMC.org/schoolofradiography
Prgm Dir: Brenda Schuette, MS RT(R)(M)(QM)
Tel: 443 849-2463   *Fax:* 443 849-2866
E-mail: bschuette@gbmc.org

Johns Hopkins Hospital
Radiography Prgm
600 N Wolfe St
Blalock B179
Baltimore, MD 21287
www.radiologycareers.rad.jhmi.edu

**Community College of Baltimore County -
    Essex Campus**
Radiography Prgm
7201 Rossville Blvd
Baltimore County, MD 21237-9987
www.ccbcmd.edu/allied_health/radiography

Allegany College of Maryland
Radiography Prgm
12401 Willowbrook Rd SE
Cumberland, MD 21502-2596
www.allegany.edu

Hagerstown Community College
Radiography Prgm
11400 Robinwood Dr
Hagerstown, MD 21742-6590
www.hagerstowncc.edu

Prince George's Community College
Radiography Prgm
301 Largo Rd
Largo, MD 20774-2199
http://academic.pgcc.edu/alliedhealth
Prgm Dir: Angela Dopkowski Anderson, MA
    RT(R)(CT)(QM)
Tel: 301 322-0699   *Fax:* 301 386-7528
E-mail: aanderson@pgcc.edu

Wor-Wic Community College
Radiography Prgm
32000 Campus Dr
Salisbury, MD 21804

Holy Cross Hospital
Radiography Prgm
1500 Forest Glen Rd
Silver Spring, MD 20910

Montgomery College
Radiography Prgm
7600 Takoma Ave
Takoma Park, MD 20912

Washington Adventist Hospital
Radiography Prgm
7600 Carroll Ave
Takoma Park, MD 20912

Chesapeake College
Radiography Prgm
PO Box 8
Wye Mills, MD 21679
www.chesapeake.edu

Massachusetts

Middlesex Community College - Bedford
Radiography Prgm
Springs Rd
Bedford, MA 01730
www.mxctc.commnet.edu/index.shtml

Bunker Hill Community College
Radiography Prgm
Medical Imaging Program
250 New Rutherford Ave
Boston, MA 02129-2925
www.bhcc.mass.edu
Prgm Dir: Donna Misrati, MBA RT(R)(CT)
Tel: 617 228-2197   *Fax:* 617 228-3380
E-mail: dmisrati@bhcc.mass.edu

Mass College of Pharmacy & Health Sciences
Radiography Prgm
179 Longwood Ave
Boston, MA 02115
www.mcphs.edu/academics/programs/
    radiologic_sciences/bs_radiography/

MEDICAL IMAGING & RADIATION THERAPY

MGH Institute of Health Professions
Radiography Prgm
Charlestown Navy Yard
36 1st Ave
Boston, MA 02129-4557
www.mghihp.edu

Roxbury Community College
Radiography Prgm
1234 Columbus Ave
Boston, MA 02120
www.rcc.mass.edu/nursing

Massasoit Community College
Radiography Prgm
One Massasoit Blvd
Brockton, MA 02302
www.massasoit.mass.edu

North Shore Community College
Radiography Prgm
One Ferncroft Rd, PO Box 3340
Danvers, MA 01923-0840
www.northshore.edu
Prgm Dir: Christine E Wiley, MEd RT(R)(M)
Tel: 978 762-4163 *Fax:* 978 762-4022
E-mail: cwiley@northshore.edu

Massachusetts Bay Community College
Radiography Prgm
19 Flagg Dr
Framingham, MA 01702
www.massbay.edu

Holyoke Community College
Radiography Prgm
303 Homestead Ave
Holyoke, MA 01040
www.hcc.mass.edu

Northern Essex Community College
Radiography Prgm
45 Franklin St
Lawrence, MA 01841-4911
www.necc.mass.edu

Regis College
Cosponsor: Lawrence Memorial
Radiography Prgm
170 Governors Ave
Medford, MA 02155
www.lmregis.org

Springfield Technical Community College
Radiography Prgm
One Armory Sq PO Box 9000
Springfield, MA 01102-9000
www.stcc.edu

Quinsigamond Community College
Radiography Prgm
670 W Boylston St
Worcester, MA 01606-2092
www.qcc.mass.edu/radiography

Michigan

Washtenaw Community College
Radiography Prgm
4800 E Huron River Dr
Ann Arbor, MI 48105-4800
www.wccnet.edu
Prgm Dir: Connie Foster, MA RT(R) RDMS
Tel: 734 973-3418 *Fax:* 734 677-5078
E-mail: cfoster@wccnet.edu

Kellogg Community College
Radiography Prgm
450 North Ave
Battle Creek, MI 49017-3397
kellogg.edu/alliedhealth/radiography
Prgm Dir: Christine L VandenBerg, BS RT(R)(MR)
Tel: 269 965-3931, Ext *Fax:* 269 565-2059
E-mail: vandenbergc@kellogg.edu

Lake Michigan College
Radiography Prgm
2755 E Napier Ave
Benton Harbor, MI 49022-1899
www.lakemichigancollege.edu

Ferris State University
Radiography Prgm
901 S State St
Big Rapids, MI 49307-9989
www.ferris.edu

Baker College of Clinton Township
Radiography Prgm
34950 Little Mack Ave
Clinton Township, MI 48035-4701
www.baker.edu

Henry Ford Community College
Radiography Prgm
Health Careers Division
5101 Evergreen Rd
Dearborn, MI 48128
www.hfcc.edu

Sinai-Grace Hospital
Radiography Prgm
6071 W Outer Dr
Detroit, MI 48235
www.sinaigrace.org
Prgm Dir: Mary Elizabeth Oras, MS RT(R)
Tel: 313 966-6866 *Fax:* 313 966-1272
E-mail: moras@dmc.org

St John Health
Radiography Prgm
St John Hospital and Med Ctr, School of Radiologic Tech
22101 Moross Rd
Detroit, MI 48236-2172
www.stjohn.org/schoolofradiology

Wayne State University
Cosponsor: Henry Ford Hospital
Radiography Prgm
259 Mack Ave
Detroit, MI 48202
www.cphs.wayne.edu
Prgm Dir: Kathleen Kath, MS RT(R)(M)
Tel: 313 916-1348 *Fax:* 313 916-3049
E-mail: kathykath@wayne.edu

Hurley Medical Center
Radiography Prgm
One Hurley Plaza
Flint, MI 48503-5993
www.hurleymc.com

Grand Rapids Community College
Radiography Prgm
143 Bostwick St NE
Grand Rapids, MI 49503

Mid Michigan Community College
Radiography Prgm
1375 S Clare Ave
Harrison, MI 48625-9447
www.midmich.edu

Jackson Community College
Radiography Prgm
2111 Emmons Rd
Jackson, MI 49201-8395

Lansing Community College
Radiography Prgm
Dept 3100 Health & Human Service Careers
 PO Box 40010
Lansing, MI 48901-7210
www.lcc.edu
Prgm Dir: Brian W Pickford, MS H E RT(R)
Tel: 517 483-5379 *Fax:* 517 483-1508
E-mail: pickforb@lcc.edu

Northern Michigan University
Radiography Prgm
Marquette, MI 49855

Baker College of Muskegon
Radiography Prgm
1903 Marquette Ave
Muskegon, MI 49442-1490
www.baker.edu

Baker College of Owosso
Radiography Prgm
1020 S Washington St
Owosso, MI 48867-4400
www.baker.edu

Port Huron Hospital
Radiography Prgm
1221 Pine Grove, PO Box 5011
Port Huron, MI 48061-5011
www.porthuronhospital.org

Beaumont Hospital - Royal Oak
Radiography Prgm
3601 W 13 Mile Rd
Royal Oak, MI 48073
www.beaumonthospitals.com
Prgm Dir: Terese A Trost, MA RT(R)
Tel: 248 551-6048 *Fax:* 248 551-5015
E-mail: ttrost@beaumont.edu

Oakland Community College - Southfield
Radiography Prgm
22322 Rutland Dr
Southfield, MI 48075-4793
www.oaklandcc.edu

Providence Hospital
Radiography Prgm
16001 W Nine Mile Rd, PO Box 2043
Southfield, MI 48037
www.stjohn.org/AlliedHealth/RadiologicTech/
Prgm Dir: Mary A Kleven, MAOM BS RT(R)(M)
Tel: 248 849-3293 *Fax:* 248 849-5397
E-mail: Mary.Kleven@stjohn.org

Delta College
Radiography Prgm
1961 Delta Rd
University Center, MI 48710

Minnesota

Riverland Community College
Radiography Prgm
1900 8th Ave NW
Austin, MN 55912
www.riverland.edu
Prgm Dir: Sandra J Nauman, MS RT(R)(M)
Tel: 507 433-0365 *Fax:* 507 433-0515
E-mail: sandra.nauman@riverland.edu

Minnesota State Community and Technical Coll - Detroit Lakes Campus
Radiography Prgm
900 Hwy 34 East
Detroit Lakes, MN 56501

Lake Superior College
Radiography Prgm
2101 Trinity Rd
Duluth, MN 55811-2741
www.lsc.edu
Prgm Dir: Britni S Hardy, MHA RT(R)
Tel: 218 733-7713   *Fax:* 218 733-7615
E-mail: b.hardy@lsc.edu

Argosy University Twin Cities Campus
Radiography Prgm
1515 Central Parkway
Eagan, MN 55121
www.argosyu.edu

Northland Community & Technical College
Radiography Prgm
2022 Central Ave NE
East Grand Forks, MN 56721-2702
www.northlandcollege.edu

Minnesota West Comm & Tech College
Radiography Prgm
311 N Spring St
Luverne, MN 56156

Dunwoody College of Technology
Radiography Prgm
818 Dunwoody Boulevard
Minneapolis, MN 55403

Saint Catherine University - Minneapolis
Radiography Prgm
601 25th Ave S
Minneapolis, MN 55454
www.stkate.edu

Veterans Affairs Medical Center
Radiography Prgm
One Veterans Dr
Minneapolis, MN 55417
www1.va.gov/minneapolis/education/educ_main.html

Mayo School of Health Sciences
Cosponsor: Mayo Clinic
Radiography Prgm
Siebens Rm 1119
200 First St SW
Rochester, MN 55905
www.mayo.edu/mshs

St Cloud Hospital
Radiography Prgm
1406 Sixth Ave N
St Cloud, MN 56303
www.centracare.com
Prgm Dir: Deanna Butcher, MA RT(R)
Tel: 320 255-5719, Ext   *Fax:* 320 255-5730
E-mail: butcherd@centracare.com

Century College
Radiography Prgm
3300 Century Ave N
White Bear Lake, MN 55110
www.century.edu

Rice Memorial Hospital
Radiography Prgm
301 Becker Ave SW
Willmar, MN 56201-3302

Minnesota State College, Southeast Technical
Radiography Prgm
1250 Homer Road
Winona, MN 55987

Mississippi

Northeast Mississippi Community College
Radiography Prgm
101 Cunningham Blvd
Booneville, MS 38829
www.nemcc.edu

Jones County Junior College
Radiography Prgm
900 S Court St
Ellisville, MS 39437
www.jcjc.edu

Itawamba Community College
Radiography Prgm
602 W Hill St
Fulton, MS 38843-0999

Mississippi Gulf Coast Community College
Radiography Prgm
PO Box 100
Gautier, MS 39553

Pearl River Community College
Radiography Prgm
5448 US Hwy 49 S
Hattiesburg, MS 39401

University of Mississippi Medical Center
Radiography Prgm
School of Health Related Professions
2500 N State St
Jackson, MS 39216-4505
shrp.umc.edu

Meridian Community College
Radiography Prgm
910 Hwy 19 N
Meridian, MS 39307
www.mcc.cc.ms.us

Mississippi Delta Community College
Radiography Prgm
PO Box 668
Moorhead, MS 38761
www.msdelta.edu
Prgm Dir: Alice K Pyles, MS RS RT(R)
Tel: 601 246-6504   *Fax:* 601 246-6507
E-mail: apyles@msdelta.edu

Hinds Community College
Radiography Prgm
PMB 10458
Raymond, MS 39154-9799
www.hindscc.edu
Prgm Dir: Stephen C Compton, MSEd RT(R)
Tel: 601 376-4826   *Fax:* 601 376-4962
E-mail: sccompton@hindscc.edu

Copiah-Lincoln Community College
Radiography Prgm
PO Box 649
Wesson, MS 39191
www.colin.edu/careertech/Radiology

Missouri

Southeast Missouri Hospital Coll of Nursing
Radiography Prgm
2001 William St, 2nd Floor
Cape Girardeau, MO 63703
www.sehcollege.org

University of Missouri
Radiography Prgm
School of Health Professions
605 Lewis Hall
Columbia, MO 65211
healthprofessions.missouri.edu/cpd/RS

Sanford-Brown College
Radiography Prgm
Fenton Campus
1345 Smizer Mill Rd
Fenton, MO 63026

Nichols Career Center
Radiography Prgm
605 Union St
Jefferson City, MO 65101
www.nicholscareercenter.org

Missouri Southern State University
Radiography Prgm
3950 E Newman Rd
Joplin, MO 64801-1595
www.mssu.edu

Avila University
Radiography Prgm
11901 Wornall Rd
Kansas City, MO 64145-9990

Colorado Technical University
Radiography Prgm
520 E 19th Ave
Kansas City, MO 64116

Metropolitan Community College - Penn Valley
Radiography Prgm
3444 Broadway
Kansas City, MO 64111
www.mcckc.edu

Research Medical Center
Radiography Prgm
2316 E Meyer Blvd
Kansas City, MO 64132-1199
http://researchmedicalcenter.com

Saint Luke's Hospital
Radiography Prgm
4401 Wornall Rd
Kansas City, MO 64111
www.saint-lukes.org

Mineral Area College
Radiography Prgm
PO Box 1000
5270 Flat River Rd
Park Hills, MO 63601
www.mineralarea.edu

Rolla Technical Center
Radiography Prgm
500 Forum Dr
Rolla, MO 65401-3699

State Fair Community College
Radiography Prgm
3201 W 16th St
Sedalia, MO 65301

Cox Medical Centers
Cosponsor: Cox College
Radiography Prgm
1423 N Jefferson Ave
Springfield, MO 65802
www.coxcollege.edu

Mercy Hospital Springfield
Radiography Prgm
1235 E Cherokee St
Springfield, MO 65804-2263
www.mercy.net/springfieldmo
Prgm Dir: Joan Hedrick, MEd RT(R)(M)
Tel: 417 820-2982   *Fax:* 417 820-3427
E-mail: Joan.Hedrick@mercy.net

Hillyard Technical Center
Radiography Prgm
3434 Faraon St
St Joseph, MO 64506

Moberly Area Community College
Radiography Prgm
615 South New Ballas Rd
St Louis, MO 63141
www.stjohnsmercy.org

St Louis Community College - Forest Park
Radiography Prgm
5600 Oakland Ave
St Louis, MO 63110
www.stlcc.edu

Nebraska

Mary Lanning Memorial Healthcare
Radiography Prgm
715 N St Joseph Ave
Hastings, NE 68901
www.mlmh.org
Prgm Dir: Cristi L Engel, MSRS RT(R)(CV)
Tel: 402 461-5170   *Fax:* 402 461-5059
E-mail: cengel@mlmh.org

Southeast Community College
Radiography Prgm
8800 O St
Lincoln, NE 68520
www.southeast.edu

Alegent Health
Radiography Prgm
7500 Mercy Rd
Omaha, NE 68124
www.alegent.com

Clarkson College
Radiography Prgm
101 S 42nd St
Omaha, NE 68131-2739
clarksoncollege.edu
Prgm Dir: Ellen L Collins, MS RT(R)(M)
Tel: 402 552-6140   *Fax:* 402 552-6019
E-mail: collins@clarksoncollege.edu

Nebraska Methodist College
Radiography Prgm
720 North 87th St
Omaha, NE 68114

University of Nebraska Medical Center
Radiography Prgm
984545 Nebraska Medical Center
Omaha, NE 68198-4545
www.unmc.edu/alliedhealth/rste

Regional West Medical Center
Radiography Prgm
4021 Ave B
Scottsbluff, NE 69361
www.rwmc.net/SORT
Prgm Dir: Daniel R Gilbert, MSEd
   RT(R)(CV)(MR)(CT)(QM)
Tel: 308 630-1155   *Fax:* 308 630-1983
E-mail: gilberd@rwmc.net

Nevada

Great Basin College
Radiography Prgm
1500 College Parkway
Elko, NV 89801

Pima Medical Institute
Radiography Prgm
3333 E Flamingo Rd
Las Vegas, NV 89121
www.pima.edu

University of Nevada - Las Vegas
Radiography Prgm
4505 Maryland Pkwy
Las Vegas, NV 89154-3017
www.unlv.edu

New Hampshire

NHTI, Concord's Community College
Radiography Prgm
31 College Dr
Concord, NH 03301-7412
www.nhti.edu

Lebanon College
Radiography Prgm
15 Hanover St
Lebanon, NH 03766
www.lebanoncollege.edu

New Jersey

Cooper University Hospital
Radiography Prgm
One Cooper Plaza, D-408 S
Camden, NJ 08103
www.cooperhealth.org

Middlesex County College
Radiography Prgm
2600 Woodbridge Ave, PO Box 3050
Edison, NJ 08818-3050
www.middlesexcc.edu
Prgm Dir: James M Ferrell, MPA ARRT NJLRT
Tel: 732 906-2583   *Fax:* 732 906-7784
E-mail: JFerrell@middlesexcc.edu

Englewood Hospital & Medical Center
Radiography Prgm
350 Engle St
Englewood, NJ 07631
www.englewoodhospital.com

Christ Hospital School of Radiography
Radiography Prgm
176 Palisade Ave
Jersey City, NJ 07306
christhospital.org

Brookdale Community College
Radiography Prgm
765 Newman Springs Rd
Lincroft, NJ 07738
www.brookdalecc.edu/pages/873.asp

Essex County College
Radiography Prgm
School of Health Related Professions
Medical Imaging Sciences, Stanley S Bergen Building
65 Bergen St
Newark, NJ 07107-1709
http://shrp.umdnj.edu

Bergen Community College
Radiography Prgm
400 Paramus Rd
Paramus, NJ 07652
www.bergen.edu

Passaic County Community College
Radiography Prgm
One College Blvd
Paterson, NJ 07505-1179
pccc.edu

Burlington County College
Radiography Prgm
601 Pemberton Browns Mills Rd
Pemberton, NJ 08068
www.bcc.edu

JFK Medical Center - Muhlenberg Schools
Radiography Prgm
Park Ave and Randolph Rd
Plainfield, NJ 07061
http://muhlenbergschools.org

County College of Morris
Radiography Prgm
214 Center Grove Rd
Randolph, NJ 07869

The Valley Hospital
Radiography Prgm
223 N Van Dien Ave
Ridgewood, NJ 07450
www.valleyhealth.com/radschool
Prgm Dir: Maureen K Wolf, MAS RT(R)(N)
Tel: 201 447-8221   *Fax:* 201 251-3280
E-mail: mwolf@valleyhealth.com

Shore Memorial Hospital
Radiography Prgm
1 E New York Ave
Somers Point, NJ 08244-2387

Mercer County Community College
Radiography Prgm
1200 Old Trenton Rd, PO Box B
Trenton, NJ 08690
www.mccc.edu

St Francis Medical Center
Radiography Prgm
601 Hamilton Ave
Trenton, NJ 08629-1986
www.stfrancismedical.com
Prgm Dir: Theresa M Levitsky, MA RT(R)(CV)(M)(QM)
Tel: 609 599-5234   *Fax:* 609 599-5529
E-mail: tlevitsky@stfrancismedical.org

Cumberland County College
Radiography Prgm
College Dr, PO Box 1500
Vineland, NJ 08362-1500

New Mexico

Pima Medical Institute - Albuquerque
Radiography Prgm
4400 Cutler Ave NE
Albuquerque, NM 87110
www.pimamedical.com

Clovis Community College
Radiography Prgm
417 Schepps Blvd
Clovis, NM 88101
www.clovis.edu

Northern New Mexico College
Radiography Prgm
921 Paseo de Onate
Espanola, NM 87532
www.nnmc.edu

Dona Ana Community College
Radiography Prgm
MSC 3DA PO Box 30001
3400 S Espina St
Las Cruces, NM 88003-8001
http://dacc.nmsu.edu

New York

Broome Community College
Radiography Prgm
1014 Upper Front St
Binghamton, NY 13901
http://sunybroome.edu
Prgm Dir: Dominick DeMichele, MSEd RT(R)(CT)
Tel: 607 778-5070   *Fax:* 607 778-5467
E-mail: demicheled@sunybroome.edu

Bronx Community College
Radiography Prgm
2155 University Ave
CP Hall Room 222
Bronx, NY 10453
www.bcc.cuny.edu
Prgm Dir: Virginia M Mishkin, MS RT (R) (M) (QM)
Tel: 718 289-5396   *Fax:* 718 289-6373
E-mail: virginia.mishkin@bcc.cuny.edu

Hostos Community College of CUNY
Radiography Prgm
500 Grand Concourse A-307
Bronx, NY 10451

New York City College of Technology
Radiography Prgm
300 Jay St
Brooklyn, NY 11201-2983

New York Methodist Hospital - Bartone Center for Allied Hlth Education
Radiography Prgm
1401 Kings Highway
Brooklyn, NY 11229
www.nymahe.org

SUNY Downstate University Hospital Brooklyn @
Radiography Prgm
339 Hicks St
Brooklyn, NY 11201
www.wehealnewyork.org

Long Island University - C W Post Campus
Radiography Prgm
720 Northern Blvd
Brookville, NY 11548-1300
www.liu.edu/radtech
Prgm Dir: James F Joyce, MS RT(R)(M)(QM)
Tel: 516 299-3075   *Fax:* 516 299-3081
E-mail: jjoyce@liu.edu

Trocaire College
Radiography Prgm
360 Choate Ave
Buffalo, NY 14220
www.trocaire.edu

Arnot Ogden Medical Center
Radiography Prgm
600 Roe Ave
Elmira, NY 14905-1676
www.arnothealth.org
Prgm Dir: Ellen R Richards, MPS RT(R)
Tel: 607 737-4289   *Fax:* 607 737-4116
E-mail: erichards@aomc.org

Glens Falls Hospital
Radiography Prgm
School of Radiologic Technology
126 South St
Glens Falls, NY 12801
www.glensfallshospital.org

St James Mercy Health System
Cosponsor: St James Mercy Hospital
Radiography Prgm
411 Canisteo St
Hornell, NY 14843
www.stjamesmercy.org

Woman's Christian Association Hospital
Radiography Prgm
207 Foote Ave
Jamestown, NY 14701-0840
www.wcahospital.org

Orange County Community College
Radiography Prgm
115 South St
Middletown, NY 10940
www.sunyorange.edu

Bellevue Hospital Center
Radiography Prgm
First Ave and 27th St, C&D Bldg, Rm D510
New York, NY 10016

Harlem Hospital Center
Radiography Prgm
506 Lenox Ave
Kountz Pavilion Rm 415
New York, NY 10037
www.harlemhospitalxrayschool.com

Robt J Hochstime Sch Rad/S Nassau Comm Hosp
Radiography Prgm
One Healthy Way
Oceanside, NY 11572
http://snch.org
Prgm Dir: Gina Collins, MPA RT(R)(M)
Tel: 516 632-4678   *Fax:* 516 632-4791
E-mail: gcollins@snch.org

CVPH Medical Center
Radiography Prgm
75 Beekman St
Plattsburgh, NY 12901
cvph.org
Prgm Dir: Douglas E Osborn, MSHA RT(R)
Tel: 518 562-7510   *Fax:* 518 562-7486
E-mail: dosborn@cvph.org

St John's University
Radiography Prgm
8000 Utopia Pkwy
Queens, NY 11439
www.stjohns.edu

Peconic Bay Medical Center School of Radiologic Technology
Radiography Prgm
1300 Roanoke Ave
Room 4303
Riverhead, NY 11901
Prgm Dir: Frank A Zaleski, MBA RT (R)
Tel: 631 548-6183   *Fax:* 631 548-6751
E-mail: fzaleski@pbmedicalcenter.org

Monroe Community College
Radiography Prgm
1000 E Henrietta Rd
Rochester, NY 14623-5780
www.monroecc.edu
Prgm Dir: Eileen M Doyle, MPA RT(R)
Tel: 585 292-2379   *Fax:* 585 292-3834
E-mail: edoyle@monroecc.edu

Mercy Medical Center
Radiography Prgm
PO Box 9024
1000 N Village Ave
Rockville Centre, NY 11571-9024

Niagara County Community College
Radiography Prgm
3111 Saunders Settlement Rd
Sanborn, NY 14132

North Country Community College
Radiography Prgm
23 Santanoni Ave, PO Box 89
Saranac Lake, NY 12983-0089
www.nccc.edu
Prgm Dir: Elizabeth Ann Wasson, MS RT(R)(M)
Tel: 518 891-2915, Ext   *Fax:* 518 891-2915
E-mail: ewasson@nccc.edu

SUNY Upstate Medical University
Radiography Prgm
Medical Imaging Sciences Program
750 E Adams St
Syracuse, NY 13210

Faxton - St Luke's Healthcare
Radiography Prgm
Champlain Ave, PO Box 479
Utica, NY 13503-0479
www.mvnhealth.com

St Elizabeth Medical Center
Radiography Prgm
2209 Genesee St
Utica, NY 13501
www.stemc.org

Westchester Community College
Radiography Prgm
75 Grasslands Rd
Valhalla, NY 10595-1698

St Joseph's Medical Center
Radiography Prgm
127 S Broadway
Yonkers, NY 10701
www.saintjosephs.org

North Carolina

Asheville-Buncombe Technical Comm College
Radiography Prgm
340 Victoria Rd
Asheville, NC 28801
www.abtech.edu
Prgm Dir: Debra Reese, MPH RT(R)
Tel: 828 254-1921, Ext   *Fax:* 828 281-9846
E-mail: debrajreese@abtech.edu

South College - Asheville
Radiography Prgm
29 Turtle Creek Drive
Asheville, NC 28803
www.southcollegenc.edu

University of North Carolina - Chapel Hill
Radiography Prgm
CB 7130 Suite 3050 Bondurant Hall
Chapel Hill, NC 27599-7130
www.med.unc.edu/ahs/radisci

Carolinas College of Health Sciences
Radiography Prgm
PO Box 32861
1200 Blythe Blvd
Charlotte, NC 28232-2861
www.CarolinasCollege.edu

Presbyterian Healthcare
Radiography Prgm
200 Hawthorne Ln, PO Box 33549
Charlotte, NC 28233-3549
www.presbyterian.org
Prgm Dir: Elizabeth S Shields, MHA RT(R)
Tel: 704 384-5104   *Fax:* 704 384-5717
E-mail: esshields@novanthealth.org

Fayetteville Technical Community College
Radiography Prgm
PO Box 35236
Fayetteville, NC 28303-0236
www.faytechcc.edu

Pitt Community College
Radiography Prgm
PO Drawer 7007, Hwy 11 S
Greenville, NC 27835-7007
www.pittcc.edu

Vance-Granville Community College
Radiography Prgm
PO Box 917
Henderson, NC 27536

Catawba Valley Community College
Radiography Prgm
2550 Hwy 70 SE
Hickory, NC 28602
www.cvcc.edu

Caldwell Comm College & Tech Institute
Radiography Prgm
2855 Hickory Blvd
Hudson, NC 28638

Guilford Technical Community College
Radiography Prgm
PO Box 309
601 High Point Rd
Jamestown, NC 27282

Lenoir Community College
Radiography Prgm
PO Box 188
Kinston, NC 28502-0188

Carteret Community College
Radiography Prgm
3505 Arendell St
Morehead City, NC 28557-2989
www.carteret.edu

Wilkes Regional Medical Center
Radiography Prgm
1508 West D St, PO Box 609
North Wilkesboro, NC 28659
www.wilkesregional.com

Sandhills Community College
Radiography Prgm
3395 Airport Rd
Pinehurst, NC 28374
www.sandhills.edu

Wake Technical Community College
Radiography Prgm
9101 Fayetteville Rd
Raleigh, NC 27603-5696
www.waketech.edu

Edgecombe Community College
Radiography Prgm
225 Tarboro St
Rocky Mount, NC 27801
www.edgecombe.edu

Rowan-Cabarrus Community College
Radiography Prgm
PO Box 1595
Salisbury, NC 28145-1595
www.rowancabarrus.edu

Cleveland Community College
Radiography Prgm
137 S Post Rd
Shelby, NC 28152
www.clevelandcommunitycollege.edu

Johnston Community College
Radiography Prgm
PO Box 2350
Smithfield, NC 27577-2350
www.johnstoncc.edu

Southwestern Community College
Radiography Prgm
447 College Dr
Sylva, NC 28779

Cape Fear Community College
Radiography Prgm
411 N Front St
Wilmington, NC 28401

Forsyth Technical Community College
Radiography Prgm
2100 Silas Creek Pkwy
Winston-Salem, NC 27103

North Dakota

Medcenter One
Radiography Prgm
300 N 7th St
Bismarck, ND 58506-5525

Sanford Medical Center/Sanford Health
Radiography Prgm
801 N Broadway
Fargo, ND 58122
www.meritcare.com

Trinity Health
Radiography Prgm
407 3rd St NE
Minot, ND 58701
www.trinityhealth.org

Ohio

Akron Children's Hospital
Radiography Prgm
One Perkins Square
Akron, OH 44308
www.akronchildrens.org
Prgm Dir: David L Whipple, MEd RT(R)
Tel: 330 543-8849, Ext 3   *Fax:* 330 543-8282
E-mail: dwhipple@chmca.org

Kent State University
Radiography Prgm
3300 Lake Rd West
Ashtabula, OH 44004

University of Cincinnati
Radiography Prgm
9555 Plainfield Rd
Blue Ash, OH 45236
www.rwc.uc.edu

Aultman College of Nursing and Health Science
Radiography Prgm
2600 Sixth St SW
Canton, OH 44710
www.aultman.org

Mercy Medical Center
Radiography Prgm
1320 Mercy Dr NW
Canton, OH 44708
www.cantonmercy.org
Prgm Dir: Gary F Greathouse, MS RT(R)
Tel: 330 489-1273, Ext   *Fax:* 330 588-4593
E-mail: gary.greathouse@cantonmercy.org

Collins Career Center
Radiography Prgm
11627 State Route 243
Chesapeake, OH 45619
www.collins-cc.edu

Xavier University
Radiography Prgm
3800 Victory Pkwy
Cincinnati, OH 45207-7332
www.xavier.edu
Prgm Dir: Donna J Endicott, MEd RT(R)
Tel: 513 745-3358   *Fax:* 513 745-3246
E-mail: endicott@xavier.edu

Columbus State Community College
Radiography Prgm
550 E Spring St
GR389
Columbus, OH 43216
www.cscc.edu/radiography

Sinclair Community College
Radiography Prgm
444 W Third St
Dayton, OH 45402-1460
www.sinclair.edu/departments/rat

Lorain County Community College
Radiography Prgm
1005 N Abbe Rd, HS223
Elyria, OH 44035
www.lorainccc.edu
Prgm Dir: Jeffrey J Walmsley, MEd RT(R)(QM)
Tel: 440 366-7197   *Fax:* 440 366-4116
E-mail: jwalmsle@lorainccc.edu

Cleveland Clinic Health System /Euclid Hospital
Radiography Prgm
18901 Lakeshore Blvd
Euclid, OH 44119
www.cchseast.org/schools

Kettering College of Medical Arts
Radiography Prgm
3737 Southern Blvd
Kettering, OH 45429
http://kcma.edu

Lakeland Community College
Radiography Prgm
7700 Clocktower Dr
Kirtland, OH 44094-5198
www.lakelandcc.edu/academic/sh/rad

Rhodes State College
Radiography Prgm
4240 Campus Dr
Lima, OH 45804-3597

North Central State College
Radiography Prgm
2441 Kenwood Circle, PO Box 698
Mansfield, OH 44901-0698
www.ncstatecollege.edu

Marietta Memorial Hospital
Radiography Prgm
401 Matthew St
Marietta, OH 45750
Prgm Dir: Paul E Richards, Jr, MA RT(R)
Tel: 740 374-8716, Ext   *Fax:* 740 373-7496
E-mail: prichards@wscc.edu

Marion Technical College
Radiography Prgm
1467 Mt Vernon Ave
Marion, OH 43302-5694
www.mtc.edu

Sanford-Brown College
Radiography Prgm
Middleburg Heights, OH 44130

Central Ohio Technical College
Radiography Prgm
1179 University Dr
Newark, OH 43055-1767
www.cotc.edu

Cuyahoga Community College
Radiography Prgm
Western Campus
11000 Pleasant Valley Rd
Parma, OH 44130-5199
www.tri-c.edu/programs/healthcareers/radiography/
   Pages/default.aspx
Prgm Dir: Elizabeth Gildone
Tel: 216 987-5264   *Fax:* 216 987-5066
E-mail: elizabeth.gildone@tri-c.edu

Shawnee State University
Radiography Prgm
940 Second St
Portsmouth, OH 45662-4344
www.shawnee.edu
Prgm Dir: William W Sykes, MBA
   RT(R)(M)(CT)(MR)(QM)
Tel: 740 351-3253   *Fax:* 740 351-3354
E-mail: bsykes@shawnee.edu

University of Rio Grande
Cosponsor: Rio Grande Community College
Radiography Prgm
PO Box 500
Rio Grande, OH 45674

Kent State University - Salem Campus
Radiography Prgm
2491 State Route 45 South
Salem, OH 44460-9412
www.salem.kent.edu
Prgm Dir: Janice J Gibson, MEd RT(R)
Tel: 330 337-4223   *Fax:* 330 337-4255
E-mail: jjgibso1@kent.edu

Eastern Gateway Community College
Radiography Prgm
4000 Sunset Blvd
Steubenville, OH 43952-3598
www.jcc.edu

Mercy College of Northwest Ohio
Radiography Prgm
2221 Madison Ave
Toledo, OH 43624-1132
www.mercycollege.edu

Owens Community College
Radiography Prgm
PO Box 10,000
Toledo, OH 43699-1947
www.owens.edu

Fortis College-Westerville
Radiography Prgm
Westerville, OH 43081

Zane State College
Radiography Prgm
1555 Newark Rd
Zanesville, OH 43701
www.zanestate.edu

Oklahoma

Western Oklahoma State College
Radiography Prgm
2801 N Main
Altus, OK 73521-1397
www.wosc.edu

Autry Technology Center
Radiography Prgm
1201 W Willow
Enid, OK 73703
www.autrytech.com

Great Plains Technology Center
Radiography Prgm
4500 W Lee Blvd
Lawton, OK 73505
www.greatplains.edu/rad
Prgm Dir: Carrie L Baxter, MEd RT(R)(M)(CT)
Tel: 580 250-5577   *Fax:* 580 250-5583
E-mail: cbaxter@greatplains.edu
Notes: The program does not award degrees but has a
agreement for transferring credits earned to the
college for an AAS in Radiologic Technology program.

Rose State College
Radiography Prgm
6420 SE 15th St
Health Sciences Division
Midwest City, OK 73110-2799
www.rose.edu/students.hsdiv/rad_prog/

Bacone College
Radiography Prgm
2299 Old Bacone Rd
Muskogee, OK 74403-1568
www.bacone.edu

Indian Capital Technology Center
Radiography Prgm
2403 N 41st St E
Muskogee, OK 74403-1799

Metro Tech Health Careers Center
Radiography Prgm
1720 Springlake Dr
Oklahoma City, OK 73111
www.metrotech.org

Univ of Oklahoma Health Sciences Center
Radiography Prgm
801 NE 13th St, CHB-451
PO Box 26901
Oklahoma City, OK 73126

Carl Albert State College
Radiography Prgm
1507 S McKenna
Poteau, OK 74953
www.carlalbert.edu

Southwestern Oklahoma State University
Radiography Prgm
409 E Mississippi
Sayre, OK 73662-1236
www.swosu.edu/sayre
Prgm Dir: Chris Stufflebean, MBA RT(R)
Tel: 580 928-5533, Ext   *Fax:* 580 928-5533
E-mail: chris.stufflebean@swosu.edu

Meridian Technology Center
Radiography Prgm
1312 S Sangre Rd
Stillwater, OK 74074-1841
www.meridian-technology.com

Tulsa Community College
Radiography Prgm
909 S Boston Ave
Tulsa, OK 74119-7263
www.tulsacc.edu
Prgm Dir: Benedict J Middleton, MS RT(R)
Tel: 918 595-7012   *Fax:* 918 595-7091
E-mail: rmiddlet@tulsacc.edu

Tulsa Technology Center
Radiography Prgm
801 E 91st St
Tulsa, OK 74132
www.tulsatech.org

Oregon

Portland Community College
Radiography Prgm
12000 SW 49th Ave, PO Box 19000
Portland, OR 97280-0990
www.pcc.edu/academ/radtech

Pennsylvania

Northampton Community College
Radiography Prgm
3835 Green Pond Rd
Bethlehem, PA 18020
www.northampton.edu
Prgm Dir: Zoland Z Zile III (retiring 6, MS RT(R)(QM)
Tel: 610 861-5387   *Fax:* 610 861-4581
E-mail: zzile@northampton.edu

**Bradford Regional Medical Center /Upper
   Allegheny Health System**
Radiography Prgm
116 Interstate Pkwy
Bradford, PA 16701
http://BRMC.com

Harcum College
Radiography Prgm
750 Montgomery Ave
Bryn Mawr, PA 19010-3158
harcum.edu

Holy Spirit Hospital
Radiography Prgm
503 N 21st St
Camp Hill, PA 17011-2288
www.hsh.org/healthcare-education/
Prgm Dir: Kevin L Otto, MS RT(R)
Tel: 717 763-2123   *Fax:* 717 972-4640
E-mail: kotto@hsh.org

Clearfield Hospital
Radiography Prgm
809 Turnpike Ave, PO Box 992
Clearfield, PA 16830
www.clearfieldhospital.org

Misericordia University
Radiography Prgm
Medical Imaging Program
301 Lake St
Dallas, PA 18612-1098
www.misericordia.edu/mi
Prgm Dir: Elaine Halesey, EdD RT(R)(QM)
Tel: 570 674-6480   *Fax:* 570 674-1497
E-mail: ehalesey@misericordia.edu

Geisinger Medical Center
Radiography Prgm
100 North Academy Ave
Danville, PA 17822-2007
www.geisinger.org

Fortis Institute-Erie
Radiography Prgm
5757 W 26th St
Erie, PA 16505

Gannon University
Radiography Prgm
109 University Square
Erie, PA 16541-0001
www.gannon.edu
Prgm Dir: Cynthia L Liotta, MS RT(R)(CT)
Tel: 814 871-5644   *Fax:* 814 871-5662
E-mail: liotta@gannon.edu

Conemaugh Valley Memorial Hospital
Radiography Prgm
1086 Franklin St
Johnstown, PA 15905-4398
http://ww.conemaugh.org/SchoolofRadTech
Prgm Dir: Gloria J Mongelluzzo, MEd RT(R)(M)
Tel: 814 534-9582   *Fax:* 814 534-5649
E-mail: gmongell@conemaugh.org

Armstrong County Memorial Hospital
Radiography Prgm
One Nolte Dr
Kittanning, PA 16201
www.acmh.org
Prgm Dir: Glenna Kanish, MAEd RTRM
Tel: 724 543-8206   *Fax:* 724 543-8652
E-mail: kanishg@acmh.org

Harrisburg Area Community College
Radiography Prgm
1641 Old Philadelphia Pike
Lancaster, PA 17602
www.hacc.edu

Lancaster Gen Coll of Nursing & Hlth Sciences
Radiography Prgm
410 N Lime St
Lancaster, PA 17602
www.lancastergeneralcollege.edu

Ohio Valley General Hospital
Radiography Prgm
25 Heckel Rd
McKees Rocks, PA 15136
www.ohiovalleyhospital.org

Community College of Allegheny County
Radiography Prgm
595 Beatty Rd
Monroeville, PA 15146-1395
www.ccac.edu

Jameson Hospital
Radiography Prgm
1000 S Mercer St
New Castle, PA 16101
www.jamesonhealthsystem.com/departments/
    radiology_school.htm

Penn State University - New Kensington
Radiography Prgm
3550 Seventh St Rd Rte 780
New Kensington, PA 15068

Bucks County Community College
Radiography Prgm
275 Swamp Rd, AHB BLDG
Newtown, PA 18940
www.bucks.edu/healthcare/radiography

Albert Einstein Medical Center
Radiography Prgm
5501 Old York Rd
Philadelphia, PA 19141
einsteinxray.org

Community College of Philadelphia
Radiography Prgm
1700 Spring Garden St
Philadelphia, PA 19130-3991
www.ccp.edu

Drexel University College of Medicine
Radiography Prgm
1505 Race St, MS 508
Philadelphia, PA 19102-1192
www.drexel.edu

Holy Family University
Radiography Prgm
Grant and Frankford Aves
9701 Frankford Ave
Philadelphia, PA 19114
www.holyfamily.edu

Penn Medicine - Hospital of the U of Penn
Radiography Prgm
3400 Spruce St Basement Donner Building
RT Education Program - Radiology
Philadelphia, PA 19104
www.uphs.upenn.edu/radiology/educ/RTed/

St Christopher Hospital School of Rad Tech
Radiography Prgm
Erie Ave at Front
Philadelphia, PA 19134
Prgm Dir: Dorothy Gray, MHS RT(R)
Tel: 215 427-6751   *Fax:* 215 427-5171
E-mail: Dorothy.Gray@tenethealth.com

Thomas Jefferson University
Radiography Prgm
901 Walnut St
Philadelphia, PA 19107-5233
www.jefferson.edu/health_professions/
    Radiologic_Sciences/
Prgm Dir: Matthew Marquess, MBA RT(T)
Tel: 215 503-1434   *Fax:* 215 503-1031
E-mail: matthew.marquess@jefferson.edu

Sanford-Brown Institute
Radiography Prgm
421 7th Ave
Pittsburgh, PA 15219
www.sanfordbrown.edu

Montgomery County Community College
Radiography Prgm
101 College Dr
Pottstown, PA 19464
www.mc3.edu/academics/programs/rt.aspx

Reading Hospital & Medical Center
Radiography Prgm
PO Box 16052
Reading, PA 19612-6052
www.readinghospital.org

Mansfield University
Radiography Prgm
One Guthrie Square
Sayre, PA 18840

Penn State University - Schuylkill Haven
Radiography Prgm
200 University Dr
Schuylkill Haven, PA 17972-0308
www.psu.edu

Johnson College
Radiography Prgm
3427 N Main Ave
Scranton, PA 18508-1495

UPMC Northwest
Radiography Prgm
100 Fairfield Dr
Seneca, PA 16346
www.upmc.edu

Sharon Regional Health System
Radiography Prgm
740 E State St
Sharon, PA 16146-3395
www.sharonregional.com/schoolradiation.htm

Crozer-Keystone Medical Center
Radiography Prgm
One Medical Center Blvd
Upland, PA 19013

Washington Hospital
Radiography Prgm
155 Wilson Ave
Washington, PA 15301
washingtonhospital.org
Prgm Dir: Karen C Williams, MA RT(R)(QM)
Tel: 724 223-3326   *Fax:* 724 250-4417
E-mail: kwilliams@washingtonhospital.org

Pennsylvania College of Technology
Radiography Prgm
One College Ave
Williamsport, PA 17701-5799
www.pct.edu

Abington Memorial Hospital
Radiography Prgm
2500 Maryland Rd
Willow Grove, PA 19090-1284
www.amh.org

York Hospital/WellSpan Health
Radiography Prgm
37 Monument Rd, Ste 101
York, PA 17403
www.wellspan.org/body.cfm?id=306

Puerto Rico

Universidad Central del Caribe
Radiography Prgm
PO Box 60327
Bayamon, PR 00960-6032
www.uccaribe.edu

Inter American University of Puerto Rico
Radiography Prgm
PO Box 5100
San German, PR 00683-9801
www.sg.inter.edu

University of Puerto Rico
Radiography Prgm
GPO Box 5067
San Juan, PR 00936-5067

Rhode Island

Community College of Rhode Island
Radiography Prgm
Flanagan Campus
1762 Louisquisset Pike
Lincoln, RI 02865-4585
www.ccri.edu

Rhode Island Hospital
Radiography Prgm
3 Davol Square
Bldg A - 4th Fl
Providence, RI 02903
www.rihsdi.org
Prgm Dir: Ellen E Alexandre, MBA RT(R)
Tel: 401 528-8531   *Fax:* 401 457-0219
E-mail: ealexandre@lifespan.org

South Carolina

Aiken Technical College
Radiography Prgm
PO Drawer 696
Aiken, SC 29802-0696
www.atc.edu

AnMed Health Medical Center
Radiography Prgm
800 N Fant St
Anderson, SC 29621
anmedhealth.org
Prgm Dir: Susan Merrill, MS RT(R)
Tel: 864 512-3705   *Fax:* 864 512-1319
E-mail: susan.merrill@anmedhealth.org

Technical College of the Lowcountry
Radiography Prgm
PO Box 1288
Beaufort, SC 29901
www.tcl.edu

Trident Technical College
Radiography Prgm
7000 Rivers Ave, PO Box 118067
Charleston, SC 29423-8067
Prgm Dir: Krista R Gentry, MA RT(R)
Tel: 843 574-6077   *Fax:* 843 574-6585
E-mail: krista.gentry@tridenttech.edu

Midlands Technical College
Radiography Prgm
PO Box 2408
Columbia, SC 29202
www.midlandstech.edu

Florence-Darlington Technical College
Radiography Prgm
PO Box 100548
Florence, SC 29501-0548
www.fdtc.edu
Prgm Dir: E Yancy Wells, MA BS RT (R)
Tel: 843 676-8529 *Fax:* 843 292-0851
E-mail: Yancy.Wells@fdtc.edu

Greenville Technical College
Radiography Prgm
PO Box 5616
MS 1202
506 S Pleasantburg Drive-AH221
Greenville, SC 29607
www.gvltec.edu

Piedmont Technical College
Radiography Prgm
PO Box 1467, Emerald Rd
Greenwood, SC 29648-1467
www.ptc.edu

Horry - Georgetown Technical College
Radiography Prgm
743 Hemlock Ave
Myrtle Beach, SC 29577

Orangeburg Calhoun Technical College
Radiography Prgm
3250 St Matthews Rd
Orangeburg, SC 29118-8299
www.octech.edu
Prgm Dir: Frances W Andrews, MA Ed RT(R)
Tel: 803 535-1356 *Fax:* 803 535-1350
E-mail: andrewsf@octech.edu

York Technical College
Radiography Prgm
452 S Anderson Rd
Rock Hill, SC 29730
www.yorktech.com

Spartanburg Community College
Radiography Prgm
PO Drawer 4386
Spartanburg, SC 29305-4386
www.sccsc.edu/HHS/xray/

South Dakota

Presentation College
Radiography Prgm
1500 N Main St
Aberdeen, SD 57401
www.presentation.edu

Mitchell Technical Institute
Radiography Prgm
821 N Capital
Mitchell, SD 57301
www.mitchelltech.edu

Rapid City Regional Hospital
Radiography Prgm
353 Fairmont Blvd, PO Box 6000
Rapid City, SD 57709-6000
www.regionalhealth.com
Prgm Dir: Jerilyn Jo Powell, MS RT(R) RDMS RVT
Tel: 605 719-8433 *Fax:* 605 719-1436
E-mail: jpowell2@regionalhealth.com

Avera McKennan Hospital
Radiography Prgm
PO Box 5045
Sioux Falls, SD 57117-5045
Prgm Dir: Susan Calmus, MRRT(R)
Tel: 605 322-1720 *Fax:* 605 322-1701
E-mail: susan.calmus@avera.org

Sanford USD Medical Center
Radiography Prgm
1305 W 18th St, PO Box 5039
Sioux Falls, SD 57117-5039
sanfordhealth.org
Prgm Dir: Candace McNamara, MBA RT(R)
Tel: 605 333-7445, Ext *Fax:* 605 333-1554
E-mail: Candace.McNamara@sanfordhealth.org

Avera Sacred Heart Hospital
Radiography Prgm
501 Summit St
Yankton, SD 57078-3899
www.averasacredheart.com

Tennessee

Chattanooga State Community College
Radiography Prgm
4501 Amnicola Hwy
Chattanooga, TN 37406-1097
www.chattanoogastate.edu/allied_health/rad_tech/
  rad_tech_main.asp
Prgm Dir: Margery Sanders, MBA RT(R)(M)(QM)
Tel: 423 697-3297 *Fax:* 423 493-8771
E-mail: margery.sanders@chattanoogastate.edu

Austin Peay State University
Radiography Prgm
Clarksville, TN 37044

Columbia State Community College
Radiography Prgm
1665 Hampshire Pike
Columbia, TN 38402-1315
www.columbiastate.edu
Prgm Dir: Brenda M Coleman, MSRS RT(R)
Tel: 931 540-2745 *Fax:* 931 540-2798
E-mail: bcoleman@columbiastate.edu

Fortis Institute
Radiography Prgm
Cookeville/KIMC Investments, Inc
1025 Highway 111
Cookeville, TN 38501
www.medvance.edu

East Tennessee State University
Radiography Prgm
Nave Center, 1000 Jason Witten Way
Elizabethton, TN 37643

Volunteer State Community College
Radiography Prgm
1480 Nashville Pike
Gallatin, TN 37066-3188
www.volstate.edu

Jackson State Community College
Radiography Prgm
2046 N Parkway
Jackson, TN 38301-3797
www.jscc.edu/academics/disciplines/allied-health/
  radiography.html

South College
Radiography Prgm
3904 Lonas Dr
Knoxville, TN 37909
southcollegetn.edu

University of Tennessee Medical Center
Cosponsor: University of Tennessee Medical Center at
  Knoxville
Radiography Prgm
Radiology Dept
1924 Alcoa Hwy
Knoxville, TN 37920-6999
www.utmedicalcenter.org/health_professionals/
  educational_services/radiography_technology
Prgm Dir: Clyde R Hembree, MBA RT(R)
Tel: 865 305-9005 *Fax:* 865 305-8946
E-mail: chembree@mc.utmck.edu

Baptist College of Health Sciences
Radiography Prgm
1003 Monroe Ave
Memphis, TN 38104
http://BCHS.edu

Concorde Career College - Memphis
Radiography Prgm
5100 Poplar Ave, Ste 132
Memphis, TN 38137

Methodist University Hospital
Radiography Prgm
1265 Union Ave
Memphis, TN 38104
www.methodisthealth.org
Prgm Dir: Melissa Yarbro, MBA RT(R)
Tel: 901 516-2308 *Fax:* 901 516-2870
E-mail: Melissa.Yarbro@mlh.org

Southwest Tennessee Community College
Radiography Prgm
PO Box 780
Memphis, TN 38101-0780
www.southwest.tn.edu

Fortis Institute
Radiography Prgm
Nashville/KIMC Investments Inc
3354 Perimeter Hill Dr - Suite 105
Nashville, TN 37211
www.medvance.edu

Nashville General Hospital
Radiography Prgm
1818 Albion St
Nashville, TN 37208
nashvillegeneral.org/specialized-health-sciences.php

Roane State Community College
Radiography Prgm
701 Briarcliff Ave
Oak Ridge, TN 37830
www.roanestate.edu

Texas

Hendrick Medical Center
Radiography Prgm
1900 Pine St
Abilene, TX 79601-2316
www.ehendrick.org/radiography
Prgm Dir: Richard K Bower, MEd RT(R)
Tel: 352 670-2427 *Fax:* 352 670-2990
E-mail: rbower@ehendrick.org

Amarillo College
Radiography Prgm
PO Box 447
Amarillo, TX 79178
www.actx.edu/radiography

Austin Community College
Radiography Prgm
3401 Webberville Rd
Austin, TX 78702
www.austincc.edu
Prgm Dir: Rudy L Garza, MS RT(R)
Tel: 512 223-5817 *Fax:* 512 223-5901
E-mail: rudygarz@austincc.edu

Baptist Hospitals of Southeast Texas
Radiography Prgm
PO Drawer 1591
Beaumont, TX 77704
www.mhbh.org

MEDICAL IMAGING & RADIATION THERAPY

Lamar Institute of Technology
Radiography Prgm
PO Box 10061
Beaumont, TX 77710
Prgm Dir: Brenda A Barrow, MEd RT(R)(CT)
Tel: 409 880-8848, Ext   *Fax:* 409 880-8955
E-mail: brenda.barrow@lit.edu

Coastal Bend College
Radiography Prgm
3800 Charco Rd
Beeville, TX 78102

Blinn College
Radiography Prgm
Texas A & M Health Science Center
8441 State Hwy 47-Clinial Building I
Bryan, TX 77807
www.blinn.edu/twe/radi
Prgm Dir: M Elia Flores, MEd RT(R)
Tel: 979 691-2011   *Fax:* 979 691-2410
E-mail: sflores@blinn.edu

Montgomery College
Radiography Prgm
3200 College Park Dr
Conroe, TX 77384

Del Mar College
Radiography Prgm
101 Baldwin and Ayers Sts
Corpus Christi, TX 78404

Lone Star College-CyFair
Radiography Prgm
9191 Barker-Cypress Rd
Cypress, TX 77433
http://cyfair.lonestar.edu

Baylor University Med Center
Radiography Prgm
3616 Worth St
Dallas, TX 75246

Brookhaven College
Radiography Prgm
3939 Valley View Lane, Farmers Branch
Dallas, TX 75244-4997

El Centro College
Radiography Prgm
801 Main St
Dallas, TX 75202-3604
www.elcentrocollege.edu

El Paso Community College
Radiography Prgm
PO Box 20500
El Paso, TX 79998
www.epcc.edu

Medical Education and Training Campus (METC)
Radiography Prgm
3151 Scott Rd
Suite 1316, MCCS-HCR
Fort Sam Houston, TX 78234-6137
http://radiology.amedd.army.mil

Tarrant County College
Radiography Prgm
245 E Belknap
Ft. Worth, TX 76102
www.tccd.edu/Courses_and_Programs/Program_Offerings/Radiologic_Tech.html
Prgm Dir: Mark Holt, MS RT(R)
Tel: 817 515-2407   *Fax:* 817 515-0654
E-mail: mark.holt@tccd.edu

Galveston College
Radiography Prgm
4015 Ave Q
Galveston, TX 77550-2782
www.gc.edu

MedVance Institute - Grand Prairie Campus
Cosponsor: KIMC Investments Inc.
Radiography Prgm
401 E Palace Parkway, Suite 100
Grand Prairie, TX 75050

Harris County Hosp Dist/Ben Taub Gen Hosp
Radiography Prgm
c/o Lyndon B Johnson General Hospital
5656 Kelley St
Houston, TX 77026

Houston Community College
Radiography Prgm
Coleman College for Health Sciences
1900 Pressler Dr, MC 1637-512
Houston, TX 77030
www.hccs.edu

Pima Medical Institute - Houston
Radiography Prgm
10201 Katy Fwy, Suite C
Houston, TX 77024
www.pmi.edu

Sanford-Brown College - North Loop
Radiography Prgm
2627 North Loop West, Suite 100
Houston, TX 77008

Univ of Texas M D Anderson Cancer Ctr
Radiography Prgm
1515 Holcombe Blvd, Unit 190
Houston, TX 77030

Laredo Community College
Radiography Prgm
West End Washington St
Laredo, TX 78040-4395
www.laredo.edu

Covenant Medical Center
Radiography Prgm
2002 W Loop 289
Suite 120
Lubbock, TX 79407

Angelina College
Radiography Prgm
PO Box 1768
3500 S First
Lufkin, TX 75902
www.angelina.edu
Prgm Dir: Angie L Wilcox, MEd RT(R)(CT)
Tel: 936 633-5413, Ext   *Fax:* 936 633-3207
E-mail: awilcox@angelina.edu

Northeast Texas Community College
Radiography Prgm
PO Box 1307
Mt. Pleasant, TX 75456

Odessa College
Radiography Prgm
201 W University Blvd
Odessa, TX 79764
www.odessa.edu/dept/radiology
Prgm Dir: Carrie B Nanson, MS RT(R)
Tel: 432 335-6469   *Fax:* 432 335-6873
E-mail: cnanson@odessa.edu

Paris Junior College
Radiography Prgm
2400 Clarksville St
Paris, Tx 75460
www.parisjc.edu

San Jacinto College Central
Radiography Prgm
8060 Spencer Hwy, PO Box 2007
Pasadena, TX 77501-2007
www.sjcd.edu

Baptist Health System
Radiography Prgm
8400 Datapoint Dr
Suite 226
San Antonio, TX 78229
www.bshp.edu

Howard College
Radiography Prgm
3501 N US Hwy 67
San Antonio, TX 78229
www.howardcollege.edu

St Philip's College
Radiography Prgm
1801 Martin Luther King Dr
San Antonio, TX 78203-2098

Tyler Junior College
Radiography Prgm
PO Box 9020
Tyler, TX 75711
www.tjc.edu

Citizens Medical Center
Radiography Prgm
2701 Hospital Dr
Victoria, TX 77901

McLennan Community College
Radiography Prgm
1400 College Dr
Waco, TX 76708

Weatherford College
Radiography Prgm
225 College Park Drive
Weatherford, TX 76086

Wharton County Junior College
Radiography Prgm
911 Boling Hwy, Ste J230
Wharton, TX 77488
www.wcjc.edu

Midwestern State University
Radiography Prgm
3410 Taft Blvd
Wichita Falls, TX 76308-2099
http://hs2.mwsu.edu/radsci/ra/
Prgm Dir: Donna Wright, EdD RT(R)
Tel: 940 397-4615   *Fax:* 940 397-4845
E-mail: donna.wright@mwsu.edu

Utah

Dixie State College of Utah
Radiography Prgm
225 South 700 East
St George, UT 84770
www.dixie.edu/health/radiography/

Salt Lake Community College
Radiography Prgm
Health Sciences Bldg
3491 W Wights Fort Rd
West Jordan, UT 84088

Vermont

Southern Vermont College
Radiography Prgm
982 Mansion Drive
Bennington, VT 05201

Champlain College
Radiography Prgm
163 S Willard St, PO Box 670
Burlington, VT 05402-0670
www.champlain.edu

Virginia

Piedmont Virginia Community College
Cosponsor: University of Virginia Medical Center
Radiography Prgm
Jefferson Park Ave, Radiology Box 800377
Charlottesville, VA 22908
www.med.virginia.edu

Richmond School of Health and Technology
Radiography Prgm
751 West Hundred Rd
Chester, VA 23836
www.rsht.edu

Danville Regional Medical Center /LifePoint Hospitals, Inc
Radiography Prgm
142 South Main St
Danville, VA 24541
www.danvilleregional.org

Mary Washington Hospital
Radiography Prgm
2300 Fall Hill Ave Ste 260
Fredericksburg, VA 22401
Prgm Dir: Donna Carroll , MEd RT(R)(M)
Tel: 540 741-1802   *Fax:* 540 741-3507
E-mail: Donna.Carroll@mwhc.com

Rockingham Memorial Hospital
Radiography Prgm
2010 Health Campus Drive
Harrisonburg, VA 22801-3293
www.rhcc.com
Prgm Dir: Russell Crank, MS RT(R)
Tel: 540 564-7236   *Fax:* 540 437-7962
E-mail: rcrank@rhcc.com

Central Virginia Community College
Radiography Prgm
3506 Wards Rd
Lynchburg, VA 24502-2498
www.cvcc.vccs.edu

ACT College
Radiography Prgm
8870 Rixlew Ln Ste 201
Manassas, VA 20109
www.actcollege.edu

ECPI University Medical Careers Institute
Radiography Prgm
1001 Omni Blvd, Ste 200
Newport News, VA 23606
www.medical.edu

Riverside School of Health Careers
Radiography Prgm
316 Main St
316 Main St
Newport News, VA 23601
www.riversideonline.com/rshc
Prgm Dir: Robin M Nelhuebel, MEd RN RT(R)
Tel: 757 240-2206   *Fax:* 757 240-2201
E-mail: robin.nelhuebel@rivhs.com

Southside Regional Medical Center
Radiography Prgm
Professional Schools
737 S Sycamore St
Petersburg, VA 23803
www.srmconline.com

Southwest Virginia Community College
Radiography Prgm
PO Box SVCC
Richlands, VA 24641-1510
www.sw.vccs.edu

Bon Secours St Mary's Hospital
Radiography Prgm
8550 Magellan Pkwy Ste 700
Richmond, VA 23227

Virginia Commonwealth University
Radiography Prgm
701 W Grace St, Ste 2100
Box 843057
Richmond, VA 23284-3057
www.sahp.vcu.edu/radsci

Virginia Western Community College
Radiography Prgm
3097 Colonial Ave SW
PO Box 14007
Roanoke, VA 24038

Tidewater Community College
Radiography Prgm
1700 College Crescent
Virginia Beach, VA 23453

Winchester Medical Center Inc
Radiography Prgm
1840 Amherst St
PO Box 3340
Winchester, VA 22601

Washington

Pima Medical Institute - Seattle
Radiography Prgm
9709 Third Ave NE, #400
Seattle, WA 98115
http://pmi.edu
Prgm Dir: Jacqueline M Kralik, MAL RT(R)(CT)(MR)
Tel: 206 322-6100, Ext   *Fax:* 206 324-1985
E-mail: jkralik@pmi.edu

Apollo College - Spokane
Cosponsor: Carrington Colleges
Radiography Prgm
10102 E Knox Ste 200
Spokane, WA 99206

Spokane Community College
Radiography Prgm
1810 N Greene St, MS 1090
Spokane, WA 99217
www.scc.spokane.edu

Tacoma Community College
Radiography Prgm
6501 S 19th St, Bldg 19
Tacoma, WA 98466
www.tacomacc.edu

West Virginia

Mountain State University
Radiography Prgm
Box 9003
Beckley, WV 25802-9003

Bluefield State College
Radiography Prgm
219 Rock St
Bluefield, WV 24701
www.bluefieldstate.edu
Prgm Dir: Melissa Oxley Haye, MS RT(R)
Tel: 304 327-4145   *Fax:* 304 327-4219
E-mail: mhaye@bluefieldstate.edu

United Hospital Center
Radiography Prgm
327 Medical Park Drive
Bridgeport, WV 26330
www.uhcwv.org
Prgm Dir: Rosemary Trupo, MBA RT(R)
Tel: 681 342-1871   *Fax:* 681 342-1858
E-mail: trupor@uhcwv.org

University of Charleston
Radiography Prgm
2300 MacCorkle Ave SE
Charleston, WV 25304
www.ucwv.edu

St Mary's Medical Center
Cosponsor: Marshall Community and Technical College
Radiography Prgm
School for Medical Imaging
2900 First Ave
Huntington, WV 25702
www.st-marys.org

West Virginia University Hospitals
Radiography Prgm
Medical Center Dr
Box 8062
Morgantown, WV 26506
www.wvuhradtech.com
Prgm Dir: Jay Morris, MA RT(R)(CV)
Tel: 304 598-4251   *Fax:* 304 598-4702
E-mail: morrisj@wvuhealthcare.com

Southern West Virginia Comm & Tech College
Radiography Prgm
PO Box 2900
Mount Gay, WV 25637
www.southernwv.edu
Prgm Dir: Eva M Hallis, MS RT(R)
Tel: 304 896-7335   *Fax:* 304 792-7028
E-mail: Eva.Hallis@southernwv.edu

Ohio Valley Medical Center
Radiography Prgm
2000 Eoff St
Wheeling, WV 26003

West Virginia Northern Community College
Radiography Prgm
1704 Market St
Wheeling, WV 26003

Wisconsin

Wheaton Franciscan Healthcare - St Joseph
Radiography Prgm
Brown Deer Campus 9252 North Green Bay Rd
Brown Deer, WI 53209

Lakeshore Technical College
Radiography Prgm
1290 North Ave
Cleveland, WI 53015-1414

Chippewa Valley Technical College
Radiography Prgm
620 W Clairemont Ave
Eau Claire, WI 54701-6162
www.cvtc.edu

Moraine Park Technical College
Radiography Prgm
235 N National Ave
Fond du Lac, WI 54936

Columbia St Mary's Hospitals
Radiography Prgm
School of Radiologic Technology
4425 N Port Washington Rd
Glendale, WI 53212
www.ccon.edu/SORT.htm
Notes: The program has affiliations with the University of Wisconsin Milwaukee, Concordia University, Mount Mary College, Carroll College, and Marian University, so students receive a bachelor's degree upon program completion.

Bellin College/Bellin Health Systems Inc
Radiography Prgm
3201 Eaton Rd
Green Bay, WI 54311
www.bellincollege.edu
Prgm Dir: Randy Griswold, MPA RT(R)
Tel: 920 433-6626   *Fax:* 920 433-1921
E-mail: randy.griswold@bellincollege.edu
Notes: Program is now a 4-year BS program in Radiologic Sciences to include radiography, CT, MRI, Mammography, DEXA and management

MEDICAL IMAGING & RADIATION THERAPY

Northeast Wisconsin Technical College
Radiography Prgm
2740 W Mason St
Green Bay, WI 54307-9042

Blackhawk Technical College
Radiography Prgm
6004 Prairie Rd PO Box 5009
Janesville, WI 53547
www.blackhawk.edu

Western Technical College
Radiography Prgm
PO Box C-0908
La Crosse, WI 54602
www.westerntc.edu
Prgm Dir: Doreen Olson, Assoc Dean MS OT
Tel: 608 789-4757   *Fax:* 608 785-9299
E-mail: olsond@westerntc.edu

Madison Area Technical College
Radiography Prgm
211 N Carroll St
Madison, WI 53703
www.matcmadison.edu/radiography
Prgm Dir: Kay A Parish, EdD RT(R) RDMS
Tel: 608 258-2478   *Fax:* 608 258-2480
E-mail: kparish@matcmadison.edu

University of Wisconsin Hospital and Clinics
Radiography Prgm
610 N Whitney Way, Suite 440
Madison, WI 53705
www.uwhealth.org/radtechschool
Prgm Dir: Karen L Tvedten, MEd RT(R)
Tel: 608 263-9029   *Fax:* 608 263-9208
E-mail: KTvedten@uwhealth.org

Saint Joseph's Hospital / Marshfield Clinic
Radiography Prgm
611 St Joseph Ave
Marshfield, WI 54449

Aurora St Luke's Medical Center
Radiography Prgm
180 W Grange Ave
Milwaukee, WI 53207
www.aurora.org/radtech
Prgm Dir: Cynthia Bradley, MS RT(R)(CT)(MR)
Tel: 414 747-4335   *Fax:* 414 747-4366
E-mail: cindy.bradley@aurora.org

Froedtert Hospital
Radiography Prgm
9200 W Wisconsin Ave
Milwaukee, WI 53226
Prgm Dir: Rochell Olive-Harmon, MSHSA RT(R)
Tel: 414 805-4999   *Fax:* 414 805-4990
E-mail: rharmon@froedterthealth.org

Milwaukee Area Technical College
Radiography Prgm
700 W State St
Milwaukee, WI 53233-1443
www.matc.edu

Theda Clark Regional Medical Center
Radiography Prgm
130 Second St
PO Box 2021
Neenah, WI 54957
www.thedacare.org
Prgm Dir: Troy Albrecht, MS RT(R)(CT)
Tel: 920 729-3146   *Fax:* 920 729-2118
E-mail: troy.albrecht@thedacare.org

Mercy Medical Center/Affinity Health System
Radiography Prgm
500 S Oakwood Rd
Oshkosh, WI 54904
www.affinityhealth.org

Wheaton Franciscan Healthcare - All Saints
Radiography Prgm
3801 Spring St
Racine, WI 53405

Northcentral Technical College
Radiography Prgm
1000 Campus Dr
Wausau, WI 54401-1899
www.ntc.edu

Sanford-Brown College
Radiography Prgm
6737 West Washington Street #2355
West Allis, WI 53214

Wyoming

Casper College
Radiography Prgm
125 College Dr
Casper, WY 82601
http://caspercollege.edu

Laramie County Community College
Radiography Prgm
1400 E College Dr
Cheyenne, WY 82007
www.lccc.wy.edu/programs/radiography
Prgm Dir: Starla L Mason, MS RT(R)(QM)
Tel: 307 778-1391   *Fax:* 307 778-1395
E-mail: smason@lccc.wy.edu

Radiographer

Programs*	Class Capacity	Begins	Length (months)	Award	Res. Tuition	Non-res. Tuition		Offers:† 1	2	3	4
Alabama											
DCH Regional Medical Center (Tuscaloosa)	20	Oct	24	Cert	$3,600	$3,600				•	•
Gadsden State Community College	24	Aug	21	AAS	$5,014	$10,028		•			
Arkansas											
Arkansas State Univ	40	Jun	24	Dipl, AAS, BS	$4,950	$9,900					
South Arkansas Community College (El Dorado)	12	Aug	24	AAS	$3,200	$6,100	per year		•	•	
California											
Bakersfield College	26	Jun	24	AS	$1,100	$6,900	per year			•	
California State Univ - Northridge	30	Aug	51	BS	$7,200	$20,000			•	•	
Foothill College (Los Altos Hills)	32	Aug	22	Dipl, AS						•	
Fresno City College	84	Aug	24	AS	$46	$261	per credit			•	
Harbor UCLA Medical Center (Torrance)	12	Jul	24	Cert						•	
Los Angeles City College	26	Sep	27	Dipl, AS	$2,500					•	
Moorpark College	26	Jun	24	AS	$960					•	
Colorado											
Community College of Denver - Lowry Campus	40	Aug	21	Dipl, AAS	$3,300	$11,000				•	
Memorial Hospital (Colorado Springs)	18	Aug	24	AAS	$5,000	$5,000	per year			•	
Connecticut											
Hartford Hospital	28	Sep	24	Dipl, Cert	$5,000	$5,000	per year			•	
Windham Community Memorial Hospital (Willimantic)	48	Sep	22	Cert	$8,500	$8,500				•	
Florida											
Brevard Community College (Cocoa)	32	Jun	23	AS	$4,200	$14,212				•	
Halifax Health Medical Center (Daytona Beach)	10	Jan	30	Cert, AS	$4,000	$6,576				•	
Marion County School of Radiologic Tech (Ocala)	30	Aug	22	Cert	$3,577	$9,600	per year			•	
St Vincent's Medical Center (Jacksonville)	11	Jul	24	Cert	$2,500	$2,500				•	
State College of Florida, Manatee-Sarasota (Bradenton)	30	May	23	AS/AAS	$5,167	$14,541	per year			•	
Georgia											
Armstrong Atlantic State Univ (Savannah)	25	Sep	21	BS	$6,765	$20,697			•	•	
College of Coastal Georgia (Brunswick)	15	Jun	24	AS						•	
Grady Health System (Atlanta)	25	Aug	24	Cert	$4,700	$4,700	per year			•	
Gwinnett Technical College (Lawrenceville)	68	Aug	21	AS	$3,200	$6,000				•	

*Data are shown only for programs that completed the 2011 AMA Survey of Health Professions Education Programs.

†Key to Offers: 1: Evening or weekend classes; 2: Non-English instruction; 3: Cultural competence instruction; 4: Distance education component.

Programs*	Class Capacity	Begins	Length (months)	Award	Res. Tuition	Non-res. Tuition		Offers:† 1	2	3	4
Ogeechee Technical College (Statesboro)	12	Aug	21	Dipl	$7,000	$14,000	per year			•	
Univ Hospital (Augusta)	14	Jul	24	Cert	$1,200	$1,200	per year			•	
Hawaii											
Kapiolani Community College (Honolulu)	25	Aug	23	AS	$3,450	$10,295				•	
Illinois											
Kishwaukee College (Malta)	15	Aug	22	AAS	$3,725					•	
McDonough District Hospital (Macomb)	5	Aug	24	Cert						•	
Moraine Valley Community College (Palos Hills)	47	Jun	26	AAS	$99	$249		•		•	
Rockford Memorial Hospital	10	Jun	24	Dipl, Cert	$2,000	$3,000				•	
Sauk Valley Community College (Dixon)	34	Aug	22	AAS	$3,200						
Wright College (Chicago)	45	Aug	24	AAS	$2,765	$9,065	per year				
Indiana											
Ball State Univ (Muncie)	20	May	26	AS	$7,912	$21,892	per year		•		•
Good Samaritan Hospital (Vincennes)	22	May	24	Cert	$2,500	$2,500					
Reid Hospital & Health Care Services (Richmond)	10	Sep	24	Cert	$3,600	$3,600	per year				
St Vincent Health/St Joseph Hospital (Indianapolis)	17	Aug	22	Cert	$3,000	$3,000	per year				
Iowa											
Covenant Medical Center (Waterloo)	12	Jun	24	Cert	$2,600					•	
Jennie Edmundson Memorial Hospital (Council Bluffs)	8	Aug	24	Cert	$3,000	$3,000	per year			•	
St Luke's Hospital dba Mercy/St. Luke's School of Radiologic Tech (Cedar Rapids)	12	Jul	24	Cert	$3,300	$3,300	per year			•	
Univ of Iowa Hospitals & Clinics (Iowa City)	42	Jul	24	Cert	$6,500	$6,500	per year		•		•
Kentucky											
Bowling Green Technical College	18	Aug	22	AAS	$4,688		per year				
Madisonville Community College	20	Aug	21	Assoc	$2,795						
Morehead State Univ	52	Aug	24	AAS							
Louisiana											
Lafayette General Medical Center	6	Sep	24	Cert	$4,500	$4,500	per year			•	
McNeese State Univ (Lake Charles)	26	Jan	28	BS	$4,992	$10,675	per year				
North Oaks Medical Center (Hammond)	16	Jul	24	Cert	$4,000	$4,000	per year			•	
Our Lady of Holy Cross College (New Orleans)	24	Aug	21	BS-HS, AS-RS						•	
Our Lady of the Lake College (Baton Rouge)	56	Aug	21	AS	$11,880	$11,880					
Maine											
Central Maine Medical Center College of Nursing & Health Professions (Lewiston)	23	Aug	22	Cert, Assoc, Dipl	$7,500	$7,500	per year			•	
Eastern Maine Community College (Bangor)	20	Aug	23	AS	$3,612	$7,224	per year				
Maryland											
Greater Baltimore Medical Center	12	Aug	23	Cert	$3,000	$3,000					
Prince George's Community College (Largo)	32	Aug	19	AAS	$2,544	$4,426				•	
Massachusetts											
Bunker Hill Community College (Boston)	136	Sep	21, 35	AS	$4,000	$10,000		•		•	
North Shore Community College (Danvers)	17	Sep	21	AS	$5,346	$13,002	per year			•	
Michigan											
Beaumont Hospital - Royal Oak	12	Jan Jul	24	Cert	$3,000	$3,000				•	
Kellogg Community College (Battle Creek)	22	May	24	AAS	$3,270	$5,120	per year				
Lansing Community College	66	Aug	21	AAS	$5,733	$8,182	per year			•	
Providence Hospital (Southfield)	12	Sep Oct	24	Cert	$5,000		per year			•	
Sinai-Grace Hospital (Detroit)	14	Jul	24		$2,000	$2,000	per year			•	
Washtenaw Community College (Ann Arbor)	35	May	24	AAS	$8,000	$12,000			•		•
Wayne State Univ (Detroit)	20	May	24	BS	$14,000	$14,000					
Minnesota											
Lake Superior College (Duluth)	76	Aug	27, 18	AAS					•	•	
Riverland Community College (Austin)	16	Aug	24	AAS						•	
St Cloud Hospital	8	Sep	24	Cert, BS						•	
Mississippi											
Hinds Community College (Raymond)	51	Jun	24	AS	$2,460	$3,960	per year				
Mississippi Delta Community College (Moorhead)	25	Aug	24	Dipl, AS	$1,165	$1,969				•	
Missouri											
Mercy Hospital Springfield	24	Jul	23	Cert	$2,500	$2,500	per year				
Nebraska											
Clarkson College (Omaha)	28	Aug	24	AS	$15,622	$15,622				•	
Mary Lanning Memorial Healthcare (Hastings)	28	Aug	24	Dipl, AAS	$3,000				•		•
Regional West Medical Center (Scottsbluff)	14	Aug	24	Cert	$2,000	$2,000	per year			•	
New Jersey											
Middlesex County College (Edison)	36	Sep	24	AAS	$5,000	$10,000				•	

*Data are shown only for programs that completed the 2011 AMA Survey of Health Professions Education Programs.

†Key to Offers: 1: Evening or weekend classes; 2: Non-English instruction; 3: Cultural competence instruction; 4: Distance education component.

MEDICAL IMAGING & RADIATION THERAPY

Radiographer

Programs*	Class Capacity	Begins	Length (months)	Award	Res. Tuition	Non-res. Tuition		Offers:† 1	2	3	4
St Francis Medical Center (Trenton)	8	Jul	24	Cert	$6,279	$6,279	per year			•	
The Valley Hospital (Ridgewood)	13	Sep	24	Cert, AS	$18,247	$18,247	per year			•	
New York											
Arnot Ogden Medical Center (Elmira)	7	Aug	23	Cert	$6,140	$8,550	per year			•	
Bronx Community College	40	Aug	24	AAS	$3,700	$5,700	per year			•	
Broome Community College (Binghamton)	76	Aug	21	AAS	$4,000	$7,500				•	•
CVPH Medical Center (Plattsburgh)	14	Jul	24	Cert	$8,000	$14,600	per year			•	
Long Island Univ - C W Post Campus (Brookville)	25	Sep	48	BS	$32,000	$32,000	per year			•	
Monroe Community College (Rochester)	46	Sep	21	AAS	$3,572	$7,144	per year			•	
North Country Community College (Saranac Lake)	40	Sep	23	Dipl, AAS	$3,900	$9,600				•	
Peconic Bay Medical Center School of Radiologic Technology (Riverhead)	12	Sep	24	Cert	$7,500					•	
Robt J Hochstime Sch Rad/S Nassau Comm Hosp (Oceanside)	10	Sep	24	Cert	$7,000	$7,000			•	•	
North Carolina											
Asheville-Buncombe Technical Comm College	20	Aug	21	AAS	$2,848	$10,340	per year			•	
Presbyterian Healthcare (Charlotte)	10	Jul	23	Cert	$2,100	$2,100	per year			•	
Ohio											
Akron Children's Hospital	34	Jun	24	Cert, AAS	$7,500	$7,500	per year			•	
Cuyahoga Community College (Parma)	32	Aug Jan	24	Dipl, AAS	$2,960	$3,905	per year	•		•	
Kent State Univ - Salem Campus	38	Jun	24	AAS	$7,215	$17,709				•	
Lorain County Community College (Elyria)	36	Aug	21	AAS	$3,500	$4,000	per year			•	
Marietta Memorial Hospital	42	Aug	24	Cert	$3,623	$7,245	per year			•	
Mercy Medical Center (Canton)	30	Jul	24	Dipl	$6,200	$6,200	per year				
Shawnee State Univ (Portsmouth)	21	May	24	AAS	$12,000	$18,000					
Xavier Univ (Cincinnati)	30	Aug	23	AS	$8,600	$8,600				•	
Oklahoma											
Great Plains Technology Center (Lawton)	22	Aug	22	Cert	$2,200	$3,200	per year			•	•
Southwestern Oklahoma State Univ (Sayre)	17	Aug	24	AAS	$4,000		per year			•	
Tulsa Community College	40	Jun	24	AAS							
Pennsylvania											
Armstrong County Memorial Hospital (Kittanning)	8	Jul	24	Cert	$3,200	$3,200	per year			•	
Conemaugh Valley Memorial Hospital (Johnstown)	20	Aug	20	Cert, AAS	$8,700		per year				
Gannon Univ (Erie)	18	Aug	24	Assoc	$26,000	$26,000				•	
Holy Spirit Hospital (Camp Hill)	9	Jan	24	Cert	$2,424	$2,424	per year			•	
Misericordia Univ (Dallas)	30	Aug	42	BS	$24,700	$24,700				•	
Northampton Community College (Bethlehem)	34	Aug	21	AAS	$3,933	$8,300	per credit			•	
St Christopher Hospital School of Rad Tech (Philadelphia)	19	Jul	24		$8,800	$8,800	per year			•	
Thomas Jefferson Univ (Philadelphia)	18	Sep	12	Dipl, BS, MS	$28,000					•	•
Washington Hospital	15	Sep	24	Cert	$11,000	$11,000	per year			•	
Rhode Island											
Rhode Island Hospital (Providence)	60	Jun	24, 30	Cert			per year			•	
South Carolina											
AnMed Health Medical Center (Anderson)	19	Jul	24	Cert	$2,000	$2,000	per year			•	
Florence-Darlington Technical College	46	Aug	21	AS	$1,883	$2,014					
Orangeburg Calhoun Technical College	16	Aug	24, 12	AAS	$5,331	$6,591					
Trident Technical College (Charleston)	59	May	24	Assoc	$5,175	$5,742	per year			•	•
South Dakota											
Avera McKennan Hospital (Sioux Falls)	20	Sep	24	Cert	$1,800	$1,800				•	
Rapid City Regional Hospital	10	Jun	24		$1,500	$1,500	per year			•	
Sanford USD Medical Center (Sioux Falls)	28	Jul	24	Cert	$1,500	$1,500	per year			•	
Tennessee											
Chattanooga State Community College	92	Aug	24	AAS	$3,794	$15,973	per year			•	
Columbia State Community College	28	Jul	22	AAS	$5,585	$22,340	per year			•	
Methodist Univ Hospital (Memphis)	25	May	24	Cert, Assoc	$4,000	$4,000	per year			•	
Univ of Tennessee Medical Center (Knoxville)	11	Jul	24	Cert	$3,000	$3,000	per year			•	
Texas											
Angelina College (Lufkin)	32	Aug	23	AAS	$1,728						
Austin Community College	50	Aug	24	AAS	$2,700	$11,500					•
Blinn College (Bryan)	18	Sep	21	AAS		$8,300					
Hendrick Medical Center (Abilene)	15	Apr Sep	21	Cert	$1,500	$1,500	per year				
Lamar Institute of Technology (Beaumont)	38	Jul	48	AAS	$5,399	$9,972				•	
Midwestern State Univ (Wichita Falls)	120	Sep	24	AAS							
Odessa College	16	Jul	24	Dipl, AAS	$2,130	$2,563				•	
Tarrant County College (Ft. Worth)	42	May	24	AAS	$1,800	$5,256	per year			•	•
Virginia											
Mary Washington Hospital (Fredericksburg)	28	Aug	23	Dipl, Cert	$4,250					•	

*Data are shown only for programs that completed the 2011 AMA Survey of Health Professions Education Programs.

†Key to Offers: 1: Evening or weekend classes; 2: Non-English instruction; 3: Cultural competence instruction; 4: Distance education component.

Radiographer

Programs*	Class Capacity	Begins	Length (months)	Award	Res. Tuition	Non-res. Tuition		Offers:† 1	2	3	4
Riverside School of Health Careers (Newport News)	64	Sep	18	Cert	$10,800	$10,800				•	•
Rockingham Memorial Hospital (Harrisonburg)	15	Jun	24	Cert, AAS	$3,500	$3,500				•	
Washington											
Pima Medical Institute - Seattle	30	Apr Aug Dec	24	AS	$15,000	$15,000				•	•
West Virginia											
Bluefield State College	23	May	24	AS	$5,745	$11,608	per year	•			•
Southern West Virginia Comm & Tech College (Mount Gay)	40	Aug	21	AAS	$8,000			•		•	•
United Hospital Center (Bridgeport)	15	Jun	24	Cert	$3,000	$3,000	per year			•	
West Virginia Univ Hospitals (Morgantown)	15	Jul	24	Cert	$2,000	$2,000	per year			•	
Wisconsin											
Aurora St Luke's Medical Center (Milwaukee)	18	Sep	24		$3,000	$3,000	per year			•	
Bellin College/Bellin Health Systems Inc (Green Bay)	16	Sep	4	BS	$17,000	$17,000	per year			•	
Froedtert Hospital (Milwaukee)	45	Sep	24	Cert, AAS	$5,000	$5,000	per year			•	
Madison Area Technical College	58	Aug	24	AAS	$2,866					•	
Theda Clark Regional Medical Center (Neenah)	16	Sep	24	Cert	$6,500	$6,500				•	
Univ of Wisconsin Hospital and Clinics (Madison)	16	Sep	24		$9,000	$9,000	per year			•	
Western Technical College (La Crosse)	32	Aug	23	AAS	$4,960	$8,200					
Wyoming											
Laramie County Community College (Cheyenne)	17	Aug	24	AAS	$3,402	$7,936	per year			•	

*Data are shown only for programs that completed the 2011 AMA Survey of Health Professions Education Programs.

†Key to Offers: 1: Evening or weekend classes; 2: Non-English instruction; 3: Cultural competence instruction; 4: Distance education component.

MEDICAL IMAGING & RADIATION THERAPY

Radiologist Assistant

Radiologist assistants are experienced, registered radiographers who have obtained additional education and certification that qualifies them to serve as radiologist extenders. They work under the supervision of a radiologist to provide patient care in the diagnostic imaging environment. The radiologist assistant is a radiographer certified by the American Registry of Radiologic Technologists (ARRT) who has successfully completed an advanced academic program encompassing a nationally recognized radiologist assistant curriculum and a radiologist-directed clinical preceptorship. The addition of RAs to the radiology team is intended to improve productivity and efficiency as the demand for medical imaging services continues to increase.

Career Description

Under radiologist supervision, the radiologist assistant performs patient assessment, patient management, and selected exams. The title "radiologist assistant" reflects the nature of the relationship between the radiologist and the radiologic technologist working in an advanced clinical role. The title clearly places the RA's professional role and clinical responsibilities within the radiology environment.

The RA has three major areas of responsibility:

- Takes a lead role in patient management and assessment. Duties in this area might include determining whether a patient has been appropriately prepared for a procedure, obtaining patient consent prior to beginning the examination, answering questions from the patient and his or her family, and adapting exam protocols to improve diagnostic quality. The radiologist assistant also is expected to serve as a patient advocate, ensuring that each patient receives quality care while in the radiology department or clinic.
- Performs selected radiology examinations and procedures under the supervision of a radiologist. The level of radiologist supervision varies, depending on the type of examination.
- May be responsible for evaluating image quality, making initial image observations, and forwarding those observations to the supervising radiologist. The supervising radiologist remains responsible for providing a final written report, an interpretation, or a diagnosis.

Employment Characteristics

Radiologist assistants are employed in health care facilities, including community hospitals, university medical centers, and freestanding clinics; they are also employed in settings where their responsibilities focus on education, management, and research.

Salary

Salaries and benefits vary with experience and employment location. Data from the 2008 *Radiologist Extender Salaries and Functions Survey* by the American Society of Radiologic Technologists (ASRT) indicate that the average salary for practitioners is $102,972, and the average salary of the top five percent of earners is $112,615. Some states require licensure as a condition of practice. For more information, refer to *www.asrt.org/content/RTs/Research/research.aspx.*.

Educational Programs

Length, Award. All educational programs for RAs are established at the baccalaureate degree or higher. RAs must be certified as radiographers by the ARRT before enrolling in an RA educational program. Programs may be two to three years, depending on program design, objectives, and the degree or certificate awarded. Many programs offer online learning options.

Curriculum. The curriculum of a recognized program includes an extensive component of technical and professional courses, including an emphasis on a structured, clinical preceptorship. Interested individuals should contact a particular program for information on specific courses and prerequisites.

Inquiries

Careers/Curriculum
American Society of Radiologic Technologists
15000 Central Avenue SE
Albuquerque, NM 87123
505 298-4500
E-mail: *customerinfo@asrt.org*
www.asrt.org

Certification/Registration
American Registry of Radiologic Technologists
1255 Northland Drive
St Paul, MN 55120
651 687-0048
www.arrt.org

Program Accreditation
The educational program must be offered through a postsecondary institution accredited by an institutional accreditation agency recognized by the ARRT. No programmatic accreditation exists for radiologist assistant programs at this time, although programs must be formally recognized by the ARRT in order for a graduate to become a candidate for ARRT certification as a registered radiologist assistant.

American Registry of Radiologic Technologists
1255 Northland Drive
St Paul, MN 55120
651 687-0048
www.arrt.org

Radiologist Assistant

Arkansas

University of Arkansas for Medical Sciences
Radiologist Assistant Prgm
Department of Imaging and Radiation Sciences
4301 West Markham, #563A
Little Rock, AR 72205
www.uams.edu/chrp/imaging
Prgm Dir: Dale Collins, MS RT(R)(M)(QM) RDMS RVT
Tel: 501 686-7438   *Fax:* 501 526-7975
E-mail: dcollins3@uams.edu

California

Loma Linda University
Radiologist Assistant Prgm
School of Allied Health Professions
Department of Radiation Technology
Nichol Hall Room A829
Loma Linda, CA 92350
www.llu.edu/llu/sahp/radtech/radiologistassistant.html

Connecticut

Quinnipiac University
Radiologist Assistant Prgm
275 Mount Carmel Ave
Hamden, CT 06518-1908
www.quinnipiac.edu

Massachusetts

Mass College of Pharmacy & Health Sciences
Radiologist Assistant Prgm
179 Longwood Ave
Boston, MA 02115
www.mcphs.edu/academics/programs/
    radiologic_sciences/mras/

Michigan

Wayne State University
Radiologist Assistant Prgm
Detroit, MI 48201
www.wayne.edu

New Jersey

Univ of Medicine & Dent of New Jersey
Radiologist Assistant Prgm
School of Health Related Professions, Medical Imaging
    Scienc
Stanley S Bergen Building
65 Bergen St
Newark, NJ 07107-1709
http://shrp.umdnj.edu

North Carolina

University of North Carolina
Radiologist Assistant Prgm
CB7130
UNC-CH Bondurant Hall
321-A South Columbia St
Chapel Hill, NC 27599-7130
www.med.unc.edu/ahs/radisci

Ohio

The Ohio State University
Radiologist Assistant Prgm
School of Allied Medical Professions, Division of
    Radiologic
Atwell Hall
453 W 10th Ave
Columbus, OH 43210
www.amp.osu.edu/rd/

Texas

Midwestern State University
Radiologist Assistant Prgm
Radiologic Sciences Department
3410 Taft Blvd
Wichita Falls, TX 76308-2099
http://hs2.mwsu.edu/radsci/ra/
Prgm Dir: Jeff Killion, PhD RT(R)(QM)
Tel: 940 397-4679   *Fax:* 940 397-4845
E-mail: jeff.killion@mwsu.edu

Utah

Weber State University
Radiologist Assistant Prgm
Department of Radiologic Sciences
3925 University Circle
Ogden, UT 84408-3925
www.weber.edu/radsci
Prgm Dir: Diane Newham, MS RT(R)(M)(CT)(QM)
Tel: 801 626-6057   *Fax:* 801 626-7966
E-mail: dnewham@weber.edu

Virginia

Virginia Commonwealth University
Radiologist Assistant Prgm
Department of Radiation Sciences, School of Allied
    Health Pr
PO Box 843057
701 West Grace St, Suite 2100
Richmond, VA 23284-3057
www.sahp.vcu.edu/radsci

Washington

Bellevue College
Radiologist Assistant Prgm
3000 Landerholm Circle SE
Bellevue, WA 98007-6484
www.bellevuecollege.edu/bas/radiology.asp

Radiologist Assistant

Programs*	Class Capacity	Begins	Length (months)	Award	Res. Tuition	Non-res. Tuition	Offers:† 1	2	3	4
Arkansas										
Univ of Arkansas for Medical Sciences (Little Rock)	12	Jan May Aug	21	BS	$343	$738			•	•
Texas										
Midwestern State Univ (Wichita Falls)	10	Aug Jan	24	Radiologist Assistant	$8,500	$9,500	•			•
Utah										
Weber State Univ (Ogden)	50			Cert, BS	$6,600	$6,600	•		•	•

*Data are shown only for programs that completed the 2011 AMA Survey of Health Professions Education Programs.

†Key to Offers: 1: Evening or weekend classes; 2: Non-English instruction; 3: Cultural competence instruction; 4: Distance education component.

Medicine

Includes:
- Doctor of Medicine (MD)
- Doctor of Osteopathic Medicine (DO)

Note: There are two types of physicians: MD, Doctor of Medicine; and DO, Doctor of Osteopathic Medicine. MDs also are known as allopathic physicians. Both MDs and DOs may legally use all accepted methods of treatment, including drugs and surgery, but DOs place special emphasis on the body's musculoskeletal system, preventive medicine, and holistic patient care, as well as practicing osteopathic manipulative treatment (OMT), the use of manual physical examination techniques to diagnose illness and injury and to encourage the body's natural tendency toward good health. DOs are more likely than MDs to be primary care specialists, although they can practice in all specialties; approximately 63 percent of practicing osteopathic physicians specialize in primary care areas, such as pediatrics, family medicine, obstetrics and gynecology, and internal medicine.

Career Description

Physicians, often referred to as doctors, serve a fundamental role in our society and have an effect upon all our lives. They diagnose illnesses and prescribe and administer treatment for people suffering from injury or disease. Physicians examine patients; obtain medical histories; and order, perform, and interpret diagnostic tests. They counsel patients on diet, hygiene, and preventive health care.

About one third of the nation's physicians are generalists—"primary care" doctors who provide lifelong medical services. These include internists, family physicians, and pediatricians. Generalists provide a wide range of services children and adults need. When patients' specific health needs require further treatment, generalist physicians send them to see a specialist physician.

Specialist physicians, such as neurologists, cardiologists, and ophthalmologists, differ from generalists in that they focus on treating a particular system or part of the body. They collaborate with generalist physicians to ensure that patients receive treatment for specific medical problems as well as complete and comprehensive care throughout life.

The ten largest specialties are:
- Internal medicine (158,019)
- Family medicine (84,167)
- Pediatrics (74,350)
- Obstetrics-gynecology (42,594)
- Anesthesiology (41,699)
- Psychiatry (41,592)
- Surgery (37,524)
- Emergency medicine (30,841)
- Diagnostic radiology (24,894)
- Orthopedic surgery (24,485)

(Source: AMA's *Physician Characteristics and Distribution in the US,* 2009 edition)

Employment Characteristics

Many physicians—primarily general and family practitioners, general internists, pediatricians, ob/gyns, and psychiatrists—work in private offices or clinics, often assisted by a small staff of nurses and other administrative or clinical personnel. Increasingly, all specialties of physicians are practicing in groups or health care settings, including hospitals, that provide backup coverage and allow for more time off. These physicians often work as part of a team coordinating care for a population of patients.

Other physicians work in research, academic settings, or with health maintenance organizations, pharmaceutical companies, medical device manufacturers, health insurance companies, or in corporations directing health and safety programs.

Many physicians work long, irregular hours. In 2008, 43 percent of all physicians and surgeons worked 50 or more hours a week; nine percent worked part-time. Physicians must travel frequently between office and hospital to care for their patients. Those who are on call deal with many patients' concerns over the phone and may make emergency visits to hospitals or nursing homes at all hours of the day or night.

Salary

An article in *Modern Healthcare* details the findings of the publication's 2011 Physician Compensation Survey:

Anesthesiology
Ranges from $341,853 to 520,000
Cardiology (invasive)
Ranges from $373,500 to 532,000
Cardiology (noninvasive)
Ranges from $346,266 to 457,921
Dermatology
Ranges from $316,770 to 440,092
Emergency Medicine
Ranges from $246,100 to 300,000
Family Medicine
Ranges from $162,908 to 221,196
Gastroenterology
Ranges from $355,484 to 468,571
General Surgery
Ranges from $312,310 to 431,347
Hospitalist
Ranges from $190,333 to 236,500
Internal Medicine
Ranges from $188,500 to 236,544
Neurology
Ranges from $226,630 to 305,000
Obstetrics/Gynecology
Ranges from $247,680 to 420,000
Oncology (including hematology)
Ranges from $315,000 to 457,000
Orthopedic Surgery
Ranges from $378,062 to 576,350
Pathology
Ranges from $230,000 to 356,281
Pediatrics
Ranges from $161,732 to 229,041
Plastic Surgery
Ranges from $360,000 to 450,000
Psychiatry
Ranges from $182,240 to 237,330
Radiation Oncology
Ranges from $266,900 to 519,677
Radiology
Ranges from $400,000 to 562,500

Urology
Ranges from $347,500 to 453,000

For more information, refer to *www.ama-assn.org/go/hpsalary*.

Employment Outlook

Employment of physicians and surgeons is projected to grow 24 percent from 2010 to 2020, much faster than the average for all occupations. Job growth will occur because of continued expansion of health care-related industries. The growing and aging population will drive overall growth in the demand for physician services, as consumers continue to demand high levels of care using the latest technologies, diagnostic tests, and therapies. Many medical schools are increasing their enrollments based on perceived new demand for physicians.

Despite growing demand for physicians and surgeons, some factors may temper growth. For example, new technologies allow physicians to be more productive. This means physicians can diagnose and treat more patients in the same amount of time. The rising costs of health care can also dramatically affect demand for physicians' services. Furthermore, demand for physicians' services is highly sensitive to changes in health care reimbursement policies. If changes to health coverage result in higher out-of-pocket costs for consumers, demand for physician services may decline.

Unlike their predecessors, newly trained physicians face radically different choices of where and how to practice. New physicians are much less likely to enter solo practice and more likely to take salaried jobs in group medical practices, clinics, and health networks.

Educational Programs

Length, Award. After completing a bachelor's degree, allopathic physicians complete four years of medical school, graduating with a doctor of medicine degree (MD); osteopathic physicians earn a doctor of osteopathic medicine degree (DO). (Some medical schools offer combined undergraduate and medical school programs that last seven rather than the customary eight years.) Next, allopathic physicians complete a residency program of three to five years or longer in their chosen specialty (eg, neurology, surgery, internal medicine); some also complete an additional fellowship of one to three years in a subspecialty, such as cardiology, pain medicine, or neonatal-perinatal medicine.

Following graduation, osteopathic graduates complete an approved 12-month internship, which serves as the link between predoctoral and postdoctoral clinical training and provides a year of maturation of clinical decision-making skills as a generalist physician. The internship exposes graduates to core disciplines including internal medicine, family medicine, general surgery, obstetrics/gynecology, pediatrics, and emergency medicine. Many graduates then choose to complete a residency program in a specialty area.

Prerequisites. Premedical students typically must complete undergraduate work in physics, biology, mathematics, English, and inorganic and organic chemistry. Students also take courses in the humanities and the social sciences. Some students volunteer at local hospitals or clinics to gain practical experience in the health professions. The minimum educational requirement for entry into a medical school is three years of college; most applicants, however, have at least a bachelor's degree, and many have advanced degrees. In addition, the Medical College Admission Test (MCAT) is required by most US medical schools.

The pathway is substantially similar for osteopathic physicians. Osteopathic medical school applicants typically have a bachelor's degree, with undergraduate studies that include one year each of English, biological sciences, physics, general chemistry, and organic

chemistry. Other requirements may include genetics, mathematics, and psychology. Most prospective DO students major in sciences with an emphasis in biology or chemistry; however, applicants may major in any discipline as long as they meet the minimum course and grade requirements. Applicants must also take the MCAT.

Curriculum. Students spend most of the first two years of medical school in laboratories and classrooms, taking courses such as:

- Anatomy
- Biochemistry
- Physiology
- Pharmacology
- Behavioral sciences
- Neurosciences
- Immunology
- Microbiology
- Pathology
- Medical ethics and law

They also learn to take medical histories, examine patients, and diagnose illnesses. During their last two years, students work with patients under the supervision of experienced physicians in hospitals and clinics, learning acute, chronic, preventive, and rehabilitative care. Through rotations in internal medicine, family medicine, obstetrics and gynecology, pediatrics, psychiatry, and surgery, they gain experience in diagnosing and treating illness.

Similarly, osteopathic medical students spend their first two years of school in lectures and laboratories, learning a core set of clinical examination skills and taking courses that cover the various systems of the body, including:

- Anatomy
- Physiology
- Microbiology
- Histology
- Osteopathic principles and practices (including osteopathic manipulative medicine)
- Pharmacology
- Clinical skills
- Doctor/patient communication

Many osteopathic colleges have students assigned to work with physicians beginning early in the first year. This process continues throughout the second year in conjunction with the necessary science courses. In the third and fourth years, osteopathic medical students spend time learning about and exploring the major specialties in medicine through clinical clerkships in both in-patient and ambulatory care settings.

Licensure and Certification

Licensure, which is required of physicians in all US states and jurisdictions, ensures that practicing physicians have appropriate education and training and that they abide by recognized standards of professional conduct while serving their patients. Candidates for first licensure must complete a rigorous examination (for MDs, Steps 1, 2, and 3 of the United States Medical Licensing Examination; for DOs, Levels 1, 2 and 3 of the Comprehensive Osteopathic Medical Licensing Examination) designed to assess a physician's ability to apply knowledge, concepts, and principles that are important in health and disease and that constitute the basis of safe and effective patient care. All applicants must submit proof of medical education and training and provide details about their work history. Finally, applicants may have to reveal information regarding past medical history (including the use of habit-forming drugs and emotional or mental illness), arrests, and convictions.

The majority of physicians choose to become board certified, which is an optional, voluntary process, although it is required by many hospitals and managed care organizations. Certification involves testing and assessment of knowledge, skills, and experience to determine whether a physician is qualified to provide quality patient care in a given specialty/subspecialty. Certification in medical specialties and subspecialties is offered to MDs through the 24 member boards of the American Board of Medical Specialties. In the past, physicians were required to recertify every seven to 10 years, primarily by a written examination; this process is being replaced by Maintenance of Certification, an ongoing rather than periodic process that will require the assessment and improvement of practice performance.

For osteopathic physicians, the Board of Trustees of the American Osteopathic Association (AOA), through the Bureau of Osteopathic Specialists, is the certifying body in osteopathic medicine; there are 19 certifying boards.

Inquiries

MD Education, Careers, Resources
American Medical Association
www.ama-assn.org/go/becominganmd

Association of American Medical Colleges
Careers in Medicine
2450 N Street NW
Washington, DC 20037-1126
E-mail: *careersinmedicine@aamc.org*
www.aamc.org/students/considering/careers.htm

DO Education, Careers, Resources
American Osteopathic Association
142 East Ontario Street
Chicago, IL 60611
800 621-1773 or 312 202-8000
www.osteopathic.org

American Association of Colleges of Osteopathic Medicine
5550 Friendship Blvd, Suite 310
Chevy Chase, MD 20815-7231
www.aacom.org

MD Program Accreditation
Liaison Committee on Medical Education
c/o American Medical Association
515 North State Street
Chicago, IL 60654
www.lcme.org

DO Program Accreditation
Commission on Osteopathic College Accreditation
American Osteopathic Association
142 East Ontario Street
Chicago, IL 60611
www.aoacoca.org

Note: Adapted in part from the Bureau of Labor Statistics, US Department of Labor, *Occupational Outlook Handbook,* Physicians and Surgeons, at *www.bls.gov/oco/ocos074.htm*.

Physician (allopathic)

Alabama

University of Alabama School of Medicine
Allopathic Medicine Prgm
Birmingham, AL 35294
www.ua.edu

University of South Alabama College of Medicine
Allopathic Medicine Prgm
Mobile, AL 36688
www.southalabama.edu/com

Alberta, Canada

University of Calgary
Allopathic Medicine Prgm
Faculty of Medicine
Calgary, AB T2N 4N1
faculty.med.ucalgary.ca

University of Alberta
Allopathic Medicine Prgm
Faculty of Medicine and Dentistry
Edmonton, AB T6G 2R7
www.med.ualberta.ca

Arizona

University of Arizona College of Medicine
Allopathic Medicine Prgm
1501 N Campbell Ave
PO Box 245073
Tucson, AZ 85724
www.medicine.arizona.edu

Arkansas

University of Arkansas for Medical Sciences College of Medicine
Allopathic Medicine Prgm
Little Rock, AR 72204
www.uams.edu/COM/

British Columbia, Canada

University of British Columbia
Allopathic Medicine Prgm
Faculty of Medicine
Vancouver, BC V6T 1Z3
www.med.ubc.ca

California

University of California - Davis School of Medicine
Allopathic Medicine Prgm
Davis, CA 95616
www.ucdmc.ucdavis.edu/medschool

University of CA - Irvine School of Medicine
Allopathic Medicine Prgm
Irvine, CA 92697
www.ucihs.uci.edu

University of California - San Diego
Allopathic Medicine Prgm
School of Medicine
La Jolla, CA 92093
https://meded-portal.ucsd.edu

Loma Linda University School of Medicine
Allopathic Medicine Prgm
Loma Linda, CA 92350
www.llu.edu/llu/medicine

University of California - Los Angeles David Geffen School of Medicine
Allopathic Medicine Prgm
Los Angeles, CA 90095
dgsom.healthsciences.ucla.edu

University of Southern California Keck School of Medicine
Allopathic Medicine Prgm
Los Angeles, CA 90089
www.usc.edu/schools/medicine/ksom.html

Stanford University School of Medicine
Allopathic Medicine Prgm
Palo Alto, CA 94305
med.stanford.edu

University of California - San Francisco School of Medicine
Allopathic Medicine Prgm
San Francisco, CA 94143
medschool.ucsf.edu

Colorado

University of Colorado Denver - Anschutz MC School of Medicine
Allopathic Medicine Prgm
Aurora, CO 80045
www.uchsc.edu/som

Connecticut

University of Connecticut School of Medicine
Allopathic Medicine Prgm
Farmington, CT 06032
medicine.uchc.edu

Yale University School of Medicine
Allopathic Medicine Prgm
New Haven, CT 06510
www.med.yale.edu/ysm

District of Columbia

George Washington University School of Medicine and Health Sciences
Allopathic Medicine Prgm
Washington, DC 20037
www.gwumc.edu/Smhs

Georgetown University Medical Center School of Medicine
Allopathic Medicine Prgm
Washington, DC 20007
gumc.georgetown.edu

Howard University College of Medicine
Allopathic Medicine Prgm
Washington, DC 20059
www.med.howard.edu

Florida

University of Florida College of Medicine
Allopathic Medicine Prgm
Gainesville, FL 32610
www.med.ufl.edu

Florida International University Herbert Wertheim College of Medicine
Allopathic Medicine Prgm
11200 SW 8th St
HLS II 693
Miami, FL 33199
http://medicine.fiu.edu

University of Miami Leonard M Miller School of Medicine
Allopathic Medicine Prgm
Miami, FL 33101
www.med.miami.edu

University of Central Florida College of Medicine
Allopathic Medicine Prgm
Orlando, FL 32827

Florida State University College of Medicine
Allopathic Medicine Prgm
Tallahassee, FL 32306-4300
med.fsu.edu

University of South Florida Health Morsani College of Medicine
Allopathic Medicine Prgm
Tampa, FL 33610
health.usf.edu/medicine/home.html

Georgia

Emory University School of Medicine
Allopathic Medicine Prgm
Atlanta, GA 30322
www.med.emory.edu

Morehouse School of Medicine
Allopathic Medicine Prgm
Atlanta, GA 30314
www.msm.edu

Georgia Health Sciences University Medical College of Georgia
Allopathic Medicine Prgm
Augusta, GA 30912
www.mcg.edu/som

Mercer University School of Medicine
Allopathic Medicine Prgm
Macon, GA 31207
medicine.mercer.edu

Hawaii

University of Hawaii at Manoa John A Burns School of Medicine
Allopathic Medicine Prgm
Honolulu, HI 96822
jabsom.hawaii.edu/jabsom

Illinois

Northwestern University , The Feinberg School of Medicine
Allopathic Medicine Prgm
Chicago, IL 60611
www.medschool.northwestern.edu

Rush University Rush Medical College
Allopathic Medicine Prgm
Chicago, IL 60612
www.rushu.rush.edu/health/dept.html

University of Chicago Div of the Biological Sciences Pritzker Sch of Med
Allopathic Medicine Prgm
Chicago, IL 60637
pritzker.bsd.uchicago.edu

University of Illinois at Chicago College of Medicine
Allopathic Medicine Prgm
Chicago, IL 60612
www.uic.edu/depts/mcam

Loyola University of Chicago Chicago Stritch School of Medicine
Allopathic Medicine Prgm
Maywood, IL 60153
www.meddean.luc.edu/node/83

Rosalind Franklin University of Medicine Chicago Medical School
Allopathic Medicine Prgm
North Chicago, IL 60064
www.rosalindfranklin.edu/cms

Southern Illinois University Edwardsville School of Medicine
Allopathic Medicine Prgm
Springfield, IL 62708
www.siumed.edu

Indiana

Indiana University School of Medicine
Allopathic Medicine Prgm
Indianapolis, IN 46223
www.medicine.iu.edu

Iowa

University of Iowa Roy J. and Lucille A. Carver College of Medicine
Allopathic Medicine Prgm
Iowa City, IA 52242
www.medicine.uiowa.edu

Kansas

University of Kansas Medical Center School of Medicine
Allopathic Medicine Prgm
Kansas City, KS 66103
www.kumc.edu/som

Kentucky

University of Kentucky College of Medicine
Allopathic Medicine Prgm
Lexington, KY 40536
www.mc.uky.edu/medicine

University of Louisville School of Medicine
Allopathic Medicine Prgm
Louisville, KY 40292
louisville.edu/medschool/

Louisiana

Louisiana State Univ Health Sciences Center School of Medicine
Allopathic Medicine Prgm
New Orleans, LA 70112
www.medschool.lsuhsc.edu

Tulane University School of Medicine
Allopathic Medicine Prgm
New Orleans, LA 70112
www.som.tulane.edu

LSU Health Science Center Shreveport School of Medicine
Allopathic Medicine Prgm
Shreveport, LA 71130
www.sh.lsuhsc.edu

Manitoba, Canada

University of Manitoba
Allopathic Medicine Prgm
Faculty of Medicine
Winnipeg, MB R3E 3P5
www.umanitoba.ca/faculties/medicine

Maryland

Johns Hopkins School of Medicine
Allopathic Medicine Prgm
Baltimore, MD 21205
www.hopkinsmedicine.org/som

University of Maryland, Baltimore School of Medicine
Allopathic Medicine Prgm
Baltimore, MD 21201
medschool.umaryland.edu

Uniformed Svcs Univ of the Health Sciences F. Edward Hebert School of Medicine
Allopathic Medicine Prgm
Bethesda, MD 20814
www.usuhs.mil/medschool/fehsom.html

Massachusetts

Boston University School of Medicine
Allopathic Medicine Prgm
Boston, MA 02118
www.bumc.bu.edu

Harvard Medical School
Allopathic Medicine Prgm
Boston, MA 02118
hms.harvard.edu/hms/

Tufts University School of Medicine
Allopathic Medicine Prgm
Boston, MA 02118
www.tufts.edu/med

University of Massachusetts - Boston Medical School
Allopathic Medicine Prgm
Worcester, MA 01655
www.umassmed.edu

Michigan

University of Michigan Medical School
Allopathic Medicine Prgm
Ann Arbor, MI 48109
www.med.umich.edu/medschool

Wayne State University School of Medicine
Allopathic Medicine Prgm
Detroit, MI 48202
www.med.wayne.edu

Michigan State University College of Human Medicine
Allopathic Medicine Prgm
East lansing, MI 48824
humanmedicine.msu.edu

Central Michigan University College of Medicine
Allopathic Medicine Prgm
Mount Pleasant, MI 48859

Oakland University William Beaumont School of Medicine
Allopathic Medicine Prgm
Rochester, MI 48309

Minnesota

University of Minnesota Medical School
Allopathic Medicine Prgm
Minneapolis, MN 55455
www.med.umn.edu

Mayo School of Health Sciences
Allopathic Medicine Prgm
Rochester, MN 55905
www.mayo.edu/mshs

Mississippi

University of Mississippi School of Medicine
Allopathic Medicine Prgm
Jackson, MS 38677
som.umc.edu

Missouri

University of Missouri School of Medicine
Allopathic Medicine Prgm
Columbia, MO 65212
www.muhealth.org/~medicine

University of Missouri - Kansas City School of Medicine
Allopathic Medicine Prgm
Kansas City, MO 64110
research.med.umkc.edu

Saint Louis University School of Medicine
Allopathic Medicine Prgm
St Louis, MO 63104
medschool.slu.edu

Washington University
Allopathic Medicine Prgm
St Louis School of Medicine
St Louis, MO 63110
medschool.wustl.edu

Nebraska

Creighton University School of Medicine
Allopathic Medicine Prgm
Omaha, NE 68178
www2.creighton.edu/medschool

University of Nebraska - Omaha College of Medicine
Allopathic Medicine Prgm
Omaha, NE 68182
www.unmc.edu/dept/com/

Nevada

University of Nevada - Reno School of Medicine
Allopathic Medicine Prgm
Reno, NV 89557
www.unr.edu/med/

New Hampshire

Dartmouth Medical School
Allopathic Medicine Prgm
Hanover, NH 03755
dms.dartmouth.edu

New Jersey

Rowan University Cooper Medical School
Allopathic Medicine Prgm
Camden, NJ 08103

Univ of Medicine & Dent of New Jersey Medical School
Allopathic Medicine Prgm
Newark, NJ 07107
www.umdnj.edu

UMDNJ - Robert Wood Johnson Medical School
Allopathic Medicine Prgm
Piscataway, NJ 08854
rwjms.umdnj.edu

New Mexico

University of New Mexico School of Medicine
Allopathic Medicine Prgm
Albuquerque, NM 87131
hsc.unm.edu/som

New York

Albany Medical College
Allopathic Medicine Prgm
Albany, NY 12208
www.amc.edu

SUNY Downstate Medical Center
Allopathic Medicine Prgm
College of Medicine
Brooklyn, NY 11203
www.hscbklyn.edu/college_of_medicine

University at Buffalo - SUNY
Allopathic Medicine Prgm
School of Medicine and Biomedical Sciences
Buffalo, NY 14260
www.smbs.buffalo.edu

Hofstra University Hofstra North Shore - LIJ School of Medicine
Allopathic Medicine Prgm
Hempstead, NY 11549-1010

Columbia University College of Physicians and Surgeons
Allopathic Medicine Prgm
New York, NY 10032
www.cumc.columbia.edu/dept/ps

Cornell University Weill Medical College
Allopathic Medicine Prgm
New York, NY 10021
www.med.cornell.edu

Mt Sinai School of Medicine
Allopathic Medicine Prgm
New York University
New York, NY 10029
www.mssm.edu

New York Medical College
Allopathic Medicine Prgm
New York, NY 10595
www.nymc.edu

New York University School of Medicine
Allopathic Medicine Prgm
New York, NY 10016
www.med.nyu.edu

Yeshiva University Albert Einstein College of Medicine
Allopathic Medicine Prgm
New York, NY 10033
www.yu.edu

University of Rochester
Allopathic Medicine Prgm
School of Medicine and Dentistry
Rochester, NY 14627
www.urmc.rochester.edu/smd

University at Stony Brook School of Medicine
Allopathic Medicine Prgm
Stony Brook, NY 11794
www.stonybrookmedicalcenter.org/education/som.cfm

SUNY Upstate Medical University
Allopathic Medicine Prgm
Syracuse, NY 13210
www.upstate.edu

Newfoundland, Canada

Memorial University of Newfoundland
Allopathic Medicine Prgm
Faculty of Medicine
St John's, NF A1C 5S7
www.med.mun.ca

North Carolina

University of North Carolina at Chapel Hill School of Medicine
Allopathic Medicine Prgm
Chapel Hill, NC 27514
www.med.unc.edu

Duke University Medical Center School of Medicine
Allopathic Medicine Prgm
Durham, NC 27710
medschool.duke.edu

East Carolina University Brody School of Medicine
Allopathic Medicine Prgm
Greenville, NC 27834
www.ecu.edu/med

Wake Forest University School of Medicine
Allopathic Medicine Prgm
Winston-Salem, NC 27157
www1.wfubmc.edu/school

North Dakota

University of North Dakota
Allopathic Medicine Prgm
School of Medicine and Health Sciences
Grand Forks, ND 58202
www.med.und.nodak.edu

Nova Scotia, Canada

Dalhousie University
Allopathic Medicine Prgm
Faculty of Medicine
Halifax, NS B3H 4H7
www.medicine.dal.ca

Ohio

University of Cincinnati College of Medicine
Allopathic Medicine Prgm
Cincinnati, OH 45267
www.med.uc.edu

Case Western Reserve University School of Medicine
Allopathic Medicine Prgm
Cleveland, OH 44106
casemed.case.edu

The Ohio State University
Allopathic Medicine Prgm
College of Medicine and Public Health
Columbus, OH 43210
sph.osu.edu

Wright State University Boonshoft School of Medicine
Allopathic Medicine Prgm
Dayton, OH 45401
www.med.wright.edu

Northeast Ohio Medical University and Pharmacy
Allopathic Medicine Prgm
Rootstown, OH 44272
www.neoucom.edu

University of Toledo College of Medicine
Allopathic Medicine Prgm
Toledo, OH 43614
hsc.utoledo.edu/med

Oklahoma

University of Oklahoma College of Medicine
Allopathic Medicine Prgm
Oklahoma City, OK 73190
www.medicine.ouhsc.edu

Ontario, Canada

McMaster University School of Medicine
Allopathic Medicine Prgm
Hamilton, ON L8N 3Z5
www.mcmaster.ca/

Queen's University
Allopathic Medicine Prgm
Faculty of Health Sciences
Kingston, ON K7L 3N6
meds.queensu.ca/

University of Western Ontario Schulich School of Medicine
Allopathic Medicine Prgm
London, ON N6A 5B8
www.schulich.uwo.ca/education/admissions/medicine/

University of Ottawa
Allopathic Medicine Prgm
Faculty of Medicine
Ottawa, ON K1H 8M5
www.medicine.uottawa.ca

Northern Ontario Medical School
Allopathic Medicine Prgm
Thunder Bay & Sudbury, ON P7B 5E1
www.normed.ca

University of Toronto
Allopathic Medicine Prgm
Faculty of Medicine
Toronto, ON M5S 1A6
www.facmed.utoronto.ca

Oregon

Oregon Health & Science University School of Medicine
Allopathic Medicine Prgm
Portland, OR 97239
www.ohsuhealth.com

Pennsylvania

Penn State University College of Medicine
Allopathic Medicine Prgm
Hershey, PA 17033
www.hmc.psu.edu/college

Drexel University College of Medicine
Allopathic Medicine Prgm
Philadelphia, PA 19104
www.drexelmed.edu

Temple University School of Medicine
Allopathic Medicine Prgm
Philadelphia, PA 19140
www.temple.edu/medicine

Thomas Jefferson University Jefferson Medical College
Allopathic Medicine Prgm
Philadelphia, PA 19107
www.jefferson.edu/jchp/home/

University of Pennsylvania Perelman School of Medicine
Allopathic Medicine Prgm
Philadelphia, PA 19106
www.med.upenn.edu

University of Pittsburgh School of Medicine
Allopathic Medicine Prgm
Pittsburgh, PA 15260
www.medschool.pitt.edu

The Commonwealth Medical College
Allopathic Medicine Prgm
Scranton, PA 18509

Puerto Rico

Universidad Central del Caribe School of Medicine
Allopathic Medicine Prgm
Bayamon, PR 00960
www.uccaribe.edu

San Juan Bautista School of Medicine
Allopathic Medicine Prgm
PO Box 4968
Caguas, PR 00726-4968

Ponce School of Medicine
Allopathic Medicine Prgm
Ponce, PR 00732
www.psm.edu

University of Puerto Rico School of Medicine
Allopathic Medicine Prgm
San Juan, PR 00936
www.md.rcm.upr.edu

Quebec, Canada

McGill University
Allopathic Medicine Prgm
Faculty of Medicine
Montreal, QC H3G 1Y6
www.medicine.mcgill.ca

University Laval
Allopathic Medicine Prgm
Faculty of Medicine
Quebec City, QC G1K 7P4
w3.fmed.ulaval.ca/site_fac/

University of Sherbrooke
Allopathic Medicine Prgm
Faculty of Medicine
Sherbrooke, QC J1K 2R1
www.usherbrooke.ca/medecine

University de Montreal
Allopathic Medicine Prgm
Faculty of Medicine
Trois Rivieres, QC H3C 3J7
www.umontreal.ca

Rhode Island

Warren Alpert Medical School of Brown Univ
Allopathic Medicine Prgm
Providence, RI 02912
bms.brown.edu

Saskatchewan, Canada

University of Saskatchewan College of Medicine
Allopathic Medicine Prgm
Saskatoon, SK S7N 0W3

South Carolina

Medical University of South Carolina College of Medicine
Allopathic Medicine Prgm
Charleston, SC 29425
www.musc.edu/com/COM1.shtml

MEDICINE

University of South Carolina School of Medicine
Allopathic Medicine Prgm
Columbia, SC 29208
www.med.sc.edu

University of South Carolina School of Medicine Greenville
Allopathic Medicine Prgm
Greenville, SC 29605-5611

South Dakota

University of South Dakota Sanford School of Medicine
Allopathic Medicine Prgm
Sioux Falls, SD 57105-1570
www.usd.edu/med

Tennessee

East Tennessee State University James H Quillen College of Medicine
Allopathic Medicine Prgm
Johnson City, TN 37614
com.etsu.edu

University of Tennessee Health Science Ctr College of Medicine
Allopathic Medicine Prgm
Memphis, TN 38163
www.utmem.edu/Medicine

Meharry Medical College
Allopathic Medicine Prgm
Nashville, TN 37208
www.mmc.edu

Vanderbilt University School of Medicine
Allopathic Medicine Prgm
Nashville, TN 37232
www.mc.vanderbilt.edu/medschool/

Texas

Texas A&M University Health Science Center College of Medicine
Allopathic Medicine Prgm
College Station, TX 77845
medicine.tamhsc.edu

Univ of Texas Southwestern Med Ctr
Allopathic Medicine Prgm
Southwestern Medical School
Dallas, TX 75390
www8.utsouthwestern.edu

Texas Tech Univ Health Sciences Center Paul L Foster School of Medicine
Allopathic Medicine Prgm
4800 Alberta Ave
El Paso, TX 79905
www.ttuhsc.edu/fostersom/

University of Texas Medical Branch School of Medicine
Allopathic Medicine Prgm
Galveston, TX 77550
www.utmb.edu

Baylor College of Medicine
Allopathic Medicine Prgm
Houston, TX 77030
www.bcm.edu

Univ of Texas Medical School at Houston
Allopathic Medicine Prgm
Houston, TX 77225
med.uth.tmc.edu

Texas Tech Univ Health Sciences Center School of Medicine
Allopathic Medicine Prgm
Lubbock, TX 79430
www.ttuhsc.edu/som

UT Health Science Center - San Antonio
Allopathic Medicine Prgm
San Antonio, TX 78229
www.uthscsa.edu

Utah

University of Utah School of Medicine
Allopathic Medicine Prgm
Salt Lake City, UT 84132
uuhsc.utah.edu/som/

Vermont

University of Vermont College of Medicine
Allopathic Medicine Prgm
Burlington, VT 05405
www.med.uvm.edu

Virginia

University of Virginia School of Medicine
Allopathic Medicine Prgm
PO Box 800793
Charlottesville, VA 22908
www.healthsystem.virginia.edu

Eastern Virginia Medical School
Allopathic Medicine Prgm
Medical College of Hampton Roads
Norfolk, VA 23507
www.evms.edu

Virginia Commonwealth University School of Medicine
Allopathic Medicine Prgm
1101 East Marshall St, Sanger Hall, Room 1-071
PO Box 980565
Richmond, VA 23298
www.medschool.vcu.edu

Virginia Tech Carilion School of Medicine and
Allopathic Medicine Prgm
Roanoke, VA 24016
www.vtc.vt.edu/education/index.html

Washington

University of Washington School of Medicine
Allopathic Medicine Prgm
Seattle, WA 98195
www.uwmedicine.org

West Virginia

Marshall University Joan C Edwards School of Medicine
Allopathic Medicine Prgm
Huntington, WV 25701
musom.marshall.edu

West Virginia University School of Medicine
Allopathic Medicine Prgm
Morgantown, WV 26506
www.hsc.wvu.edu/som

Wisconsin

University of Wisconsin - Madison
Allopathic Medicine Prgm
School of Medicine and Public Health
2141D Health Sciences Learning Center
750 Highland Ave
Madison, WI 53705
www.med.wisc.edu

Medical College of Wisconsin
Allopathic Medicine Prgm
Milwaukee, WI 53226
www.mcw.edu

Physician (osteopathic)

Arizona

Midwestern University - Glendale Campus
Osteopathic Medicine Prgm
Arizona College of Osteopathic Medicine
19555 N 59th Ave
Glendale, AZ 85308

AT Still University of Health Sciences
Osteopathic Medicine Prgm
College of Osteopathic Medicine-Mesa
5850 E Still Circle
Mesa, AZ 85206

California

Western Univ of Health Sciences
Osteopathic Medicine Prgm
College of Osteopathic Medicine of the Pacific
309 E Second St, College Plaza
Pomona, CA 91766-1889

Touro University Mare Island
Osteopathic Medicine Prgm
College of Osteopathic Medicine-CA
Vallejo, CA 94592

Colorado

Rocky Vista Univ Coll of Osteopathic Medicine
Osteopathic Medicine Prgm
3449 Chambers Rd, Ste B
Aurora, CO 80011

Florida

Lake Erie Coll of Osteopathic Medicine
Osteopathic Medicine Prgm
5000 Lakewood Ranch Blvd
Bradenton, FL 34211

Nova Southeastern University
Osteopathic Medicine Prgm
College of Osteopathic Medicine
3200 S University Dr
Fort Lauderdale, FL 33328

Georgia

Georgia Campus - PA Coll of Osteopathic Med
Osteopathic Medicine Prgm
625 Old Peachtree Rd
Suwanee, GA 30024

Illinois

Midwestern University
Osteopathic Medicine Prgm
Chicago College of Osteopathic Medicine
555 31st St
Downers Grove, IL 60515

Iowa

Des Moines University
Osteopathic Medicine Prgm
College of Osteopathic Medicine
3200 Grand Ave
Des Moines, IA 50312

Kentucky

Pikeville College
Osteopathic Medicine Prgm
School of Osteopathic Medicine
147 Sycamore St
Pikeville, KY 41501

Maine

University of New England
Osteopathic Medicine Prgm
College of Osteopathic Medicine
11 Hills Beach Rd
Biddeford, ME 04005

Michigan

Michigan State University
Osteopathic Medicine Prgm
College of Osteopathic Medicine
A-309 E Fee Hall
East Lansing, MI 48824

Mississippi

William Carey University
Osteopathic Medicine Prgm
College of Osteopathic Medicine
498 Tuscan Ave, WCU #27
Hattiesburg, MS 39401

Missouri

Kansas City Univ of Medicine and Bioscience
Osteopathic Medicine Prgm
College of Osteopathic Medicine
1750 Independence Ave
Kansas City, MO 64106

Kirksville College of Osteopathic Medicine
Cosponsor: AT Still University of Health Sciences
Osteopathic Medicine Prgm
800 W Jefferson
Kirksville, MO 63501

Nevada

Touro University - Nevada
Osteopathic Medicine Prgm
College of Osteopathic Medicine
874 American Pacific
Henderson, NV 89014

New Jersey

Univ of Medicine & Dent of New Jersey
Osteopathic Medicine Prgm
School of Osteopathic Medicine
Academic Center, One Medical Center Dr
Stratford, NJ 08084

New York

Touro College
Osteopathic Medicine Prgm
College of Osteopathic Medicine
2090 Adam Clayton Powell Blvd, 6th Fl
New York, NY 10027

New York Institute of Technology
Osteopathic Medicine Prgm
College of Osteopathic Medicine
PO Box 8000
Old Westbury, NY 11568

Ohio

Ohio University
Osteopathic Medicine Prgm
College of Osteopathic Medicine
Grosvenor, Irvine Halls
Athens, OH 45701

Oklahoma

Oklahoma State University
Osteopathic Medicine Prgm
College of Osteopathic Medicine
1111 W 17th St
Tulsa, OK 74107

Pennsylvania

Lake Erie Coll of Osteopathic Medicine - Erie
Osteopathic Medicine Prgm
1858 W Grandview Blvd
Erie, PA 16509

Philadelphia College of Osteopathic Medicine
Osteopathic Medicine Prgm
4170 City Ave
Philadelphia, PA 19131

Tennessee

Lincoln Memorial University
Osteopathic Medicine Prgm
DeBusk College of Osteopathic Medicine
6965 Cumberland Gap Pkwy
Harrogate, TN 37752

Texas

Univ of North Texas Hlth Sci Ctr at Ft Worth
Osteopathic Medicine Prgm
Texas College of Osteopathic Medicine
3500 Camp Bowie Blvd
Fort Worth, TX 76107-2970

Virginia

Edward Via Virginia Coll of Opteopathic Med
Osteopathic Medicine Prgm
2265 Kraft Dr
Blacksburg, VA 24060

Washington

Pacific Northwest Univ of Hlth Sci
Osteopathic Medicine Prgm
College of Osteopathic Medicine
111 University Pkwy, Suite 202
Yakima, WA 98901

West Virginia

West Virginia of Osteopathic Medicine
Osteopathic Medicine Prgm
400 N Lee St
Lewisburg, WV 24901

MEDICINE

Registered Nurse

Career Description

Nursing is the largest health care occupation, with 2.6 million Registered Nurses (RNs) in the nation's workforce in 2008, according to the US Bureau of Labor Statistics (BLS). RNs provide a variety of care services that include treating patients, educating patients and the public about various medical conditions, and providing advice and emotional support to patients' family members. RNs record patients' medical histories and symptoms, help to perform diagnostic tests and analyze results, operate medical machinery, administer treatment and medications, and help with patient follow-up and rehabilitation. RNs teach patients and their families how to manage illness or injury, including post-treatment home care needs, diet and exercise programs, and self-administration of medication and physical therapy. Some RNs also are educated to provide grief counseling to family members of critically ill patients. RNs work to promote general health by educating the public on various warning signs and symptoms of disease and where to go for help. RNs also might run health screening or immunization clinics, blood drives, and public seminars on various conditions.

RNs can specialize in one or more patient care specialties. The most common specialties can be divided into roughly four categories—by work setting or type of treatment; disease, ailment, or condition; organ or body system type; or population. RNs may combine specialties from more than one area—for example, pediatric oncology or cardiac emergency—depending on personal interest and employer needs.

RNs may specialize by work setting or by type of care provided:

- *Ambulatory care nurses* treat patients with a variety of illnesses and injuries on an outpatient basis, either in physicians' offices or in clinics or through electronic telehealth media
- *Critical care nurses* work in critical or intensive care hospital units and provide care to patients with cardiovascular, respiratory, or pulmonary failure
- *Emergency or trauma nurses* work in hospital emergency departments and treat patients with life-threatening conditions caused by accidents, heart attacks, and strokes
- *Holistic nurses* provide care such as acupuncture, massage and aroma therapy, and biofeedback, which are meant to treat patients' mental and spiritual health in addition to their physical health
- *Home health care nurses* provide at-home care for patients who are recovering from surgery, accidents, and childbirth
- *Hospice and palliative care nurses* provide care for, and help ease the pain of, terminally ill patients outside of hospitals
- *Infusion nurses* administer medications, fluids, and blood to patients through injections into patients' veins
- *Long-term care nurses* provide medical services on a recurring basis to patients with chronic physical or mental disorders
- *Medical-surgical nurses* provide basic medical care to a variety of patients in all health settings

- *Occupational health nurses* provide treatment for job-related injuries and illnesses and help employers to detect workplace hazards and implement health and safety standards
- *Perianesthesia nurses* provide preoperative and postoperative care to patients undergoing anesthesia during surgery
- *Perioperative nurses* assist surgeons by selecting and handling instruments, controlling bleeding, and suturing incisions
- *Psychiatric nurses* treat patients with personality and mood disorders
- *Radiologic nurses* provide care to patients undergoing diagnostic radiation procedures such as ultrasounds and magnetic resonance imaging
- *Rehabilitation nurses* care for patients with temporary and permanent disabilities
- *Transplant nurses* care for both transplant recipients and living donors and monitor signs of organ rejection

RNs specializing in a particular disease, ailment, or condition are employed in virtually all work settings, including hospitals, physicians' offices, outpatient treatment facilities, home health care agencies, and private practices. These specialties include:

- Addictions
- Developmental disabilities
- Diabetes management
- Genetics
- HIV/AIDS
- Oncology
- Wound, ostomy, and continence

RNs specializing in treatment of a particular organ or body system usually are employed in specialty physicians' offices or outpatient care facilities, although some are employed in hospital specialty or critical care units. These specialties include:

- Cardiology and vascular medicine
- Dermatology
- Gastroenterology
- Gynecology
- Nephrology
- Neuroscience
- Ophthalmology
- Orthopedics
- Otorhinolaryngology
- Respiratory disorders
- Urology

Finally, RNs may specialize by providing preventive and acute care in all health care settings to various segments of the population, including newborns (neonatology), children and adolescents (pediatrics), adults, and the elderly (gerontology or geriatrics). RNs also may provide basic health care to patients in correctional facilities, schools, summer camps, and the military.

Most RNs work as staff nurses, providing critical health care services along with physicians, surgeons, and other health care practi-

tioners. Some RNs choose to become advanced practice registered nurses and serve in one of four specialty roles:
- Clinical nurse specialists
- Nurse anesthetists
- Nurse midwives
- Nurse practitioners

Some nurses pursue careers that require little or no direct patient contact, although most of these positions still require an active RN license:
- Case managers
- Forensics nurses
- Infection control nurses
- Legal nurse consultants
- Nurse administrators
- Nurse educators
- Nurse informaticists
- Nurse researchers

RNs also may work as health care consultants, public policy advisors, pharmaceutical and medical supply researchers and salespersons, and medical writers and editors.

Employment Characteristics

Though most RNs (60%) still work in hospitals, nurses are employed in all types of settings in which health care is provided. Home health and public health nurses travel to patients' homes, schools, community centers, and other sites. RNs may spend considerable time walking and standing. Patients in hospitals and nursing care facilities require 24-hour care; consequently, nurses in these institutions may work nights, weekends, and holidays. RNs also may be on call—available to work on short notice. Nurses who work in office settings are more likely to work regular business hours. About 20 percent of RNs work part time.

Nursing has its hazards, especially in hospitals, nursing care facilities, and clinics, where nurses may care for individuals with infectious diseases. RNs must observe rigid, standardized guidelines to guard against disease and other dangers, such as those posed by radiation, accidental needle sticks, chemicals used to sterilize instruments, and anesthetics. In addition, they are vulnerable to back injury when moving patients, shocks from electrical equipment, and hazards posed by compressed gases. RNs who work with critically ill patients also may suffer emotional strain from observing patient suffering and from close personal contact with patients' families.

Aside from hospitals and inpatient and outpatient departments, nurses also work in physicians' offices, nursing care facilities, home health care services, employment services, government agencies, and outpatient care centers. Other employment settings include social assistance agencies and educational services, both public and private.

Salary

BLS data (available at *www.bls.gov/oes/current/oes291111.htm*) show that median annual earnings of registered nurses were $65,950 in May 2011. The lowest 10 percent earned less than $44,970 and the highest 10 percent earned more than $96,630. Median annual earnings in the industries employing the largest numbers of registered nurses in May 2009 were as follows:
- General medical and surgical hospitals $69,810
- Offices of physicians $72,890
- Home health care services $65,120
- Nursing care facilities $60,830

Many employers offer flexible work schedules, child care, educational benefits, and bonuses. Advanced practice registered nurses and those holding positions requiring master's or doctoral preparation often earn annual salaries exceeding $100,000.

For more information, refer to www.ama-assn.org/go/hpsalary.

Employment Outlook

The BLS reports that overall job opportunities for registered nurses are expected to be excellent but may vary by employment and geographic setting. Some employers report difficulty in attracting and retaining an adequate number of RNs. Employment of RNs is expected to grow much faster than the average for all occupations, and, because the occupation is very large, 581,500 new jobs are projected to be created through 2018, among the largest number of new jobs for any occupation. Additionally, hundreds of thousands of job openings will result from the need to replace experienced nurses who retire and leave the profession each year.

Employment of registered nurses is expected to grow by 26 percent from 2010-2020. Growth will be driven by technological advances in patient care, which permit a greater number of health problems to be treated, and by an increasing emphasis on preventive care. In addition, the number of older people, who are much more likely than younger people to need nursing care, is projected to grow rapidly.

Employment is expected to grow more slowly in hospitals. While the intensity of nursing care is likely to increase, requiring more nurses per patient, the number of inpatients (those who remain in the hospital for more than 24 hours) is not likely to grow by much. Patients are being discharged earlier, and more procedures are being done on an outpatient basis, both inside and outside hospitals. Rapid growth is expected in hospital outpatient facilities, such as those providing same-day surgery, rehabilitation, and chemotherapy.

More and more sophisticated procedures, once performed only in hospitals, are being performed in physicians' offices and in outpatient care centers, such as freestanding ambulatory surgical and emergency centers. Accordingly, employment is expected to grow fast in these places as health care in general expands.

Employment in nursing care facilities is expected to grow because of increases in the number of older persons, many of whom require long-term care. Many elderly patients want to be treated at home or in residential care facilities, which will drive demand for RNs in those settings. The financial pressure on hospitals to discharge patients as soon as possible should produce more admissions to nursing and residential care facilities and referrals to home healthcare. Job growth also is expected in units that provide specialized long-term rehabilitation for stroke and head injury patients, as well as units that treat Alzheimer's victims.

Employment in home health care is expected to increase in response to the growing number of older persons with functional disabilities, preference for care in the home, and technological advances that make it possible to bring increasingly complex treatments into the home. The type of care demanded will require nurses who are able to perform complex procedures.

Job prospects. Overall job opportunities are expected to be excellent for registered nurses. Employers in some parts of the country and in certain employment settings report difficulty in attracting and retaining an adequate number of RNs, primarily because of an aging RN workforce and a lack of younger workers to fill positions. Qualified applicants to nursing schools are being turned away because of a shortage of nursing faculty. The need for nursing faculty will only increase as many instructors near retirement. Despite the slower employment growth in hospitals, job opportunities should still be excellent because of the relatively high turnover of hospital nurses. To attract and retain qualified nurses, hospitals may offer signing bonuses, family-friendly work schedules, or subsidized training. Although faster employment growth is projected in physicians' offices and outpatient care centers, RNs may face greater competition for these positions, which generally offer regular working hours and more comfortable working environments. Generally, RNs with at least a bachelor's degree will have better job prospects than those without a bachelor's.

 ### Educational Programs

Award, Length. The three major educational paths to registered nursing are 1) a bachelor's of science degree in nursing (BSN), 2) an associate degree in nursing (ADN), and 3) a diploma. BSN programs, offered by colleges and universities, take about four years to complete, ADN programs, offered by community and junior colleges, take about three years to complete, and diploma programs, administered in hospitals, last about three years.

Many RNs with an ADN or diploma later enter bachelor's programs to prepare for a broader scope of nursing practice, through an RN-to-BSN and RN-to-MSN programs. In addition, accelerated BSN programs, lasting 12 to 18 months, are available for individuals who have a bachelor's or higher degree in another field and who are interested in moving quickly into nursing. Accelerated master's programs are also available to career changers and combine one year of an accelerated BSN program with two years of graduate study.

A bachelor's degree often is necessary for advanced clinical and administrative positions and is a prerequisite for admission to graduate nursing programs in research, consulting, and teaching, and all four advanced practice nursing specialties—clinical nurse specialist, nurse anesthetist, nurse midwife, and nurse practitioner. Individuals who complete a bachelor's receive more education in areas such as communication, leadership, and critical thinking, all of which are becoming more important as nursing care becomes more complex. Additionally, bachelor's degree programs offer more clinical experience in nonhospital settings.

Prerequisites. High school students considering a nursing career should take science, mathematics, and communications courses. Nurses should be caring, sympathetic, responsible, and detail oriented. They must be able to direct or supervise others, correctly assess patients' conditions, and determine when consultation is required. They need emotional stability to cope with human suffering, emergencies, and other stresses.

Curriculum. All nursing education programs include classroom instruction and supervised clinical experience in hospitals and other health care facilities. Students take courses in anatomy, physiology, microbiology, chemistry, nutrition, psychology and other behavioral sciences, and nursing. Coursework also includes the liberal arts for ADN and BSN students. Supervised clinical experience is provided in hospital departments such as pediatrics, psychiatry, maternity, and surgery. A growing number of programs include clinical experience in nursing care facilities, public health departments, home health agencies, and ambulatory clinics.

Advanced Training. All four advanced practice registered nursing specialties currently require at least a master's degree, and the profession is moving toward doctoral preparation for these roles. Most programs last about two years and require a BSN degree for admission; some programs require at least one to two years of clinical experience as an RN. Upon completion of a program, most advanced practice registered nurses become nationally certified in their area of specialty. In some states, certification in a specialty is required in order to practice that specialty.

 ### Licensure, Certification, Registration

In all states and the District of Columbia, students must graduate from an approved nursing program and pass a national licensing examination, known as the National Council Licensure Examination (NCLEX-RN), to obtain a nursing license. Nurses may be licensed in more than one state, either by examination or by the endorsement of a license issued by another state. Currently 24 states participate in the Nurse Licensure Compact Agreement, which allows nurses to practice in member states without recertifying. All states require periodic renewal of licenses, which may involve continuing education.

 ### Inquiries

Education, Careers, Resources
American Association of Colleges of Nursing
One Dupont Circle NW, Suite 530
Washington, DC 20036
www.aacn.nche.edu

American Nurses Association
8515 Georgia Avenue, Suite 400
Silver Spring, MD 20910
www.nursingworld.org

National League for Nursing
61 Broadway
New York, NY 10006
www.nln.org

Licensure
National Council of State Boards of Nursing
111 East Wacker Drive, Suite 2900
Chicago, IL 60611
www.ncsbn.org

Program Accreditation
(*Note:* The programs listed in this *Directory* are those accredited at the baccalaureate and/or master's level by the following organization.)

Commission on Collegiate Nursing Education
American Association of Colleges of Nursing
One Dupont Circle NW, Suite 530
Washington, DC 20036
www.aacn.nche.edu

Note: Adapted in part from the Bureau of Labor Statistics, U.S. Department of Labor, *Occupational Outlook Handbook,* Registered Nurses, at *www.bls.gov/oco/ocos083.htm.*

Nurse

Alabama

Auburn University
Nursing Prgm
Auburn University, AL 36849
www.nursing.auburn.edu

Samford University
Nursing Prgm
Birmingham, AL 35229
www.samford.edu

University of Alabama at Birmingham
Nursing Prgm
Birmingham, AL 35294
www.uab.edu

University of North Alabama
Nursing Prgm
College of Nursing and Allied Health
Florence, AL 35632

Univ of Alabama at Birmingham - Huntsville
Nursing Prgm
Huntsville, AL 35899
onlinenurse.nb.uah.edu

Jacksonville State University
Nursing Prgm
Jacksonville, AL 36265
www.jsu.edu/depart/nursing

Spring Hill College
Nursing Prgm
Division of Nursing
Mobile, AL 36608

University of Mobile
Nursing Prgm
Mobile, AL 36613
www.umobile.edu

University of South Alabama
Nursing Prgm
Mobile, AL 36688
www.usouthal.edu

Auburn University at Montgomery
Nursing Prgm
Montgomery, AL 36124
www.aum.edu

Stillman College
Nursing Prgm
Nursing Department
3601 Stillman Blvd, PO Box 1430
Tuscaloosa, AL 35401
www.stillman.edu

University of Alabama
Nursing Prgm
Tuscaloosa, AL 35487
www.ua.edu

Arizona

Northern Arizona University
Nursing Prgm
Flagstaff, AZ 86011
www.nau.edu/~hp/dept/nurse

Arizona State University
Nursing Prgm
Phoenix, AZ 85004
www.asu.edu

Grand Canyon University
Nursing Prgm
Phoenix, AZ 85017
www.gcu.edu/scon

University of Phoenix
Nursing Prgm
Phoenix, AZ 85040
www.universityof phoenix-online.com

University of Arizona
Nursing Prgm
College of Nursing
Tucson, AZ 85721
www.nursing.arizona.edu

Arkansas

Henderson State University
Nursing Prgm
Arkadelphia, AR 71999
www.hsu.edu

University of Central Arkansas
Nursing Prgm
Conway, AR 72035
www.uca.edu/chas/nursing.html

University of Arkansas
Nursing Prgm
Fayetteville, AR 72701
nurs.uark.edu

University of Arkansas for Medical Sciences
Nursing Prgm
Little Rock, AR 72205
nursing.uams.edu

California

Humboldt State University
Nursing Prgm
Arcata, CA 95521
www.humboldt.edu

Azusa Pacific University
Nursing Prgm
Azusa, CA 91702
www.apu.edu

California State University - Bakersfield
Nursing Prgm
Department of Nursing
Bakersfield, CA 93311

California State University - Channel Islands
Nursing Prgm
Nursing Program
One University Drive
Camarillo, CA 93012-8599
http://nursing.csuci.edu

California State University - Dominguez Hills
Nursing Prgm
Carson, CA 90747
www.csudh.edu

California State University - Chico
Nursing Prgm
Chico, CA 95929
www.csuchico.edu/nurs

California State University - East Bay
Nursing Prgm
Department of Nursing and Heath Sciences
4700 Ygnacio Valley Rd
Concord, CA 94521
www.csueastbay.edu

Vanguard University
Nursing Prgm
Nursing Program
55 Fair Drive
Costa Mesa, CA 92626-9601
www.vanguard.edu/sps/nursing

California State University - Fresno
Nursing Prgm
Fresno, CA 93740
www.csufresno.edu/nursing

Fresno Pacific University
Nursing Prgm
BSN Program
1717 South Chestnut Ave
Fresno, CA 93702
www.fresno.edu

California State University - Fullerton
Nursing Prgm
Fullerton, CA 92834
nursing.fullerton.edu

Concordia University - Irvine
Nursing Prgm
Division of Nursing
1530 Concordia West
Irvine, CA 92612-3203
www.cui.edu/nursing

University of CA - Irvine School of Medicine
Nursing Prgm
Nursing Program
233 Irvine Hall
Irvine, CA 92697-3959
www.ucihs.uci.edu/nursing/

West Coast University
Nursing Prgm
College of Nursing
151 Innovation Drive
Irvine, CA 92617-3040
www.westcoastuniversity.edu

National University
Nursing Prgm
Department of Nursing
La Jolla, CA 92037

Biola University
Nursing Prgm
Department of Nursing
13800 Biola Ave
La Mirada, CA 90639-0001
www.biola.edu

Loma Linda University
Nursing Prgm
Loma Linda, CA 92350
www.llu.edu

California State University - Long Beach
Nursing Prgm
Long Beach, CA 90840
www.csulb.edu/~nursing

California State University - Los Angeles
Nursing Prgm
School of Nursing
5151 State University Drive
Los Angeles, CA 90032-8171
www.calstatela.edu

Mount St Mary's College
Nursing Prgm
Los Angeles, CA 90049
www.msmc.la.edu

University of California - Los Angeles
Nursing Prgm
Los Angeles, CA 90032
www.nursing.ucla.edu

California State University - Northridge
Nursing Prgm
Northridge, CA 91330
www.csun.edu

NURSING

Holy Names University
Nursing Prgm
Department of Nursing
Oakland, CA 94619

Samuel Merritt University
Nursing Prgm
Oakland, CA 94609
www.samuelmerritt.edu

California Baptist University
Nursing Prgm
School of Nursing
8432 Magnolia Ave, Lambeth House, Room 7
Riverside, CA 92504-3297
www.calbaptist.edu

California State University - Sacramento
Nursing Prgm
Sacramento, CA 95819
www.hhs.csus.edu/NRS

California State University - San Bernardino
Nursing Prgm
San Bernardino, CA 92407
www.csusb.edu

Point Loma Nazarene University
Nursing Prgm
San Diego, CA 92106
www.ptloma.edu/nursing

San Diego State University
Nursing Prgm
San Diego, CA 92182
www.sdsu.edu

Univ of California San Diego Med Ctr
Nursing Prgm
San Diego, CA 92110
www.acusd.edu

San Francisco State University
Nursing Prgm
San Francisco, CA 94132
www.nursing.sfsu.edu

University of California - San Francisco
Nursing Prgm
San Francisco, CA 94117
www.usfca.edu/nursing

San Jose State University
Nursing Prgm
San Jose, CA 95192
www.sjsu.edu/nursing

California State University - San Marcos
Nursing Prgm
School of Nursing
333 South Twin Oaks Valley Rd
San Marcos, CA 92096-0001
www.csusm.edu/nursing

Dominican University of California
Nursing Prgm
San Rafael, CA 94901
www.dominican.edu

California State University - Stanislaus
Nursing Prgm
Turlock, CA 95382

Colorado

Adams State College
Nursing Prgm
208 Edgemont Blvd
Alamosa, CO 81102
www2.adams.edu/academics/bs-nursing/bs-nursing.php

American Sentinel University
Nursing Prgm
Nursing Program
2260 South Xanadu Way, Suite 310
Aurora, CO 80014
www.americansentinel.edu

University of Colorado at Colorado Springs
Nursing Prgm
Colorado Springs, CO 80917
www.web.uccs.edu/bethel

Regis University
Nursing Prgm
Denver, CO 80221
www.regis.edu

University of Colorado Denver - Anschutz MC
Nursing Prgm
Denver, CO 80045
www2.uchsc.edu/son

Colorado Mesa University
Nursing Prgm
Grand Junction, CO 81501
www.mesastate.edu

University of Northern Colorado
Nursing Prgm
Greeley, CO 80639
www.univnorthco.edu/nurses/son.html

Colorado Christian University
Nursing Prgm
Division of Nursing and Sciences
8787 West Alameda Ave
Lakewood, CO 80226
http://ww.ccu.edu

Connecticut

Western Connecticut State University
Nursing Prgm
Danbury, CT 06810
wcsu.edu

Fairfield University
Nursing Prgm
Fairfield, CT 06824
www.fairfield.edu

Sacred Heart University
Nursing Prgm
Fairfield, CT 06825
www.sacredheart.edu

Central Connecticut State University
Nursing Prgm
Department of Nursing
New Britain, CT 06050

Southern Connecticut State University
Nursing Prgm
New Haven, CT 06515
www.scsu.ctstateu.edu

University of Connecticut
Nursing Prgm
School of Nursing
231 Glenbrook Rd, Unit 2026
Storrs, CT 06269-2026
www.nursing.uconn.edu

Saint Joseph College
Nursing Prgm
West Hartford, CT 06117
www.sjc.edu

University of Hartford
Nursing Prgm
West Hartford, CT 06117
www.hartford.edu

Delaware

Delaware State University
Nursing Prgm
Dover, DE 19901
www.desu.edu/colleges/chpp/nursing

Wilmington College
Nursing Prgm
New Castle, DE 19720
www.wilmcoll.edu

University of Delaware-Christiana Care Health
Nursing Prgm
Newark, DE 19716
www.udel.edu/health

District of Columbia

Catholic University of America
Nursing Prgm
Washington, DC 20064
nursing.cua.edu

George Washington University
Nursing Prgm
School of Nursing
900 23rd St, NW, Suite 6167B
Washington, DC 20037
www.gwumc.edu/healthsci

Georgetown University Medical Center
Nursing Prgm
Washington, DC 20057
www.georgetown.edu

Howard University
Nursing Prgm
Washington, DC 20059
www.cpnahs.howard.edu

Trinity University
Nursing Prgm
Nursing Program
Washington, DC 20017
www.trinitydc.edu

Florida

Florida Atlantic University
Nursing Prgm
Boca Raton, FL 33431
www.fau.edu/nursing

University of Miami
Nursing Prgm
Coral Gables, FL 33146
www.miami.edu/nur

Nova Southeastern University
Nursing Prgm
Fort Lauderdale, FL 33328
www.nova.edu/nursing

Florida Gulf Coast University
Nursing Prgm
Fort Myers, FL 33965
www.fgcu.edu/chp/nursing

Keiser University
Nursing Prgm
RN/BSN Program
1900 West Commercial Blvd, Suite 100
Ft Lauderdale, FL 33309
www.keiseruniversity.edu/nursing-BS.php

University of Florida
Nursing Prgm
Gainesville, FL 32610
www.nursing.ufl.edu

Jacksonville University
Nursing Prgm
School of Nursing
Jacksonville, FL 32211

University of North Florida
Nursing Prgm
Jacksonville, FL 32224
www.unf.edu/coh

Remington College of Nursing
Nursing Prgm
660 Century Point, Suite 1050
Lake Mary, FL 32746
www.remingtonnursing.com

Florida Southern College
Nursing Prgm
Lakeland, FL 33801
www.flsouthern.edu

Florida International University
Nursing Prgm
College of Nursing and Health Sciences
11200 SW 8th St, AHC3- 529
Miami, FL 33199
www.fiu.edu

Barry University
Nursing Prgm
Miami Shores, FL 33161
www.barry.edu/nursing

Northwest Florida State College
Nursing Prgm
Department of Nursing and Allied Health
100 College Blvd, Building E
Niceville, FL 32578-1295
www.nwfsc.edu

University of Central Florida
Nursing Prgm
Orlando, FL 32816
www.cohpa.ucf.edu/nursing

University of West Florida
Nursing Prgm
Pensacola, FL 32514
www.uwf.edu/nursing

St Petersburg College
Nursing Prgm
Pinellas Park, FL 33781
www.spcollege.edu

Florida State University
Nursing Prgm
Tallahassee, FL 32306
www.fsu.edu

University of South Florida
Nursing Prgm
Tampa, FL 33612
hsc.usf.edu

Palm Beach Atlantic University
Nursing Prgm
West Palm Beach, FL 33416
www.pba.edu

Georgia

Emory University
Nursing Prgm
Atlanta, GA 30322
www.nursing.emory.edu

Georgia State University
Nursing Prgm
Atlanta, GA 30303
www.gsu.edu

Mercer University
Nursing Prgm
Atlanta, GA 30341
www.mercer.edu

Georgia Health Sciences University
Nursing Prgm
Augusta, GA 30912
www.mcg.edu/son/

University of West Georgia
Nursing Prgm
Carrollton, GA 30118
www.westga.edu

Columbus State University
Nursing Prgm
School of Nursing
4225 University Ave
Columbus, GA 31907-5645
www.columbusstate.edu

Brenau University
Nursing Prgm
Gainesville, GA 30501
www.brenau.edu

Kennesaw State University
Nursing Prgm
Kennesaw, GA 30144
www.kennesaw.edu

Clayton State University
Nursing Prgm
Morrow, GA 30260
healthsci.clayton.edu

Armstrong Atlantic State University
Nursing Prgm
Savannah, GA 31419
www.don.armstrong.edu

South University
Nursing Prgm
College of Nursing
709 Mall Blvd
Savannah, GA 31406-4881
www.southuniversity.edu

Georgia Southern University
Nursing Prgm
Statesboro, GA 30458
www.georgiasouthern.edu

Valdosta State University
Nursing Prgm
Valdosta, GA 31698
www.valdosta.edu/nursing

Hawaii

University of Hawaii at Manoa
Nursing Prgm
Honolulu, HI 96822
www.nursing.hawaii.edu

Idaho

Lewis-Clark State College
Nursing Prgm
Division of Nursing and Health Sciences
Lewiston, ID 83501

Northwest Nazarene University
Nursing Prgm
Nampa, ID 83686
www.nnu.edu/nursing

Idaho State University
Nursing Prgm
Pocatello, ID 83209
www.isu.edu/departments/nursing

Illinois

Aurora University
Nursing Prgm
Aurora, IL 60506
www.aurora.edu/nursing

Illinois Wesleyan University
Nursing Prgm
School of Nursing
Bloomington, IL 61702

Olivet Nazarene University
Nursing Prgm
Bourbonnais, IL 60914
www.olivet.edu

Eastern Illinois University
Nursing Prgm
600 Lincoln Ave, McAfee Room 2230
Charleston, IL 61920
www.eiu.edu/~nursing

DePaul University
Nursing Prgm
Department of Nursing
Chicago, IL 60614

Kaplan University
Nursing Prgm
School of Nursing and Health Care
Chicago, IL 60607

North Park University
Nursing Prgm
Chicago, IL 60625
www.northpark.edu

Saint Xavier University
Nursing Prgm
Chicago, IL 60655
www.sxu.edu

University of Illinois at Chicago
Nursing Prgm
Chicago, IL 60612
www.uic.edu

Lakeview College of Nursing
Nursing Prgm
Danville, IL 61832

Millikin University
Nursing Prgm
Decatur, IL 62522
www.millikin.edu

Northern Illinois University
Nursing Prgm
Dekalb, IL 60115
www.niu.edu

Chamberlain College of Nursing
Nursing Prgm
3005 Highland Parkway, 5th Floor
Downers Grove, IL 60515
www.chamberlain.edu

Southern Illinois University Edwardsville
Nursing Prgm
Edwardsville, IL 62026
www.siue.edu

Elmhurst College
Nursing Prgm
Deicke Center for Nursing Education
Elmhurst, IL 60126

MacMurray College
Nursing Prgm
Department of Nursing
Jacksonville, IL 62650

NURSING

University of St Francis
Nursing Prgm
College of Nursing and Allied Health
Joliet, IL 60435

McKendree University
Nursing Prgm
701 College Rd
Lebanon, IL 62254-1299
www.mckendree.edu

Benedictine University
Nursing Prgm
5700 College Rd, Kindlon Hall 248
Lisle, IL 60532
www.ben.edu/nursinghome/

Western Illinois University
Nursing Prgm
School of Nursing
1 University Circle, 339 Waggoner Hall
Macomb, IL 61455-1390
www.wiu.edu/nursing

Loyola University of Chicago
Nursing Prgm
Maywood, IL 60153
www.luc.edu/schools/nursing

Illinois State University
Nursing Prgm
Normal, IL 61790
www.mcn.ilstu.edu

Resurrection University
Nursing Prgm
Oak Park, IL 60302

Trinity Christian College
Nursing Prgm
Department of Nursing
Palos Heights, IL 60463

Methodist College of Nursing
Nursing Prgm
415 St Mark Court
Peoria, IL 61603
www.mcon.edu

Blessing Hospital
Nursing Prgm
Rieman Collge of Nursing
Quincy, IL 62305

Trinity College of Nursing & Health Sciences
Nursing Prgm
Rock Island, IL 61201
www.trinitycollegequ.edu

OSF Saint Anthony Medical Center
Nursing Prgm
Rockford, IL 61108
www.sacn.edu

Lewis University
Nursing Prgm
College of Nursing and Health Professions
Romeoville, IL 60446

Indiana

Anderson University
Nursing Prgm
1100 E Fifth St
Anderson, IN 46012-3462
www.anderson.edu

University of Southern Indiana
Nursing Prgm
Evansville, IN 47712
heath_p.usi.edu

University of Saint Francis
Nursing Prgm
Fort Wayne, IN 46808
www.sf.edu/nursing

Indiana University Northwest
Nursing Prgm
Gary, IN 46408
www.iun.indiana.edu

Goshen College
Nursing Prgm
Department of Nursing
Goshen, IN 46526

Huntington University
Nursing Prgm
Department of Nursing
2303 College Ave
Huntington, IN 46750-1237
www.huntington.edu

Indiana Univ-Purdue Univ-Indianapolis
Nursing Prgm
1111 Middle Drive, NU132
Indianapolis, IN 46202-5107
nursing.iupui.edu

Marian University
Nursing Prgm
Indianapolis, IN 46222
www.marian.edu

University of Indianapolis
Nursing Prgm
Indianapolis, IN 46227
www.uindy.edu

Indiana University - Kokomo
Nursing Prgm
Kokomo, IN 46904
www.iuk.indiana/edu.iuk/iuk_nursing.html

Indiana Wesleyan University
Nursing Prgm
Division of Nursing Education
Marion, IN 46953

Ball State University
Nursing Prgm
Muncie, IN 47306
www.bsu.edu/nursing

Indiana University Southeast
Nursing Prgm
Division of Nursing
New Albany, IN 47150

Indiana University South Bend
Nursing Prgm
South Bend, IN 46634
www.iusb.edu/~nursing

Valparaiso University
Nursing Prgm
College of Nursing
Valparaiso, IN 46383

Purdue University
Nursing Prgm
West Lafayette, IN 47907
www.nursing.purdue.edu

Iowa

Coe College
Nursing Prgm
Cedar Rapids, IA 52402
www.coe.edu

Mount Mercy College
Nursing Prgm
Department of Nursing
Cedar Rapids, IA 52402

St Ambrose University
Nursing Prgm
Davenport, IA 52803
web.sau.edu/nursing

Luther College
Nursing Prgm
Decorah, IA 52101
www.luther.edu/learning/dept/nursing.html

Grand View College
Nursing Prgm
Division of Nursing
Des Moines, IA 50316

Mercy College of Health Sciences
Nursing Prgm
Des Moines, IA 50309
www.mchs.edu

Clarke University
Nursing Prgm
Dubuque, IA 52001
www.clarke.edu

University of Dubuque
Nursing Prgm
Nursing Dept
Dubuque, IA 52001
www.dbq.edu/academics/nursing

Upper Iowa University
Nursing Prgm
605 Washington St, PO Box 1857
Fayette, IA 52142
www.uiu.edu/nursing

University of Iowa
Nursing Prgm
Iowa City, IA 52242
www.nursing.uiowa.edu

Northwestern College
Nursing Prgm
101 7th St SW
Orange City, IA 51041-1996
www.nwciowa.edu

Dordt College
Nursing Prgm
Nursing Department
Sioux Center, IA 51250

Briar Cliff University
Nursing Prgm
Department of Nursing
3303 Rebecca St
Sioux City, IA 51104
www.briarcliff.edu

Morningside College
Nursing Prgm
Department of Nursing Education
1501 Morningside Ave
Sioux City, IA 51106
www.morningside.edu

Allen College
Nursing Prgm
1825 Logan Ave
Gerard Hall
Waterloo, IA 50703
www.allencollege.edu

Kansas

Fort Hays State University
Nursing Prgm
Hays, KS 67601
www.fhsu.edu

University of Kansas
Nursing Prgm
Kansas City, KS 66160
www.kumc.edu/son

University of Saint Mary
Nursing Prgm
Department of Nursing
Leavenworth, KS 66048
www.stmary.edu

Bethel College
Nursing Prgm
North Newton, KS 67117
www.bethelks.edu

Mid-America Nazarene University
Nursing Prgm
Olathe, KS 66062
www.mnu.edu

Pittsburg State University
Nursing Prgm
Pittsburg, KS 66762
www.pittstate.edu/nurs

Baker University
Nursing Prgm
School of Nursing
Topeka, KS 66604

Washburn University
Nursing Prgm
Topeka, KS 66621
www.washburn.edu/sonu

Newman University
Nursing Prgm
Wichita, KS 67213
www.newman.edu

Tabor College
Nursing Prgm
Wichita, KS 67205
www.tabor.edu

Wichita State University
Nursing Prgm
Wichita, KS 67260
www.wichita.edu/nurs

Southwestern College
Nursing Prgm
Department of Nursing
Winfield, KS 67156

Kentucky

Berea College
Nursing Prgm
Berea, KY 40404
www.berea.edu

Western Kentucky University
Nursing Prgm
Bowling Green, KY 42101
www.wku.edu

Kentucky Christian University
Nursing Prgm
School of Nursing
Grayson, KY 41143

University of Kentucky
Nursing Prgm
Lexington, KY 40536
www.uky.edu

Bellarmine University
Nursing Prgm
Louisville, KY 40205
www.bellarmine.edu/lansing

Spalding University
Nursing Prgm
School of Nursing
Louisville, KY 40203

University of Louisville
Nursing Prgm
Louisville, KY 40202
www.louisville.edu/nursing

Morehead State University
Nursing Prgm
Morehead, KY 40351
www.moreheadstate.edu

Murray State University
Nursing Prgm
Murray, KY 42071
www.murraystate.edu/nursing

Eastern Kentucky University
Nursing Prgm
Richmond, KY 40475
www.eku.edu

Louisiana

Southern Univ and A&M College
Nursing Prgm
School of Nursing
Baton Rouge, LA 70813

Southeastern Louisiana University
Nursing Prgm
548 Western Ave, SLU 10781
Hammond, LA 70402

University of Louisiana at Lafayette
Nursing Prgm
College of Nursing and Allied Health Professions
104 University Circle
Lafayette, LA 70503
www.nursing.louisiana.edu

University of Louisiana at Monroe
Nursing Prgm
Monroe, LA 71209
www.ulm.edu/nursing

Louisiana State Univ Health Sciences Center
Nursing Prgm
New Orleans, LA 70112
www.lsumc.edu

Louisiana College
Nursing Prgm
Pineville, LA 71359
www.lacollege.edu

Northwestern State University
Nursing Prgm
Shreveport, LA 71101
www.nsula.edu

Nicholls State University
Nursing Prgm
Thibodaux, LA 70310
www.nicholls.edu

Maine

Husson University
Nursing Prgm
Bangor, ME 04401
www.husson.edu

University of Maine Fort Kent
Nursing Prgm
Division of Nursing
Fort Kent, ME 04743

University of Maine - Orono
Nursing Prgm
Orono, ME 04469
www.umaine.edu/nursing

University of Southern Maine
Nursing Prgm
Portland, ME 04104
www.usm.maine.edu/conhp

Saint Joseph's College of Maine
Nursing Prgm
Department of Nursing
Standish, ME 04084

Maryland

Coppin State University
Nursing Prgm
Helene Fuld School of Nursing
2500 West North Ave, HHSB, Room 429
Baltimore, MD 21216-3698
www.coppin.edu/nursing

Johns Hopkins University
Nursing Prgm
School of Nursing
Baltimore, MD 21205

University of Maryland, Baltimore
Nursing Prgm
School of Nursing
655 West Lombard St, Suite 102
Baltimore, MD 21201-1579
http://nursing.umaryland.edu/index.htm

Frostburg State University
Nursing Prgm
RN-BSN Program
101 Braddock Rd
Frostburg, MD 21532
www.frostburg.edu/nursing/

Salisbury University
Nursing Prgm
Salisbury, MD 21801
www.salisbury.edu

Stevenson University
Nursing Prgm
Nursing Division
Stevenson, MD 21153
www.vjc.edu

Towson University
Nursing Prgm
Towson, MD 21252
www.towson.edu

Massachusetts

University of Massachusetts - Amherst
Nursing Prgm
Amherst, MA 01003
www.umass.edu

Emmanuel College
Nursing Prgm
Department of Nursing
Boston, MA 02115

Mass College of Pharmacy & Health Sciences
Nursing Prgm
School of Nursing
Boston, MA 02115
www.mcphs.edu

MGH Institute of Health Professions
Nursing Prgm
36 First Ave
Boston, MA 02129-4557
www.mghihp.edu

NURSING

Northeastern University
Nursing Prgm
Boston, MA 02115
www.bouve.neu.edu/programs/nursing/

Simmons College
Nursing Prgm
Boston, MA 02115
www.simmons.edu

University of Massachusetts - Boston
Nursing Prgm
Boston, MA 02125
www.cnhs.umb.edu

Boston College
Nursing Prgm
William F Connell School of Nursing
Chestnut Hill, MA 02467

Elms College
Nursing Prgm
Department of Nursing
Chicopee, MA 01013

Fitchburg State College
Nursing Prgm
Fitchburg, MA 01420
www.fsc.edu

Framingham State University
Nursing Prgm
Department of Nursing
100 State St, HH220, PO Box 9101
Framingham, MA 01701-9101
www.framingham.edu/nursing/

University of Massachusetts - Lowell
Nursing Prgm
Lowell, MA 01854
www.uml.edu/college/she

Curry College
Nursing Prgm
Division of Nursing
Milton, MA 02186

Salem State University
Nursing Prgm
Salem, MA 01970
www.salemstate.edu

American International College
Nursing Prgm
1000 State St
Springfield, MA 01109
www.aic.edu

Worcester State College
Nursing Prgm
486 Chandler St
Worcester, MA 01602-2597
www.worcesterstatecollege.edu

Michigan

Siena Heights University
Nursing Prgm
Nursing Program
1247 Siena Heights Drive
Adrian, MI 49221-1796
www.sienaheights.edu

University of Michigan
Nursing Prgm
Ann Arbor, MI 48109
www.nursing.umich.edu

Robert B. Miller College
Nursing Prgm
School of Nursing
450 North Ave
Battle Creek, MI 49017
www.millercollege.edu

University of Detroit Mercy
Nursing Prgm
Detroit, MI 48221
www.udmercy.edu

Wayne State University
Nursing Prgm
Detroit, MI 48202
www.wayne.edu

Michigan State University
Nursing Prgm
East Lansing, MI 48824
nursing.msu.edu

University of Michigan - Flint
Nursing Prgm
Flint, MI 48502
www.umflint.edu/nursing

Calvin College
Nursing Prgm
Department of Nursing
Grand Rapids, MI 49546

Grand Valley State University
Nursing Prgm
Grand Rapids, MI 49503
www.gvsu.edu/kcon

Finlandia University
Nursing Prgm
Hancock, MI 49930
www.finlandia.edu

Hope College
Nursing Prgm
Holland, MI 49423
www.hope.edu/academic/nursing

Western Michigan University
Nursing Prgm
Kalamazoo, MI 49008
www.wmich.edu/hhs/nursing/

Madonna University
Nursing Prgm
Livonia, MI 48150
www.madonna.edu

Northern Michigan University
Nursing Prgm
Marquette, MI 49855
www.nmu.edu

Oakland University
Nursing Prgm
Rochester, MI 48309
www.oakland.edu

Spring Arbor University
Nursing Prgm
BSN Program
Spring Arbor, MI 49283

Saginaw Valley State University
Nursing Prgm
University Center, MI 48710
www.svsu.edu

Eastern Michigan University
Nursing Prgm
Ypsilanti, MI 48197
www.emich.edu

Minnesota

Bemidji State University
Nursing Prgm
Department of Nursing
Bemidji, MN 56601

Saint John's University
Cosponsor: College of Saint Benedict
Nursing Prgm
Nursing Department
PO Box 2000
Collegeville, MN 56321-9999
www.csbsju.edu/nursing

College of St Scholastica
Nursing Prgm
Duluth, MN 55811
www.css.edu

Minnesota State University - Mankato
Nursing Prgm
Mankato, MN 56001
www.mnsu.edu

Augsburg College
Nursing Prgm
Minneapolis, MN 55454
www.augsburg.edu

Capella University
Nursing Prgm
Nursing Department
225 South 6th St, 9th Floor
Minneapolis, MN 55402
www.capella.edu

University of Minnesota
Nursing Prgm
Minneapolis, MN 55455
www.nurs.umn.edu

Walden University
Nursing Prgm
School of Nursing
155 Fifth Ave South, Suite 100
Minneapolis, MN 55401-2597
www.waldenu.edu

Concordia College - Moorhead
Nursing Prgm
Moorhead, MN 56562
www.cord.edu/dept/splash/nursing

Minnesota State University - Moorhead
Nursing Prgm
Moorhead, MN 56563
www.mnstate.edu/nursing

Minnesota Intercollegiate Nursing Consortium
Nursing Prgm
Northfield, MN 55057

Saint Olaf College
Cosponsor: Minnesota Intercollegiate Nursing
Consortium
Nursing Prgm
1520 St Olaf Ave
Northfield, MN 55057-1098
www.stolaf.edu/depts/nursing/

Minnesota School of Business
Cosponsor: Globe University
Nursing Prgm
1401 West 76th St, Suite 500
Richfield, MN 55423
www.msbcollege.edu

Gustavus Adolphus College
Nursing Prgm
800 West College Ave
Saint Peter, MN 56082-1498
www.gac.edu

Crown College
Nursing Prgm
8700 College View Dr
St Bonifacius, MN 55375

St Cloud State University
Nursing Prgm
720 4th Ave South, Halenbeck Hall 339
St Cloud, MN 56301
www.stcloudstate.edu

College of St Benedict/St John's University
Nursing Prgm
St Joseph, MN 56374
www.csbsju.edu/nursing

Bethel University
Nursing Prgm
St Paul, MN 55112
www.bethel.edu

Metropolitan State University
Nursing Prgm
School of Nursing
St Paul, MN 55106

Winona State University
Nursing Prgm
Winona, MN 55987
www.winona.edu/nursing

Mississippi

Delta State University
Nursing Prgm
Cleveland, MS 38733
www.deltast.edu

Mississippi College
Nursing Prgm
200 South Capitol, Box 4037
Clinton, MS 39058
www.mc.edu

Mississippi University for Women
Nursing Prgm
Columbus, MS 39701
www.muw.edu/nursing

University of Southern Mississippi
Nursing Prgm
Hattiesburg, MS 39406
www.nursing.usm.edu

William Carey University
Nursing Prgm
498 Tuscan Ave, Box 8
Hattiesburg, MS 39401-5461
www.wmcarey.edu

University of Mississippi Medical Center
Nursing Prgm
Jackson, MS 39216
son.umc.edu

Missouri

Southeast Missouri State University
Nursing Prgm
Cape Girardeau, MO 63701
www2.semo.edu/nursing

University of Missouri
Nursing Prgm
Columbia, MO 65211
www.hsc.missouri.edu/son/docs/sonhome.html

Central Methodist University
Nursing Prgm
Fayette, MO 65248
www.centralmethodist.edu

Graceland University
Nursing Prgm
Independence, MO 64050
www.graceland.edu

Avila University
Nursing Prgm
Kansas City, MO 64145
www.avila.edu

Research College of Nursing
Nursing Prgm
2525 E Meyer Blvd, Room 100
Kansas City, MO 64132

Saint Luke's Hospital
Nursing Prgm
Kansas City, MO 64111
www.saint-lukes.org/about/slc

University of Missouri - Kansas City
Nursing Prgm
Kansas City, MO 64108
www.umkc.edu

Truman State University
Nursing Prgm
Kirksville, MO 63501
www.truman.edu

William Jewell College
Nursing Prgm
Department of Nursing
Liberty, MO 64068

College of the Ozarks
Nursing Prgm
Armstrong McDonald School of Nursing
One Opportunity Ave, PO Box 17
Point Lookout, MO 65726-0017
www.cofo.edu/nursing

Cox College of Nursing and Health Sciences
Nursing Prgm
Springfield, MO 65802

Missouri State University
Nursing Prgm
Springfield, MO 65897
www.smsu.edu/nursing

Missouri Western State University
Nursing Prgm
St Joseph, MO 64507
mwsc.edu/~nursing

Barnes-Jewish Coll of Nursing/Allied Health
Nursing Prgm
St Louis, MO 63110
www.barnesjewishcollege.edu

Maryville University
Nursing Prgm
St Louis, MO 63141
www.maryville.edu

Saint Louis University
Nursing Prgm
St Louis, MO 63104
www.slu.edu/colleges/nr

University of Missouri - St Louis
Nursing Prgm
St Louis, MO 63121
www.umsl.edu/divisions/nursing

University of Central Missouri
Nursing Prgm
Warrensburg, MO 64093
www.cmsu.edu

Montana

Montana State University
Nursing Prgm
Bozeman, MT 59717
www.montana.edu

University of Great Falls
Nursing Prgm
Department of Nursing
1301 20th St South
Great D47Falls, MT 59405
www.ugf.edu/academics/bsinnursingdegreecompletion

Carroll College
Nursing Prgm
Helena, MT 59625
www.carroll.edu

Nebraska

Union College
Nursing Prgm
Lincoln, NE 68506
www.ucollege.edu

Creighton University
Nursing Prgm
Omaha, NE 68178
www.creighton.edu

Nebraska Methodist College
Nursing Prgm
Omaha, NE 68114
www.methodistcollege.edu

University of Nebraska Medical Center
Nursing Prgm
Omaha, NE 68198
www.unmc.edu/nursing

Nevada

Nevada State College
Nursing Prgm
School of Nursing
Henderson, NV 89002

Touro University - Nevada
Nursing Prgm
Henderson, NV 89014
www.tu.edu/nursing/

University of Nevada - Las Vegas
Nursing Prgm
4505 Maryland Parkway, PO Box 453018
Las Vegas, NV 89154-3018
nursing.unlv.edu

University of Nevada - Reno
Nursing Prgm
Reno, NV 89557
www.unr.edu/osn

New Hampshire

University of New Hampshire
Nursing Prgm
Durham, NH 03824
www.unh.edu/nursing/

Saint Anselm College
Nursing Prgm
Department of Nursing
Manchester, NH 03102

Colby-Sawyer College
Nursing Prgm
New London, NH 03257
www.colby-sawyer.edu

New Jersey

Bloomfield College
Nursing Prgm
Division of Nursing
Bloomfield, NJ 07003

NURSING

SUNJ Rutgers Camden and UMDNJ
Nursing Prgm
Camden, NJ 08102
www.camden.rutgers.edu

The College of New Jersey
Nursing Prgm
Ewing, NJ 08628
www.tcnj.edu

Saint Peter's College
Nursing Prgm
School of Nursing
Jersey City, NJ 07306

Felician College
Nursing Prgm
Lodi, NJ 07644
www.felician.edu

Rutgers - SUNJ
Nursing Prgm
College of Nursing
Newark, NJ 07102

Univ of Medicine & Dent of New Jersey
Nursing Prgm
School of Nursing
65 Bergen St, Room 1141
Newark, NJ 07107
http://sn.umdnj.edu

Richard Stockton College of New Jersey
Nursing Prgm
Pomona, NJ 08240
www.stockton.edu

Seton Hall University
Nursing Prgm
South Orange, NJ 07079
nursing.shu.edu

Fairleigh Dickinson University
Nursing Prgm
Teaneck, NJ 07666
www.fdu.edu

Thomas Edison State College
Nursing Prgm
W Carey Edwards School of Nursing
101 West State St
Trenton, NJ 08608-1176
www.tesc.edu

William Paterson Univ of New Jersey
Nursing Prgm
Wayne, NJ 07470
www.wpunj.edu

Monmouth University
Nursing Prgm
Majorie K Unterberg School of Nursing and Health
   Studies
West Long Beach, NJ 07764

New Mexico

University of New Mexico
Nursing Prgm
Albuquerque, NM 87131
hsc.unm.edu/consg

Northern New Mexico College
Nursing Prgm
Department of Nursing Education
921 North Paseo de Onate
Espanola, NM 87532
http://nnmc.edu

New Mexico State University
Nursing Prgm
Las Cruces, NM 88003
www.nmsu.edu/~nursing

New Mexico Highlands University
Nursing Prgm
RN-BSN Program
Engineering Building, Room 101, Box 9000
Las Vegas, NM 87701
www.nmhu.edu

Western New Mexico University
Nursing Prgm
500 East 18th St, PO Box 680
Silver City, NM 88062
www.wnmu.edu/academic/nursing

New York

Binghamton University
Nursing Prgm
Decker School of Nursing
Binghamton, NY 13902

SUNY The College at Brockport
Nursing Prgm
Brockport, NY 14420
www.brockport.edu

CUNY Herbert H Lehman College
Nursing Prgm
Bronx, NY 10468
www.lehman.cuny.edu

Concordia College New York
Nursing Prgm
Division of Nursing
171 White Plains Rd
Bronxville, NY 10708
www.concordia-ny.edu

Long Island University - Brooklyn Campus
Nursing Prgm
Brooklyn, NY 11201
www.liu.edu

SUNY Downstate Medical Center
Nursing Prgm
Brooklyn, NY 11203
www.downstate.edu

St Francis College
Nursing Prgm
Department of Nursing
Brooklyn Heights, NY 11201

Long Island University - C W Post Campus
Nursing Prgm
Brookville, NY 11548
www.liu.edu

D'Youville College
Nursing Prgm
Buffalo, NY 14201
www.dyc.edu

University at Buffalo - SUNY
Nursing Prgm
Buffalo, NY 14214
nursing.buffalo.edu

Mercy College
Nursing Prgm
Dobbs Ferry, NY 10522
www.mercy.edu

Adelphi University
Nursing Prgm
One South Ave
Garden City, NY 11530
www.adephi.edu

Niagara University
Nursing Prgm
Department of Nursing
Lewiston, NY 140109

SUNY at New Paltz
Nursing Prgm
New Paltz, NY 12561
www.newpaltz.edu

College of New Rochelle
Nursing Prgm
New Rochelle, NY 10805
www.cnr.edu

American University of Beirut
Nursing Prgm
3 Dag Hammarskjold Plaza, 8th Floor
New York, NY 10017

Columbia University
Nursing Prgm
New York, NY 10032
www.nursing.hs.columbia.edu

CUNY Hunter College
Nursing Prgm
New York, NY 10010
www.hunter.cuny.edu

New York University
Nursing Prgm
New York, NY 10003
www.nyu.edu/education/nursing

Mt St Mary College
Nursing Prgm
Division of Nursing
Newburgh, NY 12550

New York Institute of Technology
Nursing Prgm
Department of Nursing
Northern Blvd, 500 Building, Room 506, PO Box 8000
Old D44Westbury+D53, NY 11568-8000
http://nyit.edu/nursing

Hartwick College
Nursing Prgm
Department of Nursing
Oneonta, NY 13820

Dominican College
Nursing Prgm
Orangeburg, NY 10962
www.dc.edu

**Keuka College at Niagara County Community
   College**
Nursing Prgm
Division of Nursing
Center for Professional Studies, One Keuka Business
   Park
Penn Yan, NY 14527
www.keuka.edu

SUNY College at Plattsburgh
Nursing Prgm
Department of Nursing
101 Broad St, Hawkins 0221A
Plattsburgh, NY 12901-2681
www.plattsburgh.edu

SUNY College at Plattsburgh
Nursing Prgm
Plattsburgh, NY 12901
www.plattsburgh.edu

Pace University
Nursing Prgm
Lienhard School of Nursing
Pleasantville, NY 10570

College of Mount St Viencent
Nursing Prgm
Department of Nursing
Riverdale, NY 10471

Nazareth College of Rochester
Nursing Prgm
Rochester, NY 14618
www.naz.edu

Roberts Wesleyan College
Nursing Prgm
2301 Westside Dr
Rochester, NY 14624

St John Fisher College
Nursing Prgm
Wegman's School of Nursing
Rochester, NY 14618

University of Rochester
Nursing Prgm
School of Nursing
601 Elmwood Ave, Box SON
Rochester, NY 14642-8404
www.urmc.rochester.edu/son

Molloy College
Nursing Prgm
Rockville Centre, NY 11571
www.molloy.edu

SUNY Empire State College
Nursing Prgm
Nursing Program
113 West Ave
Saratoga Springs+D55, NY 12866
www.esc.edu/nursing

Stony Brook University
Nursing Prgm
Health Science Center, Level 2, Room 236
Stony Brook, NY 11794-8240
www.hsc.stonybrook.edu

Le Moyne College
Nursing Prgm
Syracuse, NY 13214
www.lemoyne.edu/nursing

SUNY Upstate Medical University
Nursing Prgm
Syracuse, NY 13210
www.upstate

The Sage Colleges
Nursing Prgm
Troy, NY 12180
www.sage.edu

SUNY Institute of Tech - Utica/Rome
Nursing Prgm
Utica, NY 13504
www.sunyit.edu

Utica College
Nursing Prgm
Department of Nursing
1600 Burrstone Rd
Utica, NY 13502-4892
www.utica.edu/academic/hhs/nursing/homepage/
    nursing.htm

North Carolina

Lees-McRae College
Nursing Prgm
Banner Elk, NC 28604

Appalachian State University
Nursing Prgm
400 University Hall Drive, University Hall, PO Box 32151
Boone, NC 28608-2151
www.web.appstate.edu/academics/nursing.html

University of North Carolina
Nursing Prgm
Chapel Hill, NC 27599
www.unc.edu/depts/nursing

Queens University of Charlotte
Nursing Prgm
Charlotte, NC 28274
www.queens.edu/nursing/

Univ of North Carolina at Charlotte
Nursing Prgm
Charlotte, NC 28223
www.uncc.edu

Cabarrus College of Health Sciences
Nursing Prgm
401 Medical Park Dr
Concord, NC 28025
www.cabarruscollege.edu

Western Carolina University
Nursing Prgm
Cullowhee, NC 28723
www.wcu.edu

Duke University
Nursing Prgm
Durham, NC 27710
son3mc.duke.edu

Fayetteville State University
Nursing Prgm
Department of Nursing
Fayetteville, NC 28301

University of North Carolina - Greensboro
Nursing Prgm
Greensboro, NC 27402
www.uncg.edu

Lenoir - Rhyne University
Nursing Prgm
Hickory, NC 28601
www.lrc.edu

University of North Carolina - Pembroke
Nursing Prgm
Department of Nursing
Pembroke, NC 28372

Fayetteville State University
Nursing Prgm
Wilmington, NC 28403
www.uncwil.edu

University of North Carolina - Wilmington
Nursing Prgm
School of Nursing
Wilmington, NC 28403

Winston-Salem State University
Nursing Prgm
Division of Nursing
Winston-Salem, NC 27110

North Dakota

Medcenter One
Nursing Prgm
Bismarck, ND 58501
www.medcenterone.com/college/nursing.htm

University of Mary
Nursing Prgm
Bismarck, ND 58504
www.umary.edu

North Dakota State University
Nursing Prgm
Fargo, ND 58105
nursing.ndsu.nodak.edu

University of North Dakota
Nursing Prgm
Grand Forks, ND 58202
www.und.nodak.edu/dept/nursing

Ohio

Ohio Northern University
Nursing Prgm
525 South Main St
Ada, OH 45810
www.onu.edu

The University of Akron
Nursing Prgm
Akron, OH 44325
www.uakron.edu

Ashland University
Nursing Prgm
Ashland, OH 44805
www.ashland.edu

Ohio University
Nursing Prgm
Athens, OH 45701
www.ohiou.edu

Bowling Green State University
Nursing Prgm
College of Nursing
Bowling Green, OH 43403-0001
www.bgsu.edu

Malone College
Nursing Prgm
School of Nursing
Canton, OH 44709

Cedarville University
Nursing Prgm
Cedarville, OH 45314
www.cedarville.edu

College of Mt St Joseph
Nursing Prgm
College of Mount St Joseph
5701 Delhi Rd
Cincinnati, OH 45233-1670
www.msj.edu

University of Cincinnati
Nursing Prgm
Cncinnati, OH 45221
www.uc.edu

Xavier University
Nursing Prgm
Cincinnati, OH 45207
www.xu.edu

Cleveland State University
Nursing Prgm
Cleveland, OH 44115
www.scuohio.edu

Capital University
Nursing Prgm
Columbus, OH 43209
www.capital.edu

Mt Carmel College of Nursing
Nursing Prgm
127 South Davis Ave
Columbus, OH 43222
www.mccn.edu

The Ohio State University
Nursing Prgm
Columbus, OH 43210
www.acs.ohio-state.edu

Wright State University
Nursing Prgm
Dayton, OH 45435
www.wright.edu

NURSING

Defiance College
Nursing Prgm
Nursing Department
701 North Clinton St
Defiance, OH 43512
www.defiance.edu

Miami University
Nursing Prgm
Department of Nursing
1601 University Blvd
Hamilton, OH 45011-3399
www.eas.muohio.edu/departments/nsg/

Hiram College
Nursing Prgm
Department of Nursing
Teachout-Price Hall, PO Box 67
Hiram, OH 44234
www.hiram.edu

Kent State University
Nursing Prgm
Kent, OH 44242
www.kent.edu/nursing/nursing.html

Mount Vernon Nazarene University
Nursing Prgm
School of Nursing and Health Sciences
800 Martinsburg Rd
Mt Vernon, OH 43050-9500
www.mvnu.edu

Muskingum University
Nursing Prgm
Department of Nursing
163 Stormont St, Montgomery Hall
New Concord, OH 43762
www.muskingum.edu/dept/nursing/

Ursuline College
Nursing Prgm
Pepper Pike, OH 44124
www.ursuline.edu

Notre Dame College
Nursing Prgm
Division of Nursing
4545 College Rd
South Euclid, OH 44121-4293
www.notredamecollege.edu

Lourdes College
Nursing Prgm
Sylvania, OH 43560
www.lourdes.edu

Mercy College of Northwest Ohio
Nursing Prgm
Toledo, OH 43624
www.mercycollege.edu

University of Toledo Consortium
Nursing Prgm
Toledo, OH 43614

Urbana University
Nursing Prgm
Urbana, OH 43078
www.urbana.edu

Otterbein College
Nursing Prgm
Westerville, OH 43081
www.otterbein.edu/nursing

Oklahoma

Oklahoma Wesleyan University
Nursing Prgm
Division of Nursing
Bartlesville, OK 74006

Southern Nazarene University
Nursing Prgm
Bethany, OK 73008
www.snu.edu

Oklahoma Christian University
Nursing Prgm
2501 E Memorial Rd
Edmond, OK 73013

Oklahoma Baptist University
Nursing Prgm
School of Nursing
500 West University Ave
Shawnee, OK 74804
www.okbu.edu

Oral Roberts University
Nursing Prgm
Anna Vaughn School of Nursing
Tulsa, OK 74171

Oregon

George Fox University
Nursing Prgm
414 North Meridian St, #6273
Newberg, OR 97132-2697
www.georgefox.edu

Linfield College
Nursing Prgm
Portland, OR 97210
www.linfield.edu

Oregon Health & Science University
Nursing Prgm
Portland, OR 97239
www.ohsu.edu/son

University of Portland
Nursing Prgm
School of Nursing
Portland, OR 97203

Pennsylvania

Moravian College
Nursing Prgm
St Luke's Hospital School of Nursing
Bethlehem, PA 18018

Bloomsburg University
Nursing Prgm
Bloomsburg, PA 17815
www.bloomu.edu

California University of Pennsylvania
Nursing Prgm
California, PA 15419
www.cup.edu

Widener University
Nursing Prgm
Chester, PA 19013
www.widener.edu

Misericordia University
Nursing Prgm
Dallas, PA 18612
www.miseri.edu

Edinboro University of Pennsylvania
Nursing Prgm
Edinboro, PA 16444
www.edinboro.edu

Gannon University
Nursing Prgm
Erie, PA 16541
www.gannon.edu

Messiah College
Nursing Prgm
Grantham, PA 17027
www.messiah.edu

Immaculata University
Nursing Prgm
Immaculata, PA 19345
www.immaculata.edu

Indiana University of Pennsylvania
Nursing Prgm
Indiana, PA 15705
www.iup.edu

Lancaster Gen Coll of Nursing & Hlth Sciences
Nursing Prgm
410 North Lime St
Lancaster, PA 17602
www.lancastergeneralcollege.edu

St Francis University
Nursing Prgm
Loretto, PA 15940
www.francis.edu/nursing/nursinghome.shtml

Robert Morris University
Cosponsor: Allegheny Gen Hosp
Nursing Prgm
6001 University Blvd
Moon Township, PA 15108
www.rmu.edu

Drexel University College of Medicine
Nursing Prgm
Philadelphia, PA 19102
www.drexel.edu

Holy Family University
Nursing Prgm
Philadelphia, PA 19114
www.holyfamily.edu

La Salle University
Nursing Prgm
Philadelphia, PA 19141
www.lasalle.edu

Temple University
Nursing Prgm
Philadelphia, PA 19140
www.temple.edu

Thomas Jefferson University
Nursing Prgm
Philadelphia, PA 19107
tju.edu/chp

University of Pennsylvania
Nursing Prgm
School of Nursing
Philadelphia, PA 19104

Carlow University
Nursing Prgm
School of Nursing
Pittsburgh, PA 15213

Chatham University
Nursing Prgm
1 Woodland Rd, Coolidge 119
Pittsburgh, PA 15232-2826
sce.chatham.edu/programs/undergrad.cfm#bsn

Duquesne University
Nursing Prgm
Pittsburgh, PA 15282
www.nursing.duq.edu

University of Pittsburgh
Nursing Prgm
Pittsburgh, PA 15261
www.pitt.edu/~nursing

Alvernia University
Nursing Prgm
400 St Bernardine St
Reading, PA 19607
www.alvernia.edu

University of Scranton
Nursing Prgm
Scranton, PA 18510
www.scranton.edu

Eastern University
Nursing Prgm
St Davids, PA 19087
www.eastern.edu

Penn State University
Nursing Prgm
University Park, PA 16802
www.psu.edu

Villanova University
Nursing Prgm
College of Nursing
Villanova, PA 19085

Waynesburg University
Nursing Prgm
Waynesburg, PA 15370
www.waynesburg.edu

West Chester University
Nursing Prgm
West Chester, PA 19383
www.wcupa.edu

Wilkes University
Nursing Prgm
Department of Nursing
Wilkes-Barre, PA 18766

York College of Pennsylvania
Nursing Prgm
York, PA 17405
www.ycp.edu

Puerto Rico

Universidad Del Turabo
Nursing Prgm
School of Health Sciences
Gurabo, PR 00778

University of Puerto Rico
Nursing Prgm
San Juan, PR 00936
www.upr.edu

Rhode Island

University of Rhode Island
Nursing Prgm
Kingston, RI 02881
www.uri.edu

Rhode Island College
Nursing Prgm
144 Fogarty Life Science Bldg
600 Mt Pleasant Ave
Providence, RI 02908
www.ric.edu

South Carolina

University of South Carolina Beaufort
Nursing Prgm
Department of Nursing
1 University Blvd
Bluffton, SC 29909
www.uscb.edu

Medical University of South Carolina
Nursing Prgm
Charleston, SC 29425
www.musc.edu/nursing

Clemson University
Nursing Prgm
Clemson, SC 29634
www.clemson.edu

University of South Carolina
Nursing Prgm
Columbia, SC 29208
www.sc.edu/nursing

Lander University
Nursing Prgm
Department of Nursing
320 Stanley Ave
Greenwood, SC 29649
www.lander.edu/nursing/

Newberry College
Nursing Prgm
Department of Nursing
2100 College St
Newberry, SC 29108-2126
www.newberry.edu/academics/nursing.asp

South Carolina State University
Nursing Prgm
Orangeburg, SC 29117
www.scsu.edu

University of South Carolina Upstate
Nursing Prgm
1601 Greene St
Spartanburg, SC 29208-9998
www.uscupstate.edu

University of South Carolina Upstate, Mary Black School of Medicine
Nursing Prgm
Spartanburg, SC 29303

South Dakota

South Dakota State University
Nursing Prgm
Brookings, SD 57007
www3.sdstate.edu/academics/collegeofnursing/

National American University
Nursing Prgm
School of Nursing
5301 South Highway 16, Suite 200
Rapid City, SD 57701
http://national.edu

Augustana College
Nursing Prgm
Sioux Falls, SD 57197
www.augie.edu

University of Sioux Falls
Nursing Prgm
School of Nursing
1101 West 22nd St
Sioux Falls, SD 57105-1699
www.usiouxfalls.edu

Mt Marty College
Nursing Prgm
Yankton, SD 57078
www.mtmc.edu

Tennessee

King College
Nursing Prgm
School of Nursing
Bristol, TN 37620

University of Tennessee - Chattanooga
Nursing Prgm
Chattanooga, TN 37403
www.utc.edu

Tennessee Technological University
Nursing Prgm
Cookeville, TN 38505
www.tntech.edu/nursing

Union University
Nursing Prgm
Jackson, TN 38305
www.uu.edu/academcis/son

Carson-Newman College
Nursing Prgm
Jefferson City, TN 37760
www.cn.edu

East Tennessee State University
Nursing Prgm
Johnson City, TN 37614
www.etsu.edu/nursing

Tennessee Wesleyan College
Nursing Prgm
Fort Sanders Nursing Department
Knoxville, TN 37932

University of Tennessee - Knoxville
Nursing Prgm
Knoxville, TN 37996
nightingale.com.utk.edu

Bethel University
Nursing Prgm
Department of Nursing
325 Cherry Ave, PO Box 3328
McKenzie, TN 38201
www.bethelu.edu

Baptist College of Health Sciences
Nursing Prgm
Memphis, TN 38104
www.bchs.edu

University of Memphis
Nursing Prgm
Memphis, TN 38152
nursing.memphis.edu

Milligan College
Nursing Prgm
Milligan College, TN 37682
www.milligan.edu

Middle Tennessee State University
Nursing Prgm
Murfreesboro, TN 37132
www.mtsu.edu/~nursing

Belmont U/Trevecca Nazarene U Consortium
Nursing Prgm
Partners In Nursing
1900 Belmont Blvd
Nashville, TN 37212-3757

Belmont University
Nursing Prgm
Nashville, TN 37212

Trevecca Nazarene University
Nursing Prgm
877 Madison Ave, Suite 647
Nashville, TN 38163
www.trevecca.edu/schools/arts.sciences/nursing

Martin Methodist College
Nursing Prgm
433 W Madison St
Pulaski, TN 38478

NURSING

Texas

Abilene Christian University
Cosponsor: Patty Hanks Shelton School of Nursing
Nursing Prgm
205 Hardin Administration Building, ACU Box 29103
Abilene, TX 79699-9103
www.acu.edu

Hardin-Simmons University
Cosponsor: Patty Hanks Shelton School of Nursing
Nursing Prgm
2200 Hickory
Abilene, TX 79698-0001
www.hsutx.edu

McMurry University
Cosponsor: Patty Hanks Shelton School of Nursing
Nursing Prgm
1400 Sayles Blvd
Abilene, TX 79697
www.mcm.edu

Patty Hanks Shelton School of Nursing
Nursing Prgm
Abilene, TX 79601

University of Texas at Arlington
Nursing Prgm
Arlington, TX 76019
www.uta.edu

University of Texas at Austin
Nursing Prgm
Austin, TX 78701
www.utexas.edu/nursing

University of Mary Hardin-Baylor
Nursing Prgm
Belton, TX 76513
www.umhb.edu

Texas A&M University
Nursing Prgm
College of Nursing
8447 State Highway 47
Bryan, TX 77807
www.tamhsc.edu

West Texas A&M University
Nursing Prgm
Canyon, TX 79016
www.wtamu.edu

Texas A&M University - Corpus Christi
Nursing Prgm
Corpus Christi, TX 78412
www.tamucc.edu

Baylor University
Nursing Prgm
Dallas, TX 75246
www.baylor.edu/nursing

Texas Woman's University
Nursing Prgm
Denton, TX 76204
www.twu.edu

Univ of Texas - Pan American
Nursing Prgm
Edinburg, TX 78540
www.panam.edu/dept/nursing

University of Texas at El Paso
Nursing Prgm
El Paso, TX 79902
www.utep.edu

Texas Christian University
Nursing Prgm
Fort Worth, TX 76129
www.tcu.edu

University of Texas Medical Branch
Nursing Prgm
Galveston, TX 77555
www.utmb.edu

Prairie View A&M University
Nursing Prgm
Houston, TX 77030
www.pvamu.edu

University of Texas Health Sci Ctr Houston
Nursing Prgm
Houston, TX 77030
son.uth.tmc.edu

Southwestern Adventist University
Nursing Prgm
Department of Nursing
100 West Hillcrest
Keene, TX 76059
www.swau.edu

Texas Tech University
Nursing Prgm
Lubbock, TX 79430
www.ttuhsc.edu/son

East Texas Baptist University
Nursing Prgm
Marshall, TX 75670
www.etbu.edu

The University of the Incarnate Word
Nursing Prgm
San Antonio, TX 78209
www.uiw.edu

UT Health Science Center - San Antonio
Nursing Prgm
San Antonio, TX 78229
www.uthscsa.edu

Tarleton State University
Nursing Prgm
Stephenville, TX 76402
www.tarleton.edu/~nursing

Texas A&M University - Texarkana
Nursing Prgm
RN-BSN Program
Texarkana, TX 75501

University of Texas at Tyler
Nursing Prgm
Tyler, TX 75799
www.uttyler.edu

Midwestern State University
Nursing Prgm
Wichita Falls, TX 76308
www.mwsu.edu

Utah

Southern Utah University
Nursing Prgm
Cedar City, UT 84720
www.suu.edu/sci/nursing

Brigham Young University
Nursing Prgm
Provo, UT 84602
www.byu.edu

University of Utah
Nursing Prgm
Salt Lake City, UT 84112
www.nurs.utah.edu

Western Governors University
Nursing Prgm
Department of Nursing
4001 South 700 East, Suite 700
Salt Lake City, UT 84107-2533
www.wgu.edu/index.asp

Westminster College
Nursing Prgm
School of Nursing and Health Sciences
Salt Lake City, UT 84105

Vermont

University of Vermont
Nursing Prgm
Burlington, VT 05405
www.uvm.edu

Virginia

Marymount University
Nursing Prgm
Arlington, VA 22207
www.marymount.edu

University of Virginia
Nursing Prgm
Charlottesville, VA 22903
www.nursing.virginia.edu

George Mason University
Nursing Prgm
Fairfax, VA 22030
chhs.gmu.edu

Hampton University
Nursing Prgm
Hampton, VA 23668
www.hamptonu.edu

Eastern Mennonite University
Nursing Prgm
Department of Nursing
Harrisonburg, VA 22802

James Madison University
Nursing Prgm
Harrisonburg, VA 22807
www.nursing.jmu.edu

Liberty University
Nursing Prgm
Lynchburg, VA 24502
www.liberty.edu

Lynchburg College
Nursing Prgm
Lynchburg, VA 24501
www.lynchburg.edu

Old Dominion University
Nursing Prgm
Norfolk, VA 23529
www.odu.edu

Radford University
Nursing Prgm
Radford, VA 24142
www.runet.edu

Jefferson College of Health Sciences
Nursing Prgm
Roanoke, VA 24031
www.jchs.edu

Shenandoah University
Nursing Prgm
Winchester, VA 22601
www.su.edu/nursing

University of Virginia - Wise
Nursing Prgm
Department of Nursing
Wise, VA 24293

Washington

Olympic College
Nursing Prgm
Nursing Program
1600 Chester Ave
Bremerton, WA 98337-1699
www.olympic.edu

Eastern Washington University
Cosponsor: Washington State U Intercollegiate College
of Nursing
Nursing Prgm
526 5th St
Cheney, WA 99004-1619
www.ewu.edu

Northwest University
Nursing Prgm
Mark and Huldah Buntain School of Nursing
Kirkland, WA 98033

Seattle Pacific University
Nursing Prgm
Seattle, WA 98119
www.spu.edu

Seattle University
Nursing Prgm
Seattle, WA 98122
www.seattleu.edu/nurs

University of Washington
Nursing Prgm
Seattle, WA 98195
www.son.washington.edu

Gonzaga University
Nursing Prgm
Department of Nursing
Spokane, WA 99258

Washington State University
Cosponsor: Eastern Washington U, Whitworth College
Nursing Prgm
103 East Spokane Falls Blvd, PO Box 1495
Spokane, WA 99210-1495
www.nursing.wsu.edu

Whitworth University
Cosponsor: Washington State U Intercollegiate College
of Nursing
Nursing Prgm
300 West Hawthorne Rd
Spokane, WA 99251-0001
www.whitworth.edu/academic/programs/preprofessional
healthstudies/nursing/

Pacific Lutheran University
Nursing Prgm
School of Nursing
Tacoma, WA 98447

West Virginia

Bluefield State College
Nursing Prgm
Bluefield, WV 24701
www.bluefield.wvnet.edu

Fairmont State Univ
Nursing Prgm
Fairmont, WV 26554
www.fscwv.edu

West Virginia University
Nursing Prgm
Morgantown, WV 26506
www.hsc.wvuledu/son

Shepherd University
Nursing Prgm
Department of Nursing Education
304 North King St, PO Box 5000
Shepherdstown, WV 25443-5000
www.shepherd.edu

West Liberty State College
Nursing Prgm
West Liberty, WV 26074
www.westliberty.edu

Wheeling Jesuit University
Nursing Prgm
Wheeling, WV 26003
www.wju.edu

Wisconsin

University of Wisconsin - Eau Claire
Nursing Prgm
Eau Claire, WI 54701
www.uwec.edu/academics/nurs

Marian College
Nursing Prgm
School of Nursing
Fond du Lac, WI 54935

Columbia College of Nursing
Nursing Prgm
4425 North Port Washington Rd
Glendale, WI 53212
www.ccon.edu

Bellin College/Bellin Health Systems Inc
Nursing Prgm
Green Bay, WI 54305

University of Wisconsin - Green Bay
Nursing Prgm
Green Bay, WI 54311
www.uwgb.edu

Viterbo University
Nursing Prgm
La Crosse, WI 54601
www.viterbo.edu

Edgewood College
Nursing Prgm
Department of Nursing
Madison, WI 53711

University of Wisconsin - Madison
Nursing Prgm
Madison, WI 53792
www.son.wisc.edu

Silver Lake College of the Holy Family
Nursing Prgm
Department of Nursing
2406 South Alverno Rd
Manitowoc, WI 54220
www.sl.edu

Concordia University Wisconsin
Nursing Prgm
Mequon, WI 53097
www.cuw.edu

Alverno College
Nursing Prgm
3400 S 43rd St
PO Box 343922
Milwaukee, WI 53234-3922
www.alverno.edu

Cardinal Stritch University
Nursing Prgm
College of Nursing
Milwaukee, WI 53217

Marquette University
Nursing Prgm
Milwaukee, WI 53201
www.mu.edu

Milwaukee School of Engineering
Nursing Prgm
Milwaukee, WI 53202
www.msoe.edu

University of Wisconsin - Milwaukee
Nursing Prgm
Milwaukee, WI 53201
www.uwm.edu

University of Wisconsin - Oshkosh
Nursing Prgm
Oshkosh, WI 54901
www.uwosh.edu/home_pages/colleges/con

Carroll University
Nursing Prgm
Waukesha, WI 53186
www.cc.edu

Wyoming

University of Wyoming
Nursing Prgm
Laramie, WY 82071
www.uwyo.edu/nursing

Pharmacy

Includes:
- Pharmacist
- Pharmacy technician

Pharmacist

Pharmacists play a key role in the health care system through the medicine and information they provide. Although responsibilities vary among the different areas of pharmacy practice, the bottom line is that pharmacists help patients get well. Pharmacists are drug experts ultimately concerned about their patients' health and wellness.

The number of people requiring health care services has steadily increased, and this trend will likely continue. Due to many of society's changing social and health issues, pharmacists will face new challenges, including:

- Increases in average life span and the increased incidence of chronic diseases
- Increased complexity, number, and sophistication of medications and related products and devices
- Increased emphasis on primary and preventive health services, home health care, and long-term care

Career Description

Pharmacists provide information to patients about medications and their use and distribute drugs prescribed by physicians and other health practitioners . They advise physicians and other health practitioners on the selection, dosages, interactions, and side effects of medications. Pharmacists also monitor the health and progress of patients in response to drug therapy to ensure the safe and effective use of medication. Pharmacists must understand the use, clinical effects, and composition of drugs, including their chemical, biological, and physical properties. Compounding—the actual mixing of ingredients to form powders, tablets, capsules, ointments, and solutions—is a small part of a pharmacist's practice, because most medicines are produced by pharmaceutical companies in a standard dosage and drug delivery form.

About 65 percent of the nation's 269,000 pharmacists work in a community setting, such as a retail drugstore; about 22 percent work in a health care facility, such as a hospital, nursing home, mental health institution, or neighborhood health clinic.

Pharmacists in community and retail pharmacies counsel patients and answer questions about prescription drugs, including questions regarding possible side effects or interactions among various drugs. They provide information about over-the-counter drugs and make recommendations after talking with the patient. They also may give advice about the patient's diet, exercise, or stress management or about durable medical equipment and home health care supplies. In addition, they also may complete third-party insurance forms and other paperwork. Those who own or manage community pharmacies may sell non-health-related merchandise, hire and supervise personnel, and oversee the general operation of the pharmacy. Some community pharmacists provide specialized services to help patients manage conditions such as diabetes, asthma,

smoking cessation, or high blood pressure. Most community pharmacists also are trained to administer vaccinations.

Pharmacists in health care facilities dispense medications and advise the medical staff on the selection and effects of drugs. They may make sterile solutions to be administered intravenously. They also assess, plan, and monitor drug programs or regimens. Pharmacists counsel hospitalized patients on the use of drugs and on their use at home when the patients are discharged. Pharmacists also may evaluate drug-use patterns and outcomes for patients in hospitals or managed care organizations.

Pharmacists who work in home health care monitor drug therapy and prepare infusions—solutions that are injected into patients—and other medications for use in the home.

Some pharmacists specialize in specific drug therapy areas, such as intravenous nutrition support, oncology (cancer), nuclear pharmacy (used for chemotherapy), geriatric pharmacy, and psychopharmacotherapy (the treatment of mental disorders by means of drugs).

Most pharmacists keep confidential computerized records of patients' drug therapies to prevent harmful drug interactions. Pharmacists are responsible for the accuracy of every prescription that is filled, but they often rely upon pharmacy technicians and pharmacy aides to assist them in the dispensing process. Thus, the pharmacist may delegate prescription-filling and administrative tasks and supervise their completion. Pharmacists also frequently oversee student pharmacists serving as interns in preparation for graduation and licensure.

Increasingly, pharmacists are pursuing nontraditional pharmacy work. Some are involved in research for pharmaceutical manufacturers, developing new drugs and therapies and testing their effects on people. Others work in marketing or sales, providing expertise to clients on a drug's use, effectiveness, and possible side effects. Some pharmacists work for health insurance companies, developing pharmacy benefit packages and carrying out cost-benefit analyses on certain drugs. Other pharmacists work for the government, public health care services, the armed services, and pharmacy associations. Finally, some pharmacists are employed full time or part time as college faculty, teaching classes and performing research in a wide range of areas.

Employment Characteristics

Pharmacists work in clean, well-lighted, and well-ventilated areas. Many pharmacists spend most of their workday on their feet. When working with sterile or dangerous pharmaceutical products, pharmacists wear gloves and masks and work with other special protective equipment. Many community and hospital pharmacies are open for extended hours or around the clock, so pharmacists may work nights, weekends, and holidays. Consultant pharmacists may travel to nursing homes or other facilities to monitor patients' drug therapy.

About 19 percent of pharmacists worked part time in 2008. Most full-time salaried pharmacists worked approximately 40 hours a week. Some, including many self-employed pharmacists, worked more than 50 hours a week.

Salary

Data from the US Bureau of Labor Statistics from May 2011 show that wages at the 10th percentile are $84,490, the 50th percentile (median) at $113,390, and the 90th percentile at $144,090 (*www.bls.gov/oes/current/oes291051.htm*).

For more information, refer to *www.ama-assn.org/go/hpsalary*.

Employment Outlook

A shortfall of as many as 157,000 pharmacists is predicted by 2020, according to the findings of a conference sponsored by the Pharmacy Manpower Project, as detailed in *Professionally Determined Need for Pharmacy Services in 2020*. Similarly, a report of the Health Resources and Services Administration of the Department of Health and Human Services, *The Pharmacy Workforce: A Study of the Supply and Demand for Pharmacists*, concludes that the increasing demand for pharmacists' services is outpacing the current and possibly future pharmacist supply.

Accordingly, very good employment opportunities are expected for pharmacists through 2018 because the number of job openings created by employment growth and the need to replace pharmacists who leave the occupation or retire are expected to exceed the number of degrees granted in pharmacy. Enrollments in pharmacy programs are rising as more students are attracted by high salaries and good job prospects. Despite this increase in enrollments, job openings should still be more numerous than those seeking employment.

Employment of pharmacists is expected to grow by 17 percent between 2008 and 2018, which is faster than the average for all occupations. The increasing numbers of middle-aged and elderly people—who use more prescription drugs than younger people—will continue to spur demand for pharmacists throughout the projection period. In addition, as scientific advances lead to new drug products, and as an increasing number of people obtain prescription drug coverage, the need for these workers will continue to expand.

Community pharmacies are taking steps to manage an increasing volume of prescriptions. Automation of drug dispensing and greater employment of pharmacy technicians and pharmacy aides will help these establishments to dispense more prescriptions.

With its emphasis on cost control, managed care encourages the use of lower cost prescription drug distributors, such as mail-order firms and online pharmacies, for purchases of certain medications. Prescriptions ordered through the mail and via the Internet are filled in a central location and shipped to the patient at a lower cost. Mail-order and online pharmacies typically use automated technology to dispense medication and employ fewer pharmacists. If the utilization of mail-order pharmacies increases rapidly, job growth among pharmacists could be limited.

Employment of pharmacists will not grow as fast in hospitals as in other industries, because hospitals are reducing inpatient stays, downsizing, and consolidating departments. The number of outpatient surgeries is increasing, so more patients are being discharged and purchasing their medications through retail, supermarket, or mail-order pharmacies, rather than through hospitals. An aging population means that more pharmacy services will be required in nursing homes, assisted-living facilities, and home care settings.

The most rapid job growth among pharmacists is expected in these 3 settings.

New opportunities are emerging for pharmacists in managed care organizations where they analyze trends and patterns in medication use, and in pharmacoeconomics—the cost and benefit analysis of different drug therapies. Opportunities also are emerging for pharmacists trained in research and disease management—the development of new methods for curing and controlling diseases. Pharmacists also are finding jobs in research and development and in sales and marketing for pharmaceutical manufacturing firms. New breakthroughs in biotechnology will increase the potential for drugs to treat diseases and expand the opportunities for pharmacists to conduct research and sell medications. In addition, pharmacists are finding employment opportunities in pharmacy informatics, which uses information technology to improve patient care.

Educational Programs

Award, Length. The Doctor of Pharmacy (PharmD) degree requires at least two years of specific preprofessional (undergraduate) course work followed by four academic years (or three calendar years) of professional study. The PharmD degree has replaced the Bachelor of Pharmacy (BPharm) degree, which is no longer being awarded.

Prerequisites. Pharmacy colleges and schools may accept students directly from high school for both the prepharmacy and pharmacy curriculum, or after completion of the college course prerequisites. The majority of students enter a pharmacy program with three or more years of college experience. Entry requirements usually include courses in mathematics and natural sciences, such as chemistry, biology, and physics, as well as courses in the humanities and social sciences. Approximately two thirds of all colleges require applicants to take the Pharmacy College Admissions Test (PCAT).

Prospective pharmacists should have scientific aptitude, good communication skills, and a desire to help others. They also must be conscientious and pay close attention to detail, because the decisions they make affect human lives, and possess high ethical and professional standards. Other character traits of successful pharmacists include curiosity and desire and willingness to learn. Most importantly, pharmacists must enjoy working with people, be comfortable meeting them, and be willing to serve them in a variety of circumstances.

Curriculum. Student pharmacists learn about all aspects of drug therapy as well as how to communicate with patients and other health care providers about drug information and patient care. Other courses focus on professional ethics, public health, and developing and managing medication distribution systems. In addition to classroom instruction, students in PharmD programs spend about one fourth of their time learning in a variety of pharmacy practice settings under the supervision of licensed pharmacists.

Advanced Training. For individuals who want more laboratory and research experience, many colleges of pharmacy offer an MS or PhD degree after completion of the PharmD degree. Many master's and PhD degree holders do research for drug companies or teach at universities.

Other options for pharmacy graduates who are interested in further training include one-year or two-year residency programs or fellowships. Pharmacy residencies are postgraduate training programs in pharmacy practice and usually require the completion of a research study. There currently are more than 700 residency programs nationwide. Pharmacy fellowships are highly individualized programs that are designed to prepare participants to work in a specialized area of pharmacy, such as clinical practice or research laboratories. Some pharmacists who run their own pharmacy obtain a master's degree in business administration (MBA). Others may obtain a degree in public administration or public health.

Areas of graduate study include pharmaceutics and pharmaceutical chemistry (physical and chemical properties of drugs and dosage forms), pharmacology (effects of drugs on the body), toxicology and pharmacy administration.

Licensure, Certification, Registration

A license to practice pharmacy is required in all states, the District of Columbia, and all US territories. To obtain a license, the prospective pharmacist must graduate from a college of pharmacy accredited by the Accreditation Council for Pharmacy Education (ACPE) and pass an examination. All states require the North American Pharmacist Licensure Exam (NAPLEX), which tests pharmacy skills and knowledge, and 43 states and the District of Columbia require the Multistate Pharmacy Jurisprudence Exam (MPJE), which tests pharmacy law. Both exams are administered by the National Association of Boards of Pharmacy. Pharmacists in the eight states that do not require the MJPE must pass a state-specific exam that is similar to the MJPE. In addition to the NAPLEX and MPJE, some states require additional exams unique to their state. All states except California currently grant a license without extensive reexamination to qualified pharmacists who already are licensed by another state. In Florida, reexamination is not required if a pharmacist has passed the NAPLEX and MPJE within 12 years of applying for a license transfer. Many pharmacists are licensed to practice in more than one state. Most states require continuing education for license renewal.

Inquiries

Education, Careers, Resources
American Association of Colleges of Pharmacy
1727 King Street
Alexandria, VA 22314
703 739-2330, x1024
www.aacp.org/pharmacycareers

American Society of Health-System Pharmacists
7272 Wisconsin Avenue
Bethesda, MD 20814
www.ashp.org

American Pharmacists Association
2215 Constitution Avenue NW
Washington, DC 20037-2985
www.pharmacist.com/students

Licensure
National Association of Boards of Pharmacy
1600 Feehanville Drive
Mount Prospect, IL 60056
www.nabp.net

Program Accreditation
Accreditation Council for Pharmacy Education
20 North Clark Street, Suite 2500
Chicago, IL 60602
www.acpe-accredit.org

Note: Adapted in part from the Bureau of Labor Statistics, US Department of Labor, *Occupational Outlook Handbook,* Pharmacists, at *www.bls.gov/oco/ocos079.htm*.

Pharmacist

Alabama

Auburn University
Pharmacy Prgm
School of Pharmacy
217 Walker Bldg
Auburn University, AL 36849-5501
www.pharmacy.auburn.edu

Samford University
Pharmacy Prgm
School of Pharmacy
800 Lakeshore Dr
Birmingham, AL 35229
www.pharmacy.samford.edu

Arizona

Midwestern University - Glendale Campus
Pharmacy Prgm
College of Pharmacy
19555 N 59th Ave
Glendale, AZ 85308
www.midwestern.edu/pages/cpg.html

University of Arizona
Pharmacy Prgm
College of Pharmacy
PO Box 210207
1703 E Mabel St
Tucson, AZ 85721
www.pharmacy.arizona.edu

Arkansas

University of Arkansas for Medical Sciences
Pharmacy Prgm
College of Pharmacy
4301 W Markham St
Little Rock, AR 72205
www.uams.edu/cop

Harding University
Pharmacy Prgm
College of Pharmacy
915 E Market Ave
Box 12230
Searcy, AR 72149
www.harding.edu/Pharmacy/

California

University of California - San Diego
Pharmacy Prgm
9500 Gilman Dr, MC-0657
La Jolla, CA 92093-0657
www.ucsd.edu

Loma Linda University
Pharmacy Prgm
School of Pharmacy
West Hall 1316
11262 Campus ST
Loma Linda, CA 92350
www.llu.edu

University of Southern California
Pharmacy Prgm
School of Pharmacy
1985 Zonal Ave
Los Angeles, CA 90089-9121
www.usc.edu/schools/pharmacy

Western Univ of Health Sciences
Pharmacy Prgm
College of Pharmacy
309 E Second St
Pomona, CA 91766-1854
www.westernu.edu

California Northstate University
Pharmacy Prgm
College of Pharmacy
10811 International Drive
Rancho Cordova, CA 95670
www.californiacollegeofpharmacy.org

University of California - San Francisco
Pharmacy Prgm
San Francisco School of Pharmacy
521 Parnassus Ave Rm C-156
Box 0622
San Francisco, CA 94143-0622
www.pharmacy.ucsf.edu

University of the Pacific
Pharmacy Prgm
Thomas J Long School of Pharmacy and Health Sciences
3601 Pacific Ave
Stockton, CA 92350
www.pacific.edu/pharmacy/

Touro University Mare Island
Pharmacy Prgm
California College of Pharmacy
1310 Johnson Lane
Vallejo, CA 94592
www.tu.edu

Colorado

Regis University
Pharmacy Prgm
School of Pharmacy
3333 Regis Blvd
Denver, CO 80221-1099
www.regis.edu/rh.asp?page=study.pharm

University of Colorado at Denver
Pharmacy Prgm
Health Sciences Center School of Pharmacy
C-238 4200 E Ninth Ave
Denver, CO 80262
www.uchsc.edu/sop

Connecticut

St. Joseph College School of Pharmacy
Pharmacy Prgm
229 Trumbull St
Hartford, CT 06103-1501
www.sjc.edu

University of Connecticut
Pharmacy Prgm
School of Pharmacy
69 N Eagleville Rd Unit 3092
Storrs, CT 06269-3092
www.pharmacy.uconn.edu

District of Columbia

Howard University
Pharmacy Prgm
College of Pharmacy, Nursing, and Allied Health
    Sciences
School of Pharmacy
Sixth & W Sts NW
Washington, DC 20059
www.howard.edu

Florida

Nova Southeastern University
Pharmacy Prgm
College of Pharmacy
3200 S University Dr
Fort Lauderdale, FL 33328
pharmacy.nova.edu/home.html

University of Florida
Pharmacy Prgm
College of Pharmacy
Box 100484
J Hillis Miller Health Center
Gainesville, FL 32610
www.cop.ufl.edu

Florida A&M University
Pharmacy Prgm
College of Pharmacy and Pharmaceutical Sciences
New Pharmacy Bldg, Rm 333
1415 S Martin Luther King Jr Blvd
Tallahassee, FL 32307
www.famu.edu

University of South Florida
Pharmacy Prgm
School of Pharmacy
12901 Bruce B Downs Blvd, MDC30
Tampa, FL 33612
health.usf.edu/nocms/pharmacy/

Palm Beach Atlantic University
Pharmacy Prgm
Lloyd L Gregory School of Pharmacy
900 S Olive Ave
West Palm Beach, FL 33401
www.pba.edu

Georgia

University of Georgia
Pharmacy Prgm
College of Pharmacy
Athens, GA 30602-2351
www.rx.uga.edu

Mercer University
Pharmacy Prgm
College of Pharmacy and Health Sciences
3001 Mercer University Dr
Atlanta, GA 30341-4155
www.mercer.edu/pharmacy

South University
Pharmacy Prgm
School of Pharmacy
709 Mall Blvd
Savannah, GA 31406-4811
www.southuniversity.edu

Philadelphia College of Osteopathic Medicine
Pharmacy Prgm
School of Pharmacy
625 Old Peachtree Rd, NW
Suwanee, GA 30024
www.pcom.edu

Hawaii

University of Hawaii at Hilo
Pharmacy Prgm
College of Pharmacy
34 Rainbow Drive
Hilo, HI 96720
pharmacy.uhh.hawaii.edu

Idaho

Idaho State University
Pharmacy Prgm
College of Pharmacy
PO Box 8288
970 S 5th Ave
Pocatello, ID 83209
www.pharmacy.isu.edu/live/

Illinois

Chicago State University
Pharmacy Prgm
College of Pharmacy
9501 S King Drive
206 Douglas Hall
Chicago, IL 60628-1598
www.csu.edu/collegeofpharmacy/

University of Illinois at Chicago
Pharmacy Prgm
College of Pharmacy
833 S Wood St, M/C 874
Chicago, IL 60612
www.uic.edu/pharmacy/

Midwestern University
Pharmacy Prgm
Chicago College of Pharmacy
555 31st St
Downers Grove, IL 60515
www.midwestern.edu/pages/ccp.html

Southern Illinois University Edwardsville
Pharmacy Prgm
Edwardsville School of Pharmacy
Campus Box 2000
Edwardsville, IL 62026-2000
www.siue.edu/pharmacy/

Rosalind Franklin University of Medicine
Pharmacy Prgm
College of Pharmacy
3333 Green Bay Rd
North Chicago, IL 60064
rosalindfranklin.edu/collegeofpharmacy/

Henrotin Hospital Corp
Pharmacy Prgm
College of Pharmacy
1400 N Roosevelt
Schaumburg, IL 60173-4348
www.roosevelt.edu/pharmacy.aspx

Indiana

Manchester College
Pharmacy Prgm
School of Pharmacy
1818 Carew St, Ste 300
Fort Wayne, IN 46805
www.manchester.edu/pharmacy

Butler University
Pharmacy Prgm
College of Pharmacy and Health Sciences
4600 Sunset Ave
Indianapolis , IN 46208
www.butler.edu/cophs/

Purdue University
Pharmacy Prgm
School of Pharmacy and Pharmaceutical Sciences
575 Stadium Mall Dr
West Lafayette, IN 47907
www.pharmacy.purdue.edu

Iowa

Drake University
Pharmacy Prgm
College of Pharmacy and Health Sciences
2507 University Ave
Cline Hall Suite 106
Des Moines, IA 50311
www.pharmacy.drake.edu

University of Iowa
Pharmacy Prgm
College of Pharmacy
115 S Grand Ave
Iowa City, IA 52242
www.pharmacy.uiowa.edu

Kansas

University of Kansas
Pharmacy Prgm
School of Pharmacy
1251 Wescoe Hall Dr
Rm 2056 Malott Hall
Lawrence, KS 66045-7582
www.pharm.ku.edu

Kentucky

University of Kentucky
Pharmacy Prgm
College of Pharmacy
725 Rose St, Suite 327
Lexington, KY 40536-0082
www.mc.uky.edu/pharmacy/

Sullivan University - Lexington
Pharmacy Prgm
College of Pharmacy
2100 Gardiner Lane
Louisville, KY 40205
www.sullivan.edu/pharmacy

Lebanon

Lebanese American Univ School of Pharmacy
Pharmacy Prgm
PO Box 36
Byblos, Lebanon, LE
www.au.edu.lb/academics/schoools/pharmacy

Louisiana

University of Louisiana at Monroe
Pharmacy Prgm
College of Pharmacy
700 University Ave
Monroe, LA 71209-0900
www.ulm.edu

Xavier Univ of Louisiana College of Pharmacy
Pharmacy Prgm
1 Drexel Dr
New Orleans, LA 70125
www.xula.edu/pharmacy

Maine

Husson University
Pharmacy Prgm
School of Pharmacy
One College Circle
Bangor, ME 04401-2999
www.husson.edu

University of New England
Pharmacy Prgm
College of Pharmacy
716 Stevens Ave
Portland, ME 04103

Maryland

College of Notre Dame of Maryland
Pharmacy Prgm
School of Pharmacy
4701 N Charles St
Baltimore, MD 21210
www.ndm.edu/admission/schoolofpharmacy

University of Maryland Baltimore County
Pharmacy Prgm
School of Pharmacy
20 N Pine St, Rm 730
Baltimore, MD 21201-1180
www.pharmacy.umaryland.edu

University of Maryland Eastern Shore
Pharmacy Prgm
School of Pharmacy
1062 Hazel Hall
Princess Anne, MD 21853
www.umes.edu/pharmacy/

Massachusetts

Mass College of Pharmacy & Health Sciences
Pharmacy Prgm
School of Pharmacy-Boston
179 Longwood Ave
Boston, MA 02115
www.mcphs.edu

Northeastern University
Pharmacy Prgm
Bouve College of Health Sciences School of Pharmacy
360 Huntington Ave, 206 Mugar
Boston, MA 02115
www.bouve.neu.edu/pharmacy

Western New England University
Pharmacy Prgm
College of Pharmacy
1215 Wilbraham Rd
Springfield, MA 01119-2684
www.wne.edu/pharmacy

Mass College of Pharmacy & Health Sciences
Pharmacy Prgm
19 Foster St, Ste 400
Worcester, MA 01608
www.mcphs.edu

Michigan

University of Michigan
Pharmacy Prgm
College of Pharmacy
428 Church St
Ann Arbor, MI 48109-1065
www.umich.edu/~pharmacy/

Ferris State University
Pharmacy Prgm
College of Pharmacy
220 Ferris Dr
Big Rapids, MI 49307
www.pharmacy.ferris.edu

Wayne State University
Pharmacy Prgm
Eugene Applebaum College of Pharmacy and Health
  Sciences
259 Mack Ave, Suite 2620
Detroit, MI 48201
www.cphs.wayne.edu

Minnesota

University of Minnesota
Pharmacy Prgm
College of Pharmacy
308 Harvard St SE
5-130 Weaver-Densford Hall
Minneapolis, MN 55455-0343
www.pharmacy.umn.edu

Mississippi

University of Mississippi
Pharmacy Prgm
School of Pharmacy
PO Box 1848
University, MS 38677
www.olemiss.edu/depts/pharm_school

Missouri

University of Missouri - Kansas City
Pharmacy Prgm
School of Pharmacy
5100 Rockhill Rd
Kansas City, MO 64110-2718
www.umkc.edu/pharmacy

St Louis College of Pharmacy
Pharmacy Prgm
4588 Parkview Place
St Louis, MO 63110
www.stlcop.edu

Montana

University of Montana
Pharmacy Prgm
College of Health Professions and Biomedical Sciences
Skaggs School of Pharmacy
340 Skaggs Bldg
Missoula, MT 59812-1512
www.health.umt.edu

Nebraska

Creighton University
Pharmacy Prgm
Medical Center School of Pharmacy and Health
  Professions
2500 California Plaza
Omaha, NE 68178
www.spahp2.creighton.edu.admission.pharmacy

University of Nebraska Medical Center
Pharmacy Prgm
College of Pharmacy
986000 Nebraska Medical Center
Omaha, NE 68198-6000
www.unmc.edu/pharmacy/

Nevada

Roseman University of Health Sciences
Pharmacy Prgm
College of Phamacy
11 Sunset Way
Henderson, NV 89014
www.usn.edu

New Jersey

Rutgers University
Pharmacy Prgm
New Jersey Ernest Mario School of Pharmacy
William Levin Hall
160 Frelinghuysen Rd
Piscataway, NJ 08854-8020
pharmacy.rutgers.edu

New Mexico

University of New Mexico
Pharmacy Prgm
College of Pharmacy
1 University of New Mexico
MSC09-536
Albuquerque, NM 87131-5691
www.hsc.unm.edu/pharmacy

New York

**Albany College of Pharmacy and Health
  Science**
Pharmacy Prgm
106 New Scotland Ave
Albany, NY 12208
www.acp.edu

University at Buffalo - SUNY
Pharmacy Prgm
School of Pharmacy and Pharmaceutical Sciences
126 Cooke Hall
Amherst, NY 14260-1200
www.pharmacy.buffalo.edu

Long Island University - Brooklyn Campus
Pharmacy Prgm
Arnold & Marie Schwartz College of Pharmacy & Health
  Science
75 DeKalb Ave
University Plaza
Brooklyn, NY 11201
www.liu.edu

D'Youville College
Pharmacy Prgm
D'Youville College School of Pharmacy
320 Porter Ave
Buffalo, NY 14201
www.dyc.edu/academics/pharmacy/

St John's University
Pharmacy Prgm
College of Pharmacy and Allied Health Professions
8000 Utopia Pkwy
Jamaica, NY 11439
new.stjohns.edu/academics/graduate/pharmacy

Touro College
Pharmacy Prgm
College of Pharmacy
230 West 125th St
New York, NY 10027
www.touro.edu/pharmacy/

St John Fisher College
Pharmacy Prgm
Wegmans School of Pharmacy
3690 East Ave
Rochester, NY 14618
www.sjfc.edu/pharmacy

North Carolina

Campbell University
Pharmacy Prgm
School of Pharmacy
PO Box 1090
205 Day Dorm Rd, Rm 101
Buies Creek, NC 27506
www.campbell.edu/pharmacy

University of North Carolina Hospitals
Pharmacy Prgm
School of Pharmacy
Beard Hall CB 7360
Chapel Hill, NC 27599-7360
www.pharmacy.unc.edu

Wingate University
Pharmacy Prgm
School of Pharmacy
315 E Wilson St
Wingate, NC 28174
www.wingate.edu

North Dakota

North Dakota State University
Pharmacy Prgm
College of Pharmacy, Nursing and Allied Sciences
123 Sudro Hall
Fargo, ND 58105-5055
www.ndsu.edu/pharmacy

Ohio

Ohio Northern University
Pharmacy Prgm
College of Pharmacy
Ada, OH 45810
www.new.onu.edu/academics/pharmacy

Cedarville University
Pharmacy Prgm
School of Pharmacy
251 N Main St
Cedarville, OH 45314
www.cedarville.edu/pharmacy

University of Cincinnati
Pharmacy Prgm
College of Pharmacy
PO Box 670004
Cincinnati, OH 45267-0004
www.pharmacy.uc.edu

The Ohio State University
Pharmacy Prgm
College of Pharmacy
500 W 12th Ave
Columbus, OH 43210
www.pharmacy.ohio-state.edu

The University of Findlay
Pharmacy Prgm
College of Pharmacy
1000 N Main St
Findlay, OH 45840
www.findlay.edu/academics/colleges/cohp/

Northeast Ohio Medical University
Pharmacy Prgm
College of Pharmacy
4209 State Rte 44
Rootstown, OH 44272
www.neoucom.edu/pharmd

University of Toledo
Pharmacy Prgm
College of Pharmacy
2801 W Bancroft St
Toledo, OH 43606-3390
www.utpharmacy.org

Oklahoma

University of Oklahoma
Pharmacy Prgm
College of Pharmacy
1110 N Stonewall, Rm 133
PO Box 26901
Oklahoma City, OK 73190
www.oupharmacy.com

Southwestern Oklahoma State University
Pharmacy Prgm
School of Pharmacy
100 Campus Dr
Weatherford, OK 73096
www.swosu.edu/pharmacy

Oregon

Oregon State University
Pharmacy Prgm
College of Pharmacy
203 Pharmacy Bldg
Corvallis, OR 97331-3507
pharmacy.oregonstate.edu

Pacific University
Pharmacy Prgm
School of Pharmacy
2043 College Way
Forest Grove, OR 97116
www.pacificu.edu/pharmd/

Pennsylvania

Lake Erie Coll of Osteopathic Medicine - Erie
Pharmacy Prgm
School of Pharmacy
1858 W Grandview Blvd
Erie, PA 16509
my.lecom.edu/pharm

Temple University
Pharmacy Prgm
School of Pharmacy
3307 N Broad St
Philadelphia, PA 19140
www.temple.edu/pharmacy/

Thomas Jefferson University
Pharmacy Prgm
Jefferson College of Health Professions
130 S 9th St, Suite 1520
Philadelphia, PA 19107
www.jefferson.edu

University of the Sciences
Pharmacy Prgm
Philadelphia College of Pharmacy
600 S 43rd St
Philadelphia, PA 19104-4495
www.usip.edu

Duquesne University
Pharmacy Prgm
Mylan School of Pharmacy
306 Bayer Learning Center
Pittsburgh, PA 15282-1504
www.pharmacy.duq.edu

University of Pittsburgh
Pharmacy Prgm
School of Pharmacy
1104 Salk Hall
3501Terrace Ave
Pittsburgh, PA 15261
www.pharmacy.pitt.edu

Wilkes University
Pharmacy Prgm
Nesbitt College of Pharmacy & Nursing
84 West South St
Wilkes-Barre, PA 18766
www.wilkes.edu/pharm

Puerto Rico

University of Puerto Rico
Pharmacy Prgm
Medical Sciences Campus School of Pharmacy
PO Box 365067
San Juan, PR 00936-5067
www.upr.clu.edu

Rhode Island

University of Rhode Island
Pharmacy Prgm
College of Pharmacy
41 Lower College Rd
Kingston, RI 02881
www.uri.edu/pharm

South Carolina

South Carolina College of Pharmacy
Pharmacy Prgm
280 Calhoun St
PO Box 250141
Charleston, SC 29425
sccp.sc.edu

Presbyterian College
Pharmacy Prgm
School of Pharmacy
503 S Broad St
Clinton, SC 29325
http://pharmacy.presby.edu

South Dakota

South Dakota State University
Pharmacy Prgm
Box 2202C
1 Administration Lane
Brookings, SD 57007
www3.sdstate.edu/academics/collegeofpharmacy

Tennessee

Union University
Pharmacy Prgm
School of Pharmacy
1050 Union University Dr
Jackson, TN 38305
www.uu.edu/academics/sop/

East Tennessee State University
Pharmacy Prgm
College of Pharmacy
PO Box 70414
807 University Pkwy
Johnson City, TN 37614
www.etsu.edu/pharamcy

South College
Pharmacy Prgm
School of Pharmacy
3904 Lonas Drive
Knoxville, TN 37909
southcollegetn.edu/pharmacy/

University of Tennessee Health Science Ctr
Pharmacy Prgm
College of Pharmacy
847 Monroe Ave, Suite 226
Memphis, TN 38163
pharmacy.utmem.edu

Belmont University
Pharmacy Prgm
School of Pharmacy
1900 Belmont Blvd
Nashville, TN 37212
www.belmont.edu/pharmacy/

Lipscomb University
Pharmacy Prgm
College of Pharmacy
One University Park Drive
Nashville, TN 37204
pharmacy.lipscomb.edu

Texas

Texas Tech Univ Health Sciences Center
Pharmacy Prgm
School of Pharmacy
1300 S Coulter
Amarillo, TX 79106
www.ttuhsc.edu/sop/

University of Texas at Austin
Pharmacy Prgm
College of Pharmacy
1 University Station A1900
PHR 2.112
Austin, TX 78712-0120
www.utexas.edu/pharmacy/

Texas Southern University
Pharmacy Prgm
College of Pharmacy and Health Sciences
3100 Celburne St
Houston, TX 77004
www.tsu.edu

University of Houston
Pharmacy Prgm
College of Pharmacy
141 Sciences & Research Bldg 2
4800 Calhoun
Houston, TX 77204-5000
www.uh.edu/pharmacy/

Texas A&M University - Kingsville
Pharmacy Prgm
Texas A & M University Health Science Center
MSC 131, 1010 West Ave B
Kingsville, TX 78363-8202
pharmacy.tamhsc.edu

The University of the Incarnate Word
Pharmacy Prgm
Feik School of Pharmacy
4301 Broadway CPO 99
San Antonio, TX 78209
www.uiw.edu/pharmacy

Utah

University of Utah
Pharmacy Prgm
College of Pharmacy
30 South 2000 East
Salt Lake City, UT 84112-5820
www.pharmacy.utah.edu

Virginia

University of Appalachia College of Pharmacy
Pharmacy Prgm
PO Box 2858
Grundy, VA 24614
www.uacp.org

Hampton University
Pharmacy Prgm

Hampton, VA 23668
www.hamptonu.edu

Virginia Commonwealth Univ/Health System
Pharmacy Prgm
School of Pharmacy
410 N 12th St
MCV Box 980581
Richmond, VA 23298-0531
www.pharmacy.vcu.edu

Shenandoah University
Pharmacy Prgm
Bernard J Dunn School of Pharmacy
1460 University Dr
Winchester, VA 22601
www.su.edu/academic/pharmacy.asp

Washington

Washington State University
Pharmacy Prgm
College of Pharmacy
PO Box 646510
Pullman, WA 99164-6510
www.pharmacy.wsu.edu

University of Washington
Pharmacy Prgm
School of Pharmacy
H364 Health Sciences
Box 357631
Seattle, WA 98195-7631
depts.washington.edu/pha/

West Virginia

University of Charleston
Pharmacy Prgm
School of Pharmacy
2300 MacCorkle Ave SE
Charleston, WV 25304
www.ucwv.edu

West Virginia University
Pharmacy Prgm
School of Pharmacy
PO Box 9500
1136 Health Sciences North
Morgantown, WV 26506-9500
www.hsc.wvu.edu/sop

Wisconsin

University of Wisconsin - Madison
Pharmacy Prgm
School of Pharmacy
777 Highland Ave
Madison, WI 53705
www.pharmacy.wisc.edu

Concordia University Wisconsin
Pharmacy Prgm
School of Pharmacy
12800 N Lake Shore Dr
Mequon, WI 53097
www.cuw.edu

Wyoming

University of Wyoming
Pharmacy Prgm
School of Pharmacy
1000 E University Ave
Dept 3375
Laramie, WY 82071
www.uwyo.edu/pharmacy

Pharmacy Technician

Pharmacy technicians assist licensed pharmacists by performing duties that do not require the professional skills and judgment of a licensed pharmacist and assisting in those duties that require the expertise of a pharmacist. Pharmacy technicians are employed in every practice setting where pharmacy is practiced, including institutional, community, home care, long-term care, mail order, and managed care pharmacies. Technicians are also employed in education, research, and the pharmaceutical industry.

Technicians may be trained on the job or by completing a formal program. Some formal training programs meet the program accreditation standards established by the American Society of Health-System Pharmacists (ASHP).

Career Description

According to the Scope of Pharmacy Practice Project, pharmacy technicians spend their time in the following ways:

- 26 percent—collect, organize, and evaluate information to assist pharmacists in serving patients
- 21 percent—develop and manage medication distribution and control systems; about half of this time is spent preparing, dispensing, distributing, and administering medications
- Seven percent—provide drug information and education

These percentages, however, may vary widely for many reasons, including the wide range of training and qualifications of pharmacists, the use of technicians as directed by a given supervisory pharmacist, and variations in state pharmacy practice laws.

The ASHP Accreditation Standard for Pharmacy Technician Training Programs specifies that graduates of programs should be able to perform the following functions (among others):

- Assist the pharmacist in collecting, organizing, and evaluating information for direct patient care, drug use review, and departmental management
- Receive and screen prescription medication orders for completeness and accuracy
- Use pharmaceutical and medical terms, abbreviations, and symbols appropriately
- Prepare and distribute medications in a variety of health system settings
- Perform arithmetical calculations required for usual dosage determinations and solutions preparation
- Use knowledge of general chemical and physical properties of drugs in manufacturing and packaging operations
- Use knowledge of proper aseptic technique and packaging in the preparation of medications
- Collect payment and/or initiate billing for pharmacy services and goods
- Purchase pharmaceuticals, devices, and supplies according to an established plan in a variety of health systems
- Control medication, equipment, and device inventory according to an established plan in a variety of health systems
- Maintain pharmacy equipment in preparing, storing, and distributing investigational drug products
- Assist the pharmacist in monitoring the practice site and/or service area for compliance with federal, state, and local laws, regulations, and professional standards

- Assist the pharmacist in preparing, storing, and distributing investigational drug products
- Assist the pharmacist in the monitoring of drug therapy
- Assist the pharmacist in identifying patients who desire counseling on the use of medications, equipment, and devices
- Understand the use and side effects of prescription and nonprescription drugs used to treat common disease states
- Appreciate the need to adapt the delivery of pharmacy services for the culturally diverse
- Maintain confidentiality of patient information
- Communicate clearly orally and in writing
- Use computers to perform pharmacy functions
- Demonstrate ethical conduct in all activities related to the delivery of pharmacy services

Employment Characteristics

Pharmacy technicians typically provide their services in one or more of the following settings: health systems, community pharmacies, chain pharmacies, and home care pharmacies.

Salary

Data from the US Bureau of Labor Statistics for May 2011 show that wages at the 10th percentile are $20,310, the 50th percentile (median) at $28,940, and the 90th percentile at $41,880 (*www.bls.gov/oes/current/oes292052.htm*).

For more information, refer to *www.ama-assn.org/go/hpsalary*.

Educational Programs

Length, Award. Programs are generally 15 weeks or longer and consist of a minimum of 600 hours of training (contact) time. Graduates generally receive a certificate or associate of science (AS) degree.

Prerequisites. Applicants should have a high school diploma or equivalent and meet institutional entrance requirements.

Curriculum. The professional curriculum includes formal instruction in didactic, practical, and laboratory areas of pharmacy practice. The curriculum consists of various aspects of pharmacy technician training pertinent to contemporary pharmacy practice. Courses include

- Pharmacy mathematics/calculations
- Pharmacy for pharmacy technicians
- Sterile products
- Pharmaceutical care delivery systems
- Computer systems for pharmacy
- Payment for pharmacy services

Certification

After completing their training, technicians may become a Certified Pharmacy Technician (CPhT) by successfully taking the national certification examination offered by the Pharmacy Technician Certification Board (PTCE) or the Institute for the Certification of Pharmacy Technicians (ExCPT).

Registration

Note: Registration is state regulated and may or may not require completion of an approved formal educational program, a specific number of hours of on the job training, fingerprinting, and a criminal background check.

Check with your state board of pharmacy for more information: *www.nabp.net/boards-of-pharmacy/*

Continuing Education

Twenty CE hours are required every two years; one of these 20 hours must be in Pharmacy Law. Some states also require live CE. For more information, check with your state board of pharmacy.

Inquiries

Careers and Professional Organizations
American Association of Pharmacy Technicians
(AAPT)
PO Box 1447
Greensboro, NC 27402
877 368-4771
E-mail: *aapt@pharmacytechnician.com*
www.pharmacytechnician.com

National Pharmacy Technician Association
3707 FM 1960 Road West, Suite 460
Houston, TX 77068
281 866-7900 or 888 247-8700
www.pharmacytechnician.org

Certification

Institute for the Certification of Pharmacy Technicians (ICPT)
and National Healthcareer Association (NHA)
ExCPT Exam for the Certification of Pharmacy Technicians
7500 West 160th Street
Stilwell, Kansas 66085
Tech Phone: 866 391-9188
Office Phone: 913 661-6491
E-mail: *info@icptmail.org*
http://www.nationaltechexam.org/eligibility_rules.html
http://www.nationaltechexam.org/

Pharmacy Technician Certification Board
1100 15th Street NW, Suite 730
Washington, DC 20005-1707
800 363-8012
www.ptcb.org

Program Accreditation

American Society of Health System-Pharmacists
Accreditation Services Division
7272 Wisconsin Avenue
Bethesda, MD 20814
301 664-8720
E-mail: *llifshin@ashp.org*
www.ashp.org

Note: Adapted in part from the Bureau of Labor Statistics, U.S. Department of Labor, *Occupational Outlook Handbook, 2010-11 Edition*, Pharmacy Technicians and Aides, at *www.bls.gov/oco/ocos325.htm*.

Pharmacy Technician

Alabama

Wallace Community College
Pharmacy Technician Prgm
801 Main St NW
PO Box 2000
Hanceville, AL 35077
www.wallace.edu

Arizona

Pima Community College
Pharmacy Technician Prgm
8181 E Irvington Rd
Tucson, AZ 85709-4000
www.pima.edu

Arkansas

Arkansas State University - Beebe
Pharmacy Technician Prgm
1800 E Moore St
PO Box 909
Searcy, AR 72143
www.asub.edu
Prgm Dir: Janet McGregor Liles, MSHS CPhT
Tel: 501 207-6237   *Fax:* 501 207-6263
E-mail: jliles@searcy.asub.edu

California

North Orange County Community College
Pharmacy Technician Prgm
Continuing Education
1830 W Romneya Dr
Anaheim, CA 92801
www.nocccd.cc.ca.us

Carrington College California - Antioch
Pharmacy Technician Prgm
2157 Country Hills Dr
Antioch, CA 94509
www.westerncollege.edu

Carrington College California - Citrus Heights
Pharmacy Technician Prgm
7301 Greenback Lane, Ste A
Citrus Heights, CA 95621
www.westerncollege.edu

Carrington College California - Emeryville
Pharmacy Technician Prgm
1400 65th St
Emeryville, CA 94608
www.svcollege.com

North-West College - Glendale
Pharmacy Technician Prgm
124 S Glendale Ave
Glendale, CA 91205
www.northwestcollege.com

American University of Health Sciences
Pharmacy Technician Prgm
3501 Atlantic Ave
Long Beach, CA 90807
www.auhs.edu

American Career College
Pharmacy Technician Prgm
4021 Rosewood Ave 101
Los Angeles, CA 90004
www.americancareer.com

Charles Drew University of Medicine and Sci
Pharmacy Technician Prgm
1731 E 120th St
Los Angeles, CA 90059
www.cdrewu.edu

Cerritos College
Pharmacy Technician Prgm
11110 E Alondra Blvd
Norwalk, CA 90650
www.cerritos.edu/ho

Foothill College
Pharmacy Technician Prgm
Middlefield Campus
4000 Middlefield Rd, Suite I
Palo Alto, CA 94303-4739
www.foothill.edu

North-West College - Pasadena
Pharmacy Technician Prgm
530 East Union
Pasadena, CA 91101
www.northwestcollege.com

Carrington College California - Pleasant Hill
Pharmacy Technician Prgm
380 Civic Dr, Ste 300
Pleasant Hill, CA 94523
www.westerncollege.edu

North-West College - Pomona
Pharmacy Technician Prgm
134 W Holt Ave
Pomona, CA 91768
www.northwestcollege.com

Carrington College California - Sacramento
Pharmacy Technician Prgm
8909 Folsom Blvd
Sacramento, CA 95826

Charles A Jones Skills & Business Ed Center
Pharmacy Technician Prgm
5451 Lemon Hill Ave
Sacramento, CA 95824-1529
www.scusd.edu

Carrington College California - San Jose
Pharmacy Technician Prgm
6201 San Ignacio Ave
San Jose, CA 95119

Carrington College California - San Leandro
Pharmacy Technician Prgm
170 Bayfair Mall
San Leandro, CA 94578

Santa Ana College
Pharmacy Technician Prgm
1530 W 17th St
Santa Ana, CA 92706
www.sac.edu/pharmacy

Carrington College California - Stockton
Pharmacy Technician Prgm
1313 W Robinhood Dr, Ste B
Stockton, CA 95207

North-West College - West Covina
Pharmacy Technician Prgm
2121 Garvey Ave N
West Covina, CA 91790
www.northwestcollege.com

Colorado

Pikes Peak Community College
Pharmacy Technician Prgm
5675 S Academy Blvd, CC13
Colorado Springs, CO 80906

Arapahoe Community College
Pharmacy Technician Prgm
5900 S Santa Fe Dr
Littleton, CO 80160-9002
www.arapahoe.edu

Front Range Comm College
Pharmacy Technician Prgm
Westminster Campus
3645 W 112th Ave
Westminster, CO 80030
www.frontrange.edu

Florida

McFatter Technical Center
Pharmacy Technician Prgm
6500 Nova Dr
Davie, FL 33317

Everest Univ - Melbourne Campus
Pharmacy Technician Prgm
2401 N Harbor City Blvd
Melbourne, FL 32935

Pinellas Technical Education Centers - St Petersburg Campus
Pharmacy Technician Prgm
901 34th St South
St Petersburg, FL 33711
www.myptec.org

Henry W Brewster Technical Center
Pharmacy Technician Prgm
2222 N Tampa St
Tampa, FL 33602
www.brewster.edu

Georgia

Ogeechee Technical College
Pharmacy Technician Prgm
1 Joe Kennedy Blvd
Statesboro, GA 30458
www.ogeechee.tec.ga.us

Southwest Georgia Technical College
Pharmacy Technician Prgm
15689 US Hwy 19 N
Thomasville, GA 31799

Valdosta Technical College
Pharmacy Technician Prgm
4089 Val Tech Rd
Valdosta, GA 31602
www.valdostatech.edu

Southeastern Technical College
Pharmacy Technician Prgm
3001 E First St
Vidalia, GA 30474

Illinois

Malcolm X College
Pharmacy Technician Prgm
1900 W Van Buren St, Ste 3524
Chicago, IL 60612-3145
www.ccc.edu
Prgm Dir: Ronald D Grimmette, BS MAd Ed DPh
Tel: 312 850-7385   *Fax:* 312 850-7378
E-mail: rgrimmette@ccc.edu

Midwest Technical Institute - East Peoria
Pharmacy Technician Prgm
280 High Point Lane
East Peoria, IL 61611
www.Midwesttech.edu

Blessing Hospital
Pharmacy Technician Prgm
Broadway and 14th St
Quincy, IL 62301
www.blessinghospital.com

South Suburban College
Pharmacy Technician Prgm
15800 S State St
South Holland, IL 60473
www.southsuburbancollege.edu

Midwest Technical Institute - Springfield
Pharmacy Technician Prgm
2731 Farmers Market Rd
Springfield, IL 62707
www.midwesttech.edu

Indiana

Indiana University Health
Pharmacy Technician Prgm
Clarian Health Education Center
Rm 506 Wile Hall, PO Box 1367
Indianapolis, IN 46206-1397
www.clarian.org

Kansas

Hutchinson Community College
Pharmacy Technician Prgm
1300 N Plum
Hutchinson, KS 67501
www.hutchcc.edu

Kentucky

Jefferson Community and Technical College
Pharmacy Technician Prgm
727 W Chestnut
Louisville, KY 40203

St Catharine College
Pharmacy Technician Prgm
2735 Bardstown Rd
St Catharine, KY 40061

Louisiana

Louisiana State University - Alexandria
Pharmacy Technician Prgm
8100 Hwy 71 S
Alexandria, LA 71302
www.lsua.edu

Bossier Parish Community College
Pharmacy Technician Prgm
6220 E Texas St
Science and Allied Health Division
Bossier City, LA 71111
www.bpcc.edu

Delgado Community College
Pharmacy Technician Prgm
Allied Health Div
615 City Park Ave
New Orleans, LA 70119
Prgm Dir: Anne LaVance, BS CPhT
Tel: 504 671-6237   *Fax:* 504 483-4609
E-mail: alavan@dcc.edu

Maryland

Anne Arundel Community College
Pharmacy Technician Prgm
101 College Pkwy
Florestano 306B
Arnold, MD 21012
www.aacc.edu/default.cfm

Michigan

Washtenaw Community College
Pharmacy Technician Prgm
4800 E Huron River Dr
PO Box D-1
Ann Arbor, MI 48106

Henry Ford Community College
Pharmacy Technician Prgm
5101 Evergreen, HCEC Bldg
Dearborn, MI 48128-1495
www.hfcc.edu

Wayne County Community College District
Pharmacy Technician Prgm
801 W Fort St
Detroit, MI 48226

Mid Michigan Community College
Pharmacy Technician Prgm
2600 S Summerton Rd
Mount Pleasant, MI 48858

Minnesota

Northland Community & Technical College
Pharmacy Technician Prgm
2022 Central Ave NE
PO Box 111
East Grand Forks, MN 56721

**Minnesota State Comm & Tech Coll -
    Moorhead**
Pharmacy Technician Prgm
405 SW Colfax, PO Box 566
Wadena, MN 56482-0566

Century College
Pharmacy Technician Prgm
3300 Century Ave N
White Bear Lake, MN 55110
www.century.edu

Mississippi

Jones County Junior College
Pharmacy Technician Prgm
900 S Court St
Ellisville, MS 39437
www.jcjc.edu/depts/pharmacy

Montana

Univ of Montana-Missoula - College of Tech
Pharmacy Technician Prgm
909 South Ave W
Missoula, MT 59801
www.cte.umt.edu

Nebraska

Southeast Community College
Pharmacy Technician Prgm
4771 West Scott Rd
Beatrice, NE 68310
www.southeast.edu/programs/Pharm/default.aspx
Prgm Dir: Elina Pierce,
Tel: 402 228-8247, Ext   *Fax:* 402 228-2218
E-mail: epierce@southeast.edu

Nevada

Pima Medical Institute
Pharmacy Technician Prgm
3333 E Flamingo Rd
Las Vegas, NV 89121
www.pmi.edu

College of Southern Nevada
Pharmacy Technician Prgm
1421 Pullman Drive
Sparks, NV 89434
www.ccnn.edu
Prgm Dir: Adrienne M Santiago, CPhT
Tel: 775 856-2266, Ext   *Fax:* 775 856-0935
E-mail: asantiago@ccnn4u.com

North Carolina

Durham Technical Community College
Pharmacy Technician Prgm
1637 Lawson St
Durham, NC 27703
www.durhamtech.edu

Cape Fear Community College
Pharmacy Technician Prgm
411 N Front St
Wilmington, NC 28401
http://cfcc.edu/phm/

North Dakota

North Dakota State College of Science
Pharmacy Technician Prgm
800 6th St N
Wahpeton, ND 58076-0002
www.ndscs.nodak.edu

Ohio

Collins Career Center
Pharmacy Technician Prgm
11627 State Route 243
Chesapeake, OH 45619
www.collins-cc.k12.oh.us

Cuyahoga Community College
Pharmacy Technician Prgm
East Campus, Health Careers and Sciences
4250 Richmond Rd
Cleveland, OH 44122
www.tri-c.edu/ptech

Oregon

Chemeketa Community College
Pharmacy Technician Prgm
4000 Lancaster Dr NE
PO Box 14007
Salem, OR 97309-7070

Pennsylvania

Great Lakes Institute of Technology
Pharmacy Technician Prgm
5100 Peach St
Erie, PA 16509
www.glit.edu

Bidwell Training Center
Pharmacy Technician Prgm
1650 Metropolitan St
Pittsburgh, PA 15233

Sanford-Brown Institute
Pharmacy Technician Prgm
Penn Center East, Bldg 7
777 Penn Center Blvd, Suite 111
Pittsburgh, PA 15235

**Community College of Allegheny County -
    South Campus**
Pharmacy Technician Prgm
1750 Clairton Rd, Rte 885
West Mifflin, PA 15122
www.ccac.edu
Prgm Dir: Jane Coughanour, MT(ASCP) MEd
Tel: 412 469-6280
E-mail: jcoughanour@ccac.edu

South Carolina

Aiken Technical College
Pharmacy Technician Prgm
PO Box 696
Aiken, SC 29841

Trident Technical College
Pharmacy Technician Prgm
7000 Rivers Ave
PO Box 118067
Charleston, SC 29423-8067

Midlands Technical College
Pharmacy Technician Prgm
PO Box 2408
Columbia, SC 29202
www.midlandstech.edu

Greenville Technical College
Pharmacy Technician Prgm
PO Box 5616
Greenville, SC 29606-5616
www.gvltec.edu

Piedmont Technical College
Pharmacy Technician Prgm
620 North Emerald Rd
Greenwood, SC 29649
www.ptc.edu

Horry - Georgetown Technical College
Pharmacy Technician Prgm
743 Hemlock Ave
Myrtle Beach, SC 29577
www.hgtc.edu

Spartanburg Community College
Pharmacy Technician Prgm
PO Box 4386
Spartanburg, SC 29305
www.stcsc.edu

South Dakota

Western Dakota Technical Institute
Pharmacy Technician Prgm
800 Mickelson Dr
Rapid City, SD 57703

National American University
Pharmacy Technician Prgm
2801 S Kiwanis Ave
Sioux Falls, SD 57105
www.national.edu

Southeast Technical Institute
Pharmacy Technician Prgm
2320 N Career Ave
Sioux Falls, SD 57107

Tennessee

Chattanooga State Community College
Pharmacy Technician Prgm
4501 Amnicola Hwy
Chattanooga, TN 37406
www.chattanoogastate.edu

Tennessee Technology Center - Jackson
Pharmacy Technician Prgm
2468 Technology Center Dr
Jackson, TN 38301
www.jackson.tec.tn.us

Concorde Career College - Memphis
Pharmacy Technician Prgm
5100 Poplar Ave, Ste 132
Memphis, TN 38137
www.concorde.edu

Tennessee Technology Center - Memphis
Pharmacy Technician Prgm
550 Alabama Ave
Memphis, TN 38105-3604

Walters State Community College
Pharmacy Technician Prgm
500 S Davy Crockett Pkwy
Morristown, TN 37813-6899
www.ws.edu

Tennessee Technology Center - Murfreesboro
Pharmacy Technician Prgm
1303 Old Fort Pkwy
Murfreesboro, TN 37129

Tennessee Technology Center - Nashville
Pharmacy Technician Prgm
100 White Bridge Rd
Nashville, TN 37209

Texas

Austin Community College
Pharmacy Technician Prgm
3401 Webberville Rd
Austin, TX 78702

Richland College
Pharmacy Technician Prgm
12800 Abrams Rd
Dallas, TX 75243-2199
www.richlandcollege.edu/hp

El Paso Community College
Pharmacy Technician Prgm
PO Box 20500
El Paso, TX 79998
http://start.epcc.edu/health/Navigation/
    About/Pharm.aspx
Prgm Dir: Nader Rassaei
Tel: 915 831-4490   *Fax:* 915 831-4487
E-mail: nrassaei@epcc.edu

**Medical Education and Training Campus
  (METC)**
Pharmacy Technician Prgm
Attn: Pharmacy Program
3038 William Hardee Rd
Fort Sam Houston, TX 78234
www.metc.mil
Prgm Dir: Maj John Catoe, PharmD
Tel: 210 808-2201   *Fax:* 210 808-2208
E-mail: john.d.catoe.mil@mail.mil

University of Texas Medical Branch
Pharmacy Technician Prgm
Department of Pharmacy
301 Unversity Blvd
Galveston, TX 77555-0701

Lone Star College-North Harris
Pharmacy Technician Prgm
2700 W W Thorne Dr
Houston, TX 77073
www.northharriscollege.com

San Jacinto College North
Pharmacy Technician Prgm
5800 Uvalde Rd
Houston, TX 77049
www.sanjac.edu/PharmacyTech

San Jacinto College South
Pharmacy Technician Prgm
13735 Beamer Rd
Houston, TX 77089
www.sjcd.edu

Angelina College
Pharmacy Technician Prgm
3500 S First (Hwy 595
PO Box 1768
Lufkin, TX 75902-1768
www.angelina.edu

South Texas College
Pharmacy Technician Prgm
PO Box 9701
McAllen, TX 78502-9701
www.southtexascollege.edu

Lamar State College - Orange
Pharmacy Technician Prgm
410 Front St
Orange, TX 77630
www.lsco.edu

Northwest Vista College
Pharmacy Technician Prgm
3535 N Ellison Dr
San Antonio, TX 78251

USAF School of Health Care Sciences
Pharmacy Technician Prgm
382nd Training Squadron
917 Missile Rd, Suite 3
Sheppard AFB, TX 76311

Weatherford College
Pharmacy Technician Prgm
225 College Park Dr
Weatherford, TX 76086
www.wc.edu

Vernon College
Pharmacy Technician Prgm
4105 Maplewood Dr
Wichita Falls, TX 76308
www.vernoncollege.edu

Utah

Everest College
Pharmacy Technician Prgm
3280 West 3500 South
West Valley City, UT 84119-2632

Virginia

Naval School of Health Sciences
Pharmacy Technician Prgm
1001 Holcomb Rd
Portsmouth, VA 23708-5200
http://navmedmpte.med.navy.mil/nshs-sd/index.htm

Washington

Renton Technical College
Pharmacy Technician Prgm
3000 NE Fourth St
Renton, WA 98056

Spokane Community College
Pharmacy Technician Prgm
N 1810 Greene St, MS 2090
Spokane, WA 99217-5399
www.scc.spokane.edu/fac/stschritter

St Joseph Medical Center
Pharmacy Technician Prgm
1717 South J St
PO Box 2197
Tacoma, WA 98401-2197
http://fhshealth.org

West Virginia

Carver Career Center
Pharmacy Technician Prgm
4799 Midland Dr
Charleston, WV 25306
http://boe.kana.k12.wv.us/carver/

Wisconsin

Milwaukee Area Technical College
Pharmacy Technician Prgm
700 W State St
Milwaukee, WI 53233
www.matc.edu

Pharmacy Technician

Programs*	Class Capacity	Begins	Length (months)	Award	Res. Tuition	Non-res. Tuition	Offers:† 1	2	3	4
Arkansas										
Arkansas State Univ - Beebe (Searcy)	20	Aug	9	Cert, TC, AAS	$3,500	$5,000	•		•	•
Illinois										
Malcolm X College (Chicago)	25	Aug	9	Cert	$2,937	$7,590			•	
Louisiana										
Delgado Community College (New Orleans)	18	Summer Fall Spring	8, 9	Cert, CTS						
Nebraska										
Southeast Community College (Beatrice)	20	Jul	12	Dipl	$4,850	$5,600			•	•
Nevada										
College of Southern Nevada (Sparks)	15	Monthly	15	Dipl	$17,475	$17,475	•		•	•
Pennsylvania										
Community College of Allegheny County - South Campus (West Mifflin)	30	Aug	12	Cert, AS, Certificate	$4,100	$6,100	•		•	
Texas										
El Paso Community College	14	Aug Jan	8, 24	Cert, CC, AAS	$2,400	$3,220			•	•
Medical Education and Training Campus (METC) (Fort Sam Houston)	88	Varies	6	Cert						

*Data are shown only for programs that completed the 2011 AMA Survey of Health Professions Education Programs.

†Key to Offers: 1: Evening or weekend classes; 2: Non-English instruction; 3: Cultural competence instruction; 4: Distance education component.

History

The profession of physician assistant (PA) originated in the mid-1960s as medical corpsmen returned from Vietnam and sought opportunities to utilize their newly acquired skills in civilian life. Toward the end of that decade, Duke University, the University of Colorado, the University of Washington and Wake Forest University were among the colleges and universities instituting PA courses of study. The early 1970s brought a rapid growth in the number of such educational programs, which were supported initially with $6.1 million appropriated under the Health Manpower Act of 1972. The funding also supported some of the initial organization and administration of national programs for accreditation of PA educational programs, specifically those designed to prepare individuals as assistants to primary care physicians. Since 1992, the number of accredited PA programs has grown from 55 to 164. The Accreditation Review Commission on Education for the Physician Assistant (ARC-PA) accredits the program to award the professional credential "PA"; in addition, currently 90 percent of the institutions that sponsor PA programs also award an advanced academic degree with all institutions that sponsor programs after 2020 being required to award a graduate degree.

Career Description

The physician assistant is academically and clinically prepared to practice medicine as part of a team led by a doctor of medicine or osteopathy. Within the physician-PA relationship, PAs make clinical decisions and provide a broad range of diagnostic, therapeutic, preventive and health maintenance services. The clinical role of PAs includes primary and specialty care in medical and surgical practice settings. PA practice is centered on patient care and may include educational, research, and administrative activities.

The role of the physician assistant demands intelligence, sound judgment, intellectual honesty, appropriate interpersonal skills, and the capacity to react to emergencies in a calm and reasoned manner. An attitude of respect for self and others, adherence to the concepts of privilege and confidentiality in communicating with patients, and a commitment to the patient's welfare are essential attributes of the graduate PA.

Employment Characteristics

According to the 2010 Physician Assistant Census, published by the American Academy of Physician Assistants, of the 83,466 PAs in 2010, nearly 88 percent were in clinical practice. About 31 percent are practicing in primary care. Family medicine is the most common specialty for physician assistants, followed by emergency medicine, surgery and surgical subspecialties, subspecialties of internal medicine, general internal medicine, and dermatology.

The majority of physician assistants practice in ambulatory care settings. Solo and group practices employ 41 percent of all physician assistants, and hospitals, including in-patient and out-patient units, employ 47 percent, owing in part to the number of PAs working as house staff. Various government agencies employ nine percent of the PA workforce, primarily in state governments and the U.S. Department of Veterans Affairs. The remaining members of the profession practice in community health centers, managed care organizations, freestanding urgent care centers, correctional facilities and other settings.

Physician assistants work an average of 40 hours per week. The number of patient visits for physician assistants in outpatient settings averages 93 per week; in inpatient hospital settings, the average is 70.9 patient visits per week. Nearly 32 percent of physician assistants have on-call responsibilities.

Salary

Data from the US Bureau of Labor Statistics from May 2011 (available at *www.bls.gov/oes/current/oes291071.htm*) show that the mean annual wage of physician assistants was $84,470. The middle 50 percent of physician assistants earned between $88,660. The lowest 10 percent earned less than $60,690, and the highest 10 percent earned more than $120,060. Median annual wages in the industries employing the largest numbers of physician assistants in May 2011 were:

Outpatient care centers	$92,450
General medical and surgical hospitals	$91,620
Offices of physicians	$89,860
Colleges, universities and professional schools	$83,140
Federal Executive Branch	$83,590

For more information, refer to *www.ama-assn.org/go/hpsalary*.

Employment Outlook

Employment of PAs is expected to grow by 30 percent from 2010 to 2020, much faster than the average for all occupations. This rapid job growth reflects the expansion of health care and an emphasis on cost containment, which results in increasing emphasis on use of PAs. Physicians and institutions are expected to employ more PAs to provide primary care and to assist with medical and surgical procedures because PAs are cost-effective and productive members of the health care team. Physician assistants can relieve physicians of routine duties and procedures.

Educational Programs

As of March 2012, there are 164 accredited PA programs, and the prospects for continuing growth of the profession look strong, with more than 70 new programs in the pipeline and a robust applicant pool that has grown by more than 10 percent each year. PAs are educated as generalists in medicine, and their flexibility allows them to practice medicine in more than 60 medical and surgical specialties.

Length. The length of programs varies, largely owing to a difference in student selection criteria and in the educational objectives of the individual program. The most common program length is 27 months, with one year of classroom study and 15 months of clinical rotations. Approximately 20,000 students are enrolled in PA programs; in 2011, the 154 accredited PA programs together graduated more than 6,200 new PAs. For students enrolled in PA programs in 2011, the mean resident tuition was $58,000 and the mean nonresident tuition was $62,500.

Prerequisites. Although requirements differ widely, physiology is required by 89 percent of the programs, followed by general chemistry (88%), anatomy (86%), microbiology (76%), and biology

(71%). Half of the programs (50.0%) require their applicants to have prior health care experience, and 39 percent prefer it.

Applicants. The mean age of applicants is 27.6 years old; 72 percent are female, and they average 2.3 years of health care experience. A balance of study in the applied behavioral sciences and the biological sciences is advised for students who wish to qualify for admission to a PA program.

Curriculum. The curriculum includes 400 hours of basic sciences and nearly 600 hours of clinical medicine. The vast majority of programs (88%) now offer a master's degree.

Accreditation standards require competency-based curricula. The professional curriculum for PA education includes basic medical, behavioral and social sciences; clinical preparatory sciences, patient assessment and supervised clinical practice; health policy; and professional practice issues. Supervised clinical practice rotations in pediatrics, family medicine, general internal medicine, prenatal care and women's health, geriatrics, emergency medicine, psychiatry/behavioral medicine and general surgery offer advanced applied content and supervised clinical work experience in dealing with commonly encountered demands for the primary health care of individuals from infancy through childhood, adolescence and the various phases of adulthood. These experiences are provided in outpatient, emergency, inpatient and long-term care clinical settings.

Licensure

PAs receive their national certification from the National Commission on Certification of Physician Assistants (NCCPA). Only graduates of accredited PA programs are eligible to take the Physician Assistant National Certifying Examination (PANCE). Upon certification, PAs must complete a continuous six-year cycle to maintain certification. Every two years, PAs must earn and log 100 CME hours and reregister the certificate with NCCPA (second and fourth years), and, by the end of the sixth year, recertify by successfully completing the Physician Assistant National Recertifying Examination (PANRE).

All states require passage of the PANCE for state licensure. All 50 states, the District of Columbia, and all US territories that regulate health professionals, with the exception of Puerto Rico, have enacted laws regulating the practice of physician assistants. All 50 states, the District of Columbia, and the majority of U.S. territories authorize PA prescribing. In order to practice as a physician assistant, an individual must meet the state's licensing criteria and have a supervising physician.

Inquiries

Careers
American Academy of Physician Assistants
2318 Mill Road, Suite 1300
Alexandria, VA 22314
703 836-2272
E-mail: *aapa@aapa.org*
www.aapa.org

Physician Assistant Education Association
300 North Washington Street, Suite 710
Alexandria, VA 22314-2544
703 548-5538
E-mail: *info@PAEAonline.org*
www.paeaonline.org

National Certification
National Commission on Certification of Physician Assistants
12000 Findley Road, Suite 100
Johns Creek, GA 30097
678 417-8100
www.nccpa.net

Program Accreditation
Accreditation Review Commission on Education for the Physician Assistant
12000 Findley Road, Suite 150
Johns Creek, GA 30097
770 476-1224
E-mail: *arc-pa@arc-pa.org*
www.arc-pa.org

Note: Adapted in part from the Bureau of Labor Statistics, US Department of Labor, *Occupational Outlook Handbook,* Physician Assistants, at *www.bls.gov/oco/ocos081.htm*.

Physician Assistant

Alabama

University of Alabama at Birmingham
Surgical Physician Assistant Prgm
School of Health Professions
1530 3rd Ave S, SHP 482
Birmingham, AL 35294-1212
www.uab.edu/surgicalpa
Prgm Dir: Patricia Jennings, DrPH PA-C
Tel: 205 934-4432   *Fax:* 205 934-3780
E-mail: prjenn@uab.edu

University of South Alabama
Physician Assistant Prgm
Dept of Physician Asst Studies
1504 Springhill Ave, Suite 4410
Mobile, AL 36604-3273
www.southalabama.edu/alliedhealth/pa

Arizona

Midwestern University - Glendale Campus
Physician Assistant Prgm
19555 N 59th Ave
Glendale, AZ 85308
www.midwestern.edu

AT Still University of Health Sciences
Physician Assistant Prgm
5850 E Still Circle
Mesa, AZ 85206
www.ashs.edu

Arkansas

Harding University
Physician Assistant Prgm
915 E Market Ave
HU 12231
Searcy, AR 72149-2231
www.harding.edu/paprogram

California

University of Southern California
Physician Assistant Prgm
1000 S Fremont Ave, Unit 7
Bldg A6, 4th Fl
Alhambra, CA 91803

Loma Linda University
Physician Assistant Prgm
Nichol Hall, Rm 2033
Loma Linda, CA 92350
www.llu.edu/llu/sahp

Riverside County Regional Medical Center
Cosponsor: Riverside Community College
Physician Assistant Prgm
Moreno Valley Campus
16130 Lasselle St
Moreno Valley, CA 92551-2045
www.rcc.edu/morenovalley

Samuel Merritt University
Physician Assistant Prgm
450 30th St, 4th Fl, Rm 4708
Oakland, CA 94609
www.samuelmerritt.edu

Stanford University School of Medicine
Physician Assistant Prgm
Primary Care Associate Prgm
1215 Welch Rd, Suite Modular G
Palo Alto, CA 94305
http://pcap.stanford.edu

Western Univ of Health Sciences
Physician Assistant Prgm
Primary Care PA Program
309 E Second St
Pomona, CA 91766-1854
www.westernu.edu

University of California - Davis
Physician Assistant Prgm
2516 Stockton Blvd, Ste 254
Sacramento, CA 95817-2297
fnppa.ucdavis.edu

Touro University Mare Island
Physician Assistant Prgm
1310 Johnson Ln
Vallejo, CA 94592
www.tu.edu

San Joaquin Valley College - Visalia
Physician Assistant Prgm
8400 W Mineral King
Visalia, CA 93291
www.sjvc.edu/programs

Colorado

University of Colorado Denver - Anschutz MC
Physician Assistant Prgm
Child Health Associate, Physician Assistant Program
Mail Stop F543
Aurora, CO 80045
www.medschool.ucdenver.edu/paprogram
Prgm Dir: Jonathan Bowser, MS PA-C
Tel: 303 724-1338   *Fax:* 303 724-1350
E-mail: Jonathan.Bowser@ucdenver.edu

Red Rocks Community College
Physician Assistant Prgm
Campus Box 38
13300 W Sixth Ave
Lakewood, CO 80228
www.rrcc.edu/pa

Connecticut

Quinnipiac University
Physician Assistant Prgm
275 Mount Carmel Ave
Hamden, CT 06518-1908
www.quinnipiac.edu/x1040.xml

Yale University School of Medicine
Physician Assistant Prgm
Harkness Office Building, Second Floor
367 Cedar St
New Haven, CT 06510-3222
www.paprogram.yale.edu

District of Columbia

George Washington University
Physician Assistant Prgm
900 23rd St NW, Ste 6148
Washington, DC 20037
www.gwumc.edu/healthsci/programs/pa

Howard University
Physician Assistant Prgm
6th and Bryant Sts NW
Washington, DC 20059
www.howard.edu

Florida

Keiser University
Physician Assistant Prgm
1500 Northwest 49th St
Fort Lauderdale, FL 33309
www.keiseruniversity.edu/
   physical-therapist-assis-AS.php

**Nova Southeastern University - Fort
   Lauderdale**
Physician Assistant Prgm
3200 S University Dr
Fort Lauderdale, FL 33328

Nova Southeastern University - Fort Myers
Physician Assistant Prgm
3650 Colonial Court
Fort Myers, FL 33913
www.nova.edu/chcs/pa/swflorida/

University of Florida
Physician Assistant Prgm
College of Medicine
PO Box 100176
Gainesville, FL 32610-0176
www.med.ufl.edu/pap/apply

Nova Southeastern University - Jacksonville
Physician Assistant Prgm
6675 Corporate Center Parkway, Suite 112
Jacksonville, FL 32216
www.nova.edu/cah/pa/jacksonville/index.html

Dade Medical College
Physician Assistant Prgm
950 NW 20th St
Miami, FL 33127-4693

Barry University
Physician Assistant Prgm
11300 NE 2nd Ave, Box SGMS-PA
Miami Shores, FL 33161-6695
www.barry.edu

Nova Southeastern University - Orlando
Physician Assistant Prgm
4850 Millenia Blvd
Orlando, FL 32839

South University - Tampa
Physician Assistant Prgm
4401 N Himes Ave
Tampa, FL 33614
www.southuniversity.edu

Georgia

Emory University
Physician Assistant Prgm
School of Medicine
1462 Clifton Rd/Suite 280
Atlanta, GA 30322
http://emorypa.org
Prgm Dir: Dana Sayre-Stanhope, PA-C
Tel: 404 727-7827   *Fax:* 404 727-7836
E-mail: dsayres@emory.edu

Mercer University
Physician Assistant Prgm
3001 Mercer University Dr
Atlanta, GA 30341

Georgia Health Sciences University
Physician Assistant Prgm
Health Sciences Building, Rm EC-3304
987 St Sebastian Way
Augusta, GA 30912
www.mcg.edu/PhyAsst

South University
Physician Assistant Prgm
709 Mall Blvd
Savannah, GA 31406

Idaho

Idaho State University
Physician Assistant Prgm
921 S 8th Ave, Stop 8253
1021 S Red Hill Rd
Pocatello, ID 83209-8253
www.isu.edu/paprog

Illinois

Southern Illinois University Carbondale
Physician Assistant Prgm
School of Allied Health and School of Medicine
Lindegren Hall Rm 129 MC 6516
Carbondale, IL 62901-6516
http://mccoy.lib.siu.edu/~paprogram/

John H. Stroger Hospital of Cook County
Cosponsor: Malcolm X College
Physician Assistant Prgm
1900 W Van Buren
Room 3240
Chicago, IL 60612
www.ccc.edu/malcolmx

Northwestern University
Physician Assistant Prgm
710 N Lake Shore Drive
Abbott Hall, Fourth Floor
Chicago, IL 60611
www.familymedicine.northwestern.edu/pa_program/

Rush University
Physician Assistant Prgm
600 S Paulina St, 1021F
Chicago, IL 60612

Midwestern University
Physician Assistant Prgm
555 31st St
Downers Grove, IL 60515-1235
www.midwestern.edu
Prgm Dir: Sandhya Noronha, MD
Tel: 630 515-6034   *Fax:* 630 971-6402
E-mail: snoron@midwestern.edu

Rosalind Franklin University of Medicine
Physician Assistant Prgm
3333 Green Bay Rd
North Chicago, IL 60064-3095
www.rosalindfranklin.edu
Prgm Dir: Patrick Knott, PhD PA-C
Tel: 847 578-8689   *Fax:* 847 578-8690
E-mail: Patrick.Knott@RosalindFranklin.edu

Indiana

University of Saint Francis
Physician Assistant Prgm
Department of Physician Assistant Studies
2701 Spring St
Fort Wayne, IN 46808
www.sf.edu

Butler University
Physician Assistant Prgm
College of Pharmacy and Health Sciences
4600 Sunset Ave
Indianapolis, IN 46208
www.butler.edu/physician-assistant

Indiana State University
Physician Assistant Prgm
Student Services Building, Room 201
Terre Haute, IN 47809
www.indstate.edu/pa/contact-us.htm

Iowa

Des Moines University
Physician Assistant Prgm
3200 Grand Ave
Des Moines, IA 50312-4198
www.dmu.edu/chs/pa/

University of Iowa
Physician Assistant Prgm
Roy J and Lucille A Carver College of Medicine
5167 Westlawn
Iowa City, IA 52242-1100
http://paprogram.medicine.uiowa.edu

Kansas

Wichita State University
Physician Assistant Prgm
Campus Box 43
1845 N Fairmount
Wichita, KS 67260-0043
http://chp.wichita.edu/pa

Kentucky

University of Kentucky
Physician Assistant Prgm
Dept of Clinical Sciences
CT Wethington Building
900 S Limestone St Suite 205
Lexington, KY 40536-0200
www.mc.uky.edu/PA/

University of the Cumberlands
Physician Assistant Prgm
School of Health Science
7527 College Station Drive
Williamsburg, KY 40769
http://ucumberlands.edu

Louisiana

Our Lady of the Lake College
Physician Assistant Prgm
7443 Picardy Ave
Baton Rouge, LA 70808
www.ololcollege.edu

LSU Health Science Center Shreveport
Physician Assistant Prgm
1501 Kings Hwy, PO Box 33932
Shreveport, LA 71130-3932
www.sh.lsuhsc.edu/ah/

Maine

University of New England
Physician Assistant Prgm
716 Stevens Ave
Portland, ME 04103-2670
www.une.edu/chp/pa

Maryland

Anne Arundel Community College
Physician Assistant Prgm
101 College Pkwy
Arnold, MD 21012-1895
www.aacc.edu/physassist
Prgm Dir: Mary Jo Bondy, D H Ed MHS PA-C
Tel: 410 777-7392 *Fax:* 410 777-7099
E-mail: mjbondy@aacc.edu

Towson University CCBC Essex
Physician Assistant Prgm
7201 Rossville Blvd, N 317
Baltimore, MD 21237-3855
http://towson.edu/chp/pa

University of Maryland Eastern Shore
Physician Assistant Prgm
Modular 934-5 Backbone Rd
Princess Anne, MD 21853
www.umes.edu/pa

Massachusetts

Mass College of Pharmacy & Health Sciences
Physician Assistant Prgm
179 Longwood Ave
Master of Physician Assistant Studies-Boston
Boston, MA 02115
www.mcphs.edu/academics/schools/school_of_pa_bos/

Northeastern University
Physician Assistant Prgm
360 Huntington Ave, 202 Robinson
Boston, MA 02115-5000
www.northeastern.edu/bouve/programs/mphysassist/
    mphysassist.html

Springfield College
Physician Assistant Prgm
263 Alden St
Springfield, MA 01109-3797
www.spfldcol.edu

Mass College of Pharmacy & Health Sciences
Physician Assistant Prgm
Master of Physician Assistant
    Studies-Manchester/Worcester
19 Foster St, Suite 400
Worcester, MA 01608
www.mcphs.edu/academics/programs/
    physician_assistant_studies/PA_24_Man/

Michigan

University of Detroit Mercy
Physician Assistant Prgm
4001 W McNichols Rd
Detroit, MI 48221
http://healthprofessions.udmercy.edu/programs/
    paprogram/

Wayne State University
Physician Assistant Prgm
College of Pharmacy and Health Sciences
259 Mack Ave, Suite 2590
Detroit, MI 48201

Grand Valley State University
Physician Assistant Prgm
Center for Health Sciences
301 Michigan St NE, Suite 200
Grand Rapids, MI 49503
www.gvsu.edu/pas

Western Michigan University
Physician Assistant Prgm
1903 W Michigan Ave
Kalamazoo, MI 49008-5138
www.wmich.edu/hhs/pa

Central Michigan University
Physician Assistant Prgm
HPB 1222
Mount Pleasant, MI 48859
www.cmich.edu/chp/x485.xml

Minnesota

Augsburg College
Physician Assistant Prgm
2211 Riverside Ave, CB 149
Minneapolis, MN 55454
www.augsburg.edu/pa

Missouri

Missouri State University
Physician Assistant Prgm
901 S National Ave
Springfield, MO 65897
www.missouristate.edu/pas

Saint Louis University
Physician Assistant Prgm
3437 Caroline St, Suite 3025
Doisy College of Health Sciences
St. Louis, MO 63104-1111
pae.slu.edu
Prgm Dir: Anne Garanzini, MEd PA
Tel: 314 977-8521 *Fax:* 314 977-8649
E-mail: paprog@slu.edu

Montana

Rocky Mountain College
Physician Assistant Prgm
1511 Poly Dr
Billings, MT 59102-1796
http://pa.rocky.edu

Nebraska

Union College
Physician Assistant Prgm
3800 S 48th St
Lincoln, NE 68506

University of Nebraska Medical Center
Physician Assistant Prgm
984300 Nebraska Medical Center
Omaha, NE 68198-4300
www.unmc.edu/alliedhealth/pa
Prgm Dir: James E Somers, PhD PA
Tel: 402 559-9495 *Fax:* 402 559-7996
E-mail: SAHPadmissions@unmc.edu

Nevada

Touro University - Nevada
Physician Assistant Prgm
874 American Pacific Dr
Henderson, NV 89014
www.tu.edu/indexnv.php

New Hampshire

Mass College of Pharmacy & Health Sciences
Physician Assistant Prgm
1260 Elm St
Manchester, NH 03101
www.mcphs.edu/academics/programs/
    physician_assistant_studies/PA_24_Man/

Franklin Pierce College
Physician Assistant Prgm
24 Airport Rd, Suite 19
West Lebanon, NH 03784
www.franklinpierce.edu
Prgm Dir: Lisa Walker, MPAS PA-C
Tel: 603 298-6617 *Fax:* 603 899-4207
E-mail: paprogram@franklinpierce.edu

New Jersey

Univ of Medicine & Dent of New Jersey
Physician Assistant Prgm
Robert Wood Johnson Med Sch
675 Hoes Ln
Piscataway, NJ 08854-5635
www.shrp.umdnj.edu/programs/paweb
Prgm Dir: Ruth Fixelle, EdM PA-C
Tel: 732 235-4445 *Fax:* 732 235-4820
E-mail: r.fixelle@umdnj.edu

Seton Hall University
Physician Assistant Prgm
400 S Orange Ave
South Orange, NJ 07079
www.shu.edu/academics/gradmeded/
    ms-physician-assistant/

New Mexico

University of New Mexico
Physician Assistant Prgm
School of Medicine
Dept of Family and Community Medicine MSC 09 5040
1 University of New Mexico
Albuquerque, NM 87131-0001
http://hsc.unm.edu/som/fcm/pap/

University of St Francis
Physician Assistant Prgm
4401 Silver Ave SE, Ste B
Albuquerque, NM 87108

New York

Albany Medical College
Physician Assistant Prgm
Center for Physician Assistant Studies
47 New Scotland Ave MC 4
Albany, NY 12208-3412
www.amc.edu/pa
Prgm Dir: David Irvine, DHSc RPA-C
Tel: 518 262-5251   *Fax:* 518 262-0484
E-mail: irvined@mail.amc.edu

Daemen College
Physician Assistant Prgm
4380 Main St
Amherst, NY 14226-3592
www.daemen.edu

Touro College - Bay Shore
Physician Assistant Prgm
Winthrop University Hospital Ext Ctr
1700 Union Blvd
Bay Shore, NY 11706
www.touro.edu

Mercy College
Physician Assistant Prgm
Graduate Program in Physician Assistant Studies
1200 Waters Place
Bronx, NY 10461
www.mercy.edu

Long Island University - Brooklyn Campus
Physician Assistant Prgm
Division of Physician Assistant Studies
1 University Plaza
Brooklyn, NY 11201
http://liu.edu/Brooklyn/Academics/Schools/SHP/Dept/
     Physician-Assistant/Graduate-Programs/MS-PAS.aspx
Prgm Dir: Elizabeth Salzer, RPA-C MA
Tel: 718 488-1505   *Fax:* 718 246-6364
E-mail: elizabeth.salzer@liu.edu

SUNY Downstate Medical Center
Physician Assistant Prgm
450 Clarkson Ave, PO Box 1222
Brooklyn, NY 11203
www.downstate.edu/CHRP/pa/

D'Youville College
Physician Assistant Prgm
320 Porter Ave
Buffalo, NY 14201-1084
www.dyc.edu

St John's University
Physician Assistant Prgm
175-05 Horace Harding Expressway
Fresh Meadows, NY 11365

Hofstra University
Physician Assistant Prgm
113 Monroe Lecture Center
Hempstead, NY 11549-1270

York College, CUNY
Physician Assistant Prgm
94-20 Guy R Brewer Blvd, Rm 1E12
Jamaica, NY 11451
http://york.cuny.edu

City University of New York, The City College
Cosponsor: The Sophie Davis School of Biomedical
     Education
Physician Assistant Prgm
138th St and Convent Ave, Harris Hall, Ste 15
New York, NY 10031
http://portal.cuny.edu/portal/site/
     cuny/index.jsp?front_door=true

Pace University - Lenox Hill Hospital
Physician Assistant Prgm
1 Pace Plaza, Room Y-31
New York, NY 10038-1598
www.pace.edu/dyson/paprogram

Touro College
Physician Assistant Prgm
Manhattan PA Program
27-33 W 23rd St
New York, NY 10010
www.touro.edu/shs/pany

Weill Cornell Graduate School of Medical Sci
Physician Assistant Prgm
575 Lexington Ave
New York, NY 10022
www.med.cornell.edu/pa

New York Institute of Technology
Physician Assistant Prgm
Riland Center, Room 352
Northern Blvd, PO Box 8000
Old Westbury, NY 11568-8000
http://iris.nyit.edu/hpbls/pas

Clarkson University
Physician Assistant Prgm
Department of Physician Assistant Studies
PO Box 5882
Potsdam, NY 13699-5882
www.clarkson.edu/pa

Rochester Institute of Technology
Physician Assistant Prgm
153 Lomb Memorial Dr
Bldg 75 - CBET
Rochester, NY 14623
www.rit.edu/cos/medical/physician_assistant.html

Wagner College/Staten Island University
Physician Assistant Prgm
Concord Site
1034 Targee St, Spring Bldg
Staten Island, NY 10304
www.siuh.edu/conindex4.html

Stony Brook University
Physician Assistant Prgm
SHTM-HSC, L2-422
Stony Brook, NY 11794-8202
http://healthtechnology.stonybrookmedicine.edu/progra
     ms/pa/elpa
Prgm Dir: Peter Kuemmel, MS RPAC
Tel: 631 444-3190   *Fax:* 631 444-1404
E-mail: peter.kuemmel@stonybrook.edu

Le Moyne College
Physician Assistant Prgm
1419 Salt Springs Rd
Syracuse, NY 13214
www.lemoyne.edu/index.asp

SUNY Upstate Medical University
Physician Assistant Prgm
Room 1215, Weiskotten Hall
Syracuse, NY 13210
www.upstate.edu/chp/programs/pa/

North Carolina

Campbell University
Physician Assistant Prgm
191 Main St
PO Box 1090
Buies Creek, NC 27506
www.campbell.edu/paprogram

Duke University Medical Center
Physician Assistant Prgm
Department of Community and Family Medicine
DUMC 104780
Durham, NC 27710
pa.mc.duke.edu
Prgm Dir: Patricia Dieter, MPA PA-C
Tel: 919 681-3259   *Fax:* 919 681-9666
E-mail: patricia.dieter@duke.edu

Methodist University
Physician Assistant Prgm
5105 B College Center Dr
5107 College Center Dr
Fayetteville, NC 28311-1498
www.methodist.edu/paprogram

East Carolina University
Physician Assistant Prgm
College of Allied Health Sciences
Dept of Physician Assistant Studies
Health Sciences Building; Suite 4310
Greenville, NC 27834-4353
www.ecu.edu/pa

Wingate University
Physician Assistant Prgm
PO Box 159
Wingate, NC 28174
wingate.edu

Wake Forest University School of Medicine
Physician Assistant Prgm
Department of PA Studies
Medical Center Blvd
Winston-Salem, NC 27157-1006
www.wfubmc.edu/paprogram

North Dakota

University of North Dakota
Physician Assistant Prgm
School of Medicine & Health Sciences Room 4128
Family & Community Medicine
501 N Columbia Rd - Stop 9037
Grand Forks, ND 58202-9037
www.med.und.nodak.edu/physicianassistant

Ohio

University of Mount Union
Physician Assistant Prgm
1972 Clark Ave
Alliance, OH 44601
www.mountunion.edu/Academics/academic_programs/
     physician_assistant_studies/index.aspx

The University of Findlay
Physician Assistant Prgm
1000 N Main St
Findlay, OH 45840
www.findlay.edu

Kettering College of Medical Arts
Physician Assistant Prgm
3737 Southern Blvd
Kettering, OH 45429
www.kcma.edu

Marietta College
Physician Assistant Prgm
215 Fifth St
Marietta, OH 45750
www.marietta.edu/graduate/PA

Cuyahoga Community College
Cosponsor: Cleveland State University
Physician Assistant Prgm
11000 Pleasant Valley Rd
Parma, OH 44130
www.tri-c.edu/pa

University of Toledo
Physician Assistant Prgm
3015 Arlington Ave
MS1027
Toledo, OH 43614
www.utoledo.edu/med/pa/

Oklahoma

Univ of Oklahoma Health Sciences Center
Physician Assistant Prgm
PO Box 26901
Oklahoma City, OK 73190

University of Oklahoma - Tulsa
Physician Assistant Prgm
4502 E 41st St
Tulsa, OK 74135-2512

Oregon

Pacific University
Physician Assistant Prgm
222 SE 8th Ave, Ste 551
Hillsboro, OR 97123
www.pacificu.edu/pa/

Oregon Health & Science University
Physician Assistant Prgm
3181 SW Sam Jackson Park Rd, GH 219
Portland, OR 97239-3098
www.ohsu.edu/pa

Pennsylvania

DeSales University
Physician Assistant Prgm
2755 Station Ave
Center Valley, PA 18034-9568
www.desales.edu/physicianassistant

Salus University
Physician Assistant Prgm
8360 Old York Rd
Elkins Park, PA 19027

Gannon University
Physician Assistant Prgm
109 University Square
Erie, PA 16541-0001
www.gannon.edu/PROGRAMS/UNDER/phyasst.asp

Arcadia University
Physician Assistant Prgm
450 S Easton Rd
Glenside, PA 19038

Seton Hill University
Physician Assistant Prgm
Seton Hill Dr
Greensburg, PA 15601
www.setonhill.edu

Lock Haven University
Physician Assistant Prgm
417 RR St
Lock Haven, PA 17745
www.lhup.edu

St Francis University
Physician Assistant Prgm
Sullivan Hall Rm 104
PO Box 600
Loretto, PA 15940-0600
www.francis.edu/MPAShome.htm
Prgm Dir: Donna Yeisley, MEd PA-C
Tel: 814 472-3130   *Fax:* 814 472-3137
E-mail: pa@francis.edu

Drexel University College of Medicine
Physician Assistant Prgm
245 N 15th St, MS 504
Philadelphia, PA 19102
www.drexel.edu

Philadelphia College of Osteopathic Medicine
Physician Assistant Prgm
4190 City Ave
Rowland Hall
Philadelphia, PA 19131

Philadelphia University
Physician Assistant Prgm
School of Science and Health
School House Ln and Henry Ave
Philadelphia, PA 19144-5497
www.philau.edu/paprogram/
Prgm Dir: Lawrence Carey, PharmD
Tel: 215 951-2908   *Fax:* 215 951-2526
E-mail: careyl@philau.edu

Chatham University
Physician Assistant Prgm
Woodland Rd
Pittsburgh, PA 15232-2826
www.chatham.edu/departments/healthmgmt/
   graduate/pa/

Duquesne University
Physician Assistant Prgm
Rangos Sch of Health Sciences
Health Sciences Bldg, Suite 405
Pittsburgh, PA 15282
www.healthsciences.duq.edu/pa/pahome.html

University of Pittsburgh
Physician Assistant Prgm
3010 William Pitt Way
Room 224
Pittsburgh, PA 15213
www.shrs.pitt.edu/pa.aspx?id=2222

Marywood University
Physician Assistant Prgm
2300 Adams Ave
Scranton, PA 18509
www.marywood.edu/departments/PA_Program/
   program.stm

King's College
Physician Assistant Prgm
133 N River St
Wilkes-Barre, PA 18711-0851
www.kings.edu/paprog

Pennsylvania College of Technology
Physician Assistant Prgm
One College Ave #123
Williamsport, PA 17701

South Carolina

Medical University of South Carolina
Physician Assistant Prgm
PO Box 250962
151 B Rutledge Ave
Charleston, SC 29425
www.musc.edu/chp/pa

South Dakota

University of South Dakota
Physician Assistant Prgm
414 E Clark St
Vermillion, SD 57069-2390
www.usd.edu/pa

Tennessee

Lincoln Memorial University
Physician Assistant Prgm
Harrogate, TN 37752

South College
Physician Assistant Prgm
3904 Lonas Dr
Knoxville, TN 37909

Bethel University
Physician Assistant Prgm
325 Cherry Ave
Box 329
McKenzie, TN 38201
www.bethelu.edu/bethelpa/

Christian Brothers College
Physician Assistant Prgm
650 East Parkway South
Memphis, TN 38104
www.cbu.edu/PAS

Trevecca Nazarene University
Physician Assistant Prgm
333 Murfreesboro Rd
Nashville, TN 37210-2877
www.trevecca.edu/pa

Texas

Univ of Texas Southwestern Med Ctr
Physician Assistant Prgm
5323 Harry Hines Blvd, V4.114
Dallas, TX 75390-9090
www.utsouthwestern.edu

Univ of Texas - Pan American
Physician Assistant Prgm
1201 West University Dr
Edinburg, TX 78541
www.panam.edu/dept/pasp

Medical Education and Training Campus (METC)
Physician Assistant Prgm
Interservice PA Program, Academy of Health Sciences
Grad School/MCCS-HGE-PA, IPAP RM 1202
3151 Winfield Scott Rd, Suite 1216
Fort Sam Houston, TX 78234-6130
www.usarec.army.mil/armypa/

Univ of North Texas Hlth Sci Ctr at Ft Worth
Physician Assistant Prgm
Department of Physician Assistant Studies
3500 Camp Bowie Blvd
Fort Worth, TX 76107-2699
www.hsc.unt.edu
Prgm Dir: Henry Lemke, MMS PA-C
Tel: 817 735-2301   *Fax:* 817 735-2529
E-mail: hlemke@hsc.unt.edu

University of Texas Medical Branch
Physician Assistant Prgm
School of Health Professions
301 University Blvd
Galveston, TX 77555-1145
www.shp.utmb.edu/pas
Prgm Dir: Richard R Rahr, EdD PA-C
Tel: 409 772-3047   *Fax:* 409 772-9710
E-mail: rrahr@utmb.edu

PHYSICIAN ASSISTANT

Baylor College of Medicine
Physician Assistant Prgm
One Baylor Plaza-Room MS M108
Houston, TX 77030-3411
Prgm Dir: Carl E Fasser, PA
Tel: 713 798-5405   *Fax:* 713 798-6128
E-mail: cfasser@bcm.tmc.edu

Texas Tech Univ Health Sciences Center
Physician Assistant Prgm
3600 N Garfield
Midland, TX 79705
www.ttuhsc.edu/sah/mpa/
Prgm Dir: Elvin E Maxwell, Jr, MA MPAS PA-C
Tel: 432 620-9905   *Fax:* 432 620-8605
E-mail: ed.maxwell@ttuhsc.edu

UT Health Science Center - San Antonio
Physician Assistant Prgm
7703 Floyd Curl Dr MC6249
San Antonio, TX 78229-3900
www.uthscsa.edu

Utah

University of Utah Health Science Center
Cosponsor: Utah Medical Association
Physician Assistant Prgm
375 Chipeta Way Ste A
Salt Lake City, UT 84108
www.utah.edu/upap

Virginia

James Madison University
Physician Assistant Prgm
Dept of Health Sciences
MSC 4301
Harrisonburg, VA 22807
www.jmu.edu/healthsci/paweb

Eastern Virginia Medical School
Physician Assistant Prgm
651 Colley Ave
ERB Suite 342
Norfolk, VA 23507
www.evms.edu/evms-school-of-health-professions/
    physician-assistant.html
Prgm Dir: Thomas Parish, DHSc PA-C
Tel: 757 446-7158   *Fax:* 757 446-7403
E-mail: parishtg@evms.edu

Shenandoah University
Physician Assistant Prgm
MOB II, Ste 430
190 Campus Blvd
Winchester, VA 22601
www.su.edu/pa

Washington

University of Washington
Physician Assistant Prgm
MEDEX Northwest
4311 11th Ave NE, Suite 200
Seattle, WA 98105-4608
www.medex.washington.edu
Prgm Dir: Terry Scott, MPA PA-C
Tel: 206 616-4001   *Fax:* 206 616-3889
E-mail: medex@u.washington.edu

West Virginia

Mountain State University
Physician Assistant Prgm
PO Box 9003
Beckley, WV 25802-2830
www.mountainstate.edu

Alderson-Broaddus College
Physician Assistant Prgm
101 College Hill Dr
PO Box 2036
Philippi, WV 26416
www.ab.edu

Wisconsin

University of Wisconsin - La Crosse
Cosponsor: Gundersen Lutheran & Mayo School of
    Health Science
Physician Assistant Prgm
1725 State St, 4031 HSC
La Crosse, WI 54601-3767
www.uwlax.edu/pastudies

University of Wisconsin - Madison
Physician Assistant Prgm
1300 University Ave, 1135 MSC
Madison, WI 53706
www.physicianassistant.wisc.edu

Marquette University
Physician Assistant Prgm
PO Box 1881
Milwaukee, WI 53201-1881

Carroll University
Physician Assistant Prgm
101 N East Ave
Waukesha, WI 53186
www.carrollu.edu/gradprograms/physasst/admission.asp

Physician Assistant

Programs*	Class Capacity	Begins	Length (months)	Award	Res. Tuition	Non-res. Tuition		Offers:† 1 2 3 4
Alabama								
Univ of Alabama at Birmingham	54	Aug	27	MSPAS	$29,040	$41,463	per year	•
Colorado								
Univ of Colorado Denver - Anschutz MC (Aurora)	44	Jun	34	Dipl, MPAS	$15,527	$31,120	per year	• •
Georgia								
Emory Univ (Atlanta)	52	Aug	28	MMSC				• •
Illinois								
Midwestern Univ (Downers Grove)	86	Jun	27	MMS	$35,700	$35,700		•
Rosalind Franklin Univ of Medicine (North Chicago)	65	May	24	MS	$26,528	$26,528		•
Maryland								
Anne Arundel Community College (Arnold)	40	May	25	Cert	$19,675	$39,000		• •
Missouri								
Saint Louis Univ (St. Louis)	34	Aug	27	MMS	$73,800	$73,800	total tuition	•
Nebraska								
Univ of Nebraska Medical Center (Omaha)	48		28	MPAS	$13,000	$30,500	per year	•
New Hampshire								
Franklin Pierce College (West Lebanon)	24	Nov	27	MS	$36,000	$36,000		•
New Jersey								
Univ of Medicine & Dent of New Jersey (Piscataway)	50	Aug	36	MS	$20,000	$27,000		•
New York								
Albany Medical College	40	Jan	28	MS	$24,567	$24,567	per year	•
Long Island Univ - Brooklyn Campus	42	Aug	24	BS	$28,609	$28,609	per year	•
Stony Brook Univ	44	Jul	24	MS	$15,000	$23,000		•
North Carolina								
Duke Univ Medical Center (Durham)	80	Aug	24	Cert, MHS	$32,195	$32,195	per year	• •
Pennsylvania								
Philadelphia Univ	50	Jul	25	Dipl, Cert, MS	$33,000	$33,000		• •
St Francis Univ (Loretto)	55	May	24	MPAS	$40,000	$40,000		•
Texas								
Baylor College of Medicine (Houston)	40	Jul	30	MS	$16,850	$16,850		• •
Texas Tech Univ Health Sciences Center (Midland)	60	May	27	MPAS	$15,000	$30,000		• •
Univ of North Texas Hlth Sci Ctr at Ft Worth (Fort Worth)	44	Jul	34	MPAS	$10,300	$26,300		•
Univ of Texas Medical Branch (Galveston)	90	Jun	26, 48	MPAS	$13,000	$30,000		• •
Virginia								
Eastern Virginia Medical School (Norfolk)	80	Jan	27	MPA	$66,668	$70,791	per year	•
Washington								
Univ of Washington (Seattle)	120	Jun	26	Cert, BCHS, MCHS	$68,300	$68,300		• •

*Data are shown only for programs that completed the 2011 AMA Survey of Health Professions Education Programs.

†Key to Offers: 1: Evening or weekend classes; 2: Non-English instruction; 3: Cultural competence instruction; 4: Distance education component.

PHYSICIAN ASSISTANT

Podiatry

Podiatrist

Career Description
The human foot is a complex structure. It contains 26 bones—plus muscles, nerves, ligaments, and blood vessels—and is designed for balance and mobility. The 52 bones in the feet make up about one fourth of all the bones in the human body. Podiatrists, also known as doctors of podiatric medicine (DPMs), specialize in diagnosing and treating disorders, diseases, and injuries of the foot, ankle, and lower leg.

Podiatrists treat ingrown toenails, bunions, heel spurs, corns, calluses, and arch problems, ankle and foot injuries, deformities, and infections, wound care, including ulcerations, and foot complaints associated with diseases such as diabetes. To treat these problems, podiatrists prescribe drugs, order physical therapy, set fractures, and perform surgery. They also fit and prescribe corrective inserts called custom foot orthoses, apply plaster casts and strappings to correct deformities, and prescribe diabetic and custom-made shoes.

To diagnose a foot problem, podiatrists order x-rays, other radiology studies including MRIs, CTs and ultrasound exams, and laboratory tests. The foot may be the first area to show signs of serious conditions such as arthritis, diabetes, and heart disease. For example, patients with diabetes are prone to foot ulcers and infections due to poor circulation. Podiatrists consult with and refer patients to other health practitioners for management of the underlying disease when they detect symptoms of these disorders.

Employment Characteristics
Most podiatrists have a solo practice, although more are forming group practices with other podiatrists or health practitioners (multi-specialty groups.). The majority of podiatrists have a general podiatric practice that includes surgery, podiatric biomechanics, sports medicine, pediatrics, dermatology, and wound care. Podiatrists also may focus their attention on one or more of these specific areas.

Podiatrists who are in private practice are responsible for running a small business. In addition to treating patients, DPMs may hire and manage employees, order supplies, and keep records, among other tasks. Many podiatrists educate the community on the benefits of foot care through speaking engagements and other publicity.

In addition to working in their own offices, podiatrists also may spend time visiting patients in nursing homes or performing surgery at hospitals or ambulatory surgical centers. Those with private practices set their own hours, but may choose to work evenings and weekends to accommodate their patients.

Opportunities are also available in academia and management. Podiatrists may advance to become professors at colleges of podiatric medicine, department chiefs in hospitals, or general health administrators. Podiatrists can also be commissioned officers in the Armed Forces and US Public Health Service or work in the Department of Veterans Affairs or in municipal health departments.

Salary
According to the 2008 American Podiatric Medical Association (APMA) podiatric practice survey of its members, the starting salary for podiatric medical physicians ranges from $85,000 to $105,000, the overall average is $150,000, and the upper-range salaries are between $200,000 to $250,000. Podiatrists in partnerships tended to earn higher net incomes than those in solo practice. Self-employed podiatrists must provide for their own health insurance and retirement.

Data from the US Bureau of Labor Statistics from May 2011 show that wages at the 10th percentile were $55,690, the 50th percentile (median) $119,250, and the 90th percentile equal to or greater than $168,390 (*www.bls.gov/oes/current/oes291081.htm*).

For more information, see *www.apma.org/careers* or *www.ama-assn.org/go/hpsalary*.

Employment Outlook
The BLS projects that employment of podiatrists will increase by 20% from 2010 to 2020, faster than the average for all occupations. The demand for the services of podiatrists will continue to grow, with more people turning to podiatrists for foot care because of the rising number of injuries sustained by a more active and increasingly older population, along with the increase in the incidence of diabetes and obesity. Additional job openings will result from podiatrists who retire from the occupation, particularly members of the baby-boom generation.

Medicare and most private health insurance programs cover acute medical and surgical foot and ankle services, as well as diagnostic x rays and leg braces. Details of such coverage vary among plans. However, routine foot care, including the removal of corns and calluses, ordinarily is not covered unless the patient has a systemic condition that has resulted in severe circulatory problems or areas of desensitization in the legs or feet. Like dental services, podiatric care is often discretionary and, therefore, more dependent on disposable income than some other medical services.

Opportunities will be better for board-certified podiatrists, because many managed care organizations require board certification. Opportunities for newly trained podiatrists will be better in group medical practices, clinics, and health networks than in traditional solo practices. Establishing a practice will be most difficult in the areas surrounding colleges of podiatric medicine, where podiatrists are concentrated.

Educational Programs
Award, Length. Graduates receive the degree of Doctor of Podiatric Medicine (DPM) after completing the four-year graduate-level program.

Prerequisites. Admission to a college of podiatric medicine requires completion of at least 90 semester hours of undergraduate study, an acceptable grade point average, and suitable scores on the Medical College Admission Test (some colleges also may accept other similar premedical examinations). All colleges require 8 semester hours each of biology, inorganic chemistry, organic chemistry, and physics, as well as 6 hours of English. The science courses should be those designed for premedical students. Potential podiatric medical students also are evaluated on the basis of extracurricular and community activities, personal interviews, and letters of recommendation. About 95 percent of podiatric students have at least a bachelor's degree. In general, those interested in the field should possess scientific aptitude, manual dexterity, interpersonal skills, and good business sense.

Curriculum. Colleges of podiatric medicine offer a core curriculum similar to that in other schools of medicine. During the first 2 years, students receive classroom instruction in basic sciences, including anatomy, chemistry, pathology, and pharmacology. Third- and fourth-year students have clinical clerkships in private practices, hospitals, and clinics. During these clerkships, they learn how to take general and podiatric histories, perform routine physical examinations, interpret tests and findings, make diagnoses, and perform therapeutic procedures.

Advanced Training. Nearly all graduates complete a three- to four-year hospital-based residency program after receiving a DPM degree. Residents receive advanced training in podiatric medicine and surgery and serve clinical rotations in anesthesiology, internal medicine, pathology, radiology, emergency medicine, and orthopedic and general surgery.

Licensure and Certification

All states and the District of Columbia require a license for the practice of podiatric medicine. Each state defines its own licensing requirements, although many states grant reciprocity to podiatrists who are licensed in another state. Applicants for licensure must be graduates of a college of podiatric medicine accredited by the Council on Podiatric Medical Education and must pass written and oral examinations. Some states permit applicants to substitute the examination of the National Board of Podiatric Medical Examiners, given in the second and fourth years of podiatric medical college, for part or all of the written state examination. Most states also require the completion of a postdoctoral residency program of at least two years and continuing education for license renewal.

Podiatrists can achieve certification in podiatric orthopedics and primary podiatric medicine and/or podiatric surgery. Certification means that the DPM meets higher standards than those required for licensure. Each certification board requires advanced training, the completion of written and oral examinations, and experience as a practicing podiatrist. Most managed care organizations prefer to contract with board-certified podiatrists.

Inquiries

Education, Careers, Resources
American Podiatric Medical Association
9312 Old Georgetown Road
Bethesda, MD 20814-1621
www.apma.org/careers

American Association of Colleges of Podiatric Medicine
15850 Crabbs Branch Way, Suite 320
Rockville, MD 20855-2622
800 922-9266
www.aacpm.org

Licensure
National Board of Podiatric Medical Examiners
PO Box 510
Bellefonte, PA 16823
www.nbpme.info

Accreditation and Approval
Council on Podiatric Medical Education (CPME)
9312 Old Georgetown Road
Bethesda, MD 20814-1621
301 581-9200
www.cpme.org

Note: Adapted in part from the Bureau of Labor Statistics, US Department of Labor, *Occupational Outlook Handbook*, Podiatrists, at *www.bls.gov/oco/ocos075.htm*.

Podiatrist

Arizona

Midwestern University - Glendale Campus
Podiatric Medicine Prgm
Arizona Podiatric Medicine Program
19555 N 59th Ave
Glendale, AZ 85308
www.midwestern.edu/azpod

California

Samuel Merritt University
Podiatric Medicine Prgm
California School of Podiatric Medicine
370 Hawthorne Ave
Oakland, CA 94609
www.samuelmerritt.edu

Western Univ of Health Sciences
Podiatric Medicine Prgm
College of Podiatric Medicine
309 East Second St
Pomona, CA 91766
www.westernu.edu

Florida

Barry University
Podiatric Medicine Prgm
11300 NE Second Ave
Miami Shores, FL 33161
www.barry.edu/gms/podiatry

Illinois

Rosalind Franklin University of Medicine
Podiatric Medicine Prgm
Dr William M Scholl College of Podiatric Medicine
3333 Green Bay Rd
North Chicago, IL 60064
www.rosalindfranklin.edu

Iowa

Des Moines University
Podiatric Medicine Prgm
College of Podiatric Medicine and Surgery
3200 Grand Ave
Des Moines, IA 50312
www.dmu.edu/cpms

New York

New York College of Podiatric Medicinie
Podiatric Medicine Prgm
1800 Park Ave
New York, NY 10035
www.nycpm.edu

Ohio

Ohio College of Podiatric Medicine
Podiatric Medicine Prgm
10515 Carnegie Ave
Cleveland, OH 44106
www.ocpm.edu

Pennsylvania

Temple University
Podiatric Medicine Prgm
School of Podiatric Medicine
Eighth at Race St
Philadelphia, PA 19107
podiatry.temple.edu

Psychologist

Career Description

Psychologists study the human mind and human behavior. Research psychologists investigate the physical, cognitive, emotional, or social aspects of human behavior. Psychologists in health service provider fields provide mental health care in hospitals, clinics, schools, or private settings. Psychologists employed in applied settings, such as business, industry, government, or nonprofits, provide training, conduct research, design systems, and act as advocates for psychology.

Like other social scientists, psychologists formulate hypotheses and collect data to test their validity. Research methods vary with the topic under study. Psychologists sometimes gather information through controlled laboratory experiments or by administering personality, performance, aptitude, or intelligence tests. Other methods include observation, interviews, questionnaires, clinical studies, and surveys.

Psychologists apply their knowledge to a wide range of endeavors, including health and human services, management, education, law, and sports. In addition to working in a variety of settings, psychologists usually specialize in one of a number of different areas.

Clinical psychologists—who constitute the largest specialty—work most often in counseling centers, independent or group practices, hospitals, or clinics. They help mentally and emotionally disturbed clients adjust to life and may assist medical and surgical patients in dealing with illnesses or injuries. Some clinical psychologists work in physical rehabilitation settings, treating patients with spinal cord injuries, chronic pain or illness, stroke, arthritis, and neurological conditions. Others help people deal with times of personal crisis, such as divorce or the death of a loved one.

Clinical psychologists often interview patients and give diagnostic tests. They may provide individual, family, or group psychotherapy and may design and implement behavior modification programs. Some clinical psychologists collaborate with physicians and other specialists to develop and implement treatment and intervention programs for patients. Other clinical psychologists work in universities and medical schools, where they train graduate students in the delivery of mental health and behavioral medicine services. Some administer community mental health programs.

Areas of specialization within clinical psychology include:
- *Health psychologists*, who promote good health through health maintenance counseling programs designed to help people achieve goals, such as stopping smoking or losing weight
- *Neuropsychologists*, who study the relation between the brain and behavior. They often work in stroke and head injury programs
- *Geropsychologists*, who deal with the special problems faced by the elderly

Often, clinical psychologists will consult with other medical personnel regarding the best treatment for patients, especially treatment that includes medication. Clinical psychologists generally are not permitted to prescribe medication to treat patients; only psychiatrists and other medical doctors may prescribe certain medications.

In addition to clinical psychologists, other types of psychologists include:
- Counseling psychologists
- School psychologists
- Industrial-organizational psychologists
- Developmental psychologists
- Social psychologists
- Experimental or research psychologists

Employment Characteristics

A psychologist's working conditions are determined by type of practice and place of employment. Clinical psychologists in private practice have their own offices and set their own hours. They often offer evening and weekend hours to accommodate their clients. Those employed in hospitals, nursing homes, and other health care facilities may work shifts that include evenings and weekends, while those who work in schools and clinics generally work regular hours.

Increasingly, many psychologists are working as part of a team, consulting with other psychologists and professionals. Many experience pressures because of deadlines, tight schedules, and overtime. Their routine may be interrupted frequently. Travel may be required in order to attend conferences or conduct research.

Salary

Data from the US Bureau of Labor Statistics for May 2009 show that wages for clinical, counseling, and school psychologists at the 10th percentile are $39,270, the 50th percentile (median) $66,040, and the 90th percentile $109,470 (*www.bls.gov/oes/current/ oes193031.htm*).

For more information, refer to *www.ama-assn.org/go/hpsalary*.

Employment Outlook

Employment of psychologists is expected to grow 12 percent from 2008 to 2018, about as fast as the average for all occupations. Employment will grow because of increased demand for psychological services in schools, hospitals, social service agencies, mental health centers, substance abuse treatment clinics, consulting firms, and private companies.

Educational Programs

Award, Length. A doctoral degree, either a PhD or a Doctor of Psychology (PsyD) degree, generally requires five to seven years of graduate study.

Prerequisites. Competition for admission to graduate psychology programs is keen. Some universities require applicants to have an undergraduate major in psychology. Others prefer only coursework in basic psychology with courses in the biological, physical, and social sciences and in statistics and mathematics.

Aspiring psychologists who are interested in direct patient care must be emotionally stable, mature, and able to deal effectively with people. Sensitivity, compassion, good communication skills, and the ability to lead and inspire others are particularly important qualities for persons wishing to do clinical work and counseling. Research psychologists should be able to do detailed work both independently and as part of a team. Patience and perseverance are vital qualities, because achieving results in the psychological treatment of patients or in research may take a long time.

Curriculum. The PhD degree culminates in a dissertation based on original research. Courses in quantitative research methods, which include the use of computer-based analysis, are an integral part of graduate study and are necessary to complete the dissertation. The PsyD may be based on practical work and examinations rather than a dissertation. In clinical or counseling psychology, the requirements for the doctoral degree include at least a 1-year internship.

Licensure, Certification, Registration

Psychologists in independent practice or those who offer any type of patient care—including clinical, counseling, and school psychologists—must meet certification or licensing requirements in all states and the District of Columbia. Licensing laws vary by state and type of position and require licensed or certified psychologists to limit their practice to areas in which they have developed professional competence through training and experience. Clinical and counseling psychologists usually require a doctorate in psychology, the completion of an approved internship, and one to two years of professional experience. In addition, all states require that applicants pass an examination. Most state licensing boards administer a standardized test, and many supplement that with additional oral or essay questions. Some states require continuing education for licensure renewal.

The American Board of Professional Psychology (ABPP) recognizes professional achievement by awarding specialty certification, primarily in clinical psychology, clinical neuropsychology, and counseling, forensic, industrial-organizational, and school psychology. Requirements for ABPP certification include a doctorate in psychology, postdoctoral training in one's specialty, 5 years of experience, professional endorsements, and a passing grade on an examination.

Inquiries

Education, Careers, Resources
American Psychological Association, Research Office and Education Directorate
750 1st Street NE
Washington, DC 20002-4242
www.apa.org/students
www.apa.org/ed

Licensure, Certification
Association of State and Provincial Psychology Boards
PO Box 3079
Peachtree City, GA 30269
www.asppb.org

American Board of Professional Psychology
300 Drayton Street, 3rd Floor
Savannah, GA 31401
www.abpp.org

Program Accreditation/Approval
(*Note:* Listed in this *Directory* are clinical psychology programs accredited by the following organization.)

American Psychological Association, Commission on Accreditation
Office of Program Consultation and Accreditation
750 First Street, NE
Washington, DC 20002-4242
(202) 336-5979
E-mail: *apaaccred@apa.org*
www.apa.org/education/grad/program-accreditation.aspx

Note: Adapted in part from the Bureau of Labor Statistics, U.S. Department of Labor, *Occupational Outlook Handbook,* Psychologists, on the Internet at *www.bls.gov/oco/ocos056.htm.*
www.apa.org/ed.accreditation/

Psychologist

Alabama

Auburn University
Psychology (PhD) Prgm
Department of Psychology
Auburn, AL 36849

University of Alabama - Birmingham
Psychology (PhD) Prgm
Medical Psychology Program
Birmingham, AL 35294

University of Alabama - Tuscaloosa
Psychology (PhD) Prgm
Department of Psychology
Tuscaloosa, AL 35487

Arizona

Argosy University - Phoenix
Psychology (PsyD) Prgm
Phoenix, AZ 85021

Arizona State University
Psychology (PhD) Prgm
Department of Psychology
Tempe, AZ 85287

University of Arizona
Psychology (PhD) Prgm
Department of Psychology
Tucson, AZ 85721

Arkansas

University of Arkansas for Medical Sciences
Psychology (PhD) Prgm
Department of Psychology
Fayetteville, AR 72701

British Columbia, Canada

Simon Fraser University
Psychology (PhD) Prgm
Burnaby, BC V5A 1S6

University of British Columbia
Psychology (PhD) Prgm
Department of Psychology
Vancouver, BC V6T 1Z4

University of Victoria
Psychology (PhD) Prgm
Victoria, BC V8W 3P5

California

Alliant International University - Los Angeles
Psychology (PhD) Prgm
Alhambra, CA 91803

Azusa Pacific University
Psychology (PsyD) Prgm
Department of Graduate Psychology
Azusa, CA 91702

The Wright Insitute
Psychology (PsyD) Prgm
Berkeley, CA 94704

University of California - Berkeley
Psychology (PhD) Prgm
Department of Psychology
Berkeley, CA 94720

Alliant International University - Fresno
Psychology (PsyD) Prgm
Fresno, CA 93727

PSYCHOLOGY

Alliant International University - Fresno
Psychology (PhD) Prgm
Department of Psychology
Fresno, CA 93727

Biola University
Psychology (PsyD) Prgm
Rosemead School of Psychology
La Mirada, CA 90639

Biola University
Psychology (PhD) Prgm
Rosemead School of Psychology
La Mirada, CA 90639

University of La Verne
Psychology (PhD) Prgm
Department of Psychology
La Verne, CA 91750

Loma Linda University
Psychology (PsyD) Prgm
Department of Psychology
Loma Linda, CA 92350

Loma Linda University
Psychology (PsyD) Prgm
Department of Psychology
Loma Linda, CA 92350

Alliant International University - Los Angeles
Psychology (PsyD) Prgm
Los Angeles, CA 91803

Pepperdine University
Psychology (PhD) Prgm
Department of Psychology
Los Angeles, CA 90045

University of California - Los Angeles
Psychology (PhD) Prgm
Department of Psychology
Los Angeles, CA 90095

University of Southern California
Psychology (PhD) Prgm
Department of Psychology
Los Angeles, CA 90089

Stanbridge College
Psychology (PsyD) Prgm
Orange, CA 92868

Pacific Graduate School of Psychology
Cosponsor: Stanford Univ Med Sch Consortium
Psychology (PsyD) Prgm
Palo Alto, CA 94303

Pacific Graduate School of Psychology
Psychology (PhD) Prgm
Palo Alto, CA 94303

Fuller Theological Seminary
Psychology (PhD) Prgm
Graduate School of Psychology
Pasadena, CA 91101

Fuller Theological Seminary
Psychology (PsyD) Prgm
Graduate School of Psychology
Pasadena, CA 91101

John F Kennedy University
Psychology (PsyD) Prgm
Pleasant Hill, CA 94523

Biola University - San Francisco
Psychology (PsyD) Prgm
Department of Clinical Psychology
Point Richmond, CA 94804

Western Univ of Health Sciences
Psychology (PsyD) Prgm
Department of Clinical Psychology
Point Richmond, CA 94804-3547

Alliant International University - San Diego
Psychology (PsyD) Prgm
San Diego, CA 92131

Alliant International University - San Diego
Psychology (PhD) Prgm
San Diego, CA 92131

San Diego State University
Psychology (PhD) Prgm
Joint doctoral program in clinical psychology
San Diego, CA 92120

Alliant International University - San Francisco Bay
Psychology (PsyD) Prgm
San Francisco, CA 94133

California Institute of Integral Studies
Psychology (PsyD) Prgm
San Francisco, CA 94103

Fielding Graduate University
Psychology (PhD) Prgm
Department of Psychology
Santa Barbara, CA 93105

Colorado

University of Colorado at Boulder
Psychology (PhD) Prgm
Department of Psychology
Boulder, CO 80309

American Sentinel University
Psychology (PsyD) Prgm
Graduate School of Professional Psychology
Denver, CO 80208

American Sentinel University
Psychology (PhD) Prgm
Department of Psychology
Denver, CO 80208

University of Colorado at Denver
Psychology (PsyD) Prgm
Graduate School of Professional Psychology
Denver, CO 80208

University of Colorado at Denver
Psychology (PhD) Prgm
Department of Psychology
Denver, CO 80208

Connecticut

University of Hartford
Psychology (PsyD) Prgm
Graduate Institute of Professional Psychology
Hartford, CT 06105

Yale University School of Medicine
Psychology (PhD) Prgm
Department of Psychology
New Haven, CT 06520

University of Connecticut
Psychology (PhD) Prgm
Department of Psychology
Storrs, CT 06269

Delaware

University of Delaware-Christiana Care Health
Psychology (PhD) Prgm
Department of Psychology
Newark, DE 19716

District of Columbia

American University
Psychology (PhD) Prgm
Department of Psychology
Washington, DC 20016

Catholic University of America
Psychology (PhD) Prgm
Department of Psychology
Washington, DC 20064

Gallaudet University
Psychology (PhD) Prgm
Department of Psychology
Washington, DC 20002

George Washington University
Psychology (PsyD) Prgm
Center for Professional Psychology
Washington, DC 20037

George Washington University
Psychology (PhD) Prgm
Department of Psychology
Washington, DC 20052

Howard University
Psychology (PhD) Prgm
Department of Psychology
Washington, DC 20059

Florida

University of Miami
Psychology (PhD) Prgm
Department of Psychology
Coral Gables, FL 33124

Nova Southeastern University
Psychology (PhD) Prgm
Department of Psychology
Fort Lauderdale, FL 33314

Nova Southeastern University
Psychology (PsyD) Prgm
Fort Lauderdale, FL 33314

University of Florida
Psychology (PhD) Prgm
Department of Clinical and Health Psychology
Gainesville, FL 32610

Florida Institute of Technology
Psychology (PsyD) Prgm
School of Psychology
Melbourne, FL 32901

Carlos Albizu University
Psychology (PsyD) Prgm
Miami, FL 33172

University of Central Florida
Psychology (PhD) Prgm
Department of Psychology
Orlando, FL 32816

Florida State University
Psychology (PhD) Prgm
Department of Psychology
Tallahassee, FL 32306

Argosy University - Tampa
Psychology (PsyD) Prgm
Tampa, FL 33614

University of South Florida
Psychology (PhD) Prgm
Department of Psychology
Tampa, FL 33620

Georgia

University of Georgia
Psychology (PhD) Prgm
Department of Psychology
Athens, GA 30602

Argosy University - Atlanta Campus
Psychology (PsyD) Prgm
Department of Psychology
Atlanta, GA 30328

Emory University
Psychology (PhD) Prgm
Department of Psychology
Atlanta, GA 30322

Georgia State University
Psychology (PhD) Prgm
Department of Psychology
Atlanta, GA 30303

Hawaii

Argosy University - Hawaii Campus
Psychology (PsyD) Prgm
Department of Psychology
Honolulu, HI 96813

University of Hawaii at Manoa
Psychology (PhD) Prgm
Department of Psychology
Honolulu, HI 96822

Idaho

Idaho State University
Psychology (PhD) Prgm
Department of Psychology
Pocatello, ID 83209

Illinois

Southern Illinois University Carbondale
Psychology (PhD) Prgm
Department of Psychology
Carbondale, IL 62901

Univ of Illinois at Urbana-Champaign
Psychology (PhD) Prgm
Department of Psychology
Champaign, IL 61820

Adler School of Professional Psychology
Psychology (PsyD) Prgm
Department of Psychology
Chicago, IL 60601

Argosy University - Chicago Campus
Psychology (PsyD) Prgm
School of Professional Psychology
Chicago, IL 60654

Chicago School of Professional Psychology
Psychology (PsyD) Prgm
Chicago, IL 60610

DePaul University
Psychology (PhD) Prgm
Department of Psychology
Chicago, IL 60614

Illinois Institute of Technology
Psychology (PhD) Prgm
Institute of Psychology
Chicago, IL 60616

Loyola University of Chicago
Psychology (PhD) Prgm
Department of Psychology
Chicago, IL 60626

Northwestern University Medical School - Chicago
Psychology (PhD) Prgm
Department of Psychiatry and Behavioral Sciences
Chicago, IL 60611

Roosevelt University
Psychology (PsyD) Prgm
School of Psychology
Chicago, IL 60605

University of Illinois at Chicago
Psychology (PhD) Prgm
Department of Psychology
Chicago, IL 60607

Northern Illinois University
Psychology (PhD) Prgm
Department of Psychology
DeKalb, IL 60115

Northwestern University - Evanston
Psychology (PhD) Prgm
Department of Psychology
Evanston, IL 60208

Rosalind Franklin University of Medicine
Psychology (PhD) Prgm
Department of Psychology
North Chicago, IL 60064

Argosy University - Schaumburg
Psychology (PsyD) Prgm
Schaumburg, IL 60173

Wheaton College
Psychology (PsyD) Prgm
Wheaton, IL 60187

Indiana

Indiana University - Bloomington
Psychology (PsyD) Prgm
Department of Psychological and Brain Sciences
Bloomington, IN 47405

Indiana Univ-Purdue Univ-Indianapolis
Psychology (PhD) Prgm
Department of Psychology
Indianapolis, IN 46202

University of Indianapolis
Psychology (PsyD) Prgm
School of Psychological Sciences
Indianapolis, IN 46227

Indiana State University
Psychology (PhD) Prgm
Department of Psychology
Terre Haute, IN 47809

Purdue University
Psychology (PhD) Prgm
Department of Psychological Sciences
West Lafayette, IN 47907

Iowa

University of Iowa
Psychology (PhD) Prgm
Department of Psychology
Iowa City, IA 52242

Kansas

University of Kansas
Psychology (PhD) Prgm
Lawrence, KS 66045

Kentucky

University of Kentucky
Psychology (PhD) Prgm
Department of Psychology
Lexington, KY 40506

University of Louisville
Psychology (PhD) Prgm
Department of Psychology and Brain Sciences
Louisville, KY 40292

Louisiana

Louisiana State University
Psychology (PhD) Prgm
Department of Psychology
Baton Rouge, LA 70803

Maine

University of Maine - Orono
Psychology (PsyD) Prgm
Department of Psychology
Orono, ME 04469

Manitoba, Canada

University of Manitoba
Psychology (PhD) Prgm
Department of Psychology
Winnipeg, MB R3T 2N2

Maryland

Loyola University Maryland
Psychology (PhD) Prgm
Department of Psychology
Baltimore, MD 21210

University of Maryland Baltimore County
Psychology (PhD) Prgm
Department of Psychology
Baltimore, MD 21250

Uniformed Svcs Univ of the Health Sciences
Psychology (PhD) Prgm
Bethesda, MD 20814

Univ of Maryland at College Park
Psychology (PsyD) Prgm
Department of Psychology
College Park, MD 20742

Massachusetts

University of Massachusetts - Amherst
Psychology (PhD) Prgm
Department of Psychology
Amherst, MA 01003

Boston University
Psychology (PhD) Prgm
Department of Psychology
Boston, MA 02215

Massachusetts Sch of Prof Psychology Inc
Psychology (PsyD) Prgm
Boston, MA 02132

Suffolk University
Psychology (PhD) Prgm
Department of Psychology
Boston, MA 02114

University of Massachusetts - Boston
Psychology (PsyD) Prgm
Department of Psychology
Boston, MA 02125

American Career Institute
Psychology (PhD) Prgm
Department of Psychology
Cambridge, MA 02128

Clark University
Psychology (PhD) Prgm
Frances L Hiatt School of Psychology
Worcester, MA 01610

Michigan

University of Michigan
Psychology (PhD) Prgm
Department of Psychology
Ann Arbor, MI 48109

University of Detroit Mercy
Psychology (PhD) Prgm
Department of Psychology
Detroit, MI 48221

Wayne State University
Psychology (PhD) Prgm
Department of Psychology
Detroit, MI 48202

Michigan State University
Psychology (PhD) Prgm
Department of Psychology
East Lansing, MI 48824

Western Michigan University
Psychology (PhD) Prgm
Department of Psychology
Kalamazoo, MI 49008

Central Michigan University
Psychology (PhD) Prgm
Department of Psychology
Mount Pleasant, MI 48859

Eastern Michigan University
Psychology (PhD) Prgm
Department of Psychology
Ypsilanti, MI 48197

Minnesota

Argosy University Twin Cities Campus
Psychology (PsyD) Prgm
Eagan, MN 55121

University of Minnesota
Psychology (PhD) Prgm
Department of Psychology
Minneapolis, MN 55455

Mississippi

University of Southern Mississippi
Psychology (PhD) Prgm
Department of Psychology
Hattiesburg, MS 39406

Jackson State University
Psychology (PsyD) Prgm
Department of Psychology
Jackson, MS 39217

University of Mississippi
Psychology (PhD) Prgm
Department of Psychology
University, MS 38677

Missouri

University of Missouri
Psychology (PhD) Prgm
Department of Psychological Sciences
Columbia, MO 65211

University of Missouri - Kansas City
Psychology (PhD) Prgm
Department of Psychology
Kansas City, MO 64110

Forest Institute of Professional Psychology
Psychology (PsyD) Prgm
Springfield, MO 65807

Saint Louis University
Psychology (PhD) Prgm
St Louis, MO 63103

University of Missouri - St Louis
Psychology (PhD) Prgm
Department of Psychology
St Louis, MO 63121

Washington University
Psychology (PhD) Prgm
Department of Psychology
St Louis, MO 63130

Montana

University of Montana
Psychology (PhD) Prgm
Department of Psychology
Missoula, MT 59812

Nebraska

University of Nebraska - Lincoln
Psychology (PhD) Prgm
Department of Psychology
Lincoln, NE 68588

Nevada

University of Nevada - Las Vegas
Psychology (PhD) Prgm
Department of Psychology
Las Vegas, NV 89154

University of Nevada - Reno
Psychology (PhD) Prgm
Department of Psychology
Reno, NV 89557

New Brunswick, Canada

University of New Brunswick
Psychology (PhD) Prgm
Fredericton, NB E3B 6E4

New Hampshire

Antioch University New England
Psychology (PsyD) Prgm
Department of Clinical Psychology
Keene, NH 03431

New Jersey

Rutgers University
Psychology (PhD) Prgm
Department of Psychology
Piscataway, NJ 08854

Rutgers University - SUNJ
Psychology (PsyD) Prgm
Piscataway, NJ 08854

Fairleigh Dickinson University
Psychology (PhD) Prgm
School of Psychology
Teaneck-Hackensack Campus
Teaneck, NJ 07666

New Mexico

University of New Mexico
Psychology (PhD) Prgm
Department of Psychology
Albuquerque, NM 87131

New York

University at Albany/State U of New York
Psychology (PhD) Prgm
Department of Psychology
Albany, NY 12222

Binghamton University /SUNY
Psychology (PhD) Prgm
Department of Psychology
Binghamton, NY 13902

Fordham University
Psychology (PhD) Prgm
Department of Psychology
Bronx, NY 10458

Yeshiva University
Psychology (PhD) Prgm
Jack and Pearl Resnick Campus
Bronx, NY 10461

Yeshiva University
Psychology (PsyD) Prgm
Albert Einstein College of Medicine Campus
Bronx, NY 10461

Long Island University - Brooklyn Campus
Psychology (PsyD) Prgm
Department of Psychology
Brooklyn, NY 11201

Long Island University - C W Post Campus
Psychology (PsyD) Prgm
Brookville, NY 11548

University at Buffalo - SUNY
Psychology (PhD) Prgm
Department of Psychology
Buffalo, NY 14260

Adelphi University
Psychology (PhD) Prgm
Demar Institute of Advanced Psychological Studies
Garden City, NY 11530

St John's University
Psychology (PhD) Prgm
Department of Psychology
Jamaica, NY 11439

City University of New York, The City College
Psychology (PhD) Prgm
Department of Psychology
New York, NY 10038

Columbia University Teachers College
Psychology (PhD) Prgm
Department of Clinical Psychology
New York, NY 10027

New York University
Psychology (PhD) Prgm
Department of Psychology
New York, NY 10003

The New School
Psychology (PhD) Prgm
New York, NY 10003

University of Rochester
Psychology (PhD) Prgm
Department of Clinical and Social Sciences in
   Psychology
Rochester, NY 14627

State University at Stony Brook
Psychology (PhD) Prgm
Stony Brook, NY 11794

Syracuse University
Psychology (PhD) Prgm
Department of Psychology
Syracuse, NY 13244

North Carolina

University of North Carolina - Chapel Hill
Psychology (PhD) Prgm
Department of Psychology
Chapel Hill, NC 27599

Duke University
Psychology (PhD) Prgm
Department of Psychology and Neuroscience
Durham, NC 27708

University of North Carolina - Greensboro
Psychology (PhD) Prgm
Department of Psychology
Greensboro, NC 27402

North Dakota

University of North Dakota
Psychology (PhD) Prgm
Department of Psychology
Grand Forks, ND 58202

Ohio

Ohio University
Psychology (PhD) Prgm
Department of Psychology
Athens, OH 45701

Bowling Green State University
Psychology (PhD) Prgm
Department of Psychology
Bowling Green, OH 43403

University of Cincinnati
Psychology (PhD) Prgm
Department of Psychology
Cincinnati, OH 45221

Xavier University
Psychology (PsyD) Prgm
Department of Psychology
Cincinnati, OH 45207

Case Western Reserve University
Psychology (PhD) Prgm
Department of Psychology
Cleveland, OH 44106

The Ohio State University
Psychology (PhD) Prgm
Department of Psychology
Columbus, OH 43210

Wright State University
Psychology (PsyD) Prgm
School of Professional Psychology
Dayton, OH 45435

Kent State University
Psychology (PhD) Prgm
Department of Psychology
Kent, OH 44242

Miami University
Psychology (PhD) Prgm
Department of Psychology
Oxford, OH 45056

University of Toledo
Psychology (PhD) Prgm
Department of Psychology
Toledo, OH 43606

Oklahoma

Oklahoma State University
Psychology (PhD) Prgm
Department of Psychology
Stillwater, OK 74078

University of Tulsa
Psychology (PhD) Prgm
Department of Psychology
Tulsa, OK 74104

Ontario, Canada

University of Ottawa
Psychology (PhD) Prgm
School of Psychology
Ottawa, ON K1N 6N5

York University
Psychology (PhD) Prgm
Clinical Program-Adult Emphasis
Toronto, ON M3J 1P3

University of Waterloo
Psychology (PhD) Prgm
Waterloo, ON N2L 3G1

Oregon

University of Oregon
Psychology (PhD) Prgm
Department of Psychology
Eugene, OR 97403

Pacific University
Psychology (PsyD) Prgm
School of Professional Psychology
Forest Grove, OR 97116

George Fox University
Psychology (PsyD) Prgm
Graduate Department of Clinical Psychology
Newberg, OR 97132

Pennsylvania

Widener University
Psychology (PsyD) Prgm
School of Human Service Professions
Chester, PA 19013

Immaculata University
Psychology (PsyD) Prgm
Graduate Division
Immaculata, PA 19345

Indiana University of Pennsylvania
Psychology (PsyD) Prgm
Department of Psychology
Indiana, PA 15705

Chestnut Hill College
Psychology (PsyD) Prgm
Department of Professional Psychology
Philadelphia, PA 19118

Drexel University College of Medicine
Psychology (PhD) Prgm
Department of Psychology
Philadelphia, PA 19102

La Salle University
Psychology (PhD) Prgm
Department of Psychology
Philadelphia, PA 19141

Philadelphia College of Osteopathic Medicine
Psychology (PhD) Prgm
Department of Psychology
Philadelphia, PA 19131

Temple University
Psychology (PhD) Prgm
Department of Psychology
Philadelphia, PA 19122

University of Pennsylvania
Psychology (PhD) Prgm
Philadelphia, PA 19104

Duquesne University
Psychology (PhD) Prgm
Department of Psychology
Pittsburgh, PA 15282

University of Pittsburgh
Psychology (PhD) Prgm
Department of Psychology
Pittsburgh, PA 15260

Marywood University
Psychology (PhD) Prgm
Department of Psychology and Counseling
Scranton, PA 18509

Penn State University - University Park
Psychology (PhD) Prgm
Department of Psychology
University Park, PA 16802

Puerto Rico

Ponce School of Medicine
Psychology (PsyD) Prgm
Clinical Psychology Doctoral Program
Ponce, PR 00732

Carlos Albizu University
Psychology (PsyD) Prgm
San Juan, PR 00902

Carlos Albizu University
Psychology (PhD) Prgm
San Juan, PR 00902

Quebec, Canada

Concordia University
Psychology (PhD) Prgm
Department of Psychology
Montreal, QC H4B 1R6

McGill University
Psychology (PhD) Prgm
Montreal, QC H3A 1B1

Rhode Island

University of Rhode Island
Psychology (PhD) Prgm
Department of Psychology
Kingston, RI 02881

Saskatchewan, Canada

University of Saskatchewan
Psychology (PhD) Prgm
Department of Psychology
Saskatoon, SK S7N 5A5

South Carolina

University of South Carolina
Psychology (PhD) Prgm
Department of Psychology
Columbia, SC 29208

PSYCHOLOGY

South Dakota

University of South Dakota
Psychology (PhD) Prgm
Department of Psychology
Vermillion, SD 57069

Tennessee

University of Tennessee - Knoxville
Psychology (PhD) Prgm
Department of Psychology
Knoxville, TN 37996

University of Memphis
Psychology (PhD) Prgm
Department of Psychology
Memphis, TN 38152

Vanderbilt University
Psychology (PhD) Prgm
Department of Psychology
Nashville, TN 37203

Texas

University of Texas at Austin
Psychology (PhD) Prgm
Department of Psychology
Austin, TX 78712

Texas A&M University
Psychology (PhD) Prgm
Department of Psychology
College Station, TX 77843

Univ of Texas Southwestern Med Ctr
Psychology (PhD) Prgm
Division of Psychology
Dallas, TX 75390

University of North Texas
Psychology (PhD) Prgm
Department of Psychology
Denton, TX 76203

University of North Texas
Cosponsor: North Texas Health Sciences Center
(Consortium)
Psychology (PhD) Prgm
Denton, TX 76203

University of Houston
Psychology (PsyD) Prgm
Department of Psychology
Houston, TX 77204

Sam Houston State University
Psychology (PhD) Prgm
Department of Psychology and Philosophy
Huntsville, TX 77341

Texas Tech University
Psychology (PhD) Prgm
Department of Psychology
Lubbock, TX 79409

Baylor University - Waco
Psychology (PsyD) Prgm
Department of Psychology
Waco, TX 76798

Utah

Brigham Young University - Provo
Psychology (PhD) Prgm
Department of Psychology
Provo, UT 84602

University of Utah
Psychology (PhD) Prgm
Department of Psychology
Salt Lake City, UT 84112

Vermont

University of Vermont
Psychology (PhD) Prgm
Department of Psychology
Burlington, VT 05405

Virginia

Argosy University - Washington
Psychology (PsyD) Prgm
Arlington, VA 22209

Virginia Polytechnic Inst & State Univ
Psychology (PhD) Prgm
Department of Psychology
Blacksburg, VA 24061

University of Virginia
Psychology (PsyD) Prgm
Department of Psychology
Charlottesville, VA 22904

University of Virginia
Psychology (PhD) Prgm
Dept of Human Services
Curry School of Education
Charlottesville, VA 22904

George Mason University
Psychology (PhD) Prgm
Department of Psychology
Fairfax, VA 22030

Regent University
Psychology (PsyD) Prgm
School of Psychology and Counseling
Virginia Beach, VA 23464

Virginia Consortium Program in Clinical Psych
Psychology (PsyD) Prgm
Virginia Beach, VA 23453

Washington

Washington State University
Psychology (PhD) Prgm
Department of Psychology
Pullman, WA 99164

Seattle Pacific University
Psychology (PhD) Prgm
Department of Graduate Psychology
Seattle, WA 98119

University of Washington
Psychology (PhD) Prgm
Department of Psychology
Seattle, WA 98195

West Virginia

Marshall University
Psychology (PhD) Prgm
Department of Psychology
Huntington, WV 25755

West Virginia University
Psychology (PhD) Prgm
Department of Psychology
Morgantown, WV 26506

Wisconsin

University of Wisconsin - Madison
Psychology (PhD) Prgm
Department of Psychology
Madison, WI 53706

Marquette University
Psychology (PhD) Prgm
Department of Psychology
Milwaukee, WI 53201

University of Wisconsin - Milwaukee
Psychology (PhD) Prgm
Department of Psychology
Milwaukee, WI 53201

Wyoming

University of Wyoming
Psychology (PhD) Prgm
Department of Psychology
Laramie, WY 82071

Therapy and Rehabilitation

Includes:
- Athletic trainer
- Occupational therapist
- Occupational therapy assistant
- Physical therapist
- Physical therapist assistant
- Recreational therapist

Athletic Trainer

Athletic training is practiced by athletic trainers (ATs), health care professionals who collaborate with physicians to optimize activity and participation of patients and clients. Athletic training encompasses the prevention, diagnosis, and intervention of emergency, acute, and chronic medical conditions involving impairment, functional limitations, and disabilities.

History

Work on establishing standards for athletic training educational programs was initiated in 1959 by the National Athletic Trainers' Association (NATA), with the first two programs approved in 1969. By 1979, there were 23 undergraduate programs and two graduate programs approved by NATA. By 1997, NATA had approved 87 entry-level and 13 graduate athletic training educational programs.

The Board of Certification, Inc. (BOC) was incorporated in 1989 from the NATA to provide a certification program for entry-level Athletic Trainers (ATs). The BOC establishes and regularly reviews both the standards for the practice of athletic training and the continuing education requirements for BOC Certified ATs. The BOC has the only accredited certification program for ATs in the US. In 1997, the BOC office was moved from Raleigh, North Carolina to Omaha, Nebraska.

In 1989, NATA applied to the AMA Council on Medical Education (CME) for recognition of athletic training as an allied health occupation; recognition was granted in 1990. Also in 1990, an initial meeting was conducted to develop the Standards (Essentials) for accreditation of educational programs for athletic trainers; standards were subsequently adopted in 1991.

Following the separation of the AMA from the Committee on Allied Health Education and Accreditation (CAHEA), the Commission on Accreditation of Allied Health Education Programs (CAAHEP) was formed, with the Joint Review Committee for Athletic Training functioning as a Commission on Accreditation of that group. On July 1, 2006, the JRC-AT separated from CAAHEP and became the independent accreditor CAATE (Commission on Accreditation of Athletic Training Education). At this time, all CAAHEP-accredited athletic training education programs became CAATE-accredited.

Career Description

Past role delineation studies/practice analyses have concluded that the role of an athletic trainer includes, but is not limited to:
- Injury/illness prevention and wellness protection, which includes:

- Minimize risk of injury and illness of individuals and groups impacted by or involved in a specific activity through awareness, education, and intervention.
- Interpret individual and group pre-participation and other relevant screening information (e.g., verbal, observed, written) in accordance with accepted and applicable guidelines to minimize the risk of injury and illness.
- Identify and educate individual(s) and groups through appropriate communication methods (e.g., verbal, written) about the appropriate use of personal protective equipment (e.g., clothing, shoes, protective gear, and braces) by following accepted procedures and guidelines.
- Maintain physical activity, clinical treatment, and rehabilitation areas by complying with regulatory standards to minimize the risk of injury and illness.
- Monitor environmental conditions (e.g., weather, surfaces, client work-setting) using appropriate methods and guidelines to facilitate individual and group safety.
- Maintain or improve physical conditioning for the individual or group by designing and implementing programs (e.g., strength, flexibility, CV fitness) to minimize the risk of injury and illness.
- Promote healthy lifestyle behaviors using appropriate education and communication strategies to enhance wellness and minimize the risk of injury and illness.

Clinical evaluation and diagnosis, which includes:
- Obtain an individual's history through observation, interview, and/or review of relevant records to assess injury, illness, or health-related condition.
- Utilize appropriate visual and palpation techniques to determine the type and extent of the injury, illness, or health-related condition
- Utilize appropriate tests (e.g., ROM, special tests, neurological tests) to determine the type and extent of the injury, illness, or health-related condition.
- Formulate a clinical diagnosis by interpreting the signs, symptoms, and predisposing factors of the injury, illness, or health-related condition to determine the appropriate course of action.
- Educate the appropriate individual(s) about the clinical evaluation by communicating information about the injury, illness, or health-related condition to encourage compliance with recommended care.

Immediate and Emergency care, which includes:
- Coordinate care of individual(s) through appropriate communication (e.g., verbal, written, demonstrative) of assessment findings to pertinent individual(s).

- Apply appropriate immediate and emergency care procedures to prevent the exacerbation of health-related conditions to reduce the risk factors for morbidity and mortality.
- Implement appropriate referral strategies, while stabilizing and/or preventing exacerbation of the condition(s), to facilitate the timely transfer of care for health-related conditions beyond the scope of practice of the Athletic Trainer.
- Demonstrate how to implement and direct immediate care strategies (e.g., first aid, Emergency Action Plan) using established communication and administrative practices to provide effective care.

Treatment, and rehabilitation, which includes:
- Administer therapeutic and conditioning exercise(s) using appropriate techniques and procedures to aid recovery and restoration of function.
- Administer therapeutic modalities (e.g., electromagnetic, manual, mechanical) using appropriate techniques and procedures based on the individual's phase of recovery to restore functioning.
- Apply braces, splints, or other assistive devices according to appropriate practices in order to facilitate injury protection to achieve optimal functioning for the individual.
- Administer treatment for injury, illness, and/or health-related conditions using appropriate methods to facilitate injury protection, recovery, and/or optimal functioning for individual(s).
- Reassess the status of injuries, illnesses, and/or health-related conditions using appropriate techniques and documentation strategies to determine appropriate treatment, rehabilitation, and/or reconditioning and to evaluate readiness to return to a desired level of activity.
- Provide guidance and/or referral to specialist for individual(s) and groups through appropriate communication strategies (e.g., oral and education materials) to restore an individual(s) optimal functioning.

Organization and professional health and well-being, which includes:
- Apply basic internal business functions (e.g., business planning, financial operations, staffing) to support individual and organizational growth and development.
- Apply basic external business functions (e.g., marketing and public relations) to support organizational sustainability, growth, and development.
- Maintain records and documentation that comply with organizational, association, and regulatory standards to provide quality of care and to enable internal surveillance for program validation and evidence-based interventions.
- Demonstrate appropriate planning for coordination of resources (e.g., personnel, equipment, liability, scope of service) in event medical management and emergency action plans.
- Demonstrate an understanding of statutory and regulatory provisions and professional standards of the practice of Athletic Training in order to provide for the safety and welfare of individual(s) and groups
- Develop a support/referral process for interventions to address unhealthy lifestyle behaviors.

Source: *http://www.bocatc.org/images/stories/resources/ rdpa6_content_outline.pdf*

Employment Characteristics

Athletic trainers typically provide their services in one or more of the following settings: secondary schools, colleges and universities, professional athletic organizations, physician offices, hospital-based clinics, private sports

medicine, rehabilitation and therapy clinics, industrial/occupational commercial facilities, military, and performing arts.

Salary

Entry-level salaries in 2008 averaged $35,000. The average overall salary is $45,000, with the upper ranges from $55,000 to $85,000.

Data from the US Bureau of Labor Statistics (*www.bls.gov/oes/current/oes299091.htm*) from May 2009 show that wages at the 10th percentile are $26,170, the 50th percentile (median) at $42,400, and the 90th percentile at $65,970.

For more information, go to *www.ama-assn.org/go/hpsalary*.

Employment Outlook

Employment of athletic trainers is projected by the BLS to grow 30% from 2010 to 2020, much faster than the average for all occupations, because of their role in preventing injuries and reducing healthcare costs. Job growth will be concentrated in the healthcare industry, including hospitals and offices of health practitioners.

Educational Programs

Length. Baccalaureate degree programs require 4 years of study. Postbaccalaureate programs are generally 2 years.

Prerequisites. Applicants for the 4-year baccalaureate degree programs must have a high school diploma or equivalent and meet institutional entrance requirements. Applicants for postbaccalaureate programs should have a baccalaureate degree that includes appropriate course work and clinical experience, as specified by the institution.

Curriculum. The professional curriculum includes formal instruction in:
- Risk management and injury/illness prevention
- Pathology of injury/illness
- Clinical examination and diagnosis
- Acute care of injuries and illnesses
- General medical conditions and disabilities
- Therapeutic modalities
- Therapeutic exercise
- Conditioning and rehabilitative exercise and therapy
- Health care administration
- Psychosocial intervention and referral
- Medical ethics and legal issues
- Pharmacology
- Professional responsibilities

The didactic curriculum is augmented by a series of structured laboratory and clinical experiences.

Licensure, Registration, Certification

Almost all states require that athletic trainers hold the ATC® (Athletic Trainer, Certified) credential, which is issued by the Board of Certification, Inc. (BOC). The ATC credential is supported by three pillars: the BOC certification examination, BOC Standards of Practice and Disciplinary Process, and continuing competence requirements. The computer-based examination verifies that the knowledge, skills, and abilities required for competent performance as an athletic trainer have been met.

At the time of publication, 48 states have some form of athletic training regulation, of which 47 states require the BOC examination in order to obtain regulation. It is important to recognize, however, that passing the BOC examination is only a precursor to athletic training practice. Compliance with state regulatory requirements is mandatory and the only avenue to legal athletic training practice. For specific details regarding state regulation, contact the state regulatory agency.

Inquiries

Careers
National Athletic Trainers' Association, Inc
2952 Stemmons Freeway, Suite 200
Dallas, TX 75247
214 637-6282
800 TRY-NATA
214 637-2206 Fax
www.nata.org

Certification
Board of Certification, Inc (BOC)
BOC Administrative Offices
1415 Haney Street, Suite 200
Omaha, NE 68102
402 559-0091
402 561-0598 Fax
www.bocatc.org

Program Accreditation
Commission on Accreditation of Athletic Training Education (CAATE)
2201 Double Creek Drive, Suite 5006
Round Rock, TX 78664
512 733-9700
512 733-9701 Fax
E-mail: *sheila@caate.net or caateinfo@caate.net*
www.caate.net

Note: Adapted in part from the Bureau of Labor Statistics, US Department of Labor, *Occupational Outlook Handbook*, Athletic Trainers, at *www.bls.gov/oco/ocos294.htm*.

Athletic Trainer

Alabama

Samford University
Athletic Training Prgm
800 Lakeshore Dr
PO Box 292448
Birmingham, AL 35229
www.samford.edu

University of West Alabama
Athletic Training Prgm
Station 14
Livingston, AL 35470
http://at.uwa.edu

University of Mobile
Athletic Training Prgm
5735 College Pkwy
Mobile, AL 36663-0220
www.umobile.edu

Huntingdon College
Athletic Training Prgm
1500 E Fairview Ave
Montgomery, AL 36106

Troy University
Athletic Training Prgm
3212 Veterans Stadium Dr, 2nd Fl
Dept of Athletic Training Education
Troy, AL 36082

University of Alabama - Tuscaloosa
Athletic Training Prgm
Dept of Health Science
Box 870311
Tuscaloosa, AL 35487-0311
www.ches.ua.edu/atep

Arizona

Northern Arizona University
Athletic Training Prgm
PO Box 15094
Flagstaff, AZ 86011-5094
www.nau.edu/hp/at

Grand Canyon University
Athletic Training Prgm
3300 W Camelback Rd
Phoenix, AZ 85017
www.gcu.edu

Arkansas

Henderson State University
Athletic Training Prgm
HSU Box 7552
Arkadelphia, AR 71999-0001
www.hsu.edu/atep

Ouachita Baptist University
Athletic Training Prgm
Box 3700
Arkadelphia, AR 71998
www.obu.edu/atep

University of Central Arkansas
Athletic Training Prgm
Prince Center 133E
201 Donaghey Ave
Conway, AR 72035-0001
www.uca.edu/kped/athletictraining/

University of Arkansas
Athletic Training Prgm
HPER 308h
Fayetteville, AR 72701
www.uark.edu

Southern Arkansas University
Athletic Training Prgm
100 E University
PO Box 9299
Magnolia, AR 71754

Harding University
Athletic Training Prgm
HU Box 12281
Searcy, AR 72148
www.harding.edu

Arkansas State University
Athletic Training Prgm
PO Box 240
State University, AR 72467
www.clt.astate.edu/hpess/

California

Azusa Pacific University
Athletic Training Prgm
Dept of Exercise and Sport Science
701 E Foothill Blvd
Azusa, CA 91702
www.apu.edu/bas/exercisesport/atep/
Prgm Dir: Christopher Schmidt, PhD ATC
Tel: 626 815-6000   *Fax:* 626 815-5084
E-mail: cschmidt@apu.edu
Notes: The program, which incorporates a Christian perspective, equips students with a quality education to become lifelong learners and uses current research and scholarly instruction to prepare entry-level certified athletic trainers.

Vanguard University
Athletic Training Prgm
55 Fair Dr
Costa Mesa, CA 92626
www.vanguard.edu

California State University - Fresno
Athletic Training Prgm
5275 N Campus Dr (M/S SG28
Fresno, CA 93740-8018
www.csufresno.edu/kines

California State University - Fullerton
Athletic Training Prgm
PO Box 6870
800 North State College Blvd
Fullerton, CA 92834-6870
http://hdcs.fullerton.edu/at/
Prgm Dir: Robert Kersey, PhD ATC CSCS
Tel: 714 278-3430   *Fax:* 714 278-5317
E-mail: rkersey@fullerton.edu

Concordia University - Irvine
Athletic Training Prgm
1530 Concordia West
Irvine, CA 92612
www.cui.edu

University of La Verne
Athletic Training Prgm
1950 Third St
La Verne, CA 91750
www.ulv.edu/athletictraining

California State University - Long Beach
Athletic Training Prgm
Department of Kinesiology
1250 Bellflower Blvd
Long Beach, CA 90840

Loyola Marymount University
Athletic Training Prgm
One LMU Drive; North Hall 205
Department of Natural Science
Los Angeles, CA 90045
www.lmu.edu

California State University - Northridge
Athletic Training Prgm
18111 Nordhoff St
Department of Kinesiology
Northridge, CA 91330-8287
www.csun.edu

Chapman University
Athletic Training Prgm
One University Dr
Orange, CA 92866
www.chapman.edu/educ/atep

California Baptist University
Athletic Training Prgm
8432 Magnolia Ave
Department of Kinesiology
Riverside, CA 92504
www.calbaptist.edu

California State University - Sacramento
Athletic Training Prgm
CSUS 6000 J St
Sacramento, CA 95819
www.hhs.csus.edu/KHS/AthleticTraining

Point Loma Nazarene University
Athletic Training Prgm
3900 Lomaland Dr
San Diego, CA 92106

San Diego State University
Athletic Training Prgm
5500 Campanile Dr
Exercise and Nutrition Science Department
San Diego, CA 92182-7251

San Jose State University
Athletic Training Prgm
One Washington Square
Department of Kinesiology
San Jose, CA 95192-0054
www.sjsu.edu/kinesiology
Prgm Dir: KyungMo Han, PhD ATC CSCS
Tel: 408 924-3041   *Fax:* 408 924-3053
E-mail: kyungmo.han@sjsu.edu

University of the Pacific
Athletic Training Prgm
Dept of Sport Sciences
3601 Pacific Ave
Stockton, CA 95211
www.pacific.edu/Academics/Schools-and-Colleges/
    College-of-the-Pacific/Academics/
Prgm Dir: Jolene Baker, EdD ATC
Tel: 209 946-3182   *Fax:* 209 946-3225
E-mail: jbaker@pacific.edu

Colorado

Metropolitan State College of Denver
Athletic Training Prgm
Campus Box 25
PO Box 173362
Denver, CO 80217-3362

Fort Lewis College
Athletic Training Prgm
1000 Rim Dr
Durango, CO 81301-3999

Colorado Mesa University
Athletic Training Prgm
1100 North Ave
Grand Junction, CO 81501
www.mesastate.edu

University of Northern Colorado
Athletic Training Prgm
Sch of Kinesiology and Phys Ed
Butler-Hancock 124
Greeley, CO 80639

Colorado State University - Pueblo
Athletic Training Prgm
2200 Bonforte Blvd
Pueblo, CO 81001
www.colostate-pueblo.edu

Connecticut

Sacred Heart University
Athletic Training Prgm
5151 Park Ave
Fairfield, CT 06432
www.sacredheart.edu

Quinnipiac University
Athletic Training Prgm
275 Mount Carmel Ave
Hamden, CT 06518
www.quinnipiac.edu

Central Connecticut State University
Athletic Training Prgm
1615 Stanley St
New Britain, CT 06050-4010
www.ccsu.edu

Southern Connecticut State University
Athletic Training Prgm
Pelz Gymnasium
501 Crescent St
New Haven, CT 06515
www.southernct.edu/athletic_training/
Prgm Dir: Gary Morin, PhD ATC LAT
Tel: 203 392-6089   *Fax:* 203 392-6093
E-mail: moring1@southernct.edu

University of Connecticut
Athletic Training Prgm
Dept of Kinesiology
2095 Hillside Rd, U-1110
Storrs, CT 06269-1110
www.uconn.edu

Delaware

University of Delaware-Christiana Care Health
Athletic Training Prgm
Human Performance Laboratory, Fred Rust Ice Arena
541 S College Ave
Newark, DE 19716
www.udel.edu/HNES/AT/Site/

District of Columbia

George Washington University
Athletic Training Prgm
Department of Exercise Science
817 23rd St NW
Washington, DC 20052
www.gwumc.edu/exercise/html/athletic

Florida

University of Miami
Athletic Training Prgm
PO Box 248065
Coral Gables, FL 33124
www.education.miami.edu/Program/
    Programs.asp?Program_ID=78

Nova Southeastern University
Athletic Training Prgm
3301 College Ave
Fort Lauderdale, FL 33314
www.undergrad.nova.edu/divisions/mst/athletictraining/

Florida Gulf Coast University
Athletic Training Prgm
10501 FGCU Blvd South
Fort Myers, FL 33965

University of Florida
Athletic Training Prgm
Dept of Applied Physiology and Kinesiology
160 FL Gym, Box 118205
Gainesville, FL 32611-8205
www.hhp.ufl.edu/apk/undergrad/2006atweb/
    athletictraining.htm

University of North Florida
Athletic Training Prgm
1 UNF Drive
Brooks College of Health
Jacksonville, FL 32224-2673
www.unf.edu/brooks/athletic-physical/at.html

Florida Southern College
Athletic Training Prgm
111 Lake Hollingsworth Dr
Lakeland, FL 33801-5698
www.flsouthern.edu

Barry University
Athletic Training Prgm
11300 NE 2nd Ave
Miami Shores, FL 33161-6695
www.barry.edu/hpls

University of Central Florida
Athletic Training Prgm
4000 Central Florida Blvd, HPA II Room 121
Orlando, FL 32816-2205
www.cohpa.ucf.edu/Academics/Degrees.htm

University of West Florida
Athletic Training Prgm
11000 University Pkwy
Pensacola, FL 32524
www.uwf.edu

Florida State University
Athletic Training Prgm
422 Sandels Bldg, NFES
Tallahassee, FL 320306
www.fsu.edu

University of South Florida
Athletic Training Prgm
13220 USF Laurel Drive
MDC106
Tampa, FL 33612
www.usfathletictraining.com
Prgm Dir: Micki Cuppett, EdD ATC
Tel: 813 974-7831   *Fax:* 813 396-9195
E-mail: mcuppett@health.usf.edu

University of Tampa
Athletic Training Prgm
401 W Kennedy Blvd, Box 30F
Tampa, FL 33606
www.ut.edu
Prgm Dir: J C Andersen, PhD ATC PT SCS
Tel: 813 257-3162   *Fax:* 813 258-7482
E-mail: jcandersen@ut.edu

Palm Beach Atlantic University
Athletic Training Prgm
PO Box 24708
West Palm Beach, FL 33416-4708
www.pba.edu

Georgia

University of Georgia
Athletic Training Prgm
Ramsey Center, 330 River Rd
Department of Kinesiology
Athens, GA 30602
www.coe.uga.edu/kinesiology/exs/athletictraining/

North Georgia College & State University
Athletic Training Prgm
Memorial Hall
Dahlonega, GA 30597

Georgia College & State University
Athletic Training Prgm
Campus Box 65
Milledgeville, GA 31061
www2.gcsu.edu/acad_affairs/school_healthsci/
kinesiology/

Georgia Southern University
Athletic Training Prgm
PO Box 8076
Hollis Bldg
Statesboro, GA 30460-8076

Valdosta State University
Athletic Training Prgm
Dept of KSPE
Valdosta, GA 31698
www.valdosta.edu/coe/kspe/athletictraining

Hawaii

University of Hawaii at Manoa
Athletic Training Prgm
Dept of Kinesiology and Rehabilitation Science
1337 Lower Campus Rd PE/A 231
Honolulu, HI 96822
www.hawaii.edu/kls/atsm/

Idaho

Boise State University
Athletic Training Prgm
Dept of Kinesiology, K209
1910 University Dr
Boise, ID 83725
http://kinesiology.boisestate.edu/atep

University of Idaho
Athletic Training Prgm
Department of HPERD
PO Box 442401
Moscow, ID 83844-2401
www.uidaho.edu

Illinois

Aurora University
Athletic Training Prgm
School of Health and Physical Education
347 S Gladstone Ave
Aurora, IL 60506
www.aurora.edu/academics/programs-majors/
undergraduate/athletic-training/

Olivet Nazarene University
Athletic Training Prgm
1 University Ave
Bourbonnais, IL 60914-2345

Southern Illinois University Carbondale
Athletic Training Prgm
Department of Kinesiology
1075 S Normal Ave
Carbondale, IL 62901
www.siu.edu/~athtrain

Eastern Illinois University
Athletic Training Prgm
Department of Kinesiology & Sport Studies
600 Lincoln Ave, 2220 Lantz Gymnasium
Charleston, IL 61920
www.eiu.edu/~athtrain

North Park University
Athletic Training Prgm
3225 W Foster Ave
Chicago, IL 60625
www.northpark.edu

Millikin University
Athletic Training Prgm
1184 W Main
Decatur, IL 62522

Trinity International University
Athletic Training Prgm
2065 Half Day Rd
Deerfield, IL 60015
www.tiu.edu

Northern Illinois University
Athletic Training Prgm
Dept of Kinesiology & Physical Education
DeKalb, IL 60115

McKendree University
Athletic Training Prgm
701 College Rd
Lebanon, IL 62254-1299
www.mckendree.edu/athletictraining

Western Illinois University
Athletic Training Prgm
Brophy Hall 220B
One University Circle
Macomb, IL 61455
www.wiu.edu/coehs/kinesiology/
undergraduate_programs/athletic_training/

North Central College
Athletic Training Prgm
30 N Brainard
Naperville, IL 60540
http://noctrl.edu/atep

Illinois State University
Athletic Training Prgm
School of Kinesiology and Recreation
Campus Box 5120
251E SFCM
Normal, IL 61790-5120
www.kinrec.ilstu.edu/at
Prgm Dir: Jeremy Hawkins, PhD ATC
Tel: 309 438-2605 *Fax:* 309 438-5559
E-mail: jhawkin@ilstu.edu

Lewis University
Athletic Training Prgm
One University Parkway
Romeoville, IL 60446

Univ of Illinois at Urbana-Champaign
Athletic Training Prgm
331 Freer Hall
906 S Goodwin Ave
Urbana, IL 61801-3841
www.uiuc.edu

Indiana

Anderson University
Athletic Training Prgm
1100 E 5th St
Anderson, IN 46012-1362
www.anderson.edu

Indiana University - Bloomington
Athletic Training Prgm
Smith Research Center
2805 E 10th St
Bloomington, IN 47408
www.indiana.edu/~kines/undergraduate/training/shtml

University of Evansville
Athletic Training Prgm
1800 Lincoln Ave, Wallace Graves Hall 217
Evansville, IN 47722

Franklin College
Athletic Training Prgm
Spurlock Center
101 Branigin Blvd
Franklin, IN 46131
www.franklincollege.edu/athweb/training/
Prgm Dir: Kathy Taylor Remsburg, MS ATC LAT
Tel: 317 738-8135 *Fax:* 317 738-8248
E-mail: kremsburg@franklincollege.edu

DePauw University
Athletic Training Prgm
Kinesiology Department
702 S College St
Greencastle, IN 46135

University of Indianapolis
Athletic Training Prgm
1400 E Hanna Ave
Indianapolis, IN 46227
www.athtrg.uindy.edu

Indiana Wesleyan University
Athletic Training Prgm
4201 S Washington St
Recreation & Wellness Center
Marion, IN 46953
www.indwes.edu/Undergraduate/BS-Athletic-Training/
Prgm Dir: Adam J Thompson, PhD LAT ATC
Tel: 765 677-3482 *Fax:* 765 677-3485
E-mail: adam.thompson@indwes.edu

Ball State University
Athletic Training Prgm
HP 209
Muncie, IN 47306

Manchester College
Athletic Training Prgm
Box PERC
North Manchester, IN 46962
www.manchester.edu

Indiana State University
Athletic Training Prgm
Athletic Training Department
Arena Room C-06
Terre Haute, IN 47809
www.indstate.edu/athtrn

Purdue University
Athletic Training Prgm
Dept of Health & Kinesiology
800 W Stadium Ave
West Lafayette, IN 47907
www.cla.purdue.edu/hk/sportsmed

Iowa

Iowa State University
Athletic Training Prgm
225 Forker Bldg
Ames, IA 50011
www.sportsmed.athletic.iastate.edu

University of Northern Iowa
Athletic Training Prgm
003 Human Performance Center
Cedar Falls, IA 50614-0244

Coe College
Athletic Training Prgm
1220 First Ave NE
Cedar Rapids, IA 52402
www.coe.edu

Luther College
Athletic Training Prgm
700 College Dr
Decorah, IA 52101
www.luther.edu

Clarke University
Athletic Training Prgm
1550 Clarke Dr, MS 1757
Dubuque, IA 52001
www.clarke.edu

Loras College
Athletic Training Prgm
1450 Alta Vista St
Dubuque, IA 52001
http://depts.loras.edu/phe/training.html
Prgm Dir: Nathan Newman
Tel: 563 588-7211   *Fax:* 563 588-7451
E-mail: nathan.newman@loras.edu

Upper Iowa University
Athletic Training Prgm
605 Washington St
PO Box 1857
Fayette, IA 52142
www.uiu.edu

Simpson College
Athletic Training Prgm
701 North C St
Indianola, IA 50125
www.simpson.edu

University of Iowa
Athletic Training Prgm
414 FH
Iowa City, IA 52242-1020
www.hawkeyehealthcare.com/Education/venue05.htm

Graceland University
Athletic Training Prgm
1 University Place
Lamoni, IA 50140
www.graceland.edu/athletics/athletictraining_major/

Northwestern College
Athletic Training Prgm
208 8th St SW
Orange City, IA 51041-1998
www.nwciowa.edu

Central College
Athletic Training Prgm
812 University Box 6600
Pella, IA 50219
www.central.edu

Buena Vista University
Athletic Training Prgm
610 W Fourth St
Storm Lake, IA 50588
www.bvu.edu

Kansas

Benedictine College
Athletic Training Prgm
1020 N Second St
Atchison, KS 66002
www.benedictine.edu

Emporia State University
Athletic Training Prgm
1200 Commerical St, Box 4013
Emporia, KS 66801
www.emporia.edu/hper

Fort Hays State University
Athletic Training Prgm
600 Park St
Hays, KS 67601

Tabor College
Athletic Training Prgm
400 S Jefferson
Hillsboro, KS 67063
www.tabor.edu

University of Kansas
Athletic Training Prgm
1301 Sunnyside Ave
ROB 161-C
Lawrence, KS 66045
soe.ku.edu/athletic-training/

Bethany College
Athletic Training Prgm
335 E Swensson
Department of Health, Physical Education and Athletic
   Traini
Lindsborg, KS 67456
www.bethanylb.edu

Kansas State University
Athletic Training Prgm
210 Justin Hall
Department of Human Nutrition
Manhattan, KS 66506-1407
www.k-state.edu/humec/hn/athleticcover.htm
Prgm Dir: Shawna Jordan, PhD ATC LAT
Tel: 785 532-0151   *Fax:* 785 532-3132
E-mail: jordan@k-state.edu

Bethel College
Athletic Training Prgm
300 E 27th St
North Newton, KS 67117
www.bethelks.edu/academics/majors/athletic_training/

Mid-America Nazarene University
Athletic Training Prgm
2030 E College Way
Olathe, KS 66062-1899
www.mnu.edu

Kansas Wesleyan University
Athletic Training Prgm
100 E Claflin Ave
Salina, KS 67401-6196
www.kwu.edu

Sterling College
Athletic Training Prgm
125 W Cooper
Sterling, KS 67579
www.sterling.edu/athletics/athletic-training

Washburn University
Athletic Training Prgm
1700 SW College Ave
Topeka, KS 66621

Wichita State University
Athletic Training Prgm
1845 Fairmount; Box 16
Dept of Human Performance Studies
Wichita, KS 67260

Southwestern College
Athletic Training Prgm
100 College St
Winfield, KS 67156
www.sckans.edu/athletictraining

Kentucky

Georgetown College
Athletic Training Prgm
400 E College St; Hill Chapel #22
Department of Kinesiology and Health Studies
Georgetown, KY 40324
www.georgetowncollege.edu

Northern Kentucky University
Athletic Training Prgm
109 Albright Health Center
Highland Heights, KY 41099

Murray State University
Athletic Training Prgm
Dept of Wellness & Therapeutic Sciences
102A Carr Health Bldg
Murray, KY 42071
www.murraystate.edu/athletictraining.aspx

Eastern Kentucky University
Athletic Training Prgm
Moberly 109
521 Lancaster Ave
Richmond, KY 40475
www.athletictraining.eku.edu

Louisiana

Louisiana State University
Athletic Training Prgm
Department of Kinesiology
112 H P Long Fieldhouse
Baton Rouge, LA 70803
http://coe.ednet.lsu.edu/coe/Kinesiology/training.html

Southeastern Louisiana University
Athletic Training Prgm
SLU 10845
Hammond, LA 70402
www.selu.edu/khs

University of Louisiana at Lafayette
Athletic Training Prgm
225 Cajundome Blvd
Lafayette, LA 70506
http://kinesiology.louisiana.edu/Programs/ATEP/

McNeese State University
Athletic Training Prgm
PO Box 91855
MSU Dept of Human & Health Performance
Lake Charles, LA 70609
catalog.mcneese.edu/preview_program.php?catoid=
   1&poid=241&bc

Louisiana College
Athletic Training Prgm
1140 College Dr, Box 563
Pineville, LA 71359

Nicholls State University
Athletic Training Prgm
PO Box 2090
Thibodaux, LA 70310
www.nicholls.edu/athletic_training

Maine

University of New England
Athletic Training Prgm
11 Hills Beach Rd
Biddeford, ME 04005
www.une.edu

University of Southern Maine
Athletic Training Prgm
Department of Exercise, Health and Sport Sciences
Costello Complex, 37 College Ave
Gorham, ME 04038
www.usm.maine.edu/ehss
Prgm Dir: Brian Toy
Tel: 207 780-4799   *Fax:* 207 780-4745
E-mail: btoy@usm.maine.edu

University of Maine - Orono
Athletic Training Prgm
108 Lengyel Hall
Orono, ME 04469
www.umaine.edu

University of Maine at Presque Isle
Athletic Training Prgm
181 Main St
Presque Isle, ME 04769
www.umpi.maine.edu/cms/academics/atep/
     index-20050622327/
Prgm Dir: Barbara Blackstone, MSS
Tel: 207 768-9415   *Fax:* 207 768-9553
E-mail: barbara.blackstone@umpi.edu

Maryland

Frostburg State University
Athletic Training Prgm
Cordts Physical Education Center
Frostburg, MD 21532
www.frostburg.edu

Salisbury University
Athletic Training Prgm
1101 Camden Ave
Department of Health, Physical Education & Human
     Performance
Salisbury, MD 21801
www.salisbury.edu

Towson University
Athletic Training Prgm
8000 York Rd
Kinesiology Department
Towson, MD 21252
www.towson.edu

Massachusetts

Endicott College
Athletic Training Prgm
376 Hale St
Beverly, MA 01915

Boston University
Athletic Training Prgm
635 Commonwealth Ave
Boston, MA 02215
www.bu.edu/sargent
Prgm Dir: Sara Brown, MS ATC
Tel: 617 353-7507   *Fax:* 617 353-9463
E-mail: sara@bu.edu

Northeastern University
Athletic Training Prgm
301 Robinson Hall
Boston, MA 02115
www.neu.edu

Bridgewater State University
Athletic Training Prgm
Dept of MAHPLS
Tinsley Center
Bridgewater, MA 02325
www.bridgew.edu

Lasell College
Athletic Training Prgm
1844 Commonwealth Ave
Newton, MA 02466
www.lasell.edu

Merrimack College
Athletic Training Prgm
315 Turnpike St
North Andover, MA 01845
www.merrimack.edu

Salem State University
Athletic Training Prgm
352 Lafayette St
Salem, MA 01970-5353
www.salemstate.edu

Springfield College
Athletic Training Prgm
Exercise Science and Athletic Training Education
     Center
Springfield, MA 01109
http://catalog.spfldcol.edu/
     preview_program.php?catoid=26&poid=877

Westfield State College
Athletic Training Prgm
Department of Movement Science
577 Western Ave
Westfield, MA 01086-1630
www.wsc.ma.edu/mssls/AT/atraining.html

Michigan

Adrian College
Athletic Training Prgm
110 S Madison
Merillat Sport & Fitness Center #212
Adrian, MI 49221

Albion College
Athletic Training Prgm
Box 4830
Albion, MI 49224
www.albion.edu

Grand Valley State University
Athletic Training Prgm
Movement Science Dept
B2235 MAK
Allendale, MI 49401
www.gvsu.edu/move-sci/

Alma College
Athletic Training Prgm
614 W Superior St
Alma, MI 48801
www.alma.edu

University of Michigan
Athletic Training Prgm
401 Washtenaw Ave
Kinesiology Bldg
Ann Arbor, MI 48109-2214

Michigan State University
Athletic Training Prgm
105 IM Circle
East Lansing, MI 48824

Aquinas College
Athletic Training Prgm
1607 Robinson Rd SE
Sturrus Sports and Fitness Center, 114
Grand Rapids, MI 49506-1799
Prgm Dir: JoAnne Gorant, Asst Professor
Tel: 616 632-2899   *Fax:* 616 732-4548
E-mail: goranjoa@aquinas.edu

Hope College
Athletic Training Prgm
PO Box 9000
Holland, MI 49423
www.hope.edu/academic/kinesiology/

Western Michigan University
Athletic Training Prgm
Health, Physical Education and Recreation
1903 W Michigan Ave #5426
Kalamazoo, MI 49008
www.wmich.edu

Northern Michigan University
Athletic Training Prgm
Dept of HPER
1401 Presque Isle Ave
Marquette, MI 49855
www.nmu.edu

Central Michigan University
Athletic Training Prgm
HPB 1171
Mount Pleasant, MI 48859
www.chp.cmich.edu/atep

Lake Superior State University
Athletic Training Prgm
650 W Easterday Ave
Sault Ste Marie, MI 49783
www.lssu.edu

Saginaw Valley State University
Athletic Training Prgm
7400 Bay Rd
University Center, MI 48710
www.svsu.edu

Eastern Michigan University
Athletic Training Prgm
310 Porter Bldg
Ypsilanti, MI 48197
www.emich.edu

Minnesota

University of Minnesota - Duluth
Athletic Training Prgm
110 Sports and Health Center
1216 Ordean Court
Duluth, MN 55812
www.d.umn.edu/hper/undergraduate/majors/
     athletic_training/

Minnesota State University - Mankato
Athletic Training Prgm
1400 Highland Center
Mankato, MN 56001
http://ahn.mnsu.edu/athletictraining

Minnesota State University - Moorhead
Athletic Training Prgm
106 D Alex Namzek Hall
Moorhead, MN 56563

St Cloud State University
Athletic Training Prgm
720 4th Ave South, Halenbeck Hall 339
St Cloud, MN 56301
www.stcloudstate.edu

Bethel University
Athletic Training Prgm
3900 Bethel Dr
St Paul, MN 55112
www.bethel.edu

Gustavus Adolphus College
Athletic Training Prgm
800 W College Ave
St Peter, MN 56082
www.gustavus.edu/hes/atr/
Prgm Dir: Kyle Momsen, MA ATC
Tel: 507 933-6062   *Fax:* 507 933-8412
E-mail: kmomsen@gustavus.edu

Winona State University
Athletic Training Prgm
Memorial Hall 117
Winona, MN 55987-5838
www.winona.edu/athletictraining

Mississippi

Delta State University
Athletic Training Prgm
PO Box B-2
Cleveland, MS 38733

University of Southern Mississippi
Athletic Training Prgm
Dept of Human Performance & Recreation
118 College Dr, Box 5142
Hattiesburg, MS 39406-0001
www.usm.edu/athletictraining/

Missouri

Southwest Baptist University
Athletic Training Prgm
1600 University Ave
Bolivar, MO 65613
www.sbuniv.edu/cosm/at

Culver-Stockton College
Athletic Training Prgm
1 College Hill
Canton, MO 63435
www.culver.edu

Southeast Missouri State University
Athletic Training Prgm
One University Plaza MS7650
Cape Girardeau, MO 63701

Central Methodist University
Athletic Training Prgm
411 CMC Square
Fayette, MO 65248
www.centralmethodist.edu/cmacademics/athtrain/
Prgm Dir: Wade Welton, MS ATC/LAT
Tel: 660 248-6217   *Fax:* 660 248-6381
E-mail: wwelton@centralmethodist.edu

William Woods University
Athletic Training Prgm
One University Ave
Fulton, MO 65251

Truman State University
Athletic Training Prgm
Pershing Bldg
Kirksville, MO 63501
http://hes.truman.edu/atmaj

Park University
Athletic Training Prgm
8700 NW River Park Dr
Parkville, MO 64152
www.park.edu

Saint Louis University
Athletic Training Prgm
3437 Caroline Mall
Doisy College of Health Sciences
Saint Louis, MO 63104
http://at.slu.edu

Missouri State University
Athletic Training Prgm
Professional Bldg 160
901 S National Ave
Springfield, MO 65897

Lindenwood University
Athletic Training Prgm
209 S Kings Hwy
St Charles, MO 63301

University of Central Missouri
Athletic Training Prgm
Humphreys 204
Warrensburg, MO 64093
www.ucmo.edu

Montana

Montana State University Billings
Athletic Training Prgm
PE 119
1500 University Dr
Billings, MT 59101

University of Montana
Athletic Training Prgm
Health & Human Performance Dept
McGill Hall 101
Missoula, MT 59812-1055
www.soe.umt.edu/hhp/athletic_training/

Nebraska

University of Nebraska - Kearney
Athletic Training Prgm
905 W 25th St
Cushing Bldg Rm 158
Kearney, NE 68849

Nebraska Wesleyan University
Athletic Training Prgm
5000 St Paul Ave
Lincoln, NE 68504

University of Nebraska - Lincoln
Athletic Training Prgm
231 Mabel Lee Hall
Lincoln, NE 68588-0234
www.unl.edu

Creighton University
Athletic Training Prgm
6001 Dodge St; HPER 207 V
Omaha, NE 68178
www2.creighton.edu

University of Nebraska - Omaha
Athletic Training Prgm
HPER 207
6001 Dodge St
Omaha, NE 68182-0216
http://coe.unomaha.edu/hper/at/at_index.php

New Hampshire

University of New Hampshire
Athletic Training Prgm
124 Main St
Department of Kinesiology
Durham, NH 03824
http://chhs.unh.edu/kin_at/

Keene State College
Athletic Training Prgm
229 Main St
Keene, NH 03435
http://keene.edu

Colby-Sawyer College
Athletic Training Prgm
541 Main St
New London, NH 03257

Plymouth State University
Athletic Training Prgm
MSC 22
Plymouth, NH 03264

New Jersey

Rowan University
Athletic Training Prgm
201 Mullica Hill Rd
Glassboro, NJ 08028

Montclair State University
Athletic Training Prgm
1 Normal Ave
Montclair, NJ 07043
www.montclair.edu/pages/ate

Seton Hall University
Athletic Training Prgm
400 S Orange Ave
South Orange, NJ 07079
www.shu.edu/academics/gradmeded/
   ms-athletic-training/

Kean University
Athletic Training Prgm
D'Angola Gym, Morris Ave
Union, NJ 07083
www.kean.edu/~gball

William Paterson Univ of New Jersey
Athletic Training Prgm
Dept of Kinesiology
300 Pompton Rd
Wayne, NJ 07470
www.wpunj.edu/atep
Prgm Dir: Linda Gazzillo Diaz, EdD ATC
Tel: 973 720-2364   *Fax:* 973 720-2034
E-mail: gazzillol@wpunj.edu

New Mexico

University of New Mexico
Athletic Training Prgm
South Athletic Complex
Albuquerque, NM 87131
www.unm.edu/~lobotrng

New Mexico State University
Athletic Training Prgm
Box 30001, MSC 3FAC
Las Cruces, NM 88003-0001
www.nmsu.edu

New York

Alfred University
Athletic Training Prgm
1 Saxon Dr
Alfred, NY 14802
www.las.alfred.edu

SUNY The College at Brockport
Athletic Training Prgm
260 Tuttle South
Brockport, NY 14420

Long Island University - Brooklyn Campus
Athletic Training Prgm
1 University Plaza
HS 312
Brooklyn, NY 11201-8423
www.brooklyn.liu.edu/athletictraining

Canisius College
Athletic Training Prgm
2001 Main St
Buffalo, NY 14208-1098
www.canisius.edu/sportsmed/

SUNY College at Cortland
Athletic Training Prgm
PO Box 2000
Cortland, NY 13045
www.cortland.edu/kin

Hofstra University
Athletic Training Prgm
220 Hofstra University
The Dome
Hempstead, NY 11550

Ithaca College
Athletic Training Prgm
48 Hill Center
Ithaca, NY 14850
www.ithaca.edu/hshp/clinics/atclinic/atep/
Prgm Dir: Paul Geisler, Assoc Professor EdD ATC
Tel: 607 274-3006   *Fax:* 607 274-1943
E-mail: pgeisler@Ithaca.edu

Dominican College
Athletic Training Prgm
470 Western Hwy
Orangeburg, NY 10962
www.dc.edu

Marist College
Athletic Training Prgm
3399 North Rd
Department of Athletic Training
McCann Center Room 212
Poughkeepsie, NY 12601
www.marist.edu/science/athtraining

Stony Brook University
Athletic Training Prgm
School of Health Technology and Management
100 Nicolls Rd, Indoor Sports Complex
Stony Brook, NY 11794-3504
www.hsc.stonybrook.edu/shtm/at/

North Carolina

Lees-McRae College
Athletic Training Prgm
PO Box 128
191 Main St
Banner Elk, NC 28604
www.lmc.edu
Prgm Dir: Rita A Smith, Asst Professor
Tel: 828 898-8768   *Fax:* 828 898-8742
E-mail: smithr@lmc.edu

Gardner-Webb University
Athletic Training Prgm
Department of Physical Education,Wellness & Sport
   Studies
Campus 7257
Boiling Springs, NC 28017
www.gardner-webb.edu

Appalachian State University
Athletic Training Prgm
Health Leisure and Exercise Science
Boone, NC 28608
www.hles.appstate.edu

Campbell University
Athletic Training Prgm
PO Box 10
89 Pope St
Buies Creek, NC 27506

University of North Carolina - Chapel Hill
Athletic Training Prgm
211 Fetzer, CB 8700
Chapel Hill, NC 27599-8700
www.unc.edu/depts/exercise

Univ of North Carolina at Charlotte
Athletic Training Prgm
226 Belk Gymnasium
Dept of Kinesiology
Charlotte, NC 28223
www.health.uncc.edu/
   academic_programs.cfm?pname=bsat

Western Carolina University
Athletic Training Prgm
135 Moore Hall
Cullowhee, NC 28723

North Carolina Central University
Athletic Training Prgm
1801 Fayetteville St
PO Box 19542
Durham, NC 27707
www.nccu.edu

Methodist University
Athletic Training Prgm
5400 Ramsey St
Fayettesville, NC 28311

Greensboro College
Athletic Training Prgm
815 W Market St
Greensboro, NC 27401
www.greensboro.edu
Prgm Dir: Michelle Lesperance, EdD ATC LAT
Tel: 336 272-7102, Ext   *Fax:* 336 217-7249
E-mail: mlesperance@greensboro.edu

University of North Carolina - Greensboro
Athletic Training Prgm
Dept of Kinesiology
250 HHP
1408 Walker Ave
Greensboro, NC 27412
www.uncg.edu/kin/atep/
Prgm Dir: Aaron Terranova, EdD ATC
Tel: 336 334-3563   *Fax:* 336 334-3238
E-mail: abterran@uncg.edu

East Carolina University
Athletic Training Prgm
245 Ward Sports Medicine Bldg
Greenville, NC 27858
www.ecu.edu/cs-hhp/hlth/athletictr/athletetr.cfm
Prgm Dir: Katie Walsh, EdD ATC LAT
Tel: 252 737-4561   *Fax:* 252 737-1276
E-mail: walshk@ecu.edu

Lenoir - Rhyne University
Athletic Training Prgm
PO Box 7356
Hickory, NC 28603
www.lrc.edu/hlss

High Point University
Athletic Training Prgm
833 Montlieu Ave
High Point, NC 27262

Mars Hill College
Athletic Training Prgm
PO Box 6668
Mars Hill, NC 28754

University of North Carolina - Pembroke
Athletic Training Prgm
HPER Department
PO Box 1510
Pembroke, NC 28372
www.uncp.edu/hper/training

Shaw University
Athletic Training Prgm
118 East South St
Raleigh, NC 27601

Catawba College
Athletic Training Prgm
2300 W Innes St
Salisbury, NC 28144
www.catawba.edu

University of North Carolina - Wilmington
Athletic Training Prgm
601 S College Rd
Wilmington, NC 28403-5956

Barton College
Athletic Training Prgm
PO Box 5000
Wilson, NC 27893
www.barton.edu

Wingate University
Athletic Training Prgm
211A E Wilson St
Wingate, NC 28174
www.wingate.edu/academics/athletic-training

North Dakota

University of Mary
Athletic Training Prgm
7500 University Dr
Bismarck, ND 58504-9652
www.umary.edu/UM/AcademicInformation/
   Undergraduate/hps/AthleticTraining/

North Dakota State University
Athletic Training Prgm
Bentson Bunker Fieldhouse 9C
PO Box 5576
Fargo, ND 58105-5576
Prgm Dir: Pamela Hansen, EdD ATC
Tel: 701 231-8093   *Fax:* 701 231-8872
E-mail: pamela.j.hansen@ndsu.edu

University of North Dakota
Athletic Training Prgm
Division of Sports Medicine
2751 2nd Ave N Stop 9013
Grand Forks, ND 58202-9013
www.und.edu
Prgm Dir: Steven Westereng, LAT MA ATC
Tel: 701 777-3886   *Fax:* 701 777-2536
E-mail: steven.westereng@med.und.edu

Ohio

Ohio Northern University
Athletic Training Prgm
Dept of HPSS
243 Sports Center
Ada, OH 45810
www.onu.edu/athletictraining

The University of Akron
Athletic Training Prgm
Memorial Hall 77D
Akron, OH 44325-5103
www.uakron.edu/athletictraining

University of Mount Union
Athletic Training Prgm
1972 Clark Ave
Alliance, OH 44601
www.muc.edu

Ashland University
Athletic Training Prgm
916 King Rd
Arthur L & Maxine Sheets Rybolt Sport Sciences Center
Ashland, OH 44805
www.ashland.edu

Ohio University
Athletic Training Prgm
Grover Center E-188
Athens, OH 45701-2979
www.ohio.edu

Baldwin-Wallace College
Athletic Training Prgm
275 Eastland Rd
Berea, OH 44017
www.bw.edu/academics/hpe/programs/at/

Bowling Green State University
Athletic Training Prgm
Eppler Complex N217
Bowling Green, OH 43403
www.bgsu.edu

Cedarville University
Athletic Training Prgm
251 N Main St
Cedarville, OH 45314
www.cedarville.edu

College of Mt St Joseph
Athletic Training Prgm
Dept of Health Sciences
5701 Delhi Rd
Cincinnati, OH 45233-1870
www.msj.edu

University of Cincinnati
Athletic Training Prgm
PO Box 210002
Cincinnati, OH 45221-0002
www.uc.edu/athletictraining

Xavier University
Athletic Training Prgm
3800 Victory Pkwy
Cincinnati, OH 45207-6312
www.xavier.edu

Capital University
Athletic Training Prgm
Capital Center
1 College and Main
Columbus, OH 43209
www.capital.edu/1043/

The Ohio State University
Athletic Training Prgm
Athletic Training Division
453 W Tenth Ave
Columbus, OH 43210-2205
amp.osu.edu/at

Wright State University
Athletic Training Prgm
Health and Physical Education Dept
Rm 303 Nutter Center
Dayton, OH 45435

Defiance College
Athletic Training Prgm
701 N Clinton St
Defiance, OH 43512
www.defiance.edu/pages/edu_AT_home.html

The University of Findlay
Athletic Training Prgm
1000 N Main St
Findlay, OH 45840
www.findlay.edu/academics/colleges/cohp/
    academicprograms/graduate/mat/

Denison University
Athletic Training Prgm
Dept of Physical Education
Granville, OH 43023
www.denison.edu/phed/AT

Kent State University
Athletic Training Prgm
School of Exercise Leisure and Sport
Rm 161D MACC Gym Annex
Kent, OH 44242
www.kent.edu/athletictraining

Marietta College
Athletic Training Prgm
Dept of Sports Medicine
215 Fifth St
Marietta, OH 45750-4031
www.marietta.edu

Miami University
Athletic Training Prgm
KNH Dept
Oxford, OH 45056
Prgm Dir: J Brett Massie, EdD ATC
Tel: 513 529-8105   *Fax:* 513 529-5006
E-mail: massiejb@muohio.edu

Shawnee State University
Athletic Training Prgm
940 Second St
Portsmouth, OH 45662
www.shawnee.edu

Heidelberg University
Athletic Training Prgm
310 E Market St
Bareis Hall 108
Tiffin, OH 44883
www.heidelberg.edu

University of Toledo
Athletic Training Prgm
College of Health Science & Human Service
Dept of Kinesiology, 2801 W Bancroft St
Toledo, OH 43606
www.utoledo.edu/eduhshs/depts/kinesiology/
    athletictraining/
Prgm Dir: James M Rankin, PhD ATC
Tel: 419 530-2752   *Fax:* 419 530-2477
E-mail: james.rankin@utoledo.edu

Urbana University
Athletic Training Prgm
579 College Way
Urbana, OH 43078
www.urbana.edu

Otterbein College
Athletic Training Prgm
160 Center St, Rike Center
Westerville, OH 43081

Wilmington College
Athletic Training Prgm
1870 Quaker Way
Pyle Center Box 1246
c/o Larry Howard
Wilmington, OH 45177
www2.wilmington.edu/athletic-training/

Oklahoma

East Central University
Athletic Training Prgm
1100 E 14th
Ada, OK 74820

Southern Nazarene University
Athletic Training Prgm
6729 NW 39th Expressway
Bethany, OK 73008
www.snu.edu

University of Central Oklahoma
Athletic Training Prgm
100 N University Drive
Wantland Hall Box 189
Dept of Kinesiology and Health Studies
Edmond, OK 73034

Oklahoma State University
Athletic Training Prgm
180 Colvin Recreation Center
Stillwater, OK 74078
frontpage.okstate.edu/coe/atep/

University of Tulsa
Athletic Training Prgm
Chapman Hall 355
600 S College Ave
Tulsa, OK 74104-3189
www.cba.utulsa.edu/depts/athletic

Southwestern Oklahoma State University
Athletic Training Prgm
100 Campus Dr
Weatherford, OK 73096
www.swosu.edu/atep/

Oregon

Oregon State University
Athletic Training Prgm
226 Langton Hall
Corvallis, OR 97331-3302
www.hhs.oregonstate.edu

Linfield College
Athletic Training Prgm
900 SE Baker St
McMinnville, OR 97128
www.linfield.edu

George Fox University
Athletic Training Prgm
414 N Meridian St #6188
Newberg, OR 97132
www.georgefox.edu/academics/undergrad/
    departments/ath_tr/

Pennsylvania

Neumann University
Athletic Training Prgm
One Neumann Dr
Aston, PA 19014
www.neumann.edu

Bloomsburg University
Athletic Training Prgm
244 Nelsen Fieldhouse
Bloomsburg, PA 17815-1301
www.bloomu.edu

University of Pittsburgh - Bradford
Athletic Training Prgm
300 Campus Dr
Bradford, PA 16701
www.upb.pitt.edu

California University of Pennsylvania
Athletic Training Prgm
250 University Ave
California, PA 15419

East Stroudsburg University
Athletic Training Prgm
200 Prospect St
East Stroudsburg, PA 18301
www4.esu.edu

Mercyhurst University
Athletic Training Prgm
501 E 38th St
Erie, PA 16546-0001

Messiah College
Athletic Training Prgm
One College Ave
Grantham, PA 17027
www.messiah.edu

Indiana University of Pennsylvania
Athletic Training Prgm
228 Zink Hall
1190 Maple St
Indiana, PA 15705
www.hhs.iup.edu/hped

Lock Haven University
Athletic Training Prgm
113 Health Professions Building
Lock Haven, PA 17745
www.lhup.edu/athletictraining

Temple University
Athletic Training Prgm
Dept of Kinesiology
261 Pearson Hall
Philadelphia, PA 19122
www.temple.edu/chp/departments/kinesiology/
    Kine_BS.htm
Prgm Dir: Dani Moffit, PhD ATC
Tel: 215 204-8836   *Fax:* 215 214-4414
E-mail: moffitd@temple.edu

Duquesne University
Athletic Training Prgm
John G Rangos, Sr School of Health Sciences
122 Health Sciences Building
Pittsburgh, PA 15282
www.healthsciences.duq.edu/at/athome.html

University of Pittsburgh
Athletic Training Prgm
4044 Forbes Tower
Pittsburgh, PA 15260
www.shrs.pitt.edu

Alvernia University
Athletic Training Prgm
400 St Bernardine St
Reading, PA 19607

Marywood University
Athletic Training Prgm
2300 Adams Ave
Mellow Center
Scranton, PA 18509-1598

Slippery Rock University of Pennsylvania
Athletic Training Prgm
Department of Exercise and Rehabilitative Sciences
114 West Gym
Slippery Rock, PA 16057
www.sru.edu/ers

Eastern University
Athletic Training Prgm
1300 Eagle Rd
St Davids, PA 19087
www.eastern.edu

Penn State University
Athletic Training Prgm
275 Recreation Bldg
University Park, PA 16802
www.hhdev.psu.edu/kines

Waynesburg University
Athletic Training Prgm
51 W College St
Waynesburg, PA 15370

West Chester University
Athletic Training Prgm
Department of Sports Medicine
855 S New St
West Chester, PA 19383
www.wcupa.edu/_academics/healthsciences/sportsmed/

King's College
Athletic Training Prgm
133 N River St
Wilkes-Barre, PA 18711
www.kings.edu

South Carolina

Charleston Southern University
Athletic Training Prgm
9200 University Blvd
Charleston, SC 29406
www.charlestonsouthern.edu/ATEP

College of Charleston
Athletic Training Prgm
Department of Health and Human Performance
66 George St
Charleston, SC 29424
www.cofc.edu/~rozzis/at.html

University of South Carolina
Athletic Training Prgm
Blatt PE Center 218
Columbia, SC 29208
www.ed.sc.edu/pe/athletictraining/

Erskine College
Athletic Training Prgm
PO Box 338
Due West, SC 29639
www.erskine.edu
Prgm Dir: Scott DeCiantis, MS SCAT ATC
Tel: 864 379-8899   *Fax:* 864 379-2197
E-mail: deciantis@erskine.edu

Limestone College
Athletic Training Prgm
1115 College Dr
Gaffney, SC 29340
www.limesone.edu

Lander University
Athletic Training Prgm
PO Box 6026
Greenwood, SC 29649

Winthrop University
Athletic Training Prgm
216C Lois Rhame West Center
Rock Hill, SC 29733
www.winthrop.edu

South Dakota

South Dakota State University
Athletic Training Prgm
Health PE & Recreation
Box 2820
Brookings, SD 57007-1497

Dakota Wesleyan University
Athletic Training Prgm
1200 W University, Box 912
Mitchell, SD 57301
www.dwu.edu/catalog/courses/athletic_training.htm

National American University
Athletic Training Prgm
321 Kansas City St
Rapid City, SD 57701
www.national.edu

Augustana College
Athletic Training Prgm
2001 S Summit Ave
Elmen Center
Sioux Falls, SD 57197
www.augie.edu/athletictraining
Notes: Augustana is a private liberal arts institution; the
    athletic training program is a three-year sequenced
    didactic and clinical education.

Tennessee

King College
Athletic Training Prgm
1350 King College Rd
Bristol, TN 37620
atep.king.edu

University of Tennessee - Chattanooga
Athletic Training Prgm
615 McCallie Ave, Dept 6606
Chattanooga, TN 37403-2598
Prgm Dir: Marisa A Colston, PhD
Tel: 423 425-4743   *Fax:* 423 425-5214
E-mail: marisa-colston@utc.edu

Lee University
Athletic Training Prgm
1120 N Ocoee St
Cleveland, TN 37320-3450
www.leeuniversity.edu

Tusculum College
Athletic Training Prgm
60 Shiloh Rd
Greeneville, TN 37743
www.tusculum.edu

Lincoln Memorial University
Athletic Training Prgm
6965 Cumberland Gap Pkwy
Harrogate, TN 37752
www.lmunet.edu

Union University
Athletic Training Prgm
1050 Union University Dr
PO Box 1824
Jackson, TN 38305
www.uu.edu

Carson-Newman College
Athletic Training Prgm
Box 71897
MSAC Rm 1013
Jefferson City, TN 37760
www.cn.edu

Cumberland University
Athletic Training Prgm
One Cumberland Square
Lebanon, TN 37087
www.cumberland.edu

Middle Tennessee State University
Athletic Training Prgm
PO Box 96
Murfreesboro, TN 37132

Texas

Hardin-Simmons University
Athletic Training Prgm
2200 Hickory St
Box 16180
Abilene, TX 79698
www.hsutx.edu

University of Texas at Arlington
Athletic Training Prgm
Box 19259
Arlington, TX 76019
www.uta.edu/coed/kinesiology/atep

University of Texas at Austin
Athletic Training Prgm
1 University Station Stop D3700
Austin, TX 78712
www.edb.utexas.edu/atep

University of Mary Hardin-Baylor
Athletic Training Prgm
900 College St, Box 8010
Belton, TX 76513
www.umhb.edu

West Texas A&M University
Athletic Training Prgm
WTAMU Box 60216
Canyon, TX 79016
www.wtamu.edu/athletictraining

Texas A&M University - Commerce
Athletic Training Prgm
ATEP Dept of Health
Kinesiology and Sports Studies
Commerce, TX 75429-3011
www.tamu.edu

Texas A&M University - Corpus Christi
Athletic Training Prgm
6300 Ocean Drive; Unit 5820
Department of Kinesiology
Corpus Christi, TX 78412-5820
http://athletictraining

Texas Christian University
Athletic Training Prgm
PO Box 297730
3005 Stadium Dr
Fort Worth, TX 76129
www.tcuathletictraining.com

Texas Wesleyan University
Athletic Training Prgm
1201 Wesleyan St
Fort Worth, TX 76105
www.txwes.edu/athletictraining/

Texas Tech Univ Health Sciences Center
Athletic Training Prgm
3601 4th St, Stop 6226
Lubbock, TX 79430
www.ttuhsc.edu
Prgm Dir: LesLee Taylor, PhD ATC LAT
Tel: 806 743-1032   *Fax:* 806 743-3518
E-mail: leslee.taylor@ttuhsc.edu

East Texas Baptist University
Athletic Training Prgm
1209 N Grove
Marshall, TX 75670
www.etbu.edu

Stephen F Austin State University
Athletic Training Prgm
PO Box 13015-SFA Station
Nacogdoches, TX 75962-3015
www.kin.sfasu.edu

Angelo State University
Athletic Training Prgm
ASU Station #10899
2601 West Ave N
San Angelo, TX 76909
www.angelo.edu/org/sportmed

The University of the Incarnate Word
Athletic Training Prgm
4301 Broadway, CPO 472
San Antonio, TX 78209
www.uiw.edu/athp

Texas State University - San Marcos
Athletic Training Prgm
Dept of Health, Physical Education and Recreation
Jowers Center, 601 University Dr
San Marcos, TX 78666

Texas Lutheran University
Athletic Training Prgm
1000 W Court St
Seguin, TX 78155

Baylor University
Athletic Training Prgm
One Bear Place #97313
HHPR Dept
Waco, TX 76798-7313
www3.baylor.edu/HHPR/Undergraduate/Programs/
   ATSM/

Midwestern State University
Athletic Training Prgm
3410 Taft Blvd
Wichita Falls, TX 76308
www.mwsu.edu

Utah

Southern Utah University
Athletic Training Prgm
351 W University Blvd
Department of Physical Education & Human
   Performance
Cedar City, UT 84720
www.suu.edu
Prgm Dir: Ben Davidson, MS ATC
Tel: 435 586-7823   *Fax:* 435 865-8057
E-mail: davidson@suu.edu

Weber State University
Athletic Training Prgm
2801 University Circle
Ogden, UT 84408-2801
http://programs.weber.edu/athletictraining

Brigham Young University
Athletic Training Prgm
Dept of Exercise Sciences
267 SFH
Provo, UT 84602-2111

University of Utah
Athletic Training Prgm
1850 E 250 South, Room 241
Salt Lake City, UT 84112-0920
www.health.utah.edu/ess/Athletic_Training/

Vermont

University of Vermont
Athletic Training Prgm
305 Rowell Building
106 Carrigan Dr
Burlington, VT 05405
www.uvm.edu

Castleton State College
Athletic Training Prgm
Glenbrook Gym
Castleton, VT 05735
www.castleton.edu

Norwich University
Athletic Training Prgm
158 Harmon Dr
Northfield, VT 05663
www.norwich.edu

Virginia

Bridgewater College
Athletic Training Prgm
402 E College St, Box 66
Bridgewater, VA 22812
www.bridgewater.edu/StudentServices/WellnessCenter/
   FunkhouserCenter/AthleticTraining

Averett University
Athletic Training Prgm
420 W Main St
Danville, VA 24541
www.averett.edu

Emory & Henry College
Athletic Training Prgm
PO Box 947
Emory, VA 24327-0947
www.ehc.edu

Longwood University
Athletic Training Prgm
201 High St
Farmville, VA 23909
www.longwood.edu/hrk/8287.htm
Prgm Dir: Sharon Menegoni, MS ATC
Tel: 434 395-2845   *Fax:* 434 395-2472
E-mail: menegonism@longwood.edu

James Madison University
Athletic Training Prgm
Department of Health Sciences
MSC 4301
Harrisonburg, VA 22807

Liberty University
Athletic Training Prgm
Department of Health Sciences and Kinesiology
1971 University Blvd
Lynchburg, VA 24502
www.liberty.edu/academics/education/
   sport/index.cfm?PID=85

Lynchburg College
Athletic Training Prgm
1501 Lakeside Dr
Lynchburg, VA 24501
www.lynchburg.edu

George Mason University
Athletic Training Prgm
10900 University Blvd, MSN 4E5
Manassas, VA 20110-2203
rht.gmu.edu/atep/

Radford University
Athletic Training Prgm
Dept of Exercise, Sport & Health Education
PO Box 6957
Radford, VA 24142

Virginia Commonwealth University
Athletic Training Prgm
1015 W Main St; Box 842020
Department of Health and Human Performance
Richmond, VA 23284

Roanoke College
Athletic Training Prgm
221 College Lane
Salem, VA 24153
Prgm Dir: James Buriak, MS ATC
Tel: 540 375-2343   *Fax:* 540 375-2031
E-mail: buriak@roanoke.edu

Shenandoah University
Athletic Training Prgm
1460 University Dr
Winchester, VA 22601
www.su.edu

Washington

Eastern Washington University
Athletic Training Prgm
200 Physical Eductation Building; PEHR Dept
Cheney, WA 99004-2476
www.ewu.edu/x3356.xml

Washington State University
Athletic Training Prgm
Dept of Educational Leadership & Counseling Psycholgy
PEB 114
Pullman, WA 99164-1410
http://education.wsu.edu/academics/fields/athletic/

Whitworth University
Athletic Training Prgm
300 W Hawthorne Rd
Spokane, WA 99251-2501
www.whitworth.edu

West Virginia

Concord University
Athletic Training Prgm
PO Box 1000
Campus Box 77
Athens, WV 24712

West Virginia Wesleyan College
Athletic Training Prgm
59 College Ave
Buckhannon, WV 26201-2995
www.wvwc.edu
Prgm Dir: Rae Emrick, MS
Tel: 304 473-8002   *Fax:* 304 473-8349
E-mail: emrick_r@wvwc.edu

University of Charleston
Athletic Training Prgm
2300 MacCorkle Ave SE
Charleston, WV 25304
Prgm Dir: Ericka Zimmerman, EdD ATC
Tel: 304 357-4828   *Fax:* 304 357-4965
E-mail: erickazimmerman@ucwv.edu

Marshall University
Athletic Training Prgm
College of Education and Human Services
400 Hal Greer Blvd
108 Gullickson Hall
Huntington, WV 25755-2450
www.marshall.edu/coehs/essr/athletic.training/

West Virginia University
Athletic Training Prgm
PO Box 6116 Coliseum
Morgantown, WV 26506-6116
www.wvu.edu/~physed/attrain/wvattr-1.htm

Alderson-Broaddus College
Athletic Training Prgm
Box 2062
101 College Hill Dr
Philippi, WV 26416
www.ab.edu

Wheeling Jesuit University
Athletic Training Prgm
316 Washington Ave Department of Athletic Training
Wheeling, WV 26003
www.wju.edu/academics/at/

Wisconsin

University of Wisconsin - Eau Claire
Athletic Training Prgm
Dept of Kinesiology
213 McPhee Center
105 Garfield Ave
Eau Claire, WI 54702-4004
www.uwec.edu/kin

Carthage College
Athletic Training Prgm
2001 Alford Park Dr
Kenosha, WI 53140
www.carthage.edu

University of Wisconsin - La Crosse
Athletic Training Prgm
135 Mitchell Hall
La Crosse, WI 54601

University of Wisconsin - Madison
Athletic Training Prgm
2000 Observatory Dr, Rm 1037
Madison, WI 53706

Concordia University Wisconsin
Athletic Training Prgm
12800 N Lake Shore Dr
Mequon, WI 53097
www.cuw.edu

Marquette University
Athletic Training Prgm
PO Box 1881
Milwaukee, WI 53201-1881
www.marquette.edu

University of Wisconsin - Milwaukee
Athletic Training Prgm
Dept of Human Movement Sciences
Enderis 413
Milwaukee, WI 53201-0413
www.uwm.edu

University of Wisconsin - Oshkosh
Athletic Training Prgm
108A Albee Hall
800 Algoma Blvd
Oshkosh, WI 54901
www.uwosh.edu/athtrain
Prgm Dir: Robert Sipes, EdD ATC LAT CSCS
Tel: 920 424-1298   *Fax:* 920 424-7447
E-mail: sipesr@uwosh.edu

University of Wisconsin - Stevens Point
Athletic Training Prgm
129 HEC
Stevens Point, WI 54481
www.uwsp.edu/hesa/athtraining/

Carroll University
Athletic Training Prgm
100 N East Ave
Physical Therapy Building
Waukesha, WI 53186
www.carrollu.edu

Athletic Trainer

Programs*	Class Capacity	Begins	Length (months)	Award	Res. Tuition	Non-res. Tuition		Offers:† 1	2	3	4
California											
Azusa Pacific Univ	15	Jan of sophomore yr	28	BA	$28,000	$28,000	per year	•		•	
California State Univ - Fullerton	10	Aug	20	Dipl, BS	$5,472	$8,928					
San Jose State Univ	40	Aug	48	BS	$6,840	$12,792					
Univ of the Pacific (Stockton)	30	Aug	24	Dipl, BS	$35,770					•	
Connecticut											
Southern Connecticut State Univ (New Haven)	15	Sep	48	BS	$4,285	$13,866					
Florida											
Univ of South Florida (Tampa)	30	Summer	24	BSAT	$5,800	$15,390	per year			•	
Univ of Tampa	24	Aug	36	BSAT	$22,834	$22,834				•	
Illinois											
Illinois State Univ (Normal)	27	Jan	28	BS	$4,601	$7,217					
Indiana											
Franklin College	10	Aug	7	BA	$26,710	$26,710				•	
Indiana Wesleyan Univ (Marion)	50	Sep	32	BS	$21,956	$29,104	per year	•			•
Iowa											
Loras College (Dubuque) •	16	App during freshman yr	4	Dipl, BA Ath	$26,813	$26,813	per year				
Kansas											
Kansas State Univ (Manhattan)	20	Aug	30	Dipl, BS	$5,773	$15,776	per year				
Maine											
Univ of Maine at Presque Isle	15	Fall	4	BS	$6,600	$16,560				•	
Univ of Southern Maine (Gorham)	30	Sep	120	BS	$7,590	$19,950					

*Data are shown only for programs that completed the 2011 AMA Survey of Health Professions Education Programs.

†Key to Offers: 1: Evening or weekend classes; 2: Non-English instruction; 3: Cultural competence instruction; 4: Distance education component.

Athletic Trainer

Programs*	Class Capacity	Begins	Length (months)	Award	Res. Tuition	Non-res. Tuition		Offers:† 1	2	3	4
Massachusetts											
Boston Univ	125	Sep	48	BS	$40,848	$40,848				•	
Michigan											
Aquinas College (Grand Rapids)	12	Aug	36	Dipl, BS	$24,106	$24,106					
Minnesota											
Gustavus Adolphus College (St Peter)	12	Aug	3	BA	$43,800	$43,800	total tuition			•	
Missouri											
Central Methodist Univ (Fayette)	24	Aug	36	BSAT	$19,900	$19,900					
New Jersey											
William Paterson Univ of New Jersey (Wayne)	40	Jan	20	Dipl, BS	$11,464	$18,628	per year	•		•	•
New York											
Ithaca College	35	Aug	48	BS						•	
North Carolina											
East Carolina Univ (Greenville)	30	Aug	36	BS	$5,400	$13,000		•		•	•
Greensboro College	15	Sophomore year	30	BS	$25,300	$25,300	per credit		•	•	
Lees-McRae College (Banner Elk)	32	Aug	24	BS							
Univ of North Carolina - Greensboro	10	Jun	24	MSAT							
North Dakota											
North Dakota State Univ (Fargo)	12	Aug	22	Dipl, MATrg							
Univ of North Dakota (Grand Forks)	15	Aug	34	BSAT	$7,092	$16,767					
Ohio											
Miami Univ (Oxford)	60	Aug	24	BS AT	$11,443	$26,202	per year				
Univ of Toledo	20	Aug	33	BS	$7,598	$16,718	per year				
Pennsylvania											
Temple Univ (Philadelphia)	25	Sep	36, 48	Dipl, BSAT	$15,710	$26,862	per year				
South Carolina											
Erskine College (Due West)	12	Sep	36	BS	$39,000	$39,000					
Tennessee											
Univ of Tennessee - Chattanooga	20	Jul	23	Dipl, MS	$3,896	$10,663				•	
Texas											
Texas Tech Univ Health Sciences Center (Lubbock)	30	Late May/early Jun	24	MAT	$9,946	$21,527					
Utah											
Southern Utah Univ (Cedar City)	24	Aug	48	Dipl, BS	$4,736	$13,846				•	
Virginia											
Longwood Univ (Farmville)	32	Aug	30	BS	$10,512	$22,032				•	
Roanoke College (Salem)	24	Jan	30	BS							
West Virginia											
Univ of Charleston	36	Aug	30	BS	$19,500	$19,500	per year			•	
West Virginia Wesleyan College (Buckhannon)	15	Aug	36	BSAT	$23,940	$23,940	per year				
Wisconsin											
Univ of Wisconsin - Oshkosh	42	Sep	32	BS						•	

*Data are shown only for programs that completed the 2011 AMA Survey of Health Professions Education Programs.

†Key to Offers: 1: Evening or weekend classes; 2: Non-English instruction; 3: Cultural competence instruction; 4: Distance education component.

Occupational Therapist

The practice of occupational therapy means the therapeutic use of occupations, including everyday life activities, with individuals, groups, populations, or organizations to support participation, performance, and function in roles and situations in home, school, workplace, community, and other settings. Occupational therapy services are for habilitation, rehabilitation, and promoting health and wellness to those who have or are at risk for developing an illness, injury, disease, disorder, condition, impairment, disability, activity limitation, or participation restriction. Occupational therapy addresses the physical, cognitive, psychosocial, sensory-perceptual, and other aspects of performance in a variety of contexts and environments to support engagement in occupations that affect physical and mental health, well-being, and quality of life.

History
Important dates in the development of the field of occupational therapy:

1917—Founding of the National Society for the Promotion of Occupational Therapy

1921—The name of the association changed to the American Occupational Therapy Association (AOTA)

1923—Accreditation of educational programs becomes a stated function of the AOTA, and basic educational standards are developed

1933—The AOTA approaches the American Medical Association (AMA) Council on Medical Education to request cooperation in developing and improving educational programs for occupational therapists

1935—*Essentials of an Acceptable School of Occupational Therapy* adopted by the AMA House of Delegates

1958—The AOTA assumes responsibility for approval of educational programs for the occupational therapy assistant.

1990—The AOTA petitions the AMA to include accreditation of occupational therapy assistant programs in its system

1994—The AOTA Accreditation Committee changes its name to the Accreditation Council for Occupational Therapy Education (ACOTE) and becomes operational as an accrediting agency independent of the AMA; 197 previously accredited/approved and developing occupational therapy and occupational therapy assistant educational programs are transferred into the ACOTE accreditation system

1997—ACOTE opens its accreditation process to occupational therapy programs located outside the United States; the following year, ACOTE accredits its first non-US program, Queen Margaret University College in Edinburgh, Scotland.

1999—ACOTE votes that professional entry-level occupational therapy programs must be offered at the postbaccalaureate level by January 1, 2007 to receive or maintain ACOTE accreditation status.

2006—ACOTE formally adopts new Accreditation Standards for Master's-Degree-Level Educational Programs for the Occupational Therapist and new Accreditation Standards for Educational Programs for the Occupational Therapy Assistant, as well as Accreditation Standards for a Doctoral-Degree-Level Educational Program for the Occupational Therapist, effective 2008.

2008—ACOTE votes that effective July 1, 2013, all occupational therapy assistant educational programs must be offered at the associate degree level in order to retain ACOTE accreditation.

Career Description
Occupational therapy services are based on evaluation and assessment methods, including making skilled observations and using standardized and nonstandardized tests and measurements to identify areas for occupational therapy services.

The practice of occupational therapy includes:

A. Evaluation of factors affecting activities of daily living (ADL), instrumental activities of daily living (IADL), rest and sleep, education, work, play, leisure, and social participation, including:
   1. Client factors, including body functions (such as neuromusculoskeletal, sensory and pain, visual, mental, perceptual, cognitive) and body structures (such as cardiovascular, digestive, nervous, integumentary, genitourinary systems, and structures related to movement), values, beliefs, and spirituality.
   2. Habits, routines, roles, rituals, and behavior patterns.
   3. Physical and social environments, as well as cultural, personal, temporal, and virtual contexts and activity demands that affect performance.
   4. Performance skills, including sensory perceptual, motor and praxis, emotional regulation, cognitive and communication, and social skills.

B. Methods or approaches selected to direct the process of interventions, such as:
   1. Establishment, remediation, or restoration of a skill or ability that has not yet developed, is impaired, or is in decline.
   2. Compensation, modification, or adaption of activity or environment to enhance performance, or to prevent injuries, disorders, or other conditions
   3. Retention and enhancing of skills and abilities without which performance in everyday life activities would decline.
   4. Promotion of health and wellness, including the use of self-management strategies, to enable or enhance performance in everyday life activities.
   5. Preventing barriers to performance and participation, including injury and disability prevention.

C. Interventions and procedures to promote or enhance safety and performance in activities of daily living (ADL), instrumental activities of daily living (IADL), rest and sleep, education, work, play, leisure, and social participation, including:
   1. Therapeutic use of occupations, exercises, and activities.
   2. Training in self-care, self-management, health management and maintenance, home management, community/work reintegration, and school activities and work performance.
   3. Development, remediation, or compensation of neuromusculoskeletal, sensory and pain, visual, mental, perceptual, and cognitive functions and behavioral skills.
   4. Therapeutic use of self, including one's personality, insights, perceptions, and judgments, as part of the therapeutic process.
   5. Education and training of individuals, including family members, caregivers, groups, populations, and others.
   6. Care coordination, case management, and transition services.
   7. Consultative services to groups, programs, organizations, or communities.

8. Modification of environments (home, work, school, or community) and adaptation of processes, including the application of ergonomic principles.

9. Assessment, design, fabrication, application, fitting, and training in seating and positioning, assistive technology, adaptive devices, and orthotic devices, and training in the use of prosthetic devices.

10. Assessment, recommendation, and training in techniques to enhance functional mobility, including management of wheelchairs and other mobility devices.

11. Low vision rehabilitation.

12. Driver rehabilitation and community mobility.

13. Management of feeding, eating, and swallowing to enable eating and feeding performance.

14. Application of physical agent modalities, and use of a range of specific therapeutic procedures (such as wound care management; interventions to enhance sensory, perceptual, and cognitive processing; and manual therapy) to enhance performance skills.

15. Facilitating the occupational performance of groups, populations, or organizations through the modification of environments and the adaptation of processes.

Employment Characteristics

The wide range of clients (individuals, organizations, and populations) served by occupational therapists is located in a variety of settings, such as hospitals, clinics, rehabilitation facilities, long-term care facilities, extended care facilities, private practices, schools, camps, the clients' own homes, and community agencies. Occupational therapists both receive referrals from and make referrals to the appropriate health, educational, or medical specialists.

Salary

The results of the 2010 AOTA Workforce Study show that the median annual salary for full-time occupational therapists was $64,722, with salaries ranging from a median of up to $90,000 in the 90th percentile to $45,000 in the 10th percentile. The median hourly wage for occupational therapists working a standard part-time schedule was $34. Compensation varied, the study noted, "according to total years in the profession, region of the country and location type (urban, suburban, or rural), highest degree held within the profession, primary work setting, AOTA membership status, and more."

Data from the US Bureau of Labor Statistics from May 2011 (available at *www.bls.gov/oes/current/oes291122.htm*) show that mean annual wages of occupational therapists were $74,970. The middle 50 percent earned $73,820. The lowest 10 percent earned $49,980, and the highest 10 percent earned $104,350. Mean annual wages in the industries employing the largest numbers of occupational therapists in May 2011 (from largest to smallest) were:

Offices of other health care practitioners	$76,190
General medical and surgical hospitals	$74,250
Elementary and secondary schools	$66,880
Nursing care facilities	$80,070
Home health care services	$85,540

For more information, refer to *www.ama-assn.org/go/hpsalary*.

Employment Outlook

Employment of occupational therapists is expected to increase by 33 percent between 2010 and 2020, much faster than the average for all occupations, according to the BLS. The increasing elderly population will drive growth in the demand for occupational therapy services. The demand for occupational therapists should continue to rise as a result of the increasing number of individuals with disabilities or limited function who require therapy services.

Educational Programs

Length. Programs at the combined baccalaureate/master's level entail four to five years of college or university preparation.

Postbaccalaureate programs leading to a master's degree are generally two to two-and-a-half years, and programs leading to a doctoral degree are generally two to three years. Following completion of all educational requirements, individuals take a national certification examination. All states also regulate the practice of occupational therapy.

Prerequisites. Prerequisites vary among programs. A baccalaureate degree is a prerequisite for most master's and all doctoral-level occupational therapy programs. A strong foundation of liberal arts and biological, physical, social, and behavioral sciences may be prerequisite to, or concurrent with, the professional education of the program curriculum.

Curriculum. Curricula of accredited occupational therapy programs are required to include the following:

- A broad foundation in the liberal arts and sciences
- Basic tenets of occupational therapy
- Occupational therapy theoretical perspectives
- The process of screening and evaluation
- The process of formulating and implementing an intervention plan
- Context of service delivery
- Management of occupational therapy services
- Use of research
- Professional ethics, values, and responsibilities
- Twenty-four weeks of fieldwork education

Doctoral-level programs have additional content requirements and an experiential component to provide students with an in-depth experience in one or more of the following:

- Clinical practice skills
- Research skills
- Administration
- Leadership
- Program and policy development
- Advocacy
- Education
- Theory development

Licensure, Registration, Certification

All states, Puerto Rico, Guam, and the District of Columbia regulate the practice of occupational therapy. Different states have various types of regulation that range from licensure, the strongest form of regulation, to title protection or trademark law, the weakest. To obtain a license, applicants must graduate from an accredited occupational therapy educational program and pass a national certification examination for occupational therapists. Those who pass the exam are awarded the title "Occupational Therapist Registered (OTR)." Some states have additional requirements for therapists who work in schools or early intervention programs. These requirements may include education-related classes, an education practice certificate, or early intervention certification requirements.

Inquiries

Careers Education
American Occupational Therapy Association
4720 Montgomery Lane
PO Box 31220
Bethesda, MD 20824-1220
301 652-2682
www.aota.org

Certification
National Board for Certification in Occupational Therapy (NBCOT)
12 South Summit Avenue, Suite 100
Gaithersburg, MD 20877-4150
301 990-7979
www.nbcot.org

Program Accreditation
Accreditation Council for Occupational Therapy Education
4720 Montgomery Lane, PO Box 31220
Bethesda, MD 20824-1220
301 652-2682
www.acoteonline.org

Note: Adapted in part from the Bureau of Labor Statistics, US Department of Labor, *Occupational Outlook Handbook,* Occupational Therapists, at *www.bls.gov/oco/ocos078.htm.*

Occupational Therapist

Alabama

University of Alabama at Birmingham
Occupational Therapy Prgm
School of Health Professions
1530 3rd Ave S, RMSB 355
Birmingham, AL 35294-1212
www.uab.edu

University of South Alabama
Occupational Therapy Prgm
Department of Occupational Therapy
5721 USA Drive North, HAHN Room 2027
Mobile, AL 36688-0002
www.southalabama.edu/alliedhealth/ot/

Alabama State University
Occupational Therapy Prgm
915 S Jackson St
PO Box 271
Montgomery, AL 36101-0271
www.alasu.edu

Tuskegee University
Occupational Therapy Prgm
Sch of Nurs & Allied Health
71-265 John A Kenney Hall, Bioethics Bldg
Tuskegee, AL 36088-1696
www.tuskegee.edu/ot
Prgm Dir: Gwendolyn Gray, Professor OT
Tel: 334 727-8695 *Fax:* 334 727-8259
E-mail: grayg@mytu.tuskegee.edu

Alaska

Creighton University University of Alaska Anchorage
Occupational Therapy Prgm
3211 Providence Drive
Anchorage, AK 99508
http://spahp2.creighton.edu/offices/occupationaltherapy
/welcome.aspx

Arizona

Midwestern University - Glendale Campus
Occupational Therapy Prgm
19555 N 59th Ave
Glendale, AZ 85308-6814
www.midwestern.edu

AT Still University of Health Sciences Arizona School of Health Sciences
Occupational Therapy Prgm
5850 E Still Circle
Mesa, AZ 85206-3618
www.atsu.edu/ashs/

Arkansas

University of Central Arkansas
Occupational Therapy Prgm
201 Donaghey Ave HSC, Ste 300, Box 5001
Conway, AR 72035-0001
www.uca.edu/ot
Prgm Dir: Linda D Musselman, PhD OTR FAOTA
Tel: 501 450-5017 *Fax:* 501 450-5568
E-mail: lmusselman@uca.edu

California

California State University - Dominguez Hills
Occupational Therapy Prgm
1000 E Victoria Blvd, Welch Hall a 320 D
Carson, CA 90747-0005
www.csudh.edu/hhs/dhs/ot
Prgm Dir: Terry Peralta-Catipon, PhD OTR/L
Tel: 310 243-2812 *Fax:* 310 516-3542
E-mail: tperalta@csudh.edu

Loma Linda University
Occupational Therapy Prgm
Sch of Allied Health Professions
Nichol Hall, Rm A901
Loma Linda, CA 92350-0001
www.llu.edu

University of Southern California
Occupational Therapy Prgm
1540 Alcazar St, CHP 133
Los Angeles, CA 90089-9003
www.usc.edu/ot

Samuel Merritt University
Occupational Therapy Prgm
450 30th St, 4th Fl
Oakland, CA 94609-3302
www.samuelmerritt.edu

San Jose State University
Occupational Therapy Prgm
Coll of Applied Sciences and Arts
One Washington Square
San Jose, CA 95192-0059
www.sjsu.edu/occupationaltherapy
Prgm Dir: Heidi McHugh Pendleton, PhD OTR/L FAOTA
Tel: 408 924-3072 *Fax:* 408 924-3088
E-mail: heidi.pendleton@sjsu.edu

Univ of St Augustine for Health Sciences - San Diego Campus
Occupational Therapy Prgm
700 Windy Point Drive
San Marcos, CA 92069
www.usa.edu

Dominican University of California
Occupational Therapy Prgm
50 Acacia Ave
San Rafael, CA 94901-2298
www.dominican.edu

Colorado

Colorado State University
Occupational Therapy Prgm
219 Occupational Therapy Bldg
Fort Collins, CO 80523-1573
www.ot.cahs.colostate.edu

Connecticut

Sacred Heart University
Occupational Therapy Prgm
5151 Park Ave
Fairfield, CT 06825-1000
www.sacredheart.edu

Quinnipiac University
Occupational Therapy Prgm
Sch of Health Sciences
275 Mt Carmel Ave, N1 - HSC
Hamden, CT 06518-0569
www.quinnipiac.edu

District of Columbia

Howard University
Occupational Therapy Prgm
Division of Allied Health Sciences
516 and Bryant Sts NW, Annex I, RM 369
Washington, DC 20059-0001
www.howard.edu

Florida

Nova Southeastern University
Occupational Therapy Prgm
Occupational Therapy Department
Health Profs Div, Coll of Allied Health and Nursing
3200 S University Dr
Fort Lauderdale, FL 33328-2018
www.nova.edu/ot

Florida Gulf Coast University
Occupational Therapy Prgm
10501 FGCU Blvd South
Fort Myers, FL 33965-6565
www.fgcu.edu/CHP/OT/otmsel/index.html
Prgm Dir: Linda Martin, PhD OTR/L FAOTA
Tel: 239 590-7556   *Fax:* 239 590-7460
E-mail: lmartin@fgcu.edu

University of Florida
Occupational Therapy Prgm
101 S Newell Dr
PO Box 100164 HSC
Gainesville, FL 32611
www.ot.phhp.ufl.edu

Florida International University
Occupational Therapy Prgm
University Park Campus, NHS 442A
11200 SW 8 St
Miami, FL 33199
Prgm Dir: Kinsuk Maitra, PhD OTR/L
Tel: 305 348-2264   *Fax:* 305 348-1240
E-mail: kinsuk.maitra@fiu.edu

Barry University
Occupational Therapy Prgm
11300 NE 2nd Ave
Miami Shores, FL 33161-6695
www.barry.edu

Univ of St Augustine for Health Sciences
Occupational Therapy Prgm
Institute of Occupational Therapy
1 University Blvd
St. Augustine, FL 32086-5783
www.usa.edu

Florida A&M University
Occupational Therapy Prgm
Lewis-Beck Building
Rm 318
Tallahassee, FL 32307-3500

Georgia

Georgia Health Sciences University
Occupational Therapy Prgm
987 St Sebastian Way
EC - 2304A
Augusta, GA 30912-0700
www.mcg.edu/sah/ot/index.html

Brenau University
Occupational Therapy Prgm
500 Washington SE
Gainesville, GA 30501
www.brenau.edu/shs/ot

Brenau University - Atlanta Campus
Occupational Therapy Prgm
School of Occupational Therapy
3139 Campus Dr # 300
Norcross, GA 30071
www.brenau.edu/home/?page_id=1638

Idaho

Idaho State University
Occupational Therapy Prgm
Campus Box 8045
Pocatello, ID 83209-8045
www.isu.edu

Illinois

Chicago State University
Occupational Therapy Prgm
9501 S King Dr, Library, Rm 132
Chicago, IL 60628-1598
www.csu.edu

Rush University
Occupational Therapy Prgm
600 S Paulina, Ste 1010
Chicago, IL 60612-3833
www.rushu.rush.edu/occuth

University of Illinois at Chicago
Occupational Therapy Prgm
1919 W Taylor St M/C 811
Chicago, IL 60612-7250
www.ahs.uic.edu/ot

Midwestern University
Occupational Therapy Prgm
College of Health Sciences
555 31st St
Downers Grove, IL 60515-1235
www.midwestern.edu

Governors State University
Occupational Therapy Prgm
College of Health Professions
University Parkway, IL 60484-0975

Indiana

University of Southern Indiana
Occupational Therapy Prgm
8600 University Blvd, HP
Evansville, IN 47712-3534
http://health.usi.edu/acadprog/ot/default.asp

Indiana University
Occupational Therapy Prgm
School of Health and Rehabilitation Sciences
1140 W Michigan St, Coleman Hall 311
Indianapolis, IN 46202-5119
www.iupui.edu
Prgm Dir: Thomas F Fisher, PhD OTR CCM FAOTA
Tel: 317 274-8006   *Fax:* 317 274-2150
E-mail: fishert@iupui.edu

University of Indianapolis
Occupational Therapy Prgm
1400 East Hanna Ave
Indianapolis, IN 46227-3697
http://ot.uindy.edu
Prgm Dir: Kate DeCleene, Director of Occupational
   Therapy
Tel: 317 788-3432   *Fax:* 317 788-3542
E-mail: decleenek@uindy.edu

Iowa

St Ambrose University
Occupational Therapy Prgm
1320 West Lombard
Davenport, IA 52804
www.sau.edu

Kansas

**University of Kansas Medical Center School of
   Health Professions**
Occupational Therapy Prgm
3033 Robinson, Mail Stop 2003
3901 Rainbow Blvd
Kansas City, KS 66160-7602
alliedhealth.kumc.edu/programs/ot
Prgm Dir: Winnie Dunn, PhD OTR FAOTA
Tel: 913 588-7195   *Fax:* 913 588-4568
E-mail: wdunn@kumc.edu

Kentucky

Spalding University
Occupational Therapy Prgm
845 S Third St
Louisville, KY 40203-2188
www.spalding.edu

Eastern Kentucky University
Occupational Therapy Prgm
Department of Occupational Therapy
Dizney 103
Richmond, KY 40475-3135
www.health.eku.edu/ots

Louisiana

**Louisiana State Univ Health Sciences Center -
   New Orleans Campus**
Occupational Therapy Prgm
Sch of Allied Health Professions
1900 Gravier St
New Orleans, LA 70112
http://alliedhealth.lsuhsc.edu/OccupationalTherapy/

**LSU Health Science Center Shreveport -
   Shreveport Campus**
Occupational Therapy Prgm
1501 Kings Hwy
Shreveport, LA 71130-3932

Maine

Husson University
Occupational Therapy Prgm
1 College Circle
3rd Floor Commons
Bangor, ME 04401-2999
health.husson.edu/ot/

**University of Southern Maine at
   Lewiston-Auburn College**
Occupational Therapy Prgm
51 Westminster St
Lewiston, ME 04240-3534
www.usm.maine.edu/lac/mot

University of New England
Occupational Therapy Prgm
11 Hills Beach Rd
Portland, ME 04103

Maryland

Towson University
Occupational Therapy Prgm
8000 York Rd
Towson, MD 21252-0001
www.towson.edu/ot

Massachusetts

Boston University Sargent College
Occupational Therapy Prgm
635 Commonwealth Ave
Boston, MA 02215-1605
www.bu.edu

Bay Path College
Occupational Therapy Prgm
588 Longmeadow St
Longmeadow, MA 01106-2212
www.baypath.edu

Tufts University
Occupational Therapy Prgm
Department of Occupational Therapy
26 Winthrop St
Medford, MA 02155-7084
ase.tufts.edu/bsot
Prgm Dir: Linda Tickle-Degnen, PhD OTR/L FAOTA
Tel: 617 627-5863   *Fax:* 617 627-3722
E-mail: Linda.Tickle_Degnen@tufts.edu

Salem State University
Occupational Therapy Prgm
352 Lafayette St
Salem, MA 01970-5353
www.salemstate.edu
Notes: Unique part-time evening OT Program for OT
Assistants to return to school to obtain a combined
BS/MS degree in OT.

American International College
Occupational Therapy Prgm
1000 State St
Springfield, MA 01109-3189
www.aic.edu/pages/1.html

Springfield College
Occupational Therapy Prgm
263 Alden St
Springfield, MA 01109-3797
www.springfieldcollege.edu/ot

Worcester State College
Occupational Therapy Prgm
486 Chandler St
Worcester, MA 01602-2597

Michigan

Wayne State University
Occupational Therapy Prgm
Eugene Applebaum College of Pharmacy and Health
Sciences
259 Mack Ave
Detroit, MI 48202-3489
www.wayne.edu

Baker College Center of Graduate Studies
Occupational Therapy Prgm
1116 W Bristol Rd
Flint, MI 48507-5508
www.baker.edu

Grand Valley State University
Occupational Therapy Prgm
College of Health Professions
301 Michigan St NE, Suite 200
Grand Rapids, MI 49503-3314
www.gvsu.edu/ot

**Western Michigan University - Grand Rapids
Campus**
Occupational Therapy Prgm
Department of Occupational Therapy
200 Ionia Ave, SW
Grand Rapids, MI 49503
www.wmich.edu/grandrapids/program/
18-Occupational_Therapy_MS.html

Western Michigan University
Occupational Therapy Prgm
1903 West Michigan Ave
Kalamazoo, MI 49008-5333
www.wmich.edu/hhs/ot
Prgm Dir: Joseph M Pellerito, PhD OTR
Tel: 269 387-7263 *Fax:* 269 387-7262
E-mail: joseph.m.pellerito@wmich.edu

Saginaw Valley State University
Occupational Therapy Prgm
Wickes 280
7400 Bay Rd
University Center, MI 48710-0001
www.svsu.edu

Eastern Michigan University
Occupational Therapy Prgm
School of Health Sciences
Marshall Bldg, Room 353
Ypsilanti, MI 48197-2239
www.emich.edu

Minnesota

College of St Scholastica
Occupational Therapy Prgm
1200 Kenwood Ave
Duluth, MN 55811-4199
www.css.edu

University of Minnesota
Occupational Therapy Prgm
MMC 368
420 Delaware St SE
Minneapolis, MN 55455-0392
www.ot.umn.edu

University of Minnesota - Rochester Campus
Occupational Therapy Prgm
Center for Allied Health Programs
300 University Square, R0869A, 111 South Broadway
Rochester, MN 55904
www.ot.umn.edu

Saint Catherine University
Occupational Therapy Prgm
2004 Randolph Ave, Mail #4141
St Paul, MN 55105-1794
www.stkate.edu/academic/maot/

Mississippi

University of Mississippi Medical Center
Occupational Therapy Prgm
2500 N State St
Jackson, MS 39216-4505
www.shrp.umsmed.edu

Missouri

University of Missouri
Occupational Therapy Prgm
510 Lewis Hall
Columbia, MO 65211-4240
www.umshp.org/ot

Rockhurst University
Occupational Therapy Prgm
1100 Rockhurst Rd
Kansas City, MO 64110-2561
www.rockhurst.edu/academic/ot

Maryville University
Occupational Therapy Prgm
650 Maryville University Dr
St Louis, MO 63141

Saint Louis University
Occupational Therapy Prgm
Doisy College of Health Sciences
3437 Caroline St, Rm 2020
St Louis, MO 63104-1111
www.slu.edu/x2400.xml

Washington University
Occupational Therapy Prgm
4444 Forest Park Ave
Campus Box 8505
St Louis, MO 63108
ot.wustl.edu
Prgm Dir: M Carolyn Baum, PhD OTR/L FAOTA
Tel: 314 286-1600 *Fax:* 314 286-1601
E-mail: baumc@wusm.wustl.edu

Nebraska

College of Saint Mary
Occupational Therapy Prgm
7000 Mercy Rd
Omaha, NE 68106-2606
www.csm.edu

Creighton University
Occupational Therapy Prgm
School of Pharmacy and Health Professions
2500 California Plaza
Omaha, NE 68178-0259
http://ot.creigton.edu

Nevada

Touro University - Nevada
Occupational Therapy Prgm
874 American Pacific Dr
Henderson, NV 89014
www.tun.touro.edu

New Hampshire

University of New Hampshire
Occupational Therapy Prgm
College of Health and Human Services
Hewitt Hall, 4 Library Way
Durham, NH 03824-3563

New Jersey

Richard Stockton College of New Jersey
Occupational Therapy Prgm
PO Box 195
Jim Leeds Rd
Calloway, NJ 08205
www.stockton.edu

Kean University
Occupational Therapy Prgm
1000 Morris Ave
PO Box 411
T-209
Hillside, NJ 07205
www.kean.edu/~ot
Prgm Dir: Laurie Knis-Matthews, PhD OT
Tel: 908 737-3379 *Fax:* 908 737-3377
E-mail: lknis@kean.edu

Seton Hall University
Occupational Therapy Prgm
School of Health and Medical Sciences
McQuaid Hall
400 S Orange Ave
South Orange, NJ 07079-2689
www.shu.edu/academics/gradmeded/
ms-occupational-therapy/

New Mexico

University of New Mexico
Occupational Therapy Prgm
School of Medicine
Health Science & Service Bldg MSC09 5240
1 University of New Mexico
Albuquerque, NM 87131-0001
http://hsc.unm.edu/som/ot/

Western New Mexico University
Occupational Therapy Prgm
Master's of Occupational Therapy Program
Allied Health
PO Box 680
Silver City, NM 88062-0680
www.wnmu.edu/academic/allied/ot/MOTWelcome.shtml

New York

Touro College - Bay Shore
Occupational Therapy Prgm
1700 Union Blvd
Bay Shore, NY 11706-7928
www.touro.edu

Long Island University - Brooklyn Campus
Occupational Therapy Prgm
One University Plaza
Brooklyn, NY 11201-5372
www.brooklyn.liu.edu/health/bsmsoccthe.html

SUNY Downstate Medical Center
Occupational Therapy Prgm
Coll of Health Related Professions
450 Clarkson Ave Box 81
Brooklyn, NY 11203-2098
www.downstate.edu/chrp/ot
Prgm Dir: Joyce Sabari, PhD OTR FAOTA
Tel: 718 270-7731   *Fax:* 718 270-7464
E-mail: joyce.sabari@downstate.edu

D'Youville College
Occupational Therapy Prgm
One D'Youville Square, 320 Porter Ave
Buffalo, NY 14201-1084
www.dyc.edu
Prgm Dir: Amy J Nwora, PhD OT
Tel: 716 829-7707   *Fax:* 716 829-8137
E-mail: nworaa@dyc.edu

University at Buffalo - SUNY
Occupational Therapy Prgm
501 Stockton Kimball Tower
3435 Main St
Buffalo, NY 14214-3079
phhp.buffalo.edu/rs/ot
Prgm Dir: Susan M Nochajski, PhD OTR
Tel: 716 829-6942   *Fax:* 716 829-3217
E-mail: nochajsk@buffalo.edu

Mercy College
Occupational Therapy Prgm
555 Broadway
Dobbs Ferry, NY 10522-1134
www.mercy.edu/acadivisions/healthprofessions/grad/
   occupational_therapy.cfm
Prgm Dir: Joan Toglia, PhD OTR
Tel: 914 674-7815   *Fax:* 914 674-7840
E-mail: jtoglia@mercy.edu

Ithaca College
Occupational Therapy Prgm
206 Smiddy Hall
Ithaca, NY 14850-7079
www.ithaca.edu/hshp/ot

York College, CUNY
Occupational Therapy Prgm
94-20 Guy R Brewer Blvd
Jamaica, NY 11451-9902
www.york.cuny.edu

Keuka College
Occupational Therapy Prgm
Division of Occupational Therapy
Keuka Park, NY 14478-0098
http://academics.keuka.edu/academics/programs/
   occupational_sciences

Columbia University
Occupational Therapy Prgm
Neurological Institute 8th Fl
710 W 168th St
New York, NY 10032-2603
www.columbiaot.org

New York University
Occupational Therapy Prgm
Steinhardt School of Culture, Education & Human
   Development
35 W 4th St, 11th Fl
New York, NY 10012-1172
www.steinhardt.nyu.edu/ot
Prgm Dir: Jane Bear-Lehman, PhD OTR FAOTA
Tel: 212 998-5825   *Fax:* 212 995-4044
E-mail: jbl285@nyu.edu

Touro College - Manhattan
Occupational Therapy Prgm
27-33 W 23rd St
New York, NY 10010
www.touro.edu

New York Institute of Technology
Occupational Therapy Prgm
Department of Occupational Therapy
PO Box 8000
Old Westbury, NY 11568-8000
www.nyit.edu

Dominican College
Occupational Therapy Prgm
470 Western Hwy
Orangeburg, NY 10962-1299
www.dc.edu
Prgm Dir: Sandra F Countee, PhD OTR/L
Tel: 845 848-6039, Ext   *Fax:* 845 398-4893
E-mail: sandra.countee@dc.edu

Stony Brook University
Occupational Therapy Prgm
Sch of Health Tech and Management
Div of Rehabilitation Sciences
Stony Brook, NY 11794-8206
www.sunysb.edu

The Sage Colleges
Occupational Therapy Prgm
65 First St
Troy, NY 12180-4115
www.sage.edu/ot

Utica College
Occupational Therapy Prgm
1600 Burrstone Rd
Utica, NY 13502-4892
www.utica.edu

North Carolina

University of North Carolina - Chapel Hill
Occupational Therapy Prgm
Ste 2050 Bondurant Hall, 301A S Columbia St
CB 7122
Chapel Hill, NC 27599-7122
www.alliedhealth.unc.edu/ocsci

East Carolina University
Occupational Therapy Prgm
College of Allied Hlth Sciences
3305 Health Sciences Building
Greenville, NC 27858-4353
www.ecu.edu/ot

Lenoir - Rhyne University
Occupational Therapy Prgm
Box 7547
Hickory, NC 28603-7547
www.lrc.edu/ot

Winston-Salem State University
Occupational Therapy Prgm
School of Health Sciences
601 Martin Luther King Jr Dr
432 F L Atkins Bldg
Winston-Salem, NC 27110-0003
www.wssu.edu

North Dakota

University of Mary
Occupational Therapy Prgm
7500 University Dr
Bismarck, ND 58504-9652
www.umary.edu
Prgm Dir: Janeene Sibla, OTD MS OTR/L
Tel: 701 255-7500, Ext   *Fax:* 701 255-7687
E-mail: jsibla@umary.edu

University of North Dakota
Occupational Therapy Prgm
Hyslop 210
2751 2nd Ave N Stop 7126
Grand Forks, ND 58202-7126

Ohio

Xavier University
Occupational Therapy Prgm
3800 Victory Pkwy
Cincinnati, OH 45207-7341

Cleveland State University
Occupational Therapy Prgm
2121 Euclid Ave
Health Sciences (HS) 101
Cleveland, OH 44115-2440
www.csuohio.edu/sciences/dept/healthsciences/
   graduate/MOT
Prgm Dir: Glenn Goodman, PhD OTR/L
Tel: 216 687-2493   *Fax:* 216 687-9316
E-mail: g.goodman@csuohio.edu

The Ohio State University
Occupational Therapy Prgm
453 West 10th St
406 Atwell Hall
Columbus, OH 43210-1234
www.amp.osu.edu/ot

The University of Findlay
Occupational Therapy Prgm
1000 N Main St
323 College St
Findlay, OH 45840-3695
www.findlay.edu

Shawnee State University
Occupational Therapy Prgm
940 Second St
Portsmouth, OH 45662-4303
www.shawnee.edu

University of Toledo
Occupational Therapy Prgm
2801 Bancroft St
Mail Stop 119
Toledo, OH 43606-3390
www.utoledo.edu/hshs/ot

Oklahoma

Univ of Oklahoma Health Sciences Center
Occupational Therapy Prgm
1200 N Stonewall
Room 3096
Oklahoma City, OK 73117
w3.ouhsc.edu/rehab
Prgm Dir: Cyndy Robinson, MS OTR/L
Tel: 405 271-2131, Ext   *Fax:* 405 271-2432
E-mail: cyndy-robinson@ouhsc.edu

**Univ of Oklahoma Health Sciences Center -
   Tulsa**
Cosponsor: Univ of Oklahoma at Schusterman
Occupational Therapy Prgm
4502 E 41st St
Tulsa, OK 74135-2512
http://w3.ouhsc.edu/rehab

Oregon

Pacific University
Occupational Therapy Prgm
190 SE 8th Ave, Suite 360
Hillsboro, OR 97123-4216
www.pacificu.edu/ot

Pennsylvania

Misericordia University
Occupational Therapy Prgm
Division of Health Sciences
301 Lake St
Dallas, PA 18612-1098
www.misericordia.edu
Prgm Dir: Grace S Fisher, EdD OTR/L
Tel: 570 674-8015   *Fax:* 570 674-3052
E-mail: gfisher@misericordia.edu

Elizabethtown College
Occupational Therapy Prgm
One Alpha Dr
Elizabethtown, PA 17022-2298
www.etown.edu

Gannon University
Occupational Therapy Prgm
109 University Square
Erie, PA 16541-0001

St Francis University
Occupational Therapy Prgm
PO Box 600
Loretto, PA 15940-0600
www.francis.edu

Philadelphia University
Occupational Therapy Prgm
School House Ln and Henry Ave
Philadelphia, PA 19144-5497
www.philau.edu/ot

Temple University
Occupational Therapy Prgm
College of Health Professions
3307 N Broad St
Philadelphia, PA 19140-5101
www.temple.edu/ot

Thomas Jefferson University
Occupational Therapy Prgm
Jefferson College of Health Professions
130 S Ninth St, Rm 810, Edison Bldg
Philadelphia, PA 19107-5233
www.jefferson.edu/main

University of the Sciences
Occupational Therapy Prgm
600 S 43rd St, Box 24
Philadelphia, PA 19104-4495
www.usp.edu

Chatham University
Occupational Therapy Prgm
Woodland Rd
Pittsburgh, PA 15232-2826
www.chatham.edu/ot

Duquesne University
Occupational Therapy Prgm
Department of Occupational Therapy
Rangos School of Health Sciences Bldg
Rm 234, 600 Forbes Ave
Pittsburgh, PA 15282
www.healthsciences.duq.edu/ot/othome.html

University of Pittsburgh
Occupational Therapy Prgm
School of Health and Rehabilitation Sciences
5012 Forbes Tower
Pittsburgh, PA 15260
www.shrs.pitt.edu/mot

Alvernia University
Occupational Therapy Prgm
400 St Bernardine St, BH 112-3
Reading, PA 19607-1799
www.alvernia.edu

University of Scranton
Occupational Therapy Prgm
Leahy Hall
800 Linden St
Scranton, PA 18510-4501
www.scranton.edu
Prgm Dir: Marlene J Morgan, EdD OTR/L
Tel: 570 941-4125   *Fax:* 570 941-4380
E-mail: morganm8@Scranton.edu

Puerto Rico

University of Puerto Rico
Occupational Therapy Prgm
Medical Sciences Campus-SHP
PO Box 365067
San Juan, PR 00936-5067
www.eps.rcm.upr.edu
Prgm Dir: Wanda I Colon, PhD OTR/L
Tel: 787 758-2525, Ext   *Fax:* 787 282-8174
E-mail: wanda.colon4@upr.edu

South Carolina

Medical University of South Carolina
Occupational Therapy Prgm
College of Health Professions
151B Rutledge Ave MSC 962
Charleston, SC 29425-9620
www.musc.edu/chp/ot

South Dakota

University of South Dakota
Occupational Therapy Prgm
414 E Clark St
Vermillion, SD 57069-2390

Tennessee

University of Tennessee Health Science Ctr
Occupational Therapy Prgm
College of Allied Health
930 Madison Ave, Suite 616
Memphis, TN 38163-0002
www.uthsc.edu/allied/ot

Milligan College
Occupational Therapy Prgm
PO Box 130
Milligan College, TN 37682
www.milligan.edu/msot/
Prgm Dir: Jeff Snodgrass, PhD MPH OTR
Tel: 423 975-8010   *Fax:* 423 975-8019
E-mail: jsnodgrass@milligan.edu

Belmont University
Occupational Therapy Prgm
School of Occupational Therapy
1900 Belmont Blvd
Nashville, TN 37212-3757
www.belmont.edu/ot
Prgm Dir: Scott McPhee, Assoc Dean
Tel: 615 460-6700   *Fax:* 615 460-6475
E-mail: scott.mcphee@belmont.edu

Tennessee State University
Occupational Therapy Prgm
College of Health Sciences
3500 John A Merritt Blvd
Nashville, TN 37209-1561
www.tnstate.edu/ot

Texas

Texas Woman's University - Dallas
Occupational Therapy Prgm
8194 Walnut Hill Lane
Dallas, TX 75231
www.twu.edu/ot

Texas Woman's University
Occupational Therapy Prgm
PO Box 425648
Denton, TX 76204-5648
www.twu.edu/ot

Univ of Texas - Pan American
Occupational Therapy Prgm
1201 W University Dr
HSHE 1.130
Edinburg, TX 78539-2999
www.utpa.edu
Prgm Dir: Shirley A Wells, MPH OTR FAOTA
Tel: 956 665-2475   *Fax:* 956 665-2476
E-mail: wellssa@utpa.edu

University of Texas at El Paso
Occupational Therapy Prgm
1101 N Campbell St
El Paso, TX 79968
www.utep.edu

University of Texas Medical Branch
Occupational Therapy Prgm
301 University Blvd
Galveston, TX 77555-1142
www.sahs.utmb.edu/programs/ot
Prgm Dir: Gretchen V M Stone, PhD OT FAOTA
Tel: 409 747-3060   *Fax:* 409 747-1615
E-mail: grstone@utmb.edu

Texas Woman's University - Denton
Occupational Therapy Prgm
1130 John Freeman Blvd
Houston, TX 77030
www.twu.edu/ot
Notes: Two satellite programs (Dallas and Houston)

Texas Tech Univ Health Sciences Center
Occupational Therapy Prgm
3601 4th St, Stop 6220
Lubbock, TX 79430-6220
www.ttuhsc.edu

UT Health Science Center - San Antonio
Occupational Therapy Prgm
Department of Occupational Therapy
7703 Floyd Curl Dr
San Antonio, TX 78229-3900
www.uthscsa.edu/shp/ot
Prgm Dir: Karin J Barnes, PhD OTR
Tel: 210 567-8890   *Fax:* 210 567-8893
E-mail: barnesk@uthscsa.edu
Notes: Currently inactive

Utah

University of Utah
Occupational Therapy Prgm
520 Wakara Way
Salt Lake City, UT 84108-1290
www.health.utah.edu/ot
Prgm Dir: Lorie Richards, PhD OTR/L
Tel: 801 585-1069   *Fax:* 801 585-1001
E-mail: lorie.richards@hsc.utah.edu

Virginia

James Madison University
Occupational Therapy Prgm
Department of Health Sciences
Coll of Integrated Sci & Tech, MSC 4301
Harrisonburg, VA 22807-0001

Radford University
Occupational Therapy Prgm
Department of Occupational Therapy
PO Box 6985
Radford, VA 24142-6985
http://radford.edu/ot

Virginia Commonwealth University
Occupational Therapy Prgm
PO Box 980008
730 E Broad St, Suite 2050
Suite 2050
Richmond, VA 23298-0008
www.sahp.vcu.edu/occu

Jefferson College of Health Sciences
Occupational Therapy Prgm
920 S Jefferson St
Roanoke, VA 24013-2222

Shenandoah University
Occupational Therapy Prgm
333 W Cork St, 5th Fl
Suite 510
Winchester, VA 22601-5195
www.su.edu/ot

Washington

University of Washington
Occupational Therapy Prgm
Department of Rehabilitation Medicine
Box 356490
Seattle, WA 98195-6490
http://depts.washington.edu/rehab/ot/

Eastern Washington University
Occupational Therapy Prgm
310 N Riverpoint Blvd
Box R
Spokane, WA 99202
www.ewu.edu/ot

University of Puget Sound
Occupational Therapy Prgm
School of Occupational Therapy
1500 N Warner St #1070
Tacoma, WA 98416-0510
www.pugetsound.edu/ot
Prgm Dir: Yvonne Swinth, PhD OTR/L
Tel: 253 879-3289   *Fax:* 253 879-2933
E-mail: yswinth@pugetsound.edu

West Virginia

West Virginia University
Occupational Therapy Prgm
School of Medicine, Robert C Byrd Health Sciences
  Center
PO Box 9139
Morgantown, WV 26506-9139
www.hsc.wvu.edu/som/ot

Wisconsin

University of Wisconsin - La Crosse
Occupational Therapy Prgm
4031 Health Science Ctr
1725 State St
La Crosse, WI 54601-9959
www.uwlax.edu/ot

University of Wisconsin - Madison
Occupational Therapy Prgm
1300 University Ave, 2110 MSC
Madison, WI 53706-1532
www.soemadison.wisc.edu/kinesiology/

Concordia University Wisconsin
Occupational Therapy Prgm
12800 N Lake Shore Dr
Mequon, WI 53097-2418
www.cuw.edu/ot

Mount Mary College
Occupational Therapy Prgm
2900 N Menomonee River Pkwy
Milwaukee, WI 53222-4597
www.mtmary.edu/ot.htm

University of Wisconsin - Milwaukee
Occupational Therapy Prgm
College of Health Sciences
PO Box 413
Milwaukee, WI 53201-0413
www.uwm.edu/CHS

Wyoming

University of North Dakota at Casper College
Occupational Therapy Prgm
LS 102
125 College Drive
Casper, WY 82601
Prgm Dir: Janet S Jedlicka, PhD OTR/L FAOTA
Tel: 701 777-2209   *Fax:* 701 777-2212
E-mail: Janet.jedlicka@med.und.edu

Occupational Therapist

Programs*	Class Capacity	Begins	Length (months)	Award	Res. Tuition	Non-res. Tuition		Offers:† 1	2	3	4
Alabama											
Tuskegee Univ	20+	Aug	24	MOT	$32,640	$40,590	per year			•	•
Arkansas											
Univ of Central Arkansas (Conway)	48	May	61	BS, MS	$7,183	$12,569				•	•
California											
California State Univ - Dominguez Hills (Carson)	70	Jan	29	MSOT	$11,000	$29,000	per credit			•	
San Jose State Univ	40	Aug	36, 25	BS, MS	$6,800					•	•
Florida											
Florida Gulf Coast Univ (Fort Myers)	32	Aug	23	MS	$10,879	$37,925				•	
Florida International Univ (Miami)	40	Aug	39, 27	MS	$16,000	$36,000				•	
Indiana											
Indiana Univ (Indianapolis)	36	Summer II	24	MS	$15,864	$31,728				•	
Univ of Indianapolis	54	Aug	30	MOT	$23,770	$23,770	per year			•	
Kansas											
Univ of Kansas Medical Center School of Health Professions (Kansas City)	34	Jun	36, 45	BS, OTD	$4,000	$9,000	per year				
Massachusetts											
Tufts Univ (Medford)	45	Sep	24	Dipl, Cert, MS, OTD	$21,428	$21,428	per year			•	
Michigan											
Western Michigan Univ (Kalamazoo)	96	Sep Jan	28	BS/MS						•	
Missouri											
Washington Univ (St Louis)	80	Aug	28, 40	Dipl, MSOT, OTD	$40,000	$40,000				•	
New Jersey											
Kean Univ (Hillside)	35	Sep	30	MS, BA/MS						•	
New York											
Dominican College (Orangeburg)	32	Sep	24, 36	BS/MS	$18,900	$18,900	per year	•		•	•
D'Youville College (Buffalo)	215	Aug	58, 34	BS MS	$21,450	$21,450				•	
Mercy College (Dobbs Ferry)	35	Sep	28	MS	$24,750	$24,750		•		•	
New York Univ	50	Sep	27, 48	MS							
SUNY Downstate Medical Center (Brooklyn)	32	Jun 2	30	Dipl, MS	$13,000	$23,000	per year			•	
Univ at Buffalo - SUNY	45	Aug	60, 24	BS MS	$7,060	$14,940	per year			•	
North Dakota											
Univ of Mary (Bismarck)	38	Aug	40	MSOT	$15,000	$15,000				•	
Ohio											
Cleveland State Univ	30	Aug	28	MOT	$19,200	$34,710	per year			•	•
Oklahoma											
Univ of Oklahoma Health Sciences Center (Oklahoma City)	32	Jun	36	MOT	$8,190	$19,657			•	•	•
Pennsylvania											
Misericordia Univ (Dallas)	65	Aug	33, 60	MS				•		•	•
Univ of Scranton	56	Sep	63	BS MS	$37,106	$37,106	total tuition			•	
Puerto Rico											
Univ of Puerto Rico (San Juan)	20	Aug	27	MS	$5,000	$5,500			•	•	
Tennessee											
Belmont Univ (Nashville)	32	Aug	33, 23	OTD, MSOT	$32,400	$32,400		•		•	•
Milligan College	31	Aug	28	MSOT	$21,000	$21,000				•	
Texas											
Univ of Texas - Pan American (Edinburg)	25	Aug	27	MS	$3,800	$14,326				•	
Univ of Texas Medical Branch (Galveston)	55	Aug	24	MOT	$3,500	$9,250			•	•	
UT Health Science Center - San Antonio	35	May	33	MOT	$6,000	$16,700				•	
Utah											
Univ of Utah (Salt Lake City)	32	Aug	33	MOT	$21,074	$44,825				•	
Washington											
Univ of Puget Sound (Tacoma)	30	Sep	28	MSOT, MOT	$36,000	$36,000				•	
Wyoming											
Univ of North Dakota at Casper College	12	May	32	Masters	$17,127	$17,127				•	

*Data are shown only for programs that completed the 2011 AMA Survey of Health Professions Education Programs.

†Key to Offers: 1: Evening or weekend classes; 2: Non-English instruction; 3: Cultural competence instruction; 4: Distance education component.

Occupational Therapy Assistant

Under the supervision of and in collaboration with an occupational therapist, the occupational therapy assistant provides services to clients focusing on participation in selected activities to restore, reinforce, and enhance performance; facilitate learning of those skills and functions essential for adaptation and participation; diminish or correct pathology; and promote and maintain health and wellness. A fundamental concern is the development and maintenance of the skill and capacity throughout the lifespan to perform with satisfaction to self and others meaningful activities and roles essential to social participation and to the mastery of self and the environment. Under the supervision of and in partnership with the occupational therapist, the occupational therapy assistant participates in the development of adaptive skills and performance capacity and is concerned with factors that promote, influence, or enhance performance, as well as those that serve as barriers or impediments to the individual's occupational performance. The occupational therapy assistant provides service to those clients whose abilities to perform meaningful activities of living are threatened or impaired by:

- Developmental deficits
- The aging process
- Poverty and cultural differences
- Physical injury or illness
- Psychological or social disability

Career Description

A contemporary entry-level occupational therapy assistant must:

- Have acquired an educational foundation in the liberal arts and sciences, including a focus on issues related to diversity
- Be educated as a generalist, with a broad exposure to the delivery models and systems utilized in settings where occupational therapy is currently practiced and where it is emerging as a service
- Have achieved entry-level competence through a combination of academic and fieldwork education
- Be prepared to work under the supervision of and in cooperation with the occupational therapist
- Be prepared to articulate and apply occupational therapy principles, intervention approaches and rationales, and expected outcomes as these relate to occupational performance of the client
- Be prepared to be a lifelong learner and keep current with best practice
- Uphold the ethical standards, values, and attitudes of the occupational therapy profession

Employment Characteristics

Occupational therapy assistants assist in the planning and implementation of treatment of a diverse population in a variety of settings, such as nursing homes, hospitals and clinics, rehabilitation facilities, long-term care facilities, extended care facilities, sheltered workshops, schools and camps, private homes, and community agencies.

Salary

The results of the 2010 AOTA Workforce Study show that the median annual salary for full-time occupational therapy assistants was $44,000, with median salaries in the 90th percentile at $63,000 and at $27,429 in the 10th percentile. The median hourly wage for occupational therapy assistants working a standard part-time schedule was $22.60. Compensation varied, the study noted, "according to total years in the profession, region of the country and location type (urban, suburban, or rural), highest degree held within the profession, primary work setting, AOTA membership status, and more."

Data from the US Bureau of Labor Statistics (available at *www.bls.gov/oes/current/oes312011.htm*) indicate that mean annual wages of occupational therapy assistants were $52,150 in May 2011. The middle 50 percent earned $52,040. The lowest 10 percent earned $33,750, and the highest 10 percent earned $71,960. Mean annual wages in the industries employing the largest numbers of occupational therapy assistants in May 2011 (from the largest to smallest) were:

Offices of other health practitioners	$53,750
Nursing care facilities	$56,120
General medical and surgical hospitals	$48,440
Elementary and secondary schools	$44,310
Home health care services	$61,050

For more information, refer to *www.ama-assn.org/go/hpsalary*.

Educational Programs

Length. Education may be acquired in either a two-year associate degree program or a one- to two-year certificate program. Effective July 1, 2013, however, occupational therapy assistant education will no longer be offered at the certificate level. These technical-level education programs are located in two-year and four-year colleges and universities, and postsecondary vocational/technical schools and institutions, and include academic and fieldwork components, as do the professional-level programs.

Prerequisites. High school diploma or equivalent. A foundation of liberal arts and biological, physical, social, and behavioral sciences may be prerequisite to, or concurrent with, the technical education of the program curriculum.

Curriculum. Curricula of accredited occupational therapy assistant programs are required to include:

- A broad foundation of the liberal arts and sciences
- Basic tenets of occupational therapy
- The process of screening and evaluation
- The process of intervention and implementation
- Context of service delivery
- Assistance in the management of occupational therapy services
- Use of professional literature
- Professional ethics, values, and responsibilities

In addition, sixteen weeks of full-time fieldwork education is required.

Licensure, Registration, Certification

All states, Puerto Rico, Guam, and the District of Columbia regulate the practice of occupational therapy. To obtain a license, applicants must graduate from an accredited occupational therapy assistant educational program and pass a national certification examination for occupational therapy assistants. Those who pass the exam are awarded the title "Certified Occupational Therapy Assistant (COTA)." Some states have additional requirements for therapists who work in schools or early intervention programs. These requirements may include education-related classes, an education practice certificate, or early intervention certification requirements.

Inquiries

Careers Education
American Occupational Therapy Association
4720 Montgomery Lane
PO Box 31220
Bethesda, MD 20824-1220
301 652-2682
www.aota.org

Certification
National Board for Certification in Occupational Therapy (NBCOT)
12 South Summit Avenue, Suite 100
Gaithersburg, MD 20877-4150
301 990-7979
www.nbcot.org

Program Accreditation
Accreditation Council for Occupational Therapy Education
4720 Montgomery Lane, PO Box 31220
Bethesda, MD 20824-1220
301 652-2682 x2914
www.acoteonline.org

Note: Adapted in part from the Bureau of Labor Statistics, US Department of Labor, *Occupational Outlook Handbook*, Occupational Therapy Assistants and Aides, at *www.bls.gov/oco/ocos166.htm*.

Occupational Therapy Assistant

Alabama

Wallace State Community College
Occupational Therapy Asst Prgm
PO Box 2000
Hanceville, AL 35077-2000
www.wallacestate.edu

Arizona

Pima Medical Institute - Mesa
Occupational Therapy Asst Prgm
957 S Dobson Rd
Mesa, AZ 85202-2903
http://mesa.pmi.edu

Brown Mackie College - Phoenix
Occupational Therapy Asst Prgm
13430 North Black Canyon Highway, Suite 190
Phoenix, AZ 85029-1348
www.brownmackie.edu/phoenix/

Brown Mackie College - Tucson
Occupational Therapy Asst Prgm
Suite 204
4585 E Speedway Blvd
Tucson, AZ 85712
www.brownmackie.edu/tucson

Pima Medical Institute - Tucson
Occupational Therapy Asst Prgm
3350 E Grant Rd, Suite 200
Tuscon, AZ 85716
www.pmi.edu

Arkansas

South Arkansas Community College
Occupational Therapy Asst Prgm
PO Box 7010
300 S West Ave
El Dorado, AR 71731-7010
www.southark.edu

Baptist Health Schools Little Rock
Cosponsor: Pulaski Technical College
Occupational Therapy Asst Prgm
11900 Colonel Glenn Rd
Little Rock, AR 72210-2820

California

Grossmont College
Occupational Therapy Asst Prgm
8800 Grossmont College Dr
El Cajon, CA 92020-1799
www.gcccd.edu

Sacramento City College
Occupational Therapy Asst Prgm
Allied Health Dept
3835 Freeport Blvd
Sacramento, CA 95822-1386

Santa Ana College
Occupational Therapy Asst Prgm
1530 W 17th St
Santa Ana, CA 92706-3398

Colorado

Pima Medical Institute - Denver
Occupational Therapy Asst Prgm
7475 Dakin St, Suite 100
Denver, CO 80221
www.pmi.edu/locations/denver.asp

Pueblo Community College
Occupational Therapy Asst Prgm
900 W Orman Ave
Pueblo, CO 81004-1499

Connecticut

Housatonic Community College
Occupational Therapy Asst Prgm
900 Lafayette Blvd
Bridgeport, CT 06604-4704

Goodwin College
Occupational Therapy Asst Prgm
One Riverside Drive
East Hartford, CT 06118-1837
www.goodwin.edu

Manchester Community College
Occupational Therapy Asst Prgm
PO Box 1046
Great Path MS 17
Manchester, CT 06045-1046
www.mcc.commnet.edu

American Institute
Occupational Therapy Asst Prgm
2279 Mount Vernon Rd
Southington, CT 06489

Lincoln College of New England
Occupational Therapy Asst Prgm
2279 Mt Vernon Rd
Southington, CT 06489

Delaware

Delaware Technical Community College - Owens Campus
Occupational Therapy Asst Prgm
PO Box 610
Georgetown, DE 19947-0610
www.dtcc.edu

Delaware Technical Community College - Wilmington
Occupational Therapy Asst Prgm
333 Shipley St
Wilmington, DE 19801-2499
www.dtcc.edu

Florida

State College of Florida, Manatee-Sarasota
Occupational Therapy Asst Prgm
5840 26th St W
Bldg 28
Bradenton, FL 34207-7046
www.scf.edu

Daytona State College, Daytona Beach Campus
Occupational Therapy Asst Prgm
1800 Business Park Blvd
Daytona Beach, FL 32114
www.keiseruniversity.edu

Keiser University - Daytona Beach Campus
Occupational Therapy Asst Prgm
1800 Business Park Blvd
Daytona Beach, FL 32114
www.keiseruniversity.edu/daytona-beach.php

Keiser University - Ft Lauderdale Campus
Occupational Therapy Asst Prgm
1500 NW 49th St
Fort Lauderdale, FL 33309
www.keiseruniversity.edu
Notes: The university has expanded the OTA program to
  3 campuses, in Jacksonville, Daytona, and Pembroke
  Pines. The program is also offered in Fort
  Lauderdale, Melbourne, Orlando, and Kendall.

Florida State College at Jacksonville
Occupational Therapy Asst Prgm
4501 Capper Rd
Jacksonville, FL 32218
www.fscj.edu

Keiser University, Jacksonville Campus
Occupational Therapy Asst Prgm
6700 Southpoint Pkwy
Jacksonville, FL 32216
www.keiseruniversity.edu

Keiser University - Melbourne Campus
Occupational Therapy Asst Prgm
900 S Babcock St
Melbourne, FL 32901
www.keiseruniversity.edu

Keiser University - Miami Campus
Occupational Therapy Asst Prgm
2101 NW 117th Ave
Miami, FL 33172
www.keiseruniversity.edu/miami.php

Florida Hospital College of Health Sciences
Occupational Therapy Asst Prgm
671 Winyah Dr
Orlando, FL 32803
www.fhchs.edu

Keiser University - Orlando Campus
Occupational Therapy Asst Prgm
5600 Lake Underhill Rd
Orlando, FL 32901
www.keiseruniversity.edu

Keiser University - Pembroke Pines Campus
Occupational Therapy Asst Prgm
12520 Pines Blvd
Pembroke Pines, FL 33027-6143
www.keiseruniversity.edu

Keiser University - Tallahassee Campus
Occupational Therapy Asst Prgm
1700 Halstead Blvd
Tallahassee, FL 32309-3489
www.keiseruniversity.edu/tallahassee.php

Keiser University - West Palm Beach Campus
Occupational Therapy Asst Prgm
2085 Vista Parkway
West Palm Beach, FL 33411-2719
www.keiseruniversity.edu/west-palm-beach.php

Polk State College
Occupational Therapy Asst Prgm
999 Ave H NE
Winter Haven, FL 33881-4299
www.polk.edu

Georgia

Darton College
Occupational Therapy Asst Prgm
2400 Gillionville Rd
Albany, GA 31707-3098
Prgm Dir: Kristen Palmer Hudgins, MS OTR/L
Tel: 229 317-6908   *Fax:* 229 317-6682
E-mail: kristen.hudgins@darton.edu

Brown Mackie College - Atlanta
Occupational Therapy Asst Prgm
4370 Peachtree Rd NE
Atlanta, GA 30319
www.brownmackie.edu/atlanta
Prgm Dir: Alisha Wright, OTR/L
Tel: 404 799-4497   *Fax:* 404 799-4569
E-mail: aliwright@brownmackie.edu

Augusta Technical College
Occupational Therapy Asst Prgm
3200 Augusta Tech Dr
1400 Building
Augusta, GA 30906-3399
www.augusta.tec.ga.us

Middle Georgia College
Occupational Therapy Asst Prgm
1100 Second St SE
Cochran, GA 31014-1599
www.mgc.edu

**Georgia Northwestern Technical College -
  Walker Campus**
Occupational Therapy Asst Prgm
PO Box 569
265 Bicentennial Trail
Rock Spring, GA 30739
www.gntc.edu
Prgm Dir: Lisa Carruth, MSEd OTR/L
Tel: 706 764-3846   *Fax:* 706 764-3718
E-mail: lcarruth@gntc.edu

Hawaii

Kapiolani Community College
Cosponsor: University of Hawaii
Occupational Therapy Asst Prgm
Health Sciences Dept
4303 Diamond Head Rd, Kauila 210C
Honolulu, HI 96816-4421

Idaho

Brown Mackie College - Boise
Occupational Therapy Asst Prgm
9050 W Overland Rd
Boise, ID 83709-6281
www.brownmakcie.edu/boise/

Illinois

Parkland College
Occupational Therapy Asst Prgm
2400 W Bradley Ave
Champaign, IL 61821-1899

Wright College
Occupational Therapy Asst Prgm
4300 N Narragansett Ave
Chicago, IL 60634-1591
wright.ccc.edu
Prgm Dir: Lisa Iffland, MS OTR/L
Tel: 773 481-8876   *Fax:* 773 481-8892
E-mail: liffland@ccc.edu

Illinois Central College
Occupational Therapy Asst Prgm
201 SW Adams St
East Peoria, IL 61615
www.icc.edu

Lewis & Clark Community College
Occupational Therapy Asst Prgm
5800 Godfrey Rd
Godfrey, IL 62035-2466

Southern Illinois Collegiate Common Market
Occupational Therapy Asst Prgm
3213 S Park Ave
Herrin, IL 62948-3711
www.siccm.com

South Suburban College
Occupational Therapy Asst Prgm
15800 S State St
South Holland, IL 60473-1262

Lincoln Land Community College
Occupational Therapy Asst Prgm
5250 Shepherd Rd
PO Box 19256
Springfield, IL 62794-9256
www.llcc.edu

Indiana

University of Southern Indiana
Occupational Therapy Asst Prgm
College of Nursing and Health Professions
8600 University Blvd, HP 2068
Evansville, IN 47712-3534
health.usi.edu/acadprog/ota/index.htm

Brown Mackie College - Fort Wayne
Occupational Therapy Asst Prgm
Fort Wayne Campus
3000 E Coliseum Blvd, Suite 100
Fort Wayne, IN 46805
www.brownmackie.edu/fortwayne

Brown Mackie College - Indianapolis
Occupational Therapy Asst Prgm
Suite 100
1200 N Meridian St
Indianapolis, IN 46204
www.brownmackie.edu/indianapolis

Brown Mackie College - Merrillville
Occupational Therapy Asst Prgm
1000 E 80th Place, Suite 205M
Merrillville, IN 46410
www.brownmackie.edu/merrillville

Brown Mackie College - South Bend
Occupational Therapy Asst Prgm
3454 Douglas Rd
South Bend, IN 46635
www.brownmackie.edu

Iowa

Kirkwood Community College
Occupational Therapy Asst Prgm
6301 Kirkwood Blvd SW, PO Box 2068
Cedar Rapids, IA 52406-9973
www.kirkwood.edu/alliedhealth
Prgm Dir: Nichelle Cline, MPA OTR/L
Tel: 319 398-5566, Ext   *Fax:* 319 398-1293
E-mail: ncline@kirkwood.edu

Kansas

Brown Mackie College - Kansas City
Occupational Therapy Asst Prgm
9705 Lenexa Drive
Lenexa, KS 66215-1345
www.brownmackie.edu/kansascity/

Brown Mackie College - Salina
Occupational Therapy Asst Prgm
2106 South 9th St
Salina, KS 67401-7307
www.brownmackie.edu/salina/

Washburn University
Occupational Therapy Asst Prgm
1700 SW College Ave
Topeka, KS 66621-0001
www.washburn.edu/main/index.html

Newman University
Occupational Therapy Asst Prgm
3100 McCormick Ave
Wichita, KS 67213-2097
www.newmanu.edu

Kentucky

Brown Mackie College - Northern Kentucky
Occupational Therapy Asst Prgm
309 Buttermilk Pike
Fort Mitchell, KY 41017
www.brownmackie.edu/northernkentucky

Brown Mackie College - Louisville (Hopkinsville)
Occupational Therapy Asst Prgm
4001 Ft Campbell Blvd
Hopkinsville, KY 42240
www.brownmackie.edu/hopkinsville/

Brown Mackie College - Louisville
Occupational Therapy Asst Prgm
3605 Fern Valley Rd
Louisville, KY 40219-1916
www.brownmackie.edu/hopkinsville

Jefferson Community and Technical College
Occupational Therapy Asst Prgm
109 E Broadway St
Louisville, KY 40202-2005

Madisonville Community College
Occupational Therapy Asst Prgm
750 N Laffoon St
Madisonville, KY 42431-1636
www.madcc.kctcs.edu

Louisiana

Bossier Parish Community College
Occupational Therapy Asst Prgm
6220 E Texas St
Bossier City, LA 71111
www.bpcc.edu

University of Louisiana at Monroe
Occupational Therapy Asst Prgm
College of Health Sciences
700 University Ave, Rm 111 Caldwell Hall
Monroe, LA 71209-9000

Delgado Community College
Occupational Therapy Asst Prgm
City Park Campus
615 City Park Ave
New Orleans, LA 70119-4399
www.dcc.edu

Maine

Kennebec Valley Community College
Occupational Therapy Asst Prgm
92 Western Ave
Fairfield, ME 04937-1367
www.kvcc.me.edu

Maryland

Comm Coll of Baltimore County - Catonsville
Occupational Therapy Asst Prgm
800 S Rolling Rd
Catonsville, MD 21228-9987
www.ccbcmd.edu

Allegany College of Maryland
Occupational Therapy Asst Prgm
12401 Willowbrook Rd SE
Cumberland, MD 21502-2596
www.allegany.edu

Massachusetts

North Shore Community College
Occupational Therapy Asst Prgm
One Ferncroft Rd, PO Box 3340
Danvers, MA 01923-0840
www.northshore.edu
Prgm Dir: Maureen S Nardella, MS OTR/L
Tel: 978 762-4176   *Fax:* 978 762-4022
E-mail: maureen.nardella@northshore.edu

Bristol Community College
Occupational Therapy Asst Prgm
777 Elsbree St
Fall River, MA 02720-9960
www.BristolCommunityCollege.edu

Springfield Technical Community College
Occupational Therapy Asst Prgm
One Armory Sq, Ste 1
PO Box 9000
Springfield, MA 01102-9000
www.stcc.edu
Prgm Dir: Marianne Joyce, MA OTR/L
Tel: 413 755-4881   *Fax:* 413 755-4764
E-mail: mjoyce@stcc.edu

Quinsigamond Community College
Occupational Therapy Asst Prgm
670 W Boylston St
Worcester, MA 01606-2092
www.qcc.mass.edu

Michigan

Baker College of Allen Park
Occupational Therapy Asst Prgm
4500 Enterprise Drive
Allen Park, MI 48101-3033
www.baker.edu

Robert B. Miller College
Occupational Therapy Asst Prgm
2100 West Thompson Rd
Fenton, MI 48430-9798
www.mcc.edu

Grand Rapids Community College
Occupational Therapy Asst Prgm
143 Bostwick St NE
Grand Rapids, MI 49503-3295

Baker College of Muskegon
Occupational Therapy Asst Prgm
1903 Marquette Ave
Muskegon, MI 49442-1490
www.baker.edu
Prgm Dir: Matthew Mekkes, MSOT OTR
Tel: 231 777-5289   *Fax:* 231 777-5291
E-mail: matthew.mekkes@baker.edu

Macomb Community College
Occupational Therapy Asst Prgm
14500 E Twelve Mile Rd
Warren, MI 48088-3896
www.macomb.edu

Minnesota

Anoka Technical College
Occupational Therapy Asst Prgm
1355 W Hwy 10
Anoka, MN 55303-1590
www.ank.tec.mn.us

Northland Community & Technical College
Occupational Therapy Asst Prgm
2022 Central Ave NE
East Grand Forks, MN 56721-2702
Prgm Dir: Cassie Hilts, MOT OTR/L
Tel: 218 793-2589   *Fax:* 218 793-2862
E-mail: cassie.hilts@northlandcollege.edu

Saint Catherine University - Minneapolis
Occupational Therapy Asst Prgm
601 25th Ave S
Minneapolis, MN 55454-1494
www.stkate.edu/ota
Prgm Dir: Marianne F Christiansen, MA OTR/L FAOTA
Tel: 651 690-7772   *Fax:* 651 690-7849
E-mail: mfchristiansen@stkate.edu

Mississippi

Pearl River Community College
Occupational Therapy Asst Prgm
5448 US Hwy 49 S
Hattiesburg, MS 39401-7806
www.prcc.edu

Holmes Community College
Occupational Therapy Asst Prgm
Ridgeland Campus
412 W Ridgeland Ave
Ridgeland, MS 39157
www.holmescc.edu

Itawamba Community College
Occupational Therapy Asst Prgm
2176 S Eason Blvd
Tupelo, MS 38804
www.iccms.edu/programs/ota/

Missouri

Missouri Health Professions Consortium
Occupational Therapy Asst Prgm
203 Clark Hall
Columbia, MO 65211
www.mhpc.missouri.edu

Brown Mackie College - St. Louis
Occupational Therapy Asst Prgm
2 Soccer Park Rd
Fenton, MO 63026-2564
www.brownmackie.edu/st-louis/

Sanford-Brown College - Hazelwood Campus
Occupational Therapy Asst Prgm
75 Village Square
Hazelwood, MO 63042
www.sanford-brown.edu

Metropolitan Community College - Penn Valley
Occupational Therapy Asst Prgm
3201 SW Trafficway
Kansas City, MO 64111-2412

Ozarks Technical Community College
Occupational Therapy Asst Prgm
1001 E Chestnut Expressway
Springfield, MO 65802-3625
www.otc.edu

South Howell County Ambulance District
Occupational Therapy Asst Prgm
11333 Big Bend Blvd
St Louis, MO 631222-579
www.stlcc.edu/programs

St Louis Community College - Meramec
Occupational Therapy Asst Prgm
11333 Big Bend Blvd
St Louis, MO 63122-5799
www.stlcc.edu
Prgm Dir: Cynthia R Ballentine, MSOT OTR/L
Tel: 314 984-7364   *Fax:* 314 984-7250
E-mail: cballentine@stlcc.edu

National American University
Occupational Therapy Asst Prgm
4601 Mid Rivers Mall Drive
St Peters, MO 63376-0975
www.stchas.edu/divisions/msh/otaindex.shtml

St Charles Community College
Occupational Therapy Asst Prgm
4601 Mid Rivers Mall Dr
PO Box 76975
St. Peters, MO 63376-0975
www.stchas.edu
Prgm Dir: Francesca Woods, MA OTR/L
Tel: 636 922-8638   *Fax:* 636 922-8478
E-mail: fwoods@stchas.edu

Nebraska

Central Community College
Occupational Therapy Asst Prgm
3134 West Highway 34
PO Box 4903
Grand Island, NE 68802-4903
www.cccneb.edu/ota/

Nevada

College of Southern Nevada
Occupational Therapy Asst Prgm
West Charleston Campus
6375 W Charleston Blvd, WCL
Las Vegas, NV 89146-1139
www.csn.edu

New Hampshire

River Valley Community College
Occupational Therapy Asst Prgm
One College Dr
Claremont, NH 03743-9707
www.claremont.nhctc.edu

New Mexico

Brown Mackie College - Albuquerque
Occupational Therapy Asst Prgm
10500 Copper Ave, NE
Albuquerque, NM 87123-1845
www.brownmackie.edu/Albuquerque/

Eastern New Mexico University - Roswell
Occupational Therapy Asst Prgm
Div of Health
52 University Blvd 88203
PO Box 6000
Roswell, NM 88202-6000
www.roswell.enmu.edu

Western New Mexico University
Occupational Therapy Asst Prgm
PO Box 680
Silver City, NM 88062-0680

New York

Maria College
Occupational Therapy Asst Prgm
700 New Scotland Ave
Albany, NY 12208-1798
www.mariacollege.edu
Prgm Dir: Scott L Homer, MS OTR/L
Tel: 518 438-3111, Ext   *Fax:* 518 453-1366
E-mail: shomer@mariacollege.edu

Suffolk County Community College - Michael J Grant Campus
Occupational Therapy Asst Prgm
1001 Crooked Hill Rd, MA 308
Brentwood, NY 11717-1092
www.sunysuffolk.edu
Prgm Dir: Lisa E Hubbs, MS OTR/L
Tel: 631 851-6335   *Fax:* 631 851-6854
E-mail: hubbsl@sunysuffolk.edu

Mercy College
Occupational Therapy Asst Prgm
555 Broadway
Dobbs Ferry, NY 10522-1134
www.mercy.edu/pages/863.asp

Jamestown Community College
Occupational Therapy Asst Prgm
525 Falconer St
PO Box 20
Jamestown, NY 14702-0020
www.sunyjcc.edu/ota

LaGuardia Community College
Occupational Therapy Asst Prgm
31-10 Thomson Ave
Long Island City, NY 11101-3083
www.lagcc.cuny.edu

Orange County Community College
Occupational Therapy Asst Prgm
115 South St
Middletown, NY 10940-6404
www.sunyorange.edu

Touro College
Occupational Therapy Asst Prgm
Main Campus
27 W 23rd St
New York, NY 11010
www.touro.edu/shs

Rockland Community College
Occupational Therapy Asst Prgm
145 College Rd
Suffern, NY 10901-3699
www.sunyrockland.edu

Erie Community College
Occupational Therapy Asst Prgm
6205 Main St
Williamsville, NY 14221-7095
www.ecc.edu
Prgm Dir: Betsy Jones, MSEd OTR/L
Tel: 716 851-1320   *Fax:* 716 851-1267
E-mail: jones@ecc.edu

North Carolina

Cabarrus College of Health Sciences
Occupational Therapy Asst Prgm
401 Medical Park Dr
Concord, NC 28025-3959
www.cabarruscollege.edu

Durham Technical Community College
Occupational Therapy Asst Prgm
1637 Lawson St
Durham, NC 27703-5023
www.durhamtech.edu

Pitt Community College
Occupational Therapy Asst Prgm
PO Drawer 7007
Greenville, NC 27835-7007

Cape Fear Community College
Occupational Therapy Asst Prgm
411 N Front St
Wilmington, NC 28401-3993
http://cfcc.edu
Prgm Dir: Deborah A Amini, EdD OTR/L CHT
Tel: 910 362-7096   *Fax:* 910 362-7087
E-mail: damini@cfcc.edu

North Dakota

North Dakota State College of Science
Occupational Therapy Asst Prgm
Mayme Green Allied Health Facility
800 6th St N
Wahpeton, ND 58076-0002
www.ndscs.nodak.edu

Ohio

Brown Mackie College - Akron
Occupational Therapy Asst Prgm
755 White Pond Drive, Suite 101
Akron, OH 44320
www.brownmackie.edu/akron/

Kent State University - Ashtabula Campus
Occupational Therapy Asst Prgm
3300 Lake Rd West
Ashtabula, OH 44004
www.ashtabula.kent.edu/Academics/degrees/otat.cfm

Stark State College
Occupational Therapy Asst Prgm
6200 Frank Ave NW
Canton, OH 44720-7299
www.starkstate.edu

Cincinnati State Tech & Comm College
Occupational Therapy Asst Prgm
3520 Central Pkwy
Cincinnati, OH 45223-2690
www.cincinnatistate.edu

Cuyahoga Community College
Occupational Therapy Asst Prgm
2900 Community College Ave
Cleveland, OH 44115-3196
www.tri-c.edu/otat
Prgm Dir: Hector L Merced, MS OTR/L
Tel: 216 987-4498   *Fax:* 216 987-4386
E-mail: hector.merced@tri-c.edu

Sinclair Community College
Occupational Therapy Asst Prgm
444 W Third St
Dayton, OH 45402-1460
www.sinclair.edu

Kent State University
Occupational Therapy Asst Prgm
400 E Fourth St
East Liverpool, OH 43920-3497
www.eliv.kent.edu/academics/eastliverpool/ocat/
    index.cfm
Prgm Dir: Harriett Bynum, MS OTR/L
Tel: 330 382-7426   *Fax:* 330 382-7564
E-mail: hbynum@kent.edu

Brown Mackie College - Findlay
Occupational Therapy Asst Prgm
1700 Fostoria Ave
Findlay, OH 45840

Rhodes State College
Occupational Therapy Asst Prgm
4240 Campus Dr
Lima, OH 45804-3597
www.rhodesstate.edu

North Central State College
Occupational Therapy Asst Prgm
PO Box 698
2441 Kenwood Circle
Mansfield, OH 44901-0698
www.ncstatecollege.edu

Marion Technical College
Occupational Therapy Asst Prgm
1467 Mt Vernon Ave
Marion, OH 43302-5694
www.mtc.edu

Shawnee State University
Occupational Therapy Asst Prgm
940 Second St
Portsmouth, OH 45662-4303
www.shawnee.edu

Owens Community College
Occupational Therapy Asst Prgm
Toledo Campus Oregon Rd
PO Box 10,000
Toledo, OH 43699-1947
www.owens.edu

Zane State College
Occupational Therapy Asst Prgm
1555 Newark Rd
Zanesville, OH 43701-2694
www.zanestate.edu/
    occupationaltherapistassistantaas.htm

Oklahoma

SW Oklahoma St Univ/Caddo Kiowa Tech Ctr
Occupational Therapy Asst Prgm
PO Box 190
Fort Cobb, OK 73038

Oklahoma City Community College
Occupational Therapy Asst Prgm
Health Professions Division
7777 S May Ave
Oklahoma City, OK 73159-4444

Murray State College
Occupational Therapy Asst Prgm
One Murray Campus
Tishomingo, OK 73460
Prgm Dir: Kahlila Fowler, OTD OTR/L CEAS
Tel: 580 371-2371, Ext   *Fax:* 580 371-2667
E-mail: kfowler@mscok.edu

Brown Mackie College - Tulsa
Occupational Therapy Asst Prgm
4608 South Garnett Rd, Ste 110
Tulsa, OK 74146-5207
www.brownmackie.edu/tulsa/

Tulsa Community College - Metro Campus
Occupational Therapy Asst Prgm
Allied Hlth Services Div
909 S Boston Ave
Tulsa, OK 74119-2095
www.tulsacc.edu

Oregon

Linn-Benton Community College
Occupational Therapy Asst Prgm
6500 Pacific Blvd SW
Albany, OR 97321
www.linnbenton.edu

Pennsylvania

Harcum College
Occupational Therapy Asst Prgm
750 Montgomery Ave
Bryn Mawr, PA 19010-3476
www.harcum.edu

Penn State University - DuBois
Occupational Therapy Asst Prgm
College Place
DuBois, PA 15801-3199
www.psu.edu

Community College of Allegheny County - Boyce Campus
Occupational Therapy Asst Prgm
595 Beatty Rd
Monroeville, PA 15146-1395
www.ccac.edu

Penn State University - Mont Alto
Occupational Therapy Asst Prgm
Campus Dr
Mont Alto, PA 17237-9703
www.ma.psu/OTA
Notes: Satellite programs in Reading, PA

Mercyhurst University
Occupational Therapy Asst Prgm
16 W Division St
North East, PA 16428

Philadelphia University
Occupational Therapy Asst Prgm
Continuing and Professional Studies
4201 Henry Ave
Philadelphia, PA 19144-5497
www.philau.edu/continuinged/
Prgm Dir: Marianne Dahl, MBA OTR/L
Tel: 215 951-2900   *Fax:* 215 951-5300
E-mail: dahlm@philau.edu

Kaplan Career Institute - ICM Campus
Occupational Therapy Asst Prgm
10 Wood St
Pittsburgh, PA 15222-1977
www.kci-pittsburgh.com

Penn State University - Berks
Occupational Therapy Asst Prgm
PO Box 7009
Tulpehoeken Rd
Reading, PA 19610-6009
www.psu.edu

Lehigh Carbon Community College
Occupational Therapy Asst Prgm
4525 Education Park Dr
Schnecksville, PA 18078-2598
www.lccc.edu

Pennsylvania College of Technology
Occupational Therapy Asst Prgm
One College Ave
Williamsport, PA 17701-5799
www.pct.edu

Puerto Rico

University of Puerto Rico at Humacao
Occupational Therapy Asst Prgm
Call Box 860
Humacao, PR 00792
Prgm Dir: Carlos Galiano, PhD OTR/L
Tel: 787 850-9392   *Fax:* 787 850-9434
E-mail: carlos.galiano@upr.edu

Rhode Island

Community College of Rhode Island
Occupational Therapy Asst Prgm
Newport County Campus
One John H Chafee Blvd
Newport, RI 02840
www.ccri.edu

New England Institute of Technology
Occupational Therapy Asst Prgm
2500 Post Rd
Warwick, RI 02886-2251
www.neit.edu

South Carolina

Trident Technical College
Occupational Therapy Asst Prgm
PO Box 118067
Charleston, SC 29423-8067
www.tridenttech.edu

Greenville Technical College - Greer Campus
Occupational Therapy Asst Prgm
MS 3011
506 S Pleasantburg Dr, PO Box 5616
Greenville, SC 29606-5616
www.gvltec.edu
Prgm Dir: Beth Todd, MHSA OTR/L
Tel: 864 250-3033   *Fax:* 864 848-2038
E-mail: beth.todd@gvltec.edu

South Dakota

Lake Area Technical Institute
Occupational Therapy Asst Prgm
230 11th St NE
Watertown, SD 57201-0730
www.lakeareatech.edu

Tennessee

Nashville State Community College
Occupational Therapy Asst Prgm
120 White Bridge Rd
Nashville, TN 37209-4515
www.nscc.edu

Roane State Community College
Occupational Therapy Asst Prgm
701 Briarcliff Ave
Oak Ridge, TN 37830

Texas

Amarillo College
Occupational Therapy Asst Prgm
PO Box 447
Amarillo, TX 79178-0001
www.actx.edu/occup_therapy

Austin Community College
Occupational Therapy Asst Prgm
Eastview Campus
3401 Webberville Rd
Austin, TX 78702

Panola College
Occupational Therapy Asst Prgm
1109 W Panola St
Carthage, TX 75633-2397
www.panola.edu

Del Mar College
Occupational Therapy Asst Prgm
Dept of Allied Health
101 Baldwin and Ayers Sts
Corpus Christi, TX 78404-3897

Navarro College
Occupational Therapy Asst Prgm
3200 W 7th Ave
Corsicana, TX 75110-4818
www.navarrocollege.edu

Anamarc College
Occupational Therapy Asst Prgm
3210 Dyer St
El Paso, TX 79930-6230
www.anamarc.edu

Medical Education and Training Campus (METC)
Occupational Therapy Asst Prgm
Academy of Health Sciences
3151 Scott Rd, Suite 1230
Fort Sam Houston, TX 78234-6138

Houston Community College
Occupational Therapy Asst Prgm
Coleman College for Health Sciences
1900 Pressler Dr
Houston, TX 77030-3717
www.hccs.edu
Prgm Dir: Beverly Broussard-solomon, BA OTR/L
Tel: 713 718-7393   *Fax:* 713 718-6495
E-mail: beverly.solomon@hccs.edu

Lone Star College - Kingwood
Occupational Therapy Asst Prgm
20000 Kingwood Dr
Kingwood, TX 77339-3801
www.lonestar.edu
Prgm Dir: Norma Alicia Ticas, OTR M Ed
Tel: 281 312-1464   *Fax:* 281 312-1490
E-mail: norma.ticas@lonestar.edu

Laredo Community College
Occupational Therapy Asst Prgm
West End Washington St
Laredo, TX 78040-4395
www.laredo.edu

South Texas College
Occupational Therapy Asst Prgm
Nursing/Allied Health Division
1101 E Vermont, PO Box 9701
McAllen, TX 78501-9701
www.southtexascollege.edu/nah/program ota.htm
Prgm Dir: Espy J Brattin, OTR MEd
Tel: 956 872-3149   *Fax:* 956 872-3163
E-mail: ebrattin@southtexascollege.edu

St Philip's College
Occupational Therapy Asst Prgm
1801 Martin Luther King Dr
San Antonio, TX 78203-2098
www.alamo.edu/spc/acad/ahd/ota/otaprogam.aspx

Lone Start College - Tomball
Occupational Therapy Asst Prgm
30555 Tomball Pkwy
Tomball, TX 77375-4036
www.lonestar.edu/tomballota

Utah

Salt Lake Community College
Occupational Therapy Asst Prgm
Mail Code: JC
3491 W Wights Fort Rd
West Jordan, UT 84088
www.slcc.edu/ota
Prgm Dir: Barb Kloetzke, BS COTA/L CAPS
Tel: 801 957-6265   *Fax:* 801 957-6353
E-mail: barb.kloetzke@slcc.edu

Virginia

Southwest Virginia Community College at Virginia Highlands Community College
Occupational Therapy Asst Prgm
100 VHCC Drive
PO Box 828
Abingdon, VA 24212
www.sw.edu/msht/ota/

Southwest Virginia Community College
Occupational Therapy Asst Prgm
PO Box SVCC
Richlands, VA 24641-1101
www.sw.edu/msht/healthtech/htprograms.htm

Jefferson College of Health Sciences
Occupational Therapy Asst Prgm
PO Box 13186
101 Elm Ave
Roanoke, VA 24013-2222
www.jchs.edu

Tidewater Community College
Occupational Therapy Asst Prgm
Virginia Beach Campus
1700 College Crescent
Virginia Beach, VA 23453
www.tcc.edu

Washington

Green River Community College
Occupational Therapy Asst Prgm
12401 SE 320th St
Auburn, WA 98092-3622
www.greenriver.edu

Lake Washington Institute of Technology
Occupational Therapy Asst Prgm
Allied Health Programs
11605 132nd Ave NE
Kirkland, WA 98034-8506
www.lwtc.edu

Pima Medical Institute - Renton
Occupational Therapy Asst Prgm
555 S Renton Village Place, #400
Renton, WA 98057
www.pmi.edu/locations/renton.asp

Bates Technical College
Occupational Therapy Asst Prgm
1101 S Yakima Ave
Tacoma, WA 98406-4895
www.bates.ctc.edu

West Virginia

Mountain State University
Occupational Therapy Asst Prgm
PO Box AG
Beckley, WV 25802-2830
www.mountainstate.edu/majors/whystudy/ota/

Wisconsin

Fox Valley Technical College
Occupational Therapy Asst Prgm
1825 N Bluemound Dr, PO Box 2277
Appleton, WI 54912-2277
www.fvtc.edu

Wisconsin Indianhead Technical College - Ashland Campus
Occupational Therapy Asst Prgm
2100 Beaser Ave
Ashland, WI 54806-3699
www.witc.edu/pgmpages/ota

Western Technical College
Occupational Therapy Asst Prgm
400 Seventh St N, PO Box C-908
La Crosse, WI 54602-0908
www.westerntc.edu

Madison Area Technical College
Occupational Therapy Asst Prgm
211 N Carroll St
Madison, WI 53703-2285
www.matcmadison.edu

Milwaukee Area Technical College
Occupational Therapy Asst Prgm
700 W State St
Milwaukee, WI 53233-1443
www.matc.edu
Prgm Dir: Susan Heitman, ME OTR
Tel: 414 297-6882   *Fax:* 414 297-6851
E-mail: heitmasm@matc.edu

Wyoming

Casper College
Occupational Therapy Asst Prgm
125 College Dr
Casper, WY 82601-9958
www.caspercollege.edu
Prgm Dir: Marla J Wonser, MSOT OTR/L
Tel: 307 268-2867   *Fax:* 307 268-3034
E-mail: mwonser@caspercollege.edu

THERAPY AND REHABILITATION

Occupational Therapy Assistant

Programs*	Class Capacity	Begins	Length (months)	Award	Res. Tuition	Non-res. Tuition		Offers:† 1	2	3	4
Georgia											
Brown Mackie College - Atlanta	35	Feb Aug	24	AAS	$37,600	$37,600				•	
Darton College (Albany)	22	Aug	24	AS						•	
Georgia Northwestern Technical College - Walker Campus (Rock Spring)	20	Jul	24	AAS	$3,747		per year				
Illinois											
Wright College (Chicago)	24	Aug	28	Dipl, AAS	$2,492	$4,860	per year			•	
Iowa											
Kirkwood Community College (Cedar Rapids)	24	Aug	22	AAS						•	
Massachusetts											
North Shore Community College (Danvers)	36	Sep	14, 18	AS	$5,670	$13,790	per credit			•	
Springfield Technical Community College	12	Sep	18	AS	$4,776	$11,386	per year				
Michigan											
Baker College of Muskegon	20	Sep	28	AAS	$10,800		per year	•		•	•
Minnesota											
Northland Community & Technical College (East Grand Forks)	24	Jan	21	AAS	$5,400	$5,400	per year			•	
Saint Catherine Univ - Minneapolis	24	Sep	18	AAS	$18,000	$18,000				•	
Missouri											
St Charles Community College (St. Peters)	24	Aug	24	AAS						•	
St Louis Community College - Meramec	24	Aug	21	AAS	$2,948	$4,489	per year			•	
New York											
Erie Community College (Williamsville)	64	Sep	24	AAS	$3,600	$7,200					
Maria College (Albany)	48	late Aug	18, 32	AAS	$10,000	$10,000	per year	•		•	•
Suffolk County Community College - Michael J Grant Campus (Brentwood)	24	Aug Sep	21	AAS	$3,990	$7,980	per year			•	
North Carolina											
Cape Fear Community College (Wilmington)	24	Aug	21	AAS	$2,000	$8,000				•	•
Ohio											
Cuyahoga Community College (Cleveland)	30	May	24	AAS	$6,385	$8,292				•	
Kent State Univ (East Liverpool)	50	Aug	21	AAS	$5,288	$13,248				•	•
Oklahoma											
Murray State College (Tishomingo)	12-	Aug	26	AAS						•	
Pennsylvania											
Philadelphia Univ	30	Sep	23	AS	$17,000	$17,000		•		•	•
Puerto Rico											
Univ of Puerto Rico at Humacao	35	Aug	24	Dipl, AS	$3	$7	per credit	•	•		
South Carolina											
Greenville Technical College - Greer Campus	32	Aug	21	AAS						•	•
Texas											
Houston Community College	21	Aug	12	Cert	$5,700	$8,800				•	
Lone Star College - Kingwood	24	Jan	20	AAS	$5,500	$9,000				•	
South Texas College (McAllen)	21	Sep	24	AAS	$4,300					•	•
Utah											
Salt Lake Community College (West Jordan)	24	Fall	24	AAS	$3,052	$9,604				•	•
Wisconsin											
Milwaukee Area Technical College	26	Aug	18	AAS	$1,883	$2,722				•	•
Wyoming											
Casper College	24	Aug	26	AS	$1,136	$3,544				•	•

*Data are shown only for programs that completed the 2011 AMA Survey of Health Professions Education Programs.

†Key to Offers: 1: Evening or weekend classes; 2: Non-English instruction; 3: Cultural competence instruction; 4: Distance education component.

Physical Therapist

The physical therapist provides services to many different kinds of patients/clients, from those recovering from accidents or illness and people with disabilities to world-class athletes. Physical therapists help improve patients' strength and mobility, relieve pain, and prevent or limit permanent physical disabilities. Physical therapists take a personal and direct approach to meeting an individual's health goals, working closely with the patient and other health care practitioners. They provide the patient and the patient's family with instruction and home programs to ensure that healing continues after direct patient care has ended.

Physical therapists also work to keep people well and safe from injury, emphasizing the importance of fitness and conditioning and showing people how to avoid injuries at work or play. Physical therapy promotes optimal physical performance and enables health-conscious people to increase their overall fitness level and muscular strength and endurance.

History

The American Women's Physical Therapeutic Association was formed in 1921. It was later known as the American Physiotherapy Association, then became the American Physical Therapy Association (APTA) in the late 1940s.

Recognition and accreditation of programs in physical therapy has existed since 1928. In the early years, the process was overseen by the APTA; then the American Medical Association (AMA) provided these services; and later the APTA and AMA collaborated to accredit physical therapy programs. In 1979, the Commission on Accreditation in Physical Therapy Education (CAPTE) was recognized by USDE as an independent agency, and in 1982 AMA ceased accrediting physical therapy programs. Since 1982, CAPTE has been the only recognized accrediting agency in physical therapy.

Career Description

The physical therapist is able to evaluate a patient's:
- Aerobic capacity and endurance
- Joint motion
- Muscle strength and endurance
- Posture
- Pain
- Functional ability
- Muscle tone and reflexes
- Appearance and stability of walking
- Need and use of braces and artificial limbs
- Function of the heart and lungs
- Integrity of sensation and perception
- Integrity and health of skin
- Performance of activities required in daily living
- Developmental activities

Physical therapy techniques include:
- Therapeutic exercise
- Mobilization/manipulation and range-of-motion exercises
- Cardiovascular endurance training
- Relaxation exercises
- Therapeutic massage
- Biofeedback
- Training in activities of daily living
- Wound debridement

- Pulmonary physical therapy
- Ambulation training

Modalities, including traction, ultrasound, diathermy, electrotherapy, cryotherapy, hydrotherapy, and laser therapy, also can be applied during the treatment program.

Employment Characteristics

Physical therapists work in hospitals as well as:
- Private physical therapy offices
- Community health centers
- Corporate or industrial health centers
- Sports facilities
- Research institutions
- Rehabilitation centers
- Nursing homes
- Home health agencies
- Schools
- Pediatric centers
- Colleges and universities

Salary

Average annual income for physical therapists is approximately $75,000, depending on geographic location and practice setting. Physical therapists have the potential to earn more than $100,000 annually. Data from the US Bureau of Labor Statistics (BLS) for May 2011 show that wages at the 10th percentile were $54,710, the 50th percentile (median) at $78,270, and the 90th percentile at $110,670 (*www.bls.gov/oes/current/oes291123.htm*). Median annual wages in the industries employing the largest numbers of physical therapists in May 2009 were:

- Home health care services $89,150
- Nursing care facilities $83,220
- Offices of physicians $80,220
- Offices of other health practitioners $78,120
- General medical and surgical hospitals $78,710

For more information, refer to *www.ama-assn.org/go/hpsalary*.

Employment Outlook

Employment of physical therapists is expected to grow by 30 percent from 2010 to 2020, much faster than the average for all occupations. The increasing elderly population will drive growth in the demand for physical therapy services. The elderly population is particularly vulnerable to chronic and debilitating conditions that require therapeutic services. Also, the baby-boom generation is entering the prime age for heart attacks and strokes, increasing the demand for cardiac and physical rehabilitation. Medical and technological developments will permit a greater percentage of trauma victims and newborns with birth defects to survive, creating additional demand for rehabilitative care. In addition, growth may result from advances in medical technology and the use of evidence-based practices, which could permit the treatment of an increasing number of disabling conditions that were untreatable in the past.

In addition, the federally mandated Individuals with Disabilities Education Act guarantees that students have access to services from physical therapists and other therapeutic and rehabilitative services. Demand for physical therapists will continue in schools.

Opportunities also exist for physical therapists from minority groups, who are in great demand but short supply in all aspects of the profession. When physical therapists and their clients share a common language and similar background, the effectiveness of treatment is enhanced.

Educational Programs

Award, Length. All physical therapist education programs culminate in a post-baccalaureate degree. In 2009, there were 212 physical therapist education programs. Of these accredited programs, 12 awarded master's degrees, 200 awarded doctoral degrees. Master's degree programs typically are two to two-and-a-half years in length; doctoral degree programs last three years.

Prerequisites. Candidates should have a high overall grade point average (GPA) and a high GPA in prerequisite coursework. Volunteer experience as a physical therapy aide, letters of recommendation from physical therapists or science teachers, and excellent writing and interpersonal skills are also highly valued.

Curriculum. Educational programs include foundational science courses, such as biology, anatomy, physiology, cellular histology, exercise physiology, neuroscience, biomechanics, pharmacology, pathology, and radiology/imaging, as well as behavioral science courses, such as evidence-based practice and clinical reasoning. Some of the clinically-based courses include medical screening, examination tests and measures, diagnostic process, therapeutic interventions, outcomes assessment, and practice management. In addition to classroom and laboratory instruction, students receive supervised clinical experience.

Licensure, Certification, and Registration

After graduating from an accredited education program, physical therapist candidates must pass a state-administered national exam. Other requirements for physical therapy practice vary from state to state according to physical therapy practice acts or state regulations that govern physical therapy. For more information, contact the state licensing boards.

Inquiries

Careers, Education, and Certification
American Physical Therapy Association
1111 North Fairfax Street
Alexandria, VA 22314-1488
800 999-2782 or 703 684-2782
www.apta.org

Program Accreditation
Commission on Accreditation in Physical Therapy Education
1111 North Fairfax Street
Alexandria, VA 22314
703 684-2782
www.apta.org/capte

Note: Adapted in part from the Bureau of Labor Statistics, US Department of Labor, *Occupational Outlook Handbook,* Physical Therapists, at *www.bls.gov/oco/ocos080.htm*.

Physical Therapist

Alabama

University of Alabama at Birmingham
Physical Therapy Prgm
Department of Physical Therapy RMSB 360X
1530 Third Ave S
Birmingham, AL 35294-1212
www.uab.edu/pt

University of South Alabama
Physical Therapy Prgm
Dept of Physical Therapy
1504 Springhill Ave, Rm 1214
Mobile, AL 36604
www.southalabama.edu/alliedhealth/pt

Alabama State University
Physical Therapy Prgm
PO Box 271
915 S Jackson St
Montgomery, AL 36101-0271
www.alasu.edu

Arizona

Northern Arizona University
Physical Therapy Prgm
CU Box 15105
Flagstaff, AZ 86011
http://jan.ucc.nau.edu/~hp-p/pt

Franklin Pierce University
Physical Therapy Prgm
140 North Litchfield Rd
Goodyear, AZ 85338

AT Still University of Health Sciences
Cosponsor: Arizona School of Health Sciences
Physical Therapy Prgm
5850 E Still Circle
Mesa, AZ 85206
www.atsu.edu

Arkansas

University of Central Arkansas
Physical Therapy Prgm
Dept of Physical Therapy
201 Donaghey, PTC 300
Conway, AR 72035-0001

Arkansas State University
Physical Therapy Prgm
PO Box 910
State University, AR 72467-0910
http://pt.astate.edu

California

Azusa Pacific University
Physical Therapy Prgm
901 E Alosta Ave
Azusa, CA 91702-7000
www.apu.edu

California State University - Fresno
Physical Therapy Prgm
2345 E San Ramon Ave, MS-MH29
Fresno, CA 93740-8031
www.csufresno.edu/physicaltherapy

Loma Linda University
Physical Therapy Prgm
Dept of Physical Therapy
School of Allied Health Professions
Loma Linda, CA 92350
www.llu.edu/llu/sahp/pt

California State University - Long Beach
Physical Therapy Prgm
College of Health and Human Services
1250 Bellflower Blvd
Long Beach, CA 90840
www.csulb.edu

Mount St Mary's College
Physical Therapy Prgm
Dept of Physical Therapy
10 Chester Place
Los Angeles, CA 90007-2598
www.msmc.la.edu/pt

University of Southern California
Physical Therapy Prgm
Biokinesiology and Physical Therapy
1540 E Alcazar St, CHP 155
Los Angeles, CA 90089
www.usc.edu/pt

California State University - Northridge
Physical Therapy Prgm
Department of Physical Therapy
18111 Nordhoff St
Northridge, CA 91330-8411
http://hhd.csun.edu/pt

Samuel Merritt University
Physical Therapy Prgm
450 30th St
Oakland, CA 94609
www.samuelmerritt.edu

Chapman University
Physical Therapy Prgm
Department of Physical Therapy
One University Dr
Orange, CA 92866
www.chapman.edu

Western Univ of Health Sciences
Physical Therapy Prgm
Department of Physical Therapy Education
309 E Second St
Pomona, CA 91766-1854
www.westernu.edu

California State University - Sacramento
Physical Therapy Prgm
College of Health and Human Services
6000 J St
Sacramento, CA 95819-6020
www.hhs.csus.edu/pt

University of California - San Francisco
Cosponsor: San Francisco State Univ
Physical Therapy Prgm
1318 7th Ave
San Francisco, CA 94143-0736

University of St Augustine for Health Science
Physical Therapy Prgm
Institute of Physical Therapy
700 Windy Point Drive
San Macros, CA 92069
www.usa.edu

University of the Pacific
Physical Therapy Prgm
Dept of Physical Therapy
3601 Pacific Ave
Stockton, CA 95211
www.pacific.edu

Colorado

University of Colorado Denver - Anschutz MC
Physical Therapy Prgm
Ed 2 South, Bldg L28, Room 3106
13121 E 17th Ave - PO Box 6508
Aurora, CO 80045
www.uchsc.edu/pt

Regis University
Physical Therapy Prgm
3333 Regis Blvd G-9
Denver, CO 80221-1099
www.regis.edu/dpt

Connecticut

Sacred Heart University
Physical Therapy Prgm
5151 Park Ave
Fairfield, CT 06825-1000
www.sacredheart.edu

Quinnipiac University
Physical Therapy Prgm
School of Health Sciences
Mt Carmel Ave
Hamden, CT 06518

University of Connecticut
Physical Therapy Prgm
School of Allied Health Professions
358 Mansfield Rd, Unit 2101
Storrs, CT 06269-2101

University of Hartford
Physical Therapy Prgm
200 Bloomfield Ave
West Hartford, CT 06117-1599
www.hartford.edu

Delaware

University of Delaware-Christiana Care Health
Physical Therapy Prgm
Dept of Physical Therapy
301 McKinly Laboratory
Newark, DE 19716
www.udel.edu/pt

District of Columbia

George Washington University
Physical Therapy Prgm
School of Medicine and Health Sciences
900 23rd St NW, Suite 6145
Washington, DC 20037
www.gwumc.edu/healthsci/programs/dpt/

Howard University
Physical Therapy Prgm
Coll of Pharmacy, Nursing and Allied Health
6th and Bryant Sts NW
Washington, DC 20059
www.howard.edu

Florida

University of Miami
Physical Therapy Prgm
School of Medicine
5915 Ponce de Leon Blvd, 5th Fl
Coral Gables, FL 33146

Nova Southeastern University
Physical Therapy Prgm
Health Professions Division
3200 S University Dr
Fort Lauderdale, FL 33328

Florida Gulf Coast University
Physical Therapy Prgm
10501 FGCU Blvd South
Fort Myers, FL 33965-6565
www.fgcu.edu/chp/pt

University of Florida
Physical Therapy Prgm
Dept of Physical Therapy
Box 100154 HSC
Gainesville, FL 32610-0154
www.phhp.ufl.edu

University of North Florida
Physical Therapy Prgm
College of Health
4567 St Johns Bluff Rd S
Jacksonville, FL 32224
www.unf.edu/coh/cohphysi.htm

Florida International University
Physical Therapy Prgm
Dept of Physical Therapy, College of Nursing Health
    Sciences
11200 SW 8th St
Miami, FL 33199
www.physicaltherapy.fiu.edu

University of Central Florida
Physical Therapy Prgm
HPA-1, Ste 256
Orlando, FL 32816-2205

Univ of St Augustine for Health Sciences
Physical Therapy Prgm
1 University Blvd
St Augustine, FL 32086-5783
www.usa.edu

Florida A&M University
Physical Therapy Prgm
School of Allied Health Sciences
Rm 223 Ware-Rhaney Bldg
Tallahassee, FL 32307-3500
www.famu.edu

University of South Florida
Physical Therapy Prgm
12901 Bruce B Downs Blvd, MDC 77
Tampa, FL 33612
www.hsc.usf.edu

Georgia

Emory University
Physical Therapy Prgm
1441 Clifton Rd NE, Ste 180
Atlanta, GA 30322
www.rehabmed.emory.edu/pt

Georgia State University
Physical Therapy Prgm
Division of Physical Therapy
PO Box 4019
Atlanta, GA 30302-4019
www.gsu.edu

Georgia Health Sciences University
Physical Therapy Prgm
Dept of Physical Therapy
Augusta, GA 30912-0800
www.mcg.edu/sah/pt

North Georgia College & State University
Physical Therapy Prgm
Barnes Hall Rm A-8
Dahlonega, GA 30597
www.ngcsu.edu

Armstrong Atlantic State University
Physical Therapy Prgm
11935 Abercorn St
Savannah, GA 31419-1997
www.pt.armstrong.edu

Idaho

Idaho State University
Physical Therapy Prgm
Dept of Physical and Occupational Therapy
Kasiska College of Health Professions, Box 8045
Pocatello, ID 83209
www.isu.edu

Illinois

Northwestern University
Physical Therapy Prgm
Feinberg School of Medicine
645 N Michigan Ave, Suite 1100
Chicago, IL 60611-2814

University of Illinois at Chicago
Physical Therapy Prgm
College of Applied Health Sciences
1919 W Taylor St, M/C 898
Chicago, IL 60612
www.ahs.uic.edu/pt.

Northern Illinois University
Physical Therapy Prgm
School of Allied Health Professions
DeKalb, IL 60115
www.chhs.niu.edu/ahp/pt/

Midwestern University
Physical Therapy Prgm
College of Health Sciences
555 31st St
Downers Grove, IL 60515
www.midwestern.edu

Rosalind Franklin University of Medicine
Physical Therapy Prgm
College of Health Professions
3333 Green Bay Rd
North Chicago, IL 60064
www.rosalindfranklin.edu

Bradley University
Physical Therapy Prgm
Dept of Physical Therapy and Health Science
1501 W Bradley Ave
Peoria, IL 61625

Governors State University
Physical Therapy Prgm
1 University Parkway
University Park, IL 60466
www.govst.edu

Indiana

University of Evansville
Physical Therapy Prgm
1800 Lincoln Ave
Evansville, IN 47722
http://pt.evansville.edu

Indiana University
Physical Therapy Prgm
1140 W Michigan St, CF 326
Indianapolis, IN 46202-5119
www.dpt.indiana.edu

University of Indianapolis
Physical Therapy Prgm
Krannert School of Physical Therapy
1400 E Hanna Ave
Indianapolis, IN 46227-3697

Iowa

St Ambrose University
Physical Therapy Prgm
518 W Locust
Davenport, IA 52803
www.sau.edu

Des Moines University
Physical Therapy Prgm
College of Health Sciences
3200 Grand Ave
Des Moines, IA 50312
www.dmu.edu/PT

Clarke University
Physical Therapy Prgm
1550 Clarke Dr
Dubuque, IA 52001-3198
www.clarke.edu

University of Iowa
Physical Therapy Prgm
Carver College of Medicine
1-252 Medical Education Bldg
Iowa City, IA 52242-1190
www.medicine.uiowa.edu/physicaltherapy

Kansas

University of Kansas Medical Center
Physical Therapy Prgm
3056 Robinson Hall
3901 Rainbow Blvd
Kansas City, KS 66160-7601
www.kumc.edu/SAH/pted

Wichita State University
Physical Therapy Prgm
College of Health Professions
Ahlberg Hall, 1845 N Fairmont
Wichita, KS 67260-0043
www.wichita.edu

Kentucky

University of Kentucky
Physical Therapy Prgm
900 S Limestone Ave, CHS Bldg, Rm 204
Lexington, KY 40536-0200

Bellarmine University
Physical Therapy Prgm
Lansing School of Nursing and Health Science
2001 Newburg Rd
Louisville, KY 40205
www.bellarmine.edu/pt

Louisiana

Louisiana State Univ Health Sciences Center
Physical Therapy Prgm
1900 Gravier St
New Orleans, LA 70112
www.alliedhealth.lsuhsc.edu/physicaltherapy

LSU Health Science Center Shreveport
Physical Therapy Prgm
School of Allied Health Professions
1501 Kings Hwy, PO Box 33932
Shreveport, LA 71130-3932
www.sh.lsushc.edu/ah

Maine

Husson University
Physical Therapy Prgm
1 College Circle
Bangor, ME 04401
www.husson.edu

University of New England
Physical Therapy Prgm
Dept of Physical Therapy
716 Stevens Ave
Portland, ME 04103
www.une.edu/chp/pt

Maryland

University of Maryland, Baltimore
Physical Therapy Prgm
School of Medicine
Department of Physical Therapy and Rehabilitation
  Science
100 Penn St, Rm 115
Baltimore, MD 21201
www.pt.umaryland.edu

University of Maryland Eastern Shore
Physical Therapy Prgm
Dept of Physical Therapy
Hazel Hall Rm 2093
Princess Anne, MD 21853
www.umes.edu/pt

Massachusetts

Boston University
Physical Therapy Prgm
Sargent Coll of Hlth and Rehab Sciences
635 Commonwealth Ave
Boston, MA 02215
www.bu.edu

MGH Institute of Health Professions
Physical Therapy Prgm
Charlestown Navy Yard
36 1st Ave
Boston, MA 02129
www.mghihp.edu

Northeastern University
Physical Therapy Prgm
360 Huntington Ave
Rm 6 Robinson Hall
Boston, MA 02115
www.neu.edu

Simmons College
Physical Therapy Prgm
School for Health Studies
300 The Fenway
Boston, MA 02115
www.simmons.edu

University of Massachusetts - Lowell
Physical Therapy Prgm
Weed Hall, 3 Solomont Way Ste 5
Lowell, MA 01854-5124
www.uml.edu/college/she/PT

American International College
Physical Therapy Prgm
1000 State St
Springfield, MA 01109-983
www.aic.edu/pages/1.html

Springfield College
Physical Therapy Prgm
Dept of Physical Therapy
263 Alden St
Springfield, MA 01109
www.spfldcol.edu/pt

Michigan

Andrews University
Physical Therapy Prgm
Dept of Physical Therapy
Berrien Springs, MI 49104-0420
www.andrews.edu

Wayne State University
Physical Therapy Prgm
2248 EACPHS
Detroit, MI 48202
www.wayne.edu

University of Michigan - Flint
Physical Therapy Prgm
School of Health Professions and Studies
303 E Kearsley St
Flint, MI 48502-2186
www.umflint.edu/pt

Grand Valley State University
Physical Therapy Prgm
301 Michigan St NE, Ste 200
Grand Rapids, MI 49503
www.gvsu.edu/pt

Central Michigan University
Physical Therapy Prgm
1220 Health Professions Building
Mount Pleasant, MI 48859
www.chp.cmich.edu/pt

Oakland University
Physical Therapy Prgm
School of Health Sciences
Rochester, MI 48309-4401
www.oakland.edu/shs/pt

Minnesota

College of St Scholastica
Physical Therapy Prgm
Graduate Studies Adm Asst
1200 Kenwood Ave
Duluth, MN 55811
www.css.edu

Saint Catherine University - Minneapolis
Physical Therapy Prgm
601 25th Ave S
Minneapolis, MN 55454
www.stkate.edu/dpt

University of Minnesota
Physical Therapy Prgm
Box 388
420 Delaware St SE
Minneapolis, MN 55455
www.physther.umn.edu

Mayo School of Health Sciences
Physical Therapy Prgm
200 First St SW
Rochester, MN 55905
www.mayo.edu/mshs/pt-career.html

Mississippi

University of Mississippi Medical Center
Physical Therapy Prgm
School of Health Related Professions
2500 N State St
Jackson, MS 39216-4505
http://shrp.umc.edu

Missouri

Southwest Baptist University
Physical Therapy Prgm
1600 University Ave
Bolivar, MO 65613-2496
www.sbuniv.edu/pt

University of Missouri
Physical Therapy Prgm
School of Health Professions
106 Lewis Hall
Columbia, MO 65211
www.umshp.org/pt

Rockhurst University
Physical Therapy Prgm
1100 Rockhurst Rd
Kansas City, MO 64110
www.rockhurst.edu/pt

Missouri State University
Physical Therapy Prgm
901 S National Ave
Springfield, MO 65804-0089
www.missouristate.edu/PhysicalTherapy

Maryville University
Physical Therapy Prgm
650 Maryville University Dr
St Louis, MO 63141
www.maryville.edu

Saint Louis University
Physical Therapy Prgm
Health Sciences Center
3437 Caroline St
St Louis, MO 63104-1111
www.slu.edu/x260.xml

Washington University
Physical Therapy Prgm
School of Medicine, Campus Box 8502
4444 Forest Park Blvd, Suite 1101
St Louis, MO 63108
http://pt.wustl.edu

Montana

University of Montana
Physical Therapy Prgm
School of Physical Therapy and Rehabilitation Science
Skaggs Bldg 135
Missoula, MT 59812
www.health.umt.edu

Nebraska

Creighton University
Physical Therapy Prgm
School of Pharmacy and Health Professions
2500 California Plaza
Omaha, NE 68178
http://pt.creighton.edu

University of Nebraska Medical Center
Physical Therapy Prgm
984420 Nebraska Medical Center
Omaha, NE 68198-4420
www.unmc.edu/physicaltherapy

Nevada

University of Nevada - Las Vegas
Physical Therapy Prgm
4505 Maryland Pkwy
Box 453029
Las Vegas, NV 89154-3029
www.unlv.edu

New Hampshire

Franklin Pierce College
Physical Therapy Prgm
5 Chenell Dr
Concord, NH 03301
www.fpc.edu

New Jersey

Univ of Medicine & Dent of New Jersey
Physical Therapy Prgm
65 Bergen St, SSB 319
PO Box 1709
Newark, NJ 07101-1709
www.shrp.umdnj.edu/physicaltherapy

Richard Stockton College of New Jersey
Physical Therapy Prgm
Jim Leeds Rd
Pomona, NJ 08240
www.stockton.edu/~mpt

Seton Hall University
Physical Therapy Prgm
400 S Orange Ave
South Orange, NJ 07079-2689
www.shu.edu

SUNJ Rutgers Camden and UMDNJ
Physical Therapy Prgm
Primary Care Center, Ste 2105
40 E Laurel Rd
Stratford, NJ 08084
www.umdnj.edu/shrpweb/programs/mpt

New Mexico

University of New Mexico
Physical Therapy Prgm
Health Sciences Center
1 University of New Mexico
MSC09 5230
Albuquerque, NM 87131-0001
http://hsc.unm.edu/som/physther

New York

Daemen College
Physical Therapy Prgm
4380 Main St
Amherst, NY 14226-3592

Long Island University - Brooklyn Campus
Physical Therapy Prgm
Zeckendorf Health Sciences Center
One University Plaza
Brooklyn, NY 11201-5372
www.brooklyn.liu.edu

SUNY Downstate Medical Center
Physical Therapy Prgm
450 Clarkson Ave, Box 16
Brooklyn, NY 11203-2098
www.downstate.edu

D'Youville College
Physical Therapy Prgm
One D'Youville Sq
320 Porter Ave
Buffalo, NY 14201-1084
www.dyc.edu

University at Buffalo - SUNY
Physical Therapy Prgm
Department of Rehabilitation Science
515 Kimball Tower, 3435 Main St
Buffalo, NY 14214-3079
www.sphhp.buffalo.edu/rs

Mercy College
Physical Therapy Prgm
555 Broadway
Dobbs Ferry, NY 10522
http://grad.mercy.edu/physicaltherapy

Ithaca College
Physical Therapy Prgm
Dept of Physical Therapy
335 Smiddy Hall
Ithaca, NY 14850-7183
http://departments.ithaca.edu/pt

Columbia University
Physical Therapy Prgm
710 W 168th St, 8th Fl
New York, NY 10032
www.columbiaphysicaltherapy.org

CUNY Hunter College
Physical Therapy Prgm
425 E 25th St
New York, NY 10010
www.hunter.cuny.edu/schoolhp/pt

New York University
Physical Therapy Prgm
380 2nd Ave, 4th Fl
New York, NY 10010
http://steinhardt.nyu.edu/pt

Touro College
Physical Therapy Prgm
27 W 23rd St, 6th Fl
New York, NY 10010-4202
www.touro.edu/shs/pt/pt.asp

New York Institute of Technology
Physical Therapy Prgm
Northern Blvd
Box 8000
Old Westbury, NY 11568-8000

Dominican College
Physical Therapy Prgm
470 Western Hwy
Orangeburg, NY 10962-1299
www.dc.edu

Clarkson University
Physical Therapy Prgm
PO Box 5880
Potsdam, NY 13699-5880
www.clarkson.edu

Nazareth College of Rochester
Physical Therapy Prgm
4245 East Ave
Rochester, NY 14618-3790
www.naz.edu/dept/physical_therapy

CUNY College of Staten Island
Physical Therapy Prgm
2800 Victory Blvd
Staten Island, NY 10314
www.csi.cuny.edu

Stony Brook University
Physical Therapy Prgm
Sch of Health Tech and Management
Health Sciences Center
Stony Brook, NY 11794-8201
www.hsc.stonybrook.edu

SUNY Upstate Medical University
Physical Therapy Prgm
College of Health Professions
750 E Adams St
Syracuse, NY 13210

The Sage Colleges
Physical Therapy Prgm
Sage Graduate School, Dept of Physical Therapy
45 Ferry St
Troy, NY 12180
www.sage.edu

Utica College
Physical Therapy Prgm
Health and Human Studies Division
1600 Burrstone Rd
Utica, NY 13502-4892
http://utica.edu/academic/gce/pt

New York Medical College
Physical Therapy Prgm
Rm 302, School of Public Health
Valhalla, NY 10595
www.nymc.edu

North Carolina

University of North Carolina - Chapel Hill
Physical Therapy Prgm
Div of Physical Therapy
Medical School Wing E, CB 7135
Chapel Hill, NC 27599-7135
www.med.unc.edu/mahp/physical

Western Carolina University
Physical Therapy Prgm
312 Moore Bldg
Cullowhee, NC 28723-9646
www.wcu.edu

Duke University Medical Center
Physical Therapy Prgm
PO Box 3965
Durham, NC 27710
http://dpt.dukehealth.org

Elon University
Cosponsor: Alamance Regional Medical Center
Physical Therapy Prgm
Campus Box 2085
Elon, NC 27244-2010
www.elon.edu/home/

East Carolina University
Physical Therapy Prgm
Dept of Physical Therapy
School of Allied Health Sciences
Greenville, NC 27858-4353
www.ecu.edu/pt

Winston-Salem State University
Physical Therapy Prgm
601 Martin Luther King Jr Dr
Winston-Salem, NC 27110

North Dakota

University of Mary
Physical Therapy Prgm
7500 University Dr
Bismarck, ND 58504-9652
www.umary.edu

University of North Dakota
Physical Therapy Prgm
School of Medicine
PO Box 9037, 501 N Columbia Rd
Grand Forks, ND 58202-9037

Ohio

Ohio University
Physical Therapy Prgm
School of Physical Therapy
W290 Grover Center
Athens, OH 45701
www.ohiou.edu/phystherapy

College of Mt St Joseph
Physical Therapy Prgm
5701 Delhi Rd
Cincinnati, OH 45233-1672
www.msj.edu

University of Cincinnati
Physical Therapy Prgm
College of Allied Health Science
PO Box 670394
Cincinnati, OH 45267-0394
www.cahs.uc.edu/departments/physicalt.cfm

Cleveland State University
Physical Therapy Prgm
Dept of Health Sciences HS 122
2121 Euclid Ave
Cleveland, OH 44115-2407
http://sciences.csuohio.edu/departments/health/

The Ohio State University
Physical Therapy Prgm
516 Atwell Hall
453 W Tenth Ave
Columbus, OH 43210
www.osu.edu

University of Dayton
Physical Therapy Prgm
300 College Park
Dayton, OH 45469-1210
www.udayton.edu

The University of Findlay
Physical Therapy Prgm
1000 N Main St
Findlay, OH 45840
www.findlay.edu

Walsh University
Physical Therapy Prgm
2020 East Maple St
North Canton, OH 44720-3396
www.walsh.edu

University of Toledo
Physical Therapy Prgm
4416 Collier Bldg
3015 Arlington Ave
Toledo, OH 43614
http://hsc.utoledo.edu/healthsciences/pt/index.html

Youngstown State University
Physical Therapy Prgm
B080 Cushwa Hall
Youngstown, OH 44555-2558
http://bchhs.ysu.edu/dpt/dpt.html

Oklahoma

Langston University
Physical Therapy Prgm
School of Physical Therapy
PO Box 1500
Langston, OK 73050
www.lunet.edu

Univ of Oklahoma Health Sciences Center
Physical Therapy Prgm
College of Allied Health, Rm 235
PO Box 26901
Oklahoma City, OK 73190
www.ah.ouhsc.edu/main

Ontario, Canada

University of Western Ontario
Physical Therapy Prgm
Faculty of Health Sciences
Elborn College, Rm 1588
1201 Western Rd
London, ON N6G 1H1
www.uwo.ca/fhs/pt

University of Toronto
Physical Therapy Prgm
160 - 500 University Ave, 8th Fl
Toronto, ON MSG 1V7
www.utoronto.ca/pt

Oregon

Pacific University
Physical Therapy Prgm
School of Physical Therapy
222 SE 8th Ave, Suite 333
Hillsboro, OR 97123
www.pacificu.edu

Pennsylvania

Lebanon Valley College
Physical Therapy Prgm
101 N College Ave
Annville, PA 17003-0501
www.lvc.edu/physical-therapy/index.aspx

Neumann University
Physical Therapy Prgm
Division of Nursing and Health Sciences
1 Neumann Dr
Aston, PA 19014-1298
www.neumann.edu

Widener University
Physical Therapy Prgm
One University Plaza
Chester, PA 19013
www.widener.edu/ipte

Misericordia University
Physical Therapy Prgm
301 Lake St
Dallas, PA 18612-1098
www.misericordia.edu

Gannon University
Physical Therapy Prgm
Coll of Sciences, Engineering and Health
109 University Square
Erie, PA 16541-0001
www.gannon.edu/programs

Arcadia University
Physical Therapy Prgm
Dept of Physical Therapy
450 S Easton Rd
Glenside, PA 19038-3295
www.arcadia.edu/academic/default.aspx?id=1007

St Francis University
Physical Therapy Prgm
PO Box 600
Loretto, PA 15940-0600
www.francis.edu

Drexel University College of Medicine
Physical Therapy Prgm
Physical Therapy and Rehabilitation Sciences
Mail Stop 502, 245 N 15th St
Philadelphia, PA 19102
www.drexel.edu/cnhp/depts/rehab/programs/dpt

Temple University
Physical Therapy Prgm
College of Health Professions
3307 N Broad St
Philadelphia, PA 19140
www.temple.edu/pt

Thomas Jefferson University
Physical Therapy Prgm
College of Health Professions
130 S Ninth St, Suite 830 Edison
Philadelphia, PA 19107-5233
www.tju.edu

University of the Sciences
Physical Therapy Prgm
600 S 43rd St
Philadelphia, PA 19104
www.usip.edu

Chatham University
Physical Therapy Prgm
114 Dilworth Hall
Woodland Rd
Pittsburgh, PA 15232-2826
www.chatham.edu

Duquesne University
Physical Therapy Prgm
School of Health Sciences
139 Health Sciences Bldg
Pittsburgh, PA 15282
www.healthsciences.duq.edu/phyth

University of Pittsburgh
Physical Therapy Prgm
School of Health and Rehab Sciences
4019 Forbes Tower
Pittsburgh, PA 15260
www.shrs.pitt.edu/physicaltherapy

University of Scranton
Physical Therapy Prgm
800 Linden St
Scranton, PA 18510-4586
http://matrix.scranton.edu

Slippery Rock University of Pennsylvania
Physical Therapy Prgm
Graduate School of Physical Therapy
PT Building
Slippery Rock, PA 16057
www.sru.edu

Puerto Rico

University of Puerto Rico
Physical Therapy Prgm
Medical Sciences Campus
PO Box 365067
San Juan, PR 00936-5067
http://cprsweb.rcm.upr.edu/terapiafisica.asp

Rhode Island

University of Rhode Island
Physical Therapy Prgm
Independence Square II
25 West Independence Way
Kingston, RI 02881-0180
www.ptp.uri.edu

South Carolina

Medical University of South Carolina
Physical Therapy Prgm
Dept of Rehabilitation Sciences
PO Box 250965
Charleston, SC 29425
www.musc.edu/pt

University of South Carolina
Physical Therapy Prgm
School of Public Health
Columbia, SC 29208
www.sph.sc.edu/dpt/programstudy-postdpt.htm

South Dakota

University of South Dakota
Physical Therapy Prgm
Dept of Physical Therapy
414 E Clark St
Vermillion, SD 57069
www.usd.edu

Tennessee

University of Tennessee - Chattanooga
Physical Therapy Prgm
615 McCallie Ave
Chattanooga, TN 37403
www.utc.edu/physicaltherapy

East Tennessee State University
Physical Therapy Prgm
Box 70624
Johnson City, TN 37614
www.etsu.edu/cpah/physther

University of Tennessee Health Science Ctr
Physical Therapy Prgm
930 Madison Ave
Suite 640
Memphis, TN 38163
www.utmem.edu

Belmont University
Physical Therapy Prgm
1900 Belmont Blvd
Nashville, TN 37212-3757
www.belmont.edu/pt

Tennessee State University
Physical Therapy Prgm
3500 John A Merritt Blvd, Box 9564
Nashville, TN 37209
www.tnstate.edu

Texas

Hardin-Simmons University
Physical Therapy Prgm
2200 Hickory St
Box 16065 HSU Station
Abilene, TX 79698-6065
www.hsutx.edu/academics/graduate/programs/
	physicaltherapy

University of St Augustine for Health Science
Physical Therapy Prgm
5401 LaCrosse Ave
Austin, TX 78739

Univ of Texas Southwestern Med Ctr
Physical Therapy Prgm
Southwestern Allied Health Sciences Sch
5323 Harry Hines Blvd
Dallas, TX 75390-8876
www.utsouthwestern.edu/pt

University of Texas at El Paso
Physical Therapy Prgm
1101 N Campbell
El Paso, TX 79902-0581

US Army-Baylor University
Physical Therapy Prgm
3151 Scott Rd, Ste 1230
Fort Sam Houston, TX 78234-6138
www.cs.amedd.army.mil

University of Texas Medical Branch
Physical Therapy Prgm
School of Allied Health Sciences
301 University Blvd
Galveston, TX 77555-1144
www.sahs.utmb.edu/programs/pt

Texas Woman's University
Physical Therapy Prgm
School of Physical Therapy
6700 Fannin St
Houston, TX 77030
www.twu.edu/pt

Texas Tech Univ Health Sciences Center
Physical Therapy Prgm
3601 Fourth St
Lubbock, TX 79430
www.ttuhsc.edu/SAH

Angelo State University
Physical Therapy Prgm
2601 West Ave N
ASU Station 10923
San Angelo, TX 76909-0923
www.angelo.edu/dept/physical_therapy

UT Health Science Center - San Antonio
Physical Therapy Prgm
7703 Floyd Curl Dr MSC 6247
San Antonio, TX 78229-3900
www.uthscsa.edu/sah/pt

Texas State University - San Marcos
Physical Therapy Prgm
Health Science Center
601 University Dr
San Marcos, TX 78666
www.health.txstate.edu/pt

United Kingdom

Robert Gordon University
Physical Therapy Prgm
Faculty of Health and Social Care
Garthdee Rd
Garthdee Aberdeen, UK AB10 7QG
www.rgu.ac.uk/prospectus/disp_pgProspectusEntry.cfm?
	CourseID=MSHSPH

Utah

University of Utah
Physical Therapy Prgm
Div of Physical Therapy
520 Wakara Way
Salt Lake City, UT 84108-1290
www.health.utah.edu/pt

Vermont

University of Vermont
Physical Therapy Prgm
College of Nursing and Health Sciences
305 Rowell Bldg, 106 Carrigan Dr
Burlington, VT 05405-0068
www.uvm.edu/~cnhs

Virginia

Marymount University
Physical Therapy Prgm
2807 N Glebe Rd
Arlington, VA 22207-4299
www.marymount.edu

Hampton University
Physical Therapy Prgm
Department of Physical Therapy
Phenix Hall Rm 216
Hampton, VA 23668

Old Dominion University
Physical Therapy Prgm
School of Physical Therapy
129 Wm B Spong Jr Hall
Norfolk, VA 23529-0288
www.odu.edu/dpt

Virginia Commonwealth Univ/Health System
Physical Therapy Prgm
Medical College of Virginia Campus
Box 980224
Richmond, VA 23298-0224
www.vcu.edu/pt

Shenandoah University
Physical Therapy Prgm
333 W Cork St
Winchester, VA 22601
www.su.edu/pt

Washington

University of Washington
Physical Therapy Prgm
Physical Therapy CC-902, Rehab Medicine
1959 NE Pacific St, Box 356490
Seattle, WA 98195-6490
www.depts.washington.edu/rehab/education

Eastern Washington University
Physical Therapy Prgm
310 N Riverpoint Blvd
Box T, Rm 270
Spokane, WA 99202-0002
www.ewu.edu/pt

University of Puget Sound
Physical Therapy Prgm
1500 N Warner
CMB 1070
Tacoma, WA 98416
www.ups.edu/pt

West Virginia

West Virginia University
Physical Therapy Prgm
School of Medicine, Robert C Byrd Health Sciences
    Center
PO Box 9226
Morgantown, WV 26506-9226
www.hsc.wvu.edu/som/pt

Wheeling Jesuit University
Physical Therapy Prgm
316 Washington Ave
Wheeling, WV 26003

Wisconsin

University of Wisconsin - La Crosse
Physical Therapy Prgm
4033 Health Science Ctr
1725 State St
La Crosse, WI 54601
www.uwlax.edu/pt

University of Wisconsin - Madison
Physical Therapy Prgm
5173 Medical Sciences Center
1300 University Ave
Madison, WI 53706-1532
www.orthorehab.wisc.edu/pt

Concordia University Wisconsin
Physical Therapy Prgm
12800 N Lake Shore Dr
Mequon, WI 53092-7699

Marquette University
Physical Therapy Prgm
PO Box 1881
Milwaukee, WI 53201-1881
www.marquette.edu/chs/pt

University of Wisconsin-Milwaukee
Physical Therapy Prgm
PO Box 413
Milwaukee, WI 53201-1041
www.dpt.uwm.edu

Carroll University
Physical Therapy Prgm
100 N East Ave
Waukesha, WI 53186
www.cc.edu

Physical Therapist Assistant

Career Description
Physical therapist assistants work under the supervision of a physical therapist. Their duties include assisting the physical therapist by providing selected interventions within the plan of care, training patients in exercises and activities of daily living, conducting treatments, using special equipment, administering modalities and other treatment procedures, and reporting to the physical therapist on the patient's responses.

Employment Characteristics
Physical therapist assistants work in:
- Hospitals
- Private physical therapy offices
- Community health centers
- Corporate or industrial health centers
- Sports facilities
- Research institutions
- Rehabilitation centers
- Nursing homes
- Home health agencies
- Schools
- Pediatric centers
- Colleges and universities

Salary
Data from the US Bureau of Labor Statistics for May 2011 shows that wages at the 10th percentile were $32,030, the 50th percentile (median) at $51,040, and the 90th percentile at $71,200 (*www.bls.gov/oes/current/oes312021.htm*).

For more information, refer to *www.ama-assn.org/go/hpsalary*.

Educational Programs
Length. These associate's degree programs—usually offered in a community or junior college—are 2 years long.

Prerequisites. Successful completion of high school courses in social sciences, biology, mathematics, physics, English, and chemistry is encouraged but not required.

Curriculum. The curriculum includes one year of general education and one year of technical courses and clinical experience.

Inquiries

Careers, Education, and Certification
American Physical Therapy Association
1111 North Fairfax Street
Alexandria, VA 22314-1488
800 999-2782 or 703 684-2782
www.apta.org

Program Accreditation
Commission on Accreditation in Physical Therapy Education
1111 North Fairfax Street
Alexandria, VA 22314
703 684-2782
www.apta.org/capte

Physical Therapist Assistant

Alabama

Jefferson State Community College
Physical Therapist Assistant Prgm
Center for Health and Biological Sciences
4600 Valleydale Rd
Birmingham, AL 35242
www.jeffstateonline.com

Calhoun Community College
Physical Therapist Assistant Prgm
PO Box 2216
Decatur, AL 35609

Wallace Community College
Physical Therapist Assistant Prgm
1141 Wallace Dr
Dothan, AL 36303
www.wallace.edu

Wallace State Community College
Physical Therapist Assistant Prgm
PO Box 2000
Hanceville, AL 35077-2000
www.wallacestate.edu

Bishop State Community College
Physical Therapist Assistant Prgm
1365 Martin Luther King Ave
Mobile, AL 36603-5362
www.bishop.edu/health/pta.htm

South University
Physical Therapist Assistant Prgm
5355 Vaughn Rd
Montgomery, AL 36116-1120
www.southuniversity.edu

Arizona

Mohave Community College
Physical Therapist Assistant Prgm
1977 Acoma Blvd, West
Lake Havasu City, AZ 86403
www.mohave.edu

Carrington College
Physical Therapist Assistant Prgm
1300 South Country Club Drive
Mesa, AZ 85210

Pima Medical Institute
Physical Therapist Assistant Prgm
957 S Dobson Rd
Mesa, AZ 85202

GateWay Community College
Physical Therapist Assistant Prgm
108 N 40th St
Phoenix, AZ 85034
http://healthcare.gatewaycc.edu/Programs/
    PhysicalTherapistAssistant

Pima Medical Institute
Physical Therapist Assistant Prgm
Tucson Campus
3350 E Grant Rd
Tucson, AZ 85716

Arkansas

NorthWest Arkansas Community College
Physical Therapist Assistant Prgm
One College Dr
Bentonville, AR 72712-5091
www.nwacc.edu

South Arkansas Community College
Physical Therapist Assistant Prgm
300 West Ave
PO Box 7010
El Dorado, AR 71730
www.southark.edu

Arkansas Tech University - Ozark Campus
Physical Therapist Assistant Prgm
1700 Helberg Lane
Ozark, AR 72949

Arkansas State University
Physical Therapist Assistant Prgm
Department of Health Professions
PO Box 910
State University, AR 72467
www.astate.edu

California

Loma Linda University
Physical Therapist Assistant Prgm
School of Allied Health Professions
Nichol Hall, Rm 1911
Loma Linda, CA 92350
www.llu.edu/llu/sahp/pt/pta.htm

Ohlone College
Physical Therapist Assistant Prgm
Ohlone Community College Dist
Newark Ohlone Center, 35753 Cedar Blvd
Newark, CA 94560
www.ohlone.edu/instr/phys_ther

Concorde Career College
Physical Therapist Assistant Prgm
12412 Victory Blvd
North Hollywood, CA 91606
www.concorde.edu

Cerritos College
Physical Therapist Assistant Prgm
Health Occupations Div
11110 Alondra Blvd
Norwalk, CA 90650
www.cerritos.edu

Sacramento City College
Physical Therapist Assistant Prgm
Science and Allied Health
3835 Freeport Blvd
Sacramento, CA 95822
www.scc.losrios.edu/~sah/physther

San Diego Mesa College
Physical Therapist Assistant Prgm
7250 Mesa College Dr
San Diego, CA 92111-4998

Colorado

Pima Medical Institute - Denver
Physical Therapist Assistant Prgm
7475 Dakin St, Suite 100
Denver, CO 80221-6915
www.pmi.edu/locations/denver.asp

Morgan Community College
Physical Therapist Assistant Prgm
17800 Rd 20
Fort Morgan, CO 80701
www.morgancc.edu

Arapahoe Community College
Physical Therapist Assistant Prgm
2500 W College Dr, PO Box 9002
Littleton, CO 80160-9002
www.arapahoe.edu/deptprgrms/pta

Pueblo Community College
Physical Therapist Assistant Prgm
900 W Orman Ave
Pueblo, CO 81004
www.pueblocc.edu

Connecticut

Norwalk Community College
Physical Therapist Assistant Prgm
188 Richards Ave
Norwalk, CT 06854-1655
www.ncc.commnet.edu

Naugatuck Valley Community College
Physical Therapist Assistant Prgm
750 Chase Pkwy
Waterbury, CT 06708
www.nvcc.commnet.edu/allied_health

Delaware

Delaware Technical Community College - Owens Campus
Physical Therapist Assistant Prgm
PO Box 610
Georgetown, DE 19947
www.dtcc.edu/owens

Delaware Technical Community College - Wilmington
Physical Therapist Assistant Prgm
333 Shipley St
Wilmington, DE 19801
www.wilmington.dtcc.edu/wilmington/ah/pta.html

Florida

State College of Florida, Manatee-Sarasota
Physical Therapist Assistant Prgm
5840 26th St W
Bradenton, FL 34207
www.mccfl.edu

Broward College
Physical Therapist Assistant Prgm
Ctr for Health Science Education ll
1000 Coconut Creek Blvd
Coconut Creek, FL 33066
www.broward.edu

Daytona State College, Daytona Beach Campus
Physical Therapist Assistant Prgm
1200 International Speedway Blvd
Daytona Beach, FL 32120-2811

Keiser University
Physical Therapist Assistant Prgm
1500 NW 49th St
Fort Lauderdale, FL 33309
www.keisercollege.edu

Indian River State College
Physical Therapist Assistant Prgm
3209 Virginia Ave
Fort Pierce, FL 34981-5596
www.ircc.edu

Florida State College at Jacksonville
Physical Therapist Assistant Prgm
4501 Capper Rd
Jacksonville, FL 32218-4499
www.fccj.edu

Lake City Community College
Physical Therapist Assistant Prgm
149 SE College Place
Lake City, FL 32025

Dade Medical College
Physical Therapist Assistant Prgm
MDCC Medical Campus
950 NW 20th St
Miami, FL 33127
www.mdc.edu

College of Central Florida
Physical Therapist Assistant Prgm
PO Box 1388
Ocala, FL 34478-1388
www.cf.edu

Gulf Coast State College
Physical Therapist Assistant Prgm
5230 W US Hwy 98
Panama City, FL 32401-1041
http://health.gulfcoast.edu

Seminole State College
Physical Therapist Assistant Prgm
100 Weldon Blvd
Sanford, FL 32773-6199

St Petersburg College
Physical Therapist Assistant Prgm
PO Box 13489
St Petersburg, FL 33733
www.spcollege.edu/hec/pta

Pensacola State College
Physical Therapist Assistant Prgm
Warrington Campus
5555 W Hwy 98
Warrington, FL 32507

South University
Physical Therapist Assistant Prgm
West Palm Beach Campus
1760 N Congress Ave
West Palm Beach, FL 33409

Polk State College
Physical Therapist Assistant Prgm
999 Ave H NE
Winter Haven, FL 33881
www.polk.edu

Georgia

Chattahoochee Technical College North Metro
Physical Therapist Assistant Prgm
5198 Ross Rd
Acworth, GA 30102
www.chattahoocheetech.edu

Darton College
Physical Therapist Assistant Prgm
2400 Gillionville Rd
Albany, GA 31707
www.darton.edu

Athens Technical College
Physical Therapist Assistant Prgm
800 US Hwy 29 N
Athens, GA 30601-1500
www.athenstech.org

South University
Physical Therapist Assistant Prgm
709 Mall Blvd
Savannah, GA 31406
www.southuniversity.edu

Hawaii

Kapiolani Community College
Physical Therapist Assistant Prgm
4303 Diamond Head Rd
Health Sciences Dept, Kauila 122
Honolulu, HI 96816
www.kcc.hawaii.edu

Idaho

Idaho State University
Physical Therapist Assistant Prgm
College of Technology
Campus Box 8380
Pocatello, ID 83209-8380
www.isu.edu/departments/PTA

Illinois

Southwestern Illinois College
Physical Therapist Assistant Prgm
2500 Carlyle Rd
Belleville, IL 62221
www.southwestern.cc.il.us/

Southern Illinois University Carbondale
Physical Therapist Assistant Prgm
SIU Clinical Ctr, 4602
Carbondale, IL 62901-4602
www.siu.edu

Kaskaskia College
Physical Therapist Assistant Prgm
27210 College Rd
Centralia, IL 62801

Morton College
Physical Therapist Assistant Prgm
3801 S Central Ave
Cicero, IL 60804
www.morton.edu

Oakton Community College
Physical Therapist Assistant Prgm
1600 E Golf Rd
Des Plaines, IL 60016
www.oakton.edu/acad/dept/pta

Lake Land College
Physical Therapist Assistant Prgm
LLC Kluthe Center
1204 Network Center Dr
Effingham, IL 62401
www.lakeland.cc.il.us

Elgin Community College
Physical Therapist Assistant Prgm
Community College District 509
1700 Spartan Drive, HBT 122
Elgin, IL 60123-3719
http://elgin.edu

College of DuPage
Physical Therapist Assistant Prgm
IC 1028, 425 Fawell Blvd
Glen Ellyn, IL 60137-6599
www.cod.edu

Kankakee Community College
Physical Therapist Assistant Prgm
100 College Drive
Kankakee, IL 60901
www.kcc.edu

Black Hawk College
Physical Therapist Assistant Prgm
6600 34th Ave
Moline, IL 61265-5899
www.bhc.edu

Illinois Central College
Physical Therapist Assistant Prgm
201 SW Adams St
Peoria, IL 61635-0001
www.icc.edu

Fox College
Physical Therapist Assistant Prgm
18020 Oak Park Ave
Tinley Park, IL 60477

Indiana

University of Evansville
Physical Therapist Assistant Prgm
1800 Lincoln Ave
Evansville, IN 47722
www.evansville.edu

Brown Mackie College - Fort Wayne
Physical Therapist Assistant Prgm
3000 E Coliseum Blvd
Fort Wayne, IN 46805
www.brownmackie.edu

University of Saint Francis
Physical Therapist Assistant Prgm
2701 Spring St
Fort Wayne, IN 46808

Ivy Tech Community College
Physical Therapist Assistant Prgm
1440 E 35th Ave
Gary, IN 46409
www.ivytech.edu

University of Indianapolis
Physical Therapist Assistant Prgm
Krannert School of Physical Therapy
1400 E Hanna Ave
Indianapolis, IN 46227-3697
http://pt.uindy.edu/pta

Ivy Tech Community College - Muncie
Physical Therapist Assistant Prgm
4301 S Cowan Rd
Muncie, IN 47302

Brown Mackie College - Fort Wayne
Physical Therapist Assistant Prgm
1030 E Jefferson Blvd
South Bend, IN 46617
www.brownmackie.edu

Vincennes University
Physical Therapist Assistant Prgm
Health Occupations Dept
Vincennes, IN 47591
www.vinu.edu

Iowa

Kirkwood Community College
Physical Therapist Assistant Prgm
6301 Kirkwood Blvd SW
Cedar Rapids, IA 52406
www.kirkwood.edu

Mercy College of Health Sciences
Physical Therapist Assistant Prgm
928 6th Ave
Des Moines, IA 50309-1239
www.mchs.edu/acad_as_pt_assist.cfm

North Iowa Area Community College
Physical Therapist Assistant Prgm
500 College Dr
Mason, IA 50401
www.niacc.edu

Indian Hills Community College
Physical Therapist Assistant Prgm
Health Occupations Division
Ottumwa Campus, 525 Grandview
Ottumwa, IA 52501
www.indianhills.edu

Western Iowa Tech Community College
Physical Therapist Assistant Prgm
4647 Stone Ave, PO Box 5199
Sioux City, IA 51102-5199

Kansas

Colby Community College
Physical Therapist Assistant Prgm
1255 South Range
Colby, KS 67701
www.colbycc.edu

Hutchinson Community College
Physical Therapist Assistant Prgm
Davis Hall
1300 N Plum
Hutchinson, KS 67502
www.hutchcc.edu/pta

Kansas City Kansas Community College
Physical Therapist Assistant Prgm
PO Box 12951
7250 State Ave
Kansas City, KS 66112-9978
www.kckcc.cc.ks.us

Washburn University
Physical Therapist Assistant Prgm
School of Applied Studies
1700 SW College Ave
Topeka, KS 66621

Kentucky

Hazard Community & Technical College
Cosponsor: Southeast Kentucky Community & Technical
College
Physical Therapist Assistant Prgm
One Community College Dr
Hazard, KY 41701-2402
www.hazard.kctcs.edu

Jefferson Community and Technical College
Physical Therapist Assistant Prgm
109 E Broadway St
Louisville, KY 40202-2005
www.jefferson.kctcs.edu

Madisonville Community College
Physical Therapist Assistant Prgm
750 N Laffoon St
Madisonville, KY 42431-9185
www.madcc.kctcs.edu

**West Kentucky Community & Technical
College**
Physical Therapist Assistant Prgm
PO Box 7380
Paducah, KY 42002-7380
http://allied.westkentucky.kctcs.edu/pta

Somerset Community College
Physical Therapist Assistant Prgm
808 Monticello St
Somerset, KY 42501
www.somerset.kctcs.edu

Louisiana

Our Lady of the Lake College
Physical Therapist Assistant Prgm
7443 Picardy Ave
Baton Rouge, LA 70808
www.ololcollege.edu

Bossier Parish Community College
Physical Therapist Assistant Prgm
6220 E Texas St
Bossier City, LA 71111
www.bpcc.edu

Delgado Community College
Physical Therapist Assistant Prgm
615 City Park Ave
New Orleans, LA 70119-4399
www.dcc.edu

Louisiana College
Physical Therapist Assistant Prgm
1140 College Drive, Box 531
Pineville, LA 71359
http://lacollege.edu/alliedhealth/index.aspx

Maine

Kennebec Valley Community College
Physical Therapist Assistant Prgm
92 Western Ave
Fairfield, ME 04937-1367
www.kvcc.me.edu/pta

Maryland

Chesapeake Area Consortium for Higher Educ
Physical Therapist Assistant Prgm
101 College Pkwy
Arnold, MD 21012

Baltimore City Community College
Physical Therapist Assistant Prgm
Nursing Bldg Rm 302
2901 Liberty Heights Ave
Baltimore, MD 21215
www.bccc.edu

Allegany College of Maryland
Physical Therapist Assistant Prgm
12401 Willowbrook Rd SE
Cumberland, MD 21502-2596

Montgomery College
Physical Therapist Assistant Prgm
7600 Takoma Ave
Takoma Park, MD 20912
www.montgomerycollege.edu

Carroll Community College
Physical Therapist Assistant Prgm
1601 Washington Rd
Westminster, MD 21157
www.carrollcc.edu

Massachusetts

Bay State College
Physical Therapist Assistant Prgm
122 Commonwealth Ave
Boston, MA 02116
www.baystate.edu

North Shore Community College
Physical Therapist Assistant Prgm
One Ferncroft Rd
Danvers, MA 01923-4093
www.northshore.edu

Mount Wachusett Community College
Physical Therapist Assistant Prgm
444 Green St
Gardner, MA 01440-1000
www.mwcc.mass.edu

Berkshire Community College
Physical Therapist Assistant Prgm
1350 West St
Pittsfield, MA 01201-5786
www.berkshirecc.edu/pta

Springfield Technical Community College
Physical Therapist Assistant Prgm
One Armory Sq, Ste 1
PO Box 9000
Springfield, MA 01102
www.stcc.edu

Michigan

Washtenaw Community College
Physical Therapist Assistant Prgm
Occupational Education Building, Room 102
4800 East Huron River Drive
Ann Arbor, MI 48104-4939

Kellogg Community College
Physical Therapist Assistant Prgm
450 North Ave
Battle Creek, MI 49017
www.kellogg.edu/pta

Delta College
Physical Therapist Assistant Prgm
6263 Mackinaw Rd, P-172
Bay City, MI 48710-0001
www.delta.edu/health/pta/index.html

Macomb Community College
Physical Therapist Assistant Prgm
44575 Garfield Rd
Clinton Township, MI 48038-1139
www.macomb.edu

Henry Ford Community College
Cosponsor: Oakwood Healthcare System, Inc
Physical Therapist Assistant Prgm
5101 Evergreen Rd
Dearborn, MI 48128
www.hfcc.edu

Mott Community College - Southern Lakes Branch Campus
Physical Therapist Assistant Prgm
2100 W Thompson Rd
Fenton, MI 48430
www.mcc.edu/slbc/sbc_index.shtml

Baker College of Flint
Physical Therapist Assistant Prgm
1050 W Bristol Rd
Flint, MI 48507-5508
www.baker.edu

Finlandia University
Physical Therapist Assistant Prgm
601 Quincy St
Hancock, MI 49930-1882
www.finlandia.edu

Mid Michigan Community College
Physical Therapist Assistant Prgm
Doan Center
2600 S Summerton
Mt Pleasant, MI 48858

Baker College of Muskegon
Physical Therapist Assistant Prgm
1903 Marquette Ave
Muskegon, MI 49442
www.baker.edu

Delta College
Physical Therapist Assistant Prgm
Rm P-172
University Center, MI 48710
www.delta.edu

Minnesota

Anoka Ramsey Community College
Physical Therapist Assistant Prgm
11200 Mississippi Blvd NW
Coon Rapids, MN 55433
www.anokaramsey.edu

Lake Superior College
Physical Therapist Assistant Prgm
2101 Trinity Rd
Duluth, MN 55811
www.lsc.edu/Programs/HealthCareers/
    PhysicalTherapistAssistant

Northland Community & Technical College
Physical Therapist Assistant Prgm
2022 Central Ave NE
East Grand Forks, MN 56721

Saint Catherine University - Minneapolis
Physical Therapist Assistant Prgm
601 25th Ave S
Minneapolis, MN 55454
www.stkate.edu

Mississippi

Itawamba Community College
Physical Therapist Assistant Prgm
Dept of Applied Science and Technology
602 W Hill St
Fulton, MS 38843
www.iccms.edu

Pearl River Community College - Hattiesburg
Physical Therapist Assistant Prgm
5448 US Hwy 49 S
Hattiesburg, MS 39401
www.prcc.edu

Hinds Community College
Physical Therapist Assistant Prgm
Nursing Applied Health Center
1750 Chadwick Dr
Jackson, MS 39204-3490
www.hindscc.edu

Meridian Community College
Physical Therapist Assistant Prgm
910 Hwy 19 N
Meridian, MS 39307-5890
www.mcc.cc.ms.us

Missouri

Linn State Technical College
Physical Therapist Assistant Prgm
Capital Region Medical Center
Southwest Campus, 1432 Southwest Blvd
Jefferson City, MO 65101
www.linnstate.edu

Metropolitan Community College - Penn Valley
Physical Therapist Assistant Prgm
3201 SW Trafficway
Kansas City, MO 64111-2764
www.mcckc.edu

Ozarks Technical Community College
Physical Therapist Assistant Prgm
1001 E Chestnut Expressway
Springfield, MO 65802
www.otc.edu

Missouri Western State University
Physical Therapist Assistant Prgm
4525 Downs Dr, JGM 304
St Joseph, MO 64507-2294

St Louis Community College - Meramec
Physical Therapist Assistant Prgm
11333 Big Bend Blvd
St Louis, MO 63122
www.stlcc.edu

Montana

Montana State University
Physical Therapist Assistant Prgm
2100 16th Ave South
Great Falls, MT 59405-4907
www.msugf.edu

Nebraska

Southeast Community College
Physical Therapist Assistant Prgm
8800 O St
Lincoln, NE 68520

Northeast Community College
Physical Therapist Assistant Prgm
801 E Benjamin Ave, PO Box 469
Norfolk, NE 68702-0469
www.northeastcollege.com

Clarkson College
Physical Therapist Assistant Prgm
101 S 42nd St
Omaha, NE 68131-2739
www.clarksoncollege.edu

Nebraska Methodist College
Physical Therapist Assistant Prgm
720 North 87th St
Omaha, NE 68114

Nevada

College of Southern Nevada
Physical Therapist Assistant Prgm
6375 W Charleston Blvd
Las Vegas, NV 89146
www.ccsn.edu

New Hampshire

River Valley Community College
Physical Therapist Assistant Prgm
One College Dr
Claremont, NH 03743-9707
www.claremont.nhctc.edu/index.html

Hesser College
Physical Therapist Assistant Prgm
3 Sundial Ave
Manchester, NH 03103
www.hesser.edu

New Jersey

Essex County College
Physical Therapist Assistant Prgm
303 University Ave
Newark, NJ 07102
www.essex.edu

Bergen Community College
Physical Therapist Assistant Prgm
400 Paramus Rd, Rm S 336
Paramus, NJ 07652-1595
www.bergen.edu

Union County College
Physical Therapist Assistant Prgm
Plainfield Campus
232 E Second St
Plainfield, NJ 07060
www.ucc.edu

Mercer County Community College
Physical Therapist Assistant Prgm
1200 Old Trenton Rd, PO Box B
Trenton, NJ 08690
www.mccc.edu

New Mexico

San Juan College
Physical Therapist Assistant Prgm
4601 College Blvd
Farmington, NM 87402-4699
www.sanjuancollege.edu/pta

New York

Genesee Community College
Physical Therapist Assistant Prgm
One College Rd
Batavia, NY 14020-9704

Broome Community College
Physical Therapist Assistant Prgm
PO Box 1017
Decker Health Science Bldg 217C
Binghamton, NY 13902
www.sunybroome.edu

Kingsborough Community College
Cosponsor: The City Univ of NY
Physical Therapist Assistant Prgm
2001 Oriental Blvd
Brooklyn, NY 11235-2398

Villa Maria College of Buffalo
Physical Therapist Assistant Prgm
240 Pine Ridge Rd
Buffalo, NY 14225
www.villa.edu

SUNY at Canton
Physical Therapist Assistant Prgm
34 Cornell Dr
Canton, NY 13617-1096
www.canton.edu

Nassau Community College
Physical Therapist Assistant Prgm
One Education Dr
Garden City, NY 11530
www.ncc.edu

Herkimer County Community College
Physical Therapist Assistant Prgm
100 Reservoir Rd
Herkimer, NY 13350
www.herkimer.edu/academics/math/degrees/pta.htm

LaGuardia Community College
Physical Therapist Assistant Prgm
31-10 Thomson Ave E 300 R
Long Island City, NY 11101
www.lagcc.cuny.edu/ptaprogram

Orange County Community College
Physical Therapist Assistant Prgm
115 South St
Middletown, NY 10940
www.sunyorange.edu

New York University
Physical Therapist Assistant Prgm
School of Continuing and Prof Studies
594 Broadway, Rm 400
New York, NY 10012
www.nyu.edu

Touro College
Physical Therapist Assistant Prgm
27 W 23rd St
New York, NY 10010-4202
www.touro.edu/shs/pta.asp

Niagara County Community College
Physical Therapist Assistant Prgm
Div of Life Sciences
3111 Saunders Settlement Rd
Sanborn, NY 14132
www.niagaracc.suny.edu

**Suffolk County Community College -
    Ammerman Campus**
Physical Therapist Assistant Prgm
Dept of Education, Health and Human Services
533 College Rd
Selden, NY 11784
www.sunysuffolk.edu

Onondaga Community College
Physical Therapist Assistant Prgm
4941 Onondaga Rd
Syracuse, NY 13215
www.sunyocc.edu

North Carolina

South College - Asheville
Physical Therapist Assistant Prgm
140 Sweeten Creek Rd
Asheville, NC 28803-3152
www.southcollegenc.edu

Central Piedmont Community College
Physical Therapist Assistant Prgm
PO Box 35009
Charlotte, NC 28235
www.cpcc.edu

Surry Community College
Physical Therapist Assistant Prgm
630 South Main St
Dobson, NC 27017-7843
www.surry.cc.nc.us/

Fayetteville Technical Community College
Physical Therapist Assistant Prgm
PO Box 35236
Fayetteville, NC 28303
www.faytechcc.edu

Caldwell Comm College & Tech Institute
Physical Therapist Assistant Prgm
2855 Hickory Blvd
Hudson, NC 28638
www.caldwell.cc.nc.us

Guilford Technical Community College
Physical Therapist Assistant Prgm
601 High Point Rd, PO Box 309
Jamestown, NC 27282
www.gtcc.edu

Nash Community College
Physical Therapist Assistant Prgm
522 N Old Carriage Rd
PO Box 7488
Rocky Mount, NC 27804-0488
www.nashcc.edu

Southwestern Community College
Physical Therapist Assistant Prgm
447 College Dr
Sylva, NC 28779
www.southwest.cc.nc.us

Martin Commuity College
Physical Therapist Assistant Prgm
1161 Kehukee Park Rd
Williamston, NC 27892
www.martincc.edu

North Dakota

Williston State College
Physical Therapist Assistant Prgm
PO Box 1326, 1410 University Ave
Williston, ND 58802-1326

Ohio

Kent State University - Ashtabula Campus
Physical Therapist Assistant Prgm
3325 W 13th St
Ashtabula, OH 44004
www.ashtabula.kent.edu

Stark State College
Physical Therapist Assistant Prgm
Health Technologies Div
6200 Frank Ave NW
Canton, OH 44720
www.starkstate.edu

University of Cincinnati
Physical Therapist Assistant Prgm
Department of Rehabilitation Sciences
College of Allied Health Sciences, French East Building
3202 Eden Ave
Cincinnati, OH 45267-0394
www.cahs.uc.edu

Cuyahoga Community College
Physical Therapist Assistant Prgm
2900 Community College Ave, MHCS 126
Cleveland, OH 44115
www.tri-c.edu/pta

Sinclair Community College
Physical Therapist Assistant Prgm
444 W Third St, Rm 3340
Dayton, OH 45402
www.sinclair.edu

Kent State University - East Liverpool Campus
Physical Therapist Assistant Prgm
400 E Fourth St
East Liverpool, OH 43920-3497
www.kent.edu

Lorain County Community College
Physical Therapist Assistant Prgm
1005 N Abbe Rd
Elyria, OH 44035
www.lorainccc.edu

Rhodes State College
Physical Therapist Assistant Prgm
4240 Campus Dr
Lima, OH 45804
www.rhodesstate.edu

North Central State College
Physical Therapist Assistant Prgm
2441 Kenwood Circle, PO Box 698
Mansfield, OH 44901-0698
www.ncstatecollege.edu

Washington State Community College
Physical Therapist Assistant Prgm
710 Colegate Dr
Marietta, OH 45750
www.wscc.edu

Marion Technical College
Physical Therapist Assistant Prgm
1467 Mt Vernon Ave
Marion, OH 43302-5694
http://mtc.edu

Hocking College
Physical Therapist Assistant Prgm
3301 Hocking Pkwy SEO 309
Nelsonville, OH 45764
www.hocking.edu

Shawnee State University
Physical Therapist Assistant Prgm
940 2nd St
Portsmouth, OH 45662
www.shawnee.edu

Clark State Community College
Physical Therapist Assistant Prgm
PO Box 570
Springfield, OH 45501-0570
www.clarkstate.edu

Owens Community College
Physical Therapist Assistant Prgm
PO Box 10,000
30335 Oregon Rd
Toledo, OH 43699
www.owens.edu/academic_dept/health_tech/pta

Professional Skills Institute
Physical Therapist Assistant Prgm
20 Arco Dr
Toledo, OH 43607-1947
www.proskills.com

Zane State College
Physical Therapist Assistant Prgm
1555 Newark Rd
Zanesville, OH 43701
www.zanestate.edu

Oklahoma

SW Oklahoma St Univ/Caddo Kiowa Tech Ctr
Physical Therapist Assistant Prgm
PO Box 190
Fort Cobb, OK 73038
www.caddokiowa.com

Northeastern Oklahoma A&M College
Physical Therapist Assistant Prgm
Health Sciences Division
200 I St NE
Miami, OK 74354
www.neoam.edu

Oklahoma City Community College
Physical Therapist Assistant Prgm
7777 S May Ave
Oklahoma City, OK 73159
www.okc.cc.ok.us/

Carl Albert State College
Physical Therapist Assistant Prgm
1507 S McKenna
Poteau, OK 74953-5208
www.carlalbert.edu

Murray State College
Physical Therapist Assistant Prgm
One Murray Campus, NAH 116
Tishomingo, OK 73460
www.mscok.edu/~grobinson/PTAFolder/PTAhome.htm

Tulsa Community College
Physical Therapist Assistant Prgm
909 S Boston Ave
Tulsa, OK 74119
www.tulsacc.edu

Oregon

Mt Hood Community College
Physical Therapist Assistant Prgm
26000 SE Stark St
Gresham, OR 97030
www.mhcc.edu

Pennsylvania

Harcum College
Physical Therapist Assistant Prgm
750 Montgomery Ave
Bryn Mawr, PA 19010
www.harcum.edu

Butler County Community College
Physical Therapist Assistant Prgm
PO Box 1203
Butler, PA 16003-1203

California University of Pennsylvania
Physical Therapist Assistant Prgm
Coll of Ed and Human Serv, Dept of Hlth Sci & Sport Studies
250 University Ave
California, PA 15419-1394

Mount Aloysius College
Physical Therapist Assistant Prgm
7373 Admiral Peary Hwy
Cresson, PA 16630

Penn State University - DuBois
Physical Therapist Assistant Prgm
College Place
DuBois, PA 15801
www.ds.psu.edu/AcademicAffairs/Programs/PTA

Penn State University - Hazleton
Physical Therapist Assistant Prgm
76 University Dr
Hazleton, PA 18202

Community College of Allegheny County
Physical Therapist Assistant Prgm
595 Beatty Rd
Monroeville, PA 15146
www.ccac.edu

Penn State University - Mont Alto Campus
Physical Therapist Assistant Prgm
Campus Dr
Mont Alto, PA 17237-9703
www.ma.psu.edu/~pt

Mercyhurst University
Physical Therapist Assistant Prgm
North East Campus
16 W Division St
North East, PA 16428
www.mercyhurst.edu

Lehigh Carbon Community College
Physical Therapist Assistant Prgm
4525 Education Park Dr
Schnecksville, PA 18078-2598
www.lccc.edu

Penn State University - Shenango Campus
Physical Therapist Assistant Prgm
147 Shenango Ave
Sharon, PA 16146
www.shenango.psu.edu

Central Pennsylvania College
Physical Therapist Assistant Prgm
Campus on College Hill and Valley Rds
Summerdale, PA 17093-0309
www.centralpenn.edu

University of Pittsburgh - Titusville
Physical Therapist Assistant Prgm
504 E Main St
Titusville, PA 16354-2097
www.upt.pitt.edu/upt_pta

Puerto Rico

University of Puerto Rico at Humacao
Physical Therapist Assistant Prgm
CUH Postal Station
100 Carr 908
Humacao, PR 00791-4300
www.uprh.edu

Ponce Technological University College
Physical Therapist Assistant Prgm
Univ of Puerto Rico Regl Coll Admin
PO Box 7186
Ponce, PR 00732

Rhode Island

Community College of Rhode Island
Physical Therapist Assistant Prgm
1 John H Chafee Blvd
Newport, RI 02840
www.ccri.edu

South Carolina

Trident Technical College
Physical Therapist Assistant Prgm
PO Box 118067 AH-M
Charleston, SC 29423-8067
www.tridenttech.edu

Midlands Technical College
Physical Therapist Assistant Prgm
PO Box 2408
Columbia, SC 29202
www.midlandstech.edu

Greenville Technical College
Physical Therapist Assistant Prgm
PO Box 5616
Greenville, SC 29606-5616
www.gvltec.edu

South Dakota

Lake Area Technical Institute
Physical Therapist Assistant Prgm
230 11th St NE, PO Box 730
Watertown, SD 57201-0730
www.lakeareatech.edu

Tennessee

Chattanooga State Community College
Physical Therapist Assistant Prgm
4501 Amnicola Hwy
Chattanooga, TN 37406-1097
www.chattanoogastate.edu

Volunteer State Community College
Physical Therapist Assistant Prgm
1480 Nashville Pike
Gallatin, TN 37066
www.volstate.edu

Jackson State Community College
Physical Therapist Assistant Prgm
2046 N Parkway St
Jackson, TN 38301-3797
www.jscc.edu

South College
Physical Therapist Assistant Prgm
3904 Lonas Dr
Knoxville, TN 37909
www.southcollegetn.edu

Southwest Tennessee Community College
Physical Therapist Assistant Prgm
Union Ave Campus
737 Union Ave
Memphis, TN 38103-3322
www.southwest.tn.edu

Walters State Community College
Physical Therapist Assistant Prgm
500 S Davy Crockett Pkwy
Morristown, TN 37813-6899
www.ws.edu

Roane State Community College
Physical Therapist Assistant Prgm
701 Briarcliff Ave
Oak Ridge, TN 37830
www.roanestate.edu

Texas

Amarillo College
Physical Therapist Assistant Prgm
PO Box 447
Amarillo, TX 79178
www.actx.edu

Austin Community College
Physical Therapist Assistant Prgm
Eastview Campus
3401 Webberville Rd
Austin, TX 78702
www.austincc.edu/health/ptha

Blinn College
Physical Therapist Assistant Prgm
PO Box 6030
Bryan, TX 77805-6030
www.blinn.edu

Montgomery College
Physical Therapist Assistant Prgm
3200 College Park Dr
Conroe, TX 77384-4077
www.nhmccd.edu

Del Mar College
Physical Therapist Assistant Prgm
Div of Occupational Education and Tech
West Campus
Corpus Christi, TX 78404-3897

El Paso Community College
Physical Therapist Assistant Prgm
Rio Grande Campus, PO Box 20500
El Paso, TX 79998
www.epcc.edu

Houston Community College
Physical Therapist Assistant Prgm
Coleman College for Health Sciences
1900 Pressler Dr
Houston, TX 77030-3799
www.hccs.edu

San Jacinto College South
Physical Therapist Assistant Prgm
13735 Beamer Rd
Houston, TX 77089-6099

Tarrant County College - Northeast Campus
Physical Therapist Assistant Prgm
828 Harwood Rd
Hurst, TX 76054
www.tccd.edu/pta

Kilgore College
Physical Therapist Assistant Prgm
1100 Broadway
Kilgore, TX 75662
www.kilgore.edu/physical_therapist.asp

Laredo Community College
Physical Therapist Assistant Prgm
West End Washington St
Campus Box 153
Laredo, TX 78040
www.laredo.edu

South Texas College
Physical Therapist Assistant Prgm
PO Box 9701
McAllen, TX 78502-9701
www.stcc.cc.tx.us/nah

Odessa College
Physical Therapist Assistant Prgm
201 W University Blvd
Odessa, TX 79764
www.odessa.edu/dept/pta

St Philip's College
Physical Therapist Assistant Prgm
1801 Martin Luther King Dr
San Antonio, TX 78203-2098

McLennan Community College
Physical Therapist Assistant Prgm
1400 College Dr
Waco, TX 76708
www.mclennan.edu

Wharton County Junior College
Physical Therapist Assistant Prgm
911 Boling Hwy
Wharton, TX 77488
www.wcjc.edu

Utah

Provo College
Physical Therapist Assistant Prgm
1450 West 820 North
Provo, UT 84601
http://provocollege.edu

Salt Lake Community College
Physical Therapist Assistant Prgm
PO Box 30808
4600 S Redwood Rd
Salt Lake City, UT 84130-0808
www.slcc.edu

Virginia

Jefferson College of Health Sciences
Physical Therapist Assistant Prgm
Community Hospital of Roanoke Valley
PO Box 13186, 920 S Jefferson St
Roanoke, VA 24031-3186
www.jchs.edu

Northern Virginia Community College
Physical Therapist Assistant Prgm
6699 Springfield Center Dr
Springfield, VA 22150
www.nvcc.edu

Tidewater Community College
Physical Therapist Assistant Prgm
1700 College Crescent, Bldg E, Rm E101
Virginia Beach, VA 23453
www.tcc.edu

Wytheville Community College
Physical Therapist Assistant Prgm
1000 E Main St
Wytheville, VA 24382
www.wcc.vccs.edu

Washington

Green River Community College
Physical Therapist Assistant Prgm
Health Sciences Div, Mailstop OE-14
12401 SE 320th St
Auburn, WA 98002-3699
www.greenriver.edu/ProgramInformation/PhysicalThera
    pistAssistant.htm

Whatcom Community College
Physical Therapist Assistant Prgm
237 W Kellogg Rd
Bellingham, WA 98226

Spokane Falls Community College
Physical Therapist Assistant Prgm
3410 W Fort George Wright Dr
MS3190
Spokane, WA 99224-5288
http://spokanefalls.edu/PTA

West Virginia

Mountain State University
Physical Therapist Assistant Prgm
PO Box 9003
S Kanawha St
Beckley, WV 25801
www.mountainstate.edu

THERAPY AND REHABILITATION

Fairmont State Univ
Cosponsor: Pierpont Community & Technical College
Physical Therapist Assistant Prgm
Caperton Center
501 W Main St
Clarksburg, WV 26301
http://fairmontstate.edu

Mountwest Community & Technical College
Physical Therapist Assistant Prgm
2000 7th Ave
Cabell Hall #208
Huntington, WV 25755

Wisconsin

Northeast Wisconsin Technical College
Physical Therapist Assistant Prgm
2740 W Mason St
Green Bay, WI 54307

Blackhawk Technical College
Physical Therapist Assistant Prgm
6004 Prairie Rd, County Trunk G
Janesville, WI 53547-5009

Gateway Technical College
Physical Therapist Assistant Prgm
3520 30th Ave
Kenosha, WI 53144
www.gtc.edu

Western Technical College
Physical Therapist Assistant Prgm
304 N Sixth St, PO Box C-908
La Crosse, WI 54602-0908
www.westerntc.edu

Milwaukee Area Technical College
Physical Therapist Assistant Prgm
Health Occupations Div
700 W State St
Milwaukee, WI 53233
www.milwaukee.tec.wi.us

Recreational Therapist

Note: Recreational therapy is defined as "a treatment service designed to restore, remediate and rehabilitate a person's level of functioning and independence in life activities, to promote health and wellness as well as reduce or eliminate the activity limitations and restriction to participation in life situations caused by an illness or disabling condition" (American Therapeutic Recreation Association [ATRA], 2009). Recreational therapy, an aspect of therapeutic recreation, is a skilled therapy provided as active treatment (as defined by the Centers for Medicare and Medicaid Services). Recreational therapy, which was recognized as an allied health discipline by the Commission on Accreditation of Allied Health Education Programs (CAAHEP) at its 2010 annual meeting, is part of the broader field of therapeutic recreation, which also encompasses trained professionals dedicated to providing outcome-based recreation services to all citizens.

Career Description

Recreational therapists are professionally trained practitioners who:
- Individually assess the patient or consumer
- Plan intervention programs
- Implement safe and effective evidence-based recreational therapy interventions
- Evaluate the effectiveness of intervention programs
- Manage recreational therapy practice

Recreational therapists provide individualized and group recreational therapy interventions for individuals experiencing limitations in life activities and community participation as a result of a disabling condition, illness or disease, aging, and/or developmental factors, including those at risk. Recreational therapists use a variety of educational, behavioral, recreational, and activity-oriented strategies with clients to enhance functional performance and improve positive lifestyle behaviors designed to increase independence, effective community participation, and well-being. Recreational therapists are effective members of treatment teams in health care and community-based health care and human service agencies.

The day-to-day work experience of recreational therapists can vary dramatically, depending on the setting and clients they serve. The recreational therapist works with the client, family, members of the treatment team, and others to design and implement an individualized treatment or program plan, depending on the setting. During a typical day, a recreational therapist will respond to physician orders for assessment and treatment, conduct individualized assessments, and provide individual and group-based interventions to address treatment goals for patients on their caseload. Treatment interventions might include a stress management group or use of various relaxation and other techniques including, but not limited to:
- Progressive muscle relaxation
- Guided imagery
- Deep breathing
- Biofeedback-based relaxation techniques
- A high or low ropes course or initiatives interventions
- Adapted sports
- Manual, visual, and expressive arts
- Horticulture

- A therapeutic outing designed to meet specific goals for community integration
- A family intervention
- A therapeutic exercise or aquatic therapy session.

Recreational therapists also verbally process intervention experiences with patients to enhance the impact the activity experience has on achieving treatment goals. In a typical day the recreational therapist will also document interventions provided, note patient progress, or develop a discharge plan with a plan for aftercare.

In addition to providing treatment, recreational therapists in clinical settings assist patients/clients to improve integration and community participation, including participation in recreation, after discharge from a health care facility. This includes addressing such issues as limited knowledge of opportunities, transportation resources, inaccessible facilities attitudinal barriers, and legislation that affects people with disabling conditions. Professional activities may also include developing appropriate support groups, advocacy, and social networking strategies.

Employment Characteristics

In clinical settings, such as hospitals, psychiatric or skilled nursing facilities, substance abuse programs, and rehabilitation centers, recreational therapists treat and rehabilitate individuals with specific medical, social, and behavioral problems, usually in cooperation with physicians; nurses; psychologists; social workers; and speech, physical, and occupational therapists. In long-term, continuing care or residential facilities, recreational therapists may be involved in providing treatment as well as activities designed to maintain functioning and enhance the life quality of residents. In community settings, therapeutic recreation specialists work in adult care, outpatient programming, adaptive sports and recreation programs, home health, private consulting, developmental disabilities services, and other health and human services. Therapeutic recreation specialists working in parks and recreation services facilitate the inclusive recreation services for individuals with disabling conditions.

Recreational therapists should have assessed competency (knowledge, skill and ability) in the following recreational therapy content areas:
- Foundations of professional practice
- Recreation and leisure services
- Individualized patient/client assessment
- Planning treatment interventions
- Implementing treatment interventions
- Evaluating treatment/programs
- Managing recreational therapy practice

Recreational therapists should also have assessed competency (knowledge skill and ability) in the following support content areas as a foundation of understanding health and human functioning:
- Anatomy and physiology
- Kinesiology or biomechanics
- Human growth and development (lifecycle)
- Psychology
- Cognitive or educational psychology
- Abnormal psychology
- Disabling conditions

Many may also have support content in:

- Counseling
- Group dynamics and leadership
- First aid and safety
- Motor skill learning
- Pharmacology
- Health care organization and delivery
- Legal aspects of health care

Knowledge of disabling conditions; physical, social, cognitive, and affective development and functioning; and the application of therapeutic activities are essential in adapting activities to individual needs.

Salary

As of 2009, salary for therapeutic recreation specialists with the Certified Therapeutic Recreation Specialist® (CTRS) credential averaged $30,000 (starting), $39,000 (overall average), and $52,000 to $62,000 (upper ranges) (see *www.nctrc.org*). Data from the US Bureau of Labor Statistics (BLS) for May 2011 show that wages at the 10th percentile were $25,620, the 50th percentile (median) at $41,060, and the 90th percentile at $65,040 (*www.bls.gov/oes/current/oes291125.htm*).

For more information, refer to *www.ama-assn.org/go/hpsalary* and *www.nctrc.org*.

Employment Outlook

Recreational therapists held about 23,300 jobs in 2010. About 40 percent were in hospitals and 30 percent were in skilled nursing and residential/transitional facilities. Others were in mental health centers, adult day care programs, correctional facilities, and substance abuse centers. About seven percent of therapeutic recreation specialists work in community parks and recreation and approximately five percent were self-employed, generally contracting with long-term care facilities or community agencies to develop and oversee programs (*www.nctrc.org, www.bls.gov/oco/ocos082.htm*).

Projections from the BLS show that employment of recreational therapists is expected to increase 17 percent from 2010 to 2020, faster than the average for all occupations. Job growth will stem from the therapy needs of the aging population. With age comes an inevitable decrease in physical ability and, in some cases, mental ability, which can be limited or managed with recreation therapy. In nursing care facilities, employment will grow faster than the occupation as a whole as the number of older adults continues to grow. (*www.bls.gov/oco/ocos082.htm*)

Education Programs

Length. A bachelor's degree with a major in recreational therapy or therapeutic recreation or recreation with a specialization in recreational therapy or therapeutic recreation is required for national certification. Specific requirements can be obtained from the National Council for Therapeutic Recreation Certification (see *www.nctrc.org*)

Curriculum. In addition to recreational therapy courses in aspects of clinical practice (assessment, planning, implementing, and evaluating recreational therapy services), foundations of professional practice, management of recreational therapy practice, modality/interventions skills, and recreation and leisure services, students study human anatomy and physiology, , human growth and development, psychology, abnormal psychology, and human services supportive coursework. These content areas are required by the National Council for Therapeutic Recreation Certification. In addition, the Commission on Accreditation of Allied Health Edu-

cation Programs requires kinesiology and educational psychology. Additional content areas studied for the degree may also include motor skill learning, counseling, group dynamics and leadership, first aid and safety, pharmacology, health care organization and delivery, and legal aspects of health care. In addition, an internship under the supervision of a certified therapeutic recreation specialist or a licensed recreational therapist (who has held the credential at least one year prior to supervising the intern) is required. Refer to the NCTRC website to review curriculum standards changes, effective January 1, 2012 and 2013. (*www.nctrc.org*)

Licensure, Certification, and Registration

Some states regulate the recreational therapy profession through licensure, certification, or registration of titles. Licensure is required in New Hampshire, North Carolina, Oklahoma, and Utah. These states require individuals to make application to their state boards and meet designated competencies in order to provide safe and effective consumer services. Washington requires state registration and California requires state certification. For more information on state licensure requirements, contact:

Office of Licensed Allied Health Professionals, New Hampshire
(603) 271-8389
www.nh.gov/alliedhealth
North Carolina Board of Recreational Therapy Licensure
(336) 212-1133
www.ncbrtl.org
Oklahoma Board of Medical Licensure and Supervision
(405) 848-6841
Utah Division of Occupational and Professional Licensure
(801) 530-6628

National certification is available through the National Council for Therapeutic Recreation Certification (NCTRC), which awards the title of Certified Therapeutic Recreation Specialist (CTRS).

Career Planning Publications

The ATRA and the CAAHEP Committee on Accreditation of Recreational Therapy Education (CARTE) provide valuable information on curricula and faculty in recreational therapy or therapeutic recreation programs that prepare professionals for recreational therapy practice. These sources identify the degree levels offered and accreditation status of each program. For inclusive recreation services, contact the Inclusion and Accessibility Network of the National Recreation and Park Association.

Inquiries

Careers in Recreational Therapy
American Therapeutic Recreation Association
629 North Main Street
Hattiesburg, MS 39401
(601) 450-2872
www.atra-online.com

Careers in Inclusive Recreation Services
National Recreation and Park Association
Inclusion and Accessibility Network
22377 Belmont Ridge Road
Ashburn, VA 20148-4501
(703) 858-2151
(800 626-NRPA—membership information and other services
E-mail: *ntrs@nrpa.org*

Certification
National Council for Therapeutic Recreation Certification
7 Elmwood Drive
New City, NY 10956
(845) 639-1439
E-mail: *nctrc@nctrc.org*
www.nctrc.org

Program Accreditation: Recreational Therapy
Commission on Accreditation of Allied Health Education Programs
  (CAAHEP) in collaboration with:
Committee on Accreditation of Recreational Therapy Education
(CARTE)
1361 Park Street
Clearwater, FL 33756
(727) 210-2350
(727) 210-2354 Fax

Recreational Therapist

North Carolina

Western Carolina University
Recreational Therapy Prgm
106A Moore Building
Cullowhee, NC 28723

Veterinary Medicine

Includes:
- Veterinarian

- Veterinary technologist and technician

Veterinarian

Career Description

Veterinarians play a major role in the health care of pets, livestock, and zoo, sporting, and laboratory animals. Some veterinarians use their skills to protect humans against diseases carried by animals and conduct clinical research on human and animal health problems. Others work in basic research, broadening the scope of fundamental theoretical knowledge, and in applied research, developing new ways to use knowledge.

Veterinarians diagnose animal health problems; vaccinate against diseases, such as distemper and rabies; medicate animals suffering from infections or illnesses; treat and dress wounds; set fractures; perform surgery; and advise owners about animal feeding, behavior, and breeding.

Veterinarians who treat animals use medical equipment such as stethoscopes, surgical instruments, and diagnostic equipment, including radiographic and ultrasound equipment. Veterinarians working in research use a full range of sophisticated laboratory equipment.

Most veterinarians perform clinical work in private practices. More than 50 percent of these veterinarians predominately or exclusively treat small animals. Small-animal practitioners usually care for companion animals, such as dogs and cats, but also treat birds, reptiles, rabbits, and other animals that can be kept as pets. About one fourth of all veterinarians work in mixed animal practices, where they see pigs, goats, sheep, and some nondomestic animals in addition to companion animals.

A small number of private-practice veterinarians work exclusively with large animals, mostly horses or cows; some also care for various kinds of food animals. These veterinarians usually drive to farms or ranches to provide veterinary services for herds or individual animals. Much of this work involves preventive care to maintain the health of the animals. These veterinarians test for and vaccinate against diseases and consult with farm or ranch owners and managers regarding animal production, feeding, and housing issues. They also treat and dress wounds, set fractures, and perform surgery, including cesarean sections on birthing animals. Veterinarians euthanize animals when necessary. Other veterinarians care for zoo, aquarium, or laboratory animals.

In addition to self-employment in a solo or group practice and working as salaried employees of another practice, veterinarians are employed by the federal government, state and local governments, colleges of veterinary medicine, medical schools, research laboratories, animal food companies, and pharmaceutical companies. A few veterinarians work for zoos, but most veterinarians caring for zoo animals are private practitioners who contract with the zoos to provide services, usually on a part-time basis. In addition, many veterinarians hold faculty positions in colleges and universities.

Employment Characteristics

Currently approximately 60,000 veterinarians actively practice in the United States, with 80 percent in a solo or group practice. Veterinarians often work long hours. Those in group practices may take turns being on call for evening, night, or weekend work; solo practitioners may work extended and weekend hours, responding to emergencies or squeezing in unexpected appointments. The work setting often can be noisy.

Veterinarians in large-animal practice spend time driving between their office and farms or ranches. They work outdoors in all kinds of weather and may have to treat animals or perform surgery under unsanitary conditions. When working with animals that are frightened or in pain, veterinarians risk being bitten, kicked, or scratched.

Veterinarians working in nonclinical areas, such as public health and research, have working conditions similar to those of other professionals in those lines of work. In these cases, veterinarians enjoy clean, well-lit offices or laboratories and spend much of their time dealing with people rather than animals.

Some veterinarians are involved in food safety. Veterinarians who are livestock inspectors check animals for transmissible diseases, advise owners on the treatment of their animals and may quarantine animals. Veterinarians who are meat, poultry, or egg product inspectors examine slaughtering and processing plants, check live animals and carcasses for disease, and enforce government regulations regarding food purity and sanitation.

Veterinarians can contribute to human as well as animal health. A number of veterinarians work with physicians and scientists as they research ways to prevent and treat various human health problems. For example, veterinarians contributed greatly in conquering malaria and yellow fever, solved the mystery of botulism, produced an anticoagulant used to treat some people with heart disease, and defined and developed surgical techniques for humans, such as hip and knee joint replacements and limb and organ transplants. Today, some determine the effects of drug therapies, antibiotics, or new surgical techniques by testing them on animals.

At its 2007 annual meeting, the American Medical Association (AMA) House of Delegates voted to adopt new policy supporting more educational and research collaborations between the medical and veterinary professions to help with assessing, treating, and preventing cross-species disease transmission. Benefits of current collaborative efforts include rabies control efforts and foodborne illness evaluations. "Many infectious diseases can infect both humans and animals," said AMA Board Member Duane M Cady, MD. "New infections continue to emerge and with threats of cross-species disease transmission and pandemic in our global health environment, the time has come for the human and veterinary medical professions to work closer together for the greater protection of the public health in the 21st Century."

Salary

Data from the US Bureau of Labor Statistics (BLS) for May 2009 show that wages at the 10th percentile are $50,480, the 50th percentile (median) at $82,900, and the 90th percentile at $141,680 (*www.bls.gov/oes/current/oes291131.htm*).

According to a survey by the American Veterinary Medical Association, average starting salaries of veterinary medical college graduates in 2008 varied by type of practice as follows:

- Small animals, exclusively $64,744
- Large animals, exclusively $62,424
- Small animals, predominantly $61,753
- Mixed animals $58,522
- Large animals, predominantly $57,745
- Equine (horses) $41,636

For more information, refer to *www.ama-assn.org/go/hpsalary*.

Employment Outlook

BLS projects that employment of veterinarians will increase 36 percent through 2020, much faster than the average for all occupations. Veterinarians usually practice in animal hospitals or clinics and care primarily for small pets. Recent trends indicate particularly strong interest in cats as pets. Faster growth of the cat population is expected to increase the demand for feline medicine and veterinary services, while demand for veterinary care for dogs should continue to grow at a more modest pace.

Because many pet owners consider their pets as members of the family, they are becoming more aware of the availability of advanced care and are more willing to pay for intensive veterinary care than owners in the past. Furthermore, the number of pet owners purchasing pet insurance is rising, increasing the likelihood that considerable money will be spent on veterinary care.

More pet owners also will take advantage of nontraditional veterinary services, such as cancer treatment and preventive dental care. Modern veterinary services have caught up to human medicine; certain procedures, such as hip replacement, kidney transplants, and blood transfusions, which were once only available for humans, are now available for animals.

Continued support for public health and food and animal safety, national disease control programs, and biomedical research on human health problems will contribute to the demand for veterinarians, although the number of positions in these areas is smaller than the number in private practice. Homeland security also may provide opportunities for veterinarians involved in efforts to maintain abundant food supplies and minimize animal diseases in the United States and in foreign countries.

Excellent job opportunities are expected because there are only 28 accredited schools of veterinary medicine in the United States, resulting in a limited number of graduates—about 2,500—each year. At the same time, admission to veterinary school is competitive.

New graduates continue to be attracted to companion-animal medicine because they usually prefer to deal with pets and to live and work near heavily populated areas, where most pet owners live. Employment opportunities are very good in cities and suburbs but even better in rural areas because fewer veterinarians compete to work there.

Beginning veterinarians may take positions requiring evening or weekend work to accommodate the extended hours of operation that many practices are offering. Some veterinarians take salaried positions in retail stores offering veterinary services. Self-employed veterinarians usually have to work hard and long to build a sufficient client base.

The number of jobs for farm-animal veterinarians is likely to grow more slowly than the number of jobs for companion-animal veterinarians. Nevertheless, job prospects should be excellent for farm-animal veterinarians because of their lower earnings and because many veterinarians do not want to work outside or in rural or isolated areas.

Veterinarians with training in food safety and security, animal health and welfare, and public health and epidemiology should have the best opportunities for a career in the federal government.

Educational Programs

Award, Length. Graduates earn a Doctor of Veterinary Medicine (DVM or VMD) degree from a four-year program at an accredited college of veterinary medicine.

Prerequisites. Prerequisites for admission vary. For example, many colleges do not require a bachelor's degree for entrance, but all require a significant number of credit hours—ranging from 45 to 90 semester hours—at the undergraduate level. Nonetheless, most of the students admitted have completed an undergraduate program, and those without a bachelor's degree face a difficult task gaining admittance. Competition for admission to veterinary school is keen. The number of accredited veterinary colleges has remained largely the same since 1983, whereas the number of applicants has risen significantly. Only about one in three applicants was accepted in 2004; approximately 80 percent of entering students are female.

Students interested in a career in veterinary medicine should perform well in general science and biology in junior high school and pursue a strong science, mathematics, and biology program in high school. Before applying to veterinary college/school, students must successfully complete university-level preveterinary undergraduate course work. Each college or school of veterinary medicine establishes its own preveterinary requirements, but typically these include demonstrating basic language and communication skills and completion of courses in the social sciences, humanities, mathematics, biology, chemistry, and physics.

In addition to satisfying preveterinary course requirements, applicants must submit test scores from the Graduate Record Examination (GRE), the Veterinary College Admission Test (VCAT), or the Medical College Admission Test (MCAT), depending on the preference of the college to which they are applying. Currently, 22 schools require the GRE, four require the VCAT, and two accept the MCAT.

In admittance decisions, some veterinary medical colleges place heavy consideration on a candidate's veterinary and animal experience. Formal experience, such as work with veterinarians or scientists in clinics, agribusiness, research, or some area of health science, is particularly advantageous. Less formal experience, such as working with animals on a farm or ranch or at a stable or animal shelter, also is helpful. Students must demonstrate ambition and an eagerness to work with animals.

Prospective veterinarians must have good manual dexterity, as well as an inquiring mind, keen powers of observation, and aptitude and interest in the biological sciences. Veterinarians must maintain a lifelong interest in scientific learning. They should have an affinity for animals and the ability to get along with their owners and express compassion. Veterinarians who intend to go into private practice should possess excellent communication, managerial, leadership, and business skills, because they will need to manage their practice and employees successfully and promote, market, and sell their services.

Curriculum. Veterinary medical colleges typically require classes in:

- Organic and inorganic chemistry
- Physics

- Biochemistry
- General biology
- Animal biology
- Animal nutrition
- Genetics
- Vertebrate embryology
- Cellular biology
- Microbiology
- Zoology
- Systemic physiology

Some programs require calculus; some require only statistics, college algebra and trigonometry, or precalculus. Most veterinary medical colleges also require core courses, including some in English or literature, the social sciences, and the humanities. Increasingly, courses in practice management and career development are becoming a standard part of the curriculum, to provide a foundation of general business knowledge for new graduates.

Advanced Training. Veterinary specialties—such as pathology, internal medicine, dentistry, nutrition, ophthalmology, surgery, radiology, preventive medicine, and laboratory animal medicine—are usually in the form of a two-year internship. Interns receive a small salary but usually find that their internship experience leads to a higher beginning salary relative to those of other starting veterinarians. Veterinarians who seek board certification in a specialty also must complete a three- to four-year residency program that provides intensive training in specialties such as internal medicine, oncology, radiology, surgery, dermatology, anesthesiology, neurology, cardiology, ophthalmology, and exotic small-animal medicine.

Licensure

All states and the District of Columbia require that veterinarians be licensed before they can practice. The only exemptions are for veterinarians working for some federal agencies and some state governments. Licensing is controlled by the states and is not strictly uniform, although all states require the successful completion of the DVM degree—or equivalent education—and a passing grade on a national board examination. The Educational Commission for Foreign Veterinary Graduates (ECFVG) grants certification to individuals trained outside the United States who demonstrate that they meet specified requirements for the English language and for clinical proficiency. ECFVG certification fulfills the educational requirement for licensure in all states. Applicants for licensure satisfy the examination requirement by passing the North American Veterinary Licensing Exam (NAVLE), an eight-hour computer-based examination consisting of 360 multiple-choice questions covering all aspects of veterinary medicine. Administered by the National Board of Veterinary Medical Examiners (NBVME), the NAVLE includes visual materials

designed to test diagnostic skills and constituting 10 percent of the total examination.

The majority of states also require candidates to pass a state jurisprudence examination covering state laws and regulations. Some states do additional testing on clinical competency as well. There are few reciprocal agreements between states, making it difficult for a veterinarian to practice in a different state without first taking that state's examination.

Nearly all states have continuing education requirements for licensed veterinarians. Requirements differ by state and may involve attending a class or otherwise demonstrating knowledge of recent medical and veterinary advances.

Inquiries

Education, Careers, Resources
American Veterinary Medical Association
1931 North Meacham Road, Suite 100
Schaumburg, IL 60173-4360
www.avma.org

Association of American Veterinary Medical Colleges
1101 Vermont Avenue NW, Suite 710
Washington, DC 20005
www.aavmc.org

Licensure
National Board of Veterinary Medical Examiners
PO Box 1356
Bismarck, ND 58502
www.nbvme.org

Program Accreditation
American Veterinary Medical Association, Council on Education
1931 North Meacham Road, Suite 100
Schaumburg, IL 60173-4360
www.avma.org/education/cvea/about_accred.asp

Note: Adapted in part from the Bureau of Labor Statistics, US Department of Labor, *Occupational Outlook Handbook,* Veterinarians, at *www.bls.gov/oco/ocos076.htm.*

Veterinarian

Alabama

Auburn University
Veterinary Medicine Prgm
College of Veterinary Medicine
104 J E Greene Hall
Auburn University, AL 36849
www.vetmed.auburn.edu

Tuskegee University
Veterinary Medicine Prgm
School of Veterinary Medicine
Tuskegee, AL 36088
tuskegee.edu

Alberta, Canada

University of Calgary
Veterinary Medicine Prgm
Faculty of Veterinary Medicine
Calgary, AB T2N 4N1

California

University of California - Davis
Veterinary Medicine Prgm
Davis, CA 95616
www.vetmed.ucdavis.edu

Western Univ of Health Sciences
Veterinary Medicine Prgm
College of Veterinary Medicine
309 E Second St, College Plaza
Pomona, CA 91766
www.westernu.edu/cvm.html

Colorado

Colorado State University
Veterinary Medicine Prgm
College of Veterinary Medicine
Fort Collins, CO 80523
www.cvmbs.colostate.edu

Florida

University of Florida
Veterinary Medicine Prgm
College of Veterinary Medicine
PO Box 100125
Gainesville, FL 32610
www.vetmed.ufl.edu

Georgia

University of Georgia
Veterinary Medicine Prgm
College of Veterinary Medicine
Athens, GA 30602
www.vet.uga.edu

Illinois

Univ of Illinois at Urbana-Champaign
Veterinary Medicine Prgm
College of Veterinary Medicine
2001 S Lincoln Ave
Urbana, IL 61802
www.cvm.uiuc.edu

Indiana

Purdue University
Veterinary Medicine Prgm
School of Veterinary Medicine
1240 Lynn Hall
West Lafayette, IN 47907
www.vet.purdue.edu

Iowa

Iowa State University
Veterinary Medicine Prgm
College of Veterinary Medicine
Ames, IA 50011
www.vetmed.iastate.edu

Kansas

Kansas State University
Veterinary Medicine Prgm
College of Veterinary Medicine
Manhattan, KS 66506
www.vet.ksu.edu

Louisiana

Louisiana State University
Veterinary Medicine Prgm
School of Veterinary Medicine
Baton Rouge, LA 70803
www.vetmed.lsu.edu

Massachusetts

Tufts University
Veterinary Medicine Prgm
School of Veterinary Medicine
200 Westboro Rd
North Grafton, MA 01536
www.tufts.edu/vet

Michigan

Michigan State University
Veterinary Medicine Prgm
College of Veterinary Medicine
G-100 Veterinary Medical Center
East Lansing, MI 48824
cvm.msu.edu

Minnesota

University of Minnesota
Veterinary Medicine Prgm
College of Veterinary Medicine
1365 Gortner Ave
St Paul, MN 55108
www.cvm.umn.edu

Mississippi

Mississippi State University
Veterinary Medicine Prgm
College of Veterinary Medicine
Mississippi State, MS 39762
www.cvm.msstate.edu

Missouri

University of Missouri
Veterinary Medicine Prgm
College of Veterinary Medicine
Columbia, MO 65211
www.cvm.missouri.edu

New York

Cornell University
Veterinary Medicine Prgm
College of Veterinary Medicine
Ithaca, NY 14853
www.vet.cornell.edu

North Carolina

North Carolina State University
Veterinary Medicine Prgm
College of Veterinary Medicine
4700 Hillsborough St
Raleigh, NC 27606
www.cvm.ncsu.edu

Ohio

The Ohio State University
Veterinary Medicine Prgm
College of Veterinary Medicine
1900 Coffey Rd
Columbus, OH 43210
www.vet.ohio-state.edu

Oklahoma

Oklahoma State University
Veterinary Medicine Prgm
College of Veterinary Medicine
Stillwater, OK 74078
www.cvm.okstate.edu

Ontario, Canada

University of Guelph
Veterinary Medicine Prgm
Ontario Veterinary College
Guelph, ON N1G 2W1
www.ovc.uoguelph.ca/

Oregon

Oregon State University
Veterinary Medicine Prgm
College of Veterinary Medicine
Corvallis, OR 97331
www.vet.orst.edu

Pennsylvania

University of Pennsylvania
Veterinary Medicine Prgm
School of Veterinary Medicine
3800 Spruce St
Philadelphia, PA 19104
www.vet.upenn.edu

Prince Edward Island, Canada

University of Prince Edward Island
Veterinary Medicine Prgm
Atlantic Veterinary College
550 University Ave
Charlottetown, PE C1A 4P3
www.upei.ca/~avc

Quebec, Canada

University de Montreal
Veterinary Medicine Prgm
College of Veterinary Medicine
CP 5000
Montreal, QC H3C 3J7
www.medvet.umontreal.ca

Saskatchewan, Canada

University of Saskatchewan
Veterinary Medicine Prgm
Western College of Veterinary Medicine
52 Campus Dr
Saskatoon, SK S7N 0W3
www.usask.ca/wcvm

Tennessee

University of Tennessee Medical Center
Veterinary Medicine Prgm
College of Veterinary Medicine
2407 River Dr
Knoxville, TN 37996
www.vet.utk.edu

Texas

Texas A&M University
Veterinary Medicine Prgm
College of Veterinary Medicine and Biomedical Sciences
College Station, TX 77843
www.cvm.tamu.edu

Virginia

Virginia Polytechnic Inst & State Univ
Veterinary Medicine Prgm
Virginia-Maryland Regional College of Veterinary
  Medicine
Blacksburg, VA 24061
www.vetmed.vt.edu

Washington

Washington State University
Veterinary Medicine Prgm
College of Veterinary Medicine
Pullman, WA 99164
www.vetmed.wsu.edu

Wisconsin

University of Wisconsin - Madison
Veterinary Medicine Prgm
School of Veterinary Medicine
2015 Linden Dr W
Madison, WI 53706
www.vetmed.wisc.edu

VETERINARY MEDICINE

Veterinary Technologist and Technician

Career Description

Owners of pets and other animals today expect state-of-the-art veterinary care. To provide this service, veterinarians use the skills of veterinary technologists and technicians, who perform many of the same duties for a veterinarian that a nurse would for a physician, including routine laboratory and clinical procedures. Although specific job duties vary by employer, there often is little difference between the tasks carried out by technicians and by technologists, despite some differences in formal education and training. As a result, most workers in this occupation are called technicians.

Veterinary technologists and technicians typically conduct clinical work in a private practice under the supervision of a veterinarian—often performing various medical tests along with treating and diagnosing medical conditions and diseases in animals. For example, they may perform laboratory tests such as urinalysis and blood counts, assist with dental prophylaxis, prepare tissue samples, take blood samples, or assist veterinarians in a variety of tests and analyses in which they often utilize various items of medical equipment, such as test tubes and diagnostic equipment. While most of these duties are performed in a laboratory setting, many are not. For example, some veterinary technicians obtain and record patients' case histories, expose and develop x rays, and provide specialized nursing care. In addition, experienced veterinary technicians may discuss a pet's condition with its owners and train new clinic personnel. Veterinary technologists and technicians assisting small-animal practitioners usually care for companion animals, such as cats and dogs, but can perform a variety of duties with mice, rats, sheep, pigs, cattle, monkeys, birds, fish, and frogs. Very few veterinary technologists work in mixed animal practices where they care for both small companion animals and larger, nondomestic animals.

Besides working in private clinics and animal hospitals, veterinary technologists and technicians may work in research facilities, where they may administer medications orally or topically, prepare samples for laboratory examinations, and record information on an animal's genealogy, diet, weight, medications, food intake, and clinical signs of pain and distress. Some may be required to sterilize laboratory and surgical equipment and provide routine postoperative care. At research facilities, veterinary technologists typically work under the guidance of veterinarians, physicians, and other laboratory technicians. Some veterinary technologists vaccinate newly admitted animals and occasionally are required to euthanize seriously ill, severely injured, or unwanted animals.

While the goal of most veterinary technologists and technicians is to promote animal health, some contribute to human health as well. Veterinary technologists occasionally assist veterinarians as they work with other scientists in medical-related fields such as gene therapy and cloning. Some find opportunities in biomedical research, wildlife medicine, the military, livestock management, or pharmaceutical sales.

Employment Characteristics

People who love animals get satisfaction from working with and helping them. Some of the work, however, may be unpleasant, physically and emotionally demanding, and sometimes dangerous. At times, veterinary technicians must clean cages and lift, hold, or restrain animals, risking exposure to bites or scratches. These workers must take precautions when treating animals with germicides or insecticides. The work setting can be noisy.

Veterinary technologists and technicians who witness abused animals or who euthanize unwanted, aged, or hopelessly injured animals may experience emotional stress. Those working for humane societies and animal shelters often deal with the public, some of whom might react with hostility to any implication that the owners are neglecting or abusing their pets. Such workers must maintain a calm and professional demeanor while they enforce the laws regarding animal care. In some animal hospitals, research facilities, and animal shelters, a veterinary technician is on duty 24 hours a day, which means that some may work night shifts. Most full-time veterinary technologists and technicians work about 40 hours a week, although some work 50 or more hours a week.

Veterinary technologists and technicians held about 80,000 jobs in 2008. Most worked in veterinary services. The remainder worked in boarding kennels, animal shelters, stables, grooming salons, zoos, and local, state, and federal agencies.

Salary

Data from the US Bureau of Labor Statistics (BLS) for May 2011 show that wages at the 10th percentile are $20,880, the 50th percentile (median) at $30,140, and the 90th percentile at $44,740 (*www.bls.gov/oes/current/oes292056.htm*).

For more information, refer to *www.ama-assn.org/go/hpsalary*.

Employment Outlook

The BLS projects that employment of veterinary technologists and technicians is expected to grow 52 percent through 2020, much faster than the average for all occupations. Pet owners are becoming more affluent and more willing to pay for advanced veterinary care because many of them consider their pet to be part of the family. This growing affluence and view of pets will continue to increase the demand for veterinary care. The vast majority of veterinary technicians work at private clinical practices under veterinarians. As the number of veterinarians grows to meet the demand for veterinary care, so will the number of veterinary technicians needed to assist them.

The number of pet owners who take advantage of veterinary services for their pets is expected to grow over the projection period, increasing employment opportunities. The availability of advanced veterinary services, such as preventive dental care and surgical procedures, also will provide opportunities for workers specializing in those areas as they will be needed to assist licensed veterinarians. The growing number of cats kept as companion pets is expected to boost the demand for feline medicine and services. Further demand for these workers will stem from the desire to replace veterinary assistants with more highly skilled technicians in animal clinics and hospitals, shelters, boarding kennels, animal control facilities, and humane societies.

Continued support for public health, food and animal safety, and national disease control programs, as well as biomedical research on human health problems, also will contribute to the demand for veterinary technologists, although the number of positions in these areas is fewer than in private practice.

Excellent job opportunities are expected because of the relatively few veterinary technology graduates each year. The number of two-year programs has recently grown to about 160, but due to small class sizes, fewer than 3,800 graduates are anticipated each year, a number that is not expected to meet demand. Additionally, many veterinary technicians remain in the field less than 10 years, so the need to replace workers who leave the occupation each year also will produce many job opportunities.

Veterinary technologists also will enjoy excellent job opportunities due to the relatively low number of graduates from four-year programs—about 500 annually. However, unlike veterinary technicians who usually work in private clinical practice, veterinary technologists will have better opportunities for research jobs in a variety of settings, including biomedical facilities, diagnostic laboratories, wildlife facilities, drug and food manufacturing companies, and food safety inspection facilities.

Despite the relatively few number of graduates each year, keen competition is expected for veterinary technician jobs in zoos and aquariums, due to expected slow growth in facility capacity, low turnover among workers, the limited number of positions, and the fact that the work in zoos and aquariums attracts many candidates.

Employment of veterinary technicians and technologists is relatively stable during periods of economic recession. Layoffs are less likely to occur among veterinary technologists and technicians than in some other occupations because animals will continue to require medical care.

Educational Programs

Award, Length. Most entry-level veterinary technicians have a two-year degree, usually an associate's degree, from an accredited community college program in veterinary technology. Veterinary technology programs, in contrast, culminate in a four-year bachelor's degree.

Prerequisites. Persons interested in careers as veterinary technologists and technicians should take as many high school science, biology, and math courses as possible. Science courses taken beyond high school, in an associate's or bachelor's degree program, should emphasize practical skills in a clinical or laboratory setting. Because veterinary technologists and technicians often deal with pet owners, communication skills are very important. In addition, technologists and technicians should be able to work well with others, because teamwork with veterinarians is common. Organizational ability and attention to detail also are important.

On-the-job Training. Technologists and technicians usually begin work as trainees in routine positions under a veterinarian's direct supervision. Entry-level workers whose training or educational background encompasses extensive hands-on experience with a variety of laboratory equipment, including diagnostic and medical equipment, usually require a shorter period of on-the-job training. As they gain experience, technologists and technicians take on more responsibility and carry out more assignments under only general veterinary supervision. Some eventually may become supervisors.

VETERINARY MEDICINE

Licensure, Certification, Registration

Graduation from a veterinary technology program accredited by the American Veterinary Medical Association (AVMA) allows students to take the credentialing exam in any state in the country. Each state regulates veterinary technicians and technologists differently; however, all states require them to pass a credentialing exam following coursework. Passing the state exam assures the public that the technician or technologist has sufficient knowledge to work in a veterinary clinic or hospital. Candidates are tested for competency through an examination that includes oral, written, and practical portions and that is regulated by the state Board of Veterinary Examiners or the appropriate state agency. Depending on the state, candidates may become registered, licensed, or certified. Most states, however, use the National Veterinary Technician (NVT) exam. Prospects usually can have their passing scores transferred from one state to another, so long as both states utilize the same exam.

Employers recommend American Association for Laboratory Animal Science (AALAS) certification for those seeking employment in a research facility. AALAS offers certification for three levels of technician competence, with a focus on three principal areas—animal husbandry, facility management, and animal health and welfare. Those seeking certification must satisfy a combination of education and experience requirements prior to taking an exam. Work experience must be directly related to the maintenance, health, and well-being of laboratory animals and must be gained in a laboratory animal facility as defined by AALAS. The levels of certification, from lowest to highest, are Assistant Laboratory Animal Technician (ALAT), Laboratory Animal Technician (LAT), and Laboratory Animal Technologist (LATG).

Inquiries

Education, Careers, Resources
American Veterinary Medical Association
1931 North Meacham Road, Suite 100
Schaumburg, IL 60173-4360
www.avma.org

Certification
American Association for Laboratory Animal Science
9190 Crestwyn Hills Drive
Memphis, TN 38125
www.aalas.org

Program Accreditation
American Veterinary Medical Association
Committee on Veterinary Technician Education and Activities
1931 North Meacham Road, Suite 100
Schaumburg, IL 60173-4360
www.avma.org/education/cvea/about_accred.asp
www.avma.org/education/cvea/cvtea_process.asp#

Note: Adapted in part from the Bureau of Labor Statistics, US Department of Labor, *Occupational Outlook Handbook,* Veterinary Technologists and Technicians, at *www.bls.gov/oco/ocos183.htm.*

411

Veterinary Technician

Arizona

Penn Foster College
Veterinary Technician Prgm
14624 N Scottsdale Rd, Ste 310
Scottsdale, AZ 85254
www.pennfostercollege.edu

California

Carrington College California - Pleasant Hill
Veterinary Technician Prgm
380 Civic Dr, Ste 300
Pleasant Hill, CA 94523
www.westerncollege.com/ph_campus.asp

Carrington College California - San Jose
Veterinary Technician Prgm
6201 San Ignacio Ave
San Jose, CA 95119
www.westerncollege.edu

Carrington College California - Stockton
Veterinary Technician Prgm
1313 W Robinhood Dr, Ste B
Stockton, CA 95207
www.westerncollege.com

Massachusetts

Holyoke Community College
Veterinary Technician Prgm
303 Homestead Ave
Holyoke, MA 01040
www.hcc.mass.edu

Michigan

Macomb Community College
Veterinary Technician Prgm
Center Campus
44575 Garfield Rd
Clinton Township, MI 48044
www.macomb.cc.mi.us

Minnesota

Argosy University Twin Cities Campus
Veterinary Technician Prgm
1515 Central Parkway
Eagan, MN 55121
www.argosy.edu

Nebraska

Northeast Community College
Veterinary Technician Prgm
801 E Benjamin Ave
Norfolk, NE 68702
www.northeastcollege.com

Vatterott College - Omaha Campus
Veterinary Technician Prgm
11818 I St
Omaha, NE 68137
www.vatterott-college.com

New Jersey

Northern NJ Consortium
Veterinary Technician Prgm
400 Paramus Rd
Paramus, NJ 07652

Veterinary Technologist

Alabama

Jefferson State Community College
Veterinary Technology Prgm
2601 Carson Rd
Birmingham, AL 35215
www.jeffstateonline.com/vet_tech/

Arizona

Mesa Community College
Veterinary Technology Prgm
Animal Health
1833 W Southern Ave
Mesa, AZ 85202
www.mc.maricopa.edu

Carrington College
Veterinary Technology Prgm
1515 E Indian School Rd
Phoenix, AZ 85014
www.anthem.edu

Kaplan College
Veterinary Technology Prgm
13610 N Black Canyon Hwy
Suite 104
Phoenix, AZ 85029
www.longtechnicalcollege.com

Pima Community College
Veterinary Technology Prgm
8181 E Irvington Rd
Tucson, AZ 85709
www.pima.edu

Arkansas

Arkansas State University - Beebe
Veterinary Technology Prgm
1000 Iowa St
PO Box 1000
Beebe, AR 72012
www.asub.edu

California

Carrington College California - Citrus Heights
Veterinary Technology Prgm
7301 Greenback Lane, Ste A
Citrus Heights, CA 95621
www.westerncollege.edu

Foothill College
Veterinary Technology Prgm
12345 El Monte Rd
Los Altos Hills, CA 94022
www.foothill.fhda.edu

Yuba Community College
Veterinary Technology Prgm
2088 N Beale Rd
Marysville, CA 95901
www.yccd.edu/yuba/vettech/

California State Polytechnic University
Veterinary Technology Prgm
College of Agriculture
Animal Health Technology Program
3801 W Temple Ave
Pomona, CA 91768
www.csupomona.edu

Carrington College California - Sacramento
Veterinary Technology Prgm
8909 Folsom Blvd
Sacramento, CA 95826
www.westerncollege.com/ph_campus.asp

Cosumnes River Community College
Veterinary Technology Prgm
8401 Center Pkwy
Sacramento, CA 95823

Hartnell Community College
Veterinary Technology Prgm
Animal Health Technology Program
156 Homestead Ave
Salinas, CA 93901
www.hartnell.cc.ca.us

Carrington College California - San Leandro
Veterinary Technology Prgm
170 Bayfair Mall
San Leandro, CA 94578
www.westerncollege.com/ph_campus.asp

Mt San Antonio College
Veterinary Technology Prgm
Animal Health Technology Program
1100 N Grand Ave
Walnut, CA 91789
www.mtsac.edu

Los Angeles Pierce College
Veterinary Technology Prgm
6201 Winnetka Ave
Woodland Hills, CA 91371
www.macrohead.com/rvt

Colorado

Bel-Rea Institute of Animal Technology
Veterinary Technology Prgm
1681 S Dayton St
Denver, CO 80231
www.bel-rea.com

Community College of Denver
Veterinary Technology Prgm
1070 Alton Way
Bldg 849
Denver, CO 80230
www.ccd.rightchoice.org

Front Range Comm College
Veterinary Technology Prgm
4616 S Shields
Fort Collins, CO 80526
www.frcc.cc.co.us

Colorado Mountain College
Veterinary Technology Prgm
Spring Valley Campus
3000 County Rd 114
Glenwood Springs, CO 81601
www.coloradomtn.edu

Connecticut

Northwestern Connecticut Comm College
Veterinary Technology Prgm
Park Place E
Winsted, CT 06098
www.nwctc.commnet.edu/vettech/

Delaware

Delaware Technical Community College - Owens Campus
Veterinary Technology Prgm
PO Box 610 Route 18
Georgetown, DE 19947
www.dtcc.edu

Florida

Brevard Community College
Veterinary Technology Prgm
1519 Clearlake Rd
Cocoa, FL 32922
www.brevard.cc.fl.us

Dade Medical College
Veterinary Technology Prgm
Medical Center Campus
950 NW 20th St
Miami, FL 33127
www.mdcc.edu/medical/aht/vettech

St Petersburg College
Veterinary Technology Prgm
Box 13489
St Petersburg, FL 33733
www.spcollege.edu/hec/vt

Georgia

Athens Technical College
Veterinary Technology Prgm
800 US Hwy 29 N
Athens, GA 30601
www.athenstech.edu

Fort Valley State University
Veterinary Technology Prgm
1005 State University Dr
Fort Valley, GA 31030
www.fvsu.edu

Gwinnett Technical College
Veterinary Technology Prgm
5150 Sugarloaf Prkwy
Lawrenceville, GA 30043
www.gwinnetttechnicalcollege.com

Ogeechee Technical College
Veterinary Technology Prgm
1 Joe Kennedy Blvd
Statesboro, GA 30458

Idaho

College of Southern Idaho
Veterinary Technology Prgm
315 Falls Ave
Twin Falls, ID 83303
www.csi.id.us

Illinois

Parkland College
Veterinary Technology Prgm
2400 W Bradley Ave
Champaign, IL 61821
www.parkland.edu

Joliet Junior College
Veterinary Technology Prgm
Agriculture Sciences Dept
1215 Houbolt Rd
Joliet, IL 60431
www.jjc.cc.il.us

Indiana

International Business College - Ft Wayne
Veterinary Technology Prgm
The Vet Tech Instutite
5699 Coventry Lane
Fort Wayne, IN 46804
www.vettechinstitute.edu/camp_wayne.php

Purdue University
Veterinary Technology Prgm
School of Veterinary Medicine
West Lafayette, IN 47907
www.vet.purdue.edu/vettech

Iowa

Des Moines Area Community College
Veterinary Technology Prgm
2805 SW Snyder Dr, Ste 505
Ankeny, IA 50023
www.dmacc.edu

Kirkwood Community College
Veterinary Technology Prgm
Animal Health Program
6301 Kirkwood Blvd SW
Cedar Rapids, IA 52406
www.kirkwood.edu

Iowa Western Community College
Veterinary Technology Prgm
2700 College Rd, PO Box 4C
Council Bluffs, IA 51502
http://iwcc.cc.ia.us/programs/departments/
    veterinary-tech.asp

Kansas

Colby Community College
Veterinary Technology Prgm
1255 S Range
Colby, KS 67701
www.colbycc.edu

Kentucky

Morehead State University
Veterinary Technology Prgm
25 MSU Farm Dr
Morehead, KY 40351
www.morehead-st.edu

Murray State University
Veterinary Technology Prgm
Animal Health
Dept of Agriculture
100 AHT Center
Murray, KY 42071
www.mursuky.edu

Louisiana

Delgado Community College
Veterinary Technology Prgm
615 City Park Ave
Bldg 4, Rm 301
New Orleans, LA 70119
www.dcc.edu

Northwestern State University
Veterinary Technology Prgm
Dept of Life Sciences
225 Bienvenu Hall
New Orleans, LA 71497
www.nsula.edu

Maine

Univ of Maine Augusta (Bangor)
Veterinary Technology Prgm
85 Texas Ave
217 Belfast Hall
Bangor, ME 04401
www.uma.maine.edu/bangor

Maryland

Community College of Baltimore County - Essex Campus
Veterinary Technology Prgm
7201 Rossville Blvd
Baltimore, MD 21237
www.ccbcmd.edu

Massachusetts

North Shore Community College
Veterinary Technology Prgm
1 Ferncroft Rd
Danvers, MA 01923
www.northshore.edu

Becker College
Veterinary Technology Prgm
964 Main St
Leicester, MA 01524
www.beckercollege.com

Mt Ida College
Veterinary Technology Prgm
777 Dedham St
Newton, MA 02459
www.mountida.edu

Michigan

Baker College of Cadillac
Veterinary Technology Prgm
9600 E 13th St
Cadillac, MI 49601
www.baker.edu

Michigan State University
Veterinary Technology Prgm
College of Veterinary Medicine
A-10 Veterinary Medical Center
East Lansing, MI 48824
www.cvm.msu.edu/vettech

Baker College of Flint
Veterinary Technology Prgm
1050 W Bristol Rd
Flint, MI 48507
www.baker.edu

Baker College of Jackson
Veterinary Technology Prgm
2800 Springport Rd
Jackson, MI 49202
www.baker.edu

Baker College of Muskegon
Veterinary Technology Prgm
1903 Marquette Ave
Muskegon, MI 49442
www.baker.edu

Baker College of Port Huron
Veterinary Technology Prgm
3403 Lapeer Rd
Port Huron, MI 48060
www.baker.edu

Minnesota

Minnesota School of Business - Blaine
Veterinary Technology Prgm
3680 Pheasant Ridge Dr NE
Blaine, MN 55449
www.msbcollege.edu

Duluth Business University
Veterinary Technology Prgm
4724 Mike Colalillo Dr
Duluth, MN 55807
www.dbumn.edu

Minneapolis Business College - Plymouth
Veterinary Technology Prgm
1455 County Rd, 101 North
Plymouth, MN 55447
www.msbcollege.edu

Rochester Community & Technical College
Veterinary Technology Prgm
Animal Health Technology Program
851 30th Ave SE
Rochester, MN 55904
www.rctc.edu

Minnesota School of Business - Shakopee
Veterinary Technology Prgm
1200 Shakopee Town Square
Shakopee, MN 55379
www.msbcollege.edu

Minnesota School of Business - Waite Park
Veterinary Technology Prgm
1201 2nd St South
Waite Park, MN 56387
www.msbcollege.edu

Ridgewater College - Willmar Campus
Veterinary Technology Prgm
2101 15th Ave, NW
Willmar, MN 56201
www.ridgewater.mnscu.edu

Globe University - Woodbury
Veterinary Technology Prgm
8089 Globe Dr
Woodbury, MN 55125
www.globecollege.edu

Mississippi

Hinds Community College
Veterinary Technology Prgm
1100 PMB 11160
Raymond, MS 39154
www.hindscc.edu/Departments/Agriculture/
    VeterinaryTech.aspx

Northwest Mississippi Community College
Veterinary Technology Prgm
4975 Hwy 51 N
Senatobia, MS 38668
www.northwestms.edu

Missouri

Jefferson College
Veterinary Technology Prgm
1000 Viking Dr
Hillsboro, MO 63050
www.jeffco.edu

Maple Woods Community College
Veterinary Technology Prgm
2601 NE Barry Rd
Kansas City, MO 64156
www.mcckc.edu

Crowder College
Veterinary Technology Prgm
601 LaClede Ave
Neosho, MO 64850
www.crowder.edu

Nebraska

Nebraska College of Technical Agriculture
Veterinary Technology Prgm
RR3 Box 23A
Curtis, NE 69025
www.ncta.unl.edu

Nevada

College of Southern Nevada
Veterinary Technology Prgm
6375 W Charleston Blvd
Las Vegas, NV 89146
www.ccsn.nevada.edu

Pima Medical Institute
Veterinary Technology Prgm
3333 E Flamingo Rd
Las Vegas, NV 89121
www.pmi.edu

Truckee Meadows Community College
Veterinary Technology Prgm
7000 Dandini Blvd
Reno, NV 89512

New Hampshire

New Hampshire Comm Tech College - Stratham
Veterinary Technology Prgm
277 Portsmouth Ave
Stratham, NH 03885
www.nhctc.edu

New Jersey

Camden County College
Veterinary Technology Prgm
Animal Science Technology
PO Box 200
Blackwood, NJ 08012
www.camdencc.edu

New Mexico

Central New Mexico Community College
Veterinary Technology Prgm
525 Buena Vista SE
Albuquerque, NM 87106

San Juan College
Veterinary Technology Prgm
Distance Learning
4601 College Blvd
Farmington, NM 87402
www.sjc.cc.nm.us/pages/1.asp

New York

Alfred State College - SUNY
Veterinary Technology Prgm
Agriculture Science Building
Alfred, NY 14801
www.alfredstate.edu

Suffolk County Community College - Grant Campus
Veterinary Technology Prgm
Western Campus
Crooked Hill Rd
Brentwood, NY 11717
www.sunysuffolk.edu

Medaille College
Veterinary Technology Prgm
18 Agassiz Cr
Buffalo, NY 14214
www.medaille.edu

SUNY at Canton
Veterinary Technology Prgm
School of Science, Health, and Professional Studies
34 Cornell Dr
Canton, NY 13617
www.canton.edu

SUNY - Delhi
Veterinary Technology Prgm
156 Farnsworth Hall
Delhi, NY 13753
www.delhi.edu

Mercy College
Veterinary Technology Prgm
555 Broadway
Dobbs Ferry, NY 10522
www.mercy.edu/acadivisions/natscivettech/VetTech.cfm

LaGuardia Community College
Veterinary Technology Prgm
31-10 Thomson Ave
Long Island City, NY 11101
www.lagcc.cuny.edu

SUNY Ulster
Veterinary Technology Prgm
Cottekill Rd
Stone Ridge, NY 12484
www.sunyulster.edu

North Carolina

Asheville-Buncombe Technical Comm College
Veterinary Technology Prgm
340 Victoria Rd
Asheville, NC 28801
www.abtech.edu/ah/vet

Gaston College - Dallas
Veterinary Technology Prgm
201 Hwy 321 S
Dallas, NC 28034
www.gaston.cc.nc.us

Central Carolina Community College
Veterinary Technology Prgm
1105 Kelley Dr
Sanford, NC 27330
www.ccarolina.cc.nc.us

North Dakota

North Dakota State University
Veterinary Technology Prgm
NDSU Dept 2230
PO Box 6050
Fargo, ND 58108
http://vettech.ndsu.nodak.edu

Ohio

UC Raymond Walters College - Blue Ash
Veterinary Technology Prgm
9555 Plainfield Rd
Blue Ash, OH 45236
www.rwc.uc.edu

Bradford School
Veterinary Technology Prgm
2469 Stelzer Rd
Columbus, OH 43219
www.bradfordschoolcolumbus.edu

Columbus State Community College
Veterinary Technology Prgm
550 E Spring St
Columbus, OH 43216
www.cscc.edu

Cuyahoga Community College
Veterinary Technology Prgm
11000 Pleasant Valley Rd
Parma, OH 44130
www.tri-c.cc.oh.us

Stautzenberger College - Strongsville
Veterinary Technology Prgm
12925 Pearl Rd
Strongsville, OH 44136
www.sctoday.edu/strongsville/veterinary.php

Stautzenberger College
Veterinary Technology Prgm
5355 Southwyck
Toledo, OH 43614
www.stautzen.com

Oklahoma

Oklahoma State University
Veterinary Technology Prgm
900 N Portland Ave
Oklahoma City, OK 73107
www.osuokc.edu

Murray State College
Veterinary Technology Prgm
One Murray Campus
Tishomingo, OK 73460
www.msc.cc.ok.us

Tulsa Community College
Veterinary Technology Prgm
7505 W 41st St
Tulsa, OK 74107
www.tulsacc.edu

Ontario, Canada

University of Guelph
Veterinary Technology Prgm
Ridgetown College
Main St E
Ridgetown, ON N0P 2C0
www.ridgetownc.on.ca

Oregon

Portland Community College
Veterinary Technology Prgm
PO Box 19000
Portland, OR 97219
www.pcc.edu

Pennsylvania

Lehigh Carbon Community College
Cosponsor: Northampton Community College
Veterinary Technology Prgm
3835 Green Pond Rd
Bethlehem, PA 18020
www.lccc.edu

Harcum College
Veterinary Technology Prgm
750 Montgomery Ave
Bryn Mawr, PA 19010
www.harcum.edu

Wilson College
Veterinary Technology Prgm
1015 Philadelphia Ave
Chambersburg, PA 17201
www.wilson.edu

Manor College
Veterinary Technology Prgm
700 Fox Chase Rd
Jenkintown, PA 19046
www.manorvettech.com

Sanford-Brown Institute - Pittsburgh
Veterinary Technology Prgm
421 7th Ave
Pittsburgh, PA 15219
www.westernschool.com

Vet Tech Institute
Veterinary Technology Prgm
125 Seventh St
Pittsburgh, PA 15222
www.vettechinstitute.com

Johnson College
Veterinary Technology Prgm
3427 N Main Ave .
Scranton, PA 18508
www.johnsoncollege.com

Puerto Rico

University of Puerto Rico
Veterinary Technology Prgm
Medical Sciences Campus
PO Box 365067
San Juan, PR 00936
www.cprsweb.rcm.upr.edu

South Carolina

Trident Technical College
Veterinary Technology Prgm
1001 S Live Oak Dr
Moncks Corner, SC 29461
www.tridenttech.edu

Piedmont Technical College
Veterinary Technology Prgm
2100 College St
Newberry, SC 29108
www.newberry.edu

Tri-County Technical College
Veterinary Technology Prgm
PO Box 587
Pendleton, SC 29670
www.tctc.edu

South Dakota

National American University
Veterinary Technology Prgm
321 Kansas City St
Rapid City, SD 57701
www.national.edu/veterinary_tech.html

Tennessee

Columbia State Community College
Veterinary Technology Prgm
PO Box 1315
Health Sciences 105
Columbia, TN 38401
www.coscc.cc.tn.us

Lincoln Memorial University
Veterinary Technology Prgm
Cumberland Gap Pkwy
LMU Box 1659
Harrogate, TN 37752
www.lmunet.edu

Texas

Sul Ross State University
Veterinary Technology Prgm
School of Agriculture and Natural Resource Sciences
PO Box C-114
Alpine, TX 79830
www.sulross.edu

Cedar Valley College
Veterinary Technology Prgm
3030 N Dallas Ave
Lancaster, TX 75134
www.ollie.dcccd.edu/vettech

Midland College
Veterinary Technology Prgm
3600 N Garfield
Midland, TX 79705
www.midland.edu

Palo Alto College
Veterinary Technology Prgm
1400 W Villaret Blvd
San Antonio, TX 78224
www.accd.edu

Lone Start College - Tomball
Veterinary Technology Prgm
30555 Tomball Pkwy
Tomball, TX 77375
www.tc.nhmccd.cc.tx.us

McLennan Community College
Veterinary Technology Prgm
1400 College Dr
Waco, TX 76708
www.mclennan.edu./departments/workforce/vtech/

Utah

Utah Career College
Veterinary Technology Prgm
1902 West 7800 South
West Jordan, UT 84088
www.utahcollege.com

Vermont

Vermont Technical College
Veterinary Technology Prgm

Randolph Center, VT 05061
www.vtc.vcs.edu

Virginia

Northern Virginia Community College
Veterinary Technology Prgm
Loudoun Campus
1000 Harry Flood Byrd Hwy
Sterling, VA 20164
www.nv.cc.va.us

Blue Ridge Community College
Veterinary Technology Prgm
Box 80
Weyers Cave, VA 24486
www.br.cc.va.us

Washington

Pierce College
Veterinary Technology Prgm
9401 Farwest Dr SW
Lakewood, WA 98498
www.pierce.ctc.edu

Pima Medical Institute - Seattle
Veterinary Technology Prgm
9709 Third Ave NE, Suite 400
Seattle, WA 98115
www.pmi.edu

Yakima Valley Community College
Veterinary Technology Prgm
PO Box 22520
Yakima, WA 98907
www.yvcc.edu

VETERINARY MEDICINE

West Virginia

Fairmont State Univ
Cosponsor: Pierpont Community & Technical College
Veterinary Technology Prgm
1201 Locust Ave
Fairmont, WV 26554
www.fscwv.edu

Wisconsin

Madison Area Technical College
Veterinary Technology Prgm
3550 Anderson St
Madison, WI 53704
www.madions.tec.wi.us/matc

Wyoming

Eastern Wyoming College
Veterinary Technology Prgm
3200 West C St
Torrington, WY 82240
http://ewc.wy.edu

Vision-Related Professions

Includes:
- Ophthalmic medical technician
- Ophthalmic dispensing optician
- Optometrist

- Orientation and mobility specialist
- Orthoptist
- Teacher of the visually impaired
- Vision rehabilitation therapist

Ophthalmic Medical Technician

Career Description

Ophthalmic medical technicians are skilled professionals who perform ophthalmic (eye care) procedures under the direction or supervision of an ophthalmologist (eye doctor). They are employed primarily by ophthalmologists, but may be employed by hospitals, clinics, or physician groups. An ophthalmic medical technician cannot replace the ophthalmologist or diagnose patients, but assists the physician by collecting data, administering treatment, assisting in ophthalmic surgical procedures, and supervising patients.

The following are additional duties and tasks an ophthalmic medical technician will perform:

- Take patient medical histories
- Instruct patients about medications, tests, and procedures
- Perform vision and diagnostic tests
- Assist the ophthalmologist with patient procedures
- Coordinate patient scheduling
- Supervise and train other ophthalmic medical technicians
- Perform office management and clerical duties
- Maintain ophthalmic instruments
- Maintain and sterilize ophthalmic surgical instruments

Certification

The ophthalmic medical technician is the Standard Occupational Classification (SOC) listing for all three certification levels offered by the Joint Commission of Allied Health Personnel in Ophthalmology® (JCAHPO®). The three JCAHPO certification levels are:

1. **Certified Ophthalmic Assistant® (COA®)** provide support services to the Ophthalmologist. COAs are an important member of the eye care team, supplying vital information to the ophthalmologist who is treating the patient.
2. **Certified Ophthalmic Technician® (COT®)** are trained to perform many skilled tasks and have a strong knowledge base for work in the eye care field. COTs are dedicated to their profession and have invested time and effort in pursuit of their education. COTs work under the supervision and direction of an ophthalmologist to perform ophthalmic clinical duties. They are trained to do all COA level tasks, plus they have more responsibilities, technical skills, and experience than a COA.
3. **Certified Ophthalmic Medical Technologist® (COMT®)** are highly skilled and trained eye care professionals. Through intense study, work experience, and training, they have demonstrated a commitment to this profession. COMTs work under the supervision and direction of an ophthalmologist to perform ophthalmic clinical duties. They are trained for all the general responsibilities of COAs and COTs, and trained for additional

duties as well as providing instruction and supervision to other ophthalmic medical personnel. COMTs are expected to perform at a higher level of expertise than COTs and to exercise considerable clinical technical judgment.

Salary

According to the Association of Technical Personnel in Ophthalmology (ATPO) 2011 National Salary & Benefits Report for Ophthalmic Medical Personnel, salaries for an ophthalmic medical technician vary depending on level of training, experience, level of JCAHPO certification, location, and supervisory responsibilities.

Starting Salaries = (entry/COA level) $42,500
Overall Salaries = (intermediate/COT level) $52,500
Upper Ranges = (advanced/COMT level) $60,200

Employment Outlook

- Employment of ophthalmic medical technicians remains one of the leading industries for job growth. According to the U.S. Department of Labor, employment of medical technicians in fields such as ophthalmology ranks third on the list of 30 Fastest-Growing Occupations in the United States.
- One explanation for the positive growth in the field of ophthalmology is a sharp rise in patient numbers due to the aging population. Given that, older Americans tend to utilize more health care services and develop vision related problems later in life.
- For more than a decade, a shortage of qualified ophthalmic medical technicians has existed in communities nationwide. It is estimated there is a need for an additional 6,000 ophthalmic medical technicians in the United States alone.

Educational Programs

Length. Programs are generally less than one year for the ophthalmic assistant program, one year for the ophthalmic technician program, and two years for the ophthalmic medical technologist program.

Prerequisite. High school diploma or equivalent is required for the ophthalmic assistant and technician programs, and two years of college education is required for the ophthalmic medical technologist program.

Curriculum. In accredited educational programs, students will learn about the anatomy, physiology, and diseases of the eye as well as patient procedures and clinical skills. Students will use the skills and knowledge they gain in the classroom and apply them to hands-on supervised clinical training.

Graduates of accredited educational programs are eligible to take the National JCAHPO Certification exams. There are three levels of accredited educational programs, which are designed to prepare students to achieve one of the three levels of JCAHPO Certification.

Program Types

Ophthalmic Assistant

- The ophthalmic assistant programs are generally less than one year and may or may not have a clinical (hands-on) training component. Graduates of an ophthalmic non-clinical assistant program must complete 500 hours of work experience to be eligible to take the JCAHPO COA exam. Graduates of an ophthalmic clinical assistant program are eligible to take the COA exam after completing the program.

Ophthalmic Technician

- The ophthalmic technician programs are one year. Graduates of an ophthalmic technician program are eligible to take the JCAHPO COT exam after completing the program.

Ophthalmic Medical Technologist

- The ophthalmic medical technologist programs are two years with already completing two years of undergraduate-study work. Graduates of an ophthalmic medical technologist program are eligible to take the JCAHPO COMT exam after completing the program.

For those individuals who cannot or prefer not to attend a formal educational program, the American Academy of Ophthalmology (AAO)-and the Joint Commission on Allied Health Personnel in Ophthalmology® (JCAHPO®)offer independent study courses.

Inquiries

Careers and Certification

Joint Commission on Allied Health Personnel in Ophthalmology® (JCAHPO®)
2025 Woodlane Drive
St Paul, MN 55125-2998
800 284-3937 or 651 731-2944
E-mail: *jcahpo@jcahpo.org*
www.jcahpo.org
www.discovereyecareers.org

Association of Technical Personnel in Ophthalmology (ATPO)
2025 Woodlane Drive
St Paul, MN 55125-2998
800 482-4858 or 651 731-7245
E-mail: *atpomembership@jcahpo.org*
www.atpo.org

Program Accreditation

Commission on Accreditation of Ophthalmic Medical Programs (CoA-OMP)
2025 Woodlane Drive
St Paul, MN 55125-2998
651 731-7244
E-mail: *coa-omp@jcahpo.org*
www.coa-omp.org

Ophthalmic Assistant

Alberta, Canada

Southern Alberta Institute of Technology
Ophthalmic Assistant Prgm
1301 16th Ave NW
Calgary, AB T2M 0L4
www.sait.ca
Prgm Dir: Jennifer Hogan,
Tel: 403 284-8004   *Fax:* 403 284-8171
E-mail: jennifer.hogan@sait.ca

District of Columbia

Georgetown University Medical Center
Ophthalmic Assistant Prgm
Ophthalmic Medical Personnel Training Program
3800 Reservoir Rd, NW
Washington, DC 20007
www.georgetownuniversityhospital.org/omp
Prgm Dir: Anna Kiss, BS COMT
Tel: 202 444-4862   *Fax:* 202 444-4978
E-mail: abk26@georgetown.edu

Louisiana

Delgado Community College
Ophthalmic Assistant Prgm
Allied Health Division
615 City Park Ave, Bldg 4
New Orleans, LA 70119-4399
www.dcc.edu
Prgm Dir: Francesa Langlow, BS COA
Tel: 504 483-4003   *Fax:* 504 483-4609
E-mail: fmorel@dcc.edu

New Jersey

Univ of Medicine & Dent of New Jersey
Ophthalmic Assistant Prgm
Ophthalmic Allied Health Program
Institute of Ophthalmology and Visual Science
90 Bergen St, PO Box 1709
Newark, NJ 07107
www.umdnj.edu
Prgm Dir: Barbara F Churchill, COT
Tel: 973 972-2036   *Fax:* 973 972-2068
E-mail: churchbf@umdnj.edu

North Carolina

Caldwell Comm College & Tech Institute
Ophthalmic Assistant Prgm
Ophthalmic Medical Assistant Program
2855 Hickory Blvd
Hudson, NC 28638
www.cccti.edu/healthsci/oma/OMA.asp
Prgm Dir: Barbara T Harris, PA-C MBA COA
Tel: 828 726-2356   *Fax:* 828 726-2489
E-mail: bharris@cccti.edu

Ohio

Stark State College
Ophthalmic Assistant Prgm
6200 Frank Ave NW
Canton, OH 44720
www.starkstate.edu
Prgm Dir: Geraldine Todaro,
Tel: 330 966-5458   *Fax:* 330 966-6586
E-mail: gtodaro@starkstate.edu

Mercy College of Northwest Ohio
Ophthalmic Assistant Prgm
Ophthalmic Technology Certificate Program
2221 Madison Ave
Toledo, OH 43604
www.mercycollege.edu
Prgm Dir: Tina Broadway, COT OSA
Tel: 419 251-1329
E-mail: tina.broadway@mercycollege.edu

Oklahoma

Tulsa Technology Center
Ophthalmic Assistant Prgm
Vision Care Technology, Health Careers Centers
3420 S Memorial Dr
Tulsa, OK 74145
www.tulsatech.com
Prgm Dir: Julie Shew-Baker, MEd COT OSA
Tel: 918 828-1245
E-mail: Julie.shewbaker@tulsatech.edu

Ontario, Canada

Centennial College
Ophthalmic Assistant Prgm
941 Progress Ave
Scarborough, ON M1G 3T8
www.centennialcollege.ca
Prgm Dir: Barbara Dickson,
Tel: 416 289-5000   *Fax:* 416 694-5589
E-mail: tdyer@centennialcollege.ca

Saudi Arabia

King Khaled Eye Specialist Hospital
Ophthalmic Assistant Prgm
PO Box 7191
Riyadh, Saudi Arabia, SA 11462
Prgm Dir: Dina Al Ismail, BSN COMT
E-mail: send2dina@gmail.com

South Carolina

Trident Technical College
Ophthalmic Assistant Prgm
Ophthalmic Clinical Assistant (AH-P)
PO Box 118067
Charleston, SC 29423-8067
www.tridenttech.edu/15680.htm
Prgm Dir: Krissa Drentlaw, BS COT
Tel: 843 722-5507   *Fax:* 843 937-5352
E-mail: krissa.drentlaw@tridenttech.edu

Texas

**Medical Education and Training Campus
   (METC)**
Ophthalmic Assistant Prgm
300-P3 Eye Specialty Course
Physician Extenders Branch
2751 McIndoe Rd, Bldg 1158 South
Fort Sam Houston, TX 78234
www.cs.amedd.army.mil/eye/default.htm
Prgm Dir: MAJ Garry Hughes, MD
Tel: 210 295-4442   *Fax:* 210 295-4304
E-mail: tiffany.reid@amedd.army.mil

Tyler Junior College
Ophthalmic Assistant Prgm
Vision Care Technology
PO Box 9020
Tyler, TX 75711-9020
www.tjc.edu/vision
Prgm Dir: Steve Robbins, ABOC NCLC
Tel: 903 510-2020   *Fax:* 903 510-4928
E-mail: srob@tjc.edu

Vermont

Center for Technology - Essex
Ophthalmic Assistant Prgm
3 Educational Dr
Essex Junction, VT 05452
Prgm Dir: Anne Harris, COMT
Tel: 802 879-5558
E-mail: aharris@ccsuvt.org

Washington

Renton Technical College
Ophthalmic Assistant Prgm
3000 NE Fourth St
Renton, WA 98056
www.rtc.edu
Prgm Dir: Larry Bovard, COT
Tel: 425 235-2470, Ext 7926   *Fax:* 425 235-5836
E-mail: lbovard@rtc.edu

Wisconsin

Madison Area Technical College
Ophthalmic Assistant Prgm
Ophthalmic Clinical Assistant Program
3550 Anderson St
Madison, WI 53704
http://matcmadison.edu
Prgm Dir: Ann Hayden-Finger, BS CPOT
Tel: 608 246-6472
E-mail: ahaydenfinder@matcmadison.edu

Alberta, Canada

Alberta Health Services - Rockyview Hospital
Ophthalmic Med Technologist Prgm
Calgary Ophthalmic Medical Technology Program
Ophthalmology Clinic
7007-14th Street SW
Calgary, AB T2V 1P9
www.calgaryhealthregion.ca/ophthalmic/
Prgm Dir: Colleen Schreiber, COMT OC(C) CRA
Tel: 403 943-8526   *Fax:* 403 943-3392
E-mail: colleen.schreiber1@AlbertaHealthServices.ca

Arkansas

University of Arkansas for Medical Sciences
Ophthalmic Med Technologist Prgm
Jones Eye Institute
4301 W Markham St #523
Little Rock, AR 72205-7199
www.uams.edu/chrp/omt
Prgm Dir: Suzanne Hansen, MEd COMT
Tel: 501 526-5880   *Fax:* 501 686-7037
E-mail: OMT@uams.edu

Colorado

Pima Medical Institute - Denver
Ophthalmic Technician Prgm
7475 Dakin St
Denver, CO 80221
www.pmi.edu
Prgm Dir: Wendy Stanton, COT
Tel: 303 426-1800   *Fax:* 303 430-4048
E-mail: wstanton@pmi.edu

District of Columbia

Georgetown University Medical Center
Ophthalmic Med Technologist Prgm
Ophthalmic Medical Personnel Training Program
3800 Reservoir Rd, NW
Washington, DC 20007
www.georgetownuniversityhospital.org/omp
Prgm Dir: Anna Kiss, BS COMT
Tel: 202 444-4862   *Fax:* 202 444-4978
E-mail: abk26@georgetown.edu

Georgetown University Medical Center
Ophthalmic Technician Prgm
Ophthalmic Medical Personnel Training Program
Center for Sight, Dept Ophthalmology
3800 Reservoir Rd NW, LL PHC
Washington, DC 20007
www.georgetownuniversityhospital.org/omp
Prgm Dir: Anna Kiss, BS COMT
Tel: 202 444-4862   *Fax:* 202 444-1417
E-mail: abk26@georgetown.edu

Fiji

Pacific Eye Institute
Ophthalmic Technician Prgm
GPO Box 18641
Suva, Fiji Islands, FI
www.pacificeyeinstitute.org
Prgm Dir: John Szetu, MD
Tel: 679 368-4075   *Fax:* 697 332-4360
E-mail: resource@pacificeyeinstitute.org

Florida

Florida State College at Jacksonville
Ophthalmic Technician Prgm
4501 Capper Rd
North Campus
Jacksonville, FL 32218
www.fccj.edu
Prgm Dir: Pattie Lamell, MEd COMT
Tel: 904 713-4548
E-mail: plamell@fscj.edu

Georgia

Emory University
Ophthalmic Technician Prgm
Medical Science in Ophthalmic Technology
1365-B Clifton Rd NE 2nd Floor
Atlanta, GA 30322
www.eyecenter.emory.edu/education/
   ophthalmic_tech_training.htm
Prgm Dir: Jeff Horton, MMSc COMT
Tel: 404 778-4425   *Fax:* 404 778-4143
E-mail: jeff.horton@emory.edu

Emory University
Ophthalmic Med Technologist Prgm
1365-B Clifton Rd NE, 2nd Floor
Atlanta, GA 30322
www.eyecenter.emory.edu/
   masters_medical_science.htm
Prgm Dir: Jeff Horton, MMSc COMT
Tel: 404 778-4425   *Fax:* 404 778-4143
E-mail: jeff.horton@emory.edu

Illinois

Triton College
Ophthalmic Technician Prgm
2000 N Fifth Ave
River Grove, IL 60171
www.triton.edu
Prgm Dir: Debra Baker, MA COMT
Tel: 708 456-0300, Ext 3442   *Fax:* 708 583-3121
E-mail: dbaker1@triton.edu

Minnesota

St. Catherine University
Ophthalmic Technician Prgm
601 25th Ave South
Minneapolis, MN 55454
www.stkate.edu/academic/ophthalmic/
Prgm Dir: Aaron Shukla, PhD COMT
Tel: 651 690-8846   *Fax:* 651 690-7849
E-mail: avshukla@stkate.edu

Regions Hospital
Ophthalmic Med Technologist Prgm
School of Ophthalmic Medical Technology
864 Terrace Court
St Paul, MN 55130
www.regionshospital.com
Prgm Dir: Kristine A Fey, COMT
Tel: 651-254-3000   *Fax:* 651-778-2319
E-mail: kristine.a.fey@healthpartners.com

Regions Hospital
Ophthalmic Technician Prgm
School of Ophthalmic Medical Technology
864 Terrace Court
St. Paul, MN 55130
www.stkate.edu/academic/ophthalmic/
Prgm Dir: Kristine Fey, COMT
Tel: 651 254-3000   *Fax:* 651 778-2319
E-mail: kristine.a.fey@healthpartners.com

New Jersey

Camden County College
Ophthalmic Technician Prgm
PO Box 200 College Dr
Blackwood, NJ 08012
www.camdencc.edu
Prgm Dir: Patrick Goughary,
Tel: 856 227-7200, Ext 5058
E-mail: PGoughary@camdencc.edu

North Carolina

Duke University Medical Center
Ophthalmic Technician Prgm
School of Medicine
Ophthalmic Medical Technician Training Program
Box 3802
Durham, NC 27710
www.dukeeye.org/education
Prgm Dir: Jo Legacki, COMT
Tel: 919 681-9157   *Fax:* 919 681-9801
E-mail: joanne.legacki@duke.edu

Northwest Territories, Canada

Stanton Territorial Health Authority
Ophthalmic Med Technologist Prgm
Stanton Eye Clinic
Goga Cho Bldg, 47th St
PO Box 10
Yellowknife, NT X1A 2N1
Prgm Dir: Kent Rose, COMT
Tel: 867 873-9285   *Fax:* 867 920-7992
E-mail: kent_rose@gov.nt.ca

Nova Scotia, Canada

IWK Health Centre
Cosponsor: Dalhousie University
Ophthalmic Med Technologist Prgm
Clinical Vision Science Program
Eye Clinic, 6th Floor, 5850/5980 University Ave
PO Box 9700
Halifax, NS B3K 6R8
www.dal.ca/cvs
Prgm Dir: Karen McMain, OC(C) COMT
Tel: 902-470-8959   *Fax:* 902 470-7207
E-mail: karen.mcmain@iwk.nshealth.ca

Ontario, Canada

Kingston Ophthalmic Training Centre
Ophthalmic Technician Prgm
Department of Ophthalmology
Hotel Dieu Hospital
166 Brock Street
Kingston, ON K7L 5G2
www.hoteldieu.com/ophthalmic/KOTC.html
Prgm Dir: Craig Simms, COMT CDOS ROUB
Tel: 613 544-3400, Ext 2421   *Fax:* 613 544-3991
E-mail: simmsc@hdh.kari.net

University of Ottawa
Ophthalmic Med Technologist Prgm
Honours BS in Ophthalmic Medical Technology
The Ottawa Hospital
General Campus, 501 Smyth Rd
Ottawa, ON K1H 8L6
www.eyeinstitute.net/omtpbrochure.html
Prgm Dir: Carla Barbery, BSc COMT ROUB
Tel: 613 737-8362   *Fax:* 613 737-8836
E-mail: cbarbery@ottawahospital.on.ca

Oregon

Portland Community College
Ophthalmic Technician Prgm
705 N Killingsworth St
Portland, OR 97217
www.pcc.edu/omt
Prgm Dir: Joanne M Harris, COT
Tel: 971 722-5666   *Fax:* 971 722-5257
E-mail: jmharris@pcc.edu

Puerto Rico

University of Puerto Rico
Ophthalmic Technician Prgm
Medical Sciences Campus
PO Box 365067
San Juan, PR 00936-5067
http://cprsweb.rcm.upr.edu
Prgm Dir: Mercedes Rivera, MAEd COT
Tel: 787 758-2525, Ext 1935   *Fax:* 787 758-0636
E-mail: mercedes.rivera4@upr.edu

Tennessee

Volunteer State Community College
Ophthalmic Technician Prgm
1480 Nashville Pike
Annex Building 400, Rm 104a
Gallatin, TN 37066
www.volstate.edu
Prgm Dir: Alisha Cornish, OD COT
Tel: 615 230-3723   *Fax:* 615 230-3251
E-mail: alisha.cornish@volstate.edu

Texas

San Jacinto College Central
Ophthalmic Technician Prgm
Vision Care Technology
8060 Spencer Hwy
Health Science
Pasadena, TX 77505
www.sanjac.edu
Prgm Dir: Debra Clarke, COT
Tel: 281 478-3606   *Fax:* 281 478-2754
E-mail: debra.clarke@sjcd.edu

Virginia

Old Dominion University /Eastern Virginia Medical School
Ophthalmic Technician Prgm
Lions Center for Sight
600 Gresham Dr
Norfolk, VA 23507
www.evms.edu/ophthalmology/optech
Prgm Dir: Lori Wood, COMT
Tel: 757 38-83747   *Fax:* 757 388-2109
E-mail: optech@evms.edu

Old Dominion University /Eastern Virginia Medical School
Ophthalmic Med Technologist Prgm
Lions Center for Sight
600 Gresham Dr
Norfolk, VA 23507
www.evms.edu/ophthalmology/optech
Prgm Dir: Lori Wood, COMT
Tel: 757 388-3747   *Fax:* 757 388-2109
E-mail: optech@evms.edu

Ophthalmic Dispensing Optician

Includes:
- Ophthalmic dispensing optician
- Ophthalmic laboratory technician

Ophthalmic dispensing opticians adapt and fit corrective eyewear, including eyeglasses and contact lenses, as prescribed by an ophthalmologist or optometrist. They help customers select appropriate frames, then prepare work orders for ophthalmic laboratory technicians, who grind and insert lenses into frames. The dispensing optician then adjusts the finished eyewear to fit customer needs.

Career Description

The ophthalmic dispensing optician combines an understanding of the human eye and vision with customer service skills to order the production of corrective eyewear, aid the patient/customer in selecting appropriate, aesthetically pleasing frames, and adjust the frames to fit the customer's face.

Chief duties of the dispensing optician:
- Analyze and interpret prescriptions
- Communicate effectively with patient/customer
- Determine facial and eye measurements
- Identify the human eye structure, function, and pathology
- Assist the customer in selecting appropriate frames and lenses by assessing individual patient needs
- Use an ophthalmologist's or optometrist's prescription to prepare work orders for the ophthalmic laboratory technician
- Deliver prescription eyewear/vision aids and instruct customers in use and care
- Maintain patient/customer records and address complaints
- Provide follow-up services, including eyewear adjustment, repair, and replacement
- Explain theory of refraction
- Identify procedures associated with dispensing artificial eyes and low vision aids, when appropriate
- Adapt, dispense, and fit contact lenses
- Assist in various business duties, including frame and lens inventory, supply and equipment maintenance, and patient insurance/claim forms submission and record keeping
- Apply rules for equipment safety

Employment Characteristics

Dispensing opticians work 40-hour weeks in retail stores, some of which may offer one-stop eye examinations, frames, and on-the-spot lens grinding and fitting, or are self-employed in other optical field areas, such as sales/marketing. Other dispensing opticians provide their eye care services in conjunction with optometrists and ophthalmologists at eye care centers.

Salary

Data from the US Bureau of Labor Statistics (BLS) for May 2011 show that wages at the 10th percentile were $20,920, the 50th percentile (median) at $33,100, and the 90th percentile at $51,620 (*www.bls.gov/oes/current/oes292081.htm*). Median annual wages in the industries employing the largest numbers of dispensing opticians (from largest to smallest) were:

- General merchandise stores $36,700
- Offices of physicians $35,540
- Health and personal care stores $36,300
- Department stores $29,150
- Offices of other health professionals $32,770

For more information, refer to *www.ama-assn.org/go/hpsalary*.

Employment Outlook

The BLS projects that employment is expected to rise 29 percent through 2020, faster than the average for all occupations. Middle age is a time when many individuals use corrective lenses for the first time, and elderly persons generally require more vision care than others. As the share of the population in these older age groups increases and as people live longer, more opticians will be needed to provide service to them. In addition, awareness of the importance of regular eye exams is increasing across all age groups, especially children and those over the age of 65. Recent trends indicate a movement toward a "low vision" society, where a growing number of people view things that are closer in distance, such as computer monitors, over the course of an average day. This trend is expected to increase the need for eye care services. Fashion also influences demand. Frames come in a growing variety of styles, colors, and sizes, encouraging people to buy more than one pair.

Somewhat moderating the need for optician services is the increasing use of laser surgery to correct vision problems. Although the surgery remains relatively more expensive than eyewear, patients who successfully undergo this surgery may not require glasses or contact lenses for several years. Also, new technology is allowing workers to make the measurements needed to fit glasses and therefore allowing dispensing opticians to work faster, limiting the need for more workers.

Overall, the need to replace dispensing opticians who retire or leave the occupation will result in very good job prospects. Employment opportunities for opticians in offices of optometrists—the largest employer—will be particularly good.

Job opportunities also will be good at general merchandise stores, because this segment is expected to experience much faster than average growth, as well as high turnover due to less favorable working conditions, such as long hours and mandatory weekend shifts.

Nonetheless, the number of job openings overall will be somewhat limited because the occupation is small. Also, dispensing opticians are vulnerable to changes in the business cycle because eyewear purchases often can be deferred for a time. Job prospects will be best for those who have certification and those who have completed a formal opticianry program. Job candidates with extensive knowledge of new technology, including new refraction systems, framing materials, and edging techniques, should also experience favorable conditions.

Educational Programs

Length. Ophthalmic dispensing optician degree programs require two years of study.

Prerequisites. A high school diploma or its equivalent is generally required for entrance into a program. Ophthalmic dispensing optician students should be familiar with the principles of physics, biology, algebra, and geometry.

Curriculum. Ophthalmic dispensing opticianry educational programs include instruction in geometrical optics; ophthalmic optics; anatomy of the eye; and the use of optical instruments, machinery, and tools.

Inquiries

Careers
American Board of Opticianry
6506 Loisdale Road, #209
Springfield, VA 22150
703 719-5800
www.abo-ncle.org

National Academy of Opticianry
8401 Corporate Drive, Suite 605
Landover, MD 20785
(800 229-4828
www.nao.org

National Federation of Opticianry Schools
2800 Springport Road
Jackson, MI 49202
517 990-6945
www.nfos.org

Opticians Association of America
441 Carlisle Drive
Herndon VA 20170
703 437 8780
www.oaa.org

Program Accreditation
Commission on Opticianry Accreditation (COA)
PO Box 592
Canton, NY 13617
703 468-0566
Email: *director@COAccreditation.com*
www.COAccreditation.com

Note: Adapted in part from the Bureau of Labor Statistics, US Department of Labor, *Occupational Outlook Handbook, 2010-2011 Edition*, Opticians, Dispensing, at www.bls.gov/oco/ocos098.htm.

Ophthalmic Dispensing Optician

Connecticut

Middlesex Community College
Ophthalmic Dispensing Optician Prgm
Ophthalmic Design and Dispensing
100 Training Hill Rd
Middletown, CT 06457
www.mxcc.commnet.edu

Florida

Dade Medical College
Ophthalmic Dispensing Optician Prgm
Vision Care Technology/Opticianry
950 NW 20th St
Miami, FL 33127
www.mdc.edu

Hillsborough Community College
Ophthalmic Dispensing Optician Prgm
4001 Tampa Bay Blvd
Tampa, FL 33630
www.hccfl.edu

Georgia

Georgia Piedmont Technical College
Ophthalmic Dispensing Optician Prgm
495 N Indian Creek Dr
Clarkston, GA 30021
www.dekalbtech.org

Ogeechee Technical College
Ophthalmic Dispensing Optician Prgm
One Joe Kennedy Blvd
Statesboro, GA 30458
www.ogeecheetech.edu

Indiana

Indiana University
Ophthalmic Dispensing Optician Prgm
800 E Atwater Ave
Optician/Technician
Bloomington, IN 47405
www.opt.indiana.edu/opttech/

Michigan

Baker College of Jackson
Ophthalmic Dispensing Optician Prgm
2800 Springport Rd
Jackson, MI 49202-1299
www.baker.edu/departments/healthsci/jackson/
    opticianry.cfm

Nevada

College of Southern Nevada
Ophthalmic Dispensing Optician Prgm
6375 W Charleston Blvd
Las Vegas, NV 89146
www.ccsn.edu

New Jersey

Camden County College
Ophthalmic Dispensing Optician Prgm
PO Box 200, College Dr
Blackwood, NJ 08012
www.camdencc.edu

Essex County College
Ophthalmic Dispensing Optician Prgm
303 University Ave
Newark, NJ 07102
www.essex.edu

Raritan Valley Community College
Ophthalmic Dispensing Optician Prgm
Ophthalmic Science Program
PO Box 3300
Somerville, NJ 08876
www.raritanval.edu

New Mexico

Southwestern Indian Polytechnic Institute
Ophthalmic Dispensing Optician Prgm
Optical Technology
9169 Coors Rd NW
Albuquerque, NM 87184
www.sipi.bia.edu

New York

New York City College of Technology
Ophthalmic Dispensing Optician Prgm
Department of Vision Care Technology
300 Jay St
Brooklyn, NY 11201

TCI College of Technology
Ophthalmic Dispensing Optician Prgm
320 W 31st St
New York, NY 10001
www.interboro.com

Erie Community College - North Campus
Ophthalmic Dispensing Optician Prgm
6205 Main St
Williamsville, NY 14221-7095

North Carolina

Durham Technical Community College
Ophthalmic Dispensing Optician Prgm
1637 Lawson St
Durham, NC 27703
www.durhamtech.edu

Tennessee

Roane State Community College
Ophthalmic Dispensing Optician Prgm
Opticianry
276 Patton Ln
Harriman, TN 37748
www.roanestate.edu

Texas

Tyler Junior College
Ophthalmic Dispensing Optician Prgm
Vision Care Technology
PO Box 9020
Tyler, TX 75711-9020
www.tjc.edu

Virginia

J Sargeant Reynolds Community College
Ophthalmic Dispensing Optician Prgm
Opticianry Department
PO Box 85622
Richmond, VA 23285-5622
www.reynolds.edu

Washington

Seattle Central Community College
Ophthalmic Dispensing Optician Prgm
1701 Broadway
Seattle, WA 98122
http://seattlecentral.org

Ophthalmic Laboratory Technician

Virginia

Tri-Service Optician School (TOPS)
Ophthalmic Laboratory Technician Prgm
160 Main Rd, Ste 350 Naval Weapons Station
Yorktown, VA 23691-9984

VISION-RELATED PROFESSIONS

Optometrist

Career Description

Doctors of optometry (ODs) or optometrists examine, diagnose, treat, and manage diseases, injuries, and disorders of the visual system, the eye, and associated structures as well as identify related systemic conditions affecting the eye.

Doctors of optometry prescribe medications, low vision rehabilitation, vision therapy, spectacle lenses, and contact lenses and perform certain surgical procedures.

Optometrists counsel their patients regarding surgical and nonsurgical options that meet their visual needs related to their occupations, avocations, and lifestyles.

An optometrist has completed preprofessional undergraduate education in a college or university and four years of professional education at a college of optometry, leading to the doctor of optometry (OD) degree. Some optometrists complete an optional residency in a specific area of practice.

Optometrists are eye health care professionals state-licensed to diagnose and treat diseases and disorders of the eye and visual system.

Employment Characteristics

Most optometrists are in general practice. Some specialize in work with the elderly, children, or partially sighted persons who need specialized visual devices. Others develop and implement ways to protect workers' eyes from on-the-job strain or injury. Some specialize in contact lenses, low vision, sports vision, or vision therapy. A few teach optometry, perform research, or consult.

Most optometrists are private practitioners who also handle the business aspects of running an office, such as developing a patient base, hiring employees, keeping paper and electronic records, and ordering equipment and supplies. Optometrists who operate franchise optical stores also may have some of these duties.

Optometrists work in places—usually their own offices—that are clean, well lighted, and comfortable. Most full-time optometrists work about 40 hours a week. Many work weekends and evenings to suit the needs of patients, and are increasingly available for emergency calls as well.

Salary

The average net income from the primary practice of optometry was $130,856 in 2009, according to a recent AOA census of member optometrists.
Data from the US Bureau of Labor Statistics (BLS) from May 2011 show that wages at the 10th percentile were $51,690, the 50th percentile (median) $94,690, and the 75th percentile $183,980 (*www.bls.gov/oes/current/oes291041.htm*).

For more information, refer to *www.ama-assn.org/go/hpsalary*.

Employment Outlook

The BLS projects that employment of optometrists will grow 33 percent through 2020, much faster than the average for all occupations. A growing population that recognizes the importance of good eye care will increase demand for optometrists. Also, an increasing number of health insurance plans that include vision care should generate more job growth.

As the population ages, there will likely be more visits to optometrists and ophthalmologists because of the onset of vision problems that occur at older ages, such as cataracts, glaucoma, and macular degeneration. In addition, increased incidences of diabetes and hypertension in the general population as well as in the elderly will generate greater demand for services as these diseases often affect eyesight.

Employment of optometrists would grow more rapidly if not for productivity gains expected to allow each optometrist to see more patients. These expected gains stem from greater use of optometric assistants and other support personnel, who can reduce the amount of time optometrists need with each patient.

The increasing popularity of laser surgery to correct some vision problems was previously thought to have an adverse effect on the demand for optometrists as patients often do not require eyeglasses afterward. Optometrists, however, will still be needed to provide preoperative and postoperative care for laser surgery patients, therefore laser eye surgery will likely have little to no impact on the employment of optometrists.

Excellent job opportunities are expected over the next decade because there are only 21 schools of optometry in the US, resulting in a limited number of graduates—about 1,330—each year. This number is not expected to keep pace with demand. However, admission to optometry school is competitive.

In addition to job growth, the need to replace optometrists who retire will also create many employment opportunities. According to the American Optometric Association, nearly one quarter of practicing optometrists are approaching retirement age. As they begin to retire, many opportunities will arise, particularly in individual and group practices.

Educational Programs

Award, Length. The Doctor of Optometry (OD) degree requires completion of a four-year program at an accredited school or college of optometry.

Prerequisites. Each optometry school has slightly different admission requirements. Some schools or colleges require a four-year undergraduate degree, and many others strongly recommend it. All require at least three years of undergraduate study at an accredited college or university. Most optometry students hold a bachelor's or higher degree.

Admission requirements for most schools include general courses in biology, physics, and chemistry, in addition to organic chemistry, biochemistry, biology, microbiology (all with labs), calculus, statistics, English, psychology, social sciences, and other humanities. Because a strong background in science is important, many applicants to optometry school major in a science such as biology or chemistry, while other applicants major in another subject and take many science courses offering laboratory experience. Applicants must take the Optometry Admissions Test (OAT), which is designed to measure general academic ability and comprehension of scientific information.

Admission to optometry school is competitive. Applicants are encouraged to take the examination well in advance of intended enrollment. Most applicants take the test after their sophomore or junior year after taking courses in biology, general and organic chemistry, and physics. Some applicants are accepted to optometry school after three years of college and complete their bachelor's degree while attending optometry school.

Most schools also consider an applicant's exposure to optometry, such as becoming acquainted with at least one optometrist, as being of vital importance. Generally, schools and colleges of optometry admit students who have demonstrated strong academic commitment and who exhibit the potential to excel in deductive reasoning, interpersonal communication, and empathy.

Curriculum. Optometry programs include courses in the basic health sciences (anatomy, physiology, pathology, biochemistry, pharmacology, and public health), optics, and the vision sciences, as well as laboratory and clinical training in diagnosing and treating eye disease.

Residency and Advanced Training. Optometrists wishing to teach or conduct research may study for a master's or PhD degree in areas emphasizing the visual and ocular system. One-year postgraduate clinical residency programs are available for optometrists who wish to obtain advanced clinical competence, although residency training is not required to be licensed as an optometrist. Areas for residency programs include the following:

- Family practice optometry
- Primary eye care
- Cornea and contact lenses
- Geriatric optometry
- Pediatric optometry
- Low vision rehabilitation
- Vision therapy and rehabilitation
- Ocular disease
- Refractive and ocular surgery
- Community health optometry

Licensure, Certification, Registration

All states and the District of Columbia require that optometrists be licensed. Applicants for a license must have an OD degree from an accredited optometry school and must pass both a written national board examination and a national or state clinical board examination. The written and clinical examinations of the National Board of Examiners in Optometry usually are taken during the student's academic career.

Many states also require applicants to pass an examination on relevant state laws. Licenses are renewed every one to three years, with continuing education credits required for renewal in all states.

Inquiries

Education, Careers, Resources
American Optometric Association
243 North Lindbergh Blvd
St Louis, MO 63141-7881
800 365-2219
www.aoa.org

Association of Schools and Colleges of Optometry
6110 Executive Blvd, Suite 420
Rockville, MD 20852
301 231-5944
www.opted.org

Licensure
National Board of Examiners in Optometry
200 South College Street, #2010
Charlotte, NC 28202
www.optometry.org

Program Accreditation
Accreditation Council on Optometric Education, American
   Optometric Association
243 North Lindbergh Blvd
St Louis, MO 63141-7881
800 365-2219
E-mail: *acoe@aoa.org*
www.theacoe.org

Note: Adapted in part from the Bureau of Labor Statistics, US Department of Labor, *Occupational Outlook Handbook, 2010-11 Edition*, Optometrists, at *www.bls.gov/oco/ocos073.htm*.

Optometrist

Alabama

University of Alabama at Birmingham
Optometry Prgm
School of Optometry
1716 University Blvd
Birmingham, AL 35294
www.uab.edu

Arizona

Midwestern University - Glendale Campus
Optometry Prgm
College of Optometry
19555 N 59th Ave
Glendale, AZ 85308
www.midwestern.edu

California

University of California - Berkeley
Optometry Prgm
School of Optometry
350 Minor Hall MC 2020
Berkeley, CA 94720
spectacle.berkeley.edu

Southern California College of Optometry
Optometry Prgm
2575 Yorba Linda Blvd
Fullerton, CA 92831
www.scco.edu

Western Univ of Health Sciences
Optometry Prgm
309 E Second St
Pomona, CA 91766-1854
www.westernu.edu

Florida

Nova Southeastern University
Optometry Prgm
College of Optometry
3200 S University Dr
Fort Lauderdale, FL 33328
www.nova.edu

Illinois

Illinois College of Optometry
Optometry Prgm
3241 S Michigan Ave
Chicago, IL 60616
www.ico.edu

Indiana

Indiana University - Bloomington
Optometry Prgm
School of Optometry
800 E Atwater Ave
Bloomington, IN 47405
www.opt.indiana.edu

Massachusetts

New England College of Optometry
Optometry Prgm
424 Beacon St
Boston, MA 02115
www.neco.edu

VISION-RELATED PROFESSIONS

Mass College of Pharmacy & Health Sciences
Optometry Prgm
19 Foster St, Ste 400
Worcester, MA 01608
www.mcphs.edu

Michigan

Ferris State University - Michigan College of Optometry
Optometry Prgm
1310 Cramer Circle
Big Rapids, MI 49307
www.ferns.edu/mco

Missouri

University of Missouri - St Louis
Optometry Prgm
College of Optometry
One University Blvd
331 Marillac Hall
St Louis, MO 63121
umsl.edu/divisions/optometry

New York

SUNY - State College of Optometry
Optometry Prgm
33 W 42nd St
New York, NY 10036-8003
www.sunyopt.edu

Ohio

The Ohio State University
Optometry Prgm
College of Optometry
338 W 10th Ave
Columbus, OH 43210
www.optometry.osu.edu

Oklahoma

Northeastern State University
Optometry Prgm
Oklahoma College of Optometry
1001 N Grand Ave
Tahlequah, OK 74464
arapaho.nsuok.edu/~optometry

Ontario, Canada

University of Waterloo
Optometry Prgm
School of Optometry
Waterloo, ON N2L 3G1
www.optometry.uwaterloo.ca

Oregon

Pacific University
Optometry Prgm
College of Optometry
2043 College Way
Forest Grove, OR 97116
www.opt.pacificu.edu

Pennsylvania

Salus University
Optometry Prgm
Pennsylvania College of Optometry
Elkins Park Campus
8360 Old York Rd
Elkins Park, PA 19027
www.pco.edu

Puerto Rico

Inter American University of Puerto Rico
Optometry Prgm
School of Optometry
118 Eleanor Roosevelt St
Bayamon, PR 00957
www.optonet.inter.edu

Quebec, Canada

University de Montreal
Optometry Prgm
Ecole d'Optometrie
3744 Jean-Brillant, Suite 260-7
Montreal, QC H3T 1P1
www.opto.umontreal.ca

Tennessee

Southern College of Optometry
Optometry Prgm
1245 Madison Ave
Memphis, TN 38104
www.sco.edu

Texas

University of Houston
Optometry Prgm
College of Optometry
505 J Davis Armistead Bldg
Houston, TX 77204
www.opt.uh.edu

The University of the Incarnate Word
Optometry Prgm
9729 Datapoint
Suite 100
San Antonio, TX 78229
http://optometry.uiw.edu

Orientation and Mobility Specialist

Career Description

Orientation and mobility specialists teach people who are blind or visually impaired the skills and concepts they need to travel independently and safely at home, in the classroom, in their communities, and wherever they may want to go.

Orientation and Mobility Instruction is a sequential process in which visually impaired individuals are taught to utilize their remaining senses to determine their position within their environment and to negotiate safe movement from one place to another. The skills involved in this teaching include but are not limited to:

- Concept development, which includes body image, spatial, temporal, positional, directional. and environmental concepts
- Motor development, including motor skills needed for balance, posture, and gait, as well as the use of adaptive devices and techniques to assist those with multiple disabilities
- Sensory development, which includes visual, auditory, vestibular, kinesthetic, tactile, olfactory, and proprioceptive senses, and the interrelationships of these systems
- Residual vision stimulation and training
- Human guide technique
- Upper and lower protective techniques
- Locating dropped objects
- Trailing
- Squaring-off
- Cane techniques
- Soliciting/declining assistance
- Following directions
- Utilizing landmarks
- Search patterns
- Compass directions
- Route planning
- Analysis and identification of intersections and traffic patterns
- Use of traffic control devices
- Techniques for crossing streets
- Techniques for travel in indoor environments, outdoor residential, small and large business districts, mall travel, and rural areas

- Problem solving
- Use of public transportation
- Evaluation with sun filters for the reduction of glare
- Instructional use of low vision devices

Salary

According to the Association for Education and Rehabilitation of the Blind and Visually Impaired, the average full-time salary for orientation and mobility specialists is $46,564.

For more information, refer to *www.ama-assn.org/go/hpsalary*.

Inquiries

Careers/Curriculum
Association for Education and Rehabilitation of the Blind and Visually Impaired
1703 North Beauregard Street, Suite 440
Alexandria, VA 22311-1744
703 671-4500
www.aerbvi.org

Certification
Academy for Certification of Vision Rehabilitation and Education Professionals
300 North Commerce Park Loop, #200
Tucson, AZ 85745
520 887-6816
E-mail: *info@acvrep.org*
www.acvrep.org

Program Accreditation
Association for Education and Rehabilitation of the Blind and Visually Impaired
1703 North Beauregard Street, Suite 440
Alexandria, VA 22311-1744
703 671-4500
www.aerbvi.org

Orientation and Mobility Specialist

Arizona

University of Arizona
Orientation and Mobility Specialist Prgm
PO Box 210069
Tucson, AZ 85721
www.arizona.edu

Arkansas

University of Arkansas at Little Rock
Orientation and Mobility Specialist Prgm
2801 S University Ave
Little Rock, AR 72204
www.ualr.edu/orientationandmobility

California

California State University - Los Angeles
Orientation and Mobility Specialist Prgm
5151 State University Dr
Los Angeles, CA 90032
www.calstatela.edu

San Francisco State University
Orientation and Mobility Specialist Prgm
1600 Holloway Ave
San Francisco, CA 94132
www.sfsu.edu/~mobility

Colorado

University of Northern Colorado
Orientation and Mobility Specialist Prgm
NCLID, McKee Hall Campus Box 146
Greeley, CO 80639
http://vision.unco.edu

Florida

Florida State University
Orientation and Mobility Specialist Prgm
205 Stone Bldg
Tallahassee, FL 32306-4459
www.careersinblindness.com

Illinois

Northern Illinois University
Orientation and Mobility Specialist Prgm
Dept of Teaching and Learning
DeKalb, IL 60115
www.cedu.niu.edu/tlrn/visualdisabilities

Kentucky

University of Louisville
Orientation and Mobility Specialist Prgm
Louisville, KY 40292
www.louisville.edu

Massachusetts

University of Massachusetts - Boston
Orientation and Mobility Specialist Prgm
Boston, MA 02125
www.cnhs.umb.edu

Michigan

Western Michigan University
Orientation and Mobility Specialist Prgm
Dept of Blindness and Low Vision Studies
Mail Stop 5218
Kalamazoo, MI 49008
www.wmich.edu/hhs/blvs/

New Mexico

New Mexico State University
Orientation and Mobility Specialist Prgm
Las Cruces, NM 88003
www.nmsu.edu

New York

CUNY Hunter College
Cosponsor: The Lavelle Fund for the Blind, Inc
Orientation and Mobility Specialist Prgm
695 Park Ave, 916 W
New York, NY 10021
www.hunter.cuny.edu/education/deptsprograms/
    chart.shtml

New Zealand

Massey University
Orientation and Mobility Specialist Prgm
School of Health Sciences
Private Bag 11222
Palmerston North, NZ 04410
www.massey.ac.nz

North Carolina

North Carolina Central University
Orientation and Mobility Specialist Prgm
712 Cecil St
Durham, NC 27707

Ontario, Canada

Mohawk College
Orientation and Mobility Specialist Prgm
411 Elgin St
Brantford, ON N3T 5V2

Pennsylvania

Salus University
Orientation and Mobility Specialist Prgm
Dept of Graduate Studies
8360 Old York Rd
Elkins Park, PA 19027
www.pco.edu

University of Pittsburgh
Orientation and Mobility Specialist Prgm
Vision Studies Specialization
5316 WWPH
Pittsburgh, PA 15260

South Carolina

South Carolina State University
Orientation and Mobility Specialist Prgm
Dept of Human Services
PO Box 7417, 300 College St
Orangeburg, SC 29117

Texas

Texas Tech University
Orientation and Mobility Specialist Prgm
Personnel Preparation/Visual Impairment
Box 41071
Lubbock, TX 79409-1071

Stephen F Austin State University
Orientation and Mobility Specialist Prgm
13019 SFA Station
Nacogdoches, TX 75962
www.sfasu.edu/hs/O&M.htm

Career Description

Orthoptics involves the evaluation and treatment of disorders of vision, eye movements, and eye alignment in children and adults. The orthoptist performs a series of diagnostic tests and measurements on patients with visual disorders, including lazy eye, strabismus (misaligned eyes), and double vision. Through interpretation of testing procedures and clinical evaluation, the orthoptist helps the ophthalmologist design a treatment plan, which may involve treatment by the orthoptist, surgical treatment by the ophthalmologist, or some combination of the two.

Employment Characteristics

The orthoptist is the liaison between ophthalmologist and patient, assisting in the explanation and execution of the treatment. Orthoptists work in a variety of professional settings:

- As a consultant, the orthoptist may travel to several offices or clinics to see patients or work as a professional advisor to vision-related community agencies.
- An orthoptist may serve as a director of state or local vision screening programs.
- Academic opportunities also exist for individuals who want to offer clinical expertise and instruction to orthoptic students, medical students, and resident physicians. Orthoptists may also participate in clinical research and in the presentation and publication of scientific papers.

Orthoptists possess diagnostic ability, technical understanding, and therapeutic skills. In addition, orthoptists should be able to work well with young children, who make up a large portion of orthoptic patients. It is not uncommon for these young patients to have physical, mental, or emotional disabilities.

Salary

Orthoptists receive compensation at the high end of that earned by other health professionals, including physical therapists and physician assistants.

For more information, refer to *www.ama-assn.org/go/hpsalary*.

Educational Programs

Length. Orthoptist programs require two years of postgraduate study.

Prerequisites. A baccalaureate degree is required; however, exceptions are considered on an individual basis. The Graduate Record Examination is not required.

Curriculum. Lectures, textbooks, journal publications, and proceedings from scientific ophthalmology symposia and conferences form the basis of the didactic teaching. Primary subject areas include:

- Anatomy
- Neuroanatomy
- Physiology
- Pharmacology
- Ophthalmic optics
- Diagnostic testing and measurement
- Orthoptic treatment
- Systemic disease and ocular motor disorders
- Principles of surgery and basic ophthalmic examination techniques
- Genetics
- Child development
- Learning disabilities
- Clinical research methods
- Medical writing

In most programs, preparation and presentation of scientific papers are usually required during the second year of education.

Programs are typically structured around an eight-hour day. On average, an orthoptic student will evaluate more than 1,500 patients and observe many more during the course of study. Extensive clinical experience is part of every program.

Inquiries

Inquiries regarding a career in orthoptics, certification, and program accreditation (brochures about the profession are available upon request)

Leslie France, CO, Executive Director
American Orthoptic Council
3914 Nakoma Rd
Madison, WI 53711
608 233-5383
E-mail: *lufranceco@att.net*
www.orthoptics.org

American Association of Certified Orthoptists
Bruce Furr, CO, President
E-mail: *bfurr@umich.edu*
www.orthoptics.org

Orthoptist

British Columbia, Canada

British Columbia's Children's Hospital
Orthoptist Prgm
Dept of Ophthamology A135E
4480 Oak St
Vancouver, BC V6H 3N1

California

Childrens Hospital Los Angeles
Orthoptist Prgm
4650 Sunset Blvd
Los Angeles, CA 90027
www.chla.usc.edu

Illinois

Children's Memorial Hospital of Chicago
Orthoptist Prgm
Division of Ophthalmology
2300 Children's Plaza, Box 70
Chicago, IL 60614-3394
www.childrensmemorial.org

Iowa

University of Iowa Hospitals & Clinics
Orthoptist Prgm
Dept of Opthalmology and Visual Sciences
200 Hawkins Dr
Iowa City, IA 52242
webeye.ophth.uiowa.edu/dept/orthoptc/orthop.htm

Maryland

Greater Baltimore Medical Center
Orthoptist Prgm
Department of Ophthalmology
PPW Suite 505
6569 N Charles St
Baltimore, MD 21204
Prgm Dir: Cheryl McCarus, CO COMT OSA
Tel: 443 849-8097 *Fax:* 443 849-2648
E-mail: cmccarus@gbmc.org

Michigan

W K Kellogg Eye Center
Orthoptist Prgm
University of Michigan Orthoptic Program
1000 Wall St
Ann Arbor, MI 48105

Minnesota

St. Catherine University
Orthoptist Prgm
Pediatric Ophthalmology Dept
601 25th Ave S, Old Main Bldg, Room 401
Minneapolis, MN 55454
www.stkate.edu/academic/orthoptics/
Notes: Due to staffing changes, the program is not
    currently accepting students

University of Minnesota
Orthoptist Prgm
Dept of Ophthalmology
516 Delaware St SE MMC 493
Minneapolis, MN 55455
med.umn.edu/ophthalmology/training/orthoptic/
    home.html

New York

University at Buffalo - SUNY
Cosponsor: Ross Eye Institute
Orthoptist Prgm
Dept of Ophthalmology
Ira G Ross Eye Institute, 1176 Main St
Buffalo, NY 14209
www.rosseye.com
Prgm Dir: Kyle Arnoldi, COMT CO
Tel: 716 881-7914, Ext 14 *Fax:* 716 887-2991
E-mail: kylea@buffalo.edu

New York Eye & Ear Infirmary
Orthoptist Prgm
Allied Health School in Ophthalmology
310 E 14th St
New York, NY 10003
www.nyee.edu

Nova Scotia, Canada

IWK Health Centre
Cosponsor: Dalhousie University
Orthoptist Prgm
Clinical Vision Science Program
5850 University Ave, PO Box 9700
IWK Hospital
Halifax, NS B3J 3G9
http://cus.healthprofesions.dal.ca

Oklahoma

Orthoptic Teaching Program of Tulsa
Orthoptist Prgm
4606 East 67th St
Suite 400
Tulsa, OK 74136
www.ou.edu/tulsa/

Ontario, Canada

Hospital for Sick Children
Orthoptist Prgm
555 University Ave Rm M109
Toronto, ON M5G 1X8

Oregon

Oregon Health & Science University
Orthoptist Prgm
Department of Ophthalmology
3375 SW Terwilliger Blvd
Portland, OR 97239-4197
www.ohsu.edu

Saskatchewan, Canada

Saskatoon Health Region Orthoptic Program
Orthoptist Prgm
701 Queen St
Saskatoon, SK S7K 5T6
www.orthoptics.ca

Tennessee

Hamilton Eye Institute
Orthoptist Prgm
UTHSC 956 Court Ave, Room D-222
Memphis, TN 38163
www.eye.uthsc.edu

Vanderbilt Eye Institute
Orthoptist Prgm
Tennessee Lions Eye Center
2311 Pierce Ave
Nashville, TN 37232
www.vanderbilthealth.com/eyeinstitute/

Wisconsin

University of Wisconsin Hospital and Clinics
Orthoptist Prgm
Dept of Ophthalmology & Visual Services
2880 University Ave, Room 223
Madison, WI 53705-9030
uwhealth.org
Prgm Dir: Jacqueline Shimko, BGS CO
Tel: 608 263-7189 *Fax:* 608 263-4247
E-mail: jw.shimko@hosp.wisc.edu

Orthoptist

Programs*	Class Capacity	Begins	Length (months)	Award	Res. Tuition	Non-res. Tuition	Offers:† 1	2	3	4
Maryland										
Greater Baltimore Medical Center	2	Sep	24	Cert	$2,500	$2,500	•			
New York										
Univ at Buffalo - SUNY	4	Sep	24, 12	Cert	$3,000					
Wisconsin										
Univ of Wisconsin Hospital and Clinics (Madison)	1	Jul	24	Cert	$1,200	$1,200 per year	•			

*Data are shown only for programs that completed the 2011 AMA Survey of Health Professions Education Programs.

†Key to Offers: 1: Evening or weekend classes; 2: Non-English instruction; 3: Cultural competence instruction; 4: Distance education component.

Teacher of the Visually Impaired

Career Description

Teachers of the visually impaired (or VI teachers) are specialized teachers with unique competencies to meet the diverse needs of the visually impaired.

VI teachers work within the special education system but address the unique needs of children with visual impairments. In addition to working with the children (usually in a one-to-one relationship), VI teachers work closely with other teachers, parents, and other people and organizations in the community. VI teachers are specialists at translating medical information into educational practices.

VI teachers understand basic diagnostic information about vision and visual impairments. They take information on a student's visual diagnosis and conduct a functional vision evaluation and a learning media assessment. Based on those sources of information, VI teachers develop a plan to best teach the student and work with others to address instructional needs, including basic core curriculum and student-specific needs.

Specific duties of a VI teacher might include:

- Teaching a toddler to enjoy playing with a variety of toys
- Teaching a young child how to read and write Braille
- Teaching students how to make a favorite snack
- Working with other educators and paraprofessionals to modify materials to address the impact of the visual impairment

VI teachers are certified by states thought the educator certification systems. Depending on the state, VI teachers can be certified with a bachelors degree, a post-bachelors certification, and/or a masters degree. Teachers must have a degree in education or special education.

Inquiries

Careers/Curriculum
Association for Education and Rehabilitation of the Blind and Visually Impaired
1703 North Beauregard Street, Suite 440
Alexandria, VA 22311-1744
703 671-4500
www.aerbvi.org

Certification
Academy for Certification of Vision Rehabilitation and Education Professionals
300 North Commerce Park Loop, #200
Tucson, AZ 85745
520 887-6816
E-mail: *info@acvrep.org*
www.acvrep.org

Program Accreditation
Association for Education and Rehabilitation of the Blind and Visually Impaired
1703 North Beauregard Street, Suite 440
Alexandria, VA 22311-1744
703 671-4500
www.aerbvi.org

Teacher of the Visually Impaired

Arizona

University of Arizona
Teacher of the Visually Impaired Prgm
Education Bldg, Rm 412
PO Box 210069
Tucson, AZ 85721

Florida

Florida State University
Teacher of the Visually Impaired Prgm
205 Stone Bldg
Tallahassee, FL 32306

Illinois

Northern Illinois University
Teacher of the Visually Impaired Prgm
Department of Teaching and Learning
DeKalb, IL 60115

Michigan

Michigan State University
Teacher of the Visually Impaired Prgm
313 Erickson Hall
East Lansing, MI 48824

Missouri

Missouri State University
Teacher of the Visually Impaired Prgm
901 S National Ave
Springfield, MO 65897

New Mexico

New Mexico State University
Teacher of the Visually Impaired Prgm
MSC 3SPE
PO Box 30001
Las Cruces, NM 88003

Pennsylvania

Salus University
Teacher of the Visually Impaired Prgm
Elkins Park Campus
8360 Old York Rd
Elkins Park, PA 19027

Tennessee

Vanderbilt University
Cosponsor: Peabody College of Optometry
Teacher of the Visually Impaired Prgm
Box 328
Nashville, TN 37203

Vision Rehabilitation Therapist

Career Description

- Vision rehabilitation therapists (formerly rehabilitation teachers) instruct persons with vision impairment in the use of compensatory skills and assistive technology that will enable them to live safe, productive, and independent lives. Specific responsibilities include
- Assessing and evaluating learners' needs in home, work, and community environments
- Developing and implementing instructional programs, case management, and record keeping
- Helping persons with visual impairment identify and use local and national resources
- Facilitate psychosocial adjustment to blindness and vision loss

Employment Characteristics

Vision rehabilitation therapists work in organizations that enhance vocational opportunities, independent living, and educational development of persons with vision loss. This may include working in center-based or itinerant settings, including clients' homes and workplaces. Vision rehabilitation therapists provide individualized programs of instruction that accommodate the unique needs of specialized groups, including persons who are aging, deaf-blind, or disabled.

Salary

According to the Association for Education and Rehabilitation of the Blind and Visually Impaired, the average full-time salary for vision rehabilitation therapists is $37,055.

For more information, refer to *www.ama-assn.org/go/hpsalary*.

Inquiries

Careers/Curriculum
Association for Education and Rehabilitation of the Blind and Visually Impaired
1703 North Beauregard Street, Suite 440
Alexandria, VA 22311-1744
703 671-4500
www.aerbvi.org

Certification
Academy for Certification of Vision Rehabilitation and Education Professionals
300 North Commerce Park Loop, #200
Tucson, AZ 85745
520 887-6816
E-mail: *info@acvrep.org*
www.acvrep.org

Program Accreditation
Association for Education and Rehabilitation of the Blind and Visually Impaired
1703 North Beauregard Street, Suite 440
Alexandria, VA 22311-1744
703 671-4500
www.aerbvi.org

Vision Rehabilitation Therapist

Arkansas

University of Arkansas at Little Rock
Vision Rehabilitation Therapy Prgm
Dept of CARE
2801 S University Ave
Little Rock, AR 72204-1099
www.ualr.edu/rehdept

Florida

Florida State University
Vision Rehabilitation Therapy Prgm
205 Stone Bldg
Tallahassee, FL 32306-4489
www.careersinblindness.com

Illinois

Northern Illinois University
Vision Rehabilitation Therapy Prgm
Dept of Teaching and Learning
DeKalb, IL 60115
www.cedu.niu.edu/tlrn/visualdisabilities

Michigan

Western Michigan University
Vision Rehabilitation Therapy Prgm
Dept of Blindness and Low Vision Studies
3413 Sangren Hall
Kalamazoo, MI 49008-5218

New York

CUNY Hunter College
Vision Rehabilitation Therapy Prgm
Dept of Special Education
695 Park Ave
New York, NY 10065
www.hunter.cuny.edu/education/programs/bvi_rehab/

Ontario, Canada

Mohawk College
Vision Rehabilitation Therapy Prgm
11 Elgin St
Brantford, ON N3T 5V2
www.mohawkc.on.ca

Pennsylvania

Salus University
Vision Rehabilitation Therapy Prgm
Dept of Graduate Studies in Vision Impairment
8360 Old York Rd
Elkins Park, PA 19027-1598
www.pco.edu

Section II

Institutions Sponsoring Accredited Programs

Alabama

Andalusia

Lurleen B Wallace Community College
Seth Hammett, MBA, President
PO Box 1418
Andalusia, AL 36420
205 222-6591
Type: Junior or Comm Coll
Control: State, County, or Local Govt
• Diagnostic Med Sonography (General) Prgm
• Emergency Med Tech-Paramedic Prgm
• Surgical Technology Prgm

Auburn University

Auburn University
Edward Richardson, President
107 Sanford Hall
Auburn University, AL 36849
334 844-4650
Type: 4-year Coll or Univ
Control: State, County, or Local Govt
• Audiologist Prgm
• Counseling Prgm
• Dietetics-Didactic Prgm
• Music Therapy Prgm
• Nursing Prgm
• Pharmacy Prgm
• Psychology (PhD) Prgm
• Rehabilitation Counseling Prgm
• Speech-Language Pathology Prgm
• Veterinary Medicine Prgm

Bay Minette

James H Faulkner State Community College
Gary L Branch, President
1900 Hwy 31 S
Bay Minette, AL 36507-2619
334 580-2100
Type: Junior or Comm Coll
Control: State, County, or Local Govt
• Dental Assistant Prgm
• Emergency Med Tech-Paramedic Prgm
• Surgical Technology Prgm

Bessemer

Lawson State Community College
Bessemer, AL 35022
• Dental Assistant Prgm

Birmingham

Fortis Institute - Birmingham
Birmingham, AL 35211
• Dental Hygiene Prgm

Jefferson State Community College
Judy M Merritt, PhD, President
2601 Carson Rd
Birmingham, AL 35215
205 983-5920
Type: Junior or Comm Coll
Control: State, County, or Local Govt
• Clin Lab Technician/Med Lab Technician Prgm
• Emergency Med Tech-Paramedic Prgm
• Physical Therapist Assistant Prgm
• Radiography Prgm
• Veterinary Technology Prgm

Samford University
Thomas E Corts, PhD, President
800 Lakeshore Dr
Birmingham, AL 35229
205 870-5727
Type: 4-year Coll or Univ
Control: Nonprofit (Private or Religious)
• Athletic Training Prgm
• Dietetics-Didactic Prgm
• Music Therapy Prgm
• Nursing Prgm
• Pharmacy Prgm

University of Alabama at Birmingham
Carol Garrison, PhD, President
AB 1070
1530 3rd Ave S
Birmingham, AL 35294-0110
205 934-4636
Type: 4-year Coll or Univ
Control: State, County, or Local Govt
• Clin Lab Scientist/Med Technologist Prgm
• Cytotechnology Prgm
• Dietetic Internship Prgm
• Genetic Counseling Prgm
• Music Therapy Prgm
• Nuclear Medicine Technology Prgm
• Nursing Prgm
• Occupational Therapy Prgm
• Optometry Prgm
• Physical Therapy Prgm
• Rehabilitation Counseling Prgm
• Respiratory Care Prgm
• Surgical Physician Assistant Prgm

Decatur

Calhoun Community College
Marilyn Beck, EdD, President
PO Box 2216 Hwy 31 N
Decatur, AL 35609
256 306-2500
Type: Junior or Comm Coll
Control: State, County, or Local Govt
• Clin Lab Technician/Med Lab Technician Prgm
• Dental Assistant Prgm
• Emergency Med Tech-Paramedic Prgm
• Physical Therapist Assistant Prgm
• Surgical Technology Prgm

Dothan

Flowers Hospital
L Keith Granger, BS, President
PO Box 6907
Dothan, AL 36302
334 793-5000
Type: Hosp or Med Ctr: 100-299 Beds
Control: For Profit
• Surgical Technology Prgm

Wallace Community College
Linda Young, EdD, President
1141 Wallace Dr
Dothan, AL 36303
800 543-2426
Type: Junior or Comm Coll
Control: State, County, or Local Govt
• Emergency Med Tech-Paramedic Prgm
• Medical Assistant Prgm
• Pharmacy Technician Prgm
• Physical Therapist Assistant Prgm
• Radiography Prgm
• Respiratory Care Prgm

Florence

University of North Alabama
Florence, AL 35632
Type: 4-year Coll or Univ
Control: State, County, or Local Govt
• Music Therapy Prgm
• Nursing Prgm

Gadsden

Gadsden State Community College
Darryl Harrison, President
PO Box 227
1001 George Wallace Dr
Gadsden, AL 35902-0227
256 549-8221
Type: Junior or Comm Coll
Control: State, County, or Local Govt
• Clin Lab Technician/Med Lab Technician Prgm
• Emergency Med Tech-Paramedic Prgm
• Radiography Prgm

Hanceville

Wallace State Community College
Vicki Hawsey, EdD, President
Commerce Bldg 801 Main St N W
PO Box 2000
Hanceville, AL 35077-2000
256 352-8130
Type: Junior or Comm Coll
Control: State, County, or Local Govt
• Clin Lab Technician/Med Lab Technician Prgm
• Dental Assistant Prgm
• Dental Hygiene Prgm
• Diagnostic Med Sonography (General) Prgm
• Emergency Med Tech-Paramedic Prgm
• Medical Assistant Prgm
• Occupational Therapy Asst Prgm
• Physical Therapist Assistant Prgm
• Polysomnographic Technology Prgm
• Radiography Prgm
• Respiratory Care Prgm

Huntsville

Crestwood Medical Center
One Hospital Dr SE
Huntsville, AL 35801
Type: Acad Health Ctr/Med Sch
Control: Nonprofit (Private or Religious)
• Radiography Prgm

Huntsville Hospital
David Spillers, MHA, CEO
101 Sivley Rd
Huntsville, AL 35801
256 265-8123
Type: Hosp or Med Ctr: 500 Beds
Control: State, County, or Local Govt
• Radiography Prgm

Oakwood College
Benjamin F Reaves, President
Huntsville, AL 35896
205 726-7000
Type: 4-year Coll or Univ
Control: Nonprofit (Private or Religious)
• Dietetic Internship Prgm

Univ of Alabama at Birmingham - Huntsville
Frank A Franz, MD, President
301 Sparkman Dr
Huntsville, AL 35899-1911
256 890-6150
Type: 4-year Coll or Univ
Control: State, County, or Local Govt
• Music Therapy Prgm
• Nursing Prgm

Jacksonville

Jacksonville State University
Harold J McGee, President
Jacksonville, AL 36265
205 782-5781
Type: 4-year Coll or Univ
Control: State, County, or Local Govt
• Music Therapy Prgm
• Nursing Prgm

Livingston

University of West Alabama
Richard Holland, PhD, President
Station 1
Livingston, AL 35470
205 652-3527
Type: 4-year Coll or Univ
Control: State, County, or Local Govt
• Athletic Training Prgm

Marion

Judson College
302 Bibb Street
Marion, AL 36756
• Music Therapy Prgm

Mobile

Bishop State Community College
Yvonne Kennedy, PhD, President
351 N Broad St
Mobile, AL 36603-5898
205 690-6416
Type: Junior or Comm Coll
Control: State, County, or Local Govt
• Emergency Med Tech-Paramedic Prgm
• Physical Therapist Assistant Prgm

Fortis College
Mobile, AL 36609
• Dental Assistant Prgm

Spring Hill College
Mobile, AL 36608
Type: 4-year Coll or Univ
Control: Nonprofit (Private or Religious)
• Nursing Prgm

University of Mobile
Mark R Foley, PhD, President
5735 College Pkwy
Mobile, AL 36663-0220
251 442-2201
Type: 4-year Coll or Univ
Control: State, County, or Local Govt
• Athletic Training Prgm
• Music Therapy Prgm
• Nursing Prgm

University of South Alabama
V Gordon Moulton, MBA, President
307 N University Blvd
AD Room 122
Mobile, AL 36688-0002
251 460-6111
Type: Acad Health Ctr/Med Sch
Control: State, County, or Local Govt
• Allopathic Medicine Prgm
• Audiologist Prgm
• Emergency Med Tech-Paramedic Prgm
• Music Therapy Prgm
• Nursing Prgm
• Occupational Therapy Prgm
• Physical Therapy Prgm
• Physician Assistant Prgm
• Radiation Therapy Prgm
• Radiography Prgm
• Respiratory Care Prgm
• Speech-Language Pathology Prgm

Virginia College

Madeline Little, President, South Region
5901 Airport Blvd
Mobile, AL 36608
251 343-7227
Type: Vocational or Tech Sch
Control: For Profit
• Diagnostic Med Sonography (General/Vascular) Prgm
• Surgical Technology Prgm (3)

Montevallo

University of Montevallo
Robert M McChesney, President
Station 6001
Montevallo, AL 35115
205 665-6000
Type: 4-year Coll or Univ
Control: State, County, or Local Govt
• Counseling Prgm
• Dietetics-Didactic Prgm
• Music Therapy Prgm
• Speech-Language Pathology Prgm

Montgomery

Alabama State Department of Education
Montgomery, AL 36130-2101
Control: State, County, or Local Govt
• Dietetic Internship Prgm

Alabama State University
William H Harris, PhD, President
915 S Jackson St
Montgomery, AL 36101-0271
334 229-4200
Type: 4-year Coll or Univ
Control: State, County, or Local Govt
• Music Therapy Prgm
• Occupational Therapy Prgm
• Physical Therapy Prgm

Auburn University at Montgomery
John Veres, PhD
PO Box 244023
Chancellor's Office
Montgomery, AL 36124
334 244-3602
Type: 4-year Coll or Univ
Control: State, County, or Local Govt
• Clin Lab Scientist/Med Technologist Prgm
• Cytotechnology Prgm
• Nursing Prgm

Baptist Medical Center South
Russell Tyner, BA MHA, CEO
2105 East South Boulevard
Montgomery, AL 36111
334 273-4400
Type: Hosp or Med Ctr: 300-499 Beds
Control: Nonprofit (Private or Religious)
• Clin Lab Scientist/Med Technologist Prgm

Huntingdon College
J Cameron West, ThM MDiv, President
1500 E Fairview Ave
Montgomery, AL 36106
334 833-4409
Type: 4-year Coll or Univ
Control: Nonprofit (Private or Religious)
• Athletic Training Prgm
• Music Therapy Prgm

South University
Victor Biebighauser, BA, President
5355 Vaughn Rd
Montgomery, AL 36116-1120
334 395-8800
Type: 4-year Coll or Univ
Control: For Profit
• Medical Assistant Prgm
• Physical Therapist Assistant Prgm

Trenholm State Technical College
Sam Munnerlyn, MA, President
1225 Air Base Blvd
Montgomery, AL 36108
334 420-4200
Type: Vocational or Tech Sch
Control: State, County, or Local Govt
• Dental Assistant Prgm
• Diagnostic Med Sonography (General) Prgm
• Emergency Med Tech-Paramedic Prgm
• Medical Assistant Prgm
• Radiography Prgm

Muscle Shoals

Northwest-Shoals Community College
Humphrey Lee, EdD, President
PO Box 2545
Muscle Shoals, AL 35662
256 331-5200
Type: Junior or Comm Coll
Control: State, County, or Local Govt
• Emergency Med Tech-Paramedic Prgm

Normal

Alabama A&M University
Robert R Jennings, EdD, President
PO Box 1357
Normal, AL 35762
205 851-5000
Type: 4-year Coll or Univ
Control: State, County, or Local Govt
• Dietetics-Didactic Prgm
• Rehabilitation Counseling Prgm
• Speech-Language Pathology Prgm

Opelika

Southern Union State Community College
Amelia Pearson, EdD, President
1701 LaFayette Pkwy
Opelika, AL 36801
334 745-6437
Type: Junior or Comm Coll
Control: State, County, or Local Govt
• Emergency Med Tech-Paramedic Prgm
• Radiography Prgm
• Surgical Technology Prgm

Rainsville

Northeast Alabama Community College
David Campbell, PhD, President
PO Box 159
Rainsville, AL 35986-0159
256 228-6001
Type: Junior or Comm Coll
Control: State, County, or Local Govt
• Emergency Med Tech-Paramedic Prgm

Spanish Fort

Institute of Ultrasound Diagnostics
Smyth R Gill, BA, CFO
31214 Coleman Lane
Ste A
Spanish Fort, AL 36527
251 621-8668
Type: Vocational or Tech Sch
Control: For Profit
• Diagnostic Med Sonography (General) Prgm

Sumiton

Bevill State Community College
Harold Wade, EdD, President
PO Box 800
Sumiton, AL 35148-0800
205 648-3271
Type: Junior or Comm Coll
Control: State, County, or Local Govt
• Emergency Med Tech-Paramedic Prgm
• Surgical Technology Prgm

Troy

Troy University
Jack Hawkins, Jr, PhD, Chancellor
University Ave
Troy, AL 36082
334 670-3200
Type: 4-year Coll or Univ
Control: State, County, or Local Govt
• Athletic Training Prgm
• Counseling Prgm (2)
• Music Therapy Prgm
• Rehabilitation Counseling Prgm

Tuscaloosa

DCH Regional Medical Center
Bryan N Kindred, MBA, President/CEO
809 University Blvd E
Tuscaloosa, AL 35401
205 759-7177
Type: Hosp or Med Ctr: 500 Beds
Control: State, County, or Local Govt
• Radiography Prgm

Shelton State Community College
Mark Heinrich, EdD, President
9500 Old Greensboro Rd
Tuscaloosa, AL 35405
205 391-2472
Type: Junior or Comm Coll
Control: State, County, or Local Govt
• Respiratory Care Prgm

Stillman College
Tuscaloosa, AL 35401
Type: 4-year Coll or Univ
Control: Nonprofit (Private or Religious)
• Music Therapy Prgm
• Nursing Prgm

University of Alabama
Robert Witt, PhD, President
PO Box 870100
Tuscaloosa, AL 35487
205 348-5100
Type: 4-year Coll or Univ
Control: State, County, or Local Govt
• Allopathic Medicine Prgm
• Athletic Training Prgm
• Counseling Prgm
• Dentistry Prgm
• Dietetics-Coordinated Prgm
• Dietetics-Didactic Prgm
• Medical Librarian Prgm
• Music Therapy Prgm
• Nursing Prgm
• Psychology (PhD) Prgm (2)
• Rehabilitation Counseling Prgm
• Speech-Language Pathology Prgm

Tuskegee

Tuskegee University
Gilbert L Rochon, PhD, President
308 Kresge Ctr
Office of the President/Kresge Building
Tuskegee, AL 36088-1677
334 727-8501
Type: 4-year Coll or Univ
Control: Nonprofit (Private or Religious)
• Clin Lab Scientist/Med Technologist Prgm
• Dietetics-Didactic Prgm
• Occupational Therapy Prgm
• Veterinary Medicine Prgm

Alaska

Anchorage

University of Alaska Anchorage
Frances Ulmer, JD, Chancellor
3211 Providence Dr
ADM 217
Anchorage, AK 99508-4614
907 786-1437
Type: 4-year Coll or Univ
Control: State, County, or Local Govt
• Clin Lab Scientist/Med Technologist Prgm
• Clin Lab Technician/Med Lab Technician Prgm
• Dental Assistant Prgm
• Dental Hygiene Prgm
• Dietetic Internship Prgm
• Dietetics-Didactic Prgm
• Medical Assistant Prgm
• Music Therapy Prgm

Fairbanks

University of Alaska - Fairbanks
Steve Jones, PhD, Chancellor
320 Signers Hall
Fairbanks, AK 99775-7500
907 474-7112
Type: 4-year Coll or Univ
Control: State, County, or Local Govt
• Dental Hygiene Prgm
• Emergency Med Tech-Paramedic Prgm
• Medical Assistant Prgm
• Music Therapy Prgm

INSTITUTIONS

Alberta, Canada

Calgary

Alberta Health Services - Rockyview Hospital
Calgary, AB T2V 1P9
• Ophthalmic Med Technologist Prgm

Southern Alberta Institute of Technology
1301 16th Avenue NW
Calgary, AB T2M 0L4
Type: Vocational or Tech Sch
Control: Other
• Ophthalmic Assistant Prgm

University of Calgary
Calgary, AB T2N 4N1
Type: 4-year Coll or Univ
Control: State, County, or Local Govt
• Allopathic Medicine Prgm
• Pathologists' Assistant Prgm
• Veterinary Medicine Prgm

Edmonton

University of Alberta
Indira Samarasekera, PhD, President
Edmonton, AB T6G 2M7
Type: 4-year Coll or Univ
Control: Nonprofit (Private or Religious)
• Allopathic Medicine Prgm
• Medical Librarian Prgm

Arizona

Chandler

Chandler-Gilbert Community College
Maria L Hesse, EdD, President
2626 East Pecos Rd
Chandler, AZ 85225
480 732-7075
Type: Acad Health Ctr/Med Sch
Control: For Profit
• Dietetic Technician-AD Prgm

Coolidge

Central Arizona College
Kathleen Arns, PhD, President
Woodruff at Overfield Rd
Coolidge, AZ 85228
602 426-4444
Type: Junior or Comm Coll
Control: State, County, or Local Govt
• Dietetic Technician-AD Prgm
• Medical Assistant Prgm
• Radiography Prgm

Flagstaff

Northern Arizona University
Haeger John, PhD, President
PO Box 4092
Flagstaff, AZ 86011
928 523-3232
Type: 4-year Coll or Univ
Control: State, County, or Local Govt
• Athletic Training Prgm
• Counseling Prgm
• Dental Hygiene Prgm
• Nursing Prgm
• Physical Therapy Prgm
• Speech-Language Pathology Prgm

Glendale

Midwestern University - Glendale Campus
Kathleen H Goeppinger, PhD, President and CEO
19555 N 59th Ave
Glendale, AZ 85308
623 572-3400
Type: Acad Health Ctr/Med Sch
Control: Nonprofit (Private or Religious)
• Dentistry Prgm
• Occupational Therapy Prgm
• Optometry Prgm
• Osteopathic Medicine Prgm
• Perfusion Prgm
• Pharmacy Prgm
• Physician Assistant Prgm
• Podiatric Medicine Prgm

Goodyear

Franklin Pierce University
140 N Litchfield Rd
Goodyear, AZ 85338
• Physical Therapy Prgm

Kingman

Mohave Community College
Thomas C Henry, PhD, Chancellor
1971 Jagerson Ave
Kingman, AZ 86401
928 757-0800
Type: Junior or Comm Coll
Control: State, County, or Local Govt
• Dental Hygiene Prgm
• Emergency Med Tech-Paramedic Prgm
• Physical Therapist Assistant Prgm
• Surgical Technology Prgm

Mesa

Arizona Medical Training Institute
1530 North Country Club, Suite 11
Mesa, AZ 85201
• Phlebotomy Prgm

Carrington College - Mesa
Mesa, AZ 85210
• Dental Hygiene Prgm

East Valley Institute of Technology
Mesa, AZ 85201
Type: Vocational or Tech Sch
• Surgical Technology Prgm

Mesa Community College
Wayne Giles, EdD, President
1833 W Southern Ave
Mesa, AZ 85205
480 461-7299
Type: Junior or Comm Coll
Control: State, County, or Local Govt
• Dental Hygiene Prgm
• Veterinary Technology Prgm

Phoenix

Argosy University
Phoenix, AZ 85021
Type: 4-year Coll or Univ
Control: For Profit
• Psychology (PsyD) Prgm

Brookline College - Phoenix
2445 W Dunlap Ave, Suite 100
Phoenix, AZ 85021
Type: 4-year Coll or Univ
Control: For Profit
• Clin Lab Technician/Med Lab Technician Prgm

Brown Mackie College - Phoenix
Connie Scollard, Campus President
13430 North Black Canyon Highway
Phoenix, AZ 85029
480 375-2357
• Occupational Therapy Asst Prgm

Carrington College
Thomas A Bloom, PhD, President
7600 North 16th Street, Suite 16
Phoenix, AZ 85020
• Physical Therapist Assistant Prgm
• Radiography Prgm
• Veterinary Technology Prgm

DeVry University - Phoenix
2149 W. Dunlap Avenue
Phoenix, AZ 85021
Type: 4-year Coll or Univ
Control: For Profit
• Clin Lab Scientist/Med Technologist Prgm

Fortis College - Phoenix
Phoenix, AZ 85006
• Dental Hygiene Prgm

GateWay Community College
Eugene Giovannini, EdD, President
108 N 40th St
Phoenix, AZ 85034
602 286-8000
Type: Junior or Comm Coll
Control: State, County, or Local Govt
• Diagnostic Med Sonography (General) Prgm
• Neurodiagnostic Tech Prgm
• Nuclear Medicine Technology Prgm
• Physical Therapist Assistant Prgm
• Polysomnographic Technology Prgm
• Radiation Therapy Prgm
• Radiography Prgm
• Respiratory Care Prgm
• Surgical Technology Prgm

Grand Canyon University
Gil Stafford, PhD, President
PO Box 111097
Phoenix, AZ 85061-1097
602 249-3300
Type: 4-year Coll or Univ
Control: Nonprofit (Private or Religious)
- Athletic Training Prgm
- Nursing Prgm

Kaplan College
Debra Thibodeaux, MBA, Executive Director
13610 N Black Canyon Hwy 104
Phoenix, AZ 85029
602 548-1955
Type: Vocational or Tech Sch
Control: For Profit
- Medical Assistant Prgm
- Respiratory Care Prgm
- Veterinary Technology Prgm

Paradise Valley Community College
Mary Kay Kickels, President
18401 N 32nd St
Phoenix, AZ 85032
602 787-6610
Type: Acad Health Ctr/Med Sch
Control: For Profit
- Dietetic Technician-AD Prgm

Paradise Valley Unified School District
20621 N 32nd St
Phoenix, AZ 85032
602 493-2600
Type: Acad Health Ctr/Med Sch
Control: State, County, or Local Govt
- Dietetic Internship Prgm

Phoenix College
Anna Solley, EdD, President
1202 W Thomas Rd
Phoenix, AZ 85013
602 285-7364
Type: Junior or Comm Coll
Control: State, County, or Local Govt
- Clin Lab Technician/Med Lab Technician Prgm
- Dental Assistant Prgm
- Dental Hygiene Prgm
- Histotechnician Prgm

Southwestern DI Consortium
Poenix Indian Medical Center
Phoenix, AZ 85016
Type: Consortium
Control: Nonprofit (Private or Religious)
- Dietetic Internship Prgm

University of Phoenix
Laura Palmer Noone, PhD JD, President
4615 E Elwood St
PO Box 52076
Phoenix, AZ 85040
480 966-9577
Type: 4-year Coll or Univ
Control: For Profit
- Counseling Prgm
- Nursing Prgm

Prescott

Yavapai County Health Department
930 Division St
Prescott, AZ 86301
602 771-3122
Type: Nonhosp HC Facil, BB, or Lab
Control: State, County, or Local Govt
- Emergency Med Tech-Paramedic Prgm
- Radiography Prgm

Scottsdale

Penn Foster College
Richard W Ferrin, PhD, President
14300 N Northsight Blvd
Scottsdale, AZ 85254
480 947-6644
Type: 4-year Coll or Univ
Control: State, County, or Local Govt
- Veterinary Technician Prgm

Tempe

Arizona State University
Michael M Crow, PhD, President
PO Box 877705
Office of the President, Mail Code 7705
Tempe, AZ 85287-7705
480 965-8972
Type: 4-year Coll or Univ
Control: State, County, or Local Govt
- Audiologist Prgm
- Clin Lab Scientist/Med Technologist Prgm
- Counseling Prgm
- Dietetic Internship Prgm
- Dietetics-Didactic Prgm
- Music Therapy Prgm
- Nursing Prgm
- Psychology (PhD) Prgm
- Speech-Language Pathology Prgm

Blood Systems Laboratories
Tempe, AZ 85282
Type: Nonhosp HC Facil, BB, or Lab
- Specialist in BB Tech Prgm

Maricopa County Dept of Public Health
Office of Nutrition Services
1414 W Broadway Ste 237
Tempe, AZ 85282
602 966-3090
Type: Nonhosp HC Facil, BB, or Lab
Control: State, County, or Local Govt
- Dietetic Internship Prgm

Rio Salado College
Linda M Thor, President
2323 W 14th St
Tempe, AZ 85281-6950
480 517-8000
Type: Junior or Comm Coll
Control: State, County, or Local Govt
- Dental Assistant Prgm
- Dental Hygiene Prgm

Tucson

Brown Mackie College - Tucson
Holly Helscher, PhD, President
4585 E Speedway Blvd
Tucson, AZ 85712
520 319-3300
Type: Junior or Comm Coll
Control: For Profit
- Occupational Therapy Asst Prgm

Carondelet St Mary's Hospital
Morrisons Custom Management Company
1601 W St Mary's Rd
Tucson, AZ 85745
520 622-5833
Type: Hosp or Med Ctr: 100-299 Beds
Control: Nonprofit (Private or Religious)
- Dietetic Internship Prgm

Pima Community College
Roy Flores, PhD, Chancellor
4905 E Broadway
Pima Community College District Office
Tucson, AZ 85709-1005
520 206-4500
Type: Junior or Comm Coll
Control: State, County, or Local Govt
- Clin Lab Technician/Med Lab Technician Prgm
- Dental Assistant Prgm
- Dental Hygiene Prgm
- Dental Lab Technician Prgm
- Emergency Med Tech-Paramedic Prgm
- Pharmacy Technician Prgm
- Radiography Prgm
- Respiratory Care Prgm
- Surgical Technology Prgm
- Veterinary Technology Prgm

Pima Medical Institute
Richard L Luebke, Jr, BS, President
40 N Swan, Suite 100
Tucson, AZ 85711
520 326-1600
Type: Vocational or Tech Sch
Control: For Profit
- Occupational Therapy Asst Prgm (2)
- Physical Therapist Assistant Prgm (2)
- Radiography Prgm (2)
- Respiratory Care Prgm (2)

University of Arizona
Robert Shelton, PhD, President
Adminstration Bldg Rm 712
Tucson, AZ 85721-0066
520 621-5511
Type: 4-year Coll or Univ
Control: State, County, or Local Govt
- Allopathic Medicine Prgm
- Audiologist Prgm
- Dietetic Internship Prgm
- Dietetics-Didactic Prgm
- Medical Librarian Prgm
- Music Therapy Prgm
- Nursing Prgm
- Orientation and Mobility Specialist Prgm
- Perfusion Prgm
- Pharmacy Prgm
- Psychology (PhD) Prgm
- Rehabilitation Counseling Prgm
- Speech-Language Pathology Prgm
- Teacher of the Visually Impaired Prgm

Yuma

Arizona Western College
Don Schoening, PhD, President
PO Box 929
Yuma, AZ 85366-0929
Type: 4-year Coll or Univ
Control: State, County, or Local Govt
• Radiography Prgm

Arkansas

Arkadelphia

Henderson State University
Charles Dunn, PhD, President
HSU Box 7532
Arkadelphia, AR 71999-0001
870 230-5091
Type: 4-year Coll or Univ
Control: State, County, or Local Govt
• Athletic Training Prgm
• Counseling Prgm
• Dietetics-Didactic Prgm
• Nursing Prgm

Ouachita Baptist University
Andrew Westmoreland, EdD, President
410 Ouachita Ct
OBU Box 3753
Arkadelphia, AR 71998
870 245-5000
Type: 4-year Coll or Univ
Control: Nonprofit (Private or Religious)
• Athletic Training Prgm
• Dietetics-Didactic Prgm
• Music Therapy Prgm

Batesville

Univ of Arkansas Comm Coll - Batesville
Deborah Frazier, EdD, Chancellor
PO Box 3350
Batesville, AR 72501
870 793-7581
Type: Junior or Comm Coll
Control: State, County, or Local Govt
• Emergency Med Tech-Paramedic Prgm

Beebe

Arkansas State University - Beebe
Eugene McKay, PhD, Chancellor
PO Box 1000
Beebe, AR 72012
501 882-8857
Type: Junior or Comm Coll
Control: State, County, or Local Govt
• Clin Lab Technician/Med Lab Technician Prgm
• Emergency Med Tech-Paramedic Prgm
• Pharmacy Technician Prgm
• Veterinary Technology Prgm

Bentonville

NorthWest Arkansas Community College
Rebecca Paneitz, PhD, President
One College Dr
Bentonville, AR 72712-5091
479 619-4251
Type: Junior or Comm Coll
Control: State, County, or Local Govt
• Emergency Med Tech-Paramedic Prgm
• Physical Therapist Assistant Prgm
• Respiratory Care Prgm

Blytheville

Arkansas Northeastern College
Robin Myers, EdD, President
PO Box 1109
Blytheville, AR 72316
870 762-1020
Type: Junior or Comm Coll
Control: State, County, or Local Govt
• Dental Assistant Prgm
• Emergency Med Tech-Paramedic Prgm

Conway

Hendrix College
1600 Washington Avenue
Conway, AR 72032
• Music Therapy Prgm

University of Central Arkansas
Lu Hardin, JD, President
Wingo Hall, Ste 207
201 Donaghey Ave
Conway, AR 72035
501 450-3170
Type: 4-year Coll or Univ
Control: State, County, or Local Govt
• Athletic Training Prgm
• Dietetic Internship Prgm
• Dietetics-Didactic Prgm
• Music Therapy Prgm
• Nursing Prgm
• Occupational Therapy Prgm
• Physical Therapy Prgm
• Speech-Language Pathology Prgm

El Dorado

South Arkansas Community College
Barbara Jones, PhD, President and CEO
PO Box 7010
300 S West Ave
El Dorado, AR 71731-7010
870 862-8131
Type: Junior or Comm Coll
Control: State, County, or Local Govt
• Clin Lab Technician/Med Lab Technician Prgm
• Emergency Med Tech-Paramedic Prgm
• Occupational Therapy Asst Prgm
• Phlebotomy Prgm
• Physical Therapist Assistant Prgm
• Radiography Prgm
• Surgical Technology Prgm

Fayetteville

University of Arkansas
John White, PhD, Chancellor
Adminstration Bldg
Fayetteville, AR 72701
479 575-4148
Type: 4-year Coll or Univ
Control: State, County, or Local Govt
• Athletic Training Prgm
• Counseling Prgm
• Dietetics-Didactic Prgm
• Music Therapy Prgm
• Nursing Prgm
• Rehabilitation Counseling Prgm
• Speech-Language Pathology Prgm

Forrest City

East Arkansas Community College
Coy Grace, President
1700 Newcastle Rd
Forrest City, AR 72335
870 633-4480
Type: Junior or Comm Coll
Control: State, County, or Local Govt
• Emergency Med Tech-Paramedic Prgm

Fort Smith

University of Arkansas - Fort Smith
Paul Beran, PhD, Chancellor
5201 Grand Ave
PO Box 3649
Fort Smith, AR 72913
479 788-7004
Type: 4-year Coll or Univ
Control: State, County, or Local Govt
• Dental Hygiene Prgm
• Diagnostic Med Sonography (General) Prgm
• Music Therapy Prgm
• Radiography Prgm
• Surgical Technology Prgm

Harrison

North Arkansas College
Jeffery R Olson, PhD, President
1515 Pioneer Dr
Harrison, AR 72601-5599
870 391-3212
Type: Junior or Comm Coll
Control: State, County, or Local Govt
• Clin Lab Technician/Med Lab Technician Prgm
• Emergency Med Tech-Paramedic Prgm
• Radiography Prgm
• Surgical Technology Prgm

Helena

Phillips Community College/U of Arkansas
Steven Murray, EdD, Chancellor
PO Box 785
1000 Campus Dr
Helena, AR 72342
870 338-6474
Type: Junior or Comm Coll
Control: State, County, or Local Govt
• Clin Lab Technician/Med Lab Technician Prgm
• Phlebotomy Prgm

Hope

Univ of Arkansas Comm Coll - Hope
Welch Charles, EdD, Chancellor
PO Box 140
2500 S Main
Hope, AR 71801
870 777-5722
Type: Junior or Comm Coll
Control: State, County, or Local Govt
• Emergency Med Tech-Paramedic Prgm

Hot Springs

National Park Community College
Sally Carder, PhD, President
101 College Dr
Hot Springs, AR 71913-9174
501 760-4200
Type: Junior or Comm Coll
Control: State, County, or Local Govt
• Clin Lab Technician/Med Lab Technician Prgm
• Emergency Med Tech-Paramedic Prgm
• Radiography Prgm

Little Rock

Baptist Health Schools Little Rock
Russell D Harrington, Jr, FACHE, President
9601 Lile Dr Hwy 630 Exit 7
Little Rock, AR 72205
501 202-2000
Type: Hosp or Med Ctr: 500 Beds
Control: Nonprofit (Private or Religious)
• Clin Lab Scientist/Med Technologist Prgm
• Histotechnician Prgm
• Nuclear Medicine Technology Prgm
• Occupational Therapy Asst Prgm
• Polysomnographic Technology Prgm
• Radiography Prgm
• Surgical Technology Prgm

Central Arkansas Radiation Therapy Inst
Janice Burford, CEO, President
PO Box 55050
Little Rock, AR 72215
501 664-8573
Type: Nonhosp HC Facil, BB, or Lab
Control: Nonprofit (Private or Religious)
• Radiation Therapy Prgm

Saint Vincent Health System
Peter Banko, CEO
Two St Vincent Circle
Little Rock, AR 72205-5499
501 552-3910
Type: Consortium
Control: Nonprofit (Private or Religious)
• Radiography Prgm

University of Arkansas at Little Rock
Joel Anderson, Chancellor
2801 S University Ave
Little Rock, AR 72204
501 569-3000
Type: 4-year Coll or Univ
Control: State, County, or Local Govt
• Audiologist Prgm
• Music Therapy Prgm
• Orientation and Mobility Specialist Prgm
• Rehabilitation Counseling Prgm
• Speech-Language Pathology Prgm
• Vision Rehabilitation Therapy Prgm

University of Arkansas for Medical Sciences
Richard Pierson, Chancellor
4301 W Markham #557
Little Rock, AR 72205
501 686-5662
Type: Acad Health Ctr/Med Sch
Control: State, County, or Local Govt
• Allopathic Medicine Prgm
• Clin Lab Scientist/Med Technologist Prgm
• Cytotechnology Prgm
• Dental Hygiene Prgm
• Diagnostic Med Sonography (General) Prgm
• Dietetic Internship Prgm
• Emergency Med Tech-Paramedic Prgm
• Genetic Counseling Prgm
• Medical Dosimetry Prgm
• Nuclear Medicine Technology Prgm
• Nursing Prgm
• Ophthalmic Med Technologist Prgm
• Pharmacy Prgm
• Psychology (PhD) Prgm
• Radiography Prgm (3)
• Radiologist Assistant Prgm
• Respiratory Care Prgm (2)
• Surgical Technology Prgm

Magnolia

Southern Arkansas University
David F Rankin, PhD CFA, President
100 E University
Magnolia, AR 71753-5000
870 235-4001
Type: 4-year Coll or Univ
Control: State, County, or Local Govt
• Athletic Training Prgm
• Music Therapy Prgm

Monticello

U of Arkansas at Monticello Coll of Tech
H Jack Lassiter, PhD, Chancellor
346 University Dr
PO Box 3596
Monticello, AR 71656
870 460-1020
Type: 4-year Coll or Univ
Control: State, County, or Local Govt
• Emergency Med Tech-Paramedic Prgm
• Music Therapy Prgm

North Little Rock

Pulaski Technical College
Dan Bakke, EdD, President
3000 W Scenic Rd
North Little Rock, AR 72118
501 812-2216
Type: Junior or Comm Coll
Control: State, County, or Local Govt
• Dental Assistant Prgm

Ozark

Arkansas Tech University - Ozark Campus
Jo Alice Blondin, PhD, Chancellor
1700 Helberg Lane
Ozark, AR 72949
479 667-2117
Type: 4-year Coll or Univ
Control: State, County, or Local Govt
• Emergency Med Tech-Paramedic Prgm
• Physical Therapist Assistant Prgm

Pine Bluff

Southeast Arkansas College
Phil E Shirley, PhD, President
1900 Hazel St
Pine Bluff, AR 71603
870 543-5907
Type: Junior or Comm Coll
Control: State, County, or Local Govt
• Emergency Med Tech-Paramedic Prgm
• Phlebotomy Prgm
• Radiography Prgm
• Respiratory Care Prgm
• Surgical Technology Prgm

University of Arkansas at Pine Bluff
Lawrence A Davis, Chancellor
1200 N University Dr
Pine Bluff, AR 71601
501 575-8470
Type: 4-year Coll or Univ
Control: State, County, or Local Govt
• Dietetics-Didactic Prgm
• Music Therapy Prgm

Pocahontas

Black River Technical College
Richard Gaines, MS, Director
PO Box 468
Pocahontas, AR 72455
870 248-4000
Type: Vocational or Tech Sch
Control: State, County, or Local Govt
• Dietetic Technician-AD Prgm
• Emergency Med Tech-Paramedic Prgm
• Respiratory Care Prgm

Russellville

Arkansas Tech University
Robert Charles Brown, PhD, President
Administration 210
1605 Coliseum Dr
Russellville, AR 72801
479 968-0237
Type: 4-year Coll or Univ
Control: State, County, or Local Govt
• Medical Assistant Prgm

Searcy

Harding University
David B Burks, President
915 E Market Ave
HU 12256
Searcy, AR 72149-2256
501 279-4274
Type: 4-year Coll or Univ
Control: Nonprofit (Private or Religious)
• Athletic Training Prgm
• Dietetics-Didactic Prgm
• Pharmacy Prgm
• Physician Assistant Prgm
• Speech-Language Pathology Prgm

Springdale

Northwest Technical Institute
George Burch, EdD, President
PO Box 2000
709 S Old Missouri Rd
Springdale, AR 72765
479 751-8824
Type: Vocational or Tech Sch
Control: State, County, or Local Govt
• Surgical Technology Prgm

State University

Arkansas State University
Administration, PO Box 600
State University, AR 72467-0010
870 972-3465
Type: 4-year Coll or Univ
Control: Nonprofit (Private or Religious)
• Athletic Training Prgm
• Clin Lab Scientist/Med Technologist Prgm
• Clin Lab Technician/Med Lab Technician Prgm
• Counseling Prgm
• Diagnostic Med Sonography (General) Prgm
• Dietetics-Coordinated Prgm
• Magnetic Resonance Technologist Prgm
• Music Therapy Prgm
• Physical Therapist Assistant Prgm
• Physical Therapy Prgm
• Radiation Therapy Prgm
• Radiography Prgm
• Rehabilitation Counseling Prgm
• Speech-Language Pathology Prgm

British Columbia, Canada

Burnaby

Simon Fraser University
Burnaby, BC V5A 1S6
Type: 4-year Coll or Univ
Control: State, County, or Local Govt
• Psychology (PhD) Prgm

Lake Country

CanScribe Career Centre
223 3121 Hill Rd
Lake Country, BC V4V 1G1
Type: Acad Health Ctr/Med Sch
Control: For Profit
• Medical Transcriptionist Prgm

Langley

Trinity Western University
7600 Glover Rd
Langley, BC V2Y 1Y1
604 888-7511
Type: 4-year Coll or Univ
Control: Nonprofit (Private or Religious)
• Counseling Prgm

Vancouver

British Columbia's Children's Hospital
4480 Oak St
Vancouver, BC V6N 3V4
604 875-2111
Type: Hosp or Med Ctr: 100-299 Beds
Control: State, County, or Local Govt
• Orthoptist Prgm

University of British Columbia
Stephen J Toope, PhD, President
T325-Third Floor-Koerner Pavillion
2211 Westbrook Mall
Vancouver, BC V6T 1Z1
Type: 4-year Coll or Univ
Control: State, County, or Local Govt
• Allopathic Medicine Prgm
• Genetic Counseling Prgm
• Medical Librarian Prgm
• Psychology (PhD) Prgm

Victoria

University of Victoria
Victoria, BC V8W 3P5
Type: 4-year Coll or Univ
Control: State, County, or Local Govt
• Psychology (PhD) Prgm

California

Alameda

College of Alameda
George Herring, PhD, President
555 Atlantic Ave
Alameda, CA 94501
510 748-2262
Type: Junior or Comm Coll
Control: State, County, or Local Govt
• Dental Assistant Prgm

Alhambra

Everest College - Alhambra
Melody Rider, BA, School President
2215 Mission Rd
Alhambra, CA 91803
626 979-4940
Type: Vocational or Tech Sch
Control: For Profit
• Medical Assistant Prgm

Platt College Los Angeles, LLC
Alhambra, CA 91803
Type: Vocational or Tech Sch
• Diagnostic Med Sonography (General) Prgm

Anaheim

Everest College
Staci Mall, BA MA, School President
511 N Brookhurst St, Ste 300
Anaheim, CA 92801
714 953-6500
Type: Vocational or Tech Sch
Control: For Profit
• Medical Assistant Prgm (2)

North Orange County Community College
Jerome Hunter, PhD, Chancellor
1830 W Romneya Dr
Anaheim, CA 92801
714 808-4797
Type: 4-year Coll or Univ
Control: State, County, or Local Govt
• Pharmacy Technician Prgm

Angwin

Pacific Union College
D Malcolm Maxwell, President
Angwin, CA 94508
707 965-6311
Type: 4-year Coll or Univ
Control: Nonprofit (Private or Religious)
• Music Therapy Prgm

Aptos

Cabrillo College
Brian King, PhD, President/Superintendent
6500 Soquel Dr
Aptos, CA 95003
831 479-6306
Type: Junior or Comm Coll
Control: State, County, or Local Govt
• Dental Hygiene Prgm
• Medical Assistant Prgm
• Radiography Prgm

Arcata

Humboldt State University
Rollin C Richmond, PhD, President
1 Harpst St
Arcata, CA 95521
707 826-3311
Type: 4-year Coll or Univ
Control: State, County, or Local Govt
• Nursing Prgm

Azusa

Azusa Pacific University
Jon R Wallace, DBA, President
901 E Alosta Ave
Azusa, CA 91702
626 812-3031
Type: 4-year Coll or Univ
Control: Nonprofit (Private or Religious)
• Athletic Training Prgm
• Music Therapy Prgm
• Nursing Prgm
• Physical Therapy Prgm
• Psychology (PsyD) Prgm

Bakersfield

Bakersfield College
Greg A Chamberlain, PhD, President
1801 Panorama Dr
Bakersfield, CA 93305
661 395-4211
Type: Junior or Comm Coll
Control: State, County, or Local Govt
• Emergency Med Tech-Paramedic Prgm
• Radiography Prgm

California State University - Bakersfield
Thomas Arciniega, PhD, President
9001 Stockdale Hwy
Bakersfield, CA 93311
805 833-2241
Type: 4-year Coll or Univ
Control: State, County, or Local Govt
• Nursing Prgm

Clinica Sierra Vista
1430 Truxtun Ave, Ste 120
Bakersfield, CA 93301-3834
Type: Acad Health Ctr/Med Sch
Control: Nonprofit (Private or Religious)
• Dietetic Internship Prgm

Belmont

Notre Dame de Namur University
Jack Oblack, President
Ralston Ave
Belmont, CA 94002
415 593-1601
Type: 4-year Coll or Univ
Control: Nonprofit (Private or Religious)
• Art Therapy Prgm

Berkeley

The Wright Insitute
Berkeley, CA 94704
Type: Acad Health Ctr/Med Sch
Control: For Profit
• Psychology (PsyD) Prgm

University of California - Berkeley
Robert Berdahl, Chancellor
Berkeley, CA 94720
510 642-6000
Type: 4-year Coll or Univ
Control: State, County, or Local Govt
• Dietetics-Didactic Prgm
• Optometry Prgm
• Psychology (PhD) Prgm

Burlingame

Mills-Peninsula Health Services
Robert W Merwin, MS, CEO
1501 Trousdale Dr
Burlingame, CA 94010
650 696-5678
Type: Hosp or Med Ctr: 300-499 Beds
Control: Nonprofit (Private or Religious)
• Radiography Prgm

Camarillo

California State University - Channel Islands
Camarillo, CA 93012-8599
Type: 4-year Coll or Univ
Control: State, County, or Local Govt
• Nursing Prgm

Carson

California State University - Dominguez Hills
Mildred Garcia, EdD, President
1000 E Victoria St
Carson, CA 90747-9960
310 243-3696
Type: 4-year Coll or Univ
Control: State, County, or Local Govt
• Clin Lab Scientist/Med Technologist Prgm
• Music Therapy Prgm
• Nursing Prgm
• Occupational Therapy Prgm
• Orthotist/Prosthetist Prgm

Chico

California State University - Chico
Manuel A Esteban, President
Chico, CA 95929-0222
916 898-5871
Type: 4-year Coll or Univ
Control: State, County, or Local Govt
• Dietetic Internship Prgm
• Dietetics-Didactic Prgm
• Emergency Med Tech-Paramedic Prgm
• Music Therapy Prgm
• Nursing Prgm
• Speech-Language Pathology Prgm

Chula Vista

Pima Medical Institute
Richard L Luebke, Jr, CEO
780 Bay Blvd, Ste 101
Chula Vista, CA 91910
619 425-3200
Type: Vocational or Tech Sch
Control: Nonprofit (Private or Religious)
• Occupational Therapy Asst Prgm
• Radiography Prgm
• Respiratory Care Prgm

Southwestern College
Neil Yoneji, MS, Interim Supt/President
900 Otay Lakes Rd
Chula Vista, CA 91910
619 482-6301
Type: Junior or Comm Coll
Control: State, County, or Local Govt
• Clin Lab Technician/Med Lab Technician Prgm
• Dental Hygiene Prgm
• Emergency Med Tech-Paramedic Prgm
• Surgical Technology Prgm

Colton

Arrowhead Regional Medical Center
Patrick Petre, Director
400 N Pepper Ave
Colton, CA 92324-1819
909 580-6150
Type: Hosp or Med Ctr: 300-499 Beds
Control: State, County, or Local Govt
• Clin Lab Scientist/Med Technologist Prgm
• Radiography Prgm

Commerce

Los Angeles County EMS Agency
Cathy Chidester, MSN, Assistant Director
5555 Ferguson Dr, Ste 220
Commerce, CA 90022
323 890-7545
Type: Junior or Comm Coll
Control: State, County, or Local Govt
• Emergency Med Tech-Paramedic Prgm

Concord

Gurnick Academy of Medical Arts
Concord, CA
• Radiography Prgm

Mt Diablo Adult Education
Joanne Durkee, Director of Adult Educ
1266 San Carlos Ave
Concord, CA 94518
925 685-7340
Type: Vocational or Tech Sch
Control: Nonprofit (Private or Religious)
• Surgical Technology Prgm

Costa Mesa

Career Networks Institute
Jim Buffington, BA, President
3420 Bristol St, Ste 209
Costa Mesa, CA 92626
714 568-1566
Type: Vocational or Tech Sch
Control: For Profit
• Surgical Technology Prgm

Orange Coast College
Robert Dees, PhD, President
2701 Fairview Rd
Costa Mesa, CA 92628-5005
714 432-5712
Type: Junior or Comm Coll
Control: State, County, or Local Govt
• Cardiovascular Tech (Invasive/Noninvasive) Prgm
• Dental Assistant Prgm
• Diagnostic Med Sonography (General) Prgm
• Dietetic Technician-AD Prgm
• Medical Assistant Prgm
• Neurodiagnostic Tech Prgm
• Polysomnographic Technology Prgm
• Radiography Prgm
• Respiratory Care Prgm

Vanguard University
Murray Dempster, PhD, President
55 Fair Dr
Costa Mesa, CA 92626
714 556-3610
Type: 4-year Coll or Univ
Control: Nonprofit (Private or Religious)
• Athletic Training Prgm
• Nursing Prgm

Culver City

West Los Angeles College
Frank Quiambao, President
9000 Overland Ave
Culver City, CA 90230
310 287-4200
Type: Junior or Comm Coll
Control: State, County, or Local Govt
• Dental Hygiene Prgm

Cupertino

De Anza College
Brian Murphy, President
21250 Stevens Creek Blvd
Cupertino, CA 95014
408 864-8705
Type: Junior or Comm Coll
Control: State, County, or Local Govt
• Clin Lab Technician/Med Lab Technician Prgm

Cypress

Cypress College
Michael Kasler, PhD, President
9200 Valley View St
Cypress, CA 90630
714 484-7000
Type: Junior or Comm Coll
Control: State, County, or Local Govt
• Dental Assistant Prgm
• Dental Hygiene Prgm
• Diagnostic Med Sonography (General) Prgm
• Radiography Prgm

Duarte

City of Hope
Virgina Opipare, MD, EVP and COO
1500 E Duarte Rd
Duarte, CA 91010
626 359-8111
Type: Hosp or Med Ctr: 300-499 Beds
Control: Nonprofit (Private or Religious)
• Radiation Therapy Prgm

El Cajon

Grossmont College
Sunita Cooke, PhD, President
8800 Grossmont College Dr
El Cajon, CA 92020
619 644-7100
Type: Junior or Comm Coll
Control: State, County, or Local Govt
• Cardiovascular Tech (Invasive/Vasc/Echo)
  Prgm
• Occupational Therapy Asst Prgm
• Respiratory Care Prgm

Encino

Phillips Graduate Institute
Lisa Porche-Burke, PhD, President
5445 Balboa Blvd
Encino, CA 91316-1509
818 386-5600
Type: 4-year Coll or Univ
Control: Nonprofit (Private or Religious)
• Art Therapy Prgm

Eureka

College of the Redwoods
Casey Crabill, President
Tompkins Hill Rd
Eureka, CA 95501
707 445-6700
Type: Junior or Comm Coll
Control: State, County, or Local Govt
• Dental Assistant Prgm
• Emergency Med Tech-Paramedic Prgm

North Coast Emergency Medical Services
Larry Karsteadt, MS, Executive Director
3340 Glenwood St
Eureka, Ca 95501
707 445-2081
Type: Vocational or Tech Sch
Control: State, County, or Local Govt
• Emergency Med Tech-Paramedic Prgm

Folsom

Folsom Lake College
10 College Parkway
Folsom, CA 95630
Type: Junior or Comm Coll
Control: State, County, or Local Govt
• Clin Lab Technician/Med Lab Technician Prgm

Foster City

California EMS Academy Inc
Nancy L Black, RN MS, President
1098 Foster City Blvd
Ste 106 PMB 708
Foster City, CA 94404
866 577-9197
Type: Vocational or Tech Sch
Control: State, County, or Local Govt
• Emergency Med Tech-Paramedic Prgm

Fremont

Ohlone College
Douglas Treadway, PhD,
  Superintendent/President
43600 Mission Blvd
PO Box 3909
Fremont, CA 94539
510 659-6200
Type: Junior or Comm Coll
Control: State, County, or Local Govt
• Physical Therapist Assistant Prgm
• Respiratory Care Prgm

Fresno

Alliant International University
Fresno, CA 93727
Type: 4-year Coll or Univ
Control: Nonprofit (Private or Religious)
• Psychology (PhD) Prgm (3)
• Psychology (PsyD) Prgm (4)

California Institute of Medical Science, Inc
1901 E Shields, Suite B-118
Fresno, CA 93726
• Phlebotomy Prgm

California State University - Fresno
John D Welty, EdD, President
5241 N Maple Ave
Fresno, CA 93740-0080
559 278-2423
Type: 4-year Coll or Univ
Control: State, County, or Local Govt
• Athletic Training Prgm
• Counseling Prgm
• Dietetic Internship Prgm
• Dietetics-Didactic Prgm
• Music Therapy Prgm
• Nursing Prgm
• Physical Therapy Prgm
• Rehabilitation Counseling Prgm
• Speech-Language Pathology Prgm

Community Regional Medical Center
Bruce Perry, President
PO Box 1232
Fresno, CA 93715
209 442-3911
Type: Hosp or Med Ctr: 300-499 Beds
Control: Nonprofit (Private or Religious)
• Diagnostic Med Sonography (General/Cardiac)
  Prgm

Fresno City College
Ned Doffoney, PhD, President
1101 E University Ave
Fresno, CA 93741
559 442-8244
Type: Junior or Comm Coll
Control: State, County, or Local Govt
• Dental Hygiene Prgm
• Emergency Med Tech-Paramedic Prgm
• Radiography Prgm
• Respiratory Care Prgm
• Surgical Technology Prgm

Fresno County Paramedic Program
Brad Maggy, MPA, Interim Director
1221 Fulton Mall
Fresno, CA 93721
559 445-3200
Type: Junior or Comm Coll
Control: State, County, or Local Govt
• Emergency Med Tech-Paramedic Prgm

Fresno Pacific University
Fresno, CA 93702
Type: 4-year Coll or Univ
Control: Nonprofit (Private or Religious)
• Nursing Prgm

Fullerton

California State University - Fullerton
Milton A Gordon, PhD, President
PO Box 6810
Fullerton, CA 92834-6810
714 278-3456
Type: 4-year Coll or Univ
Control: State, County, or Local Govt
• Athletic Training Prgm
• Nursing Prgm
• Speech-Language Pathology Prgm

Southern California College of Optometry
Lesley Walls, OD MD, President
2575 Yorba Linda Blvd
Fullerton, CA 92831
714 870-7226
Type: Junior or Comm Coll
Control: Nonprofit (Private or Religious)
• Optometry Prgm

Gardena

Everest College - Gardena
Bill Wherritt, President
1045 W Redondo Beach Blvd, Ste 275
Gardena, CA 90247
310 527-7105
Type: Vocational or Tech Sch
Control: For Profit
• Medical Assistant Prgm

Glendale

Glendale Career College
Serjik Kesachekian, MBA, Campus Director
1015 Grandview Ave
Glendale, CA 91201
818 956-4915
Type: Vocational or Tech Sch
Control: For Profit
• Surgical Technology Prgm

Glendora

Citrus College
Michael J Viera, PhD, President/Superintendent
1000 W Foothill
Glendora, CA 91740
818 963-0323
Type: Junior or Comm Coll
Control: State, County, or Local Govt
• Dental Assistant Prgm

Hayward

California State University - East Bay
Norma S Rees, President
25800 Carlos Bee Blvd
Hayward, CA 94542
510 881-3086
Type: 4-year Coll or Univ
Control: State, County, or Local Govt
• Music Therapy Prgm
• Nursing Prgm
• Speech-Language Pathology Prgm

Chabot College
Celia Barbarena, EdD, President
25555 Hesperian Blvd
PO Box 5001
Hayward, CA 94545-5001
510 786-6640
Type: Junior or Comm Coll
Control: State, County, or Local Govt
• Dental Hygiene Prgm
• Medical Assistant Prgm

Life Chiropractic College West
25001 Industrial Blvd
Hayward, CA 94545
Type: Acad Health Ctr/Med Sch
Control: For Profit
• Chiropractic Prgm

Imperial

Imperial Valley Community College
Paul Pai, EdD, President
380 E Aten Rd
Imperial, CA 92251
760 355-6219
Type: Junior or Comm Coll
Control: State, County, or Local Govt
• Emergency Med Tech-Paramedic Prgm

Irvine

Concordia University - Irvine
Jacob Preus, STM ThD, President
1530 Concordia West
Irvine, CA 92612
949 854-8002
Type: 4-year Coll or Univ
Control: Nonprofit (Private or Religious)
• Athletic Training Prgm
• Nursing Prgm

Stanbridge College
Yasith Weerasuriya, Chief Executive Officer
2041 Business Center Drive, #107
Irvine, CA 92612
949 794-9090
• Psychology (PsyD) Prgm

University of CA - Irvine School of Medicine
Michael V Drake, MD, Chancellor
510 Administration
Campus Dr
Irvine, CA 92697
949 824-5111
Type: Acad Health Ctr/Med Sch
Control: State, County, or Local Govt
• Allopathic Medicine Prgm
• Genetic Counseling Prgm
• Nursing Prgm

West Coast University
Irvine, CA 92617-3040
Type: 4-year Coll or Univ
Control: For Profit
• Dental Hygiene Prgm
• Nursing Prgm

Irwindale

Premiere Career College
Fe Ludovico-Aragon, MD, Executive Director
12901 Ramona Blvd
Irwindale, CA 91706
626 814-2080
Type: Vocational or Tech Sch
Control: For Profit
• Surgical Technology Prgm

Public Health Foundation Enterprises
WIC Program
12781 Schabarum Ave
Irwindale, CA 91706-6802
818 856-6376
Type: Nonhosp HC Facil, BB, or Lab
Control: Nonprofit (Private or Religious)
• Dietetic Internship Prgm

Kentfield

College of Marin
Frances White, PhD, Superintendent/President
835 College Ave
Kentfield, CA 94904
415 457-8811
Type: Junior or Comm Coll
Control: State, County, or Local Govt
• Dental Assistant Prgm

La Jolla

National University
La Jolla, CA 92037
Type: 4-year Coll or Univ
Control: Nonprofit (Private or Religious)
• Nursing Prgm

University of California - San Diego
Marye Anne Fox, PhD, Chancellor
9500 Gilman Dr MC 0005
La Jolla, CA 92093-0657
858 534-3135
Type: 4-year Coll or Univ
Control: State, County, or Local Govt
• Allopathic Medicine Prgm
• Pharmacy Prgm

La Mirada

Biola University
La Mirada, CA 90639
Type: 4-year Coll or Univ
Control: State, County, or Local Govt
• Music Therapy Prgm
• Nursing Prgm
• Psychology (PhD) Prgm
• Psychology (PsyD) Prgm (2)

La Puente

Hacienda LaPuente Adult Education
Alan Kern, MA, Adult School Director
Willow Campus
14101 E Nelson Ave
La Puente, CA 91746-2640
626 933-3915
Type: Consortium
Control: Nonprofit (Private or Religious)
• Dental Assistant Prgm

La Verne

University of La Verne
Stephen Morgan, EdD, President
1950 Third St
La Verne, CA 91750
909 593-4900
Type: 4-year Coll or Univ
Control: State, County, or Local Govt
• Athletic Training Prgm
• Psychology (PhD) Prgm

Lancaster

Antelope Valley College
Steve Buffalo, PhD, President
3041 W Ave K, Admin Bldg
Lancaster, CA 93534
805 943-3241
Type: 4-year Coll or Univ
Control: State, County, or Local Govt
• Radiography Prgm

University of Antelope Valley (UAV)
Lancaster, CA 93534
Type: 4-year Coll or Univ
• Emergency Med Tech-Paramedic Prgm

Livermore

National College of Technical Instruction
Floyd Graves, VP Admin & Support Serv
7575 Southfront Rd
Livermore, CA 94550
800 827-0111
Type: Vocational or Tech Sch
Control: For Profit
• Emergency Med Tech-Paramedic Prgm (6)

Loma Linda

Loma Linda University
Richard H Hart, MD Dr PH, Chancellor, CEO
Office of the President
Magan Hall, Room 111
Loma Linda, CA 92354
909 558-1000
Type: Acad Health Ctr/Med Sch
Control: Nonprofit (Private or Religious)
• Allopathic Medicine Prgm
• Clin Lab Scientist/Med Technologist Prgm
• Cytotechnology Prgm
• Dental Hygiene Prgm
• Dentistry Prgm
• Diagnostic Med Sonography (General) Prgm
• Dietetics-Coordinated Prgm
• Medical Dosimetry Prgm
• Nursing Prgm
• Occupational Therapy Prgm
• Pharmacy Prgm
• Physical Therapist Assistant Prgm
• Physical Therapy Prgm
• Physician Assistant Prgm
• Psychology (PsyD) Prgm (2)
• Radiation Therapy Prgm
• Radiography Prgm
• Radiologist Assistant Prgm
• Respiratory Care Prgm
• Speech-Language Pathology Prgm

Long Beach

American University of Health Sciences
Kim Dang, PhD, President/Owner
3501 Atlantic Ave
Long Beach, CA 90807
562 988-2278
Type: 4-year Coll or Univ
Control: For Profit
• Pharmacy Technician Prgm

California State University - Long Beach
F King Alexander, PhD, President
1250 Bellflower Blvd SS/AD 300
Long Beach, CA 90840-0115
562 985-4121
Type: 4-year Coll or Univ
Control: State, County, or Local Govt
• Athletic Training Prgm
• Dietetic Internship Prgm
• Dietetics-Didactic Prgm
• Kinesiotherapy Prgm
• Music Therapy Prgm
• Nursing Prgm
• Physical Therapy Prgm
• Radiation Therapy Prgm
• Speech-Language Pathology Prgm

Los Altos Hills

Foothill College
Judy Miner, Ed D, President
12345 El Monte Rd
Los Altos Hills, CA 94022
650 949-7200
Type: Junior or Comm Coll
Control: State, County, or Local Govt
• Dental Assistant Prgm
• Dental Hygiene Prgm
• Diagnostic Med Sonography (General) Prgm
• Emergency Med Tech-Paramedic Prgm
• Pharmacy Technician Prgm
• Radiography Prgm
• Respiratory Care Prgm
• Veterinary Technology Prgm

Los Angeles

American Career College
David A Pyle, President
4021 Rosewood Ave 101
Los Angeles, CA 90004
Type: Vocational or Tech Sch
Control: For Profit
• Pharmacy Technician Prgm
• Surgical Technology Prgm (2)

California State University - Los Angeles
James M Rosser, President
5151 State University Dr
Los Angeles, CA 90032
323 343-4690
Type: 4-year Coll or Univ
Control: State, County, or Local Govt
• Audiologist Prgm
• Counseling Prgm
• Dietetics-Coordinated Prgm
• Dietetics-Didactic Prgm
• Nursing Prgm
• Orientation and Mobility Specialist Prgm
• Rehabilitation Counseling Prgm
• Speech-Language Pathology Prgm

Career Colleges of America
Ron Scheachter Meisel, MS, CEO
1801 N La Cienega Blvd #301
Los Angeles, CA 90035
310 287-9001
Type: Vocational or Tech Sch
Control: For Profit
• Surgical Technology Prgm (2)

Cedars Sinai Medical Center
Thomas Priselac, Exec Vice Pres
8700 Beverly Blvd
Los Angeles, CA 90048
310 855-6211
Type: Hosp or Med Ctr: 500 Beds
Control: Nonprofit (Private or Religious)
• Cytogenetic Technology Prgm

Center for Child Development/Disabilities/UAP
Walter W Noce, Jr, MPH, President, CEO
4650 Sunset Blvd
Los Angeles, CA 90027
213 669-2301
Type: Hosp or Med Ctr: 300-499 Beds
Control: Nonprofit (Private or Religious)
• Dietetic Internship Prgm

Charles Drew University of Medicine and Sci
Susan Kelly, MD, President/COO
1731 E 120th St
Los Angeles, CA 90059
323 563-4800
Type: Acad Health Ctr/Med Sch
Control: Nonprofit (Private or Religious)
• Diagnostic Med Sonography (General) Prgm
• Pharmacy Technician Prgm
• Radiography Prgm

Childrens Hospital Los Angeles
4650 Sunset Blvd, Mailstop 88
Los Angeles, CA 90027
323 361-5697
Type: Hosp or Med Ctr: 300-499 Beds
Control: Nonprofit (Private or Religious)
• Orthoptist Prgm

Cleveland Chriractic College of Los Angeles
590 N Vermont Ave
Los Angeles, CA 90004
Type: Acad Health Ctr/Med Sch
Control: For Profit
• Chiropractic Prgm

East Los Angeles Education and Career Center
2100 Marengo St
Los Angeles, CA 90033
213 223-1283
Type: Vocational or Tech Sch
Control: State, County, or Local Govt
• Radiography Prgm

Everest College - Los Angeles
Johnny Arellano, President
3640 Wilshire Blvd
Ste 500
Los Angeles, CA 90010
213 388-9950
Type: Vocational or Tech Sch
Control: For Profit
• Medical Assistant Prgm

Greater LA Cytotechnology Training Consortium
Sheldon King, MD, Interim Med Ctr Dir
Administration 17-165 CHS
10833 Le Conte Ave
Los Angeles, CA 90024-1730
310 825-5041
Type: Consortium
Control: State, County, or Local Govt
• Cytotechnology Prgm

Los Angeles City College
Jamillah Moore, PhD, Interim President
855 N Vermont Ave
Los Angeles, CA 90029
323 953-4000
Type: Junior or Comm Coll
Control: State, County, or Local Govt
- Dental Lab Technician Prgm
- Dietetic Technician-AD Prgm
- Radiography Prgm

Los Angeles County+USC Healthcare Network
Douglas D Bagley, MS, Interim Exec Dir
1200 N State St, Rm 112
Los Angeles, CA 90033
213 226-6501
Type: Hosp or Med Ctr: 500 Beds
Control: State, County, or Local Govt
- Dietetic Internship Prgm

Loyola Marymount University
Robert B Lawton, SJ, President
1 LMU Dr
Los Angeles, CA 90045
310 338-2700
Type: 4-year Coll or Univ
Control: Nonprofit (Private or Religious)
- Art Therapy Prgm
- Athletic Training Prgm
- Music Therapy Prgm

Mount St Mary's College
Jacqueline Powers Doud, PhD, President
Chalon Campus
12001 Chalon Rd
Los Angeles, CA 90049-1599
310 954-4000
Type: 4-year Coll or Univ
Control: Nonprofit (Private or Religious)
- Nursing Prgm
- Physical Therapy Prgm

UCLA Medical Center, Department of Pathology
Jonathan Braun, MD, Chairman
10833 Le Conte Avenue, 13-222A, CHS
Department of Pathology
Los Angeles, CA 90095
310 794-7953
Type: Acad Health Ctr/Med Sch
Control: State, County, or Local Govt
- Emergency Med Tech-Paramedic Prgm

University of California - Los Angeles
Albert Carnesale, Chancellor
Box 951405, Murphy Hall 2147
Los Angeles, CA 90095-1405
Type: 4-year Coll or Univ
Control: State, County, or Local Govt
- Allopathic Medicine Prgm
- Dentistry Prgm
- Medical Librarian Prgm
- Nursing Prgm
- Psychology (PhD) Prgm

University of Southern California
C.L. Max Nikias, PhD, President
University Park Campus
110 Bovard, ADM-110
Los Angeles, CA 90089-0012
213 740-2111
Type: 4-year Coll or Univ
Control: Nonprofit (Private or Religious)
- Allopathic Medicine Prgm
- Dental Hygiene Prgm
- Dentistry Prgm
- Music Therapy Prgm
- Occupational Therapy Prgm
- Pharmacy Prgm
- Physical Therapy Prgm
- Physician Assistant Prgm
- Psychology (PhD) Prgm

VA Greater Los Angeles Healthcare System
Kenneth J Clark, MA JD, Director
11301 Wilshire Blvd
Los Angeles, CA 90073
310 268-3132
Type: Dept of Veterans Affairs
Control: Fed Govt
- Dietetic Internship Prgm

Malibu

Pepperdine University
David Davenport, President
24255 Pacific Coast Hwy
Malibu, CA 90263
310 456-4000
Type: 4-year Coll or Univ
Control: Nonprofit (Private or Religious)
- Dietetics-Didactic Prgm
- Psychology (PhD) Prgm

Marysville

Yuba Community College
Paul Mendoza, President
2088 N Beale Rd
Marysville, CA 95901
916 741-6716
Type: Junior or Comm Coll
Control: State, County, or Local Govt
- Radiography Prgm
- Veterinary Technology Prgm

Merced

Merced College
Benjamin Duran, PhD, President/Superintendent
3600 M St
Merced, CA 95348-2898
209 384-6101
Type: Junior or Comm Coll
Control: State, County, or Local Govt
- Diagnostic Med Sonography (General/Cardiac) Prgm
- Radiography Prgm

Mission Viejo

Saddleback College
Dixie Bullock, RN MN, President
28000 Marguerite Pkwy
Mission Viejo, CA 92692
949 582-4500
Type: Junior or Comm Coll
Control: State, County, or Local Govt
- Emergency Med Tech-Paramedic Prgm

Modesto

Modesto Junior College
Richard Rose, PhD, President
435 College Ave
Modesto, CA 95350-9977
209 575-6067
Type: Junior or Comm Coll
Control: State, County, or Local Govt
- Dental Assistant Prgm
- Medical Assistant Prgm
- Respiratory Care Prgm

Monterey

Monterey Peninsula College
Doug Garrison, EdD, Superintendent/Pres
980 Fremont St
Monterey, CA 93940
831 646-4060
Type: Junior or Comm Coll
Control: State, County, or Local Govt
- Dental Assistant Prgm

Monterey Park

East Los Angeles College
Ernest H Moreno, MA, President
1301 Avenida Cesar Chavez
Monterey Park, CA 91754
323 265-8662
Type: Junior or Comm Coll
Control: State, County, or Local Govt
- Respiratory Care Prgm

Moorpark

Moorpark College
Pam Eddinger, PhD, President
7075 Campus Rd
Moorpark, CA 93021
805 378-1400
Type: Junior or Comm Coll
Control: State, County, or Local Govt
- Radiography Prgm

Moreno Valley

Riverside County Regional Medical Center
Salvatore Rotella, PhD, President
Moreno Valley Campus
16130 Lasselle St
Moreno Valley, CA 92551-2045
951 571-6166
Type: Acad Health Ctr/Med Sch
Control: State, County, or Local Govt
- Physician Assistant Prgm

INSTITUTIONS

Napa

Napa State Hospital
2100 Napa Vallejo Hwy
Napa, CA 94558
707 253-5428
Type: Hosp or Med Ctr: 100-299 Beds
Control: Nonprofit (Private or Religious)
• Dietetic Internship Prgm

Napa Valley College
Diane Carey, PhD, President/Superintendent
2277 Napa Vallejo Hwy
Napa, CA 94558
707 253-3360
Type: Junior or Comm Coll
Control: State, County, or Local Govt
• Emergency Med Tech-Paramedic Prgm
• Respiratory Care Prgm

North Hollywood

Kaplan College
Steven A Bagley, MA, Interim President
6180 Laurel Canyon Blvd
Ste 101
North Hollywood, CA 91606
818 763-2563
Type: 4-year Coll or Univ
Control: For Profit
• Radiography Prgm
• Respiratory Care Prgm

Northridge

California State University - Northridge
Jolene Koester, PhD, President
18111 Nordhoff St
Northridge, CA 91330
818 677-2121
Type: 4-year Coll or Univ
Control: State, County, or Local Govt
• Athletic Training Prgm
• Counseling Prgm
• Dietetic Internship Prgm
• Dietetics-Didactic Prgm
• Music Therapy Prgm
• Nursing Prgm
• Physical Therapy Prgm
• Radiography Prgm
• Speech-Language Pathology Prgm

Norwalk

Cerritos College
Noelia Vela, EdD, President/Superintendent
11110 E Alondra Blvd
Norwalk, CA 90650
562 860-2451
Type: Junior or Comm Coll
Control: State, County, or Local Govt
• Dental Assistant Prgm
• Dental Hygiene Prgm
• Pharmacy Technician Prgm
• Physical Therapist Assistant Prgm

Oakland

Holy Names University
Oakland, CA 94619
Type: 4-year Coll or Univ
Control: Nonprofit (Private or Religious)
• Nursing Prgm

Merritt College
Evelyn Wesley, PhD, President
12500 Campus Dr
Oakland, CA 94619
510 436-2414
Type: Junior or Comm Coll
Control: State, County, or Local Govt
• Dietetic Technician-AD Prgm
• Radiography Prgm

Samuel Merritt University
Sharon Diaz, PhD, President
3100 Telegraph Avenue
Ste 2840
Oakland, CA 94609-3108
510 869-6511
Type: 4-year Coll or Univ
Control: Nonprofit (Private or Religious)
• Nursing Prgm
• Occupational Therapy Prgm
• Physical Therapy Prgm
• Physician Assistant Prgm
• Podiatric Medicine Prgm

TPMG Regional Laboratory
Patricia Conolly
1950 Franklin St
Oakland, CA 94612
510 987-4101
Type: Hosp or Med Ctr: 100-299 Beds
Control: Nonprofit (Private or Religious)
• Histotechnician Prgm

Oceanside

MiraCosta College
Oceanside, CA 92056
Type: Junior or Comm Coll
• Surgical Technology Prgm

Orange

Chapman University
James L Doti, PhD, President
One University Dr
Orange, CA 92866
714 997-6611
Type: 4-year Coll or Univ
Control: Nonprofit (Private or Religious)
• Athletic Training Prgm
• Music Therapy Prgm
• Physical Therapy Prgm
• Speech-Language Pathology Prgm

Univ of California Irvine Med Ctr
Mark Laret, Executive Director
UCI Medical Ctr
101 City Dr S
Orange, CA 92868-3298
714 456-5678
Type: Acad Health Ctr/Med Sch
Control: State, County, or Local Govt
• Clin Lab Scientist/Med Technologist Prgm

Oroville

Butte College
Diana Van Der Ploeg, PhD, President
3536 Butte Campus Dr
Oroville, CA 95965
530 895-2484
Type: Junior or Comm Coll
Control: State, County, or Local Govt
• Emergency Med Tech-Paramedic Prgm
• Respiratory Care Prgm

Oxnard

Oxnard College
Steven F Arvizu, PhD, President
4000 S Rose Ave
Oxnard, CA 93033-6699
805 986-5800
Type: Junior or Comm Coll
Control: State, County, or Local Govt
• Dental Hygiene Prgm

Palo Alto

Pacific Graduate School of Psychology
Palo Alto, CA 94303
Type: Acad Health Ctr/Med Sch
Control: For Profit
• Psychology (PhD) Prgm
• Psychology (PsyD) Prgm

VA Palo Alto Health Care System
Elizabeth Joyce Freeman, Director
3801 Miranda Ave
Palo Alto, CA 94304
650 493-5000
Type: Hosp or Med Ctr: 500 Beds
Control: Nonprofit (Private or Religious)
• Nuclear Medicine Technology Prgm

Pasadena

Fuller Theological Seminary
Pasadena, CA 91101
Type: Acad Health Ctr/Med Sch
Control: For Profit
• Psychology (PhD) Prgm
• Psychology (PsyD) Prgm

Pasadena City College
Paulette Purfumo, PhD, President
1570 E Colorado Blvd
Pasadena, CA 91106
626 585-7123
Type: Junior or Comm Coll
Control: State, County, or Local Govt
• Dental Assistant Prgm
• Dental Hygiene Prgm
• Dental Lab Technician Prgm
• Medical Assistant Prgm
• Radiography Prgm

Patton

Patton State Hospital
3102 E Highland Ave
Patton, CA 92369
909 425-7297
Type: Nonhosp HC Facil, BB, or Lab
Control: Nonprofit (Private or Religious)
• Dietetic Internship Prgm

Pleasant Hill

Diablo Valley College
Judy Walters, PhD, President
321 Golf Club Rd
Pleasant Hill, CA 94523
925 685-1230
Type: Junior or Comm Coll
Control: State, County, or Local Govt
• Clin Lab Technician/Med Lab Technician Prgm
• Dental Assistant Prgm
• Dental Hygiene Prgm

John F Kennedy University
Pleasant Hill, CA 94523
Type: 4-year Coll or Univ
Control: Nonprofit (Private or Religious)
• Psychology (PsyD) Prgm

Pomona

American Red Cross Blood Services
100 Red Cross Way
Pomona, CA 91768
Type: Nonhosp HC Facil, BB, or Lab
Control: Nonprofit (Private or Religious)
• Specialist in BB Tech Prgm

California State Polytechnic University
Bob H Suzuki, President
3801 W Temple Ave
Pomona, CA 91768
909 869-2000
Type: 4-year Coll or Univ
Control: State, County, or Local Govt
• Dietetic Internship Prgm
• Dietetics-Didactic Prgm
• Veterinary Technology Prgm

Western Univ of Health Sciences
Philip Pumerantz, PhD, President
309 E Second St
Pomona, CA 91766-1854
909 469-5200
Type: Acad Health Ctr/Med Sch
Control: Nonprofit (Private or Religious)
• Dentistry Prgm
• Optometry Prgm
• Osteopathic Medicine Prgm
• Pharmacy Prgm
• Physical Therapy Prgm
• Physician Assistant Prgm
• Podiatric Medicine Prgm
• Psychology (PsyD) Prgm
• Veterinary Medicine Prgm

Porterville

Porterville Development Center
Porterville, CA 93258
209 782-2753
Type: Nonhosp HC Facil, BB, or Lab
Control: Nonprofit (Private or Religious)
• Dietetic Internship Prgm

Rancho Cordova

California Northstate University
Rancho Cordova, CA 95670
• Pharmacy Prgm

Rancho Cucamonga

Chaffey College
Henry Shannon, PhD, Superintendent/President
5885 Haven Ave
Rancho Cucamonga, CA 91737
909 941-2100
Type: Junior or Comm Coll
Control: State, County, or Local Govt
• Dental Assistant Prgm
• Dietetic Technician-AD Prgm
• Radiography Prgm

Rancho Mirage

Eisenhower Memorial Hospital
Aubrey G Serfling, MBA MA, President/CEO
39000 Bob Hope Dr
Rancho Mirage, CA 92270
760 340-3911
Type: Hosp or Med Ctr: 100-299 Beds
Control: Nonprofit (Private or Religious)
• Clin Lab Scientist/Med Technologist Prgm

Redding

Shasta College
Gary Lewis, Superintendent/President
PO Box 496006
Redding, CA 96049-6006
530 225-4600
Type: Junior or Comm Coll
Control: State, County, or Local Govt
• Dental Hygiene Prgm

Redlands

University of Redlands
Stuart Dorsey, President
PO Box 3080
1200 E Colton Ave
Redlands, CA 92373-0999
909 793-2121
Type: 4-year Coll or Univ
Control: Nonprofit (Private or Religious)
• Speech-Language Pathology Prgm

Redwood City

Canada College
Tom Mohr, President
4200 Farm Hill Blvd
Redwood City, CA 94061
650 306-3283
Type: Junior or Comm Coll
Control: State, County, or Local Govt
• Radiography Prgm

Reedley

Central Valley WIC Dietetic Internship
1560 E Manning Ave
Reedley, CA 93654
Type: Acad Health Ctr/Med Sch
Control: Fed Govt
• Dietetic Internship Prgm

Reseda

Everest College - Reseda
Steven R Schilling, BA MA, President
18040 Sherman Way
Reseda, CA 91335
818 774-0550
Type: Vocational or Tech Sch
Control: For Profit
• Surgical Technology Prgm

Richmond

Kaiser Permanente School of Allied Health Sci
Gwenette S Jackson, BA CRT, School
   Administrator
938 Marina Way South
Richmond, CA 94804
510 307-2412
Type: Vocational or Tech Sch
Control: Nonprofit (Private or Religious)
• Clin Lab Technician/Med Lab Technician Prgm
• Diagnostic Med Sonography (General) Prgm
• Nuclear Medicine Technology Prgm
• Radiation Therapy Prgm
• Radiography Prgm

Riverside

California Baptist University
Riverside, CA 92504-3297
Type: 4-year Coll or Univ
Control: Nonprofit (Private or Religious)
• Athletic Training Prgm
• Nursing Prgm

Moreno Valley College
Riverside, CA 92506
Type: 4-year Coll or Univ
• Dental Assistant Prgm
• Emergency Med Tech-Paramedic Prgm

Riverside Comm Coll - Moreno Valley Campus
Irving Hedrick, EdD, Interim Chancellor
16130 Lasselle
Riverside, CA 92551
951 571-6161
Type: Junior or Comm Coll
Control: State, County, or Local Govt
• Dental Hygiene Prgm
• Emergency Med Tech-Paramedic Prgm

Rohnert Park

Sonoma State University
1801 E Cotati Ave
Rohnert Park, CA 94928-3609
707 664-2880
Type: 4-year Coll or Univ
Control: State, County, or Local Govt
• Counseling Prgm

Sacramento

American River College
David Viar, EdD, President
4700 College Oak Dr
Sacramento, CA 95841
916 484-8211
Type: Junior or Comm Coll
Control: State, County, or Local Govt
• Emergency Med Tech-Paramedic Prgm
• Respiratory Care Prgm

California State University - Sacramento
Alexander Gonzalez, PhD, President
CSUS 6000 J St
Sacramento, CA 95819
916 278-7737
Type: 4-year Coll or Univ
Control: State, County, or Local Govt
- Athletic Training Prgm
- Dietetic Internship Prgm
- Dietetics-Didactic Prgm
- Emergency Med Tech-Paramedic Prgm
- Nursing Prgm
- Physical Therapy Prgm
- Rehabilitation Counseling Prgm
- Speech-Language Pathology Prgm

Carrington College California
George Montgomery, BA, CEO
8909 Folsom Blvd
Sacramento, CA 95826
916 388-2881
Type: Vocational or Tech Sch
Control: For Profit
- Dental Hygiene Prgm
- Medical Assistant Prgm (8)
- Pharmacy Technician Prgm (8)
- Surgical Technology Prgm (2)
- Veterinary Technician Prgm (3)
- Veterinary Technology Prgm (3)

Charles A Jones Skills & Business Ed Center
Kirk Williams, CEO, Principal
5451 Lemon Hill Ave
Sacramento, CA 95824-1529
Type: Acad Health Ctr/Med Sch
Control: State, County, or Local Govt
- Pharmacy Technician Prgm

Cosumnes River Community College
Francisco Rodriguez, PhD, President
8401 Center Pkwy
Sacramento, CA 95823
916 688-7321
Type: Junior or Comm Coll
Control: State, County, or Local Govt
- Medical Assistant Prgm
- Veterinary Technology Prgm

Sacramento City College
Kathryn E Jeffrey, PhD, President
3835 Freeport Blvd
Sacramento, CA 95822-1386
916 558-2100
Type: Junior or Comm Coll
Control: State, County, or Local Govt
- Dental Assistant Prgm
- Dental Hygiene Prgm
- Occupational Therapy Asst Prgm
- Physical Therapist Assistant Prgm

UC Davis Medical Center
Ann Rice
2315 Stockton Blvd
Sacramento, CA 95817
916 734-0751
Type: Acad Health Ctr/Med Sch
Control: State, County, or Local Govt
- Dietetic Internship Prgm

Univ of California Davis Health System
Ann Rice, Hospital CEO
2315 Stockton Blvd
Sacramento, CA 95817
916 453-0750
Type: Acad Health Ctr/Med Sch
Control: State, County, or Local Govt
- Clin Lab Scientist/Med Technologist Prgm

University of California - Davis
Claire Pomeroy, MD, Dean
School of Medicine
4610 X Street, Ste 3101
Sacramento, CA 95817
916 734-3578
Type: 4-year Coll or Univ
Control: State, County, or Local Govt
- Allopathic Medicine Prgm
- Dietetics-Didactic Prgm
- Physician Assistant Prgm
- Veterinary Medicine Prgm

Salinas

Hartnell Community College
Pheobe Helm, President
411 Central Ave
Salinas, CA 93901
831 755-6700
Type: Junior or Comm Coll
Control: State, County, or Local Govt
- Clin Lab Technician/Med Lab Technician Prgm
- Veterinary Technology Prgm

San Bernardino

California State University - San Bernardino
Anthony H Evans, President
5500 University Pkwy
San Bernardino, CA 92407
909 880-5000
Type: 4-year Coll or Univ
Control: State, County, or Local Govt
- Dietetics-Didactic Prgm
- Music Therapy Prgm
- Nursing Prgm
- Rehabilitation Counseling Prgm

Concorde Career College
Ron Johnson, MEd, Campus President
201 E Airport Drive
Ste 100
San Bernardino, CA 92408
909 884-8891
Type: Vocational or Tech Sch
Control: For Profit
- Dental Hygiene Prgm (3)
- Physical Therapist Assistant Prgm
- Respiratory Care Prgm
- Surgical Technology Prgm (3)

Everest College - San Bernardino
217 E Club Center Dr
San Bernardino, CA 92408
Type: Vocational or Tech Sch
Control: For Profit
- Medical Assistant Prgm

San Bruno

Skyline College
Victoria Morrow, PhD, President
3300 College Dr
San Bruno, CA 94066
650 738-4111
Type: Junior or Comm Coll
Control: State, County, or Local Govt
- Respiratory Care Prgm
- Surgical Technology Prgm

San Diego

California College San Diego
Carl Barney, CEO
2820 Camino del Rio S
San Diego, CA 92108
619 295-5785
Type: 4-year Coll or Univ
Control: For Profit
- Respiratory Care Prgm

Mueller College of Holistic Studies
Jeff Welsh, PhD MA HHP, President and CEO
4607 Park Blvd
San Diego, CA 92116
619 291-9811
Type: Vocational or Tech Sch
Control: For Profit
- Massage Therapy Prgm

Naval School of Health Sciences, San Diego
CAPT Debra M Ryken, CAPT DC USN,
    Commanding Officer
34101 Farenholt Ave
San Diego, CA 92134
619 532-7700
Type: Dept of Defense
Control: Fed Govt
- Clin Lab Technician/Med Lab Technician Prgm

Point Loma Nazarene University
Bob Brower, PhD, President
3900 Lomaland Dr
San Diego, CA 92106
619 849-2216
Type: Acad Health Ctr/Med Sch
Control: For Profit
- Athletic Training Prgm
- Dietetics-Didactic Prgm
- Music Therapy Prgm
- Nursing Prgm

San Diego Mesa College
Rita Cepeda, EdD, President
7250 Mesa College Dr
San Diego, CA 92111
619 388-2755
Type: Junior or Comm Coll
Control: State, County, or Local Govt
- Dental Assistant Prgm
- Physical Therapist Assistant Prgm
- Radiography Prgm

San Diego State University
Stephen L Weber, PhD, President
5500 Campanile Dr
San Diego, CA 92182-1518
619 594-7746
Type: 4-year Coll or Univ
Control: State, County, or Local Govt
• Athletic Training Prgm
• Audiologist Prgm
• Dietetic Internship Prgm
• Dietetics-Didactic Prgm
• Kinesiotherapy Prgm
• Nursing Prgm
• Psychology (PhD) Prgm
• Rehabilitation Counseling Prgm
• Speech-Language Pathology Prgm

Univ of California San Diego Med Ctr
Richard Liekweg, Director
200 W Arbor Dr, H-910C
San Diego, CA 92103-8970
619 543-6654
Type: Hosp or Med Ctr: 300-499 Beds
Control: State, County, or Local Govt
• Clin Lab Scientist/Med Technologist Prgm
• Diagnostic Med Sonography (General) Prgm
• Nursing Prgm

VA San Diego Healthcare System
3350 La Jolla Village Dr
San Diego, CA 92161
619 552-8585
Type: Dept of Veterans Affairs
Control: Fed Govt
• Dietetic Internship Prgm

San Francisco

California Institute of Integral Studies
San Francisco, CA 94103
Type: Acad Health Ctr/Med Sch
Control: Nonprofit (Private or Religious)
• Psychology (PsyD) Prgm

City College of San Francisco
Donald Griffin, PhD, Acting Chancellor
50 Phelan Ave
San Francisco, CA 94112
415 239-3000
Type: Junior or Comm Coll
Control: State, County, or Local Govt
• Dental Assistant Prgm
• Emergency Med Tech-Paramedic Prgm
• Medical Assistant Prgm
• Radiation Therapy Prgm
• Radiography Prgm

Everest College - San Francisco
Barbara Woosley, MA, President
814 Mission St
San Francisco, CA 94103
415 777-2500
Type: Vocational or Tech Sch
Control: For Profit
• Medical Assistant Prgm

Heald College
Nolan Miura, MBA, President/CEO
601 Montgomery
San Francisco, CA 94105
415 808-1400
Type: Vocational or Tech Sch
Control: Nonprofit (Private or Religious)
• Dental Assistant Prgm (3)
• Medical Assistant Prgm (9)

San Francisco State University
Robert A Corrigan, PhD, President
1600 Holloway Ave ADM 562
San Francisco, CA 94132
415 338-1381
Type: 4-year Coll or Univ
Control: State, County, or Local Govt
• Clin Lab Scientist/Med Technologist Prgm
• Counseling Prgm
• Dietetic Internship Prgm
• Dietetics-Didactic Prgm
• Music Therapy Prgm
• Nursing Prgm
• Orientation and Mobility Specialist Prgm
• Rehabilitation Counseling Prgm
• Speech-Language Pathology Prgm

University of California - San Francisco
Hailet Debas, MD, Chancellor
Box 0402
San Francisco, CA 94143
415 476-2401
Type: Acad Health Ctr/Med Sch
Control: State, County, or Local Govt
• Allopathic Medicine Prgm
• Dentistry Prgm
• Dietetic Internship Prgm
• Nursing Prgm
• Pharmacy Prgm
• Physical Therapy Prgm

San Jose

Institute of Medical Education
130 Park Center Plaza
San Jose, CA 95113
• Clin Lab Technician/Med Lab Technician Prgm

Palmer College of Chiropractic West
90 E Tasman Dr
San Jose, CA 95134
Type: Acad Health Ctr/Med Sch
Control: For Profit
• Chiropractic Prgm

San Jose City College
Chui Tsang, President
2100 Moorpark Ave
San Jose, CA 95128
408 298-2181
Type: Junior or Comm Coll
Control: State, County, or Local Govt
• Dental Assistant Prgm

San Jose State University
Don Kassing, MBA, Interm President
Tower Hall 206
One Washington Square
San Jose, CA 95192-0002
408 924-1177
Type: 4-year Coll or Univ
Control: State, County, or Local Govt
• Athletic Training Prgm
• Clin Lab Scientist/Med Technologist Prgm
• Dietetic Internship Prgm
• Dietetics-Didactic Prgm
• Medical Librarian Prgm
• Music Therapy Prgm
• Nursing Prgm
• Occupational Therapy Prgm
• Speech-Language Pathology Prgm

WestMed College
Veronica Shepardson, RN, School Director
1330 S Bascom Ave, Ste G
San Jose, CA 95128
408 977-0723
Type: Vocational or Tech Sch
Control: For Profit
• Emergency Med Tech-Paramedic Prgm

San Juan Capistrano

Quest Diagnostics Nichols Institute
33608 Ortega Highway
San Juan Capistrano, CA 92690
Type: Nonhosp HC Facil, BB, or Lab
Control: For Profit
• Cytogenetic Technology Prgm

San Luis Obispo

California Polytechnic State University
Warren J Baker, President
San Luis Obispo, CA 93407
805 756-1111
Type: 4-year Coll or Univ
Control: State, County, or Local Govt
• Dietetic Internship Prgm
• Dietetics-Didactic Prgm
• Music Therapy Prgm

Cuesta College
San Luis Obispo, CA 93403
Type: Junior or Comm Coll
• Emergency Med Tech-Paramedic Prgm

San Marcos

California State University - San Marcos
San Marcos, CA 92096-0001
Type: 4-year Coll or Univ
Control: State, County, or Local Govt
• Nursing Prgm
• Speech-Language Pathology Prgm

Palomar Community College
Robert Deegan, EdD, Superintendent/President
1140 W Mission Rd
San Marcos, CA 92069
760 744-1150
Type: Junior or Comm Coll
Control: State, County, or Local Govt
• Dental Assistant Prgm
• Emergency Med Tech-Paramedic Prgm

University of St Augustine for Health Science
700 Windy Point Drive
San Marcos, CA 92069
• Physical Therapy Prgm

San Mateo

College of San Mateo
Michael Claire, President
1700 W Hillsdale Blvd
San Mateo, CA 94402
415 574-6161
Type: Junior or Comm Coll
Control: State, County, or Local Govt
• Dental Assistant Prgm

San Pablo

Contra Costa College
D Candy Rose, President
2600 Mission Bell Dr
San Pablo, CA 94806
510 235-7800
Type: Junior or Comm Coll
Control: State, County, or Local Govt
• Dental Assistant Prgm

San Rafael

Dominican University of California
Joseph R Fink, PhD, President
50 Acacia Ave
San Rafael, CA 94901-2298
415 485-3200
Type: 4-year Coll or Univ
Control: State, County, or Local Govt
• Nursing Prgm
• Occupational Therapy Prgm

Santa Ana

Newbridge College
J Ramon Villanueva, School Director
1840 E 17th St, Ste 140
Santa Ana, CA 92705
714 550-8000
Type: Vocational or Tech Sch
Control: For Profit
• Surgical Technology Prgm

Santa Ana College
Erlinda Martinez, EdD, President
1530 W 17th St
Santa Ana, CA 92706-3398
714 564-6975
Type: Junior or Comm Coll
Control: State, County, or Local Govt
• Occupational Therapy Asst Prgm
• Pharmacy Technician Prgm

Santa Barbara

Fielding Graduate University
Santa Barbara, CA 93105
Type: 4-year Coll or Univ
Control: Nonprofit (Private or Religious)
• Psychology (PhD) Prgm

Santa Barbara City College
Andreea Surban, Superintendent/President
721 Cliff Dr
Santa Barbara, CA 93109-2394
805 965-0581
Type: Junior or Comm Coll
Control: State, County, or Local Govt
• Cancer Registrar Prgm
• Diagnostic Med Sonography (General) Prgm
• Radiography Prgm

Santa Barbara Cottage Hospital
Ronald Werft, President/CEO
PO Box 689 Pueblo at Bath Sts
Santa Barbara, CA 93102
805 569-7111
Type: Hosp or Med Ctr: 300-499 Beds
Control: Nonprofit (Private or Religious)
• Clin Lab Scientist/Med Technologist Prgm

Santa Clarita

College of the Canyons
26455 Rockwell Canyon Road
Santa Clarita, CA 91355
Type: Junior or Comm Coll
Control: State, County, or Local Govt
• Clin Lab Technician/Med Lab Technician Prgm

Santa Cruz

Emergency Training Services Inc
David Barbin, BS, CEO
3050 Paul Sweet Rd
Santa Cruz, CA 95065
831 476-8813
Type: Vocational or Tech Sch
Control: For Profit
• Emergency Med Tech-Paramedic Prgm

IEC Corporation
Santa Cruz, CA 95065
Type: Vocational or Tech Sch
• Emergency Med Tech-Paramedic Prgm

Santa Rosa

Santa Rosa Junior College
Robert F Agrella, EdD, Superintendent/President
1501 Mendocino Ave
Santa Rosa, CA 95401
707 527-4431
Type: Junior or Comm Coll
Control: State, County, or Local Govt
• Dental Assistant Prgm
• Dental Hygiene Prgm
• Dietetic Technician-AD Prgm
• Emergency Med Tech-Paramedic Prgm
• Radiography Prgm

Simi Valley

Simi Valley Adult School
Sondra Jones, MA, Director
3192 Los Angeles Ave
Simi Valley, CA 93065
805 579-6200
Type: Vocational or Tech Sch
Control: State, County, or Local Govt
• Respiratory Care Prgm
• Surgical Technology Prgm

Stanford

Stanford University School of Medicine
Phillip Pizzo, MD, Dean
Rm M121
Stanford, CA 94305-5302
415 723-6436
Type: Acad Health Ctr/Med Sch
Control: Nonprofit (Private or Religious)
• Allopathic Medicine Prgm
• Genetic Counseling Prgm
• Physician Assistant Prgm

Stockton

Emergency Medical Sciences Training Institute
Craig Stroup, BS EMT-P, Program Director
343 E Main St #906
Stockton, CA 95202
209 461-5550
Type: Vocational or Tech Sch
Control: Nonprofit (Private or Religious)
• Emergency Med Tech-Paramedic Prgm (2)

San Joaquin General Hospital
Richard Aldred, Hospital Director
PO Box 1020
Stockton, CA 95201
209 468-6600
Type: Hosp or Med Ctr: 100-299 Beds
Control: State, County, or Local Govt
• Radiography Prgm

University of the Pacific
Donald De Rosa, President
3601 Pacific Ave
Stockton, CA 95211
209 946-2222
Type: 4-year Coll or Univ
Control: For Profit
• Athletic Training Prgm
• Dental Hygiene Prgm
• Dentistry Prgm
• Music Therapy Prgm
• Pharmacy Prgm
• Physical Therapy Prgm
• Speech-Language Pathology Prgm

Sylmar

Olive View/UCLA Medical Center
Melinda D Anderson, CEO
14445 Olive View Dr, Rm 2C155
Sylmar, CA 91342-1495
818 364-4224
Type: Hosp or Med Ctr: 100-299 Beds
Control: State, County, or Local Govt
• Dietetic Internship Prgm

Taft

Taft College
Darnell Roe, EdD, President/Superintendent
29 Emmons Park Dr
Box 1437
Taft, CA 93268
661 763-7700
Type: Junior or Comm Coll
Control: State, County, or Local Govt
• Dental Hygiene Prgm

Torrance

El Camino College
Thomas M Fallo, Superintendent/President
16007 Crenshaw Blvd
Torrance, CA 90506
310 532-3670
Type: Junior or Comm Coll
Control: State, County, or Local Govt
• Radiography Prgm
• Respiratory Care Prgm

Harbor UCLA Medical Center
Miguel Ortiz-Marroquin, MBA, Interim CEO
1000 W Carson St Box 1
Torrance, CA 90509-2910
310 222-2101
Type: Hosp or Med Ctr: 500 Beds
Control: State, County, or Local Govt
• Nuclear Medicine Technology Prgm
• Radiography Prgm

Southern California Regional Occupational Ctr
Christine Hoffman, EdD, Superintendent
2300 Crenshaw Blvd
Torrance, CA 90501
310 224-4220
Type: Vocational or Tech Sch
Control: State, County, or Local Govt
• Medical Assistant Prgm

Turlock

California State University - Stanislaus
David P Dauwalder, PhD, Provost/VP
801 W Monte Vista Ave
Turlock, CA 95382
209 667-3203
Type: 4-year Coll or Univ
Control: State, County, or Local Govt
• Genetic Counseling Prgm
• Music Therapy Prgm
• Nursing Prgm

Ukiah

Mendocino Community College
Kathryn Lehner, MBA, President
1000 Hensley Creek Rd
Ukiah, CA 95482
707 467-1047
Type: Junior or Comm Coll
Control: State, County, or Local Govt
• Emergency Med Tech-Paramedic Prgm

Vallejo

Touro University Mare Island
Bernard Laner, President
1310 Johnson Ln
Vallejo, CA 94592
707 638-5442
Type: 4-year Coll or Univ
Control: State, County, or Local Govt
• Osteopathic Medicine Prgm
• Pharmacy Prgm
• Physician Assistant Prgm

Valley Glen

Los Angeles Valley College
Sue Carleo, EdD, President
5800 Fulton Ave
Valley Glen, CA 91401-4096
818 947-2321
Type: Junior or Comm Coll
Control: State, County, or Local Govt
• Respiratory Care Prgm

Ventura

Ventura College
Larry Claderon, EdD, President
School of Prehospital & Emergency Med
4667 Telegraph Rd
Ventura, CA 93003
805 654-6460
Type: Junior or Comm Coll
Control: State, County, or Local Govt
• Emergency Med Tech-Paramedic Prgm

Victorville

Victor Valley Community College District
Patricia Spencer, PhD, President/Superintendent
18422 Bear Valley Rd
Victorville, CA 92392-5849
760 245-4271
Type: Junior or Comm Coll
Control: State, County, or Local Govt
• Emergency Med Tech-Paramedic Prgm
• Respiratory Care Prgm

Visalia

San Joaquin Valley College
Mark Perry, President
3828 W Caldwell Ave
Visalia, CA 93277
559 734-9000
Type: Junior or Comm Coll
Control: For Profit
• Dental Hygiene Prgm (2)
• Physician Assistant Prgm
• Respiratory Care Prgm (3)
• Surgical Technology Prgm (2)

Walnut

Mt San Antonio College
John Nixon, President/CEO
1100 N Grand Ave
Walnut, CA 91789
909 594-5611
Type: Junior or Comm Coll
Control: State, County, or Local Govt
• Emergency Med Tech-Paramedic Prgm
• Histotechnician Prgm
• Radiography Prgm
• Respiratory Care Prgm
• Veterinary Technology Prgm

West Covina

East San Gabriel Valley ROP
Laurel Adler, EdD, Superintendent
1501 W Del Norte Ave
West Covina, CA 91790
626 472-5121
Type: Vocational or Tech Sch
Control: State, County, or Local Govt
• Medical Assistant Prgm

North-West College
Marsha Fuerst, President/CEO
2121 W Garvey Ave N
West Covina, CA 91790
626 960-5046
Type: Vocational or Tech Sch
Control: For Profit
• Pharmacy Technician Prgm (4)
• Surgical Technology Prgm

Whittier

Southern California Univ of Health Sciences
16200 E Amber Valley Dr
Whittier, CA 90604
Type: Acad Health Ctr/Med Sch
Control: For Profit
• Chiropractic Prgm

Woodland Hills

Los Angeles Pierce College
Robert Garber, President
6201 Winnetka Ave
Woodland Hills, CA 91371
818 719-6408
Type: 4-year Coll or Univ
Control: State, County, or Local Govt
• Veterinary Technology Prgm

Yucaipa

Crafton Hills College
Gloria Macias Harrison, MA, President
11711 Sand Canyon Rd
Yucaipa, CA 92399
909 389-3200
Type: Junior or Comm Coll
Control: State, County, or Local Govt
• Emergency Med Tech-Paramedic Prgm
• Respiratory Care Prgm

Colorado

Alamosa

Adams State College
Richard Wueste, JD, President
208 Edgemont Blvd
Richardson Hall 210
Alamosa, CO 81102-0001
719 587-7341
Type: 4-year Coll or Univ
Control: State, County, or Local Govt
• Counseling Prgm
• Music Therapy Prgm
• Nursing Prgm

Aurora

American Sentinel University
Aurora, CO 80014
• Nursing Prgm
• Psychology (PhD) Prgm
• Psychology (PsyD) Prgm

Concorde Career College - Aurora
Al Short, MA, Campus President
111 N Havana St
Aurora, CO 80010
303 861-1151
Type: Vocational or Tech Sch
Control: For Profit
• Dental Hygiene Prgm
• Radiography Prgm
• Surgical Technology Prgm

Everest College
Patricia Schlotter, MBA, President
14280 E Jewell Ave
Ste 100
Aurora, CO 80012
303 745-6244
Type: Junior or Comm Coll
Control: For Profit
• Medical Assistant Prgm (3)
• Surgical Technology Prgm

Rocky Vista Univ Coll of Osteopathic Medicine
3449 Chambers Rd, Ste B
Aurora, CO 80011
Type: Acad Health Ctr/Med Sch
Control: Nonprofit (Private or Religious)
• Osteopathic Medicine Prgm

T H Pickens Technical Center
Art Bogardus, PhD, Executive Director
Career and Technical Education
500 Airport Blvd
Aurora, CO 80011
303 344-4910
Type: Vocational or Tech Sch
Control: State, County, or Local Govt
• Dental Assistant Prgm
• Respiratory Care Prgm

University of Colorado Denver - Anschutz MC
Bruce Schroffel, MS, President
131001 E 17th Pl, Ste C-1015
F-417 PO Box 6508
Aurora, CO 80045-0508
303 724-5773
Type: Acad Health Ctr/Med Sch
Control: State, County, or Local Govt
• Allopathic Medicine Prgm
• Counseling Prgm
• Dentistry Prgm
• Diagnostic Med Sonography (General) Prgm
• Genetic Counseling Prgm
• Nursing Prgm
• Physical Therapy Prgm
• Physician Assistant Prgm

Boulder

Naropa University
Thomas Coburn, PhD, President
2130 Arapahoe Ave
Boulder, CO 80302
303 444-0202
Type: 4-year Coll or Univ
Control: Nonprofit (Private or Religious)
• Art Therapy Prgm
• Dance/Movement Therapy Prgm

University of Colorado at Boulder
Campus Box 409
Boulder, CO 80309-0409
303 492-6445
Type: 4-year Coll or Univ
Control: State, County, or Local Govt
• Audiologist Prgm
• Music Therapy Prgm
• Psychology (PhD) Prgm
• Speech-Language Pathology Prgm

Colorado Springs

IntelliTec Medical Institute
Tim Durkin
2345 N Academy Blvd
Colorado Springs, CO 90809
719 596-7400
Type: Vocational or Tech Sch
Control: For Profit
• Dental Assistant Prgm

Memorial Hospital
Lawrence McEvoy, MD, CEO
1400 East Boulder
175 S Union Ste 240
Colorado Springs, CO 80909
719 365-5000
Type: Hosp or Med Ctr: 300-499 Beds
Control: State, County, or Local Govt
• Radiography Prgm

National American University-Colorado Springs
Colorado Springs, CO 80920-5377
Type: 4-year Coll or Univ
• Medical Assistant Prgm

Penrose Hospital
Margaret Sabin, Interim CEO
Centura Health
2222 N Nevada Ave, PO Box 7021
Colorado Springs, CO 80907-7021
719 776-5000
Type: Hosp or Med Ctr: 300-499 Beds
Control: Nonprofit (Private or Religious)
• Clin Lab Scientist/Med Technologist Prgm
• Dietetic Internship Prgm

Pikes Peak Community College
Edwin Ray, PhD, VP of Educational Service
5765 S Academy Blvd
Colorado Springs, CO 80906
719 502-3100
Type: Junior or Comm Coll
Control: State, County, or Local Govt
• Dental Assistant Prgm
• Emergency Med Tech-Paramedic Prgm
• Pharmacy Technician Prgm

University of Colorado at Colorado Springs
Pam Shockley Zalabat, PhD, Chancellor
1420 Austin Bluffs Pkwy
Colorado Springs, CO 80933-7150
719 262-3000
Type: 4-year Coll or Univ
Control: State, County, or Local Govt
• Counseling Prgm
• Dietetics-Didactic Prgm
• Nursing Prgm

Denver

Bel-Rea Institute of Animal Technology
Nolan Rucker, BS MS DVM, Dean of Education
1681 S Dayton St
Denver, CO 80231
Type: Vocational or Tech Sch
Control: Nonprofit (Private or Religious)
• Veterinary Technology Prgm

Centura Health-St Anthony Hospitals
Peter Makowski, CEO, St Anthony Hospitals
4231 W 16th Ave
Denver, CO 80204
303 629-4350
Type: Hosp or Med Ctr: 500 Beds
Control: Nonprofit (Private or Religious)
• Emergency Med Tech-Paramedic Prgm
• Radiography Prgm

Community College of Aurora
Les Moroye, MA, Assoc VP
9235 E 10th Dr, Rm 118
Denver, CO 80230
303 340-7119
Type: Junior or Comm Coll
Control: State, County, or Local Govt
• Emergency Med Tech-Paramedic Prgm

Community College of Denver
Karen Bleeker, PhD, President
PO Box 173363
Denver, CO 80217
303 556-2600
Type: Junior or Comm Coll
Control: State, County, or Local Govt
• Dental Hygiene Prgm
• Medical Assistant Prgm
• Radiography Prgm
• Veterinary Technology Prgm

Denver Health Medical Center
Patricia Gabow, MD, CEO
660 Bannock St Mail Code 0278
Denver, CO 80204
303 436-6611
Type: Hosp or Med Ctr: 300-499 Beds
Control: State, County, or Local Govt
• Emergency Med Tech-Paramedic Prgm

Johnson & Wales University
7150 Montview Blvd
Denver, CO 80220
Type: 4-year Coll or Univ
Control: Nonprofit (Private or Religious)
• Dietetics-Didactic Prgm

Massage Therapy Institute of Colorado
Mark Manton, Director
1441 York St, Ste 301
Denver, CO 80206
303 329-6345
Type: Acad Health Ctr/Med Sch
Control: For Profit
• Massage Therapy Prgm

Metropolitan State College of Denver
Raymond Kieft, EdD, Interim President
Campus Box 1
PO Box 173362
Denver, CO 80217-3362
303 556-3022
Type: 4-year Coll or Univ
Control: State, County, or Local Govt
• Athletic Training Prgm
• Clin Lab Scientist/Med Technologist Prgm
• Dietetics-Didactic Prgm
• Exercise Science Prgm
• Music Therapy Prgm

National American University - Denver
Denver, CO 80222
Type: 4-year Coll or Univ
• Medical Assistant Prgm

Pima Medical Institute - Denver
Richard L Luebke, Sr, President
7475 Dakin Street, Suite 100
Denver, CO 80221
303 426-1800
Type: Vocational or Tech Sch
Control: For Profit
• Occupational Therapy Asst Prgm
• Ophthalmic Technician Prgm
• Physical Therapist Assistant Prgm
• Radiography Prgm
• Respiratory Care Prgm

Regis University
Michael J Sheeran, SJ, President
3333 Regis Blvd
Denver, CO 80221-1099
303 458-4190
Type: 4-year Coll or Univ
Control: Nonprofit (Private or Religious)
• Counseling Prgm
• Nursing Prgm
• Pharmacy Prgm
• Physical Therapy Prgm

University of Colorado at Denver
Mark Heckler, Provost
Campus Box 168
PO Box 173364
Denver, CO 80217-3364
303 556-2400
Type: 4-year Coll or Univ
Control: State, County, or Local Govt
• Counseling Prgm
• Dental Hygiene Prgm
• Pharmacy Prgm
• Psychology (PhD) Prgm
• Psychology (PsyD) Prgm

Westwood College
Natalie Williams, Campus President
7350 N Broadway
Denver, CO 80221-3653
800 992-5050
Type: Vocational or Tech Sch
Control: For Profit
• Medical Assistant Prgm

Durango

Fort Lewis College
Brad Bartel, PhD, President
1000 Rim Dr
Durango, CO 81301-3999
970 247-7100
Type: 4-year Coll or Univ
Control: State, County, or Local Govt
• Athletic Training Prgm
• Music Therapy Prgm

Eaton

Academy of Natural Therapy
123 Elm Ave
PO Box 237
Eaton, CO 80615
Type: Vocational or Tech Sch
Control: For Profit
• Massage Therapy Prgm

Englewood

HealthONE EMS
Mary White, President
501 E Hampden
Englewood, CO 80110
303 788-6484
Type: Hosp or Med Ctr: 300-499 Beds
Control: For Profit
• Emergency Med Tech-Paramedic Prgm

Tri-County Health Department
7000 E Bellview Ave, Ste 301
Englewood, CO 80111-1628
303 220-9200
Type: Nonhosp HC Facil, BB, or Lab
Control: State, County, or Local Govt
• Dietetic Internship Prgm

Fort Collins

Colorado State University
Larry Penley, PhD, President
102 Administration Bldg
Fort Collins, CO 80523
970 491-6211
Type: 4-year Coll or Univ
Control: State, County, or Local Govt
• Counseling Prgm
• Dietetics-Coordinated Prgm
• Dietetics-Didactic Prgm
• Music Therapy Prgm
• Occupational Therapy Prgm
• Veterinary Medicine Prgm

Fort Morgan

Morgan Community College
John R McKay, PhD, President
17800 Rd 20
Fort Morgan, CO 80701-4399
970 867-3081
Type: Junior or Comm Coll
Control: State, County, or Local Govt
• Physical Therapist Assistant Prgm

Glenwood Springs

Colorado Mountain College
Bob Spuhler, PhD, President
831 Grand Ave
Glenwood Springs, CO 81601
970 945-8366
Type: Junior or Comm Coll
Control: State, County, or Local Govt
• Emergency Med Tech-Paramedic Prgm
• Veterinary Technology Prgm

Grand Junction

Colorado Mesa University
Timothy Foster, JD, President
1100 North Ave
Grand Junction, CO 81501
970 248-1498
Type: 4-year Coll or Univ
Control: State, County, or Local Govt
• Athletic Training Prgm
• Emergency Med Tech-Paramedic Prgm
• Music Therapy Prgm
• Nursing Prgm
• Radiography Prgm

Mesa State College
Grand Junction, CO 81501
Type: 4-year Coll or Univ
• Emergency Med Tech-Paramedic Prgm

Greeley

Aims Community College
Marilynn Liddell, PhD, President
PO Box 69
Greeley, CO 80632
303 330-8008
Type: Junior or Comm Coll
Control: State, County, or Local Govt
• Emergency Med Tech-Paramedic Prgm
• Surgical Technology Prgm

University of Northern Colorado
Kay Norton, JD, President
Carter Hall 4000
Greeley, CO 80639
970 351-2121
Type: 4-year Coll or Univ
Control: State, County, or Local Govt
• Athletic Training Prgm
• Audiologist Prgm
• Counseling Prgm
• Dietetic Internship Prgm
• Dietetics-Didactic Prgm
• Nursing Prgm
• Orientation and Mobility Specialist Prgm
• Rehabilitation Counseling Prgm
• Speech-Language Pathology Prgm

INSTITUTIONS

Lakewood

Colorado Christian University
Lakewood, CO 80226
Type: 4-year Coll or Univ
Control: Nonprofit (Private or Religious)
• Music Therapy Prgm
• Nursing Prgm

Red Rocks Community College
Michele Haney, PhD, President
13300 W Sixth Ave
Lakewood, CO 80228-1255
303 914-6215
Type: Junior or Comm Coll
Control: State, County, or Local Govt
• Medical Assistant Prgm
• Physician Assistant Prgm
• Radiography Prgm

Littleton

Arapahoe Community College
Berton Glandon, PhD, President
5900 S Santa Fe Dr
PO Box 9002
Littleton, CO 80160-9002
303 797-5701
Type: Junior or Comm Coll
Control: State, County, or Local Govt
• Clin Lab Technician/Med Lab Technician Prgm
• Medical Assistant Prgm
• Pharmacy Technician Prgm
• Physical Therapist Assistant Prgm

Denver Seminary
Craig Williford, PhD
6399 S Santa Fe Dr
Littleton, CO 80120
303 761-2482
Type: 4-year Coll or Univ
Control: Nonprofit (Private or Religious)
• Counseling Prgm

Pueblo

Colorado State University - Pueblo
Joe Garcia, JD, President
Adm 301 - 2200 Bonforte Blvd
Pueblo, CO 81001
719 549-2306
Type: 4-year Coll or Univ
Control: State, County, or Local Govt
• Athletic Training Prgm
• Music Therapy Prgm

Colorado Technical University
Pueblo, CO 81003
Type: 4-year Coll or Univ
• Surgical Technology Prgm

Parkview Medical Center
Mike Baxter, President/CEO
400 W 16th St
Pueblo, CO 81003
719 584-4266
Type: Hosp or Med Ctr: 100-299 Beds
Control: Nonprofit (Private or Religious)
• Clin Lab Scientist/Med Technologist Prgm

Pueblo Community College
Patty Erjavec, MNM, President
900 W Orman Ave
Pueblo, CO 81004-1499
719 549-3213
Type: Junior or Comm Coll
Control: State, County, or Local Govt
• Dental Assistant Prgm
• Dental Hygiene Prgm
• Emergency Med Tech-Paramedic Prgm
• Occupational Therapy Asst Prgm
• Physical Therapist Assistant Prgm
• Polysomnographic Technology Prgm
• Respiratory Care Prgm

Rangley

Colorado Northwestern Community College
John Boyd, President
500 Kennedy Dr
Rangley, CO 81648
970 675-2261
Type: Junior or Comm Coll
Control: State, County, or Local Govt
• Dental Hygiene Prgm

Westminster

Colorado Technical Univ - Denver North
Westminster, CO 80234
Type: 4-year Coll or Univ
• Surgical Technology Prgm

Front Range Comm College
Mike Kupcho, MBA, Interim President
3645 W 112th Ave
Westminster, CO 80030
303 404-5422
Type: Junior or Comm Coll
Control: Nonprofit (Private or Religious)
• Dental Assistant Prgm
• Medical Assistant Prgm
• Pharmacy Technician Prgm
• Phlebotomy Prgm
• Veterinary Technology Prgm

Connecticut

Branford

Branford Hall Career Institute
Gary Camp, CEO
One Summit Pl
Branford, CT 06405
203 488-2525
Type: Vocational or Tech Sch
Control: For Profit
• Medical Assistant Prgm

Bridgeport

Bridgeport Hospital
Robert Trefry, President
267 Grant St
Bridgeport, CT 06610
203 384-3464
Type: Hosp or Med Ctr: 500 Beds
Control: Nonprofit (Private or Religious)
• Surgical Technology Prgm

Housatonic Community College
Anita Gliniecki, MSN, President
900 Lafayette Blvd
Bridgeport, CT 06604-4704
203 332-5224
Type: Junior or Comm Coll
Control: State, County, or Local Govt
• Occupational Therapy Asst Prgm

St Vincent's College
Martha K Shouldis, EdD, President
2800 Main St
Bridgeport, CT 06606
203 576-5578
Type: Junior or Comm Coll
Control: Nonprofit (Private or Religious)
• Medical Assistant Prgm
• Radiography Prgm

University of Bridgeport
Neil Albert Salonen, President
30 Hazel St
Bridgeport, CT 06601
203 576-4000
Type: 4-year Coll or Univ
Control: Nonprofit (Private or Religious)
• Chiropractic Prgm
• Clin Lab Scientist/Med Technologist Prgm
• Dental Hygiene Prgm

Danbury

Danbury Hospital
Frank Kelly, MBA, President/CEO
24 Hospital Ave
Danbury, CT 06810
203 739-7066
Type: Hosp or Med Ctr: 300-499 Beds
Control: Nonprofit (Private or Religious)
• Clin Lab Scientist/Med Technologist Prgm
• Dietetic Internship Prgm
• Radiography Prgm
• Surgical Technology Prgm

Western Connecticut State University
181 White St
Danbury, CT 06810-6885
203 837-8200
Type: 4-year Coll or Univ
Control: State, County, or Local Govt
• Counseling Prgm
• Music Therapy Prgm
• Nursing Prgm

Danielson

Quinebaug Valley Community College
Dianne E Williams, BS MS, President
742 Upper Maple St
Danielson, CT 06239
860 774-1160
Type: Junior or Comm Coll
Control: State, County, or Local Govt
• Medical Assistant Prgm

East Hartford

Goodwin College
Mark E Scheinberg, BA, President
One Riverside Drive, East Hartford, CT.
1 Riverside Drive
East Hartford, CT 06029
860 528-4111
Type: 4-year Coll or Univ
Control: Nonprofit (Private or Religious)
• Histotechnician Prgm
• Medical Assistant Prgm
• Occupational Therapy Asst Prgm

Fairfield

Fairfield University
1073 N Benson Rd
Fairfield, CT 06430-5195
203 254-4000
Type: 4-year Coll or Univ
Control: State, County, or Local Govt
• Counseling Prgm
• Nursing Prgm

Sacred Heart University
John Petillo, PhD, President
5151 Park Ave
Fairfield, CT 06825
203 371-7999
Type: 4-year Coll or Univ
Control: Nonprofit (Private or Religious)
• Athletic Training Prgm
• Nursing Prgm
• Occupational Therapy Prgm
• Physical Therapy Prgm

Farmington

Tunxis Community College
Cathryn L Addy, PhD, President
271 Scott Swamp Rd
Farmington, CT 06032-3187
860 255-3500
Type: Junior or Comm Coll
Control: State, County, or Local Govt
• Dental Assistant Prgm
• Dental Hygiene Prgm

Hamden

Eli Whitney Technical High School
E Paulett Moore, Director
71 Jones Rd
Hamden, CT 06514
203 397-4031
Type: Vocational or Tech Sch
Control: State, County, or Local Govt
• Surgical Technology Prgm

Quinnipiac University
John L Lahey, PhD, President
275 Mt Carmel Ave
Hamden, CT 06518-1908
203 582-8200
Type: 4-year Coll or Univ
Control: Nonprofit (Private or Religious)
• Athletic Training Prgm
• Occupational Therapy Prgm
• Pathologists' Assistant Prgm
• Perfusion Prgm
• Physical Therapy Prgm
• Physician Assistant Prgm
• Radiography Prgm
• Radiologist Assistant Prgm
• Respiratory Care Prgm

Stone Academy
William Mangini, School Director
1315 Dixwell Ave
Hamden, CT 06514
203 288-7474
Type: Vocational or Tech Sch
Control: For Profit
• Medical Assistant Prgm

Hartford

A I Prince Technical High School
William Chaffin, PhD, Principal
401 Flatbush Ave
Hartford, CT 06106
860 951-7112
Type: Vocational or Tech Sch
Control: State, County, or Local Govt
• Dental Assistant Prgm
• Surgical Technology Prgm

Capital Community College
Calvin Woodland, EdD PsyD, President
950 Main St
Hartford, CT 06103
860 906-5000
Type: Junior or Comm Coll
Control: State, County, or Local Govt
• Emergency Med Tech-Paramedic Prgm
• Medical Assistant Prgm
• Radiography Prgm

Hartford Hospital
Joseph Elliot, MHA, President/CEO
80 Seymour St
PO Box 5037
Hartford, CT 06106
860 545-5000
Type: Hosp or Med Ctr: 500 Beds
Control: Nonprofit (Private or Religious)
• Clin Lab Scientist/Med Technologist Prgm
• Radiation Therapy Prgm
• Radiography Prgm

St Francis Hospital & Medical Center
David D'Eramo, PhD, President
114 Woodland St
Hartford, CT 06105
860 714-4900
Type: Hosp or Med Ctr: 500 Beds
Control: Nonprofit (Private or Religious)
• Diagnostic Med Sonography (Cardiac) Prgm

St. Joseph College School of Pharmacy
Hartford, CT 06103-1501
Type: Junior or Comm Coll
Control: Nonprofit (Private or Religious)
• Pharmacy Prgm

Manchester

Manchester Community College
Gena Glickman, PhD, President
Great Path Mail Station 1
PO Box 1046
Manchester, CT 06045-1046
860 512-3100
Type: Junior or Comm Coll
Control: State, County, or Local Govt
• Occupational Therapy Asst Prgm
• Respiratory Care Prgm
• Surgical Technology Prgm

Middletown

Middlesex Community College
Wilfredo Nieves, EdD, President
100 Training Hill Rd
Middletown, CT 06457
860 343-5701
Type: Junior or Comm Coll
Control: State, County, or Local Govt
• Ophthalmic Dispensing Optician Prgm
• Radiography Prgm

New Britain

Central Connecticut State University
Jack Miller, EdD, President
1615 Stanley St
New Britain, CT 06050-4010
860 832-3003
Type: 4-year Coll or Univ
Control: State, County, or Local Govt
• Athletic Training Prgm
• Music Therapy Prgm
• Nursing Prgm
• Rehabilitation Counseling Prgm

Lincoln Tech Institute
Craig Avery, BS, Regional Exec Director
200 John Downey Dr
New Britain, CT 06051
860 225-8641
Type: Vocational or Tech Sch
Control: For Profit
• Dental Assistant Prgm
• Medical Assistant Prgm

New Haven

Albertus Magnus College
Julia M McNamara, PhD
700 Prospect St
New Haven, CT 06511
203 773-8529
Type: 4-year Coll or Univ
Control: Nonprofit (Private or Religious)
• Art Therapy Prgm

Gateway Community College
Dorsey Kendrick, PhD, President
60 Sargent Dr
New Haven, CT 06511
203 285-2060
Type: Junior or Comm Coll
Control: State, County, or Local Govt
• Dietetic Technician-AD Prgm
• Nuclear Medicine Technology Prgm
• Radiation Therapy Prgm
• Radiography Prgm

New Haven Sponsor Hospital
New Haven, CT 06511
Type: Consortium
• Emergency Med Tech-Paramedic Prgm

Southern Connecticut State University
Cheryl Norton, PhD, President
501 Crescent St
New Haven, CT 06515
203 397-4234
Type: 4-year Coll or Univ
Control: State, County, or Local Govt
• Athletic Training Prgm
• Counseling Prgm
• Exercise Science Prgm
• Medical Librarian Prgm
• Nursing Prgm
• Speech-Language Pathology Prgm

Yale University School of Medicine
Robert Alpern, MD, Dean
333 Cedar St
New Haven, CT 06510
203 785-4672
Type: Acad Health Ctr/Med Sch
Control: Nonprofit (Private or Religious)
• Allopathic Medicine Prgm
• Music Therapy Prgm
• Physician Assistant Prgm
• Psychology (PhD) Prgm

Yale-New Haven Hospital
20 York St GBB
New Haven, CT 06504
203 785-5074
Type: Hosp or Med Ctr: 500 Beds
Control: Nonprofit (Private or Religious)
• Diagnostic Med Sonography (General/Cardiac) Prgm
• Dietetic Internship Prgm

New London

Ridley-Lowell Business & Technical Institute
Wilfred T Weymouth, MS, President
470 Bank St
New London, CT 06320
860 443-7441
Type: Vocational or Tech Sch
Control: For Profit
• Medical Assistant Prgm

Newington

Connecticut Center for Massage Therapy
Stephen Kitts, Executive Director
75 Kitts Lane
Newington, CT 06111
860 667-1886
Type: Vocational or Tech Sch
Control: For Profit
• Massage Therapy Prgm (3)

Norwalk

Norwalk Community College
David Levinson, PhD, President
188 Richards Ave
Norwalk, CT 06854-1655
203 857-7003
Type: Junior or Comm Coll
Control: State, County, or Local Govt
• Medical Assistant Prgm
• Physical Therapist Assistant Prgm

Norwalk Hospital/Norwalk Community College
David W Osborne, MS, CEO
Maple St
Norwalk, CT 06856
203 852-2211
Type: Hosp or Med Ctr: 100-299 Beds
Control: Nonprofit (Private or Religious)
• Respiratory Care Prgm

Southington

Lincoln College of New England
Michael Diffily, PhD, Vice President for Academic Affairs
2279 Mt Vernon Rd
Southington, CT 06489
860 628-4751
Type: Vocational or Tech Sch
Control: For Profit
• Dental Assistant Prgm
• Dental Hygiene Prgm
• Dietetic Technician-AD Prgm
• Medical Assistant Prgm
• Nuclear Medicine Technology Prgm
• Occupational Therapy Asst Prgm

Stamford

Stamford Hospital
Brian G Grissler, MA, President/CEO
Shelburne Rd PO Box 9317
Stamford, CT 06904-9317
203 276-7000
Type: Hosp or Med Ctr: 300-499 Beds
Control: Nonprofit (Private or Religious)
• Radiography Prgm

Storrs

University of Connecticut
Michael Hogan, President
Gulley Hall
Unit 2048
Storrs, CT 06269
860 486-2337
Type: 4-year Coll or Univ
Control: State, County, or Local Govt
• Allopathic Medicine Prgm
• Athletic Training Prgm
• Audiologist Prgm
• Counseling Prgm
• Cytogenetic Technology Prgm
• Dentistry Prgm
• Diagnostic Molecular Scientist Prgm
• Dietetic Internship Prgm
• Dietetics-Coordinated Prgm
• Dietetics-Didactic Prgm
• Music Therapy Prgm
• Nursing Prgm
• Pharmacy Prgm
• Physical Therapy Prgm
• Psychology (PhD) Prgm
• Speech-Language Pathology Prgm

Waterbury

Naugatuck Valley Community College
Daisy De Filippis, PhD, President
750 Chase Pkwy
Waterbury, CT 06708
203 575-8044
Type: Junior or Comm Coll
Control: State, County, or Local Govt
• Physical Therapist Assistant Prgm
• Radiography Prgm
• Respiratory Care Prgm

West Hartford

American Institute
West Hartford, CT 06110
Type: Vocational or Tech Sch
• Medical Assistant Prgm
• Occupational Therapy Asst Prgm

Saint Joseph College
Winifred E Coleman, President
1678 Asylum Ave
West Hartford, CT 06117
203 232-4571
Type: 4-year Coll or Univ
Control: Nonprofit (Private or Religious)
• Dietetic Internship Prgm
• Dietetics-Didactic Prgm
• Nursing Prgm

The Hartt School
University of Hartford
West Hartford, CT 06117
• Music Therapy Prgm

University of Hartford
Walter Harrison, PhD, President
200 Bloomfield Ave
West Hartford, CT 06117-1599
860 768-4417
Type: 4-year Coll or Univ
Control: Nonprofit (Private or Religious)
• Clin Lab Scientist/Med Technologist Prgm
• Nursing Prgm
• Orthotist/Prosthetist Prgm
• Physical Therapy Prgm
• Psychology (PsyD) Prgm
• Radiography Prgm
• Respiratory Care Prgm

West Haven

University of New Haven
Lawrence J Denardis, President
300 Orange Ave
West Haven, CT 06516
203 932-7000
Type: 4-year Coll or Univ
Control: Nonprofit (Private or Religious)
• Dental Hygiene Prgm
• Dietetics-Didactic Prgm

Willimantic

Windham Community Memorial Hospital
Richard Brvenik, MA FACHE, President/CEO
112 Mansfield Ave
Willimantic, CT 06226
860 456-6800
Type: Hosp or Med Ctr: 100-299 Beds
Control: Nonprofit (Private or Religious)
• Radiography Prgm

Windham Regional Vocational Tech School
210 Birch St
Willimantic, CT 06226
203 456-3789
Type: Vocational or Tech Sch
Control: State, County, or Local Govt
• Dental Assistant Prgm

Winsted

Northwestern Connecticut Comm College
Barbara Douglass, PhD, President
Park Place E
Winsted, CT 06098
860 738-6410
Type: Junior or Comm Coll
Control: State, County, or Local Govt
• Medical Assistant Prgm
• Veterinary Technology Prgm

Delaware

Dagsboro

National Massage Therapy Institute
Dagsboro, DE 19939
Type: Acad Health Ctr/Med Sch
Control: For Profit
• Massage Therapy Prgm

Dover

Delaware State University
William B Delauder, President
Dover, DE 19901
302 739-4924
Type: 4-year Coll or Univ
Control: State, County, or Local Govt
• Dietetics-Didactic Prgm
• Nursing Prgm

Delaware Technical Community College
Orlando J George, Jr, EdD, President
PO Box 897
Dover, DE 19903
302 739-4053
Type: Junior or Comm Coll
Control: State, County, or Local Govt
• Clin Lab Technician/Med Lab Technician Prgm
• Dental Hygiene Prgm
• Diagnostic Med Sonography
  (Gen/Card/Vascular) Prgm
• Emergency Med Tech-Paramedic Prgm
• Histotechnician Prgm
• Medical Assistant Prgm
• Nuclear Medicine Technology Prgm
• Occupational Therapy Asst Prgm (2)
• Physical Therapist Assistant Prgm (2)
• Radiography Prgm (2)
• Respiratory Care Prgm (2)
• Veterinary Technology Prgm

New Castle

Wilmington College
320 Dupont Hwy
New Castle, DE 19720-6491
302 328-9401
Type: 4-year Coll or Univ
Control: State, County, or Local Govt
• Counseling Prgm
• Nursing Prgm

Newark

University of Delaware-Christiana Care Health
Patrick T Harker, PhD, President
104A Hullihen Hall
Office of the President
Newark, DE 19716
302 831-2111
Type: 4-year Coll or Univ
Control: Nonprofit (Private or Religious)
• Athletic Training Prgm
• Clin Lab Scientist/Med Technologist Prgm
• Dietetic Internship Prgm
• Dietetics-Didactic Prgm
• Music Therapy Prgm
• Nursing Prgm
• Physical Therapy Prgm
• Psychology (PhD) Prgm

District of Columbia

Washington

American University
Washington, DC 20016
Type: 4-year Coll or Univ
Control: State, County, or Local Govt
• Psychology (PhD) Prgm

Catholic University of America
Br Patrick F Ellis, FSC, President
103 Executive Bldg
Washington, DC 20064
202 319-5100
Type: 4-year Coll or Univ
Control: Nonprofit (Private or Religious)
• Medical Librarian Prgm
• Nursing Prgm
• Psychology (PhD) Prgm

Gallaudet University
I King Jordan, PhD, President
800 Florida Ave NE
Washington, DC 20002
202 651-5329
Type: 4-year Coll or Univ
Control: Nonprofit (Private or Religious)
• Audiologist Prgm
• Counseling Prgm
• Psychology (PhD) Prgm
• Speech-Language Pathology Prgm

George Washington University
Steven Knapp, Provost & VP Hlth Affairs
Office of the President
2121 I Street, NW, Ste 801
Washington, DC 20052
202 994-6500
Type: 4-year Coll or Univ
Control: Nonprofit (Private or Religious)
• Allopathic Medicine Prgm
• Art Therapy Prgm
• Athletic Training Prgm
• Clin Lab Scientist/Med Technologist Prgm
• Counseling Prgm
• Diagnostic Med Sonography
  (Gen/Card/Vascular) Prgm
• Music Therapy Prgm
• Nursing Prgm
• Physical Therapy Prgm
• Physician Assistant Prgm
• Psychology (PhD) Prgm
• Psychology (PsyD) Prgm
• Rehabilitation Counseling Prgm
• Speech-Language Pathology Prgm

Georgetown University Medical Center
Sam Wiesel, MD, Exec VP Hlth Sciences
120 Bldg D, 4000 Reservoir Dr NW
Washington, DC 20007
202 687-4601
Type: Acad Health Ctr/Med Sch
Control: Nonprofit (Private or Religious)
• Allopathic Medicine Prgm
• Nursing Prgm
• Ophthalmic Assistant Prgm
• Ophthalmic Med Technologist Prgm
• Ophthalmic Technician Prgm

Howard University
Sidney A Ribeau, President
Mordecai Wyatt Johnson Admin Bldg
2400 Sixth St NW
Washington, DC 20059
202 806-6100
Type: 4-year Coll or Univ
Control: Nonprofit (Private or Religious)
• Allopathic Medicine Prgm
• Clin Lab Scientist/Med Technologist Prgm
• Dental Hygiene Prgm
• Dentistry Prgm
• Dietetics-Coordinated Prgm
• Genetic Counseling Prgm
• Music Therapy Prgm
• Nursing Prgm
• Occupational Therapy Prgm
• Pharmacy Prgm
• Physical Therapy Prgm
• Physician Assistant Prgm
• Psychology (PhD) Prgm
• Radiation Therapy Prgm
• Speech-Language Pathology Prgm

Potomac Massage Training Institute
Demara Stamler, Executive Director
5028 Wisconsin Ave NW, LL
Washington, DC 20016-4118
202 686-7046
Type: Vocational or Tech Sch
Control: Nonprofit (Private or Religious)
• Massage Therapy Prgm

Trinity University
125 Michigan Ave NE
Washington, DC 20017
Type: 4-year Coll or Univ
Control: Nonprofit (Private or Religious)
• Nursing Prgm

University of the District of Columbia
Allen L Sessoms, PhD, President
4200 Connecticut Ave NW
Washington, DC 20008
202 274-5100
Type: 4-year Coll or Univ
Control: State, County, or Local Govt
• Dietetics-Didactic Prgm
• Respiratory Care Prgm
• Speech-Language Pathology Prgm

Washington Hospital Center
James Caldas, MHSA, President, CEO
110 Irving St NW
Washington, DC 20010
202 877-6101
Type: Hosp or Med Ctr: 500 Beds
Control: Nonprofit (Private or Religious)
• Clin Lab Scientist/Med Technologist Prgm
• Radiography Prgm

Fiji

Suva Fiji

Pacific Eye Institute
Suva Fiji, FI
• Ophthalmic Technician Prgm

Florida

Avon Park

South Florida Community College
Norman L Stephens, Jr, EdD, President
600 W College Dr
Avon Park, FL 33825-9399
863 453-6661
Type: Junior or Comm Coll
Control: State, County, or Local Govt
• Dental Assistant Prgm
• Dental Hygiene Prgm
• Radiography Prgm

Bay Pines

Bay Pines VA Medical Center
Bay Pines, FL 33744
Type: Hosp or Med Ctr: 300-499 Beds
Control: Nonprofit (Private or Religious)
• Dietetic Internship Prgm

Boca Raton

Florida Atlantic University
Frank T Brogan, MEd, President
777 Glades Rd
Boca Raton, FL 33431
561 297-3450
Type: 4-year Coll or Univ
Control: State, County, or Local Govt
• Counseling Prgm
• Music Therapy Prgm
• Nursing Prgm
• Rehabilitation Counseling Prgm
• Speech-Language Pathology Prgm

West Boca Medical Center
Richard Gold, CEO
21644 State Rd 7
Boca Raton, FL 33428
561 488-8000
Type: Hosp or Med Ctr: 100-299 Beds
Control: For Profit
• Radiography Prgm

Boynton Beach

Bethesda Memorial Hospital
Robert Hill, MHA, President
2815 S Seacrest Blvd
Boynton Beach, FL 33435
561 737-7733
Type: Hosp or Med Ctr: 300-499 Beds
Control: Nonprofit (Private or Religious)
• Radiography Prgm

Bradenton

Lake Erie Coll of Osteopathic Medicine
5000 Lakewood Ranch Blvd
Bradenton, FL 34211
Type: Acad Health Ctr/Med Sch
Control: Nonprofit (Private or Religious)
• Dentistry Prgm
• Osteopathic Medicine Prgm

Manatee Technical Institute
Mary Cantrell, PhD, Director
5603 34th St W
Bradenton, FL 34210
941 751-7900
Type: Vocational or Tech Sch
Control: State, County, or Local Govt
• Dental Assistant Prgm
• Emergency Med Tech-Paramedic Prgm
• Medical Assistant Prgm
• Surgical Technology Prgm

State College of Florida, Manatee-Sarasota
Lars A Hafner, PhD, President
5840 26th St W
PO Box 1849
Bradenton, FL 34207-7046
941 752-5201
Type: Junior or Comm Coll
Control: State, County, or Local Govt
• Dental Hygiene Prgm
• Occupational Therapy Asst Prgm
• Physical Therapist Assistant Prgm
• Radiography Prgm

Cape Coral

21st Century Oncology Inc School of Rad Tech
Daniel E Dosoretz, MD ABR, CEO
1419 SE 8th Terrace
Cape Coral, FL 33990
941 489-3420
Type: Nonhosp HC Facil, BB, or Lab
Control: For Profit
• Radiation Therapy Prgm

High Tech North-Lee County
Cape Coral, FL 33993
Type: Vocational or Tech Sch
• Surgical Technology Prgm

Clearwater

The Players School of Music
923 McMullen Booth Road
Clearwater, FL 33759
• Music Therapy Prgm

Cocoa

Brevard Community College
James A Drake, PhD, District President
1519 Clearlake Rd
Cocoa, FL 32922
321 433-7000
Type: Junior or Comm Coll
Control: State, County, or Local Govt
• Clin Lab Technician/Med Lab Technician Prgm
• Dental Assistant Prgm
• Dental Hygiene Prgm
• Emergency Med Tech-Paramedic Prgm
• Medical Assistant Prgm
• Radiography Prgm
• Surgical Technology Prgm
• Veterinary Technology Prgm

Coconut Creek

Atlantic Technical Center
Coconut Creek, FL 33063
• Dental Assistant Prgm

Coral Gables

University of Miami
Donna Shalala, PhD, President
University Station
PO Box 248006
Coral Gables, FL 33124
305 284-5155
Type: 4-year Coll or Univ
Control: Nonprofit (Private or Religious)
• Athletic Training Prgm
• Music Therapy Prgm
• Nursing Prgm
• Physical Therapy Prgm
• Psychology (PhD) Prgm

Davie

McFatter Technical Center
Mark Thomas, MS, Director
6500 Nova Dr
Davie, FL 33317
754 321-5700
Type: Vocational or Tech Sch
Control: State, County, or Local Govt
• Dental Lab Technician Prgm
• Medical Assistant Prgm
• Pharmacy Technician Prgm

Daytona Beach

Daytona State College, Daytona Beach Campus
Frank Lombardo, MS, Interm President
1200 W International Speedway Boulevard
Daytona Beach, FL 32114
386 506-3417
Type: Junior or Comm Coll
Control: State, County, or Local Govt
• Dental Assistant Prgm
• Dental Hygiene Prgm
• Emergency Med Tech-Paramedic Prgm
• Medical Assistant Prgm
• Occupational Therapy Asst Prgm
• Physical Therapist Assistant Prgm
• Respiratory Care Prgm
• Surgical Technology Prgm

Halifax Health Medical Center
Dan Lang, MHA, Administrator
303 N Clyde Morris Blvd
PO Box 2830
Daytona Beach, FL 32114
386 254-4065
Type: Hosp or Med Ctr: 500 Beds
Control: Nonprofit (Private or Religious)
• Radiography Prgm

Deland

Stetson University
H Douglas Lee, BD ThM PhD, President
421 N Woodland Blvd, Unit 8258
Deland, FL 32720-3701
386 822-7250
Type: 4-year Coll or Univ
Control: Nonprofit (Private or Religious)
• Counseling Prgm
• Music Therapy Prgm

Delray Beach

Institute of Allied Medical Professions
Thomas Haggerty, President
5150 Linton Blvd, Suite 340
Delray Beach, FL 33484
561 381-4990
Type: Acad Health Ctr/Med Sch
Control: Nonprofit (Private or Religious)
• Diagnostic Med Sonography (General/Cardiac) Prgm
• Nuclear Medicine Technology Prgm
• Radiation Therapy Prgm
• Radiography Prgm

Eustis

Lake Technical Center
Steve Hand, MEd, Director
2001 Kurt St
Eustis, FL 32726
352 742-6486
Type: Vocational or Tech Sch
Control: State, County, or Local Govt
• Emergency Med Tech-Paramedic Prgm

Fern Park

Lincoln Technical Institute
Gerald Newman, ABA, President
7275 Estapano Circle
Fern Park, FL 32730
407 673-7406
Type: Vocational or Tech Sch
Control: For Profit
• Dental Assistant Prgm

Fort Lauderdale

Broward College
J David Armstrong, Jr, PhD, President
111 E Las Olas Blvd
Fort Lauderdale, FL 33301
954 201-7401
Type: 4-year Coll or Univ
Control: State, County, or Local Govt
• Dental Assistant Prgm
• Dental Hygiene Prgm
• Diagnostic Med Sonography (General/Cardiac) Prgm
• Emergency Med Tech-Paramedic Prgm
• Medical Assistant Prgm
• Physical Therapist Assistant Prgm
• Respiratory Care Prgm

Keiser Career College
Carole Fuller, BPS, President
1900 W Commerical Blvd
Fort Lauderdale, FL 33309
954 776-4476
Type: Junior or Comm Coll
Control: For Profit
• Surgical Technology Prgm (3)

Keiser University
Arthur Keiser, PhD, Executive Vice Chancellor
1900 W Commerical Blvd Suite 100
Fort Lauderdale, FL 33309
954 275-6498
Type: 4-year Coll or Univ
Control: For Profit
• Clin Lab Technician/Med Lab Technician Prgm
• Diagnostic Med Sonography (General) Prgm (3)
• Dietetics-Coordinated Prgm
• Histotechnician Prgm (2)
• Medical Assistant Prgm
• Nursing Prgm
• Occupational Therapy Asst Prgm (8)
• Physical Therapist Assistant Prgm
• Physician Assistant Prgm
• Radiography Prgm (6)
• Surgical Technology Prgm

Nova Southeastern University
Ray Ferrero, JD, Chancellor
3301 College Ave
Fort Lauderdale, FL 33314-7796
954 262-7575
Type: 4-year Coll or Univ
Control: Nonprofit (Private or Religious)
• Anesthesiologist Asst Prgm (2)
• Athletic Training Prgm
• Audiologist Prgm
• Dentistry Prgm
• Diagnostic Med Sonography (Vascular) Prgm
• Nursing Prgm
• Occupational Therapy Prgm
• Optometry Prgm
• Osteopathic Medicine Prgm
• Pharmacy Prgm
• Physical Therapy Prgm
• Physician Assistant Prgm (4)
• Psychology (PhD) Prgm
• Psychology (PsyD) Prgm
• Speech-Language Pathology Prgm

Fort Myers

Edison State College
Kenneth P Walker, PhD, President
8099 College Pkwy SW
PO Box 60210
Fort Myers, FL 33906-6210
239 941-9211
Type: 4-year Coll or Univ
Control: State, County, or Local Govt
• Cardiovascular Tech (Invasive) Prgm
• Dental Hygiene Prgm
• Emergency Med Tech-Paramedic Prgm
• Radiography Prgm
• Respiratory Care Prgm

Florida Gulf Coast University
Wilson G Bradshaw, PhD, President
10501 FGCU Blvd S
Fort Myers, FL 33965-6565
239 590-1055
Type: 4-year Coll or Univ
Control: State, County, or Local Govt
• Athletic Training Prgm
• Clin Lab Scientist/Med Technologist Prgm
• Counseling Prgm
• Nursing Prgm
• Occupational Therapy Prgm
• Physical Therapy Prgm

Hodges University
Terry P McMahan, JD, President
8695 College Pkwy, Ste 217
Fort Myers, FL 33919
941 482-0019
Type: 4-year Coll or Univ
Control: Nonprofit (Private or Religious)
• Medical Assistant Prgm

Southwest Florida College
Don Jones, BS MBA, CEO
1685 Medical Lane
Fort Myers, FL 33907
239 939-4766
Type: 4-year Coll or Univ
Control: Nonprofit (Private or Religious)
• Clin Lab Technician/Med Lab Technician Prgm
(2)

Fort Pierce

Indian River State College
Edwin R Massey, PhD, President
3209 Virginia Ave
Fort Pierce, FL 34981-5599
772 462-7201
Type: Junior or Comm Coll
Control: State, County, or Local Govt
• Clin Lab Technician/Med Lab Technician Prgm
• Dental Assistant Prgm
• Dental Hygiene Prgm
• Dental Lab Technician Prgm
• Emergency Med Tech-Paramedic Prgm
• Medical Assistant Prgm
• Physical Therapist Assistant Prgm
• Radiography Prgm
• Respiratory Care Prgm
• Surgical Technology Prgm

Gainesville

Florida School of Massage
Gainesville, FL 32608
Type: Acad Health Ctr/Med Sch
Control: For Profit
• Massage Therapy Prgm

Santa Fe College
Jackson Sasser, PhD, President
3000 NW 83rd St
Gainesville, FL 32606-6200
352 395-5164
Type: Junior or Comm Coll
Control: State, County, or Local Govt
• Cardiovascular Tech (Invasive/Noninv/Vasc)
  Prgm
• Clin Lab Scientist/Med Technologist Prgm
• Dental Assistant Prgm
• Dental Hygiene Prgm
• Diagnostic Med Sonography (General) Prgm
• Emergency Med Tech-Paramedic Prgm
• Nuclear Medicine Technology Prgm
• Radiography Prgm
• Surgical Technology Prgm

University of Florida
Bernard Machen, PhD, President
PO Box 113150
226 Tigert Hall
Gainesville, FL 32611-3150
352 392-1311
Type: 4-year Coll or Univ
Control: State, County, or Local Govt
• Allopathic Medicine Prgm
• Athletic Training Prgm
• Audiologist Prgm
• Counseling Prgm (3)
• Dentistry Prgm
• Dietetic Internship Prgm
• Dietetics-Didactic Prgm
• Music Therapy Prgm
• Nursing Prgm
• Occupational Therapy Prgm
• Pharmacy Prgm
• Physical Therapy Prgm
• Physician Assistant Prgm
• Psychology (PhD) Prgm
• Rehabilitation Counseling Prgm
• Speech-Language Pathology Prgm
• Veterinary Medicine Prgm

Hialeah

Everest Institute-Hialeah Campus
Hialeah, FL 33012
Type: Vocational or Tech Sch
• Surgical Technology Prgm

Hollywood

Sheridan Technical Center
D Robert Boegli, Director
5400 Sheridan St
Hollywood, FL 33021
754 321-2007
Type: Vocational or Tech Sch
Control: State, County, or Local Govt
• Medical Transcriptionist Prgm
• Surgical Technology Prgm

Jacksonville

Florida State College at Jacksonville
Steven R Wallace, PhD, President
501 W State St
Jacksonville, FL 32202
904 632-3203
Type: Junior or Comm Coll
Control: State, County, or Local Govt
• Clin Lab Technician/Med Lab Technician Prgm
• Dental Assistant Prgm
• Dental Hygiene Prgm
• Dietetic Technician-AD Prgm
• Emergency Med Tech-Paramedic Prgm
• Histotechnician Prgm
• Occupational Therapy Asst Prgm
• Ophthalmic Technician Prgm
• Physical Therapist Assistant Prgm
• Respiratory Care Prgm
• Surgical Technology Prgm

Jacksonville University
Jacksonville, FL 32211
Type: 4-year Coll or Univ
Control: State, County, or Local Govt
• Nursing Prgm

Keiser University, Jacksonville Campus
George L Hanbury II, PhD, President
6675 Corporate Ctr Pkwy #115
Jacksonville, FL 32216-8088
904 245-8910
• Occupational Therapy Asst Prgm
• Radiography Prgm

Mayo Clinic Jacksonville
Michael B Wood, MD, President
4500 San Pablo Rd
Jacksonville, FL 32224
Type: Hosp or Med Ctr: 300-499 Beds
Control: Nonprofit (Private or Religious)
• Radiography Prgm

Sanford Brown Institute - Jacksonville
Jacksonville, FL 32256
• Dental Assistant Prgm
• Dental Hygiene Prgm

Shands Jacksonville Medical Center
James Burkhart, CEO
655 W Eighth St
Jacksonville, FL 32209
904 244-0411
Type: Hosp or Med Ctr: 500 Beds
Control: Nonprofit (Private or Religious)
• Radiography Prgm

St Luke's Hosp/Mayo Clinic Jacksonville
4201 Belfort Rd
Jacksonville, FL 32216-1431
904 296-3733
Type: Nonhosp HC Facil, BB, or Lab
Control: Nonprofit (Private or Religious)
• Dietetic Internship Prgm

St Vincent's Medical Center
Scott Whalen, PhD, President and CEO
1 Shircliffe Way
Jacksonville, FL 32204
904 308-8446
Type: Hosp or Med Ctr: 500 Beds
Control: Nonprofit (Private or Religious)
• Clin Lab Scientist/Med Technologist Prgm
• Diagnostic Med Sonography (General/Vascular)
  Prgm
• Nuclear Medicine Technology Prgm
• Radiography Prgm

University of North Florida
John Delaney, JD, President
Office of the President
1 University Dr
Jacksonville, FL 32224-2645
904 620-2500
Type: 4-year Coll or Univ
Control: State, County, or Local Govt
• Athletic Training Prgm
• Clin Lab Scientist/Med Technologist Prgm
• Counseling Prgm
• Dietetic Internship Prgm
• Dietetics-Didactic Prgm
• Music Therapy Prgm
• Nursing Prgm
• Physical Therapy Prgm

Virginia College-Jacksonville
Jacksonville, FL 32207
Type: Vocational or Tech Sch
• Surgical Technology Prgm

Lake City

Florida Gateway College
Lake City, FL 32025
Type: Junior or Comm Coll
• Emergency Med Tech-Paramedic Prgm

Lake City Community College
Charles Hall, EdD, President
149 SE College Place
Lake City, FL 32025
386 754-4200
Type: Junior or Comm Coll
Control: State, County, or Local Govt
• Physical Therapist Assistant Prgm

Lake Mary

Remington College of Nursing
Lake Mary, FL 32746
Type: 4-year Coll or Univ
Control: For Profit
• Nursing Prgm

Lake Worth

Palm Beach State College
Dennis P Gallon, PhD, President
4200 Congress Ave
Lake Worth, FL 33461-4796
561 868-3350
Type: Junior or Comm Coll
Control: State, County, or Local Govt
• Dental Assistant Prgm
• Dental Hygiene Prgm
• Diagnostic Med Sonography (General) Prgm
• Emergency Med Tech-Paramedic Prgm
• Medical Assistant Prgm
• Radiography Prgm
• Respiratory Care Prgm
• Surgical Technology Prgm

Lakeland

Everest Univ - Lakeland Campus
Edmund K Gross, EdD, President
995 E Memorial Blvd, Ste 110
Lakeland, FL 33801
941 686-1444
Type: 4-year Coll or Univ
Control: For Profit
• Medical Assistant Prgm

Florida Career Institute
Pamela J Corrigan, RN MEd, CEO
4222 S Florida Ave
Lakeland, FL 33813
863 646-1400
Type: Vocational or Tech Sch
Control: For Profit
• Medical Assistant Prgm

Florida Southern College
Anne Kerr, PhD, President
111 Lake Hollingsworth Dr
Lakeland, FL 33801-5698
863 680-4100
Type: 4-year Coll or Univ
Control: Nonprofit (Private or Religious)
• Athletic Training Prgm
• Nursing Prgm

Lakeland Regional Medical Center
Jack T Stephens, President/CEO
1324 Lakeland Hills Blvd
PO Box 95448
Lakeland, FL 33804
863 687-1100
Type: Hosp or Med Ctr: 500 Beds
Control: Nonprofit (Private or Religious)
• Histotechnician Prgm
• Radiography Prgm

Traviss Career Center
Kenneth Lloyd, PhD
3225 Winter Lake Rd
Lakeland, FL 33803
863 449-2700
Type: Vocational or Tech Sch
Control: State, County, or Local Govt
• Dental Assistant Prgm
• Surgical Technology Prgm

Largo

Everest Univ - Largo Campus
John Buck, BME, President
1199 East Bay Drive
Largo, FL 33770
727 725-2688
Type: 4-year Coll or Univ
Control: For Profit
• Medical Assistant Prgm

Lauderdale Lakes

Sanford-Brown Institute - Ft Lauderdale
1201 W Cypress Creek Rd
Lauderdale Lakes, FL 33309
954 308-7400
Type: Vocational or Tech Sch
Control: For Profit
• Cardiovascular Tech (Echocardiography) Prgm
• Dental Assistant Prgm
• Dental Hygiene Prgm
• Diagnostic Med Sonography (General) Prgm

Live Oak

Suwannee-Hamilton Technical Center
Live Oak, FL 32064
Type: Vocational or Tech Sch
• Surgical Technology Prgm

Maitland

Florida College of Natural Health
Dale Weiberg, Campus Director
2600 Lake Lucian Dr
Maitland, FL 33126
407 261-0319
Type: Vocational or Tech Sch
Control: For Profit
• Massage Therapy Prgm (4)

Melbourne

Everest Univ - Melbourne Campus
Mark Judge, MBA, President
2401 N Harbor City Blvd
Melbourne, FL 32935
321 253-2929
Type: 4-year Coll or Univ
Control: For Profit
• Medical Assistant Prgm
• Pharmacy Technician Prgm

Florida Institute of Technology
Melbourne, FL 32901
Type: Vocational or Tech Sch
Control: For Profit
• Psychology (PsyD) Prgm

Miami

Carlos Albizu University
Miami, FL 32172
Type: 4-year Coll or Univ
Control: Nonprofit (Private or Religious)
• Psychology (PsyD) Prgm

Dade Medical College
Ernesto Perez, President
300 NE 2nd Avenue #Wolfson 1472
Miami, FL 33132
305 237-3316
Type: 4-year Coll or Univ
Control: State, County, or Local Govt
• Clin Lab Technician/Med Lab Technician Prgm
• Dental Hygiene Prgm
• Diagnostic Med Sonography (General/Cardiac) Prgm
• Emergency Med Tech-Paramedic Prgm
• Histotechnician Prgm
• Ophthalmic Dispensing Optician Prgm
• Physical Therapist Assistant Prgm
• Physician Assistant Prgm
• Radiography Prgm (2)
• Respiratory Care Prgm
• Veterinary Technology Prgm

Educating Hands School of Massage
Iris Burman
120 SW 8th St
Miami, FL 33130
305 285-6991
Type: Vocational or Tech Sch
Control: For Profit
• Massage Therapy Prgm

Everest Institute-Kendall Campus
Miami, FL 33186
Type: Vocational or Tech Sch
• Surgical Technology Prgm

Florida International University
Mark Rosenberg, PhD, President
Office of Academic Affairs
University Park Campus
Miami, FL 33199
305 348-2111
Type: 4-year Coll or Univ
Control: State, County, or Local Govt
• Allopathic Medicine Prgm
• Counseling Prgm
• Dietetics-Coordinated Prgm
• Dietetics-Didactic Prgm
• Music Therapy Prgm
• Nursing Prgm
• Occupational Therapy Prgm
• Physical Therapy Prgm
• Speech-Language Pathology Prgm

Jackson Memorial Hospital
Eneida Roldan, MD MPH MBA, President and CEO
Jackson Health System
1611 NW 12th Ave
Miami, FL 33136-1094
305 585-6754
Type: Hosp or Med Ctr: 500 Beds
Control: State, County, or Local Govt
• Nuclear Medicine Technology Prgm
• Radiography Prgm

Lindsey Hopkins Tech Education Center
Rosa Borgen, MS, Principal
750 NW 20th St
Miami, FL 33127
305 324-6070
Type: Vocational or Tech Sch
Control: State, County, or Local Govt
• Surgical Technology Prgm

Miami Dade Comm Coll/Jackson Mem Hosp
Ira C Clark, MA, President
Jackson Memorial Hospital
1611 NW 12th Ave
Miami, FL 33136-1094
305 585-6754
Type: Consortium
Control: State, County, or Local Govt
• Radiography Prgm

Professional Training Centers
Marc A Mattia, MS RT(R)
13926 SW 47th St
Miami, FL 33175
305 220-4120
Type: Vocational or Tech Sch
Control: For Profit
• Radiography Prgm

Robert Morgan Educational Center
Greg Zawyer, MS, Principal
18180 SW 122nd Ave
Miami, FL 33177
305 253-9920
Type: Vocational or Tech Sch
Control: State, County, or Local Govt
• Dental Assistant Prgm
• Medical Assistant Prgm

University of Miami
Bernard J Fogel, MD, Vice President, Dean
1600 NW 10th Ave R-699
Miami, FL 33136
305 585-6545
Type: Acad Health Ctr/Med Sch
Control: Nonprofit (Private or Religious)
• Allopathic Medicine Prgm

Miami Beach

New World Symphony
500 17th Street
Miami Beach, FL 33139
• Music Therapy Prgm

Miami Shores

Barry University
Linda M Bevilacqua, OP, President
11300 NE 2nd Ave
Miami Shores, FL 33161-6695
305 899-3010
Type: 4-year Coll or Univ
Control: Nonprofit (Private or Religious)
• Athletic Training Prgm
• Counseling Prgm
• Histotechnology Prgm
• Nursing Prgm
• Occupational Therapy Prgm
• Perfusion Prgm
• Physician Assistant Prgm
• Podiatric Medicine Prgm

Miramar

Concorde Career Institute
Tim Vogeley, MA, Campus President
10933 Marks Way
Miramar, FL 33025
954 731-8880
Type: Vocational or Tech Sch
Control: For Profit
• Dental Assistant Prgm
• Surgical Technology Prgm (3)

Mulberry

Fortis Institute
Mulberry, FL 33860
Type: Vocational or Tech Sch
• Medical Assistant Prgm

Naples

Lorenzo Walker Institute of Technology
Jeanette Johnson, MS, Principal
3702 Estey Ave
Naples, FL 34104
239 377-0906
Type: Vocational or Tech Sch
Control: State, County, or Local Govt
• Dental Assistant Prgm
• Medical Assistant Prgm
• Surgical Technology Prgm

New Port Richey

Pasco County Health Department
10841 Little Rd
New Port Richey, FL 34654-2533
813 869-3900
Type: Nonhosp HC Facil, BB, or Lab
Control: State, County, or Local Govt
• Dietetic Internship Prgm

Pasco-Hernando Community College
Katherine M Johnson, EdD, President
10230 Ridge Rd
New Port Richey, FL 34654-5199
727 847-2727
Type: Junior or Comm Coll
Control: State, County, or Local Govt
• Dental Hygiene Prgm
• Emergency Med Tech-Paramedic Prgm

Niceville

Northwest Florida State College
Niceville, FL 32578-1295
Type: 4-year Coll or Univ
Control: State, County, or Local Govt
• Dental Assistant Prgm
• Nursing Prgm

Ocala

College of Central Florida
Charles Dassance, PhD, President
3001 SW College Rd
PO Box 1388
Ocala, FL 34474
352 854-2322
Type: Junior or Comm Coll
Control: State, County, or Local Govt
• Dental Assistant Prgm
• Emergency Med Tech-Paramedic Prgm
• Physical Therapist Assistant Prgm
• Surgical Technology Prgm

Community Technical & Adult Education Center
Samuel Lauff, Jr, MA, Administrator
1014 SW 7th Rd
Ocala, FL 34474
352 671-7200
Type: Vocational or Tech Sch
Control: State, County, or Local Govt
• Medical Assistant Prgm

Marion County School of Radiologic Tech
Deborah Jenkins, MEd, Administrator
1014 SW 7th Rd
Ocala, FL 34474-3172
352 671-7200
Type: Vocational or Tech Sch
Control: State, County, or Local Govt
• Radiography Prgm

Orange Park

Fortis College-Orange Park
Orange Park, FL 32073
Type: Junior or Comm Coll
• Surgical Technology Prgm

Orlando

Everest Univ - North Orlando Campus
Ouida B Kirby, BS, President
5421 Diplomat Circle
Orlando, FL 32810
407 628-5870
Type: 4-year Coll or Univ
Control: For Profit
• Medical Assistant Prgm

Everest University - Orlando College South
Louise Stienkeoway, PhD, President
9200 SouthPark Center Loop
Orlando, FL 32819
407 851-2525
Type: 4-year Coll or Univ
Control: For Profit
• Medical Assistant Prgm

Florida Hospital
Sandra Randolph, CEO
601 E Rollins St
Orlando, FL 32803
407 303-1574
Type: Hosp or Med Ctr: 500 Beds
Control: Nonprofit (Private or Religious)
• Phlebotomy Prgm

Florida Hospital College of Health Sciences
David E Greenlaw, DMiN, President
671 Winyah Dr
Orlando, FL 32803
407 303-7747
Type: 4-year Coll or Univ
Control: Nonprofit (Private or Religious)
• Diagnostic Med Sonography
  (Gen/Card/Vascular) Prgm
• Nuclear Medicine Technology Prgm
• Occupational Therapy Asst Prgm
• Radiography Prgm

Orlando Tech
Ferol Lynne Voltaggio, MEd, Senior Director
301 W Amelia St
Orlando, FL 32801
407 246-7060
Type: Vocational or Tech Sch
Control: State, County, or Local Govt
• Dental Assistant Prgm
• Surgical Technology Prgm

Sanford Brown Institute - Orlando
Orlando, FL 32809
• Dental Hygiene Prgm

University of Central Florida
John C Hitt, PhD, President
308 Millican Hall
4000 Central Florida Blvd
Orlando, FL 32816-0002
407 823-1823
Type: 4-year Coll or Univ
Control: State, County, or Local Govt
• Allopathic Medicine Prgm
• Athletic Training Prgm
• Clin Lab Scientist/Med Technologist Prgm
• Counseling Prgm
• Music Therapy Prgm
• Nursing Prgm
• Physical Therapy Prgm
• Psychology (PhD) Prgm
• Respiratory Care Prgm
• Speech-Language Pathology Prgm

Valencia College
Sanford C Shugart, PhD, President
PO Box 3028
Orlando, FL 32802-3028
407 299-5000
Type: Junior or Comm Coll
Control: State, County, or Local Govt
• Cardiovascular Tech (Invasive) Prgm
• Dental Hygiene Prgm
• Diagnostic Med Sonography (General) Prgm
• Emergency Med Tech-Paramedic Prgm
• Radiography Prgm
• Respiratory Care Prgm

Osprey

Sarasota District Schools
101 Old Venice Rd
Osprey, FL 34229-9023
Control: State, County, or Local Govt
• Dietetic Internship Prgm

Palm Harbor

Central Florida Institute
Alfred A McCloy, MBA, President
30522 US 19 N, Ste 200
Palm Harbor, FL 34684
727 786-4707
Type: Vocational or Tech Sch
Control: For Profit
• Cardiovascular Tech (Invasive/Noninv/Vasc)
  Prgm
• Diagnostic Med Sonography (General) Prgm
  (2)
• Polysomnographic Technology Prgm
• Surgical Technology Prgm

Panama City

Gulf Coast State College
James Kerley, PhD, President
5230 W US Hwy 98
Panama City, FL 32401-1041
850 769-1551
Type: Junior or Comm Coll
Control: State, County, or Local Govt
• Dental Assistant Prgm
• Dental Hygiene Prgm
• Emergency Med Tech-Paramedic Prgm
• Physical Therapist Assistant Prgm
• Radiography Prgm
• Surgical Technology Prgm

Pensacola

Pensacola State College
Edward Meadows, PhD, President
1000 College Blvd
Pensacola, FL 32501
850 484-1700
Type: Junior or Comm Coll
Control: State, County, or Local Govt
• Dental Hygiene Prgm
• Emergency Med Tech-Paramedic Prgm
• Medical Assistant Prgm
• Physical Therapist Assistant Prgm
• Radiography Prgm
• Surgical Technology Prgm

University of West Florida
Judy Bense, President
11000 University Pkwy
Pensacola, FL 32514-5750
850 474-2200
Type: 4-year Coll or Univ
Control: State, County, or Local Govt
• Athletic Training Prgm
• Clin Lab Scientist/Med Technologist Prgm
• Music Therapy Prgm
• Nursing Prgm

Virginia College at Penascola
Bruce G Capps, BS, President
19 W Garden St
Pensacola, FL 32501
850 916-9868
Type: Vocational or Tech Sch
Control: For Profit
• Surgical Technology Prgm

Port Charlotte

Charlotte Technical Center
Judith Willis, Director
18300 Toledo Blade Blvd
Port Charlotte, FL 33948-3399
941 255-7500
Type: Vocational or Tech Sch
Control: State, County, or Local Govt
• Dental Assistant Prgm

Port Orange

Palmer College of Chiropractic
4777 City Center Pkwy
Port Orange, FL 32129
Type: Acad Health Ctr/Med Sch
Control: For Profit
• Chiropractic Prgm

Sanford

Seminole State College
E Ann McGee, EdD, President
100 Weldon Blvd
Sanford, FL 32773
407 708-4722
Type: Junior or Comm Coll
Control: State, County, or Local Govt
• Emergency Med Tech-Paramedic Prgm
• Medical Transcriptionist Prgm
• Physical Therapist Assistant Prgm
• Respiratory Care Prgm

Sarasota

Sarasota County Technical Institute
Bruce Andersen, MA, Director
4748 Beneva Rd
Sarasota, FL 34233-1798
813 924-1365
Type: Vocational or Tech Sch
Control: State, County, or Local Govt
• Emergency Med Tech-Paramedic Prgm
• Surgical Technology Prgm

Sarasota Memorial Hospital
1700 S Tamiami Trail
Sarasota, FL 34239-3555
813 917-1080
Type: Hosp or Med Ctr: 500 Beds
Control: Nonprofit (Private or Religious)
• Dietetic Internship Prgm

Sarasota School of Massage Therapy
Joe Lubow, BS LMT, Director
1932 Ringling Blvd
Sarasota, FL 34236
941 957-0577
Type: Vocational or Tech Sch
Control: For Profit
• Massage Therapy Prgm

St Augustine

First Coast Technical College
Christine Cothron, President
2980 Collins Ave
St Augustine, FL 32095-1919
904 824-4401
Type: Vocational or Tech Sch
Control: State, County, or Local Govt
• Emergency Med Tech-Paramedic Prgm
• Medical Assistant Prgm

Univ of St Augustine for Health Sciences
Wanda Nitsch, PhD PT, President
1 University Blvd
St Augustine, FL 32086
904 826-0084
Type: Acad Health Ctr/Med Sch
Control: For Profit
• Occupational Therapy Prgm (2)
• Physical Therapy Prgm

St Petersburg

Bayfront Medical Center
Sue S Brody, MHA, President/CEO
701 Sixth St S
St Petersburg, FL 33701
727 823-1234
Type: Hosp or Med Ctr: 500 Beds
Control: Nonprofit (Private or Religious)
• Clin Lab Scientist/Med Technologist Prgm

Pinellas Technical Education Centers
Dennis Jauch, EdD, Chief Operating Officer
901 34th St South
St Petersburg, FL 33711-2298
727 893-2500
Type: Vocational or Tech Sch
Control: State, County, or Local Govt
• Dental Assistant Prgm
• Pharmacy Technician Prgm
• Surgical Technology Prgm

St Petersburg College
Carl Kuttler, Provost, Health Educ Ctr
PO Box 13489
St Petersburg, FL 33733
727 341-3245
Type: 4-year Coll or Univ
Control: State, County, or Local Govt
• Clin Lab Technician/Med Lab Technician Prgm
• Dental Hygiene Prgm
• Emergency Med Tech-Paramedic Prgm
• Nursing Prgm
• Orthotist/Prosthetist Prgm
• Physical Therapist Assistant Prgm
• Radiography Prgm
• Respiratory Care Prgm
• Veterinary Technology Prgm

Transfusion Med Acad Ctr FL Blood Svcs
German F Leparc, MD, Chief Medical Officer
10100 Dr Martin Luther King Jr St N
St Petersburg, FL 33716-3806
727 568-5433
Type: Nonhosp HC Facil, BB, or Lab
Control: Nonprofit (Private or Religious)
• Specialist in BB Tech Prgm

Tallahassee

Florida A&M University
James Ammons, PhD, President
400 Lee Hall
Tallahassee, FL 32307-3100
850 599-3225
Type: 4-year Coll or Univ
Control: State, County, or Local Govt
• Occupational Therapy Prgm
• Pharmacy Prgm
• Physical Therapy Prgm
• Respiratory Care Prgm

Florida Department of Education
325 W Gaines St, Rm 1032
Tallahassee, FL 32399-0400
Type: Acad Health Ctr/Med Sch
Control: State, County, or Local Govt
• Dietetic Internship Prgm

Florida State University
T K Wetherell, PhD, President
211 WES
Tallahassee, FL 32306
850 644-2525
Type: 4-year Coll or Univ
Control: State, County, or Local Govt
• Allopathic Medicine Prgm
• Art Therapy Prgm
• Athletic Training Prgm
• Counseling Prgm
• Dietetic Internship Prgm
• Dietetics-Didactic Prgm
• Medical Librarian Prgm
• Music Therapy Prgm
• Nursing Prgm
• Orientation and Mobility Specialist Prgm
• Psychology (PhD) Prgm
• Rehabilitation Counseling Prgm
• Speech-Language Pathology Prgm
• Teacher of the Visually Impaired Prgm
• Vision Rehabilitation Therapy Prgm

Lively Technical Center
Jean Ferguson, MS, Principal
500 N Appleyard Dr
Tallahassee, FL 32304
904 487-7401
Type: Vocational or Tech Sch
Control: State, County, or Local Govt
• Medical Assistant Prgm

Tallahassee Community College
William Law, PhD, President
444 Appleyard Dr
Tallahassee, FL 32304
850 201-8660
Type: Junior or Comm Coll
Control: State, County, or Local Govt
• Dental Assistant Prgm
• Dental Hygiene Prgm
• Emergency Med Tech-Paramedic Prgm
• Respiratory Care Prgm

Tampa

Argosy University
Tampa, FL 33614
Type: 4-year Coll or Univ
Control: For Profit
• Psychology (PsyD) Prgm

Erwin Technical Center
James Rich, Principal
2010 E Hillsborough Ave
Tampa, FL 33610-8299
813 231-1800
Type: Vocational or Tech Sch
Control: State, County, or Local Govt
• Dental Assistant Prgm
• Medical Assistant Prgm
• Neurodiagnostic Tech Prgm

Everest Univ - Brandon Campus
Stan Banks, II, BS, President
3924 Coconut Palm Dr
Tampa, FL 33619
813 621-0041
Type: 4-year Coll or Univ
Control: For Profit
• Medical Assistant Prgm
• Radiography Prgm
• Surgical Technology Prgm

Everest Univ - Tampa
Thomas M Barlow, President
3319 W Hillsborough Ave
Tampa, FL 33614
813 879-6000
Type: 4-year Coll or Univ
Control: For Profit
• Medical Assistant Prgm

Henry W Brewster Technical Center
Janice Carter Collier, Prinicpal
2222 N Tampa St
Tampa, FL 33602
Type: Vocational or Tech Sch
Control: State, County, or Local Govt
• Pharmacy Technician Prgm

Hillsborough Community College
Gwendolyn Stephenson, PhD, President
PO Box 31127
39 Columbia Dr (Davis Island)
Tampa, FL 33631-3127
813 253-7050
Type: Junior or Comm Coll
Control: State, County, or Local Govt
• Dental Assistant Prgm
• Dental Hygiene Prgm
• Diagnostic Med Sonography (General) Prgm
• Dietetic Technician-AD Prgm
• Emergency Med Tech-Paramedic Prgm
• Nuclear Medicine Technology Prgm
• Ophthalmic Dispensing Optician Prgm
• Radiation Therapy Prgm
• Radiography Prgm
• Respiratory Care Prgm

James A Haley Veteran's Hospital
13000 N Bruce B Downs Blvd
Tampa, FL 33612-4745
813 972-2000
Type: Hosp or Med Ctr: 300-499 Beds
Control: Fed Govt
• Dietetic Internship Prgm

Tampa General Hospital
Ron Hytoff, MD, President, CEO
PO Box 1289
1 Tampa General Circle
Tampa, FL 33606
813 844-7662
Type: Hosp or Med Ctr: 500 Beds
Control: Nonprofit (Private or Religious)
• Clin Lab Scientist/Med Technologist Prgm

University of South Florida
Judith Genshaft, PhD, President
ADM 241
Tampa, FL 33620
813 974-2791
Type: 4-year Coll or Univ
Control: State, County, or Local Govt
• Allopathic Medicine Prgm
• Athletic Training Prgm
• Audiologist Prgm
• Counseling Prgm
• Medical Librarian Prgm
• Music Therapy Prgm
• Nursing Prgm
• Pharmacy Prgm
• Physical Therapy Prgm
• Psychology (PhD) Prgm
• Rehabilitation Counseling Prgm
• Speech-Language Pathology Prgm

University of Tampa
Ronald Vaughn, PhD, President
401 W Kennedy Blvd
Tampa, FL 33606
813 253-6201
Type: 4-year Coll or Univ
Control: Nonprofit (Private or Religious)
• Athletic Training Prgm
• Music Therapy Prgm

West Palm Beach

MedVance Institute
John Hopkins, PhD, CEO/President
KIMC Investments, Medvance Institute
1401 Forum Way
West Palm Beach, FL 33401
561 832-3535
Type: Vocational or Tech Sch
Control: For Profit
• Clin Lab Technician/Med Lab Technician Prgm
  (2)
• Radiography Prgm (3)
• Surgical Technology Prgm (2)

Palm Beach Atlantic University
David W Clark, PhD, President
PO Box 24708
West Palm Beach, FL 33416-4708
561 803-2302
Type: 4-year Coll or Univ
Control: Nonprofit (Private or Religious)
• Athletic Training Prgm
• Music Therapy Prgm
• Nursing Prgm
• Pharmacy Prgm

South University
Tracey Schoonmaker, President
1760 N Congress Ave
West Palm Beach, FL 33409
561 697-9200
Type: 4-year Coll or Univ
Control: For Profit
• Physical Therapist Assistant Prgm
• Physician Assistant Prgm

Winter Haven

Polk State College
Eileen Holden, EdD, President
999 Ave H NE
Winter Haven, FL 33881-4299
863 297-1098
Type: Junior or Comm Coll
Control: State, County, or Local Govt
• Cardiovascular Tech (Invasive) Prgm
• Diagnostic Med Sonography (General) Prgm
• Emergency Med Tech-Paramedic Prgm
• Occupational Therapy Asst Prgm
• Physical Therapist Assistant Prgm
• Radiography Prgm

Winter Park

Fortis College-Winter Park
Winter Park, FL 32789
Type: Vocational or Tech Sch
• Medical Assistant Prgm

Rollins College
1000 Holt Ave
Winter Park, FL 32789-4499
407 646-2000
Type: 4-year Coll or Univ
Control: Nonprofit (Private or Religious)
• Counseling Prgm
• Music Therapy Prgm

Winter Park Tech
Diane Culpepper, PhD, Director
901 Webster Ave
Winter Park, FL 32789
407 622-2915
Type: Vocational or Tech Sch
Control: State, County, or Local Govt
• Medical Assistant Prgm
• Medical Transcriptionist Prgm

Georgia

Acworth

Chattahoochee Technical College North Metro
Steve Dougherty, MA, President
5198 Ross Rd
Acworth, GA 30102
770 975-4126
Type: Vocational or Tech Sch
Control: State, County, or Local Govt
• Medical Assistant Prgm
• Physical Therapist Assistant Prgm
• Radiography Prgm

Albany

Albany Technical College
Anthony Parker, PhD, President
1704 S Slappey Blvd
Albany, GA 31701-3514
229 430-3500
Type: Vocational or Tech Sch
Control: State, County, or Local Govt
• Dental Assistant Prgm
• Medical Assistant Prgm
• Radiography Prgm
• Surgical Technology Prgm

Darton College
Peter J Sireno, EdD, President
2400 Gillionville Rd
Albany, GA 31707
229 317-6846
Type: Junior or Comm Coll
Control: State, County, or Local Govt
• Cardiovascular Tech (Invasive/Echo) Prgm
• Clin Lab Technician/Med Lab Technician Prgm
• Dental Hygiene Prgm
• Histotechnician Prgm
• Occupational Therapy Asst Prgm
• Physical Therapist Assistant Prgm
• Respiratory Care Prgm

Athens

Athens Technical College
Flora Tydings, EdD, President
800 US Hwy 29 N
Athens, GA 30601
706 355-5000
Type: Junior or Comm Coll
Control: State, County, or Local Govt
• Dental Assistant Prgm
• Dental Hygiene Prgm
• Diagnostic Med Sonography (General) Prgm
• Physical Therapist Assistant Prgm
• Radiography Prgm
• Respiratory Care Prgm
• Surgical Technology Prgm
• Veterinary Technology Prgm

University of Georgia
Michael F Adams, PhD, President
Administration Bldg
Athens, GA 30602
706 542-1214
Type: 4-year Coll or Univ
Control: State, County, or Local Govt
• Athletic Training Prgm
• Counseling Prgm
• Dietetic Internship Prgm
• Dietetics-Didactic Prgm
• Music Therapy Prgm
• Pharmacy Prgm
• Psychology (PhD) Prgm
• Speech-Language Pathology Prgm
• Veterinary Medicine Prgm

Atlanta

Argosy University
Atlanta, GA 30328
Type: 4-year Coll or Univ
Control: For Profit
• Psychology (PsyD) Prgm

Atlanta Technical College
Alvetta Peterson-Thomas, EdS, President
1560 Metropolitan Parkway SW
Atlanta, GA 30310
404 225-4400
Type: Vocational or Tech Sch
Control: State, County, or Local Govt
- Dental Assistant Prgm
- Dental Hygiene Prgm
- Dental Lab Technician Prgm
- Medical Assistant Prgm

Brown Mackie College - Atlanta
Daniel Summer, Campus President
4370 Peachtree Road
Atlanta, GA 30319
404 799-4500
- Occupational Therapy Asst Prgm

Div of Pub Hlth/Georgia Dept of Hum Res
2 Peachtree St NE
Atlanta, GA 30303-3141
404 657-2884
Type: Nonhosp HC Facil, BB, or Lab
Control: State, County, or Local Govt
- Dietetic Internship Prgm

Emory University
James W Wagner, PhD, President
408 Administration Bldg
Atlanta, GA 30322
404 727-6012
Type: 4-year Coll or Univ
Control: Nonprofit (Private or Religious)
- Allopathic Medicine Prgm
- Anesthesiologist Asst Prgm
- Genetic Counseling Prgm
- Nursing Prgm
- Ophthalmic Med Technologist Prgm
- Ophthalmic Technician Prgm
- Physical Therapy Prgm
- Physician Assistant Prgm
- Psychology (PhD) Prgm
- Radiography Prgm

Emory University Hospital
John D Henry, Sr, FACHE, CEO
1364 Clifton Rd NE, Rm B216
Atlanta, GA 30322
404 712-4881
Type: Hosp or Med Ctr: 500 Beds
Control: Nonprofit (Private or Religious)
- Dietetic Internship Prgm

Emory University System of Health Care
John D Henry Sr, FACHE, Administrator
1364 Clifton Rd NE, Rm B216
Atlanta, GA 30322
404 712-7397
Type: Hosp or Med Ctr: 500 Beds
Control: Nonprofit (Private or Religious)
- Clin Lab Scientist/Med Technologist Prgm

Georgia Institute of Technology
Gary Schuster, PhD, Interim President
225 North Ave NW
Atlanta, GA 30332-0325
404 894-5051
Type: 4-year Coll or Univ
Control: State, County, or Local Govt
- Orthotist/Prosthetist Prgm

Georgia State University
Carl V Patton, PhD, President
PO Box 3999
300 Alumni Hall
Atlanta, GA 30302-3999
404 651-2560
Type: 4-year Coll or Univ
Control: State, County, or Local Govt
- Counseling Prgm
- Dietetic Internship Prgm
- Dietetics-Coordinated Prgm
- Dietetics-Didactic Prgm
- Exercise Physiology - Applied Prgm
- Exercise Science Prgm
- Music Therapy Prgm
- Nursing Prgm
- Physical Therapy Prgm
- Psychology (PhD) Prgm
- Rehabilitation Counseling Prgm
- Respiratory Care Prgm
- Speech-Language Pathology Prgm

Grady Health System
Pamela Stephenson, Esq, President/CEO
80 Jesse Hill Jr Dr, SE
PO Box 26189
Atlanta, GA 30303-3050
404 616-4252
Type: Hosp or Med Ctr: 500 Beds
Control: State, County, or Local Govt
- Diagnostic Med Sonography (General) Prgm
- Radiation Therapy Prgm
- Radiography Prgm

Institute of Allied Medical Professions
Thomas Haggerty, President
5673 Peachtree Dunwoody Rd
Ste 450
Atlanta, GA 30342
Type: Acad Health Ctr/Med Sch
Control: For Profit
- Radiation Therapy Prgm

Morehouse School of Medicine
John E Maupin, Jr, DDS MBA, President
720 Westview Dr SW
Atlanta, GA 30310
Type: Acad Health Ctr/Med Sch
Control: Nonprofit (Private or Religious)
- Allopathic Medicine Prgm

Morrison Chartwells
Atlanta, GA 30342
- Dietetic Internship Prgm

Sanford-Brown Institute
Glenn W Alderson, BA, Executive Director
1140 Hammond Dr, Ste 1150
Atlanta, GA 30328
770 350-0009
Type: Vocational or Tech Sch
Control: For Profit
- Diagnostic Med Sonography (General) Prgm

Westwood College
Khaliffa Alshammiry, MD MS, Executive Director
2309 Parklake Dr NE
Atlanta, GA 30345
404 962-2990
Type: Junior or Comm Coll
Control: For Profit
- Medical Assistant Prgm (2)

Augusta

Augusta Area Dietetic Internship
Larry Read, CEO, Univ Hlth Care Syst
University Hospital
1350 Walton Way (10)
Augusta, GA 30901-2629
706 774-8045
Type: Hosp or Med Ctr: 300-499 Beds
Control: Nonprofit (Private or Religious)
- Dietetic Internship Prgm

Augusta Technical College
Terry D Elam, MEd, President
3200 Augusta Tech Dr
Augusta, GA 30906
706 771-4005
Type: Vocational or Tech Sch
Control: State, County, or Local Govt
- Cardiovascular Tech (Invasive/Noninv/Vasc) Prgm
- Dental Assistant Prgm
- Medical Assistant Prgm
- Occupational Therapy Asst Prgm
- Respiratory Care Prgm
- Surgical Technology Prgm

Georgia Health Sciences University
James Thompson, MD, Interim President
1120 15th St, Rm AA-311
Augusta, GA 30912
706 721-2301
Type: Acad Health Ctr/Med Sch
Control: State, County, or Local Govt
- Allopathic Medicine Prgm
- Clin Lab Scientist/Med Technologist Prgm
- Dental Hygiene Prgm
- Dentistry Prgm
- Diagnostic Med Sonography (General) Prgm
- Medical Illustrator Prgm
- Nuclear Medicine Technology Prgm
- Nursing Prgm
- Occupational Therapy Prgm
- Physical Therapy Prgm
- Physician Assistant Prgm
- Radiation Therapy Prgm
- Respiratory Care Prgm

University Hospital
J Larry Read, MBA, President/CEO
1350 Walton Way
Augusta, GA 30901
706 722-9011
Type: Hosp or Med Ctr: 500 Beds
Control: Nonprofit (Private or Religious)
- Radiography Prgm

Virginia College-Augusta
Augusta, GA 30909
Type: Vocational or Tech Sch
- Surgical Technology Prgm

Brunswick

College of Coastal Georgia
Valerie Hepburn, PhD, President
3700 Altama Ave
Brunswick, GA 31520-3644
912 279-5705
Type: 4-year Coll or Univ
Control: State, County, or Local Govt
- Clin Lab Technician/Med Lab Technician Prgm
- Radiography Prgm

Carrollton

University of West Georgia
Beheruz N Sethna, President
Carrollton, GA 30118-0001
770 836-6500
Type: 4-year Coll or Univ
Control: State, County, or Local Govt
• Counseling Prgm
• Music Therapy Prgm
• Nursing Prgm
• Speech-Language Pathology Prgm

Clarkesville

North Georgia Technical College
Steve Dougherty, MS, President
PO Box 65
1500 Hwy 197 North
Clarkesville, GA 30523
706 754-7701
Type: Vocational or Tech Sch
Control: State, County, or Local Govt
• Clin Lab Technician/Med Lab Technician Prgm
• Medical Assistant Prgm (2)

Clarkston

Georgia Piedmont Technical College
Clarkston, GA 30021
Type: Vocational or Tech Sch
• Medical Assistant Prgm

Georgia Piedmont Technical College
Robin Hoffman, PhD, President
495 N Indian Creek Dr
Clarkston, GA 30021
404 297-9522
Type: Vocational or Tech Sch
Control: State, County, or Local Govt
• Clin Lab Technician/Med Lab Technician Prgm
• Medical Assistant Prgm
• Ophthalmic Dispensing Optician Prgm

Cochran

Middle Georgia College
W. Michael Stoy, PhD, President
1100 Second St SE
Cochran, GA 31014-1599
478 934-3011
Type: Junior or Comm Coll
Control: State, County, or Local Govt
• Occupational Therapy Asst Prgm

Columbus

Columbus State University
Frank D Brown, PhD, President
4225 University Ave
Columbus, GA 31907-5645
706 568-2211
Type: 4-year Coll or Univ
Control: State, County, or Local Govt
• Counseling Prgm
• Music Therapy Prgm
• Nursing Prgm

Columbus Technical College
J Robert Jones, EdS, President
928 Manchester Expwy
Columbus, GA 31904-6572
706 649-1837
Type: Vocational or Tech Sch
Control: State, County, or Local Govt
• Dental Assistant Prgm
• Dental Hygiene Prgm
• Medical Assistant Prgm
• Radiography Prgm
• Surgical Technology Prgm

Dacula

Gwinnett County Fire and Emergency Services
Dacula, GA 30019
Type: Consortium
• Emergency Med Tech-Paramedic Prgm

Dahlonega

North Georgia College & State University
David Potter, PhD, President
Prince Memorial Hall
Dahlonega, GA 30597
706 864-1993
Type: 4-year Coll or Univ
Control: State, County, or Local Govt
• Athletic Training Prgm
• Physical Therapy Prgm

Decatur

DeKalb Medical Center
Eric Norwood, MHA, CEO
2701 N Decatur Rd
Decatur, GA 30033
404 501-5206
Type: Hosp or Med Ctr: 300-499 Beds
Control: Nonprofit (Private or Religious)
• Radiography Prgm

Georgia Perimeter College
Jacquelyn M Belcher, President
3251 Panthersville Rd
Decatur, GA 30034
404 244-2365
Type: Junior or Comm Coll
Control: State, County, or Local Govt
• Dental Hygiene Prgm

Dublin

Oconee Fall Line Technical College
Randall L Peters, MA, President
560 Pinehill Rd
Dublin, GA 31021
478 275-6590
Type: Vocational or Tech Sch
Control: State, County, or Local Govt
• Medical Assistant Prgm
• Radiography Prgm
• Respiratory Care Prgm

Fort Valley

Fort Valley State University
Larry E Rivers, PhD, President
1005 State University Dr
Fort Valley, GA 31030-4313
478 825-6315
Type: 4-year Coll or Univ
Control: State, County, or Local Govt
• Dietetics-Didactic Prgm
• Rehabilitation Counseling Prgm
• Veterinary Technology Prgm

Gainesville

Brenau University
Wanda Saed, PhD, President
500 Washington SE
Gainesville, GA 30501
770 534-6110
Type: 4-year Coll or Univ
Control: For Profit
• Nursing Prgm
• Occupational Therapy Prgm (2)

Griffin

Southern Crescent Technical College
Robert Arnold, EdD, CEO
501 Varsity Rd
Griffin, GA 30223
770 228-7365
Type: Vocational or Tech Sch
Control: State, County, or Local Govt
• Dental Assistant Prgm
• Medical Assistant Prgm
• Respiratory Care Prgm
• Surgical Technology Prgm

Kennesaw

Kennesaw State University
Daniel Papp, President
1000 Chastain Rd
Kennesaw, GA 30144-5591
770 423-6033
Type: 4-year Coll or Univ
Control: State, County, or Local Govt
• Cytogenetic Technology Prgm
• Music Therapy Prgm
• Nursing Prgm

LaFayette

Dalton State College
John Schwenn, PhD, President
650 College Drive
LaFayette, GA 30720-3778
706 272-4438
Type: 4-year Coll or Univ
Control: State, County, or Local Govt
• Clin Lab Technician/Med Lab Technician Prgm
• Medical Assistant Prgm
• Phlebotomy Prgm
• Radiography Prgm

LaGrange

West Georgia Technical College
Perrin Alford, MBA, Interim President
One College Circle
LaGrange, GA 30240
706 845-4323
Type: Vocational or Tech Sch
Control: State, County, or Local Govt
• Radiography Prgm

Lawrenceville

Gwinnett Technical College
Sharon Bartels, ABJ MEd, President
5150 Sugarloaf Parkway
Lawrenceville, GA 30043
678 226-6602
Type: Junior or Comm Coll
Control: State, County, or Local Govt
• Dental Assistant Prgm
• Emergency Med Tech-Paramedic Prgm
• Medical Assistant Prgm
• Radiography Prgm
• Respiratory Care Prgm
• Surgical Technology Prgm
• Veterinary Technology Prgm

Macon

Central Georgia Technical College
Ronald D Natale II, PhD, President
3300 Macon Tech Dr
Macon, GA 31206
478 757-3501
Type: Vocational or Tech Sch
Control: State, County, or Local Govt
• Clin Lab Technician/Med Lab Technician Prgm
• Dental Hygiene Prgm
• Surgical Technology Prgm

Macon State College
David Bell, PhD, President
100 College Station Dr
Macon, GA 31206-5145
478 471-2700
Type: 4-year Coll or Univ
Control: State, County, or Local Govt
• Respiratory Care Prgm

Mercer University
William D Underwood, President
Macon, GA 31207
478 301-2500
Type: 4-year Coll or Univ
Control: Nonprofit (Private or Religious)
• Allopathic Medicine Prgm
• Nursing Prgm
• Pharmacy Prgm
• Physician Assistant Prgm

Miller-Motte Technical College - Macon
(McCann School of Business & Technology)
175 Tom Hill Senior Road
Macon, GA 31210
Type: Vocational or Tech Sch
Control: For Profit
• Clin Lab Technician/Med Lab Technician Prgm

Marietta

Chattahoochee Technical College
Kary Porter, BBA, Acting President
980 S Cobb Dr
Marietta, GA 30060
770 528-4500
Type: Vocational or Tech Sch
Control: State, County, or Local Govt
• Clin Lab Technician/Med Lab Technician Prgm
• Medical Assistant Prgm
• Surgical Technology Prgm

Everest College-Marietta
Marietta, GA 30067
Type: Vocational or Tech Sch
• Surgical Technology Prgm

Life University
Sid E Williams, President
1269 Barclay Cir
Marietta, GA 30060
404 424-0554
Type: 4-year Coll or Univ
Control: Nonprofit (Private or Religious)
• Chiropractic Prgm
• Dietetic Internship Prgm
• Dietetics-Didactic Prgm

Milledgeville

Georgia College & State University
Dorothy Leland, President
Milledgeville, GA 31061
478 445-4444
Type: 4-year Coll or Univ
Control: State, County, or Local Govt
• Athletic Training Prgm
• Music Therapy Prgm

Morrow

Clayton State University
Thomas K Harden, EdD, President
2000 Clayton State Blvd
Morrow, GA 30260
678 466-4300
Type: 4-year Coll or Univ
Control: State, County, or Local Govt
• Dental Hygiene Prgm
• Nursing Prgm

Moultrie

Moultrie Technical College
Tina Anderson, EdD, President
800 Veterans Pkwy N
Moultrie, GA 31788
229 891-7000
Type: Vocational or Tech Sch
Control: State, County, or Local Govt
• Medical Assistant Prgm
• Radiography Prgm
• Surgical Technology Prgm

Oakwood

Lanier Technical College
Michael Moye, EdD, President
2990 Landrum Education Dr
Oakwood, GA 30566-0058
770 531-6300
Type: Vocational or Tech Sch
Control: State, County, or Local Govt
• Clin Lab Technician/Med Lab Technician Prgm
• Dental Assistant Prgm
• Dental Hygiene Prgm
• Medical Assistant Prgm (3)
• Radiography Prgm
• Surgical Technology Prgm

Riverdale

Southern Regional Medical Center
11 Upper Riverdale Rd SW
Riverdale, GA 30274-2600
770 991-8053
Type: Hosp or Med Ctr: 300-499 Beds
Control: Nonprofit (Private or Religious)
• Dietetic Internship Prgm

Rock Spring

Georgia Northwestern Technical College
Jeff King, EdD, Interim President
PO Box 569
265 Bicentennial Trail
Rock Spring, GA 30739
706 764-3530
Type: Vocational or Tech Sch
Control: State, County, or Local Govt
• Medical Assistant Prgm
• Occupational Therapy Asst Prgm
• Surgical Technology Prgm

Rome

Georgia Highlands College
Randy Pierce, President
3175 Cedartown Hwy SE
Rome, GA 30161
706 802-5000
Type: Junior or Comm Coll
Control: State, County, or Local Govt
• Dental Hygiene Prgm

Georgia Northwestern Technical College
Craig McDaniel, EdD, President
One Maurice Culberson Dr
Rome, GA 30161
706 295-6927
Type: Vocational or Tech Sch
Control: State, County, or Local Govt
• Dental Assistant Prgm
• Diagnostic Med Sonography
  (Gen/Card/Vascular) Prgm
• Emergency Med Tech-Paramedic Prgm
• Medical Assistant Prgm
• Radiation Therapy Prgm
• Radiography Prgm
• Respiratory Care Prgm

Savannah

Armstrong Atlantic State University
Thomas Jones, PhD, President
11935 Abercorn St
Savannah, GA 31419-1997
912 344-2821
Type: 4-year Coll or Univ
Control: State, County, or Local Govt
- Clin Lab Scientist/Med Technologist Prgm
- Dental Hygiene Prgm
- Nuclear Medicine Technology Prgm
- Nursing Prgm
- Physical Therapy Prgm
- Radiation Therapy Prgm
- Radiography Prgm
- Respiratory Care Prgm
- Speech-Language Pathology Prgm

Savannah Technical College
Terry D Elam, BA M Ed, Interim President
5717 White Bluff Rd
Savannah, GA 31405-5521
912 443-3495
Type: Vocational or Tech Sch
Control: State, County, or Local Govt
- Dental Assistant Prgm
- Dental Hygiene Prgm
- Medical Assistant Prgm
- Surgical Technology Prgm

South University
John South, Chancellor
709 Mall Blvd
Savannah, GA 31406
912 201-8000
Type: 4-year Coll or Univ
Control: For Profit
- Anesthesiologist Asst Prgm
- Medical Assistant Prgm
- Nursing Prgm
- Pharmacy Prgm
- Physical Therapist Assistant Prgm
- Physician Assistant Prgm

Smyrna

Fortis College
Smyrna, GA
- Dental Assistant Prgm
- Dental Hygiene Prgm

Statesboro

Georgia Southern University
Bruce F Grube, PhD, President
PO Box 8033
Marvin Pittman Admin Bldg
Statesboro, GA 30460-8033
912 681-5211
Type: 4-year Coll or Univ
Control: State, County, or Local Govt
- Athletic Training Prgm
- Dietetics-Didactic Prgm
- Music Therapy Prgm
- Nursing Prgm

Ogeechee Technical College
Dawn Cartee, EdD, President
One Joe Kennedy Blvd
Statesboro, GA 30458
912 681-5500
Type: Vocational or Tech Sch
Control: State, County, or Local Govt
- Cancer Registrar Prgm
- Dental Assistant Prgm
- Diagnostic Med Sonography (General/Cardiac) Prgm
- Medical Assistant Prgm
- Ophthalmic Dispensing Optician Prgm
- Pharmacy Technician Prgm
- Radiography Prgm
- Surgical Technology Prgm
- Veterinary Technology Prgm

Suwanee

Georgia Campus - PA Coll of Osteopathic Med
625 Old Peachtree Rd
Suwanee, GA 30024
Type: Acad Health Ctr/Med Sch
Control: Nonprofit (Private or Religious)
- Osteopathic Medicine Prgm

Thomasville

Southwest Georgia Technical College
Glenn Deibert, EdD, President
15689 US Hwy 19 North
Thomasville, GA 31792
229 225-5069
Type: Vocational or Tech Sch
Control: State, County, or Local Govt
- Clin Lab Technician/Med Lab Technician Prgm
- Medical Assistant Prgm
- Pharmacy Technician Prgm
- Respiratory Care Prgm
- Surgical Technology Prgm

Thomas University
Gary Bonvillian, PhD, President
Forbes Bldg
1501 Millpond Rd
Thomasville, GA 31792
229 226-1621
Type: 4-year Coll or Univ
Control: Nonprofit (Private or Religious)
- Clin Lab Scientist/Med Technologist Prgm
- Rehabilitation Counseling Prgm

Valdosta

Valdosta State University
Ronald M Zaccari, PhD, President
West Hall
Valdosta, GA 31698
229 333-5952
Type: 4-year Coll or Univ
Control: State, County, or Local Govt
- Athletic Training Prgm
- Music Therapy Prgm
- Nursing Prgm
- Speech-Language Pathology Prgm

Valdosta Technical College
F D Toth, President
4089 Valtech Rd
PO Box 928
Valdosta, GA 31602
229 333-2100
Type: Vocational or Tech Sch
Control: State, County, or Local Govt
- Pharmacy Technician Prgm

Wiregrass Georgia Technical College
Valdosta, GA 316030928
Type: Vocational or Tech Sch
- Clin Lab Technician/Med Lab Technician Prgm
- Dental Assistant Prgm
- Dental Hygiene Prgm
- Surgical Technology Prgm

Vidalia

Southeastern Technical College
Cathryn T Mitchell, EdD, President
3001 E First St
Vidalia, GA 30474
912 538-3101
Type: Vocational or Tech Sch
Control: State, County, or Local Govt
- Clin Lab Technician/Med Lab Technician Prgm
- Dental Hygiene Prgm
- Medical Assistant Prgm
- Pharmacy Technician Prgm
- Radiography Prgm
- Surgical Technology Prgm

Waco

West Georgia Technical College
Skip Sullivan, EdD, President
176 Murphy Campus Blvd
Waco, GA 30182
770 537-7976
Type: Vocational or Tech Sch
Control: State, County, or Local Govt
- Clin Lab Technician/Med Lab Technician Prgm
- Dental Hygiene Prgm
- Medical Assistant Prgm
- Radiography Prgm
- Surgical Technology Prgm

Warner Robins

Middle Georgia Technical College
Ivan Allen, EdD, President
80 Cohen Walker Dr
Warner Robins, GA 31088
478 988-6833
Type: Vocational or Tech Sch
Control: State, County, or Local Govt
- Dental Hygiene Prgm
- Radiography Prgm
- Surgical Technology Prgm

Waycross

Okefenokee Technical College
Gail Thaxton, EdD, President
1701 Carswell Ave
Waycross, GA 31503
912 287-5828
Type: Vocational or Tech Sch
Control: State, County, or Local Govt
• Clin Lab Technician/Med Lab Technician Prgm
• Medical Assistant Prgm
• Radiography Prgm
• Surgical Technology Prgm

Guam

GMF Barrigada

Guam Community College
Herominiano Delos Santos, EdD, President
PO Box 23069
GMF Barrigada, GU 96921
671 735-5636
Type: Junior or Comm Coll
Control: State, County, or Local Govt
• Medical Assistant Prgm (2)

Hawaii

Hilo

University of Hawaii at Hilo
Hilo, HI 96720
Type: 4-year Coll or Univ
Control: State, County, or Local Govt
• Pharmacy Prgm

Honolulu

Argosy University
Honolulu, HI 96813
Type: 4-year Coll or Univ
Control: For Profit
• Psychology (PsyD) Prgm

Heald College - Honolulu Campus
Evelyn A Schemmel, BS, Executive Director
1500 Kapiolani Blvd
Honolulu, HI 96814
808 955-1500
Type: Junior or Comm Coll
Control: For Profit
• Dental Assistant Prgm
• Medical Assistant Prgm

Kapiolani Community College
Leon Richards, PhD, Chancellor
4303 Diamond Head Rd
Ilima Bldg, Rm 213
Honolulu, HI 96816-4421
808 734-9000
Type: Junior or Comm Coll
Control: State, County, or Local Govt
• Clin Lab Technician/Med Lab Technician Prgm
• Medical Assistant Prgm
• Occupational Therapy Asst Prgm
• Phlebotomy Prgm
• Physical Therapist Assistant Prgm
• Radiography Prgm
• Respiratory Care Prgm
• Surgical Technology Prgm

University of Hawaii at Manoa
David McClain, Interim Chancellor
2444 Dole Street
Bachman Hall 202
Honolulu, HI 96822
808 956-8207
Type: 4-year Coll or Univ
Control: State, County, or Local Govt
• Allopathic Medicine Prgm
• Athletic Training Prgm
• Clin Lab Scientist/Med Technologist Prgm
• Dental Hygiene Prgm
• Dietetics-Didactic Prgm
• Medical Librarian Prgm
• Music Therapy Prgm
• Nursing Prgm
• Psychology (PhD) Prgm
• Rehabilitation Counseling Prgm
• Speech-Language Pathology Prgm

Kahului

Maui Community College
310 Kaahumana Ave
Kahului, HI 96732
808 984-3500
Type: Junior or Comm Coll
Control: State, County, or Local Govt
• Dental Assistant Prgm

University of Hawaii Maui College
Kahului, HI 96732
• Dental Hygiene Prgm

Idaho

Boise

Boise State University
Robert Kustra, PhD, President
1910 University Dr
Boise, ID 83725-1000
208 426-1491
Type: 4-year Coll or Univ
Control: State, County, or Local Govt
• Athletic Training Prgm
• Counseling Prgm
• Diagnostic Med Sonography (General) Prgm
• Music Therapy Prgm
• Radiography Prgm
• Respiratory Care Prgm

Brown Mackie College - Boise
Steven Kalina, Campus President
9050 W Overland Rd
Suite 100
Boise, ID 83709-6281
208 321-8760
Type: Junior or Comm Coll
Control: For Profit
• Occupational Therapy Asst Prgm

Carrington College of Boise
Lois Hine, RN PhD, Executive Director
1200 N Liberty St
Boise, ID 83704
208 672-0710
Type: Vocational or Tech Sch
Control: For Profit
• Dental Assistant Prgm
• Dental Hygiene Prgm

College of Western Idaho
Boise, ID 83725-2005
Type: Junior or Comm Coll
• Dental Assistant Prgm
• Surgical Technology Prgm

Coeur d'Alene

North Idaho College
Priscilla Bell, PhD, President
1000 W Garden Ave
Coeur d'Alene, ID 83814
208 769-3300
Type: Junior or Comm Coll
Control: State, County, or Local Govt
• Radiography Prgm

Idaho Falls

Eastern Idaho Technical College
William Robertson, MEd, President
1600 South 2500 East
Idaho Falls, ID 83404-5788
208 524-3000
Type: Vocational or Tech Sch
Control: State, County, or Local Govt
• Medical Assistant Prgm
• Surgical Technology Prgm

Lewiston

Lewis-Clark State College
Dene Thomas, PhD, President
500 8th Ave
Lewiston, ID 83501
208 792-2216
Type: 4-year Coll or Univ
Control: State, County, or Local Govt
• Medical Assistant Prgm
• Nursing Prgm

Moscow

University of Idaho
Steven Daley-Laursen, PhD, President
PO Box 443151
Moscow, ID 83844-3151
208 885-6365
Type: 4-year Coll or Univ
Control: State, County, or Local Govt
• Athletic Training Prgm
• Counseling Prgm
• Dietetics-Coordinated Prgm
• Music Therapy Prgm
• Rehabilitation Counseling Prgm

Nampa

Northwest Nazarene University
Richard A Hagood, President
623 Holly St
Nampa, ID 83686-5897
208 467-8011
Type: 4-year Coll or Univ
Control: State, County, or Local Govt
• Counseling Prgm
• Music Therapy Prgm
• Nursing Prgm

Pocatello

Idaho State University
Arthur C Vailas, PhD, President
921S, 8th Ave Stop 8310
Administration B
Pocatello, ID 83209
208 282-3440
Type: 4-year Coll or Univ
Control: State, County, or Local Govt
• Audiologist Prgm
• Clin Lab Scientist/Med Technologist Prgm
• Counseling Prgm
• Dental Hygiene Prgm
• Dietetic Internship Prgm
• Dietetics-Didactic Prgm
• Emergency Med Tech-Paramedic Prgm
• Medical Assistant Prgm
• Music Therapy Prgm
• Nursing Prgm
• Occupational Therapy Prgm
• Pharmacy Prgm
• Physical Therapist Assistant Prgm
• Physical Therapy Prgm
• Physician Assistant Prgm
• Psychology (PhD) Prgm
• Speech-Language Pathology Prgm

Rexburg

Brigham Young University
Rexburg, ID 83460-1690
Type: 4-year Coll or Univ
• Emergency Med Tech-Paramedic Prgm
• Medical Assistant Prgm

Twin Falls

College of Southern Idaho
Jerry Beck, EdD, President
315 Falls Ave
PO Box 1238
Twin Falls, ID 83303-1238
208 732-6728
Type: Junior or Comm Coll
Control: State, County, or Local Govt
• Dental Hygiene Prgm
• Emergency Med Tech-Paramedic Prgm
• Medical Assistant Prgm
• Radiography Prgm
• Surgical Assistant Prgm
• Surgical Technology Prgm
• Veterinary Technology Prgm

Illinois

Aurora

Aurora University
Rebecca L Sherrick, PhD, President
347 S Gladstone Ave
Aurora, IL 60506-4892
630 844-5476
Type: 4-year Coll or Univ
Control: Nonprofit (Private or Religious)
• Athletic Training Prgm
• Nursing Prgm

Belleville

Southwestern Illinois College
Georgia Costello, PhD, President
2500 Carlyle Ave
Belleville, IL 62221-5899
618 235-2770
Type: Junior or Comm Coll
Control: State, County, or Local Govt
• Clin Lab Technician/Med Lab Technician Prgm
• Medical Assistant Prgm
• Physical Therapist Assistant Prgm
• Radiography Prgm
• Respiratory Care Prgm

Bloomington

Illinois Wesleyan University
Bloomington, IL 61702
Type: 4-year Coll or Univ
Control: Nonprofit (Private or Religious)
• Music Therapy Prgm
• Nursing Prgm

Bourbonnais

Olivet Nazarene University
John C Bowling, EdD, President
One University Ave
Bourbonnais, IL 60914
815 939-5011
Type: 4-year Coll or Univ
Control: Nonprofit (Private or Religious)
• Athletic Training Prgm
• Dietetics-Didactic Prgm
• Music Therapy Prgm
• Nursing Prgm

Carbondale

Southern Illinois University Carbondale
Samuel Goldman, PhD, Interim Chancellor
116 Anthony Hall, MC 6801
Carbondale, IL 62901
618 453-2341
Type: 4-year Coll or Univ
Control: State, County, or Local Govt
• Athletic Training Prgm
• Counseling Prgm
• Dental Hygiene Prgm
• Diagnostic Med Sonography (General) Prgm
• Dietetic Internship Prgm
• Dietetics-Didactic Prgm
• Medical Dosimetry Prgm
• Music Therapy Prgm
• Physical Therapist Assistant Prgm
• Physician Assistant Prgm
• Psychology (PhD) Prgm
• Radiation Therapy Prgm
• Rehabilitation Counseling Prgm
• Respiratory Care Prgm
• Speech-Language Pathology Prgm

Carterville

John A Logan College
Robert Mees, PhD, President
700 Logan College Rd
Carterville, IL 62918
618 985-2828
Type: Junior or Comm Coll
Control: Nonprofit (Private or Religious)
• Dental Assistant Prgm
• Dental Hygiene Prgm
• Diagnostic Med Sonography (Cardiac) Prgm

Centralia

Kaskaskia College
James Underwood, EdD, President
27210 College Rd
Centralia, IL 62801
618 545-3000
Type: Junior or Comm Coll
Control: State, County, or Local Govt
• Dental Assistant Prgm
• Physical Therapist Assistant Prgm
• Radiography Prgm
• Respiratory Care Prgm

Champaign

Parkland College
Thomas Ramage, EdD, President
2400 W Bradley Ave
Champaign, IL 61821-1899
217 351-2231
Type: Junior or Comm Coll
Control: State, County, or Local Govt
• Dental Hygiene Prgm
• Dietetic Technician-AD Prgm
• Occupational Therapy Asst Prgm
• Radiography Prgm
• Respiratory Care Prgm
• Surgical Technology Prgm
• Veterinary Technology Prgm

Univ of Illinois at Urbana-Champaign
Richard Herman, PhD, Chancellor
317 Swanlund Admin
MC 304
Champaign, IL 61801
217 333-6290
Type: 4-year Coll or Univ
Control: State, County, or Local Govt
• Athletic Training Prgm
• Audiologist Prgm
• Dietetic Internship Prgm
• Dietetics-Didactic Prgm
• Medical Librarian Prgm
• Music Therapy Prgm
• Psychology (PhD) Prgm
• Rehabilitation Counseling Prgm
• Speech-Language Pathology Prgm
• Veterinary Medicine Prgm

Charleston

Eastern Illinois University
William Perry, PhD, President
600 Lincoln Ave
Charleston, IL 61920
217 581-2011
Type: 4-year Coll or Univ
Control: State, County, or Local Govt
• Athletic Training Prgm
• Counseling Prgm
• Dietetic Internship Prgm
• Dietetics-Didactic Prgm
• Music Therapy Prgm
• Nursing Prgm
• Speech-Language Pathology Prgm

Chicago

Adler School of Professional Psychology
Ray Crossman, PhD, President
65 E Wacker Pl, Ste 2100
Chicago, IL 60601-7203
312 201-5900
Type: 4-year Coll or Univ
Control: Nonprofit (Private or Religious)
• Art Therapy Prgm
• Psychology (PsyD) Prgm

American Health Information Management Assoc
233 N Michigan Ave
Chicago, IL 60601
Control: For Profit
• Cancer Registrar Prgm

Argosy University
Chicago, IL 60654
Type: 4-year Coll or Univ
Control: For Profit
• Psychology (PsyD) Prgm (2)

Chicago School of Massage Therapy
Jason Scholte, President
17 N State, 5th Fl
Chicago, IL 60602
312 753-7900
Type: Vocational or Tech Sch
Control: For Profit
• Massage Therapy Prgm (2)

Chicago School of Professional Psychology
Chicago, IL 60610
Type: Acad Health Ctr/Med Sch
Control: Nonprofit (Private or Religious)
• Psychology (PsyD) Prgm

Chicago State University
Wayne Watson, PhD, President
9501 S King Dr
Chicago, IL 60628-1598
773 995-2400
Type: 4-year Coll or Univ
Control: State, County, or Local Govt
• Counseling Prgm
• Occupational Therapy Prgm
• Pharmacy Prgm

Children's Memorial Hospital of Chicago
Patrick M Magoon, President and CEO
2300 Children's Plaza, Box 70
Chicago, IL 60614-3394
773 880-4000
Type: Hosp or Med Ctr: 500 Beds
Control: Nonprofit (Private or Religious)
• Orthoptist Prgm

Columbia College
Warrick L Carter, PhD, President
600 S Michigan
Chicago, IL 60605-9988
Type: 4-year Coll or Univ
Control: State, County, or Local Govt
• Dance/Movement Therapy Prgm

DePaul University
Rev John Richardson, President
25 E Jackson Blvd
Chicago, IL 60604
312 341-8000
Type: 4-year Coll or Univ
Control: Nonprofit (Private or Religious)
• Music Therapy Prgm
• Nursing Prgm
• Psychology (PhD) Prgm

Henrotin Hospital Corp
Edward E Bruun, President
111 W Oak St
Chicago, IL 60610
312 440-7801
Type: Hosp or Med Ctr: 300-499 Beds
Control: Nonprofit (Private or Religious)
• Pharmacy Prgm

Illinois College of Optometry
Arol Augsburger, OD MS, President
3241 S Michigan Ave
Chicago, IL 60616
312 949-7400
Type: Junior or Comm Coll
Control: Nonprofit (Private or Religious)
• Optometry Prgm

Illinois Institute of Technology
Lewis M Collens, President
3300 S Federal St
Chicago, IL 60616
312 567-3000
Type: 4-year Coll or Univ
Control: Nonprofit (Private or Religious)
• Psychology (PhD) Prgm
• Rehabilitation Counseling Prgm

John H. Stroger Hospital of Cook County
Ghingo W Brooks
1900 W Van Buren St
Room 1100
Chicago, IL 60612
312 850-7037
• Physician Assistant Prgm

Kaplan University
Chicago, IL 60607
Type: 4-year Coll or Univ
Control: For Profit
• Medical Assistant Prgm
• Nursing Prgm

Kennedy-King College
Wayne Watson, President
6800 S Wentworth Ave
Chicago, IL 60621
773 602-5229
Type: Junior or Comm Coll
Control: State, County, or Local Govt
• Dental Hygiene Prgm

Loyola University of Chicago
John J Piderit, President
820 N Michigan Ave
Chicago, IL 60611
312 915-6000
Type: 4-year Coll or Univ
Control: Nonprofit (Private or Religious)
• Allopathic Medicine Prgm
• Clin Lab Scientist/Med Technologist Prgm
• Dietetic Internship Prgm
• Nursing Prgm
• Psychology (PhD) Prgm

Malcolm X College
Zerrie D Campbell, MS MA, President
1900 W Van Buren St
Chicago, IL 60612
312 850-7037
Type: Junior or Comm Coll
Control: State, County, or Local Govt
• Pharmacy Technician Prgm
• Radiography Prgm
• Respiratory Care Prgm
• Surgical Technology Prgm

National Latino Education Institute
Mary Gonzalez-Koenig, President
2011 W Pershing Rd
Chicago, IL 60608
773 247-0707
Type: Acad Health Ctr/Med Sch
Control: Nonprofit (Private or Religious)
• Medical Assistant Prgm

North Park University
David L Parkyn, President
3225 W Foster Ave
Chicago, IL 60625
773 244-5710
Type: 4-year Coll or Univ
Control: Nonprofit (Private or Religious)
• Athletic Training Prgm
• Nursing Prgm

Northeastern Illinois University
5500 N St Louis Ave
Chicago, IL 60625-4699
773 583-4050
Type: 4-year Coll or Univ
Control: State, County, or Local Govt
- Counseling Prgm
- Music Therapy Prgm
- Rehabilitation Counseling Prgm

Northwestern Memorial Hospital
Dean Harrison, MBA, President and CEO
251 E Huron St
Feinberg 3-710
Chicago, IL 60611
312 926-3007
Type: Hosp or Med Ctr: 500 Beds
Control: Nonprofit (Private or Religious)
- Diagnostic Med Sonography (General) Prgm
- Nuclear Medicine Technology Prgm
- Radiation Therapy Prgm
- Radiography Prgm

Olive Harvey College
Valerie R Roberson, PhD, Interim President
10001 S Woodlawn Ave
Chicago, IL 60628
773 291-6313
Type: Junior or Comm Coll
Control: State, County, or Local Govt
- Respiratory Care Prgm

Robert Morris University
Michael Viollt, President
401 S State St
Chicago, IL 60605
312 935-6600
Type: 4-year Coll or Univ
Control: Nonprofit (Private or Religious)
- Medical Assistant Prgm (2)
- Surgical Technology Prgm

Roosevelt University
Charles R Middleton, PhD, President
430 S Michigan Ave
Chicago, IL 60605-1394
312 341-3500
Type: 4-year Coll or Univ
Control: Nonprofit (Private or Religious)
- Counseling Prgm
- Psychology (PsyD) Prgm

Rush University
Larry J Goodman, MD, President
Suite 140-143 AAC
600 South Paulina Street
Chicago, IL 60612-3833
312 942-7073
Type: Acad Health Ctr/Med Sch
Control: Nonprofit (Private or Religious)
- Allopathic Medicine Prgm
- Clin Lab Scientist/Med Technologist Prgm
- Diagnostic Med Sonography (Vascular) Prgm
- Occupational Therapy Prgm
- Perfusion Prgm
- Physician Assistant Prgm
- Specialist in BB Tech Prgm

Rush University Medical Center
Larry Goodman, MD, President and CEO
1725 W Harrison St, Ste 364
Chicago, IL 60612
312 942-7073
Type: Acad Health Ctr/Med Sch
Control: Nonprofit (Private or Religious)
- Audiologist Prgm
- Dietetic Internship Prgm
- Speech-Language Pathology Prgm

Saint Xavier University
Richard A Yanikoski, President
3700 W 103rd St
Chicago, IL 60655
312 298-3561
Type: 4-year Coll or Univ
Control: Nonprofit (Private or Religious)
- Nursing Prgm
- Speech-Language Pathology Prgm

School of the Art Institute of Chicago
Lisa Wainwright, PhD, Dean of Faculty
37 S Wabash Ave
Chicago, IL 60603
312 899-1291
Type: 4-year Coll or Univ
Control: Nonprofit (Private or Religious)
- Art Therapy Prgm

St Augustine College
Andrew Sund, MS, President
1333-45 W Argyle St
Chicago, IL 60640
773 878-7502
Type: Junior or Comm Coll
Control: Nonprofit (Private or Religious)
- Respiratory Care Prgm

University of Chicago
Chicago, IL 60637
Type: 4-year Coll or Univ
Control: Nonprofit (Private or Religious)
- Allopathic Medicine Prgm

University of Illinois at Chicago
R Michael Tanner, PhD, Provost
University Hall
601 S Morgan St M/C 105
Chicago, IL 60612-7128
312 413-3450
Type: 4-year Coll or Univ
Control: State, County, or Local Govt
- Allopathic Medicine Prgm
- Dentistry Prgm
- Dietetics-Coordinated Prgm
- Dietetics-Didactic Prgm
- Medical Illustrator Prgm
- Nursing Prgm
- Occupational Therapy Prgm
- Pharmacy Prgm
- Physical Therapy Prgm
- Psychology (PhD) Prgm

Westwood College
Lou Pagano, MS, Executive Director
8501 W Higgins Rd
Chicago, IL 60631
847 928-1710
Type: Vocational or Tech Sch
Control: For Profit
- Medical Assistant Prgm (2)

Wright College
Charles P Guengerich, PhD, President
4300 N Narragansett Ave
Chicago, IL 60634
773 777-7900
Type: Junior or Comm Coll
Control: State, County, or Local Govt
- Occupational Therapy Asst Prgm
- Radiography Prgm

Chicago Heights

Prairie State College
Eric Radkte, MA, Interim President
202 S Halsted
Chicago Heights, IL 60411
708 709-3500
Type: Junior or Comm Coll
Control: State, County, or Local Govt
- Dental Hygiene Prgm
- Surgical Technology Prgm

Cicero

Morton College
Brent Knight, PhD, President
3801 S Central Ave
Cicero, IL 60804
708 656-8000
Type: Junior or Comm Coll
Control: State, County, or Local Govt
- Massage Therapy Prgm
- Physical Therapist Assistant Prgm

Collinsville

Sanford-Brown College - Collinsville
1101 Eastport Plaza Drive
Collinsville, IL 62234
Type: Vocational or Tech Sch
Control: For Profit
- Clin Lab Technician/Med Lab Technician Prgm

Danville

Danville Area Community College
Alice M Jacobs, PhD, President
2000 E Main St
Danville, IL 61832
217 443-8848
Type: Junior or Comm Coll
Control: State, County, or Local Govt
- Radiography Prgm

Lakeview College of Nursing
Danville, IL 61832
Type: Acad Health Ctr/Med Sch
Control: Nonprofit (Private or Religious)
- Nursing Prgm

Decatur

Millikin University
Douglas E Zemke, President
1184 W Main
Decatur, IL 62522
800 373-7733
Type: 4-year Coll or Univ
Control: Nonprofit (Private or Religious)
- Athletic Training Prgm
- Music Therapy Prgm
- Nursing Prgm

INSTITUTIONS

Richland Community College
Gayle Saunders, PhD, President
1 College Park
Decatur, IL 62521-8512
217 875-7200
Type: Junior or Comm Coll
Control: State, County, or Local Govt
• Medical Transcriptionist Prgm
• Surgical Technology Prgm

Deerfield

Trinity International University
Gregory L Waybright, PhD, President
2065 Half Day Rd
Deerfield, IL 60015
Type: 4-year Coll or Univ
Control: State, County, or Local Govt
• Athletic Training Prgm

DeKalb

Northern Illinois University
John Peters, PhD, President
Altgeld 300A
DeKalb, IL 60115
815 753-9500
Type: 4-year Coll or Univ
Control: State, County, or Local Govt
• Athletic Training Prgm
• Audiologist Prgm
• Clin Lab Scientist/Med Technologist Prgm
• Counseling Prgm
• Dietetic Internship Prgm
• Dietetics-Didactic Prgm
• Music Therapy Prgm
• Nursing Prgm
• Orientation and Mobility Specialist Prgm
• Physical Therapy Prgm
• Psychology (PhD) Prgm
• Rehabilitation Counseling Prgm
• Speech-Language Pathology Prgm
• Teacher of the Visually Impaired Prgm
• Vision Rehabilitation Therapy Prgm

Des Plaines

Oakton Community College
Margaret B Lee, PhD, President
1600 E Golf Rd
Des Plaines, IL 60016
847 635-1801
Type: Junior or Comm Coll
Control: State, County, or Local Govt
• Clin Lab Technician/Med Lab Technician Prgm
• Physical Therapist Assistant Prgm

Dixon

Sauk Valley Community College
George J Mihel, EdD, President
173 IL Rte 2
Dixon, IL 61021-9110
815 288-5511
Type: Junior or Comm Coll
Control: State, County, or Local Govt
• Radiography Prgm

Downers Grove

Advocate Good Samaritan Hospital
Downers Grove, IL 60515
Type: Hosp or Med Ctr d Beds
• Emergency Med Tech-Paramedic Prgm

Chamberlain College of Nursing
Downers Grove, IL 60515
Type: 4-year Coll or Univ
Control: For Profit
• Nursing Prgm

Midwestern University
Kathleen H Goepplinger, PhD, President
555 31st St
Downers Grove, IL 60515-1235
630 515-7300
Type: Acad Health Ctr/Med Sch
Control: Nonprofit (Private or Religious)
• Dentistry Prgm
• Occupational Therapy Prgm
• Osteopathic Medicine Prgm
• Pharmacy Prgm
• Physical Therapy Prgm
• Physician Assistant Prgm

East Peoria

Illinois Central College
John S Erwin, President
One College Dr
East Peoria, IL 61635-0001
309 694-5520
Type: Junior or Comm Coll
Control: State, County, or Local Govt
• Clin Lab Technician/Med Lab Technician Prgm
• Dental Hygiene Prgm
• Medical Assistant Prgm
• Occupational Therapy Asst Prgm
• Physical Therapist Assistant Prgm
• Radiography Prgm
• Respiratory Care Prgm
• Surgical Technology Prgm

Edwardsville

Southern Illinois University Edwardsville
Vaughn Vandegrift, PhD, Chancellor
Box 1151
Edwardsville, IL 62026
618 650-2475
Type: 4-year Coll or Univ
Control: State, County, or Local Govt
• Allopathic Medicine Prgm
• Art Therapy Prgm
• Counseling Prgm
• Dentistry Prgm
• Music Therapy Prgm
• Nursing Prgm
• Pharmacy Prgm
• Speech-Language Pathology Prgm

Elgin

Elgin Community College
David Sam, PhD, President
1700 Spartan Dr
Elgin, IL 60123-7193
847 214-7374
Type: Junior or Comm Coll
Control: State, County, or Local Govt
• Clin Lab Technician/Med Lab Technician Prgm
• Dental Assistant Prgm
• Histotechnician Prgm
• Massage Therapy Prgm
• Physical Therapist Assistant Prgm
• Radiography Prgm
• Surgical Technology Prgm

Elmhurst

Elmhurst College
Elmhurst, IL 60126
Type: 4-year Coll or Univ
Control: Nonprofit (Private or Religious)
• Nursing Prgm

Evanston

NorthShore University Health System
J P Gallagher, President/CEO
Hospitals and Clinics, Evanston Hospital
2650 Ridge Ave
Evanston, IL 60201
847 570-2005
Type: Acad Health Ctr/Med Sch
Control: Other
• Clin Lab Scientist/Med Technologist Prgm

Northwestern University
Henry S Bienen, PhD, President
2299 Sheridan Rd
Evanston, IL 60201
708 491-7456
Type: 4-year Coll or Univ
Control: Nonprofit (Private or Religious)
• Allopathic Medicine Prgm
• Audiologist Prgm
• Genetic Counseling Prgm
• Music Therapy Prgm
• Orthotist/Prosthetist Prgm
• Physical Therapy Prgm
• Physician Assistant Prgm
• Psychology (PhD) Prgm (2)
• Speech-Language Pathology Prgm

St Francis Hospital
Jeffrey Murphy, CEO
355 Ridge Ave
Evanston, IL 60202
847 492-4000
Type: Hosp or Med Ctr: 300-499 Beds
Control: Nonprofit (Private or Religious)
• Radiography Prgm

Freeport

Highland Community College
Freeport, IL 61032-9973
Type: Junior or Comm Coll
• Medical Assistant Prgm

Galesburg

Carl Sandburg College
Thomas A Schmidt, MBA, President
2400 Tom L Wilson Blvd
Galesburg, IL 61401
309 344-2518
Type: Junior or Comm Coll
Control: State, County, or Local Govt
• Dental Hygiene Prgm

Glen Ellyn

College of DuPage
Harold D McAninich, PhD, President
425 Fawell Blvd
Glen Ellyn, IL 60137
630 942-2800
Type: Junior or Comm Coll
Control: State, County, or Local Govt
• Dental Hygiene Prgm
• Diagnostic Med Sonography (General/Vascular) Prgm
• Medical Assistant Prgm
• Nuclear Medicine Technology Prgm
• Physical Therapist Assistant Prgm
• Radiography Prgm
• Surgical Technology Prgm

Godfrey

Lewis & Clark Community College
Dale T Chapman, EdD, President
5800 Godfrey Rd
Godfrey, IL 62035-2466
618 468-2000
Type: Junior or Comm Coll
Control: State, County, or Local Govt
• Dental Assistant Prgm
• Dental Hygiene Prgm
• Occupational Therapy Asst Prgm

Grayslake

College of Lake County
Girard Weber, PhD, Interim President
19351 W Washington St
Grayslake, IL 60085
847 543-2000
Type: Junior or Comm Coll
Control: State, County, or Local Govt
• Dental Hygiene Prgm
• Medical Assistant Prgm
• Phlebotomy Prgm
• Radiography Prgm
• Surgical Technology Prgm

Harvey

Ingalls Memorial Hospital
One Ingalls Dr
Harvey, IL 60426
708 333-2300
Type: Hosp or Med Ctr: 300-499 Beds
Control: Nonprofit (Private or Religious)
• Dietetic Internship Prgm

Herrin

Southern Illinois Collegiate Common Market
Mary J Sullivan, PhD, Executive Director
3213 S Park Ave
Herrin, IL 62948
618 942-6902
Type: Consortium
Control: State, County, or Local Govt
• Clin Lab Technician/Med Lab Technician Prgm
• Occupational Therapy Asst Prgm
• Surgical Technology Prgm

Hines

Edward Hines Jr. VA Hospital
Nathan Geraths, Director
Fifth Ave and Roosevelt Rd
PO Box 5000
Hines, IL 60141-3030
708 202-2153
Type: Dept of Veterans Affairs
Control: Fed Govt
• Clin Lab Scientist/Med Technologist Prgm
• Dietetic Internship Prgm

Ina

Rend Lake College
468 N Ken Gray Pkwy
Ina, IL 62846
Type: Junior or Comm Coll
Control: State, County, or Local Govt
• Radiography Prgm

Jacksonville

MacMurray College
Jacksonville, IL 62650
Type: 4-year Coll or Univ
Control: Nonprofit (Private or Religious)
• Nursing Prgm

Joliet

Joliet Junior College
Gena Proulx, PhD, President
1215 Houbolt Rd
Joliet, IL 60431
815 280-2207
Type: Junior or Comm Coll
Control: State, County, or Local Govt
• Veterinary Technology Prgm

University of St Francis
Connie Bauer, PhD, Provost
500 Wilcox St
Joliet, IL 60435
815 740-3369
Type: 4-year Coll or Univ
Control: Nonprofit (Private or Religious)
• Nursing Prgm

Kankakee

Kankakee Community College
Larry Huffman, Interim President
100 College Drive
Kankakee, IL 60901-0888
815 802-8110
Type: Junior or Comm Coll
Control: State, County, or Local Govt
• Clin Lab Technician/Med Lab Technician Prgm
• Physical Therapist Assistant Prgm
• Respiratory Care Prgm

Lebanon

McKendree University
James M Dennis, PhD, President
701 College Rd
Lebanon, IL 62254-1299
618 537-6936
Type: 4-year Coll or Univ
Control: Nonprofit (Private or Religious)
• Athletic Training Prgm
• Nursing Prgm

Lincoln

Midwest Technical Institute
Brian Huff, President
405 N Limit St
PO Box 506
Lincoln, IL 62656
217 735-3105
Type: Vocational or Tech Sch
Control: For Profit
• Medical Assistant Prgm
• Pharmacy Technician Prgm (2)

Lisle

Benedictine University
William J Carroll, President
5700 College Rd
Lisle, IL 60532
708 960-1500
Type: 4-year Coll or Univ
Control: Nonprofit (Private or Religious)
• Dietetic Internship Prgm
• Dietetics-Didactic Prgm
• Nursing Prgm

Lombard

National University of Health Sciences
James F Winterstein, DC, President
200 E Roosevelt Rd
Lombard, IL 60148
630 889-6604
Type: Acad Health Ctr/Med Sch
Control: Nonprofit (Private or Religious)
• Chiropractic Prgm
• Massage Therapy Prgm

Macomb

McDonough District Hospital
Stephen R Hopper, MS, President
525 E Grant St
Macomb, IL 61455
309 833-4101
Type: Hosp or Med Ctr: 100-299 Beds
Control: State, County, or Local Govt
• Radiography Prgm

Western Illinois University
Al Goldfarb, PhD, President
209 Sherman Hall
1 University Circle
Macomb, IL 61455
309 298-1824
Type: 4-year Coll or Univ
Control: State, County, or Local Govt
• Athletic Training Prgm
• Counseling Prgm
• Dietetics-Didactic Prgm
• Music Therapy Prgm
• Nursing Prgm
• Speech-Language Pathology Prgm

Malta

Kishwaukee College
Thomas Choice, PhD, President
21193 Malta Rd
Malta, IL 60150
815 825-2086
Type: Junior or Comm Coll
Control: State, County, or Local Govt
• Massage Therapy Prgm
• Radiography Prgm

Mattoon

Lake Land College
Scott Lensink, MBA, President
5001 Lake Land Blvd
Mattoon, IL 61938-9366
217 234-5253
Type: Junior or Comm Coll
Control: State, County, or Local Govt
• Dental Hygiene Prgm
• Physical Therapist Assistant Prgm

Maywood

Loyola University Medical Center
Anthony Barbato, MD, Executive Vice President
2160 S First Ave
Maywood, IL 60153
708 216-9000
Type: Hosp or Med Ctr: 500 Beds
Control: Nonprofit (Private or Religious)
• Emergency Med Tech-Paramedic Prgm

Moline

Black Hawk College
Keith Miller, PhD, President
6600 34th Ave
Moline, IL 61265-5899
309 796-1311
Type: Junior or Comm Coll
Control: State, County, or Local Govt
• Physical Therapist Assistant Prgm

Naperville

North Central College
Harold R Wilde, PhD, President
30 N Brainard
Naperville, IL 60540
630 637-5454
Type: 4-year Coll or Univ
Control: Nonprofit (Private or Religious)
• Athletic Training Prgm

Normal

Heartland Community College
1500 W Raab Road
Normal, IL 61761
Type: Junior or Comm Coll
Control: State, County, or Local Govt
• Radiography Prgm

Illinois State University
C Alvin Bowman, PhD, President
1000 President's Office
418 Hovey Hall
Normal, IL 61790-1000
309 438-5677
Type: 4-year Coll or Univ
Control: State, County, or Local Govt
• Athletic Training Prgm
• Audiologist Prgm
• Clin Lab Scientist/Med Technologist Prgm
• Dietetic Internship Prgm
• Dietetics-Didactic Prgm
• Music Therapy Prgm
• Nursing Prgm
• Speech-Language Pathology Prgm

North Chicago

Rosalind Franklin University of Medicine
K Michael Welch, MBChB FRCP, President/CEO
3333 Green Bay Rd
North Chicago, IL 60064
847 578-3300
Type: Acad Health Ctr/Med Sch
Control: Nonprofit (Private or Religious)
• Allopathic Medicine Prgm
• Pathologists' Assistant Prgm
• Pharmacy Prgm
• Physical Therapy Prgm
• Physician Assistant Prgm
• Podiatric Medicine Prgm
• Psychology (PhD) Prgm

Oak Park

Resurrection University
Oak Park, IL 60302
Type: Acad Health Ctr/Med Sch
Control: Nonprofit (Private or Religious)
• Nursing Prgm

Oglesby

Illinois Valley Community College
Jean Goodnow, President
815 N Orlando Smith Ave
Oglesby, IL 61348-9691
815 224-2720
Type: Junior or Comm Coll
Control: State, County, or Local Govt
• Dental Assistant Prgm

Olney

Olney Central College
Jackie Davis, EdD, President
305 N West St
Olney, IL 62450
618 395-7777
Type: Junior or Comm Coll
Control: State, County, or Local Govt
• Radiography Prgm

Palatine

Harper College
Robert Breuder, PhD, President
1200 W Algonquin Rd
Palatine, IL 60067
847 925-6000
Type: Junior or Comm Coll
Control: State, County, or Local Govt
• Dental Hygiene Prgm
• Diagnostic Med Sonography (General/Cardiac) Prgm
• Dietetic Technician-AD Prgm
• Medical Assistant Prgm
• Radiography Prgm

Palos Heights

Trinity Christian College
Palos Heights, IL 60463
Type: 4-year Coll or Univ
Control: Nonprofit (Private or Religious)
• Nursing Prgm

Palos Hills

Moraine Valley Community College
Vernon Crawley, PhD, President/CEO
9000 W College Pkwy
President's Office
Palos Hills, IL 60465
708 974-4300
Type: Junior or Comm Coll
Control: State, County, or Local Govt
• Medical Assistant Prgm
• Phlebotomy Prgm
• Polysomnographic Technology Prgm
• Radiography Prgm
• Respiratory Care Prgm

Peoria

Bradley University
David Broski, President
1501 W Bradley Ave
Peoria, IL 61625
309 676-7611
Type: 4-year Coll or Univ
Control: Nonprofit (Private or Religious)
• Counseling Prgm
• Dietetic Internship Prgm
• Dietetics-Didactic Prgm
• Physical Therapy Prgm

Methodist College of Nursing
Peoria, IL 61603
Type: 4-year Coll or Univ
Control: Nonprofit (Private or Religious)
• Nursing Prgm

Midstate College
R Dale Bunch, President
411 W Northmoor Rd
Peoria, IL 61614
309 692-4092
Type: 4-year Coll or Univ
Control: For Profit
• Medical Assistant Prgm

OSF Saint Francis Medical Center
Keith Steffen, Administrator
530 NE Glen Oak Ave
Peoria, IL 61637
309 655-2439
Type: Hosp or Med Ctr: 500 Beds
Control: Nonprofit (Private or Religious)
• Clin Lab Scientist/Med Technologist Prgm
• Dietetic Internship Prgm
• Histotechnician Prgm
• Radiography Prgm

Quincy

Blessing Hospital
Maureen Kahn, RN MHA, President/CEO
Broadway at 11th St
PO Box 7005
Quincy, IL 62301
217 223-8400
Type: Hosp or Med Ctr: 300-499 Beds
Control: Nonprofit (Private or Religious)
• Clin Lab Technician/Med Lab Technician Prgm
• Nursing Prgm
• Pharmacy Technician Prgm
• Radiography Prgm

John Wood Community College
William M Simpson, EdD, President
1301 S 48th St
Quincy, IL 62305
217 224-6500
Type: Junior or Comm Coll
Control: State, County, or Local Govt
• Surgical Technology Prgm

River Forest

Concordia University
Manfred Booa, PhD, Acting President
7400 Augusta
River Forest, IL 60305-1499
708 771-8300
Type: Vocational or Tech Sch
Control: Nonprofit (Private or Religious)
• Counseling Prgm

Dominican University
Donna M Carroll, President
7900 W Division
River Forest, IL 60305
708 366-2490
Type: 4-year Coll or Univ
Control: Nonprofit (Private or Religious)
• Dietetics-Coordinated Prgm
• Dietetics-Didactic Prgm
• Medical Librarian Prgm

River Grove

Triton College
Patricia Granados, EdD, President
2000 N Fifth Ave
River Grove, IL 60171
708 456-0300
Type: Junior or Comm Coll
Control: State, County, or Local Govt
• Diagnostic Med Sonography (General) Prgm
• Nuclear Medicine Technology Prgm
• Ophthalmic Technician Prgm
• Radiography Prgm
• Respiratory Care Prgm
• Surgical Technology Prgm

Rock Island

Trinity College of Nursing & Health Sciences
Carol Dwyer, RN MSN MM, President
2122 25th Ave
Rock Island, IL 61201
309 779-2256
Type: 4-year Coll or Univ
Control: Nonprofit (Private or Religious)
• Nursing Prgm
• Radiography Prgm
• Surgical Technology Prgm

Rockford

OSF Saint Anthony Medical Center
David Schertz, CEO/President
5666 E State St
Rockford, IL 61108
815 226-2000
Type: Hosp or Med Ctr: 100-299 Beds
Control: Nonprofit (Private or Religious)
• Nursing Prgm

Rock Valley College
Jack J Becherer, EdD, President
3301 N Mulford Rd
Rockford, IL 61114-5699
815 654-4260
Type: Junior or Comm Coll
Control: State, County, or Local Govt
• Dental Hygiene Prgm
• Respiratory Care Prgm
• Surgical Technology Prgm

Rockford Career College
James Devaney, PhD, CEO
730 N Church
Rockford, IL 61103
815 965-8616
Type: Vocational or Tech Sch
Control: For Profit
• Medical Assistant Prgm

Rockford Memorial Hospital
Gary Kaatz, MS, President
2400 N Rockton Ave
Rockford, IL 61103
815 971-5000
Type: Hosp or Med Ctr: 300-499 Beds
Control: Nonprofit (Private or Religious)
• Radiography Prgm

Swedish American Hospital
William Gorski, MD, President/CEO
1401 E State St
Rockford, IL 61104-2298
815 968-4400
Type: Hosp or Med Ctr: 300-499 Beds
Control: Nonprofit (Private or Religious)
• Emergency Med Tech-Paramedic Prgm
• Radiation Therapy Prgm
• Radiography Prgm

Romeoville

Lewis University
Brother James Gaffney, FSC, President
One University Pkwy
Romeoville, IL 60446
815 838-0500
Type: 4-year Coll or Univ
Control: State, County, or Local Govt
• Athletic Training Prgm
• Nursing Prgm

Rosemont

Northwestern College
Lawrence W Schumacher, BA, President
9700 W Higgins Rd, Ste 750
Rosemont, IL 60018
847 318-8550
Type: Junior or Comm Coll
Control: For Profit
• Medical Assistant Prgm (3)
• Radiography Prgm

Skokie

Everest College
Jeanette Prickett, JD, Campus President
9811 Woods Dr
Skokie, IL 60077
847 470-0277
Type: Vocational or Tech Sch
Control: For Profit
• Medical Assistant Prgm (3)

Sanford Brown College - Skokie
Skokie, IL 60007
• Dental Hygiene Prgm

South Holland

South Suburban College
George T Dammer, MS, President
15800 S State St
South Holland, IL 60473-1262
708 596-2000
Type: Junior or Comm Coll
Control: State, County, or Local Govt
• Medical Assistant Prgm
• Occupational Therapy Asst Prgm
• Pharmacy Technician Prgm
• Phlebotomy Prgm

Springfield

Lincoln Land Community College
Charlotte Warren, PhD, President
5250 Shepherd Rd
PO Box 19256
Springfield, IL 62794-9256
217 786-2273
Type: Junior or Comm Coll
Control: State, County, or Local Govt
• Occupational Therapy Asst Prgm
• Radiography Prgm

St John's Hospital
Robert Ritz, FACHE, Exec Vice President
800 E Carpenter
Springfield, IL 62769
217 544-6464
Type: Consortium
Control: Nonprofit (Private or Religious)
• Clin Lab Scientist/Med Technologist Prgm
• Neurodiagnostic Tech Prgm
• Respiratory Care Prgm

University of Illinois at Springfield
Richard Ringeisen, PhD, Chancellor
One University Plaza
Springfield, IL 62703
217 206-6634
Type: 4-year Coll or Univ
Control: State, County, or Local Govt
• Clin Lab Scientist/Med Technologist Prgm
• Counseling Prgm

Sugar Grove

Waubonsee Community College
Christine J Sobek, EdD, President
Rte 47 at Waubonsee Dr
Sugar Grove, IL 60554
630 466-7900
Type: Junior or Comm Coll
Control: State, County, or Local Govt
• Medical Assistant Prgm
• Surgical Technology Prgm

Tinley Park

Fox College
18020 Oak Park Avenue
Tinley Park, IL 60477
• Physical Therapist Assistant Prgm

University Park

Governors State University
Elaine Maimon, PhD, President
1 University Pkwy
University Park, IL 60466
708 534-4130
Type: 4-year Coll or Univ
Control: State, County, or Local Govt
• Counseling Prgm
• Occupational Therapy Prgm
• Physical Therapy Prgm
• Speech-Language Pathology Prgm

Wheaton

Wheaton College
Wheaton, IL 60187
Type: 4-year Coll or Univ
Control: State, County, or Local Govt
• Psychology (PsyD) Prgm

Indiana

Alexandria

Alexandria School of Scientific Therapeutics
Herbert Hobbs, CEO
809 S Harrison
PO Box 287
Alexandria, IN 46001
765 724-9152
Type: Acad Health Ctr/Med Sch
Control: For Profit
• Massage Therapy Prgm

Anderson

Anderson University
James L Edwards, PhD, President
1100 E 5th St
Anderson, IN 46012
765 641-4011
Type: 4-year Coll or Univ
Control: Nonprofit (Private or Religious)
• Athletic Training Prgm
• Nursing Prgm

Beech Grove

St Francis Hospital & Health Centers
Robert J Brody, MHA, President/CEO
1600 Albany St
Beech Grove, IN 46107
317 783-8133
Type: Hosp or Med Ctr: 500 Beds
Control: Nonprofit (Private or Religious)
• Clin Lab Scientist/Med Technologist Prgm
• Emergency Med Tech-Paramedic Prgm

Bloomington

Indiana University - Bloomington
Adam Herbert, PhD, President
President's Office, Bryan Hall
Bloomington, IN 47405
812 855-4613
Type: 4-year Coll or Univ
Control: State, County, or Local Govt
• Athletic Training Prgm
• Audiologist Prgm
• Counseling Prgm
• Dietetics-Didactic Prgm
• Optometry Prgm
• Psychology (PsyD) Prgm
• Speech-Language Pathology Prgm

Pelham - Ball Memorial Consortium
Bloomington, IN 47401
Type: Vocational or Tech Sch
• Emergency Med Tech-Paramedic Prgm

Columbus

Columbus Area Career Connection/Ivy Tech St
Christy Ross, BS CDA, Instructor, Director
230 S Marr Rd
Columbus, IN 47201
812 376-4202
Type: Vocational or Tech Sch
Control: Nonprofit (Private or Religious)
• Dental Assistant Prgm

Columbus Regional Hospital
Douglas J Leonard, Vice President
2400 E 17th St
Columbus, IN 47201
812 376-5439
Type: Hosp or Med Ctr: 300-499 Beds
Control: State, County, or Local Govt
• Radiography Prgm

Corydon

Harrison County Hospital Paramedic Consortium
Corydon, IN 47112
Type: Consortium
• Emergency Med Tech-Paramedic Prgm

Crown Point

St Anthony Medical Center
Seth C R Warren, MBA, President
1201 S Main St
Crown Point, IN 46307
219 757-6132
Type: Hosp or Med Ctr: 100-299 Beds
Control: Nonprofit (Private or Religious)
• Diagnostic Med Sonography (Cardiac) Prgm
• Emergency Med Tech-Paramedic Prgm

Decatur

Adams Memorial Hospital
Decatur, IN 46733
Type: Hosp or Med Ctr d Beds
• Emergency Med Tech-Paramedic Prgm

Elkhart

Elkhart General Hospital
Greg Lintjer, President
600 E Blvd
Elkhart, IN 46514
574 293-8961
Type: Hosp or Med Ctr: 300-499 Beds
Control: State, County, or Local Govt
• Emergency Med Tech-Paramedic Prgm

Evansville

University of Evansville
Stephen G Jennings, President
1800 Lincoln Ave
Evansville, IN 47722
812 488-2151
Type: 4-year Coll or Univ
Control: Nonprofit (Private or Religious)
• Athletic Training Prgm
• Music Therapy Prgm
• Physical Therapist Assistant Prgm
• Physical Therapy Prgm

University of Southern Indiana
H Ray Hoops, PhD, President
8600 University Blvd
Evansville, IN 47712-3534
812 464-1756
Type: 4-year Coll or Univ
Control: State, County, or Local Govt
• Dental Assistant Prgm
• Dental Hygiene Prgm
• Diagnostic Med Sonography
  (Gen/Card/Vascular) Prgm
• Dietetics-Didactic Prgm
• Nursing Prgm
• Occupational Therapy Asst Prgm
• Occupational Therapy Prgm
• Radiography Prgm
• Respiratory Care Prgm

Fort Wayne

Brown Mackie College - Fort Wayne
James C Bishop, MBA, Campus President
3000 East Coliseum Boulevard
Fort Wayne, IN 46802
260 484-4400
Type: Junior or Comm Coll
Control: For Profit
• Medical Assistant Prgm (2)
• Occupational Therapy Asst Prgm
• Physical Therapist Assistant Prgm (2)
• Surgical Technology Prgm (2)

Indiana Univ - Purdue Univ Ft Wayne
Michael A Wartell, PhD, Chancellor
2101 Coliseum Blvd E
Fort Wayne, IN 46805
260 481-6103
Type: 4-year Coll or Univ
Control: State, County, or Local Govt
• Dental Assistant Prgm
• Dental Hygiene Prgm
• Dental Lab Technician Prgm
• Music Therapy Prgm
• Radiography Prgm

International Business College
Jim C Zillman, President
5699 Coventry Ln
Fort Wayne, IN 46804
260 459-4500
Type: Vocational or Tech Sch
Control: For Profit
• Medical Assistant Prgm
• Veterinary Technology Prgm

Medtech College-Fort Wayne
Fort Wayne, IN 46804
Type: Vocational or Tech Sch
• Clin Lab Technician/Med Lab Technician Prgm
• Medical Assistant Prgm

Parkview Hospital
Sue Ehinger, MD, COO
2200 Randallia Dr
Fort Wayne, IN 46805
260 373-3606
Type: Hosp or Med Ctr: 500 Beds
Control: Nonprofit (Private or Religious)
• Clin Lab Scientist/Med Technologist Prgm

St Joseph Medical Center
Allen V Rupiper, CEO
700 Broadway
Fort Wayne, IN 46802
219 425-3690
Type: Hosp or Med Ctr: 300-499 Beds
Control: Nonprofit (Private or Religious)
• Clin Lab Scientist/Med Technologist Prgm

University of Saint Francis
Sr M Elise Kriss, OSF PhD, President
2701 Spring St
Fort Wayne, IN 46808
260 434-3101
Type: 4-year Coll or Univ
Control: Nonprofit (Private or Religious)
• Nursing Prgm
• Physical Therapist Assistant Prgm
• Physician Assistant Prgm
• Radiography Prgm
• Surgical Technology Prgm

Franklin

Franklin College
Jay Moseley, PhD, President
101 Branigin Boulevard
Old Main
Franklin, IN 46131
317 738-8010
Type: 4-year Coll or Univ
Control: State, County, or Local Govt
• Athletic Training Prgm

Gary

Indiana University Northwest
Bruce Bergland, PhD, Chancellor
3400 Broadway
Gary, IN 46368
219 980-6700
Type: 4-year Coll or Univ
Control: State, County, or Local Govt
• Dental Assistant Prgm
• Dental Hygiene Prgm
• Nursing Prgm
• Radiation Therapy Prgm
• Radiography Prgm
• Respiratory Care Prgm

Methodist Hospitals Inc
Ian E McFadden, President/CEO
Northlake Campus
600 Grant St
Gary, IN 46402
219 886-4602
Type: Hosp or Med Ctr: 500 Beds
Control: Nonprofit (Private or Religious)
• Emergency Med Tech-Paramedic Prgm

Goshen

Goshen College
Goshen, IN 46526
Type: 4-year Coll or Univ
Control: Nonprofit (Private or Religious)
• Nursing Prgm

Greencastle

DePauw University
Robert G Bottoms, D Min, President
313 S Locust
Administration Bldg
Greencastle, IN 46135
765 658-4055
Type: 4-year Coll or Univ
Control: Nonprofit (Private or Religious)
• Athletic Training Prgm
• Music Therapy Prgm

Greenfield

Hancock Regional Hospital
Robert Keen, PhD, President and CEO
801 N State St
Greenfield, IN 46140
317 462-0457
Type: Hosp or Med Ctr: 100-299 Beds
Control: For Profit
• Radiography Prgm

Greenwood

MedTech College-Greenwood
Greenwood, IN 46221
Type: Vocational or Tech Sch
• Clin Lab Technician/Med Lab Technician Prgm
• Medical Assistant Prgm

Hammond

St Margaret Mercy Healthcare Centers
Tom Gryzbek, President/CEO
Mercy Healthcare Ctrs
5454 Hohman Ave
Hammond, IN 46320
219 932-2300
Type: Hosp or Med Ctr: 300-499 Beds
Control: Nonprofit (Private or Religious)
• Clin Lab Scientist/Med Technologist Prgm

Huntington

Huntington University
Huntington, IN 46750-1237
Type: 4-year Coll or Univ
Control: Nonprofit (Private or Religious)
• Nursing Prgm

Indianapolis

Brown Mackie College - Indianapolis
Lisa Ramirez, MBA, Campus President
1200 N Meridian Street, Suite 100
Indianapolis, IN 46204
317 554-8310
Type: Junior or Comm Coll
Control: For Profit
• Occupational Therapy Asst Prgm

Butler University
Indianapolis, IN 46208
Type: 4-year Coll or Univ
Control: Nonprofit (Private or Religious)
• Pharmacy Prgm
• Physician Assistant Prgm

Community Health Network
William E Corley, President
1500 N Ritter Ave
Indianapolis, IN 46219
317 355-5529
Type: Hosp or Med Ctr: 500 Beds
Control: Other
• Emergency Med Tech-Paramedic Prgm
• Radiography Prgm

Harrison College
Kenneth J Konesco, President
550 E Washington St
Indianapolis, IN 46204
317 264-5656
Type: Vocational or Tech Sch
Control: For Profit
• Clin Lab Technician/Med Lab Technician Prgm
• Medical Assistant Prgm (10)
• Surgical Technology Prgm (2)

Indiana Blood Center
Byron Buhner, AB MS, President/CEO
3450 N Meridian St
Indianapolis, IN 46208
317 916-5001
Type: Hosp or Med Ctr: 300-499 Beds
Control: Nonprofit (Private or Religious)
• Specialist in BB Tech Prgm

Indiana University
Charles R Bantz, PhD, Chancellor and Vice Pres
355 Lansing Street
AO Room 104 B
Indianapolis, IN 46202-2896
317 274-4417
Type: 4-year Coll or Univ
Control: State, County, or Local Govt
• Allopathic Medicine Prgm
• Clin Lab Scientist/Med Technologist Prgm
• Cytotechnology Prgm
• Dental Assistant Prgm
• Dental Hygiene Prgm
• Dentistry Prgm
• Dietetic Internship Prgm
• Emergency Med Tech-Paramedic Prgm
• Genetic Counseling Prgm
• Histotechnician Prgm
• Medical Dosimetry Prgm
• Medical Librarian Prgm
• Music Therapy Prgm
• Nuclear Medicine Technology Prgm
• Occupational Therapy Prgm
• Ophthalmic Dispensing Optician Prgm
• Pathologists' Assistant Prgm
• Physical Therapy Prgm
• Radiation Therapy Prgm
• Radiography Prgm
• Respiratory Care Prgm

Indiana University Health
Daniel F Evans, JD, President/CEO
PO Box 1367
Indianapolis, IN 46206-1367
317 962-5900
Type: Hosp or Med Ctr: 500 Beds
Control: Nonprofit (Private or Religious)
• Clin Lab Scientist/Med Technologist Prgm
• Counseling Prgm
• Emergency Med Tech-Paramedic Prgm (2)
• Neurodiagnostic Tech Prgm
• Pharmacy Technician Prgm
• Respiratory Care Prgm
• Surgical Technology Prgm

Indiana Univ-Purdue Univ-Indianapolis
Charles R Bantz, Chancellor
425 University Blvd
Cavanaugh Hall 441
Indianapolis, IN 46202
Type: 4-year Coll or Univ
Control: State, County, or Local Govt
• Music Therapy Prgm
• Nursing Prgm
• Psychology (PhD) Prgm

International Business Coll - Indianapolis
Eric Stovall, President
7205 Shadeland Station
Indianapolis, IN 46256
317 841-6400
Type: Vocational or Tech Sch
Control: For Profit
• Dental Assistant Prgm
• Medical Assistant Prgm

Ivy Tech Community College
Thomas J Snyder, MBA, President
50 W Fall Creek Pkwy North Dr
Indianapolis, IN 46208
317 921-4800
Type: Junior or Comm Coll
Control: State, County, or Local Govt
• Clin Lab Technician/Med Lab Technician Prgm (3)
• Dental Assistant Prgm (4)
• Dental Hygiene Prgm (2)
• Emergency Med Tech-Paramedic Prgm (6)
• Medical Assistant Prgm (17)
• Phlebotomy Prgm
• Physical Therapist Assistant Prgm (2)
• Radiation Therapy Prgm
• Radiography Prgm (3)
• Respiratory Care Prgm (6)
• Surgical Technology Prgm (8)

Kaplan College
Barri Shirk, BA MS, Executive Directror
7302 Woodland Dr
Indianapolis, IN 46278-1736
317 299-6001
Type: Vocational or Tech Sch
Control: For Profit
• Dental Assistant Prgm
• Medical Assistant Prgm

Marian University
Daniel A Felicetti, PhD, President
3200 Cold Spring Rd
Indianapolis, IN 46222
317 929-0237
Type: 4-year Coll or Univ
Control: Nonprofit (Private or Religious)
• Nursing Prgm

MedTech College-Indianapolis
Indianapolis, IN 46250
Type: Vocational or Tech Sch
• Clin Lab Technician/Med Lab Technician Prgm
• Medical Assistant Prgm

National College - Indianapolis
Indianapolis, IN 46250
Type: Junior or Comm Coll
• Medical Assistant Prgm

St Vincent Hosp & Health Care Ctr
Douglas French, President
2001 W 86th St
Indianapolis, IN 46260
317 338-7073
Type: Hosp or Med Ctr: 500 Beds
Control: Nonprofit (Private or Religious)
• Emergency Med Tech-Paramedic Prgm

University of Indianapolis
Beverly J Pitts, EdD, President
1400 E Hanna Ave
Indianapolis, IN 46227-3697
317 788-3211
Type: 4-year Coll or Univ
Control: Nonprofit (Private or Religious)
• Athletic Training Prgm
• Exercise Science Prgm
• Music Therapy Prgm
• Nursing Prgm
• Occupational Therapy Prgm
• Physical Therapist Assistant Prgm
• Physical Therapy Prgm
• Psychology (PsyD) Prgm

Kokomo

Howard Regional Health System
Kokomo, IN 46902
Type: Hosp or Med Ctr d Beds
• Emergency Med Tech-Paramedic Prgm

Indiana University - Kokomo
Ruth J Person, PhD, Chancellor
2300 S Washington St
Kokomo, IN 46902
765 453-2000
Type: 4-year Coll or Univ
Control: State, County, or Local Govt
• Nursing Prgm
• Radiography Prgm

St Vincent Health/St Joseph Hospital
Darcy Burthay, MSN RN, President
1907 W Sycamore St
Kokomo, IN 46901
317 452-5611
Type: Consortium
Control: Nonprofit (Private or Religious)
• Radiography Prgm

Lowell

In Training Inc College of Adult Education
182 Deanna Drive
Lowell, IN 46356
• Phlebotomy Prgm

Madison

King's Daughters' Hospital & Health Services
Roger J Allman, MHA, President/CEO
One King's Daughters' Dr, PO Box 447
Madison, IN 47250
812 265-5211
Type: Hosp or Med Ctr: 100-299 Beds
Control: Nonprofit (Private or Religious)
• Radiography Prgm

Marion

Indiana Wesleyan University
Henry Smith, PhD, President
4201 S Washington St
Marion, IN 46953
765 677-2100
Type: 4-year Coll or Univ
Control: Nonprofit (Private or Religious)
• Athletic Training Prgm
• Counseling Prgm
• Nursing Prgm

Merrillville

Brown Mackie College - Merrillville
Shalisa Powell, MA Ed, Campus President
1000 E 80th Place, Suite 205M
Merrillville, IN 46410
219 381-2227
• Occupational Therapy Asst Prgm
• Surgical Technology Prgm

Everest College
Mary Klinefelter, President
707 E 80th Pl, Ste 200
Merrillville, IN 46410
219 756-6811
Type: Vocational or Tech Sch
Control: State, County, or Local Govt
• Surgical Technology Prgm

Muncie

Ball Memorial Hospital/PA Labs,Inc.
Michael Haley, President
2401 W University Ave
Muncie, IN 47303-3499
765 747-3251
Type: Hosp or Med Ctr: 300-499 Beds
Control: Nonprofit (Private or Religious)
• Clin Lab Scientist/Med Technologist Prgm

Ball State University
Jo Ann Gora, PhD, President
Administration Bldg 101
Muncie, IN 47306
317 285-5555
Type: 4-year Coll or Univ
Control: State, County, or Local Govt
• Athletic Training Prgm
• Audiologist Prgm
• Counseling Prgm
• Dietetic Internship Prgm
• Dietetics-Didactic Prgm
• Music Therapy Prgm
• Nursing Prgm
• Radiography Prgm
• Rehabilitation Counseling Prgm
• Speech-Language Pathology Prgm

New Albany

Indiana University Southeast
New Albany, IN 47150
Type: 4-year Coll or Univ
Control: State, County, or Local Govt
• Nursing Prgm

North Manchester

Manchester College
Jo Young Switzer, PhD, President
Manchester College Box PRES
North Manchester, IN 46962
219 982-5050
Type: 4-year Coll or Univ
Control: Nonprofit (Private or Religious)
• Athletic Training Prgm
• Pharmacy Prgm

Richmond

Reid Hospital & Health Care Services
Barry S MacDowell, MHA, President
1401 Chester Blvd
Richmond, IN 47374
765 983-3122
Type: Hosp or Med Ctr: 100-299 Beds
Control: Nonprofit (Private or Religious)
• Radiography Prgm

South Bend

Brown Mackie College - South Bend
Louise Stienkeoway, MBA, Campus President
3454 Douglas Road
South Bend, IN 46635
574 237-0774
• Occupational Therapy Asst Prgm

Indiana University South Bend
Una Mae Reck, PhD, Chancellor
1700 Mishawaka Ave, Box 7111
South Bend, IN 46634
574 237-4220
Type: 4-year Coll or Univ
Control: State, County, or Local Govt
• Counseling Prgm
• Dental Hygiene Prgm
• Nursing Prgm
• Radiography Prgm

Ivy Tech Community College - North Central
Virginia Calvin, EdD, Chancellor
220 Dean Johnson Blvd
South Bend, IN 46601
574 289-7001
Type: Junior or Comm Coll
Control: State, County, or Local Govt
• Emergency Med Tech-Paramedic Prgm

St Mary of the Woods

St Mary of the Woods College
Joan Lescinski, President
St Mary of the Woods, IN 47876
812 535-5154
Type: 4-year Coll or Univ
Control: Nonprofit (Private or Religious)
• Music Therapy Prgm

Terre Haute

Indiana State University
Dan Bradley, PhD, President
Parsons Hall Room 208
Terre Haute, IN 47809
812 237-4000
Type: 4-year Coll or Univ
Control: State, County, or Local Govt
• Athletic Training Prgm
• Counseling Prgm
• Dietetics-Coordinated Prgm
• Music Therapy Prgm
• Physician Assistant Prgm
• Psychology (PhD) Prgm
• Speech-Language Pathology Prgm

Valparaiso

Valparaiso University
Valparaiso, IN 46383
Type: 4-year Coll or Univ
Control: Nonprofit (Private or Religious)
• Music Therapy Prgm
• Nursing Prgm

Vincennes

Good Samaritan Hospital
Matthew Bailey, MHA, President and CEO
520 S Seventh St
Vincennes, IN 47591
812 885-3195
Type: Hosp or Med Ctr: 100-299 Beds
Control: State, County, or Local Govt
• Clin Lab Scientist/Med Technologist Prgm
• Radiography Prgm

Vincennes University
Richard E Helton, PhD, President
1002 First St N
Vincennes, IN 47591
812 888-4201
Type: Junior or Comm Coll
Control: State, County, or Local Govt
• Emergency Med Tech-Paramedic Prgm
• Physical Therapist Assistant Prgm
• Surgical Technology Prgm

West Lafayette

Purdue University
France A Cordova, PhD, President
Hovde Hall
West Lafayette, IN 47907
765 494-9708
Type: 4-year Coll or Univ
Control: State, County, or Local Govt
• Athletic Training Prgm
• Audiologist Prgm
• Counseling Prgm
• Dietetics-Coordinated Prgm
• Dietetics-Didactic Prgm
• Nursing Prgm
• Pharmacy Prgm
• Psychology (PhD) Prgm
• Speech-Language Pathology Prgm
• Veterinary Medicine Prgm
• Veterinary Technology Prgm

Iowa

Ames

Iowa State University
Gregory Geoffroy, PhD, President
2035 President
117 Beardshear
Ames, IA 50011
515 294-2042
Type: 4-year Coll or Univ
Control: State, County, or Local Govt
• Athletic Training Prgm
• Dietetic Internship Prgm
• Dietetics-Didactic Prgm
• Music Therapy Prgm
• Veterinary Medicine Prgm

Anamosa

Carlson College of Massage Therapy
Ruth Carlson
11809 County Rd
Box 28
Anamosa, IA 52205
319 462-3402
Type: Acad Health Ctr/Med Sch
Control: For Profit
• Massage Therapy Prgm

Ankeny

Des Moines Area Community College
Robert Denson, JD, President
Bldg 22
2006 S Ankeny Blvd
Ankeny, IA 50023
515 964-6638
Type: Junior or Comm Coll
Control: State, County, or Local Govt
• Clin Lab Technician/Med Lab Technician Prgm
• Dental Assistant Prgm
• Dental Hygiene Prgm
• Medical Assistant Prgm
• Respiratory Care Prgm
• Surgical Technology Prgm
• Veterinary Technology Prgm

Bettendorf

Eastern Iowa Community College
Bettendorf, IA
• Dental Assistant Prgm

Scott Community College
Thomas Coley, PhD, President
500 Belmont Rd
Bettendorf, IA 52722
563 441-4061
Type: Junior or Comm Coll
Control: State, County, or Local Govt
• Cancer Registrar Prgm
• Neurodiagnostic Tech Prgm
• Radiography Prgm

Calmar

Northeast Iowa Community College
Penelope Wills, PhD, President
1625 Hwy 150 S
PO Box 400
Calmar, IA 52132
563 562-3263
Type: Junior or Comm Coll
Control: State, County, or Local Govt
• Dental Assistant Prgm
• Radiography Prgm
• Respiratory Care Prgm

Cedar Falls

Kaplan University - Cedar Falls
Cedar Falls, IA 50613-6309
Type: 4-year Coll or Univ
• Medical Assistant Prgm

University of Northern Iowa
Benjamin Allen, PhD, President
Seerley Hall
Cedar Falls, IA 50614-0002
319 273-2566
Type: 4-year Coll or Univ
Control: State, County, or Local Govt
• Athletic Training Prgm
• Counseling Prgm
• Music Therapy Prgm
• Speech-Language Pathology Prgm

Cedar Rapids

Coe College
James Phifer, PhD, President
1220 First Ave NE
Cedar Rapids, IA 52402
319 399-8686
Type: 4-year Coll or Univ
Control: Nonprofit (Private or Religious)
• Athletic Training Prgm
• Nursing Prgm

Kaplan University - Cedar Rapids
Cedar Rapids, IA 52404
Type: 4-year Coll or Univ
• Medical Assistant Prgm

Kirkwood Community College
Mick Starcevich, EdD, President
6301 Kirkwood Blvd SW
PO Box 2068
Cedar Rapids, IA 52406-9973
319 398-5501
Type: Junior or Comm Coll
Control: State, County, or Local Govt
• Dental Assistant Prgm
• Dental Hygiene Prgm
• Dental Lab Technician Prgm
• Emergency Med Tech-Paramedic Prgm
• Medical Assistant Prgm
• Neurodiagnostic Tech Prgm
• Occupational Therapy Asst Prgm
• Physical Therapist Assistant Prgm
• Respiratory Care Prgm
• Surgical Technology Prgm
• Veterinary Technology Prgm

Mount Mercy College
Cedar Rapids, IA 52402
Type: 4-year Coll or Univ
Control: Nonprofit (Private or Religious)
• Nursing Prgm

St Luke's Hospital
Theodore Townsend, MD, President/CEO
PO Box 3026
1026 A Avenue NE
Cedar Rapids, IA 52402
319 369-7203
Type: Hosp or Med Ctr: 300-499 Beds
Control: Nonprofit (Private or Religious)
• Clin Lab Scientist/Med Technologist Prgm
• Radiography Prgm

Council Bluff

Kaplan University - Council Bluffs
Council Bluff, IA 51503
Type: 4-year Coll or Univ
• Medical Assistant Prgm

Council Bluffs

Iowa Western Community College
Dan Kinney, PhD, President
2700 College Rd Box 4-C
Council Bluffs, IA 51502-3004
712 325-3200
Type: Junior or Comm Coll
Control: State, County, or Local Govt
• Dental Assistant Prgm
• Dental Hygiene Prgm
• Medical Assistant Prgm
• Surgical Technology Prgm
• Veterinary Technology Prgm

Jennie Edmundson Memorial Hospital
Steven P Baumert, MPA PT, President and CEO
933 E Pierce St
Council Bluffs, IA 51501
712 396-6222
Type: Hosp or Med Ctr: 100-299 Beds
Control: Nonprofit (Private or Religious)
• Radiography Prgm

Davenport

Kaplan University, Davenport Campus
Mark Garland, PhD, Campus President
1801 E Kimberly Rd, Ste 1
Davenport, IA 52807
563 355-3500
Type: Vocational or Tech Sch
Control: For Profit
• Medical Assistant Prgm

Palmer College of Chiropractic
1000 Brady St
Davenport, IA 52803
Type: Acad Health Ctr/Med Sch
Control: For Profit
• Chiropractic Prgm

St Ambrose University
Sister Joan Lescinski, CJS PhD, President
518 W Locust St
Ambrose Hall
Davenport, IA 52803
563 333-6213
Type: 4-year Coll or Univ
Control: Nonprofit (Private or Religious)
• Nursing Prgm
• Occupational Therapy Prgm
• Physical Therapy Prgm
• Speech-Language Pathology Prgm

Decorah

Luther College
Richard L Torgerson, PhD, President
700 College Dr
Decorah, IA 52101
563 387-1001
Type: 4-year Coll or Univ
Control: Nonprofit (Private or Religious)
• Athletic Training Prgm
• Nursing Prgm

Des Moines

Des Moines University
Terry Branstad, DSC, President
3440 Grand Ave
Des Moines, IA 50312
515 271-1500
Type: 4-year Coll or Univ
Control: Nonprofit (Private or Religious)
• Osteopathic Medicine Prgm
• Physical Therapy Prgm
• Physician Assistant Prgm
• Podiatric Medicine Prgm

Drake University
David Maxwell, President
25th St and University Ave
Des Moines, IA 50311
515 271-2011
Type: 4-year Coll or Univ
Control: Nonprofit (Private or Religious)
• Pharmacy Prgm
• Rehabilitation Counseling Prgm

Grand View College
Des Moines, IA 50316
Type: 4-year Coll or Univ
Control: Nonprofit (Private or Religious)
• Nursing Prgm

Iowa Methodist Med Ctr/Iowa Hlth - Des Moines
Eric Crowell, MS MHA, President and CEO
1200 Pleasant St
Des Moines, IA 50309-1453
515 241-6201
Type: Hosp or Med Ctr: 500 Beds
Control: Nonprofit (Private or Religious)
• Radiography Prgm

Kaplan University - Des Moines
Des Moines, IA 50323
Type: 4-year Coll or Univ
• Medical Assistant Prgm

Mercy College of Health Sciences
Barbara Quijano Decker, JD, President
928 Sixth Ave
Des Moines, IA 50309
515 643-6601
Type: 4-year Coll or Univ
Control: Nonprofit (Private or Religious)
• Diagnostic Med Sonography (General/Cardiac) Prgm
• Medical Assistant Prgm
• Nuclear Medicine Technology Prgm
• Nursing Prgm
• Physical Therapist Assistant Prgm
• Polysomnographic Technology Prgm
• Radiography Prgm
• Surgical Technology Prgm

Mercy Medical Center - Des Moines
David Vellinga, CEO
1111 6th Ave
Des Moines, IA 50314
515 247-4278
Type: Hosp or Med Ctr: 500 Beds
Control: Nonprofit (Private or Religious)
• Clin Lab Scientist/Med Technologist Prgm
• Emergency Med Tech-Paramedic Prgm

Vatterott College - Des Moines Campus
Pamela Belll, President
6100 Thornton Ave
Ste 290
Des Moines, IA 50321
515 309-9000
Type: Vocational or Tech Sch
Control: For Profit
• Dental Assistant Prgm

Dubuque

Clarke University
Joanne Burrows, PhD, President
1550 Clarke Dr
Dubuque, IA 52001-3198
563 588-6300
Type: 4-year Coll or Univ
Control: Nonprofit (Private or Religious)
• Athletic Training Prgm
• Nursing Prgm
• Physical Therapy Prgm

Loras College
James E Collins, President
1450 Alta Vista
Dubuque, IA 52004-0178
563 588-7647
Type: 4-year Coll or Univ
Control: State, County, or Local Govt
• Athletic Training Prgm

University of Dubuque
2000 University Ave
Dubuque, IA 52001
Type: 4-year Coll or Univ
Control: Nonprofit (Private or Religious)
• Nursing Prgm

Estherville

Iowa Lakes Community College
Mike Hupfer, BSE JD, President
19 S 7th St
Estherville, IA 51334-2295
712 362-0438
Type: Junior or Comm Coll
Control: State, County, or Local Govt
• Medical Assistant Prgm
• Surgical Technology Prgm

Fayette

Upper Iowa University
Alan Walker, PhD, President
605 Washington St
PO Box 1857
Fayette, IA 52142
563 425-5201
Type: 4-year Coll or Univ
Control: Nonprofit (Private or Religious)
• Athletic Training Prgm
• Nursing Prgm

Fort Dodge

Iowa Central Community College
Dan Kinney, PhD, President
330 Ave M
One Triton Circle
Fort Dodge, IA 50501
800 362-2793
Type: Junior or Comm Coll
Control: State, County, or Local Govt
• Clin Lab Technician/Med Lab Technician Prgm
• Dental Hygiene Prgm
• Medical Assistant Prgm
• Radiography Prgm

Indianola

Simpson College
John Byrd, President
701 North C St
Hillman Hall
Indianola, IA 50125
515 961-1611
Type: 4-year Coll or Univ
Control: State, County, or Local Govt
• Athletic Training Prgm

Iowa City

University of Iowa
Sally Mason, PhD, President
101 Jessup Hall
Iowa City, IA 52242
319 335-3549
Type: 4-year Coll or Univ
Control: State, County, or Local Govt
- Allopathic Medicine Prgm
- Athletic Training Prgm
- Audiologist Prgm
- Counseling Prgm
- Dentistry Prgm
- Medical Librarian Prgm
- Music Therapy Prgm
- Nursing Prgm
- Pharmacy Prgm
- Physical Therapy Prgm
- Physician Assistant Prgm
- Psychology (PhD) Prgm
- Rehabilitation Counseling Prgm
- Speech-Language Pathology Prgm

University of Iowa Hospitals & Clinics
Kenneth Kates, CEO
200 Hawkins Dr 1353 JCP
Iowa City, IA 52242-1059
319 356-3155
Type: Hosp or Med Ctr: 500 Beds
Control: State, County, or Local Govt
- Diagnostic Med Sonography
  (Gen/Card/Vascular) Prgm
- Dietetic Internship Prgm
- Emergency Med Tech-Paramedic Prgm
- Nuclear Medicine Technology Prgm
- Orthoptist Prgm
- Perfusion Prgm
- Radiation Therapy Prgm
- Radiography Prgm

Iowa Falls

Ellsworth Community College
Iowa Falls, IA 50126-1163
Type: Junior or Comm Coll
- Medical Assistant Prgm

Lamoni

Graceland University
John Sellars, PhD, President
1 University Place
Lamoni, IA 50140
641 784-5111
Type: 4-year Coll or Univ
Control: Nonprofit (Private or Religious)
- Athletic Training Prgm

Marshalltown

Marshalltown Community College
Tim A Wynes, JD, President
3702 S Center St
Marshalltown, IA 50158
515 752-4643
Type: Junior or Comm Coll
Control: State, County, or Local Govt
- Dental Assistant Prgm

Mason City

Kaplan University - Mason City
Mason City, IA 50401
Type: 4-year Coll or Univ
- Medical Assistant Prgm

Mercy Medical Center - North Iowa
James Fitzpatrick, CHE, President/CEO
1000 Fourth St SW
Mason City, IA 50401
800 637-2994
Type: Hosp or Med Ctr: 300-499 Beds
Control: Nonprofit (Private or Religious)
- Radiography Prgm

North Iowa Area Community College
Michael Morrison, PhD, President
500 College Dr
Mason City, IA 50401
515 421-4200
Type: Junior or Comm Coll
Control: State, County, or Local Govt
- Medical Assistant Prgm
- Physical Therapist Assistant Prgm

Orange City

Northwestern College
Bruce Murphy, PhD, President
101 7th St SW
Orange City, IA 51041-1996
712 707-7100
Type: 4-year Coll or Univ
Control: Nonprofit (Private or Religious)
- Athletic Training Prgm
- Nursing Prgm

Ottumwa

Indian Hills Community College
Jim Lindenmayer, PhD, President
525 Grandview Ave, Building 1
Ottumwa, IA 52501
641 683-5185
Type: Junior or Comm Coll
Control: State, County, or Local Govt
- Clin Lab Technician/Med Lab Technician Prgm
- Clinical Assisting Prgm
- Emergency Med Tech-Paramedic Prgm
- Physical Therapist Assistant Prgm
- Radiography Prgm

Pella

Central College
David Roe, PhD, President
812 University Box 6300
Pella, IA 50219
641 628-5269
Type: 4-year Coll or Univ
Control: Nonprofit (Private or Religious)
- Athletic Training Prgm

Sioux Center

Dordt College
Carl E Zylstra, PhD, President
498 4th Ave NE
Sioux Center, IA 51250
712 722-6002
Type: 4-year Coll or Univ
Control: Nonprofit (Private or Religious)
- Nursing Prgm

Sioux City

Briar Cliff University
Sioux City, IA 51104
Type: 4-year Coll or Univ
Control: Nonprofit (Private or Religious)
- Nursing Prgm

Mercy Medical Center - Sioux City
Robert Peebles, President/CEO
801 Fifth St
Sioux City, IA 51101
712 279-2018
Type: Hosp or Med Ctr: 100-299 Beds
Control: Nonprofit (Private or Religious)
- Clin Lab Scientist/Med Technologist Prgm

Morningside College
Sioux City, IA 51106
Type: 4-year Coll or Univ
Control: Nonprofit (Private or Religious)
- Nursing Prgm

St. Luke's College/St. Luke's Regl Med Ctr
Peter Thoreen, MBA, President, CEO
2720 Stone Park Blvd
Sioux City, IA 51104
712 279-3207
Type: Vocational or Tech Sch
Control: Nonprofit (Private or Religious)
- Clin Lab Scientist/Med Technologist Prgm
- Phlebotomy Prgm
- Radiography Prgm
- Respiratory Care Prgm

Western Iowa Tech Community College
Robert Dunker, PhD, President
4647 Stone Ave
PO Box 5199
Sioux City, IA 51102-5199
712 274-6400
Type: Junior or Comm Coll
Control: State, County, or Local Govt
- Dental Assistant Prgm
- Emergency Med Tech-Paramedic Prgm
- Medical Assistant Prgm
- Physical Therapist Assistant Prgm
- Surgical Technology Prgm

Storm Lake

Buena Vista University
Fredrick V Moore, President
610 W Fourth St
Storm Lake, IA 50588
712 749-2103
Type: 4-year Coll or Univ
Control: State, County, or Local Govt
- Athletic Training Prgm

Waterloo

Allen College
Jerry Durham, PhD, Chancellor
1825 Logan Ave
Waterloo, IA 50703
319 226-2015
Type: 4-year Coll or Univ
Control: Nonprofit (Private or Religious)
- Clin Lab Scientist/Med Technologist Prgm
- Nuclear Medicine Technology Prgm
- Nursing Prgm
- Radiography Prgm

Covenant Medical Center
Raymond Burfeind, President
3421 W Ninth St
Waterloo, IA 50702
319 236-4111
Type: Hosp or Med Ctr: 300-499 Beds
Control: Nonprofit (Private or Religious)
• Radiography Prgm

Hawkeye Community College
Greg Schmitz, PhD, President
1501 E Orange Rd
PO Box 8015
Waterloo, IA 50704-8015
319 296-2320
Type: Junior or Comm Coll
Control: State, County, or Local Govt
• Clin Lab Technician/Med Lab Technician Prgm
• Dental Assistant Prgm
• Dental Hygiene Prgm
• Respiratory Care Prgm

Waverly

Wartburg College
Jack Ohle, President
902 12th St NW
Waverly, IA 50677
319 352-0979
Type: 4-year Coll or Univ
Control: Nonprofit (Private or Religious)
• Music Therapy Prgm

West Burlington

Southeastern Community College
Beverly Simone, President
1500 W Agency Rd
PO Box 180
West Burlington, IA 52655-0180
319 752-2731
Type: Junior or Comm Coll
Control: State, County, or Local Govt
• Emergency Med Tech-Paramedic Prgm
• Medical Assistant Prgm
• Respiratory Care Prgm

Kansas

Arkansas City

Cowley County Community College
Patrick J McAtee, PhD, President
PO Box 1147
Arkansas City, KS 67005
800 593-2222
Type: Junior or Comm Coll
Control: State, County, or Local Govt
• Emergency Med Tech-Paramedic Prgm

Atchison

Benedictine College
Daniel Carey, PhD, President
1020 N Second St
Atchison, KS 66002-1499
913 367-5340
Type: 4-year Coll or Univ
Control: State, County, or Local Govt
• Athletic Training Prgm

Coffeyville

Coffeyville Community College
Howard G Bass, PhD, President
400 W 11th St
Coffeyville, KS 67337
620 251-7700
Type: Junior or Comm Coll
Control: State, County, or Local Govt
• Emergency Med Tech-Paramedic Prgm
• Medical Assistant Prgm

Colby

Colby Community College
Lynn Krider, PhD, President
1255 S Range
Colby, KS 67701
785 462-3984
Type: Junior or Comm Coll
Control: State, County, or Local Govt
• Physical Therapist Assistant Prgm
• Veterinary Technology Prgm

Emporia

Emporia State University
Michael Lane, PhD, President
1200 Commercial St, Box 4001
Emporia, KS 66801
620 341-5551
Type: 4-year Coll or Univ
Control: State, County, or Local Govt
• Art Therapy Prgm
• Athletic Training Prgm
• Counseling Prgm
• Medical Librarian Prgm
• Rehabilitation Counseling Prgm

Flint Hills Technical College
Dean Hollenbeck, PhD, President
3301 W 18th Ave
Emporia, KS 66801
620 341-1306
Type: Vocational or Tech Sch
Control: State, County, or Local Govt
• Dental Assistant Prgm
• Dental Hygiene Prgm
• Emergency Med Tech-Paramedic Prgm

Garden City

Garden City Community College
Carol Ballantyne, PhD, President
801 Campus Dr
Garden City, KS 67846
620 276-9602
Type: Junior or Comm Coll
Control: State, County, or Local Govt
• Emergency Med Tech-Paramedic Prgm

Goodland

Northwest Kansas Technical College
Kenneth Clouse, MS, President
1209 Harrison St
PO Box 668
Goodland, KS 67735-0668
785 890-3641
Type: Vocational or Tech Sch
Control: State, County, or Local Govt
• Medical Assistant Prgm

Great Bend

Barton County Community College
Carl Heilman, PhD, President
245 NE 30th Rd
Great Bend, KS 67530-9283
620 792-9301
Type: Junior or Comm Coll
Control: State, County, or Local Govt
• Clin Lab Technician/Med Lab Technician Prgm
• Emergency Med Tech-Paramedic Prgm

Hays

Fort Hays State University
Lawrence Gould, PhD, Provost
600 Park St
Hays, KS 67601
785 628-4000
Type: 4-year Coll or Univ
Control: State, County, or Local Govt
• Athletic Training Prgm
• Music Therapy Prgm
• Nursing Prgm
• Radiography Prgm
• Speech-Language Pathology Prgm

Hillsboro

Tabor College
Jules Glanzer, DMin, President
400 S Jefferson
Hillsboro, KS 67063
620 947-3121
Type: 4-year Coll or Univ
Control: Nonprofit (Private or Religious)
• Athletic Training Prgm
• Nursing Prgm

Hutchinson

Hutchinson Community College
Edward E Berger, EdD, President
1300 N Plum St
Hutchinson, KS 67501
620 665-3505
Type: Junior or Comm Coll
Control: State, County, or Local Govt
• Emergency Med Tech-Paramedic Prgm
• Pharmacy Technician Prgm
• Physical Therapist Assistant Prgm
• Radiography Prgm
• Surgical Technology Prgm

Kansas City

Kansas City Community College
Shirley Wendel, PhD, Consortial Comm Chair
7250 State Ave
Kansas City, KS 66112
913 288-7126
Type: Consortium
Control: State, County, or Local Govt
• Respiratory Care Prgm

Kansas City Kansas Community College
Thomas R Burke, PhD, President
7250 State Ave
PO Box 12951
Kansas City, KS 66112-9978
913 288-7123
Type: Junior or Comm Coll
Control: State, County, or Local Govt
• Emergency Med Tech-Paramedic Prgm
• Physical Therapist Assistant Prgm

University of Kansas Medical Center
Bob Page, Exec Vice Chancellor
3901 Rainbow Blvd, Mail Stop 3011
3015 Murphy Administration Bldg MS 1049
Kansas City, KS 66160
913 588-7332
Type: Acad Health Ctr/Med Sch
Control: State, County, or Local Govt
• Allopathic Medicine Prgm
• Clin Lab Scientist/Med Technologist Prgm
• Cytotechnology Prgm
• Diagnostic Med Sonography
  (Gen/Card/Vascular) Prgm
• Diagnostic Molecular Scientist Prgm
• Dietetic Internship Prgm
• Nuclear Medicine Technology Prgm
• Occupational Therapy Prgm
• Physical Therapy Prgm
• Respiratory Care Prgm

Lawrence

University of Kansas
Robert E Hemenway, Chancellor
3031 Dole Ctr
Lawrence, KS 66045
785 864-0630
Type: 4-year Coll or Univ
Control: State, County, or Local Govt
• Athletic Training Prgm
• Audiologist Prgm
• Music Therapy Prgm
• Nursing Prgm
• Pharmacy Prgm
• Psychology (PhD) Prgm
• Speech-Language Pathology Prgm

Leavenworth

University of Saint Mary
4100 S 4th St
Leavenworth, KS 66048
Type: 4-year Coll or Univ
Control: Nonprofit (Private or Religious)
• Nursing Prgm

Lenexa

Brown Mackie College - Kansas City
Susan Naples, PhD, Campus President
9705 Lenexa Drive
Lenexa, KS 66215-1345
913 768-1900
Type: Junior or Comm Coll
Control: For Profit
• Occupational Therapy Asst Prgm

Liberal

Seward County Community College
Duane Dunn, EdD, President
PO Box 1137
Liberal, KS 67905
620 417-1010
Type: Junior or Comm Coll
Control: State, County, or Local Govt
• Clin Lab Technician/Med Lab Technician Prgm
• Respiratory Care Prgm
• Surgical Technology Prgm

Lindsborg

Bethany College
Lindsborg, KS 67456
Type: 4-year Coll or Univ
Control: Nonprofit (Private or Religious)
• Athletic Training Prgm

Manhattan

Kansas State University
Jon Wefald, President
Anderson Hall
Manhattan, KS 66506-5301
913 532-6221
Type: 4-year Coll or Univ
Control: State, County, or Local Govt
• Athletic Training Prgm
• Dietetics-Coordinated Prgm
• Dietetics-Didactic Prgm
• Music Therapy Prgm
• Speech-Language Pathology Prgm
• Veterinary Medicine Prgm

North Newton

Bethel College
Barry Bartel, JD, President
300 E 27th St
North Newton, KS 67117
316 283-2500
Type: 4-year Coll or Univ
Control: Nonprofit (Private or Religious)
• Athletic Training Prgm
• Nursing Prgm

Olathe

Mid-America Nazarene University
Edwin H Robinson, PhD MRE, President
2030 E College Way
Olathe, KS 66062
913 782-3750
Type: 4-year Coll or Univ
Control: State, County, or Local Govt
• Athletic Training Prgm
• Nursing Prgm

Oveland Park

Cleveland Chiropractic College of Kansas City
10850 Lowell Ave
Oveland Park, KS 66210
Type: Acad Health Ctr/Med Sch
Control: For Profit
• Chiropractic Prgm

Overland Park

Johnson County Community College
Terry Calaway, EdD, Interim President
12345 College Blvd
Overland Park, KS 66210-1299
913 469-8500
Type: Junior or Comm Coll
Control: State, County, or Local Govt
• Dental Hygiene Prgm
• Emergency Med Tech-Paramedic Prgm
• Polysomnographic Technology Prgm
• Respiratory Care Prgm

National American University - Overland Park
Overland Park, KS 66212-5451
Type: 4-year Coll or Univ
• Medical Assistant Prgm

Parsons

Labette Community College
George Knox, EdD, President
200 S 14th St
Parsons, KS 67357
620 421-6700
Type: Junior or Comm Coll
Control: State, County, or Local Govt
• Radiography Prgm
• Respiratory Care Prgm

Pittsburg

Pittsburg State University
Thomas Bryant
1701 S Broadway
Pittsburg, KS 66762-7500
316 231-7000
Type: 4-year Coll or Univ
Control: State, County, or Local Govt
• Counseling Prgm
• Music Therapy Prgm
• Nursing Prgm

Salina

Brown Mackie College - Salina
Judy Holmes, MBA, Campus President
2106 South 9th Street
Salina, KS 67401
785 823-4601
• Occupational Therapy Asst Prgm

Kansas Wesleyan University
Phillip P Kerstetter, PhD, President
100 E Claflin Ave
Salina, KS 67401-6198
785 827-5541
Type: 4-year Coll or Univ
Control: Nonprofit (Private or Religious)
• Athletic Training Prgm

Salina Area Technical College
Duane Custer, Director
2562 Centennial Rd
Salina, KS 67401
785 309-3108
Type: Vocational or Tech Sch
Control: Other
• Dental Assistant Prgm

Sterling

Sterling College
Bruce Douglas, PhD, President
125 W Cooper
Sterling, KS 67579
620 278-4213
Type: 4-year Coll or Univ
Control: State, County, or Local Govt
• Athletic Training Prgm

Topeka

Baker University
Kathleen L Harr, DNSc RN, Chief Nurse
   Administrator
1500 SW Tenth St
Topeka, KS 66604
785 354-5853
Type: 4-year Coll or Univ
Control: Nonprofit (Private or Religious)
• Nursing Prgm

Washburn University
Jerry Farley, PhD, President
1700 SW College Blvd
Topeka, KS 66621
785 670-1556
Type: 4-year Coll or Univ
Control: State, County, or Local Govt
• Athletic Training Prgm
• Diagnostic Med Sonography
   (Gen/Card/Vascular) Prgm
• Music Therapy Prgm
• Nursing Prgm
• Occupational Therapy Asst Prgm
• Physical Therapist Assistant Prgm
• Radiography Prgm
• Respiratory Care Prgm
• Surgical Technology Prgm

Wichita

Newman University
Noreen Carrocci, PhD, President/CEO
3100 McCormick Ave
Wichita, KS 67213-2097
316 942-4291
Type: 4-year Coll or Univ
Control: Nonprofit (Private or Religious)
• Nursing Prgm
• Occupational Therapy Asst Prgm
• Radiography Prgm
• Respiratory Care Prgm

Wichita Area Technical College
Peter Gustaf, BS MS EMAB, President
301 S Grove
Wichita, KS 67211
316 677-9400
Type: Vocational or Tech Sch
Control: State, County, or Local Govt
• Dental Assistant Prgm
• Medical Assistant Prgm
• Surgical Technology Prgm

Wichita State University
Donald Beggs, PhD, President
1845 N Fairmont
Wichita, KS 67260-0001
316 978-3001
Type: 4-year Coll or Univ
Control: State, County, or Local Govt
• Athletic Training Prgm
• Audiologist Prgm
• Clin Lab Scientist/Med Technologist Prgm
• Dental Hygiene Prgm
• Nursing Prgm
• Physical Therapy Prgm
• Physician Assistant Prgm
• Speech-Language Pathology Prgm

Winfield

Southwestern College
W R Merriman, Jr, PhD, President
100 College St
Winfield, KS 67156
620 229-6223
Type: 4-year Coll or Univ
Control: Nonprofit (Private or Religious)
• Athletic Training Prgm
• Nursing Prgm

Kentucky

Ashland

Ashland Technical and Community College
Stu Taylor, School Director
4818 Roberts Dr
Ashland, KY 41102-9046
606 929-2055
Type: Vocational or Tech Sch
Control: State, County, or Local Govt
• Surgical Technology Prgm

Berea

Berea College
Larry D Shinn, President
Berea, KY 40404
606 986-9341
Type: 4-year Coll or Univ
Control: Nonprofit (Private or Religious)
• Nursing Prgm

Bowling Green

Bowling Green Technical College
Nathan Hodges, EdD, President
1845 Loop Dr
Bowling Green, KY 42101
270 901-1111
Type: Junior or Comm Coll
Control: State, County, or Local Govt
• Diagnostic Med Sonography (General) Prgm
• Polysomnographic Technology Prgm
• Radiography Prgm
• Respiratory Care Prgm
• Surgical Technology Prgm

Western Kentucky University
Gary A Ransdell, PhD, President
Wetherby Administration Bldg 135
Bowling Green, KY 42101-3576
270 745-4346
Type: 4-year Coll or Univ
Control: State, County, or Local Govt
• Counseling Prgm
• Dental Hygiene Prgm
• Dietetics-Didactic Prgm
• Music Therapy Prgm
• Nursing Prgm
• Speech-Language Pathology Prgm

Columbia

Lindsey Wilson College
210 Lindsey Wilson St
Columbia, KY 42728-1298
502 384-2126
Type: 4-year Coll or Univ
Control: Nonprofit (Private or Religious)
• Counseling Prgm

Edgewood

St Elizabeth Medical Center
Joseph Gross, FACHE, President/CEO
One Medical Village Dr
Edgewood, KY 41017
859 301-2111
Type: Hosp or Med Ctr: 500 Beds
Control: Nonprofit (Private or Religious)
• Clin Lab Scientist/Med Technologist Prgm

Elizabethtown

Elizabethtown Community & Technical College
Thelma White, PhD, President
620 College Street Rd
Elizabethtown, KY 42701
270 769-2371
Type: Junior or Comm Coll
Control: State, County, or Local Govt
• Radiography Prgm

Fort Mitchell

Brown Mackie College - Northern Kentucky
Christine Knouff, Campus President
309 Buttermilk Pike
Fort Mitchell, KY 41017
859 341-5627
• Occupational Therapy Asst Prgm
• Surgical Technology Prgm

Georgetown

Georgetown College
Georgetown, KY 40324
Type: 4-year Coll or Univ
Control: Nonprofit (Private or Religious)
• Athletic Training Prgm
• Medical Assistant Prgm

Grayson

Kentucky Christian University
Grayson, KY 41143
Type: 4-year Coll or Univ
Control: Nonprofit (Private or Religious)
• Nursing Prgm

Hazard

Hazard Community & Technical College
Allen Goben, PhD, President
One Community College Dr, Hwy 15 S
Hazard, KY 41701
606 436-5721
Type: Junior or Comm Coll
Control: State, County, or Local Govt
- Diagnostic Med Sonography (General/Vascular) Prgm
- Physical Therapist Assistant Prgm
- Radiography Prgm
- Surgical Technology Prgm

Henderson

Henderson Community College
Patrick Lake, EdD, President
2660 S Green St
Henderson, KY 42420
270 827-1867
Type: Junior or Comm Coll
Control: State, County, or Local Govt
- Clin Lab Technician/Med Lab Technician Prgm
- Dental Hygiene Prgm
- Medical Assistant Prgm

Highland Heights

Northern Kentucky University
James Votruba, PhD, President
Office of the President, Admin Ctr 800B
Highland Heights, KY 41099-2104
606 572-5123
Type: 4-year Coll or Univ
Control: State, County, or Local Govt
- Athletic Training Prgm
- Music Therapy Prgm
- Radiography Prgm
- Respiratory Care Prgm

Lexington

Bluegrass Community and Technical College
Augusta Julian, EdD, President/CEO
470 Cooper Dr, Oswald Bldg
Rm 209
Lexington, KY 40506-0235
859 246-6501
Type: Vocational or Tech Sch
Control: State, County, or Local Govt
- Dental Assistant Prgm
- Dental Hygiene Prgm
- Dental Lab Technician Prgm
- Medical Assistant Prgm
- Nuclear Medicine Technology Prgm
- Polysomnographic Technology Prgm
- Radiography Prgm
- Respiratory Care Prgm
- Surgical Technology Prgm

National College - Lexington
Lexington, KY 40508-2312
Type: Junior or Comm Coll
- Surgical Technology Prgm

Spencerian College
Buddy Hoskinson, MEd, Executive Director
1575 Winchester Rd
Lexington, KY 40505
859 223-9608
Type: Vocational or Tech Sch
Control: For Profit
- Cardiovascular Tech (Invasive) Prgm
- Medical Assistant Prgm (2)
- Radiography Prgm (2)
- Surgical Technology Prgm

St Joseph Health System
Gene Woods, MHA, President/CEO
One St Joseph Dr
Lexington, KY 40504
859 313-1000
Type: Hosp or Med Ctr: 300-499 Beds
Control: Nonprofit (Private or Religious)
- Radiography Prgm

Sullivan University - Lexington
James Ploskonka, PhD, Executive Director
2355 Harrodsburg Rd
Lexington, KY 40504
606 276-4357
Type: 4-year Coll or Univ
Control: For Profit
- Medical Assistant Prgm
- Pharmacy Prgm

Univ of Kentucky Hospital
Murray Clark, PhD, Assoc VP, Med Ctr
N106 Chandler Medical Center
Lexington, KY 40536-0293
859 323-2044
Type: Acad Health Ctr/Med Sch
Control: Nonprofit (Private or Religious)
- Dietetic Internship Prgm

University of Kentucky
Lee Todd, PhD, President
Administration Bldg
101 Main Building
Lexington, KY 40506
859 257-1701
Type: 4-year Coll or Univ
Control: State, County, or Local Govt
- Allopathic Medicine Prgm
- Clin Lab Scientist/Med Technologist Prgm
- Dentistry Prgm
- Dietetic Internship Prgm
- Dietetics-Coordinated Prgm
- Dietetics-Didactic Prgm
- Medical Librarian Prgm
- Music Therapy Prgm
- Nursing Prgm
- Pharmacy Prgm
- Physical Therapy Prgm
- Physician Assistant Prgm
- Psychology (PhD) Prgm
- Rehabilitation Counseling Prgm
- Speech-Language Pathology Prgm

Louisville

Bellarmine University
Joseph McGowan, VP, Academic Affairs
2001 Newburg Rd
Louisville, KY 40205
502 452-8234
Type: 4-year Coll or Univ
Control: Nonprofit (Private or Religious)
- Clin Lab Scientist/Med Technologist Prgm
- Nursing Prgm
- Physical Therapy Prgm

Brown Mackie College - Louisville
Michael Fontaine, MBA, Campus President
3605 Fern Valley Road
Louisville, KY 40219-1916
502 810-6010
Type: Junior or Comm Coll
Control: For Profit
- Occupational Therapy Asst Prgm (2)
- Surgical Technology Prgm

Jefferson Community and Technical College
Anthony Newberry, PhD, President
109 E Broadway
Louisville, KY 40202
502 213-5333
Type: Junior or Comm Coll
Control: State, County, or Local Govt
- Clin Lab Technician/Med Lab Technician Prgm
- Diagnostic Med Sonography (General/Vascular) Prgm
- Medical Assistant Prgm
- Nuclear Medicine Technology Prgm
- Occupational Therapy Asst Prgm
- Pharmacy Technician Prgm
- Physical Therapist Assistant Prgm
- Radiography Prgm
- Respiratory Care Prgm
- Surgical Technology Prgm

Norton Healthcare
Stephen A Williams, BA MHA, President
PO Box 35070
Louisville, KY 40202
502 629-8791
Type: Hosp or Med Ctr: 300-499 Beds
Control: Nonprofit (Private or Religious)
- Cardiovascular Tech (Echocardiography) Prgm

Spalding University
Tori Murden McClure, JD MDIV MFA, President
845 S Third St
Louisville, KY 40203-2188
502 585-9911
Type: 4-year Coll or Univ
Control: Nonprofit (Private or Religious)
- Nursing Prgm
- Occupational Therapy Prgm

University of Louisville
James Ramsey, PhD, President
Grawmeyer Hall
Health Sciences Center
Louisville, KY 40292
502 852-5417
Type: 4-year Coll or Univ
Control: State, County, or Local Govt
• Allopathic Medicine Prgm
• Art Therapy Prgm
• Audiologist Prgm
• Dental Hygiene Prgm
• Dentistry Prgm
• Music Therapy Prgm
• Nursing Prgm
• Orientation and Mobility Specialist Prgm
• Psychology (PhD) Prgm
• Speech-Language Pathology Prgm

Madisonville

HCC/MCC Consortium
Judith Rhoads, EdD, President
2000 College Drive
Madisonville, KY 42431
270 824-8562
Type: Consortium
Control: State, County, or Local Govt
• Clin Lab Technician/Med Lab Technician Prgm

Madisonville Community College
Judith Rhoads, EdD, President
2000 College Dr
North Campus
Madisonville, KY 42431
270 824-8562
Type: Junior or Comm Coll
Control: State, County, or Local Govt
• Occupational Therapy Asst Prgm
• Physical Therapist Assistant Prgm
• Radiography Prgm
• Respiratory Care Prgm
• Surgical Assistant Prgm
• Surgical Technology Prgm

Morehead

Maysville Comm & Tech College
Kenneth Brown, Chief Academic Officer
609 Viking Dr
Morehead, KY 40351
606 783-1538
Type: Vocational or Tech Sch
Control: State, County, or Local Govt
• Medical Assistant Prgm
• Respiratory Care Prgm
• Surgical Technology Prgm

Morehead State University
Wayne Andrews, PhD, President
201 Howell McDowell Admin Bldg
Morehead, KY 40351
606 783-2022
Type: 4-year Coll or Univ
Control: State, County, or Local Govt
• Diagnostic Med Sonography (General) Prgm
• Nursing Prgm
• Radiography Prgm
• Veterinary Technology Prgm

Mount Vernon

Laurel Technical College - Rockcastle
Donna Hopkins, MA, Principal
PO Box 275
Mount Vernon, KY 40456
606 676-9065
Type: Vocational or Tech Sch
Control: State, County, or Local Govt
• Respiratory Care Prgm

Murray

Murray State University
Randy Dunn, EdD, President
President's Office
218 Wells Hall
Murray, KY 42071
270 762-3763
Type: 4-year Coll or Univ
Control: State, County, or Local Govt
• Athletic Training Prgm
• Dietetic Internship Prgm
• Dietetics-Didactic Prgm
• Music Therapy Prgm
• Nursing Prgm
• Speech-Language Pathology Prgm
• Veterinary Technology Prgm

Owensboro

Owensboro Community & Technical College
Paula Gastenveld, PhD, President
4800 New Hartford Rd
Owensboro, KY 42303-1899
502 686-4400
Type: Junior or Comm Coll
Control: State, County, or Local Govt
• Radiography Prgm
• Surgical Technology Prgm

Owensboro Medical Health System
Jeffery Barber, CEO
811 E Parrish Ave
PO Box 20007
Owensboro, KY 42304-0007
270 688-2001
Type: Hosp or Med Ctr: 300-499 Beds
Control: Nonprofit (Private or Religious)
• Clin Lab Scientist/Med Technologist Prgm

Paducah

West Kentucky Community & Technical College
Barbara Veazey, PhD RN, President/CEO
PO Box 7380
4810 Alben Barkley Dr
Paducah, KY 42002-7380
270 534-3082
Type: Junior or Comm Coll
Control: State, County, or Local Govt
• Clin Lab Technician/Med Lab Technician Prgm
• Dental Assistant Prgm
• Diagnostic Med Sonography (General) Prgm
• Physical Therapist Assistant Prgm
• Polysomnographic Technology Prgm
• Radiography Prgm
• Respiratory Care Prgm
• Surgical Technology Prgm

Pikeville

Pikeville College
Harold H Smith, President
214 Sycamore St
Pikeville, KY 41501-119
606 432-9200
Type: 4-year Coll or Univ
Control: Nonprofit (Private or Religious)
• Osteopathic Medicine Prgm

Pineville

Southeast Kentucky Comm & Tech College
W Bruce Ayers, EdD, President
3300 US 25E South
Pineville, KY 40977
606 248-2118
Type: Junior or Comm Coll
Control: State, County, or Local Govt
• Clin Lab Technician/Med Lab Technician Prgm
• Radiography Prgm
• Respiratory Care Prgm
• Surgical Technology Prgm

Prestonsburg

Big Sandy Community & Technical College
George D Edwards, PhD, President/CEO
1 Bert T Combs Dr
Prestonsburg, KY 41653
888 641-4132
Type: Junior or Comm Coll
Control: State, County, or Local Govt
• Dental Hygiene Prgm
• Respiratory Care Prgm

Richmond

Eastern Kentucky University
Douglas Whitlock, PhD, President
Coates Box 1A Admin Bldg Rm 107
521 Lancaster Ave
Richmond, KY 40475
859 622-2977
Type: 4-year Coll or Univ
Control: State, County, or Local Govt
• Athletic Training Prgm
• Clin Lab Scientist/Med Technologist Prgm
• Clin Lab Technician/Med Lab Technician Prgm
• Counseling Prgm
• Dietetic Internship Prgm
• Dietetics-Didactic Prgm
• Emergency Med Tech-Paramedic Prgm
• Music Therapy Prgm
• Nursing Prgm
• Occupational Therapy Prgm
• Speech-Language Pathology Prgm

Somerset

Somerset Community College
Jo Marshall, PhD, President
808 Monticello St
Somerset, KY 42501
606 451-6602
Type: Junior or Comm Coll
Control: State, County, or Local Govt
• Clin Lab Technician/Med Lab Technician Prgm
• Physical Therapist Assistant Prgm
• Radiography Prgm
• Surgical Technology Prgm

INSTITUTIONS

St Catharine

St Catharine College
William D Huston, MA, President
2735 Bardstown Rd
St Catharine, KY 40061
859 336-5082
Type: Junior or Comm Coll
Control: Nonprofit (Private or Religious)
• Diagnostic Med Sonography
  (Gen/Card/Vascular) Prgm
• Pharmacy Technician Prgm
• Radiation Therapy Prgm
• Radiography Prgm
• Surgical Technology Prgm

Williamsburg

University of the Cumberlands
Williamsburg, KY 40769
Type: 4-year Coll or Univ
Control: Nonprofit (Private or Religious)
• Physician Assistant Prgm

Lebanon

Byblos, Lebanon

Lebanese American Univ School of Pharmacy
Joseph G Jabbra, PhD, President
PO Box 36
Byblos, Lebanon, LE
Type: 4-year Coll or Univ
Control: For Profit
• Pharmacy Prgm

Louisiana

Alexandria

Louisiana State University - Alexandria
David Manuel, Chancellor
8100 Hwy 71 S
Alexandria, LA 71302-9121
318 445-3672
Type: 4-year Coll or Univ
Control: State, County, or Local Govt
• Clin Lab Technician/Med Lab Technician Prgm
• Pharmacy Technician Prgm
• Radiography Prgm

Rapides Regional Medical Center
David Williams, President
211 Fourth St
PO Box 30101
Alexandria, LA 71301
318 769-3150
Type: Hosp or Med Ctr: 300-499 Beds
Control: For Profit
• Clin Lab Scientist/Med Technologist Prgm
• Phlebotomy Prgm

Baton Rouge

Acadiana Technical College
Joe D May, PhD, System President
265 South Foster Dr
Baton Rouge, LA 70806
225 922-1643
Type: Vocational or Tech Sch
Control: State, County, or Local Govt
• Clin Lab Technician/Med Lab Technician Prgm
• Respiratory Care Prgm
• Surgical Technology Prgm

Baton Rouge General Medical Center
William Holman, President/CEO
3600 Florida St
PO Box 2511-70821
Baton Rouge, LA 70806
225 387-7000
Type: Hosp or Med Ctr: 300-499 Beds
Control: Nonprofit (Private or Religious)
• Radiography Prgm

Blue Cliff College - Baton Rouge
Kathie Lea Love
6160 Perkins Rd, Ste 200
Baton Rouge, LA 70808-4191
225 757-3770
Type: Vocational or Tech Sch
Control: For Profit
• Massage Therapy Prgm

Fortis College
John Hopkins, CEO
9255 Interline Ave
Baton Rouge, LA 70809
225 248-1015
Type: Vocational or Tech Sch
Control: For Profit
• Clin Lab Technician/Med Lab Technician Prgm
• Radiography Prgm
• Surgical Technology Prgm

Louisiana State U Fire & Emergency Training I
Baton Rouge, LA 70820
Type: 4-year Coll or Univ
• Emergency Med Tech-Paramedic Prgm

Louisiana State Univ and A&M College
William E Davis, Chancellor
Baton Rouge, LA 70803
504 388-3202
Type: 4-year Coll or Univ
Control: State, County, or Local Govt
• Speech-Language Pathology Prgm

Louisiana State University
Mike Martin, PhD, Chancellor
156 Thomas Boyd Hall
Baton Rouge, LA 70803
225 578-6977
Type: 4-year Coll or Univ
Control: State, County, or Local Govt
• Athletic Training Prgm
• Counseling Prgm
• Dental Hygiene Prgm
• Dental Lab Technician Prgm
• Dentistry Prgm
• Dietetics-Didactic Prgm
• Medical Librarian Prgm
• Music Therapy Prgm
• Psychology (PhD) Prgm
• Veterinary Medicine Prgm

Our Lady of the Lake College
Sandra Harper, PhD, President
7434 Perkins Rd
Baton Rouge, LA 70808
225 768-1710
Type: 4-year Coll or Univ
Control: Nonprofit (Private or Religious)
• Clin Lab Scientist/Med Technologist Prgm
• Physical Therapist Assistant Prgm
• Physician Assistant Prgm
• Radiography Prgm
• Respiratory Care Prgm
• Surgical Technology Prgm

Southern Univ and A&M College
Edward Jackson, PhD, Chancellor
Baton Rouge, LA 70813
225 771-5020
Type: 4-year Coll or Univ
Control: State, County, or Local Govt
• Dietetic Internship Prgm
• Dietetics-Didactic Prgm
• Nursing Prgm
• Rehabilitation Counseling Prgm
• Speech-Language Pathology Prgm

Bossier City

Bossier Parish Community College
Jim Henderson, MS, Chancellor
6220 E Texas St
Bossier City, LA 71111
318 678-6332
Type: Junior or Comm Coll
Control: State, County, or Local Govt
• Emergency Med Tech-Paramedic Prgm
• Medical Assistant Prgm
• Occupational Therapy Asst Prgm
• Pharmacy Technician Prgm
• Phlebotomy Prgm
• Physical Therapist Assistant Prgm
• Respiratory Care Prgm
• Surgical Technology Prgm

Eunice

Louisiana State University at Eunice
William J Nunez III, PhD, Chancellor
PO Box 1129
Eunice, LA 70535
318 457-7311
Type: Junior or Comm Coll
Control: State, County, or Local Govt
• Diagnostic Med Sonography (General) Prgm
• Radiography Prgm
• Respiratory Care Prgm

Hammond

North Oaks Medical Center
James E Cathey, Jr, CEO
15790 Paul Vega MD Dr
Hammond, LA 70403
985 345-2700
Type: Hosp or Med Ctr: 300-499 Beds
Control: State, County, or Local Govt
• Dietetic Internship Prgm
• Radiography Prgm

Southeastern Louisiana University
Randay Moffett, EdD, President
SLU 10784
Hammond, LA 70402
985 549-2280
Type: 4-year Coll or Univ
Control: State, County, or Local Govt
• Athletic Training Prgm
• Counseling Prgm
• Music Therapy Prgm
• Nursing Prgm
• Speech-Language Pathology Prgm

Houma

L E Fletcher Technical Community College
F Travis Lavigne, Jr, BS MS, Chancellor
310 Saint Charles St
PO Box 5033
Houma, LA 70361
985 858-5745
Type: Vocational or Tech Sch
Control: Nonprofit (Private or Religious)
• Phlebotomy Prgm

Lacombe

Cardiovascular Technology Training Inc
James Emerson Smith III, MD, CEO
64040 Hwy 434
Lacombe, LA 70445
985 867-3100
Type: Vocational or Tech Sch
Control: For Profit
• Cardiovascular Technology Prgm

Lafayette

Acadiana Technical College - Lafayette
Lafayette, LA 70506
Type: Vocational or Tech Sch
• Surgical Technology Prgm

Lafayette General Medical Center
John J Burdin, Jr, MHA, President
1214 Coolidge Ave
PO Box 52009 OCS
Lafayette, LA 70505
318 289-7381
Type: Hosp or Med Ctr: 100-299 Beds
Control: Nonprofit (Private or Religious)
• Radiography Prgm

National EMS Academy
Lafayette, LA 70507
Type: Junior or Comm Coll
• Emergency Med Tech-Paramedic Prgm

University of Louisiana at Lafayette
Ray Authement, PhD, President
UL Drawer 41008
Lafayette, LA 70504
337 482-6203
Type: 4-year Coll or Univ
Control: State, County, or Local Govt
• Athletic Training Prgm
• Dietetic Internship Prgm
• Dietetics-Didactic Prgm
• Music Therapy Prgm
• Nursing Prgm
• Speech-Language Pathology Prgm

Lake Charles

Lake Charles Memorial Hospital
Larry Graham, President
1701 Oak Park Blvd
Lake Charles, LA 70601
337 494-3000
Type: Hosp or Med Ctr: 300-499 Beds
Control: Nonprofit (Private or Religious)
• Clin Lab Scientist/Med Technologist Prgm

McNeese State University
Robert D Hebert, PhD, President
Box 93300
4205 Ryan Street
Lake Charles, LA 70609
337 475-5556
Type: 4-year Coll or Univ
Control: State, County, or Local Govt
• Athletic Training Prgm
• Clin Lab Scientist/Med Technologist Prgm
• Dietetic Internship Prgm
• Dietetics-Didactic Prgm
• Radiography Prgm

Monroe

Career Technical College
Cheryl Lokey, Director
2319 Louisville Ave
Monroe, LA 71201
318 323-2889
Type: Vocational or Tech Sch
Control: For Profit
• Medical Assistant Prgm (2)
• Radiography Prgm
• Surgical Technology Prgm

University of Louisiana at Monroe
Nick J Bruno, PhD, President
700 University Ave, NE Station
Monroe, LA 71209-0430
318 342-1010
Type: 4-year Coll or Univ
Control: State, County, or Local Govt
• Clin Lab Scientist/Med Technologist Prgm
• Counseling Prgm
• Dental Hygiene Prgm
• Exercise Physiology - Clinical Prgm
• Exercise Science Prgm
• Music Therapy Prgm
• Nursing Prgm
• Occupational Therapy Asst Prgm
• Pharmacy Prgm
• Radiography Prgm
• Speech-Language Pathology Prgm

Natchitoches

Northwestern State University
Randall J Webb, EdD, President
Natchitoches, LA 71497
318 357-5701
Type: 4-year Coll or Univ
Control: State, County, or Local Govt
• Counseling Prgm
• Music Therapy Prgm
• Nursing Prgm
• Radiography Prgm
• Veterinary Technology Prgm

New Orleans

Delgado Community College
Deborah Lea, MEd, Interm Chancellor
615 City Park Ave
New Orleans, LA 70119
504 361-6697
Type: Junior or Comm Coll
Control: State, County, or Local Govt
• Clin Lab Technician/Med Lab Technician Prgm
• Diagnostic Med Sonography (General) Prgm
• Dietetic Technician-AD Prgm
• Emergency Med Tech-Paramedic Prgm
• Nuclear Medicine Technology Prgm
• Occupational Therapy Asst Prgm
• Ophthalmic Assistant Prgm
• Pharmacy Technician Prgm
• Phlebotomy Prgm
• Physical Therapist Assistant Prgm
• Radiation Therapy Prgm
• Radiography Prgm
• Respiratory Care Prgm
• Surgical Technology Prgm
• Veterinary Technology Prgm

Louisiana State Univ Health Sciences Center
Larry H Hollier, MD, Chancellor
433 Bolivar St
Resource Center
New Orleans, LA 70112-2223
504 568-4800
Type: Acad Health Ctr/Med Sch
Control: State, County, or Local Govt
• Allopathic Medicine Prgm
• Audiologist Prgm
• Cardiovascular Tech (Noninvasive) Prgm
• Clin Lab Scientist/Med Technologist Prgm
• Nursing Prgm
• Occupational Therapy Prgm
• Physical Therapy Prgm
• Rehabilitation Counseling Prgm
• Respiratory Care Prgm
• Speech-Language Pathology Prgm

Loyola University New Orleans
Kevin Wildes, SJ, President
6363 St Charles Ave
New Orleans, LA 70118
504 865-2011
Type: 4-year Coll or Univ
Control: Nonprofit (Private or Religious)
• Counseling Prgm
• Music Therapy Prgm

Medical Center of Louisiana
Roxanne Townsend, Acting CEO
2021 Perdido St
New Orleans, LA 70112
504 903-0283
Type: Hosp or Med Ctr: 300-499 Beds
Control: State, County, or Local Govt
• Specialist in BB Tech Prgm

Our Lady of Holy Cross College
Rev Anthony DeConcilliis, PhD, President
4123 Woodland Dr
New Orleans, LA 70131-7399
504 394-7744
Type: 4-year Coll or Univ
Control: Nonprofit (Private or Religious)
• Counseling Prgm
• Radiography Prgm
• Respiratory Care Prgm

INSTITUTIONS

Tulane University
Eamon M Kelly, President
New Orleans, LA 70118
504 865-5000
Type: 4-year Coll or Univ
Control: Nonprofit (Private or Religious)
• Allopathic Medicine Prgm
• Dietetic Internship Prgm

University of New Orleans
Timothy P Ryan, PhD, Chancellor
Lake Front
New Orleans, LA 70148-0001
504 280-6000
Type: 4-year Coll or Univ
Control: State, County, or Local Govt
• Counseling Prgm
• Music Therapy Prgm

Xavier Univ of Louisiana College of Pharmacy
Wayne Harris, BS MS PhD, Professor & Dean
1 Drexel Dr
New Orleans, LA 70125
504 520-7421
Type: Acad Health Ctr/Med Sch
Control: Nonprofit (Private or Religious)
• Pharmacy Prgm

Pineville

Louisiana College
Joe Aguillard, President
Alexandria Hall, Rm 125
Pineville, LA 71359
318 487-7401
Type: 4-year Coll or Univ
Control: State, County, or Local Govt
• Athletic Training Prgm
• Nursing Prgm
• Physical Therapist Assistant Prgm

Ruston

Louisiana Tech University
Daniel D Reneau, PhD, President
PO Box 3168
Ruston, LA 71272
318 257-3785
Type: 4-year Coll or Univ
Control: State, County, or Local Govt
• Audiologist Prgm
• Dietetic Internship Prgm
• Dietetics-Didactic Prgm
• Speech-Language Pathology Prgm

Shreveport

LSU Health Science Center Shreveport
Robert Barish, Chancellor and Dean
1501 Kings Hwy
Shreveport, LA 71130
318 675-5242
Type: Acad Health Ctr/Med Sch
Control: State, County, or Local Govt
• Allopathic Medicine Prgm
• Clin Lab Scientist/Med Technologist Prgm
• Occupational Therapy Prgm
• Physical Therapy Prgm
• Physician Assistant Prgm
• Respiratory Care Prgm
• Speech-Language Pathology Prgm

Overton Brooks VA Medical Center
George Moore, MHA, Director
510 E Stoner Ave
Shreveport, LA 71101-4295
318 990-5140
Type: Hosp or Med Ctr: 100-299 Beds
Control: Fed Govt
• Clin Lab Scientist/Med Technologist Prgm

Southern Univ at Shreveport
Ray Belton, PhD, Chancellor
3050 Martin Luther King Jr Dr
Shreveport, LA 71107-8032
318 670-6000
Type: Junior or Comm Coll
Control: State, County, or Local Govt
• Clin Lab Technician/Med Lab Technician Prgm
• Dental Hygiene Prgm
• Phlebotomy Prgm
• Radiography Prgm
• Respiratory Care Prgm
• Surgical Technology Prgm

Thibodaux

Nicholls State University
Stephen Hulbert, EdD, President
PO Box 2001
Thibodaux, LA 70310
504 448-4003
Type: 4-year Coll or Univ
Control: State, County, or Local Govt
• Athletic Training Prgm
• Dietetics-Didactic Prgm
• Nursing Prgm
• Respiratory Care Prgm

Maine

Augusta

Univ of Maine Augusta (Bangor)
Allyson Handley, MA, President
46 University Dr
Augusta, ME 04330
207 621-3000
Type: 4-year Coll or Univ
Control: State, County, or Local Govt
• Dental Assistant Prgm
• Dental Hygiene Prgm
• Veterinary Technology Prgm

University of Maine
Charles Lyons, DEd, President
46 University Dr
Augusta, ME 04330
207 621-3403
Type: 4-year Coll or Univ
Control: State, County, or Local Govt
• Nursing Prgm

Bangor

Beal College
Allen Stehle, BS, President
99 Farm Rd
Bangor, ME 04401
207 947-4591
Type: Junior or Comm Coll
Control: For Profit
• Medical Assistant Prgm

Eastern Maine Community College
Joyce B Hedlund, EdD, President
354 Hogan Rd
Bangor, ME 04401
207 974-4691
Type: Junior or Comm Coll
Control: State, County, or Local Govt
• Medical Assistant Prgm
• Radiography Prgm
• Surgical Technology Prgm

Eastern Maine Medical Center
Deborah Carey-Johnson, President, CEO
489 State St
Bangor, ME 04401
207 973-7000
Type: Hosp or Med Ctr: 300-499 Beds
Control: Nonprofit (Private or Religious)
• Clin Lab Scientist/Med Technologist Prgm

Husson University
William H Beardsley, PhD, President
One College Circle
206 Peabody Hall
Bangor, ME 04401-2999
207 973-7138
Type: 4-year Coll or Univ
Control: Nonprofit (Private or Religious)
• Nursing Prgm
• Occupational Therapy Prgm
• Pharmacy Prgm
• Physical Therapy Prgm

Biddeford

University of New England
Danielle Ripich, PhD, President
11 Hills Beach Rd
Biddeford, ME 04005-9599
207 283-0171
Type: 4-year Coll or Univ
Control: Nonprofit (Private or Religious)
• Athletic Training Prgm
• Dental Hygiene Prgm
• Occupational Therapy Prgm
• Osteopathic Medicine Prgm
• Pharmacy Prgm
• Physical Therapy Prgm
• Physician Assistant Prgm

Bridgton

New Hampshire Institute for Therapeutic Arts
Patrick Ian Cowan, PhD, Executive Director
Bridgton, ME 04009
603 882-3022
Type: Vocational or Tech Sch
Control: For Profit
• Massage Therapy Prgm

Calais

Washington County Technical College
Calais, ME 04619-9701
Type: Vocational or Tech Sch
Control: State, County, or Local Govt
• Medical Assistant Prgm

Fairfield

Kennebec Valley Community College
Barbara W Woodlee, EdD, President
92 Western Ave
Fairfield, ME 04937-1367
207 453-5129
Type: Junior or Comm Coll
Control: State, County, or Local Govt
• Diagnostic Med Sonography (General) Prgm
• Medical Assistant Prgm
• Occupational Therapy Asst Prgm
• Physical Therapist Assistant Prgm
• Radiography Prgm
• Respiratory Care Prgm

Lewiston

Central Maine Medical Center
Peter Chalke, MHA, President
300 Main St
Lewiston, ME 04240
207 795-2700
Type: Hosp or Med Ctr: 100-299 Beds
Control: Nonprofit (Private or Religious)
• Nuclear Medicine Technology Prgm
• Radiography Prgm

Orono

University of Maine - Orono
Robert Kennedy, PhD, President
5703 Alumni Hall, Rm 200
Orono, ME 04469
207 581-1512
Type: 4-year Coll or Univ
Control: State, County, or Local Govt
• Athletic Training Prgm
• Dietetic Internship Prgm
• Dietetics-Didactic Prgm
• Nursing Prgm
• Psychology (PsyD) Prgm
• Speech-Language Pathology Prgm

Portland

Maine Medical Center
Vincent Conti, President
22 Bramhall St
Portland, ME 04102
207 871-2491
Type: Hosp or Med Ctr: 500 Beds
Control: Nonprofit (Private or Religious)
• Surgical Technology Prgm

University of Southern Maine
Selma Botman, PhD, President
96 Falmouth St, PO Box 9300
Portland, ME 04104-9300
207 780-4480
Type: 4-year Coll or Univ
Control: State, County, or Local Govt
• Athletic Training Prgm
• Counseling Prgm
• Exercise Science Prgm
• Music Therapy Prgm
• Nursing Prgm
• Occupational Therapy Prgm
• Rehabilitation Counseling Prgm

Presque Isle

University of Maine at Presque Isle
Donald Zillman, PhD, President
181 Main St
22 Preble Hall
Presque Isle, ME 04769
207 768-9623
Type: 4-year Coll or Univ
Control: State, County, or Local Govt
• Athletic Training Prgm
• Clin Lab Technician/Med Lab Technician Prgm

South Portland

Southern Maine Community College
James Ortiz, EdD, President
Fort Rd
South Portland, ME 04106
207 741-5500
Type: Junior or Comm Coll
Control: State, County, or Local Govt
• Dietetic Technician-AD Prgm
• Radiation Therapy Prgm
• Radiography Prgm
• Respiratory Care Prgm

Standish

Saint Joseph's College of Maine
Standish, ME 04084
Type: 4-year Coll or Univ
Control: Nonprofit (Private or Religious)
• Nursing Prgm

Waldoboro

Downeast School of Massage
Nancy W Dail, BA LMT NCTMB, Director
99 Moose Meadow Lane
Waldoboro, ME 04572
207 832-5531
Type: Acad Health Ctr/Med Sch
Control: For Profit
• Massage Therapy Prgm

Manitoba, Canada

Winnipeg

Massage Therapy College of Manitoba
Garth Beddome, BA RMT, Director
Winnipeg, MB R3G 1C3
204 772-8999
Type: Acad Health Ctr/Med Sch
Control: For Profit
• Massage Therapy Prgm

University of Manitoba
770 Bannatyne Ave
Winnipeg, MB R3E 0W3
Type: 4-year Coll or Univ
Control: Nonprofit (Private or Religious)
• Allopathic Medicine Prgm
• Psychology (PhD) Prgm

Maryland

Arnold

Anne Arundel Community College
Martha A Smith, PhD, President
101 College Pkwy
Arnold, MD 21012-1875
410 777-2222
Type: Junior or Comm Coll
Control: State, County, or Local Govt
• Clin Lab Technician/Med Lab Technician Prgm
• Emergency Med Tech-Paramedic Prgm
• Medical Assistant Prgm
• Pharmacy Technician Prgm
• Physician Assistant Prgm
• Radiography Prgm

Chesapeake Area Consortium for Higher Educ
101 College Pkwy
Arnold, MD 21012
Type: Consortium
Control: Nonprofit (Private or Religious)
• Physical Therapist Assistant Prgm

Baltimore

All-State Career - Healthcare Division
Baltimore, MD 21224
• Dental Assistant Prgm

Baltimore City Community College
Richard Turner, DME, President
2901 Liberty Heights Ave
Baltimore, MD 21215-7893
410 462-7799
Type: Junior or Comm Coll
Control: State, County, or Local Govt
• Dental Hygiene Prgm
• Dietetic Technician-AD Prgm
• Physical Therapist Assistant Prgm
• Respiratory Care Prgm
• Surgical Technology Prgm

College of Notre Dame of Maryland
Baltimore, MD 21210
Type: 4-year Coll or Univ
Control: Nonprofit (Private or Religious)
• Pharmacy Prgm

Comm Coll of Baltimore County - Catonsville
Sandra Kurtinitis, PhD, President
7200 Soellers Point Rd
Baltimore, MD 21222
410 285-9993
Type: Junior or Comm Coll
Control: State, County, or Local Govt
• Occupational Therapy Asst Prgm

Coppin State University
Sadie Gregory, Interim President
2500 W North Ave
Baltimore, MD 21216
410 951-3838
Type: 4-year Coll or Univ
Control: State, County, or Local Govt
• Nursing Prgm
• Rehabilitation Counseling Prgm

Fortis Institute
Baltimore, MD 21244
Type: Vocational or Tech Sch
- Dental Hygiene Prgm
- Radiography Prgm
- Surgical Technology Prgm

Greater Baltimore Medical Center
Lawerence Merlis, MBA, President
6701 N Charles St
Baltimore, MD 21204
443 849-2121
Type: Hosp or Med Ctr: 300-499 Beds
Control: Nonprofit (Private or Religious)
- Orthoptist Prgm
- Radiography Prgm

Johns Hopkins Bayview Medical Center
4940 Eastern Ave
Baltimore, MD 21224-2735
Type: Acad Health Ctr/Med Sch
Control: Nonprofit (Private or Religious)
- Dietetic Internship Prgm
- Dietetics-Coordinated Prgm

Johns Hopkins Hospital
Ronald R Peterson, MHA, President
733 N Broadway, BRB 104
Baltimore, MD 21287
410 955-9540
Type: Hosp or Med Ctr: 500 Beds
Control: Nonprofit (Private or Religious)
- Diagnostic Med Sonography (General) Prgm
- Nuclear Medicine Technology Prgm
- Radiography Prgm
- Specialist in BB Tech Prgm

Johns Hopkins School of Medicine
Edward D Miller, Jr, MD, President, CEO
100 Medical Admin Bldg
720 N Rutland Ave
Baltimore, MD 21205
410 955-3180
Type: Acad Health Ctr/Med Sch
Control: Nonprofit (Private or Religious)
- Allopathic Medicine Prgm
- Medical Illustrator Prgm

Johns Hopkins University
Baltimore, MD 21205
Type: 4-year Coll or Univ
Control: Nonprofit (Private or Religious)
- Genetic Counseling Prgm
- Nursing Prgm

Loyola University Maryland
Brian Linnane, SJ PhD, President
4501 N Charles St
Baltimore, MD 21210
410 617-2000
Type: 4-year Coll or Univ
Control: Nonprofit (Private or Religious)
- Counseling Prgm (2)
- Psychology (PhD) Prgm
- Speech-Language Pathology Prgm

Morgan State University
Earl S Richardson, EdD, President
Coldspring Ln and Hillen Rd
1700 East Coldspring Lane
Baltimore, MD 21215
443 885-3000
Type: 4-year Coll or Univ
Control: State, County, or Local Govt
- Clin Lab Scientist/Med Technologist Prgm
- Dietetics-Didactic Prgm

University of Maryland Baltimore County
Freeman Hrabowski, PhD, President
1000 Hilltop Circle
1450 S Rolling Rd
Baltimore, MD 21250
410 455-3880
Type: 4-year Coll or Univ
Control: State, County, or Local Govt
- Diagnostic Med Sonography (Gen/Card/Vascular) Prgm
- Emergency Med Tech-Paramedic Prgm
- Pharmacy Prgm
- Psychology (PhD) Prgm

University of Maryland Medical System
22 S Greene St
Baltimore, MD 21201-1544
410 328-2561
Type: Acad Health Ctr/Med Sch
Control: State, County, or Local Govt
- Dietetic Internship Prgm
- Medical Dosimetry Prgm

University of Maryland, Baltimore
David J Ramsay, DM DPhil, President
522 West Lombard Street
The Saratoga Building, Room 03-124
Baltimore, MD 21201
410 706-0500
Type: 4-year Coll or Univ
Control: State, County, or Local Govt
- Allopathic Medicine Prgm
- Clin Lab Scientist/Med Technologist Prgm
- Dental Hygiene Prgm
- Dentistry Prgm
- Genetic Counseling Prgm
- Medical Librarian Prgm
- Nursing Prgm
- Pathologists' Assistant Prgm
- Physical Therapy Prgm
- Rehabilitation Counseling Prgm

Baltimore County

Community College of Baltimore County
Sandra Kurtinitis, PhD, President
7201 Rossville Blvd
Baltimore County, MD 21237-3898
410 780-6322
Type: Junior or Comm Coll
Control: State, County, or Local Govt
- Clin Lab Technician/Med Lab Technician Prgm
- Dental Hygiene Prgm
- Emergency Med Tech-Paramedic Prgm
- Polysomnographic Technology Prgm
- Radiation Therapy Prgm
- Radiography Prgm
- Respiratory Care Prgm
- Surgical Technology Prgm
- Veterinary Technology Prgm

Bel Air

Harford Community College
James F LaCalle, EdD, President
401 Thomas Run Rd
Bel Air, MD 21015
443 412-2493
Type: Junior or Comm Coll
Control: State, County, or Local Govt
- Histotechnician Prgm
- Medical Assistant Prgm

Bethesda

National Institutes of Health
John Gallin
10 Center Dr
CRC Building 10, Room 6-2551
Bethesda, MD 20892
301 496-4114
Type: Acad Health Ctr/Med Sch
Control: Fed Govt
- Dietetic Internship Prgm

NIH Clinical Center Department of Transfusion
John Gallin, MD, Deputy Director
10 Center Dr, CRC Building 10
Room 6-2551
Bethesda, MD 20892
301 496-4114
Type: Hosp or Med Ctr: 300-499 Beds
Control: Fed Govt
- Specialist in BB Tech Prgm

Uniformed Svcs Univ of the Health Sciences
Bethesda, MD 20814
Type: Acad Health Ctr/Med Sch
Control: Fed Govt
- Allopathic Medicine Prgm
- Psychology (PhD) Prgm

Walter Reed National Military Med Ctr
Norvell Coots, COL, Healthcare Sys Commander
8901 Rockville Pike
Bethesda, MD 20889-5600
202 782-6394
Type: Dept of Defense
Control: Fed Govt
- Clin Lab Scientist/Med Technologist Prgm
- Perfusion Prgm
- Specialist in BB Tech Prgm

College Park

Univ of Maryland at College Park
William E Kirwan, President
College Park, MD 20742
301 405-1000
Type: 4-year Coll or Univ
Control: State, County, or Local Govt
- Audiologist Prgm
- Counseling Prgm
- Dietetic Internship Prgm
- Dietetics-Didactic Prgm
- Music Therapy Prgm
- Psychology (PsyD) Prgm
- Speech-Language Pathology Prgm

Columbia

Howard Community College
Kathleen Heatherington, PhD, President
10901 Little Patuxent Parkway
Columbia, MD 21044
410 772-4820
Type: Junior or Comm Coll
Control: State, County, or Local Govt
• Cardiovascular Tech (Invasive) Prgm
• Emergency Med Tech-Paramedic Prgm

Sodexho Health Care Services, Mid Atlantic
Columbia, MD 21044
Type: Acad Health Ctr/Med Sch
Control: For Profit
• Dietetic Internship Prgm

Cumberland

Allegany College of Maryland
Gary Durr, PhD, Interim President
12401 Willowbrook Rd SE
Cumberland, MD 21502-2596
301 784-5270
Type: Junior or Comm Coll
Control: State, County, or Local Govt
• Clin Lab Technician/Med Lab Technician Prgm
• Dental Hygiene Prgm
• Massage Therapy Prgm
• Medical Assistant Prgm
• Occupational Therapy Asst Prgm
• Physical Therapist Assistant Prgm
• Radiography Prgm
• Respiratory Care Prgm

Frederick

Frederick Community College
Patricia Stanley, EdD, President
7932 Opossumtown Pike
Frederick, MD 21702
301 846-2400
Type: Junior or Comm Coll
Control: State, County, or Local Govt
• Respiratory Care Prgm
• Surgical Technology Prgm

Frostburg

Frostburg State University
Catherine R Gira, PhD, President
101 Braddock Rd
Frostburg, MD 21532
301 687-4111
Type: 4-year Coll or Univ
Control: State, County, or Local Govt
• Athletic Training Prgm
• Nursing Prgm

Hagerstown

Hagerstown Community College
Guy Altieri, EdD, President
11400 Robinwood Dr
Hagerstown, MD 21742-6590
301 790-2800
Type: Junior or Comm Coll
Control: State, County, or Local Govt
• Emergency Med Tech-Paramedic Prgm
• Radiography Prgm

Kaplan College - Hagerstown
W Christopher Motz, MEd, President
18618 Crestwood Dr
Hagerstown, MD 21742
301 739-2680
Type: Junior or Comm Coll
Control: For Profit
• Medical Assistant Prgm
• Phlebotomy Prgm

La Plata

College of Southern Maryland
8730 Mitchell Rd. PO Box 910
La Plata, MD 20646-0910
Type: Junior or Comm Coll
Control: State, County, or Local Govt
• Clin Lab Technician/Med Lab Technician Prgm

Landover

Sanford-Brown Institute - Landover
Landover, MD 20785
Type: Vocational or Tech Sch
• Diagnostic Med Sonography (General) Prgm

Largo

Prince George's Community College
Charlene Dukes, Ed D, President
301 Largo Rd
Largo, MD 20774
301 322-0400
Type: Junior or Comm Coll
Control: State, County, or Local Govt
• Nuclear Medicine Technology Prgm
• Radiography Prgm
• Respiratory Care Prgm

Linthicum

Baltimore School of Massage
Richard Rynders, Campus Director
517 Progress Dr, Ste A-L
Linthicum, MD 21090
410 636-7929
Type: Vocational or Tech Sch
Control: For Profit
• Massage Therapy Prgm

New Market

Associates in Emergency Care
Renee Joyce, RN BSN, Administrator
5628 Wellspring Court
New Market, MD 20872
301 865-8880
Type: Vocational or Tech Sch
Control: For Profit
• Emergency Med Tech-Paramedic Prgm

North East

Cecil Community College
W Stephen Pannill, EdD, President
One Seahawk Dr
North East, MD 21901
410 287-6060
Type: Junior or Comm Coll
Control: State, County, or Local Govt
• Medical Assistant Prgm

Princess Anne

University of Maryland Eastern Shore
Thelma B Thompson, PhD, President
Princess Anne, MD 21853
410 651-2200
Type: 4-year Coll or Univ
Control: State, County, or Local Govt
• Dietetic Internship Prgm
• Dietetics-Didactic Prgm
• Pharmacy Prgm
• Physical Therapy Prgm
• Physician Assistant Prgm
• Rehabilitation Counseling Prgm

Rockville

Montgomery College
Brian K Johnson, EdD, President
Central Admin Office
900 Hungerford
Rockville, MD 20850
240 567-5264
Type: Junior or Comm Coll
Control: State, County, or Local Govt
• Diagnostic Med Sonography
  (Gen/Card/Vascular) Prgm
• Music Therapy Prgm
• Physical Therapist Assistant Prgm
• Radiography Prgm
• Surgical Technology Prgm

Salisbury

Salisbury University
Janet Dudley-Eshbach, PhD, President
1101 Camden Ave
Holloway Hall
Salisbury, MD 21801
410 543-6012
Type: 4-year Coll or Univ
Control: State, County, or Local Govt
• Athletic Training Prgm
• Clin Lab Scientist/Med Technologist Prgm
• Exercise Science Prgm
• Music Therapy Prgm
• Nursing Prgm
• Respiratory Care Prgm

Wor-Wic Community College
Murray K Hoy, PhD, President
32000 Campus Dr
Salisbury, MD 21801
410 334-2800
Type: Junior or Comm Coll
Control: State, County, or Local Govt
• Radiography Prgm

Silver Spring

Holy Cross Hospital
Kevin Sexton, MHA, President and CEO
1500 Forest Glen Rd
Silver Spring, MD 20910
301 754-7000
Type: Hosp or Med Ctr: 500 Beds
Control: Nonprofit (Private or Religious)
• Radiography Prgm

INSTITUTIONS

Stevenson

Stevenson University
Kevin Manning
1525 Greenspring Valley Rd
Stevenson, MD 21153
410 486-7000
Type: 4-year Coll or Univ
Control: For Profit
• Clin Lab Scientist/Med Technologist Prgm
• Nursing Prgm

Takoma Park

Montgomery County Community College
Takoma Park, MD 20912
Type: Junior or Comm Coll
• Polysomnographic Technology Prgm

Washington Adventist Hospital
Brian Breckenridge, President
7600 Carroll Ave
Takoma Park, MD 20912
301 891-7600
Type: Hosp or Med Ctr: 300-499 Beds
Control: Nonprofit (Private or Religious)
• Radiography Prgm

Washington Adventist University
Randall Wisbey, PhD, President
7600 Flower Ave
Takoma Park, MD 20912
301 891-4128
Type: 4-year Coll or Univ
Control: Nonprofit (Private or Religious)
• Respiratory Care Prgm

Timonium

Institute of Health Sciences
Timonium, MD 21093
Type: Acad Health Ctr/Med Sch
• Neurodiagnostic Tech Prgm

Towson

Fortis College - Towson
Sheila Kell, Director
700 York Rd
Towson, MD 21204
410 337-5155
Type: Vocational or Tech Sch
Control: For Profit
• Dental Assistant Prgm
• Medical Assistant Prgm

Towson University
Robert Caret, PhD, President
8000 York Rd
Towson, MD 21252-0001
410 704-2356
Type: 4-year Coll or Univ
Control: State, County, or Local Govt
• Athletic Training Prgm
• Audiologist Prgm
• Music Therapy Prgm
• Nursing Prgm
• Occupational Therapy Prgm
• Physician Assistant Prgm
• Speech-Language Pathology Prgm

Westminster

Carroll Community College
Faye Pappallardo
1601 Washington Rd
Westminster, MD 21157
410 386-8255
Type: Junior or Comm Coll
Control: State, County, or Local Govt
• Physical Therapist Assistant Prgm

White Marsh

Medix School
Duncan Anderson, President and CEO
5024A Campbell Boulevard
White Marsh, MD 21236
410 633-2929
Type: Vocational or Tech Sch
Control: For Profit
• Medical Assistant Prgm

Wye Mills

Chesapeake College
Stuart M Bounds, EdD, President
PO Box 8
Wye Mills, MD 21679
410 822-5400
Type: Junior or Comm Coll
Control: State, County, or Local Govt
• Radiography Prgm
• Surgical Technology Prgm

Massachusetts

Amherst

University of Massachusetts - Amherst
John Lombardi, Chancellor
Amherst, MA 01003
413 545-0111
Type: 4-year Coll or Univ
Control: State, County, or Local Govt
• Audiologist Prgm
• Dietetic Internship Prgm
• Dietetics-Didactic Prgm
• Music Therapy Prgm
• Nursing Prgm
• Psychology (PhD) Prgm
• Speech-Language Pathology Prgm

Auburndale

Lasell College
Thomas E J De Witt, PhD, President
1844 Commonwealth Ave
Auburndale, MA 02466
617 243-2000
Type: 4-year Coll or Univ
Control: Nonprofit (Private or Religious)
• Athletic Training Prgm

Bedford

Middlesex Community College
Carole A Cowan, EdD, President
Springs Rd
Bedford, MA 01730
781 280-3100
Type: Junior or Comm Coll
Control: State, County, or Local Govt
• Dental Assistant Prgm
• Dental Hygiene Prgm
• Dental Lab Technician Prgm
• Diagnostic Med Sonography (General) Prgm
• Medical Assistant Prgm
• Radiography Prgm

Beverly

Endicott College
Richard Wylie, EdD, President
376 Hale St
Beverly, MA 01915
978 232-2000
Type: 4-year Coll or Univ
Control: Nonprofit (Private or Religious)
• Athletic Training Prgm

Boston

Bay State College
Howard E Horton, Esq, President
122 Commonwealth Ave
Boston, MA 02116
617 217-9000
Type: Junior or Comm Coll
Control: For Profit
• Physical Therapist Assistant Prgm

Berklee College of Music
Roger Brown, President
1140 Boylston St
Boston, MA 02215
617 266-1400
Type: 4-year Coll or Univ
Control: Nonprofit (Private or Religious)
• Music Therapy Prgm

Beth Israel Deaconess Medical Center
Paul Levey, President
330 Brookline Ave
Boston, MA 02215-5399
617 667-2203
Type: Hosp or Med Ctr: 500 Beds
Control: Nonprofit (Private or Religious)
• Dietetic Internship Prgm

Boston University
Robert A Brown, PhD, President
One Sherborn St
Boston, MA 02215
617 353-2200
Type: 4-year Coll or Univ
Control: Nonprofit (Private or Religious)
• Allopathic Medicine Prgm
• Athletic Training Prgm
• Dentistry Prgm
• Dietetic Internship Prgm
• Dietetics-Didactic Prgm
• Genetic Counseling Prgm
• Occupational Therapy Prgm
• Physical Therapy Prgm
• Psychology (PhD) Prgm
• Speech-Language Pathology Prgm

Brigham & Women's Hospital
Gary Gottleib, MD, CEO
75 Francis St
Boston, MA 02115-6195
617 732-5595
Type: Hosp or Med Ctr: 500 Beds
Control: Nonprofit (Private or Religious)
• Dietetic Internship Prgm

Bunker Hill Community College
Mary L Fifield, PhD, President
250 New Rutherford Ave
Boston, MA 02129-2925
617 228-2400
Type: Junior or Comm Coll
Control: State, County, or Local Govt
• Clin Lab Technician/Med Lab Technician Prgm
• Diagnostic Med Sonography (General/Cardiac) Prgm
• Radiography Prgm
• Surgical Technology Prgm

Emerson College
Jacqueline W Liebergott, President
100 Beacon St
Boston, MA 02116
617 578-8500
Type: 4-year Coll or Univ
Control: Nonprofit (Private or Religious)
• Speech-Language Pathology Prgm

Emmanuel College
Boston, MA 02115
Type: 4-year Coll or Univ
Control: Nonprofit (Private or Religious)
• Nursing Prgm

Frances Stern Nutrition Center
Thomas O'Donnell, MD, President
750 Washington St
PO Box 451
Boston, MA 02111
617 636-7655
Type: Hosp or Med Ctr: 300-499 Beds
Control: Nonprofit (Private or Religious)
• Dietetic Internship Prgm

Harvard Medical School
Boston, MA 02118
Type: Acad Health Ctr/Med Sch
Control: Nonprofit (Private or Religious)
• Allopathic Medicine Prgm
• Dentistry Prgm

Kaplan Career Institute - Boston
Boston, MA 02215
• Dental Assistant Prgm
• Dental Hygiene Prgm

Mass College of Pharmacy & Health Sciences
Charles F Monahan, Jr, BS ScD (Hon), President
179 Longwood Ave
Boston, MA 02115
617 732-2880
Type: Nonhosp HC Facil, BB, or Lab
Control: Nonprofit (Private or Religious)
• Dental Hygiene Prgm
• Nuclear Medicine Technology Prgm
• Nursing Prgm
• Optometry Prgm
• Pharmacy Prgm (2)
• Physician Assistant Prgm (2)
• Radiation Therapy Prgm
• Radiography Prgm
• Radiologist Assistant Prgm

Massachusetts General Hospital
J Robert Buchanan, MD, General Director
32 Fruit St
Boston, MA 02114
617 726-2101
Type: Hosp or Med Ctr: 500 Beds
Control: Nonprofit (Private or Religious)
• Dietetic Internship Prgm

Massachusetts Sch of Prof Psychology Inc
Boston, MA 02125
Type: Acad Health Ctr/Med Sch
Control: For Profit
• Psychology (PsyD) Prgm

MGH Institute of Health Professions
Janis Bellack, PhD RN FAAN, President
Charlestown Navy Yard
36 First Ave
Boston, MA 02129-4557
617 726-2947
Control: Nonprofit (Private or Religious)
• Nursing Prgm
• Physical Therapy Prgm
• Radiography Prgm
• Speech-Language Pathology Prgm

New England College of Optometry
Elizabeth Chen, MBA, President
424 Beacon St
Boston, MA 02115
Type: Junior or Comm Coll
Control: Nonprofit (Private or Religious)
• Optometry Prgm

Northeastern University
Joseph E Anon, PhD, President
Office of the President
716 Columbus Pl
Boston, MA 02115
617 373-2000
Type: 4-year Coll or Univ
Control: Nonprofit (Private or Religious)
• Athletic Training Prgm
• Audiologist Prgm
• Nursing Prgm
• Pharmacy Prgm
• Physical Therapy Prgm
• Physician Assistant Prgm
• Respiratory Care Prgm
• Speech-Language Pathology Prgm

Roxbury Community College
Terrence Gomes, EdD, President
1234 Columbus Ave
Boston, MA 02120
617 427-0060
Type: Junior or Comm Coll
Control: State, County, or Local Govt
• Radiography Prgm

Simmons College
Daniel Cheever, Jr, EdD, President
300 The Fenway
Boston, MA 02115
617 521-2000
Type: 4-year Coll or Univ
Control: Nonprofit (Private or Religious)
• Dietetic Internship Prgm
• Dietetics-Didactic Prgm
• Medical Librarian Prgm
• Nursing Prgm
• Physical Therapy Prgm

Suffolk University
David J Sargent, PhD, President
Beacon Hill
Boston, MA 02108-2770
617 573-8000
Type: 4-year Coll or Univ
Control: State, County, or Local Govt
• Psychology (PhD) Prgm
• Radiation Therapy Prgm

University of Massachusetts - Boston
Keith Motley, Chancellor
100 Morrissey Blvd
Boston, MA 02125
617 287-5000
Type: 4-year Coll or Univ
Control: State, County, or Local Govt
• Allopathic Medicine Prgm
• Nursing Prgm
• Orientation and Mobility Specialist Prgm
• Psychology (PsyD) Prgm
• Rehabilitation Counseling Prgm

Braintree

American Career Institute
Braintree, MA 02184
Type: 4-year Coll or Univ
• Medical Assistant Prgm
• Psychology (PhD) Prgm

Clark University
Robert Payne, PhD, Vice President
725 Granite Plaza
Braintree, MA 02184
781 794-3400
Type: 4-year Coll or Univ
Control: Nonprofit (Private or Religious)
• Psychology (PhD) Prgm

Bridgewater

Bridgewater State University
Adrian Tinsley, PhD, President
Bridgewater, MA 02325
508 697-1201
Type: 4-year Coll or Univ
Control: State, County, or Local Govt
• Athletic Training Prgm
• Counseling Prgm

Brockton

Massasoit Community College
Charles Wall, PhD, President
1 Massasoit Blvd
Brockton, MA 02301
508 588-9100
Type: Junior or Comm Coll
Control: State, County, or Local Govt
• Dental Assistant Prgm
• Medical Assistant Prgm
• Radiography Prgm
• Respiratory Care Prgm

Cambridge

Lesley University
Joseph Moore, President
29 Everett St
Cambridge, MA 02138
617 868-9600
Type: 4-year Coll or Univ
Control: Nonprofit (Private or Religious)
• Art Therapy Prgm
• Dance/Movement Therapy Prgm
• Music Therapy Prgm

Mount Auburn Hospital
Francis P Lynch, President
330 Mt Auburn St
Cambridge, MA 02238
617 492-3500
Type: Hosp or Med Ctr: 300-499 Beds
Control: Nonprofit (Private or Religious)
• Dietetic Internship Prgm

Pro EMS Center for Medics
Cambridge, MA 02138
Type: Vocational or Tech Sch
• Emergency Med Tech-Paramedic Prgm

Chestnut Hill

Boston College
Chestnut Hill, MA 02467
Type: 4-year Coll or Univ
Control: Nonprofit (Private or Religious)
• Nursing Prgm

Chicopee

Elms College
Chicopee, MA 01013
Type: 4-year Coll or Univ
Control: Nonprofit (Private or Religious)
• Nursing Prgm

Porter and Chester Institute - Chicopee
Henry Kamerzel, VP and Executive Director
134 Dulong Circle
Chicopee, MA 01022
413 593-3339
Type: Vocational or Tech Sch
Control: For Profit
• Medical Assistant Prgm

Danvers

North Shore Community College
Wayne M Burton, EdD, President
One Ferncroft Rd, PO Box 3340
Danvers, MA 01923-0840
978 762-4000
Type: Junior or Comm Coll
Control: State, County, or Local Govt
• Medical Assistant Prgm
• Occupational Therapy Asst Prgm
• Physical Therapist Assistant Prgm
• Radiography Prgm
• Respiratory Care Prgm
• Surgical Technology Prgm
• Veterinary Technology Prgm

Dorchester

Laboure College
Joseph McNabe', PhD, President
2120 Dorchester Ave
Dorchester, MA 02124-5698
617 296-8300
Type: Junior or Comm Coll
Control: Nonprofit (Private or Religious)
• Dietetic Technician-AD Prgm
• Neurodiagnostic Tech Prgm
• Radiation Therapy Prgm

Fall River

Bristol Community College
John J Sbrega, PhD, President
777 Elsbree St
Fall River, MA 02720
508 678-2811
Type: Junior or Comm Coll
Control: State, County, or Local Govt
• Clin Lab Technician/Med Lab Technician Prgm
• Dental Hygiene Prgm
• Medical Assistant Prgm
• Occupational Therapy Asst Prgm

Fitchburg

Fitchburg State College
Michael P Riccards, PhD, President
160 Pearl St
Fitchburg, MA 01420
508 665-3112
Type: 4-year Coll or Univ
Control: State, County, or Local Govt
• Nursing Prgm

Framingham

Framingham State University
Paul F Weller, President
100 State St
Framingham, MA 01701
508 620-1220
Type: 4-year Coll or Univ
Control: State, County, or Local Govt
• Dietetics-Coordinated Prgm
• Dietetics-Didactic Prgm
• Nursing Prgm

Gardner

Mount Wachusett Community College
Daniel M Asquino, PhD, President
444 Green St
Gardner, MA 01440
978 632-6600
Type: Junior or Comm Coll
Control: State, County, or Local Govt
• Clin Lab Technician/Med Lab Technician Prgm
• Dental Assistant Prgm
• Dental Hygiene Prgm
• Massage Therapy Prgm
• Medical Assistant Prgm
• Physical Therapist Assistant Prgm

Greenfield

Stillpoint Program - Greenfield Comm Coll
270 Main St
Greenfield, MA 01301
Type: Acad Health Ctr/Med Sch
Control: For Profit
• Massage Therapy Prgm

Haverhill

Northern Essex Community College
David F Hartleb, JD, President
100 Elliott Way
Haverhill, MA 01830
978 556-3855
Type: Junior or Comm Coll
Control: State, County, or Local Govt
• Dental Assistant Prgm
• Medical Assistant Prgm
• Polysomnographic Technology Prgm
• Radiography Prgm
• Respiratory Care Prgm

Holyoke

Holyoke Community College
William Messner, EdD, President
303 Homestead Ave
Holyoke, MA 01040
413 538-7000
Type: Junior or Comm Coll
Control: State, County, or Local Govt
• Radiography Prgm
• Veterinary Technician Prgm

Longmeadow

Bay Path College
Carol A Leary, PhD, President
588 Longmeadow St
Longmeadow, MA 01106
413 565-1241
Type: 4-year Coll or Univ
Control: Nonprofit (Private or Religious)
• Occupational Therapy Prgm

Lowell

University of Massachusetts - Lowell
Martin Meehan, JD, Chancellor
One University Ave
Lowell, MA 01854
978 934-2201
Type: 4-year Coll or Univ
Control: State, County, or Local Govt
• Clin Lab Scientist/Med Technologist Prgm
• Music Therapy Prgm
• Nursing Prgm
• Physical Therapy Prgm

Medford

Tufts University
Lawrence Bacow, PhD, President
Ballou Hall
Medford, MA 02155-7084
617 627-3300
Type: 4-year Coll or Univ
Control: Nonprofit (Private or Religious)
• Allopathic Medicine Prgm
• Dentistry Prgm
• Occupational Therapy Prgm
• Veterinary Medicine Prgm

Milton

Curry College
Kenneth K Quigley, Jr, President
1071 Blue Hill Ave
Milton, MA 02186
617 333-0500
Type: 4-year Coll or Univ
Control: Nonprofit (Private or Religious)
• Nursing Prgm

Newton Centre

Mt Ida College
Carol Matteson, PhD, President
School of Business
777 Dedham St
Newton Centre, MA 02459
617 928-4500
Type: 4-year Coll or Univ
Control: Nonprofit (Private or Religious)
• Dental Hygiene Prgm
• Veterinary Technology Prgm

North Adams

Charles H McCann Technical School
James J Brosnan, CAGS, Superintendent
70 Hodges Cross Rd
North Adams, MA 01247
413 663-5383
Type: Vocational or Tech Sch
Control: State, County, or Local Govt
• Dental Assistant Prgm
• Medical Assistant Prgm
• Surgical Technology Prgm

North Andover

Merrimack College
Joseph Calderone, OSA, Interim President
315 Turnpike St
North Andover, MA 01845
978 837-5111
Type: 4-year Coll or Univ
Control: Nonprofit (Private or Religious)
• Athletic Training Prgm

North Dartmouth

University of Massachusetts - Dartmouth
Jean MacCormack, EdD, Chancellor
Office of the Chancellor
Foster Administration Building
North Dartmouth, MA 02747-2300
508 999-8004
Type: 4-year Coll or Univ
Control: State, County, or Local Govt
• Clin Lab Scientist/Med Technologist Prgm

Paxton

Anna Maria College
Bernard Parker, President
Sunset Ln
Paxton, MA 01612-1198
508 849-3335
Type: 4-year Coll or Univ
Control: Nonprofit (Private or Religious)
• Music Therapy Prgm

Pittsfield

Berkshire Community College
Paul Raverta, President
1350 West St
Pittsfield, MA 01201
413 499-4660
Type: Junior or Comm Coll
Control: State, County, or Local Govt
• Physical Therapist Assistant Prgm
• Respiratory Care Prgm

Berkshire Medical Center
Diane Kelly, Chief Operating Officer
725 North St
Pittsfield, MA 01201-4124
413 395-7998
Type: Hosp or Med Ctr: 300-499 Beds
Control: Nonprofit (Private or Religious)
• Clin Lab Scientist/Med Technologist Prgm

Quincy

Quincy College
Martha Sue Harris, MEd, President
24 Saville Ave
Quincy, MA 02169
617 984-1776
Type: Junior or Comm Coll
Control: State, County, or Local Govt
• Clin Lab Technician/Med Lab Technician Prgm
• Surgical Technology Prgm

Salem

Salem State University
Patricia Maguire Meservey, PhD, President
352 Lafayette St
Salem, MA 01970-5353
978 542-6134
Type: 4-year Coll or Univ
Control: State, County, or Local Govt
• Athletic Training Prgm
• Music Therapy Prgm
• Nuclear Medicine Technology Prgm
• Nursing Prgm
• Occupational Therapy Prgm

South Easton

Southeastern Technical Institute
Luis Lopes, EdS, Superintendent
250 Foundry St
South Easton, MA 02375
508 238-1860
Type: Vocational or Tech Sch
Control: Nonprofit (Private or Religious)
• Dental Assistant Prgm
• Medical Assistant Prgm

Springfield

American International College
Vincent M Maniaci, JD, EdD, President
1000 State St
Springfield, MA 01109-3189
413 205-3202
Type: 4-year Coll or Univ
Control: Nonprofit (Private or Religious)
• Nursing Prgm
• Occupational Therapy Prgm
• Physical Therapy Prgm

Springfield College
Richard B Flynn, EdD, President
Marsh Memorial
263 Alden St
Springfield, MA 01109
413 748-3241
Type: 4-year Coll or Univ
Control: Nonprofit (Private or Religious)
• Art Therapy Prgm
• Athletic Training Prgm
• Exercise Physiology - Clinical Prgm
• Exercise Science Prgm
• Occupational Therapy Prgm
• Physical Therapy Prgm
• Physician Assistant Prgm
• Rehabilitation Counseling Prgm

Springfield Technical Community College
Ira Rubenzahl, PhD, President
2 Armory Square, Ste 1
PO Box 9000
Springfield, MA 01102-9000
413 755-4906
Type: Junior or Comm Coll
Control: State, County, or Local Govt
• Clin Lab Technician/Med Lab Technician Prgm
• Clinical Assisting Prgm
• Dental Assistant Prgm
• Dental Hygiene Prgm
• Diagnostic Med Sonography (General) Prgm
• Massage Therapy Prgm
• Medical Assistant Prgm
• Nuclear Medicine Technology Prgm
• Occupational Therapy Asst Prgm
• Physical Therapist Assistant Prgm
• Radiography Prgm
• Respiratory Care Prgm
• Surgical Technology Prgm

Western New England University
Springfield, MA 01119-2684
Type: 4-year Coll or Univ
Control: Nonprofit (Private or Religious)
• Pharmacy Prgm

Waltham

Brandeis University
Jehuda Reinharz, President
South St
Waltham, MA 02454-9110
781 736-2000
Type: 4-year Coll or Univ
Control: Nonprofit (Private or Religious)
• Genetic Counseling Prgm

Sodexho Health Care Services
153 Second Ave
Waltham, MA 02254-3730
800 926-7429
Type: Acad Health Ctr/Med Sch
Control: For Profit
• Dietetic Internship Prgm (2)

Watertown

Cortiva Institute - Muscular Therapy Inst
Mary Ann DiRoberts, President
103 Morse St
Watertown, MA 02472
617 668-1000
Type: Acad Health Ctr/Med Sch
Control: For Profit
• Massage Therapy Prgm

Wellesley Hills

Massachusetts Bay Community College
Carole Berotte Joseph, PhD, President
Wellesley Hills Campus
50 Oakland St
Wellesley Hills, MA 02481
781 230-3100
Type: Junior or Comm Coll
Control: State, County, or Local Govt
• Radiography Prgm
• Surgical Technology Prgm

West Barnstable

Cape Cod Community College
Kathleen Schatzberg, EdD, President
2240 Iyanough Rd
West Barnstable, MA 02668-1599
508 362-2131
Type: Junior or Comm Coll
Control: State, County, or Local Govt
• Dental Hygiene Prgm
• Medical Assistant Prgm

Westfield

Westfield State College
Evan Dobelle, PhD, President
Office of the President
577 Western Ave
Westfield, MA 01086-1630
413 572-5201
Type: 4-year Coll or Univ
Control: State, County, or Local Govt
• Athletic Training Prgm
• Exercise Science Prgm
• Music Therapy Prgm

Weston

Regis College
Mary Jane England, MD, President
235 Wellsley St
Weston, MA 02493
781 768-7000
Type: 4-year Coll or Univ
Control: State, County, or Local Govt
• Nuclear Medicine Technology Prgm
• Radiography Prgm

Worcester

Assumption College
Joseph H Hagan, President
500 Salisbury St
Worcester, MA 01615
508 767-7000
Type: 4-year Coll or Univ
Control: Nonprofit (Private or Religious)
• Rehabilitation Counseling Prgm

Becker College
Franklin M Loew, PhD, President
61 Sever St Box 15071
Worcester, MA 01615-0071
508 791-9241
Type: 4-year Coll or Univ
Control: Nonprofit (Private or Religious)
• Veterinary Technology Prgm

Quinsigamond Community College
Gail Carberry, EdD, President
670 W Boylston St
Worcester, MA 01606-2092
508 854-4203
Type: Junior or Comm Coll
Control: State, County, or Local Govt
• Dental Assistant Prgm
• Dental Hygiene Prgm
• Medical Assistant Prgm
• Occupational Therapy Asst Prgm
• Radiography Prgm
• Respiratory Care Prgm
• Surgical Technology Prgm

The Salter School
Charlene Keefe, BS, President
155 Ararat St
Worcester, MA 01606-3450
508 853-1074
Type: Vocational or Tech Sch
Control: For Profit
• Dental Assistant Prgm
• Medical Assistant Prgm

UMass Memorial Medical Center
John O'Brien, MD, CEO, Clinical Systems
One Biotech Park, 365 Plantation St
Worcester, MA 01655
508 856-4114
Type: Hosp or Med Ctr: 500 Beds
Control: Nonprofit (Private or Religious)
• Nuclear Medicine Technology Prgm
• Radiation Therapy Prgm

Worcester State College
Janelle Ashley, PhD, President
486 Chandler St
Worcester, MA 01602-2597
508 929-8020
Type: 4-year Coll or Univ
Control: State, County, or Local Govt
• Nursing Prgm
• Occupational Therapy Prgm
• Speech-Language Pathology Prgm

Michigan

Adrian

Adrian College
Adrian, MI 49221
Type: 4-year Coll or Univ
Control: Nonprofit (Private or Religious)
• Athletic Training Prgm

Siena Heights University
Adrian, MI 49221
Type: 4-year Coll or Univ
Control: Nonprofit (Private or Religious)
• Nursing Prgm

Albion

Albion College
Donna Randall, PhD, President
203 Ferguson Bldg
Albion, MI 49224
517 629-0210
Type: 4-year Coll or Univ
Control: Nonprofit (Private or Religious)
• Athletic Training Prgm
• Music Therapy Prgm

Allen Park

Baker College of Allen Park
Aaron Maike, President
4500 Enterprise Dr
Allen Park, MI 48101
313 425-3721
Type: 4-year Coll or Univ
Control: Nonprofit (Private or Religious)
• Medical Assistant Prgm
• Occupational Therapy Asst Prgm
• Surgical Technology Prgm

Allendale

Grand Valley State University
Thomas J Haas, PhD, President
22 Zumberge
Allendale, MI 49401-9403
616 331-2100
Type: 4-year Coll or Univ
Control: State, County, or Local Govt
• Athletic Training Prgm
• Clin Lab Scientist/Med Technologist Prgm
• Diagnostic Med Sonography
   (Gen/Card/Vascular) Prgm
• Music Therapy Prgm
• Nursing Prgm
• Occupational Therapy Prgm
• Physical Therapy Prgm
• Physician Assistant Prgm
• Radiation Therapy Prgm

Alma

Alma College
Saundra Tracy, PhD, President
614 W Superior St
Alma, MI 48801
989 463-7146
Type: 4-year Coll or Univ
Control: Nonprofit (Private or Religious)
• Athletic Training Prgm

Alpena

Alpena Community College
Olin Joynton, PhD, President
665 Johnson St
Alpena, MI 49707
989 358-7246
Type: Junior or Comm Coll
Control: State, County, or Local Govt
• Medical Assistant Prgm

Ann Arbor

Ann Arbor Institute of Massage Therapy
Jocelyn Granger, NCBTMB, Director
180 Jackson Plaza
Ste 100
Ann Arbor, MI 48103
734 677-4430
Type: Acad Health Ctr/Med Sch
Control: For Profit
• Massage Therapy Prgm

Huron Valley Ambulance
Dale J Berry, EMT-P, President, CEO
1200 State Circle
Ann Arbor, MI 48108
734 477-6262
Type: Vocational or Tech Sch
Control: Nonprofit (Private or Religious)
• Emergency Med Tech-Paramedic Prgm

University of Michigan
Mary Sue Coleman, PhD, President
2074 Fleming Adm Bldg
503 Thompson St
Ann Arbor, MI 48109-1340
734 764-6270
Type: 4-year Coll or Univ
Control: State, County, or Local Govt
• Allopathic Medicine Prgm
• Athletic Training Prgm
• Dental Hygiene Prgm
• Dentistry Prgm
• Dietetic Internship Prgm
• Dietetics-Didactic Prgm
• Genetic Counseling Prgm
• Medical Librarian Prgm
• Music Therapy Prgm
• Nursing Prgm
• Pharmacy Prgm
• Psychology (PhD) Prgm

University of Michigan Hospitals & Health Ctr
1500 E Medical Ctr Dr
Ann Arbor, MI 48109-0056
313 936-5199
Type: Hosp or Med Ctr: 100-299 Beds
Control: State, County, or Local Govt
• Dietetic Internship Prgm

W K Kellogg Eye Center
Bruce Furr, Clinical Instructor
1000 Wall St
Ann Arbor, MI 48105
734 936-8594
Control: Other
• Orthoptist Prgm

Washtenaw Community College
Larry Whitworth, EdD, President
4800 E Huron River Drive
Ann Arbor, MI 48105-4800
734 973-3491
Type: Junior or Comm Coll
Control: State, County, or Local Govt
• Dental Assistant Prgm
• Pharmacy Technician Prgm
• Physical Therapist Assistant Prgm
• Radiography Prgm

Auburn Hills

Baker College of Auburn Hills
Jeffrey M Love, President
1500 University Dr
Auburn Hills, MI 48326-2642
248 340-0600
Type: 4-year Coll or Univ
Control: Nonprofit (Private or Religious)
• Dental Assistant Prgm
• Dental Hygiene Prgm
• Diagnostic Med Sonography
  (Gen/Card/Vascular) Prgm
• Medical Assistant Prgm
• Phlebotomy Prgm

Battle Creek

Kellogg Community College
G Edward Haring, PhD, President
450 North Ave
Battle Creek, MI 49017
269 965-3931
Type: Junior or Comm Coll
Control: State, County, or Local Govt
• Clin Lab Technician/Med Lab Technician Prgm
• Dental Hygiene Prgm
• Physical Therapist Assistant Prgm
• Radiography Prgm

Robert B. Miller College
Battle Creek, MI 49017
Type: 4-year Coll or Univ
Control: Nonprofit (Private or Religious)
• Nursing Prgm
• Occupational Therapy Asst Prgm

Benton Harbor

Lake Michigan College
Randall Miller, EdD, President
2755 E Napier Ave
Benton Harbor, MI 49022-1899
269 927-8601
Type: Junior or Comm Coll
Control: State, County, or Local Govt
• Dental Assistant Prgm
• Radiography Prgm

Berkley

Beaumont Sleep Evaluation Svcs - Berkley Ctr
Berkley, MI 48072
Type: Hosp or Med Ctr d Beds
• Polysomnographic Technology Prgm

Berrien Springs

Andrews University
Niels-Erik Andreasen, PhD, President
4150 Administration Drive President's Of
Berrien Springs, MI 49104-0670
269 471-3100
Type: 4-year Coll or Univ
Control: Nonprofit (Private or Religious)
• Clin Lab Scientist/Med Technologist Prgm
• Counseling Prgm
• Dietetic Internship Prgm
• Dietetics-Didactic Prgm
• Music Therapy Prgm
• Physical Therapy Prgm

Big Rapids

Ferris State University
David Eisler, PhD, President
1201 S State St
CSS 301
Big Rapids, MI 49307-2737
231 591-2500
Type: 4-year Coll or Univ
Control: State, County, or Local Govt
• Clin Lab Scientist/Med Technologist Prgm
• Clin Lab Technician/Med Lab Technician Prgm
• Dental Hygiene Prgm
• Diagnostic Med Sonography (General) Prgm
• Nuclear Medicine Technology Prgm
• Optometry Prgm
• Pharmacy Prgm
• Radiography Prgm
• Respiratory Care Prgm

Bloomfield Hills

Oakland Community College
Timothy Meyer, PhD, Chancellor
George A Bee Administrative Ctr
2480 Opdyke Rd
Bloomfield Hills, MI 48304-2266
248 341-2115
Type: Junior or Comm Coll
Control: State, County, or Local Govt
• Dental Hygiene Prgm
• Diagnostic Med Sonography (General) Prgm
• Medical Assistant Prgm
• Radiography Prgm
• Respiratory Care Prgm
• Surgical Technology Prgm

Cadillac

Baker College of Cadillac
Robert VanDellen, PhD, President
9600 E 13th St
Cadillac, MI 49601
231 876-3100
Type: 4-year Coll or Univ
Control: Nonprofit (Private or Religious)
• Medical Assistant Prgm
• Surgical Technology Prgm
• Veterinary Technology Prgm

Centreville

Glen Oaks Community College
Gary S Wheeler, PhD, President
62249 Shimmel Rd
Centreville, MI 49032
269 467-9945
Type: Junior or Comm Coll
Control: State, County, or Local Govt
• Medical Assistant Prgm

Clinton Township

Baker College of Clinton Township
Donald Torline, MBA, President
34950 Little Mack Ave
Clinton Township, MI 48035
586 791-6610
Type: 4-year Coll or Univ
Control: Nonprofit (Private or Religious)
• Medical Assistant Prgm
• Radiography Prgm
• Surgical Technology Prgm

Dearborn

Henry Ford Community College
Gail Mee, EdD, President
5101 Evergreen Rd
Dearborn, MI 48128-1495
313 845-9218
Type: Junior or Comm Coll
Control: State, County, or Local Govt
• Medical Assistant Prgm
• Pharmacy Technician Prgm
• Physical Therapist Assistant Prgm
• Radiography Prgm
• Respiratory Care Prgm
• Surgical Technology Prgm

Detroit

DMC University Laboratories
Verdell Tolbert, MT, VP, Laboratory Services
4201 St Antoine Blvd
Detroit, MI 48201
313 993-0539
Type: Acad Health Ctr/Med Sch
Control: Nonprofit (Private or Religious)
• Clin Lab Scientist/Med Technologist Prgm
• Cytotechnology Prgm
• Histotechnician Prgm
• Phlebotomy Prgm

Harper University Hospital
Paul Broughton, President
3990 John R St
Detroit, MI 48201-2097
313 745-9375
Type: Hosp or Med Ctr: 500 Beds
Control: Nonprofit (Private or Religious)
• Dietetic Internship Prgm

Henry Ford Hospital
Anthony Armada, MBA, CEO
2799 W Grand Blvd
A-2 Administration
Detroit, MI 48202
313 876-1257
Type: Hosp or Med Ctr: 500 Beds
Control: Nonprofit (Private or Religious)
• Diagnostic Med Sonography (General) Prgm
• Dietetic Internship Prgm

Kaplan Career Institute - Dearborn Campus
Detroit, MI 48228
• Dental Assistant Prgm

Sinai-Grace Hospital
Conrad Mallett, JD, President
6071 W Outer Dr
Detroit, MI 48235
313 966-3525
Type: Hosp or Med Ctr: 300-499 Beds
Control: Nonprofit (Private or Religious)
• Radiography Prgm

University of Detroit Mercy
Rev Gerard L Stockhausen, SJ PhD, President
4001 W McNichols Rd
PO Box 19900
Detroit, MI 48221
313 993-1455
Type: 4-year Coll or Univ
Control: Nonprofit (Private or Religious)
• Counseling Prgm
• Dentistry Prgm
• Nursing Prgm
• Physician Assistant Prgm
• Psychology (PhD) Prgm

Wayne County Community College District
Curtis L Ivery, PhD, Chancellor
801 W Fort St
Detroit, MI 48226-9975
313 496-2510
Type: Junior or Comm Coll
Control: State, County, or Local Govt
• Dental Assistant Prgm
• Dental Hygiene Prgm
• Dietetic Technician-AD Prgm
• Pharmacy Technician Prgm
• Surgical Assistant Prgm
• Surgical Technology Prgm (2)

Wayne State University
Allan Gilmour, PhD, President
4200 Faculty Admin Bldg
Detroit, MI 48202-3489
313 577-2230
Type: 4-year Coll or Univ
Control: State, County, or Local Govt
• Allopathic Medicine Prgm
• Art Therapy Prgm
• Audiologist Prgm
• Clin Lab Scientist/Med Technologist Prgm
• Counseling Prgm
• Dietetics-Coordinated Prgm
• Genetic Counseling Prgm
• Medical Librarian Prgm
• Music Therapy Prgm
• Nursing Prgm
• Occupational Therapy Prgm
• Pathologists' Assistant Prgm
• Pharmacy Prgm
• Physical Therapy Prgm
• Physician Assistant Prgm
• Psychology (PhD) Prgm
• Radiation Therapy Prgm
• Radiography Prgm
• Radiologist Assistant Prgm
• Rehabilitation Counseling Prgm
• Speech-Language Pathology Prgm

East Lansing

Michigan State University
Lou Anna Simon, Provost
450 Administration Building
East Lansing, MI 48824
517 355-6560
Type: 4-year Coll or Univ
Control: State, County, or Local Govt
• Allopathic Medicine Prgm
• Athletic Training Prgm
• Clin Lab Scientist/Med Technologist Prgm
• Counseling Prgm
• Diagnostic Molecular Scientist Prgm
• Dietetic Internship Prgm
• Dietetics-Didactic Prgm
• Music Therapy Prgm
• Nursing Prgm
• Osteopathic Medicine Prgm
• Psychology (PhD) Prgm
• Rehabilitation Counseling Prgm
• Speech-Language Pathology Prgm
• Teacher of the Visually Impaired Prgm
• Veterinary Medicine Prgm
• Veterinary Technology Prgm

Ferndale

Medright Incorporated
Gail Lucas, Program Director
427 Allen
Ferndale, MI 48220
248 703-9928
Type: Acad Health Ctr/Med Sch
Control: For Profit
• Phlebotomy Prgm

Flint

Baker College Center of Graduate Studies
Michael Heberling, PhD, President
1116 W Bristol Rd
Flint, MI 48507-5508
810 766-4374
Type: 4-year Coll or Univ
Control: Nonprofit (Private or Religious)
• Occupational Therapy Prgm

Baker College of Flint
Julianne T Princinsky, EdD, President
1050 W Bristol Rd
Flint, MI 48507-5508
810 766-4036
Type: 4-year Coll or Univ
Control: Nonprofit (Private or Religious)
• Medical Assistant Prgm
• Physical Therapist Assistant Prgm
• Polysomnographic Technology Prgm
• Surgical Technology Prgm
• Veterinary Technology Prgm

Hurley Medical Center
Patrick Wardell, President/CEO
One Hurley Plaza
Flint, MI 48503
810 257-9237
Type: Hosp or Med Ctr: 300-499 Beds
Control: State, County, or Local Govt
• Clin Lab Scientist/Med Technologist Prgm
• Dietetic Internship Prgm
• Radiography Prgm

Mott Community College
M Richard Shaink, President
1401 E Court St
Flint, MI 48503
810 762-0200
Type: Junior or Comm Coll
Control: State, County, or Local Govt
• Dental Assistant Prgm
• Dental Hygiene Prgm
• Physical Therapist Assistant Prgm
• Respiratory Care Prgm

University of Michigan - Flint
Ruth Persons, MS PhD, Chancellor
303 E Kearsley St
Flint, MI 48502-2186
810 762-3322
Type: 4-year Coll or Univ
Control: State, County, or Local Govt
• Nursing Prgm
• Physical Therapy Prgm
• Radiation Therapy Prgm

Grand Rapids

Aquinas College
Harry J Knopke, PhD, President
1607 Robinson Rd SE
Grand Rapids, MI 49506-1799
616 632-2880
Type: 4-year Coll or Univ
Control: Nonprofit (Private or Religious)
• Athletic Training Prgm

Calvin College
Gaylen Byker, President
Office of the President
Spoelhof Center 390
Grand Rapids, MI 49546
616 526-6100
Type: 4-year Coll or Univ
Control: Nonprofit (Private or Religious)
• Music Therapy Prgm
• Nursing Prgm
• Speech-Language Pathology Prgm

Davenport University
Randolph Flechsig, PhD, President
415 E Fulton St
Grand Rapids, MI 49503
616 451-3511
Type: 4-year Coll or Univ
Control: Nonprofit (Private or Religious)
• Medical Assistant Prgm (4)

Grand Rapids Community College
Anne Mulder, PhD, Interim President
143 Bostwick Ave NE
Grand Rapids, MI 49503-3295
616 234-3901
Type: Junior or Comm Coll
Control: State, County, or Local Govt
• Dental Assistant Prgm
• Dental Hygiene Prgm
• Occupational Therapy Asst Prgm
• Radiography Prgm

Hancock

Finlandia University
Robert Ubbelohde, President
Quincy 601
Hancock, MI 49930-1882
906 482-6300
Type: Junior or Comm Coll
Control: Nonprofit (Private or Religious)
• Nursing Prgm
• Physical Therapist Assistant Prgm

Harrison

Mid Michigan Community College
Carol C Churchill, MA, President
1375 S Clare Ave
Harrison, MI 48625
989 386-6622
Type: Junior or Comm Coll
Control: State, County, or Local Govt
• Medical Assistant Prgm
• Pharmacy Technician Prgm
• Phlebotomy Prgm
• Physical Therapist Assistant Prgm
• Radiography Prgm

Holland

Hope College
James Bultman, EdD, President
PO Box 9000
Holland, MI 49422-9000
616 395-7780
Type: 4-year Coll or Univ
Control: Nonprofit (Private or Religious)
• Athletic Training Prgm
• Nursing Prgm

Jackson

Baker College of Jackson
Patricia Kaufman, PhD, President
2800 Springport Rd
Jackson, MI 49202
517 789-6123
Type: 4-year Coll or Univ
Control: Nonprofit (Private or Religious)
• Clin Lab Technician/Med Lab Technician Prgm
• Medical Assistant Prgm
• Ophthalmic Dispensing Optician Prgm
• Radiation Therapy Prgm
• Surgical Technology Prgm
• Veterinary Technology Prgm

Jackson Community College
Daniel J Phelan, PhD, President
2111 Emmons Rd
Jackson, MI 49201-8399
517 787-0800
Type: Junior or Comm Coll
Control: State, County, or Local Govt
• Diagnostic Med Sonography (Gen/Card/Vascular) Prgm
• Medical Assistant Prgm
• Radiography Prgm

Kalamazoo

Kalamazoo Valley Community College
Marilyn J Schlack, EdD, President
Texas Township Campus
6767 West O Ave, PO Box 4070
Kalamazoo, MI 49003-4070
269 488-4434
Type: Junior or Comm Coll
Control: State, County, or Local Govt
• Dental Hygiene Prgm
• Emergency Med Tech-Paramedic Prgm
• Medical Assistant Prgm
• Respiratory Care Prgm

Western Michigan University
Timothy J Greene, PhD, Provost and Vice President
1903 W Michigan Avenue, Mail Stop 5204
Kalamazoo, MI 49008-5204
269 387-2378
Type: 4-year Coll or Univ
Control: State, County, or Local Govt
• Athletic Training Prgm
• Audiologist Prgm
• Counseling Prgm
• Dietetic Internship Prgm
• Dietetics-Didactic Prgm
• Music Therapy Prgm
• Nursing Prgm
• Occupational Therapy Prgm (2)
• Orientation and Mobility Specialist Prgm
• Physician Assistant Prgm
• Psychology (PhD) Prgm
• Rehabilitation Counseling Prgm
• Speech-Language Pathology Prgm
• Vision Rehabilitation Therapy Prgm

Lansing

Lansing Community College
Brent Knight, EdD, President
521 N Washington Sq
8100 President's Ofc, PO Box 40010
Lansing, MI 48901-7210
517 483-1851
Type: Junior or Comm Coll
Control: State, County, or Local Govt
• Dental Hygiene Prgm
• Emergency Med Tech-Paramedic Prgm
• Histotechnician Prgm
• Radiography Prgm
• Surgical Technology Prgm

Livonia

Madonna University
Mary Francilene, President
36600 Schoolcraft Rd
Livonia, MI 48150
313 591-5000
Type: 4-year Coll or Univ
Control: Nonprofit (Private or Religious)
• Clin Lab Scientist/Med Technologist Prgm
• Dietetics-Didactic Prgm
• Nursing Prgm

Schoolcraft College
Conway A Jeffress, PhD, President
18600 Haggerty Rd
Livonia, MI 48152-2696
734 462-4400
Type: Junior or Comm Coll
Control: State, County, or Local Govt
• Medical Assistant Prgm

Marquette

Northern Michigan University
Leslie Wong, PhD, President
1401 Presque Isle Ave
Marquette, MI 49855
906 227-2242
Type: 4-year Coll or Univ
Control: State, County, or Local Govt
• Athletic Training Prgm
• Clin Lab Scientist/Med Technologist Prgm
• Clin Lab Technician/Med Lab Technician Prgm
• Clinical Assisting Prgm
• Cytogenetic Technology Prgm
• Diagnostic Molecular Scientist Prgm
• Music Therapy Prgm
• Nursing Prgm
• Radiography Prgm
• Surgical Technology Prgm

Monroe

Monroe County Community College
David Nixon, MA, President
1555 S Raisinville Rd
Monroe, MI 48161
734 384-4166
Type: Junior or Comm Coll
Control: State, County, or Local Govt
• Respiratory Care Prgm

Mount Pleasant

Central Michigan University
Michael Rao, PhD, President
106 Warriner Hall
Mount Pleasant, MI 48859
989 774-3131
Type: 4-year Coll or Univ
Control: State, County, or Local Govt
• Allopathic Medicine Prgm
• Athletic Training Prgm
• Audiologist Prgm
• Dietetic Internship Prgm
• Dietetics-Didactic Prgm
• Music Therapy Prgm
• Physical Therapy Prgm
• Physician Assistant Prgm
• Psychology (PhD) Prgm
• Speech-Language Pathology Prgm

Muskegon

Baker College of Muskegon
Lee Coggin, JD, President
1903 Marquette Ave
Muskegon, MI 49442-9982
231 777-5244
Type: 4-year Coll or Univ
Control: Nonprofit (Private or Religious)
• Medical Assistant Prgm
• Occupational Therapy Asst Prgm
• Physical Therapist Assistant Prgm
• Radiography Prgm
• Surgical Technology Prgm
• Veterinary Technology Prgm

Muskegon Community College
David Rule, PhD, President
221 S Quarterline Rd
Muskegon, MI 49442
616 777-0303
Type: Junior or Comm Coll
Control: State, County, or Local Govt
• Respiratory Care Prgm

Owosso

Baker College of Owosso
Pete Karsten, PhD, President, CEO
1020 S Washington St
Owosso, MI 48867
989 729-3431
Type: 4-year Coll or Univ
Control: Nonprofit (Private or Religious)
• Clin Lab Technician/Med Lab Technician Prgm
  (2)
• Diagnostic Med Sonography (General) Prgm
• Medical Assistant Prgm
• Phlebotomy Prgm
• Radiography Prgm

Port Huron

Baker College of Port Huron
Connie Harrison, PhD, President
3403 Lapeer Rd
Port Huron, MI 48060
810 985-7000
Type: 4-year Coll or Univ
Control: Nonprofit (Private or Religious)
• Clin Lab Technician/Med Lab Technician Prgm
• Dental Assistant Prgm
• Dental Hygiene Prgm
• Medical Assistant Prgm
• Surgical Technology Prgm
• Veterinary Technology Prgm

Lakewood School of Therapeutic Massage
Nancy Levitt, Director
1102 6th St
Port Huron, MI 48060
810 987-3959
Type: Acad Health Ctr/Med Sch
Control: For Profit
• Massage Therapy Prgm

Port Huron Hospital
Thomas D DeFauw, MHA, President
1221 Pine Grove
Port Huron, MI 48061-5011
810 987-5000
Type: Hosp or Med Ctr: 100-299 Beds
Control: Nonprofit (Private or Religious)
• Radiography Prgm

Rochester

Oakland University
Gary D Russi, PhD, President
North Foundation Hall
Rochester, MI 48063
313 370-3500
Type: 4-year Coll or Univ
Control: State, County, or Local Govt
• Allopathic Medicine Prgm
• Counseling Prgm
• Nursing Prgm
• Physical Therapy Prgm

Royal Oak

Beaumont Hospital - Royal Oak
John D Labriola, President, CEO
3601 W 13 Mile Rd
Royal Oak, MI 48073-6769
248 898-5400
Type: Hosp or Med Ctr: 500 Beds
Control: Nonprofit (Private or Religious)
• Clin Lab Scientist/Med Technologist Prgm
• Histotechnician Prgm
• Histotechnology Prgm
• Nuclear Medicine Technology Prgm
• Radiation Therapy Prgm
• Radiography Prgm

Sault Ste Marie

Lake Superior State University
Betty Youngblood, PhD, President
650 W Easterday Ave
Sault Ste Marie, MI 49783
906 635-2202
Type: 4-year Coll or Univ
Control: State, County, or Local Govt
• Athletic Training Prgm

Sidney

Montcalm Community College
Donald Burns, PhD, President
2800 College Dr
Sidney, MI 48885
517 328-1221
Type: Junior or Comm Coll
Control: State, County, or Local Govt
• Medical Assistant Prgm

Southfield

Everest Institute-Southfield
Southfield, MI 48033
Type: Vocational or Tech Sch
• Medical Assistant Prgm

National Institute of Technology
Marchelle (Mickey) Weaver, BA, President
26111 Evergreen Rd
Ste 201
Southfield, MI 48076
248 799-9933
Type: Vocational or Tech Sch
Control: For Profit
• Medical Assistant Prgm

Providence Hospital
Diane Radloff, MHA, CEO, Providence Oper Unit
16001 W Nine Mile Rd
Southfield, MI 48075
248 849-3000
Type: Hosp or Med Ctr: 300-499 Beds
Control: Nonprofit (Private or Religious)
• Diagnostic Med Sonography (General/Vascular)
  Prgm
• Radiography Prgm

Spring Arbor

Spring Arbor University
Spring Arbor, MI 49283
Type: 4-year Coll or Univ
Control: State, County, or Local Govt
• Nursing Prgm

Traverse City

Northwestern Michigan College
Timothy Nelson, MA, President
1701 E Front St
Traverse City, MI 49686
616 995-1010
Type: Junior or Comm Coll
Control: State, County, or Local Govt
• Dental Assistant Prgm

Troy

Carnegie Institute
Robert J McEachern, BA MSF, President
550 Stephenson Hwy, Ste 100-110
Troy, MI 48083
248 589-1078
Type: Vocational or Tech Sch
Control: For Profit
• Cardiovascular Tech (Invasive/Vasc/Echo)
  Prgm
• Medical Assistant Prgm
• Neurodiagnostic Tech Prgm

University Center

Delta College
Jean Goodnow, PhD, President
1961 Delta Rd
University Center, MI 48710
989 686-9201
Type: Junior or Comm Coll
Control: State, County, or Local Govt
• Dental Assistant Prgm
• Dental Hygiene Prgm
• Diagnostic Med Sonography (General) Prgm
• Physical Therapist Assistant Prgm (2)
• Radiography Prgm
• Respiratory Care Prgm
• Surgical Technology Prgm

Saginaw Valley State University
Eric R Gilbertson, JD, President
7400 Bay Rd
University Center, MI 48710-0001
989 964-4145
Type: 4-year Coll or Univ
Control: State, County, or Local Govt
• Athletic Training Prgm
• Clin Lab Scientist/Med Technologist Prgm
• Music Therapy Prgm
• Nursing Prgm
• Occupational Therapy Prgm

Warren

Macomb Community College
James Jacobs, PhD, President
14500 E Twelve Mile Rd
Building D-300
Warren, MI 48088-3896
586 445-7596
Type: Junior or Comm Coll
Control: State, County, or Local Govt
• Clin Lab Technician/Med Lab Technician Prgm
• Medical Assistant Prgm
• Nuclear Medicine Technology Prgm
• Occupational Therapy Asst Prgm
• Physical Therapist Assistant Prgm
• Respiratory Care Prgm
• Surgical Technology Prgm
• Veterinary Technician Prgm

St John Health
Patricia Maryland, PhD, President CEO
28000 Dequindre Rd
Warren, MI 48092
586 753-0710
Type: Hosp or Med Ctr: 500 Beds
Control: Nonprofit (Private or Religious)
• Clin Lab Scientist/Med Technologist Prgm
• Radiography Prgm

Ypsilanti

Eastern Michigan University
Susan W Martin, PhD, President
Ypsilanti, MI 48197-2239
734 487-1849
Type: 4-year Coll or Univ
Control: State, County, or Local Govt
• Athletic Training Prgm
• Clin Lab Scientist/Med Technologist Prgm
• Counseling Prgm
• Dietetics-Coordinated Prgm
• Music Therapy Prgm
• Nursing Prgm
• Occupational Therapy Prgm
• Orthotist/Prosthetist Prgm
• Psychology (PhD) Prgm
• Speech-Language Pathology Prgm

Minnesota

Alexandria

Alexandria Technical College
Kevin Kopischke, PhD, President
1601 Jefferson St
Alexandria, MN 56308
320 762-4404
Type: Vocational or Tech Sch
Control: State, County, or Local Govt
• Clin Lab Technician/Med Lab Technician Prgm

Anoka

Anoka Technical College
Shari Olson, PhD, Interm President
1355 W Hwy 10
Anoka, MN 55303-1590
763 576-4828
Type: Vocational or Tech Sch
Control: State, County, or Local Govt
• Medical Assistant Prgm
• Occupational Therapy Asst Prgm
• Surgical Technology Prgm

Austin

Riverland Community College
Gary Rhodes, PhD, President
1600 8th Ave NW
Austin, MN 55912
507 433-0508
Type: Junior or Comm Coll
Control: State, County, or Local Govt
• Radiography Prgm

Bemidji

Bemidji State University
Jeanine E Gangeness, RN MS, Chief Nurse
  Administrator
1500 Birchmont Dr NE
105 Deputy Hall
Bemidji, MN 56601
Type: 4-year Coll or Univ
Control: State, County, or Local Govt
• Music Therapy Prgm
• Nursing Prgm

Northwest Technical College - Bemidji
Jon E Quistgaard, PhD, President
905 Grant Ave SE
Bemidji, MN 56601
218 333-6600
Type: Vocational or Tech Sch
Control: State, County, or Local Govt
• Dental Assistant Prgm

Bloomington

Academy College
Bloomington, MN 55420
Type: 4-year Coll or Univ
• Medical Assistant Prgm

Normandale Community College
Joseph Opatz, PhD, President
9700 France Ave S
Bloomington, MN 55431
952 487-8200
Type: Junior or Comm Coll
Control: State, County, or Local Govt
• Dental Hygiene Prgm
• Dietetic Technician-AD Prgm

Northwestern Health Science University
Alfred Traina, DC
2501 W 84th St
Bloomington, MN 55431
Type: Acad Health Ctr/Med Sch
Control: For Profit
• Chiropractic Prgm
• Massage Therapy Prgm

Brainerd

Central Lakes College
Sally J Ihne, President
300 Quince St
Brainerd, MN 56401
218 828-2525
Type: Junior or Comm Coll
Control: For Profit
- Dental Assistant Prgm
- Medical Assistant Prgm

Brooklyn Park

Hennepin Technical College
Ronald Kraft, Interim President
9000 Brooklyn Blvd
Brooklyn Park, MN 55445
763 488-2414
Type: Vocational or Tech Sch
Control: State, County, or Local Govt
- Dental Assistant Prgm
- Medical Assistant Prgm

North Hennepin Community College
Ann Wynia, Interim President
7411 85th Ave N
President's Office ES24
Brooklyn Park, MN 55445
763 424-0820
Type: Junior or Comm Coll
Control: State, County, or Local Govt
- Clin Lab Technician/Med Lab Technician Prgm
- Histotechnician Prgm

Collegeville

Saint John's University
Collegeville, MN 56321
Type: 4-year Coll or Univ
Control: Nonprofit (Private or Religious)
- Nursing Prgm

Coon Rapids

Anoka Ramsey Community College
Patrick M Johns, PhD, President
11200 Mississippi Blvd NW
Coon Rapids, MN 55433
763 422-3435
Type: Junior or Comm Coll
Control: State, County, or Local Govt
- Physical Therapist Assistant Prgm

Crystal

Herzing University
John Slama, MA (Admin), President
5700 West Broadway
Crystal, MN 55428
763 535-3000
Type: Vocational or Tech Sch
Control: For Profit
- Clin Lab Technician/Med Lab Technician Prgm
- Dental Assistant Prgm
- Dental Hygiene Prgm
- Medical Assistant Prgm

Duluth

College of St Scholastica
Larry Goodwin, PhD, President
1200 Kenwood Ave
Duluth, MN 55811
218 723-6033
Type: 4-year Coll or Univ
Control: Nonprofit (Private or Religious)
- Nursing Prgm
- Occupational Therapy Prgm
- Physical Therapy Prgm

Duluth Business University
James R Gessner, President
4724 Mike Colalillo Dr
Duluth, MN 55807
218 722-4000
Type: Vocational or Tech Sch
Control: For Profit
- Medical Assistant Prgm
- Veterinary Technology Prgm

Lake Superior College
Kathleen Nelson, EdD, President
2101 Trinity Rd
Duluth, MN 55811-3399
218 733-7600
Type: Junior or Comm Coll
Control: State, County, or Local Govt
- Clin Lab Technician/Med Lab Technician Prgm
- Dental Hygiene Prgm
- Medical Assistant Prgm
- Physical Therapist Assistant Prgm
- Radiography Prgm
- Respiratory Care Prgm
- Surgical Technology Prgm

University of Minnesota - Duluth
Kathryn A Martin, Chancellor
Duluth, MN 55812
218 726-8000
Type: 4-year Coll or Univ
Control: State, County, or Local Govt
- Athletic Training Prgm
- Music Therapy Prgm
- Speech-Language Pathology Prgm

Eagan

Argosy University Twin Cities Campus
Scott Tjaden, PhD, Campus President
1515 Central Pkwy
Eagan, MN 55121
651 846-3407
Type: 4-year Coll or Univ
Control: For Profit
- Clin Lab Scientist/Med Technologist Prgm
- Clin Lab Technician/Med Lab Technician Prgm
- Dental Hygiene Prgm
- Diagnostic Med Sonography (General/Cardiac) Prgm
- Histotechnician Prgm
- Medical Assistant Prgm
- Psychology (PsyD) Prgm
- Radiation Therapy Prgm
- Radiography Prgm
- Veterinary Technician Prgm

Eveleth

Mesabi Range Community and Technical College
Eveleth, MN 55734
Type: Junior or Comm Coll
- Emergency Med Tech-Paramedic Prgm

Fergus Falls

ER Training Assoc/Greater Minn Paramedic Cons
Beth Domholdt, VP of Student Services
PO Box 1014
214 East Junius Ave
Fergus Falls, MN 56537
218 998-2739
Type: Consortium
Control: For Profit
- Emergency Med Tech-Paramedic Prgm

Minnesota State Community and Technical Coll
Ann Valentine, PhD, President
1414 College Way
Fergus Falls, MN 56537
218 736-1500
Type: Junior or Comm Coll
Control: State, County, or Local Govt
- Clin Lab Technician/Med Lab Technician Prgm
- Radiography Prgm

Hibbing

Hibbing Community College
Kenneth Simberg, MS, President
1515 E 25th St
Hibbing, MN 55746
800 224-4422
Type: Vocational or Tech Sch
Control: State, County, or Local Govt
- Clin Lab Technician/Med Lab Technician Prgm
- Dental Assistant Prgm

Inver Grove Heights

Inver Hills Community College
Cheryl Frank, PhD, President
2500 E 80th St
Inver Grove Heights, MN 55076
651 460-8641
Type: Junior or Comm Coll
Control: State, County, or Local Govt
- Emergency Med Tech-Paramedic Prgm

Mankato

Minnesota State University - Mankato
Richard Davenport, PhD, President
301 Wigley Adminstration Building
Mankato, MN 56001-8400
507 389-2463
Type: 4-year Coll or Univ
Control: State, County, or Local Govt
- Athletic Training Prgm
- Counseling Prgm
- Dental Hygiene Prgm
- Dietetics-Didactic Prgm
- Nursing Prgm
- Rehabilitation Counseling Prgm
- Speech-Language Pathology Prgm

Minneapolis

Augsburg College
Paul Pribbenow, PhD, President
2211 Riverside Ave, CB 131
Minneapolis, MN 55454
612 330-1212
Type: 4-year Coll or Univ
Control: Nonprofit (Private or Religious)
- Music Therapy Prgm
- Nursing Prgm
- Physician Assistant Prgm

Capella University
Minneapolis, MN 55402
Type: 4-year Coll or Univ
Control: Nonprofit (Private or Religious)
- Nursing Prgm

Dunwoody College of Technology
818 Dunwoody Boulevard
Minneapolis, MN 55403
Type: 4-year Coll or Univ
Control: Nonprofit (Private or Religious)
- Radiography Prgm

Fairview Health Services
Mark Eustis, President and CEO
2450 Riverside Ave
Minneapolis, MN 55455
612 672-6161
Type: Hosp or Med Ctr: 500 Beds
Control: Nonprofit (Private or Religious)
- Clin Lab Scientist/Med Technologist Prgm

Hennepin County Medical Center
Lynn Abrahamsen, Administrator
701 Park Ave S
Minneapolis, MN 55415
612 873-2343
Type: Hosp or Med Ctr: 300-499 Beds
Control: State, County, or Local Govt
- Clin Lab Scientist/Med Technologist Prgm
- Emergency Med Tech-Paramedic Prgm
- Phlebotomy Prgm

Minneapolis Community & Technical College
Phil Davis, President
1501 Hennepin Ave S
Minneapolis, MN 55403
612 659-6300
Type: Vocational or Tech Sch
Control: State, County, or Local Govt
- Dental Assistant Prgm
- Neurodiagnostic Tech Prgm
- Phlebotomy Prgm
- Polysomnographic Technology Prgm

St. Catherine University
Andrea J Lee, IHM, President
601 25th Ave. South
Minneapolis, MN 55454
651 690-8846
- Ophthalmic Technician Prgm
- Orthoptist Prgm

University of Minnesota
Robert Bruininks, PhD, President
202 Morrill Hall
100 Church St SE
Minneapolis, MN 55455
612 625-1616
Type: 4-year Coll or Univ
Control: State, County, or Local Govt
- Allopathic Medicine Prgm
- Audiologist Prgm
- Clin Lab Scientist/Med Technologist Prgm
- Dental Hygiene Prgm
- Dentistry Prgm
- Dietetics-Coordinated Prgm
- Genetic Counseling Prgm
- Music Therapy Prgm
- Nursing Prgm
- Occupational Therapy Prgm (2)
- Orthoptist Prgm
- Pharmacy Prgm
- Physical Therapy Prgm
- Psychology (PhD) Prgm
- Speech-Language Pathology Prgm
- Veterinary Medicine Prgm

University of Minnesota Med Ctr - Fairview
Mark Eustis, President
Fairview Health Services
2450 Riverside Ave
Minneapolis, MN 55454
612 672-6000
Type: Hosp or Med Ctr: 300-499 Beds
Control: Nonprofit (Private or Religious)
- Dietetic Internship Prgm
- Radiation Therapy Prgm

Veterans Affairs Medical Center
Steven Kleinglass, FACHE, Director
One Veteran's Dr, Mail Rte 114
Minneapolis, MN 55417
612 725-2000
Type: Dept of Veterans Affairs
Control: Fed Govt
- Dietetic Internship Prgm
- Radiography Prgm

Walden University
Minneapolis, MN 55401
Type: 4-year Coll or Univ
Control: For Profit
- Nursing Prgm

Moorhead

Concordia College - Moorhead
Paul J Dovre, President
Moorhead, MN 56562
218 299-3947
Type: 4-year Coll or Univ
Control: Nonprofit (Private or Religious)
- Dietetic Internship Prgm
- Dietetics-Didactic Prgm
- Nursing Prgm

Minnesota State Comm & Tech Coll - Moorhead
Ann Valentine, PhD, President
1900 28th Ave S
Moorhead, MN 56560
888 696-7282
Type: Vocational or Tech Sch
Control: State, County, or Local Govt
- Dental Assistant Prgm
- Dental Hygiene Prgm
- Pharmacy Technician Prgm

Minnesota State University - Moorhead
211C Lommen Hall
Moorhead, MN 56563
Type: 4-year Coll or Univ
Control: State, County, or Local Govt
- Athletic Training Prgm
- Counseling Prgm
- Nursing Prgm
- Speech-Language Pathology Prgm

North Mankato

South Central College
Keith Stover, MA, President
1920 Lee Blvd
PO Box 1920
North Mankato, MN 56003
507 389-7200
Type: Vocational or Tech Sch
Control: State, County, or Local Govt
- Clin Lab Technician/Med Lab Technician Prgm
- Dental Assistant Prgm
- Emergency Med Tech-Paramedic Prgm

Northfield

Minnesota Intercollegiate Nursing Consortium
Northfield, MN 55057
Type: Acad Health Ctr/Med Sch
Control: Nonprofit (Private or Religious)
- Nursing Prgm

Saint Olaf College
Northfield, MN 55057
Type: 4-year Coll or Univ
Control: Nonprofit (Private or Religious)
- Nursing Prgm

Richfield

Minnesota School of Business
Terry L Myhre, President
1401 W 76th St, Ste 500
Richfield, MN 55423-3846
612 861-2000
Type: Vocational or Tech Sch
Control: For Profit
- Nursing Prgm
- Veterinary Technology Prgm (3)

Rochester

Mayo Clinic
Denis Cortese
200 First St SW
Rochester, MN 55905
507 284-2662
Type: Hosp or Med Ctr: 300-499 Beds
Control: Nonprofit (Private or Religious)
• Clin Lab Scientist/Med Technologist Prgm
• Cytogenetic Technology Prgm
• Histotechnician Prgm
• Phlebotomy Prgm

Mayo School of Health Sciences
Denis A Cortese, MD, President/CEO
200 First St SW
Siebens 12
Rochester, MN 55905
507 284-2663
Type: Acad Health Ctr/Med Sch
Control: Nonprofit (Private or Religious)
• Allopathic Medicine Prgm
• Cytotechnology Prgm
• Diagnostic Med Sonography
  (Gen/Card/Vascular) Prgm
• Neurodiagnostic Tech Prgm
• Nuclear Medicine Technology Prgm
• Physical Therapy Prgm
• Radiation Therapy Prgm
• Radiography Prgm
• Respiratory Care Prgm

Rochester Community & Technical College
Donald Supalla, MS, President
851 30th Ave SE
Rochester, MN 55904-4999
507 285-7215
Type: Junior or Comm Coll
Control: State, County, or Local Govt
• Dental Assistant Prgm
• Dental Hygiene Prgm
• Emergency Med Tech-Paramedic Prgm
• Surgical Technology Prgm
• Veterinary Technology Prgm

St Mary's Hospital
1216 2nd St SW
Rochester, MN 55902-1906
507 255-5221
Type: Hosp or Med Ctr: 300-499 Beds
Control: Nonprofit (Private or Religious)
• Dietetic Internship Prgm

Rosemount

Dakota County Technical College
Ron Thomas, PhD, President
1300 E 145th St
Rosemount, MN 55068-2999
612 423-2200
Type: Vocational or Tech Sch
Control: State, County, or Local Govt
• Dental Assistant Prgm
• Medical Assistant Prgm

Roseville

Minneapolis Business College
David Whitman, MA, President
1711 W County Rd B
Ste 100N
Roseville, MN 55113
651 636-7406
Type: Vocational or Tech Sch
Control: For Profit
• Medical Assistant Prgm
• Veterinary Technology Prgm

National American University - Roseville
Roseville, MN 55113-4035
Type: Vocational or Tech Sch
• Medical Assistant Prgm

Rasmussen College
Kristi A Waite, President
1700 W Hwy 36, Ste 830
Roseville, MN 55133
651 636-3305
Type: Junior or Comm Coll
Control: For Profit
• Clin Lab Technician/Med Lab Technician Prgm
  (6)
• Medical Assistant Prgm (7)
• Surgical Technology Prgm (3)

St Bonifacius

Crown College
8700 College View Dr
St Bonifacius, MN 55375
Type: 4-year Coll or Univ
Control: For Profit
• Nursing Prgm

St Cloud

St Cloud Hospital
Craig Broman, President
1406 Sixth Ave N
St Cloud, MN 56303
320 255-5661
Type: Hosp or Med Ctr: 300-499 Beds
Control: Nonprofit (Private or Religious)
• Radiography Prgm

St Cloud State University
Earl Potter, President
720 Fourth Ave S
St Cloud, MN 56301
320 255-2240
Type: 4-year Coll or Univ
Control: State, County, or Local Govt
• Athletic Training Prgm
• Clin Lab Scientist/Med Technologist Prgm
• Counseling Prgm
• Music Therapy Prgm
• Nursing Prgm
• Rehabilitation Counseling Prgm
• Speech-Language Pathology Prgm

St Cloud Technical and Community College
Joyce Helens, MS, President
1540 Northway Dr
St Cloud, MN 56303
320 308-5017
Type: Vocational or Tech Sch
Control: Nonprofit (Private or Religious)
• Cardiovascular Tech (Invasive/Echo) Prgm
• Dental Assistant Prgm
• Dental Hygiene Prgm
• Diagnostic Med Sonography (General) Prgm
• Emergency Med Tech-Paramedic Prgm
• Surgical Technology Prgm

St Joseph

College of St Benedict/St John's University
Colman O'Connell, President
37 S College Ave
St Joseph, MN 56374
612 363-5011
Type: Consortium
Control: Nonprofit (Private or Religious)
• Dietetics-Didactic Prgm
• Music Therapy Prgm
• Nursing Prgm

St Paul

Bethel University
George K Brushaber, PhD, President
3900 Bethel Dr
St Paul, MN 55112
651 638-6230
Type: 4-year Coll or Univ
Control: Nonprofit (Private or Religious)
• Athletic Training Prgm
• Nursing Prgm

Metropolitan State University
St Paul, MN 55106
Type: 4-year Coll or Univ
Control: State, County, or Local Govt
• Nursing Prgm

Regions Hospital
Brock D Nelson, President/CEO
640 Jackson St
St Paul, MN 55101
651 254-2189
Type: Hosp or Med Ctr: 300-499 Beds
Control: Nonprofit (Private or Religious)
• Ophthalmic Med Technologist Prgm
• Ophthalmic Technician Prgm

Saint Catherine University
Andrea J Lee, IHM, President
2004 Randolph Ave
St Paul, MN 55105-1794
651 690-6525
Type: 4-year Coll or Univ
Control: Nonprofit (Private or Religious)
• Diagnostic Med Sonography (General) Prgm
• Dietetics-Didactic Prgm
• Exercise Science Prgm
• Occupational Therapy Asst Prgm
• Occupational Therapy Prgm
• Phlebotomy Prgm
• Physical Therapist Assistant Prgm
• Physical Therapy Prgm
• Radiography Prgm
• Respiratory Care Prgm

Saint Paul College
Donovan Schwichtenberg, PhD, President
235 Marshall Ave
St Paul, MN 55102
651 846-1335
Type: Junior or Comm Coll
Control: State, County, or Local Govt
• Clin Lab Technician/Med Lab Technician Prgm
• Respiratory Care Prgm

University of Minnesota - St Paul
1334 Eckles Ave
St Paul, MN 55108
612 624-9278
Type: 4-year Coll or Univ
Control: State, County, or Local Govt
• Dietetic Internship Prgm
• Dietetics-Didactic Prgm

St Peter

Gustavus Adolphus College
Jack Ohle, PhD, President
800 W College Ave
St Peter, MN 56082
507 933-8000
Type: 4-year Coll or Univ
Control: Nonprofit (Private or Religious)
• Athletic Training Prgm
• Nursing Prgm

Thief River Falls

Northland Community & Technical College
Anne Temte, PhD, President
1101 Highway 1 East
Thief River Falls, MN 56721-2702
218 683-8611
Type: Junior or Comm Coll
Control: State, County, or Local Govt
• Cardiovascular Tech (Invasive) Prgm
• Emergency Med Tech-Paramedic Prgm
• Medical Assistant Prgm
• Occupational Therapy Asst Prgm
• Pharmacy Technician Prgm
• Physical Therapist Assistant Prgm
• Radiography Prgm
• Respiratory Care Prgm
• Surgical Technology Prgm

White Bear Lake

Century College
Larry Litecky, PhD, President
3300 Century Ave
White Bear Lake, MN 55110
651 779-3342
Type: Junior or Comm Coll
Control: State, County, or Local Govt
• Dental Assistant Prgm
• Dental Hygiene Prgm
• Emergency Med Tech-Paramedic Prgm
• Medical Assistant Prgm
• Orthotist/Prosthetist Prgm
• Pharmacy Technician Prgm
• Radiography Prgm

Willmar

Rice Memorial Hospital
Lawrence Massa, CEO
301 Becker Ave SW
Willmar, MN 56201
320 235-4543
Type: Hosp or Med Ctr: 100-299 Beds
Control: State, County, or Local Govt
• Radiography Prgm

Ridgewater College - Willmar Campus
Douglas Allen, President
PO Box 1097
Willmar, MN 56201-1097
320 222-5220
Type: Vocational or Tech Sch
Control: State, County, or Local Govt
• Emergency Med Tech-Paramedic Prgm
• Medical Assistant Prgm
• Veterinary Technology Prgm

Winona

Minnesota State College, Southeast Technical
1250 Homer Road
Winona, MN 55987
Type: Vocational or Tech Sch
Control: State, County, or Local Govt
• Radiography Prgm

Saint Mary's University of Minnesota
William Mann, PhD, President
700 Terrace Heights #30
Winona, MN 55987
507 457-1503
Type: 4-year Coll or Univ
Control: Nonprofit (Private or Religious)
• Nuclear Medicine Technology Prgm
• Surgical Technology Prgm

Winona State University
Judith Ramaley, PhD, President
PO Box 5838
Winona, MN 55987-5838
507 457-5003
Type: 4-year Coll or Univ
Control: State, County, or Local Govt
• Athletic Training Prgm
• Clin Lab Scientist/Med Technologist Prgm
• Counseling Prgm
• Music Therapy Prgm
• Nursing Prgm

Woodbury

Globe University
Terry Myhre
8089 Globe Drive
7166 10th St N
Woodbury, MN 55125
651 730-5100
Type: 4-year Coll or Univ
Control: For Profit
• Veterinary Technology Prgm

Worthington

Minnesota West Comm & Tech College
Richard Shrubb, PhD, President
1450 Collegeway
Worthington, MN 56187
507 372-3491
Type: Vocational or Tech Sch
Control: State, County, or Local Govt
• Clin Lab Technician/Med Lab Technician Prgm
• Dental Assistant Prgm
• Medical Assistant Prgm
• Radiography Prgm
• Surgical Technology Prgm

Mississippi

Booneville

Northeast Mississippi Community College
Johnny Allen, PhD, President
101 Cunningham Blvd
Booneville, MS 38829
662 720-7226
Type: Junior or Comm Coll
Control: State, County, or Local Govt
• Clin Lab Technician/Med Lab Technician Prgm
• Dental Hygiene Prgm
• Medical Assistant Prgm
• Radiography Prgm
• Respiratory Care Prgm

Clarksdale

Coahoma Community College
Clarksdale, MS 38614
Type: Junior or Comm Coll
• Polysomnographic Technology Prgm

Cleveland

Delta State University
John Hilpert, PhD, President
Box A-1
Cleveland, MS 38733-0002
601 846-3000
Type: 4-year Coll or Univ
Control: State, County, or Local Govt
• Athletic Training Prgm
• Counseling Prgm
• Dietetics-Coordinated Prgm
• Nursing Prgm

Clinton

Mississippi College
Royce Lee, PhD, President
200 W College St
Clinton, MS 39058-0001
601 925-3000
Type: 4-year Coll or Univ
Control: Nonprofit (Private or Religious)
• Counseling Prgm
• Nursing Prgm

Columbus

Mississippi University for Women
Clyda S Rent, President
PO Box W-1340
Columbus, MS 39701
601 329-4750
Type: 4-year Coll or Univ
Control: State, County, or Local Govt
• Music Therapy Prgm
• Nursing Prgm
• Speech-Language Pathology Prgm

Decatur

East Central Community College
Phil A Suthpin, EdD, President
PO Box 129
Decatur, MS 39327
601 635-2111
Type: Junior or Comm Coll
Control: State, County, or Local Govt
• Emergency Med Tech-Paramedic Prgm
• Surgical Technology Prgm

Ellisville

Jones County Junior College
Jesse Smith, EdD, President
900 S Court St
Ellisville, MS 39437
601 477-4100
Type: Junior or Comm Coll
Control: State, County, or Local Govt
• Emergency Med Tech-Paramedic Prgm
• Pharmacy Technician Prgm
• Radiography Prgm

Fulton

Itawamba Community College
David Cole, PhD, President
602 W Hill St
Fulton, MS 38843
662 862-8001
Type: Junior or Comm Coll
Control: State, County, or Local Govt
• Diagnostic Med Sonography (General) Prgm
• Emergency Med Tech-Paramedic Prgm
• Occupational Therapy Asst Prgm
• Physical Therapist Assistant Prgm
• Radiography Prgm
• Respiratory Care Prgm
• Surgical Technology Prgm

Goodman

Holmes Community College
Glenn Boyce, EdD, President
Goodman Campus
PO Box 369
Goodman, MS 39079
662 418-9012
Type: Junior or Comm Coll
Control: State, County, or Local Govt
• Emergency Med Tech-Paramedic Prgm
• Occupational Therapy Asst Prgm
• Surgical Technology Prgm

Gulfport

Miller-Motte Technical College - Gulfport
(McCann School of Business & Technology
12121 Highway 49 North
Gulfport, MS 39503
Type: Vocational or Tech Sch
Control: For Profit
• Clin Lab Technician/Med Lab Technician Prgm

Hattiesburg

University of Southern Mississippi
Martha D Saunders, PhD, President
118 College Drive, #5001
Hattiesburg, MS 39406-5001
601 266-5001
Type: 4-year Coll or Univ
Control: State, County, or Local Govt
• Athletic Training Prgm
• Audiologist Prgm
• Clin Lab Scientist/Med Technologist Prgm
• Counseling Prgm
• Dietetic Internship Prgm
• Dietetics-Didactic Prgm
• Kinesiotherapy Prgm
• Medical Librarian Prgm
• Nursing Prgm
• Phlebotomy Prgm
• Psychology (PhD) Prgm
• Speech-Language Pathology Prgm

William Carey University
James W Edwards, PhD, President
Tuscan Ave
Hattiesburg, MS 39401-9913
601 582-6223
Type: 4-year Coll or Univ
Control: Nonprofit (Private or Religious)
• Music Therapy Prgm
• Nursing Prgm
• Osteopathic Medicine Prgm

Jackson

Jackson State University
James E Lyons, Sr, President
1440 J R Lynch St
Jackson, MS 39217
601 968-2100
Type: 4-year Coll or Univ
Control: State, County, or Local Govt
• Counseling Prgm
• Psychology (PsyD) Prgm
• Rehabilitation Counseling Prgm
• Speech-Language Pathology Prgm

Mississippi Baptist Medical Center
Mark Slyter, Exec Director
1225 N State St
Jackson, MS 39202
601 968-1000
Type: Hosp or Med Ctr: 500 Beds
Control: Nonprofit (Private or Religious)
• Clin Lab Scientist/Med Technologist Prgm

Mississippi School of Therapeutic Massage
Zercon Smith, Owner
5140 Galaxie Dr
Jackson, MS 39206
601 362-3624
Type: Acad Health Ctr/Med Sch
Control: For Profit
• Massage Therapy Prgm

University of Mississippi Medical Center
James E Keeton, MD, Vice Chancellor for Health
2500 N State St
Jackson, MS 39216-4505
601 984-1010
Type: Hosp or Med Ctr: 500 Beds
Control: State, County, or Local Govt
• Clin Lab Scientist/Med Technologist Prgm
• Cytotechnology Prgm
• Dental Hygiene Prgm
• Dentistry Prgm
• Nuclear Medicine Technology Prgm
• Nursing Prgm
• Occupational Therapy Prgm
• Physical Therapy Prgm
• Radiography Prgm

Lorman

Alcorn State University
Rudolph E Waters, Interim President
Lorman, MS 39096
601 877-6100
Type: 4-year Coll or Univ
Control: State, County, or Local Govt
• Dietetics-Didactic Prgm

Mayhew

East Mississippi Community College
Mayhew, MS 39753
Type: Junior or Comm Coll
• Emergency Med Tech-Paramedic Prgm

Meridian

Meridian Community College
Scott Elliott, PhD, President
910 Hwy 19 N
Meridian, MS 39307
601 484-8618
Type: Junior or Comm Coll
Control: State, County, or Local Govt
• Clin Lab Technician/Med Lab Technician Prgm
• Dental Assistant Prgm
• Dental Hygiene Prgm
• Physical Therapist Assistant Prgm
• Radiography Prgm
• Respiratory Care Prgm
• Surgical Technology Prgm

Mississippi State

Mississippi State University
Donald W Zacharias, President
Mississippi State, MS 39762
601 325-2131
Type: 4-year Coll or Univ
Control: State, County, or Local Govt
• Counseling Prgm
• Dietetic Internship Prgm
• Dietetics-Didactic Prgm
• Rehabilitation Counseling Prgm
• Veterinary Medicine Prgm

Moorhead

Mississippi Delta Community College
Larry G Bailey, PhD, President
PO Box 668
Moorhead, MS 38761
601 246-6300
Type: Junior or Comm Coll
Control: State, County, or Local Govt
- Clin Lab Technician/Med Lab Technician Prgm
- Dental Hygiene Prgm
- Radiography Prgm

Perkinston

Mississippi Gulf Coast Community College
Mary Graham, EdD, President
PO Box 609
Perkinston, MS 39573
601 928-5211
Type: Junior or Comm Coll
Control: State, County, or Local Govt
- Clin Lab Technician/Med Lab Technician Prgm
- Emergency Med Tech-Paramedic Prgm
- Radiography Prgm
- Respiratory Care Prgm
- Surgical Technology Prgm

Poplarville

Pearl River Community College
William Lewis, EdD, President
101 Hwy 11 N
Poplarville, MS 39470
601 403-1200
Type: Junior or Comm Coll
Control: State, County, or Local Govt
- Clin Lab Technician/Med Lab Technician Prgm
- Dental Assistant Prgm
- Dental Hygiene Prgm
- Occupational Therapy Asst Prgm
- Physical Therapist Assistant Prgm
- Radiography Prgm
- Respiratory Care Prgm
- Surgical Technology Prgm

Raymond

Hinds Community College
Vernon Clyde Muse, EdD, President
PO Box 1100
501 E Main St
Raymond, MS 39154-1100
601 857-3352
Type: Junior or Comm Coll
Control: State, County, or Local Govt
- Clin Lab Technician/Med Lab Technician Prgm
- Dental Assistant Prgm
- Diagnostic Med Sonography (General) Prgm
- Emergency Med Tech-Paramedic Prgm
- Medical Assistant Prgm
- Physical Therapist Assistant Prgm
- Radiography Prgm
- Respiratory Care Prgm
- Surgical Technology Prgm
- Veterinary Technology Prgm

Senatobia

Northwest Mississippi Community College
Gary L Spears, MEd, President
4975 Hwy 51 N
Senatobia, MS 38668
601 562-3227
Type: Junior or Comm Coll
Control: State, County, or Local Govt
- Emergency Med Tech-Paramedic Prgm
- Respiratory Care Prgm
- Veterinary Technology Prgm

Tupelo

North Mississippi Medical Center
John Heer, Jr, MS, CEO
830 S Gloster
Tupelo, MS 38801
662 377-3136
Type: Hosp or Med Ctr: 500 Beds
Control: Nonprofit (Private or Religious)
- Clin Lab Scientist/Med Technologist Prgm

University

University of Mississippi
Robert C Khayat, Chancellor
University, MS 38677
601 232-7211
Type: 4-year Coll or Univ
Control: State, County, or Local Govt
- Allopathic Medicine Prgm
- Counseling Prgm
- Dietetics-Coordinated Prgm
- Dietetics-Didactic Prgm
- Music Therapy Prgm
- Pharmacy Prgm
- Psychology (PhD) Prgm
- Speech-Language Pathology Prgm

Wesson

Copiah-Lincoln Community College
Ronnie Nettles, EdD, President
PO Box 457
Wesson, MS 39191-0457
601 643-8300
Type: Junior or Comm Coll
Control: State, County, or Local Govt
- Clin Lab Technician/Med Lab Technician Prgm
- Radiography Prgm
- Respiratory Care Prgm

Missouri

Bolivar

Southwest Baptist University
Pat Taylor, President
1600 University Ave
Bolivar, MO 65613-2597
417 328-1500
Type: 4-year Coll or Univ
Control: State, County, or Local Govt
- Athletic Training Prgm
- Music Therapy Prgm
- Physical Therapy Prgm

Canton

Culver-Stockton College
William L Fox, PhD, President
1 College Hill
Canton, MO 63435
217 231-6510
Type: 4-year Coll or Univ
Control: Nonprofit (Private or Religious)
- Athletic Training Prgm

Cape Girardeau

Cape Girardeau Career & Technology Center
Richard Payne, Director CTC
Special School Administrator
1080 S Silver Springs Rd
Cape Girardeau, MO 63703
573 334-0449
Type: Vocational or Tech Sch
Control: State, County, or Local Govt
- Emergency Med Tech-Paramedic Prgm
- Respiratory Care Prgm

Southeast Missouri Hospital Coll of Nursing
Tonya Buttry, MSN RNC, President
College of Nursing and Health Sciences
2001 William St
Cape Girardeau, MO 63703
573 334-6825
Type: Hosp or Med Ctr: 100-299 Beds
Control: Nonprofit (Private or Religious)
- Clin Lab Scientist/Med Technologist Prgm
- Radiography Prgm
- Surgical Technology Prgm

Southeast Missouri State University
Kenneth Dobbins, PhD, President
One University Plaza, Mail Stop 3300
Cape Girardeau, MO 63701
573 651-2222
Type: 4-year Coll or Univ
Control: State, County, or Local Govt
- Athletic Training Prgm
- Counseling Prgm
- Dietetic Internship Prgm
- Dietetics-Didactic Prgm
- Music Therapy Prgm
- Nursing Prgm
- Speech-Language Pathology Prgm

Chesterfield

Logan College of Chiropractic
1851 Schoettler Rd
Chesterfield, MO 63017
Type: Acad Health Ctr/Med Sch
Control: For Profit
- Chiropractic Prgm

Chillicothe

Grand River Technical School
Chillicothe, MO 64601
Type: Vocational or Tech Sch
- Emergency Med Tech-Paramedic Prgm

Columbia

Columbia Public Schools
James R Ritter, EdD, Superintendent of Schools
1818 W Worley
Columbia, MO 65203
573 886-2149
Type: Vocational or Tech Sch
Control: State, County, or Local Govt
• Surgical Technology Prgm

University of Missouri
Brady Deaton, PhD, Chancellor
105 Jesse Hall
Columbia, MO 65211
573 882-3387
Type: 4-year Coll or Univ
Control: State, County, or Local Govt
• Allopathic Medicine Prgm
• Diagnostic Med Sonography (General/Vascular) Prgm
• Dietetics-Coordinated Prgm
• Medical Librarian Prgm
• Music Therapy Prgm
• Nuclear Medicine Technology Prgm
• Nursing Prgm
• Occupational Therapy Prgm
• Physical Therapy Prgm
• Psychology (PhD) Prgm
• Radiography Prgm
• Respiratory Care Prgm
• Speech-Language Pathology Prgm
• Veterinary Medicine Prgm

Fayette

Central Methodist University
Marianne E Inman, PhD, President
411 CMC Square
Fayette, MO 65248
660 248-6221
Type: 4-year Coll or Univ
Control: Nonprofit (Private or Religious)
• Athletic Training Prgm
• Nursing Prgm

Fulton

William Woods University
Jahnae Barnett, PhD, President
One University Ave
Fulton, MO 65251
573 592-4216
Type: 4-year Coll or Univ
Control: Nonprofit (Private or Religious)
• Athletic Training Prgm

Hannibal

Hannibal Career & Technical Center
Roger McGregor, Director
4550 McMasters Ave
Hannibal, MO 63401
573 221-4430
Type: Vocational or Tech Sch
Control: State, County, or Local Govt
• Respiratory Care Prgm

Hazelwood

Sanford-Brown College - Hazelwood Campus
Athena M Seidel, MA, President
75 Village Sq
Hazelwood, MO 63042
314 687-2900
Type: Junior or Comm Coll
Control: For Profit
• Occupational Therapy Asst Prgm

Hillsboro

Jefferson College
Wayne H Watts, PhD, President
1000 Viking Dr
Hillsboro, MO 63050
Type: Acad Health Ctr/Med Sch
Control: For Profit
• Veterinary Technology Prgm

Independence

Graceland University
Independence, MO 64050
Type: 4-year Coll or Univ
Control: Nonprofit (Private or Religious)
• Nursing Prgm

National American University
Independence, MO 64057
Type: 4-year Coll or Univ
• Clin Lab Technician/Med Lab Technician Prgm
• Medical Assistant Prgm
• Occupational Therapy Asst Prgm

Jefferson City

Lincoln University
Jefferson City, MO 65101
Type: 4-year Coll or Univ
• Surgical Technology Prgm

Missouri Dept of Health & Senior Service
Office of Administration
1706 E Elm St, PO Box 687
Jefferson City, MO 65102
314 751-8145
Type: Acad Health Ctr/Med Sch
Control: State, County, or Local Govt
• Dietetic Internship Prgm

Nichols Career Center
Bert Kimble, EdD, Superintendent
609 Union
Jefferson City, MO 65101
573 659-3012
Type: Vocational or Tech Sch
Control: State, County, or Local Govt
• Dental Assistant Prgm
• Radiography Prgm

Joplin

Franklin Tech Ctr/Missouri Southern St Univ
James Simpson, PhD, School Superintendent
1717 E 15th St
Joplin, MO 64802
417 625-5200
Type: Vocational or Tech Sch
Control: State, County, or Local Govt
• Surgical Technology Prgm

Missouri Southern State University
Terri Agee, Acting President
3950 E Newman Rd
Joplin, MO 64801-1595
417 625-9328
Type: 4-year Coll or Univ
Control: State, County, or Local Govt
• Dental Hygiene Prgm
• Radiography Prgm

St John's Regional Medical Center
George Caralis, President
2727 McClelland Blvd
Joplin, MO 64804
417 625-2200
Type: Hosp or Med Ctr: 300-499 Beds
Control: Nonprofit (Private or Religious)
• Clin Lab Scientist/Med Technologist Prgm

Kansas City

ARAMARK Healthcare Kansas City
St Joseph Health System
1000 Carondelet Dr
Kansas City, MO 64114-4802
816 943-2146
Control: For Profit
• Dietetic Internship Prgm

Avila University
Thomas Gordon, JD LLM, President
11901 Wornall Rd
Kansas City, MO 64145
816 942-8400
Type: 4-year Coll or Univ
Control: Nonprofit (Private or Religious)
• Nursing Prgm
• Radiography Prgm

Colorado Technical University
Tim Gramling, MS, President
520 E 19th St
Kansas City, MO 64116
816 303-7804
Type: 4-year Coll or Univ
Control: For Profit
• Radiography Prgm
• Surgical Technology Prgm

Concorde Career College - Kansas City
Deborah Crow, MS, Campus President
3239 Broadway
Kansas City, MO 64111
816 531-5223
Type: Junior or Comm Coll
Control: For Profit
• Dental Assistant Prgm
• Dental Hygiene Prgm
• Respiratory Care Prgm

Kansas City Univ of Medicine and Bioscience
1750 Independence Ave
Kansas City, MO 64106
Type: Acad Health Ctr/Med Sch
Control: Nonprofit (Private or Religious)
• Osteopathic Medicine Prgm

Maple Woods Community College
Mern Saliman, PhD, President
2601 NE Barry Rd
Kansas City, MO 64156
816 437-3044
Type: 4-year Coll or Univ
Control: State, County, or Local Govt
• Veterinary Technology Prgm

Metropolitan Community College - Penn Valley
Bernard Franklin, PhD, President
3201 SW Trafficway
Kansas City, MO 64111-2764
816 604-4201
Type: Junior or Comm Coll
Control: State, County, or Local Govt
• Dental Assistant Prgm
• Occupational Therapy Asst Prgm
• Physical Therapist Assistant Prgm
• Radiography Prgm
• Surgical Technology Prgm

Research College of Nursing
Kansas City, MO 64132
Type: Acad Health Ctr/Med Sch
Control: For Profit
• Nursing Prgm

Research Medical Center
Kevin Hicks, MBA, CEO
2316 E Meyer Blvd
Kansas City, MO 64132-1199
816 276-4101
Control: For Profit
• Nuclear Medicine Technology Prgm
• Radiography Prgm

Rockhurst University
Thomas Curran, OSFS, President
1100 Rockhurst Rd
Kansas City, MO 64110-2561
816 501-4250
Type: 4-year Coll or Univ
Control: Nonprofit (Private or Religious)
• Occupational Therapy Prgm
• Physical Therapy Prgm
• Speech-Language Pathology Prgm

Saint Luke's Hospital
Julie Quirin, CEO
4401 Wornall Rd
Kansas City, MO 64111
816 932-3800
Type: Hosp or Med Ctr: 500 Beds
Control: Nonprofit (Private or Religious)
• Clin Lab Scientist/Med Technologist Prgm
• Diagnostic Med Sonography (General) Prgm
• Nursing Prgm
• Phlebotomy Prgm
• Radiography Prgm

University of Missouri - Kansas City
Guy Bailey, PhD, Chancellor
5115 Oak
Kansas City, MO 64110-2499
816 235-1000
Type: 4-year Coll or Univ
Control: State, County, or Local Govt
• Allopathic Medicine Prgm
• Anesthesiologist Asst Prgm
• Dental Hygiene Prgm
• Dentistry Prgm
• Music Therapy Prgm
• Nursing Prgm
• Pharmacy Prgm
• Psychology (PhD) Prgm

Kirksville

AT Still University of Health Sciences
Jack Magruder, EdD, President
800 West Jefferson Street
Kirksville, MO 63501-1443
660 626-2121
Type: Acad Health Ctr/Med Sch
Control: Nonprofit (Private or Religious)
• Audiologist Prgm
• Dentistry Prgm
• Occupational Therapy Prgm
• Osteopathic Medicine Prgm
• Physical Therapy Prgm
• Physician Assistant Prgm

Kirksville College of Osteopathic Medicine
800 W Jefferson
Kirksville, MO 63501
Type: Acad Health Ctr/Med Sch
Control: Nonprofit (Private or Religious)
• Osteopathic Medicine Prgm

Truman State University
Barbara Dixon, DMA, President
200 McClain Hall
Kirksville, MO 63501
660 785-4000
Type: 4-year Coll or Univ
Control: State, County, or Local Govt
• Athletic Training Prgm
• Music Therapy Prgm
• Nursing Prgm
• Speech-Language Pathology Prgm

Liberty

William Jewell College
Liberty, MO 64068
Type: 4-year Coll or Univ
Control: Nonprofit (Private or Religious)
• Nursing Prgm

Linn

Linn State Technical College
Donald Claycomb, PhD, President
One Technology Dr
Linn, MO 65051
573 897-5000
Type: Vocational or Tech Sch
Control: State, County, or Local Govt
• Physical Therapist Assistant Prgm

Maryville

Northwest Missouri State University
Dean L Hubbard, President
Maryville, MO 64468
816 562-1212
Type: 4-year Coll or Univ
Control: State, County, or Local Govt
• Dietetics-Didactic Prgm
• Music Therapy Prgm

Moberly

Missouri Health Professions Consortium
Evelyn Jorgensen, PhD, President and
  Representative
101 College Avenue
Moberly, MO 65270-1304
660 263-4110
• Occupational Therapy Asst Prgm

Neosho

Crowder College
Alan Marble, President
601 LaClede Ave
Neosho, MO 64850
417 455-5534
Type: Acad Health Ctr/Med Sch
Control: For Profit
• Veterinary Technology Prgm

North Kansas City

North Kansas City Hospital
David Carpenter, MS JD, President and CEO
2800 Clay Edwards Dr
North Kansas City, MO 64116
816 691-2020
Type: Hosp or Med Ctr: 300-499 Beds
Control: State, County, or Local Govt
• Clin Lab Scientist/Med Technologist Prgm

Sanford-Brown College
Dennis Townsend, MEd, Campus President
520 E 19th Ave
North Kansas City, MO 64116
816 472-7400
Type: 4-year Coll or Univ
Control: For Profit
• Diagnostic Med Sonography (General) Prgm
• Polysomnographic Technology Prgm
• Radiography Prgm
• Respiratory Care Prgm

Park Hills

Mineral Area College
Terry Barnes, President
PO Box 1000
5270 Flat River Road
Park Hills, MO 63601
573 518-2138
Type: Junior or Comm Coll
Control: State, County, or Local Govt
• Radiography Prgm

Parkville

Park University
Beverley Byers-Pevitts, PhD, President
8700 NW Riverpark Dr
Parkville, MO 64152
816 741-2000
Type: 4-year Coll or Univ
Control: Nonprofit (Private or Religious)
• Athletic Training Prgm

Point Lookout

College of the Ozarks
Jerry C Davis, President
Point Lookout, MO 65726
417 334-6411
Type: 4-year Coll or Univ
Control: Nonprofit (Private or Religious)
• Dietetics-Didactic Prgm
• Nursing Prgm

Poplar Bluff

Three Rivers Community College
Joseph Rozman, MS, President
2080 Three Rivers Blvd
Poplar Bluff, MO 63901-2393
573 840-9600
Type: Junior or Comm Coll
Control: State, County, or Local Govt
• Clin Lab Technician/Med Lab Technician Prgm

Rolla

Rolla Technical Center
Janece Martin, PhD, Director Vocational Prgms
500 Forum Dr
Rolla, MO 65401
573 458-0160
Type: Vocational or Tech Sch
Control: State, County, or Local Govt
• Diagnostic Med Sonography (General/Vascular)
  Prgm
• Radiography Prgm
• Respiratory Care Prgm
• Surgical Technology Prgm

Sedalia

State Fair Community College
Marsha Drennon, EdD, President
3201 W 16th St
Sedalia, MO 65301
660 530-5800
Type: Junior or Comm Coll
Control: State, County, or Local Govt
• Dental Hygiene Prgm
• Radiography Prgm

Springfield

Cox College of Nursing and Health Sciences
Springfield, MO 65802
Type: Acad Health Ctr/Med Sch
Control: Nonprofit (Private or Religious)
• Dietetic Internship Prgm
• Nursing Prgm

Cox Medical Centers
Robert H Bezanson, MHA, Administrator
3801 South National Ave
Springfield, MO 65807
417 269-3108
Type: Hosp or Med Ctr: 500 Beds
Control: Nonprofit (Private or Religious)
• Clin Lab Scientist/Med Technologist Prgm
• Diagnostic Med Sonography
  (Gen/Card/Vascular) Prgm
• Radiography Prgm

Drury University
Todd Parnel, PhD, Interim President
Burnham Hall 102
Springfield, MO 65802
417 873-7201
Type: 4-year Coll or Univ
Control: State, County, or Local Govt
• Music Therapy Prgm

Everest College - Springfield Campus
Gary Myers, MS, President
1010 W Sunshine
Springfield, MO 65807
417 864-7220
Type: Vocational or Tech Sch
Control: For Profit
• Medical Assistant Prgm

Forest Institute of Professional Psychology
Springfield, MO 65807
Type: Acad Health Ctr/Med Sch
Control: For Profit
• Psychology (PsyD) Prgm

Mercy Hospital Springfield
Robert Brodhead, President
1235 E Cherokee
Springfield, MO 65804
417 820-2709
Type: Hosp or Med Ctr: 500 Beds
Control: Nonprofit (Private or Religious)
• Clin Lab Scientist/Med Technologist Prgm
• Radiography Prgm

Missouri State University
Michael Nietzel, PhD, President
901 S National Ave
Springfield, MO 65897
417 836-8500
Type: 4-year Coll or Univ
Control: State, County, or Local Govt
• Athletic Training Prgm
• Audiologist Prgm
• Dietetics-Didactic Prgm
• Nursing Prgm
• Physical Therapy Prgm
• Physician Assistant Prgm
• Respiratory Care Prgm
• Speech-Language Pathology Prgm
• Teacher of the Visually Impaired Prgm

Ozarks Technical Community College
Hal Higdon, PhD, President
1001 E Chestnut Expressway
Springfield, MO 65802
417 447-2602
Type: Junior or Comm Coll
Control: State, County, or Local Govt
• Clin Lab Technician/Med Lab Technician Prgm
• Dental Assistant Prgm
• Dental Hygiene Prgm
• Emergency Med Tech-Paramedic Prgm
• Occupational Therapy Asst Prgm
• Physical Therapist Assistant Prgm
• Respiratory Care Prgm
• Surgical Technology Prgm

St Charles

Lindenwood University
James Evans, President
209 S Kings Hwy
St Charles, MO 63301
636 949-4900
Type: 4-year Coll or Univ
Control: State, County, or Local Govt
• Athletic Training Prgm

St Joseph

Hillyard Technical Center
Robert D Stewart, MS, Director
3434 Faragon St
St Joseph, MO 64506
816 671-4170
Type: Vocational or Tech Sch
Control: Nonprofit (Private or Religious)
• Diagnostic Med Sonography (General/Vascular)
  Prgm
• Radiography Prgm
• Surgical Technology Prgm

Missouri Western State University
James Scanlon, President
4525 Downs Dr
St Joseph, MO 64507
816 271-4237
Type: 4-year Coll or Univ
Control: State, County, or Local Govt
• Music Therapy Prgm
• Nursing Prgm
• Physical Therapist Assistant Prgm

North Central Missouri College
St Joseph, MO 64506
• Dental Hygiene Prgm

St Louis

Barnes-Jewish Coll of Nursing/Allied Health
Ron Evens, MD, President
306 S Kingshighway Blvd
St Louis, MO 63110
314 454-7054
Type: 4-year Coll or Univ
Control: Nonprofit (Private or Religious)
• Nursing Prgm

DVA Medical Center
Jefferson Barracks Div
One Jefferson Barracks Dr
St Louis, MO 63125
314 894-6631
Type: Dept of Veterans Affairs
Control: Fed Govt
• Dietetic Internship Prgm

Fontbonne University
Dennis Golden, President
6800 Wydown Blvd
St Louis, MO 63105
314 862-3456
Type: 4-year Coll or Univ
Control: Nonprofit (Private or Religious)
• Dietetics-Didactic Prgm
• Speech-Language Pathology Prgm

IHM Health Studies Center
Mark Corley, EMT-P, Chairman
2500 Abbott Place
St Louis, MO 63143
314 768-1000
Type: Vocational or Tech Sch
Control: For Profit
• Emergency Med Tech-Paramedic Prgm

Maryville University
Mark Lombardi, PhD, President
650 Maryville University Dr
St Louis, MO 63141-7299
314 529-9300
Type: 4-year Coll or Univ
Control: Nonprofit (Private or Religious)
• Music Therapy Prgm
• Nursing Prgm
• Occupational Therapy Prgm
• Physical Therapy Prgm
• Rehabilitation Counseling Prgm

Missouri College
Michael Vander Velde, MA, President
10121 Manchester Rd
St Louis, MO 63122
314 821-7700
Type: Vocational or Tech Sch
Control: For Profit
• Dental Assistant Prgm
• Dental Hygiene Prgm

Saint Louis University
Lawrence Biondi, Provost
221 N Grand Boulevard, DuBourg Hall
St Louis, MO 63103-2097
314 977-7780
Type: Acad Health Ctr/Med Sch
Control: Nonprofit (Private or Religious)
• Allopathic Medicine Prgm
• Athletic Training Prgm
• Clin Lab Scientist/Med Technologist Prgm
• Cytotechnology Prgm
• Dietetic Internship Prgm
• Dietetics-Didactic Prgm
• Nuclear Medicine Technology Prgm
• Nursing Prgm
• Occupational Therapy Prgm
• Physical Therapy Prgm
• Physician Assistant Prgm
• Psychology (PhD) Prgm
• Radiation Therapy Prgm
• Speech-Language Pathology Prgm

St John's Mercy Medical Center
Denny DeNarvaez, President/CEO
615 S New Ballas Rd
St Louis, MO 63141
314 251-1952
Type: Hosp or Med Ctr: 500 Beds
Control: Nonprofit (Private or Religious)
• Clin Lab Scientist/Med Technologist Prgm

St Louis College of Pharmacy
Wendy Duncan-Hewitt, PhD, Dean
4588 Parkview Place
St Louis, MO 63110
314 446-8341
Type: Acad Health Ctr/Med Sch
Control: For Profit
• Pharmacy Prgm

St Louis Community College
Morris Johnson, MSW, Interim Chancellor
5600 Oakland Ave
St Louis, MO 63110-1393
314 644-9743
Type: Junior or Comm Coll
Control: State, County, or Local Govt
• Clin Lab Technician/Med Lab Technician Prgm
• Dental Assistant Prgm
• Dental Hygiene Prgm
• Diagnostic Med Sonography (Gen/Card/Vascular) Prgm
• Dietetic Technician-AD Prgm
• Occupational Therapy Asst Prgm
• Physical Therapist Assistant Prgm
• Radiography Prgm
• Respiratory Care Prgm
• Surgical Technology Prgm

University of Missouri - St Louis
Blanche M Touhill, President
8001 Natural Bridge Rd
St Louis, MO 63121-4499
314 516-5000
Type: 4-year Coll or Univ
Control: State, County, or Local Govt
• Counseling Prgm
• Nursing Prgm
• Optometry Prgm
• Psychology (PhD) Prgm

Washington University
Mark S Wrighton, PhD, Chancellor
Brookings Dr Campus Box 1192
St Louis, MO 63130
314 935-5100
Type: Acad Health Ctr/Med Sch
Control: Nonprofit (Private or Religious)
• Allopathic Medicine Prgm
• Audiologist Prgm
• Occupational Therapy Prgm
• Physical Therapy Prgm
• Psychology (PhD) Prgm

St Peters

St Charles Community College
John McGuire, PhD, President
4601 Mid Rivers Mall Dr
PO Box 76975
St Peters, MO 63376-0975
314 922-8380
Type: Junior or Comm Coll
Control: State, County, or Local Govt
• Occupational Therapy Asst Prgm

St. Louis

Missouri Baptist University
St. Louis, MO 63141
Type: 4-year Coll or Univ
• Exercise Science Prgm

Moberly Area Community College
Jeffrey Johnston, President
615 South New Ballas Road
St. Louis, MO 63141
• Clin Lab Technician/Med Lab Technician Prgm
• Radiography Prgm

Warrensburg

University of Central Missouri
Aaron Podolefsky, PhD, President
Warrensburg, MO 64093
816 543-4111
Type: 4-year Coll or Univ
Control: State, County, or Local Govt
• Athletic Training Prgm
• Dietetics-Didactic Prgm
• Music Therapy Prgm
• Nursing Prgm
• Speech-Language Pathology Prgm

West Plains

South Central Career Center
Steve Bryant, MS EdS, Director
610 Olden
West Plains, MO 65775
417 256-6152
Type: Vocational or Tech Sch
Control: State, County, or Local Govt
• Surgical Technology Prgm

South Howell County Ambulance District
West Plains, MO 65775
Type: Consortium
• Emergency Med Tech-Paramedic Prgm
• Occupational Therapy Asst Prgm

Montana

Billings

Montana State University Billings
Ronald P Sexton, PhD, Chancellor
1500 University Dr
Billings, MT 59101
406 657-2300
Type: 4-year Coll or Univ
Control: State, County, or Local Govt
• Athletic Training Prgm
• Emergency Med Tech-Paramedic Prgm
• Music Therapy Prgm
• Rehabilitation Counseling Prgm

Rocky Mountain College
Michael Mace, MBA, President
1511 Poly Dr
Billings, MT 59102
406 657-1015
Type: 4-year Coll or Univ
Control: Nonprofit (Private or Religious)
• Physician Assistant Prgm

Bozeman

Health Works Institute
Ruth Marion, Owner-Director
111 S Grand, Annex 3
Bozeman, MT 59715
406 582-1555
Type: Vocational or Tech Sch
Control: For Profit
• Massage Therapy Prgm

Montana State University
Geoffrey Gamble, President
Bozeman, MT 59717
406 994-0211
Type: 4-year Coll or Univ
Control: State, County, or Local Govt
• Clin Lab Scientist/Med Technologist Prgm
• Counseling Prgm
• Dietetic Internship Prgm
• Dietetics-Didactic Prgm
• Music Therapy Prgm
• Nursing Prgm
• Physical Therapist Assistant Prgm

Great Falls

Montana State Univ - Great Falls Coll of Tech
Joe Schaffer, EdD, Dean
2100 16th Ave S
Great Falls, MT 59405
406 771-4310
Type: Vocational or Tech Sch
Control: State, County, or Local Govt
• Dental Assistant Prgm
• Dental Hygiene Prgm
• Dietetic Technician-AD Prgm
• Emergency Med Tech-Paramedic Prgm
• Medical Assistant Prgm
• Respiratory Care Prgm
• Surgical Technology Prgm

University of Great Falls
Great Falls, MT 59405
Type: 4-year Coll or Univ
Control: Nonprofit (Private or Religious)
• Nursing Prgm

Helena

Carroll College
Thomas J Trebon, President
1601 N Benton Ave
Helena, MT 59625
406 447-4402
Type: 4-year Coll or Univ
Control: Nonprofit (Private or Religious)
• Nursing Prgm

Kalispell

Flathead Valley Community College
Jane A Karas, PhD, President
777 Grandview Dr
Kalispell, MT 59901
406 756-3822
Type: Junior or Comm Coll
Control: State, County, or Local Govt
• Medical Assistant Prgm
• Surgical Technology Prgm

Missoula

Univ of Montana-Missoula - College of Tech
Dennis Lerum, Dean
909 S Ave W
Missoula, MT 59801
Type: 4-year Coll or Univ
Control: State, County, or Local Govt
• Pharmacy Technician Prgm

University of Montana
George Dennison, PhD, President
University Hall 109
Missoula, MT 59812
406 243-2311
Type: 4-year Coll or Univ
Control: State, County, or Local Govt
• Athletic Training Prgm
• Counseling Prgm
• Pharmacy Prgm
• Physical Therapy Prgm
• Psychology (PhD) Prgm
• Respiratory Care Prgm
• Speech-Language Pathology Prgm
• Surgical Technology Prgm

Pablo

Salish Kootenai College
Dr. Luana Ross, PhD, President
PO Box 70
52000 Hwy 93
Pablo, MT 59855
406 675-4800
Type: Junior or Comm Coll
Control: Nonprofit (Private or Religious)
• Dental Assistant Prgm

Nebraska

Curtis

Nebraska College of Technical Agriculture
Weldon Sleight, PhD, Dean
Curtis, NE 69025
308 367-5238
Type: Vocational or Tech Sch
Control: For Profit
• Veterinary Technology Prgm

Grand Island

Central Community College
Greg Smith, PhD, President
PO Box 4903
Grand Island, NE 68802-4903
308 389-6300
Type: Junior or Comm Coll
Control: State, County, or Local Govt
• Clin Lab Technician/Med Lab Technician Prgm
• Dental Assistant Prgm
• Dental Hygiene Prgm
• Emergency Med Tech-Paramedic Prgm
• Medical Assistant Prgm
• Occupational Therapy Asst Prgm

Hastings

Mary Lanning Memorial Healthcare
W Michael Kearney, MHA, Administrator
715 N St Joseph
Hastings, NE 68901
402 463-4521
Type: Hosp or Med Ctr: 100-299 Beds
Control: Nonprofit (Private or Religious)
• Radiography Prgm

Kearney

University of Nebraska - Kearney
Douglas Kristensen, JD, Chancellor
905 W 25th St
Founders Hall
Kearney, NE 68849
308 865-8208
Type: 4-year Coll or Univ
Control: State, County, or Local Govt
• Athletic Training Prgm
• Counseling Prgm
• Music Therapy Prgm
• Speech-Language Pathology Prgm

Lincoln

BryanLGH College of Health Sciences
Phylis Hollamon, MSN, President
5035 Everett St
Lincoln, NE 68506
402 481-3867
Type: 4-year Coll or Univ
Control: Nonprofit (Private or Religious)
• Cardiovascular Tech (Invasive/Noninv/Vasc) Prgm
• Diagnostic Med Sonography (General) Prgm

Kaplan University - Lincoln
Thomas Lardenoit, Director
1821 K Street
Lincoln, NE 68508
402 474-5315
Type: Junior or Comm Coll
Control: State, County, or Local Govt
• Medical Assistant Prgm

Nebraska Wesleyan University
Frederik Ohles, PhD, President
5000 St Paul Ave
Lincoln, NE 68504
402 466-2217
Type: 4-year Coll or Univ
Control: Nonprofit (Private or Religious)
• Athletic Training Prgm
• Music Therapy Prgm

Southeast Community College
Jack Huck, PhD, President
301 South 68th St. Place, Lincoln, NE 68
Lincoln, NE 68510-2449
402 323-3415
Type: Junior or Comm Coll
Control: State, County, or Local Govt
• Clin Lab Technician/Med Lab Technician Prgm
• Dental Assistant Prgm
• Dietetic Technician-AD Prgm
• Medical Assistant Prgm
• Pharmacy Technician Prgm
• Physical Therapist Assistant Prgm
• Polysomnographic Technology Prgm
• Radiography Prgm
• Respiratory Care Prgm
• Surgical Technology Prgm

Union College
David Smith, EdD, President
3800 S 48th St
Lincoln, NE 68506
402 486-2500
Type: 4-year Coll or Univ
Control: Nonprofit (Private or Religious)
• Nursing Prgm
• Physician Assistant Prgm

University of Nebraska - Lincoln
Harvey Perlman, JD, Chancellor
201 ADM
Lincoln, NE 68588-0419
402 472-2116
Type: 4-year Coll or Univ
Control: State, County, or Local Govt
- Athletic Training Prgm
- Audiologist Prgm
- Dental Hygiene Prgm
- Dietetic Internship Prgm
- Dietetics-Didactic Prgm
- Music Therapy Prgm
- Psychology (PhD) Prgm
- Speech-Language Pathology Prgm

Norfolk

Northeast Community College
Bill R Path
801 E Benjamin Ave
PO Box 469
Norfolk, NE 68702-0469
Type: Junior or Comm Coll
Control: State, County, or Local Govt
- Physical Therapist Assistant Prgm
- Veterinary Technician Prgm

North Platte

Mid-Plains Community College
Michael Chipps, PhD, President
601 W State Farm Rd
North Platte, NE 69101
308 535-3719
Type: Junior or Comm Coll
Control: State, County, or Local Govt
- Clin Lab Technician/Med Lab Technician Prgm
- Dental Assistant Prgm

Omaha

Alegent Health
Wayne A Sensor, FACHE, President/CEO
1010 N 96th St
Omaha, NE 68122
402 343-4410
Type: Hosp or Med Ctr: 300-499 Beds
Control: Nonprofit (Private or Religious)
- Radiography Prgm
- Respiratory Care Prgm

Clarkson College
Louis Burgher, MD, President
101 S 42nd St
Omaha, NE 68131-2739
402 552-3394
Type: 4-year Coll or Univ
Control: Nonprofit (Private or Religious)
- Physical Therapist Assistant Prgm
- Radiography Prgm

College of Saint Mary
Maryanne Stevens, RSM PhD, President
7000 Mercy Rd
Omaha, NE 68106
402 399-2435
Type: 4-year Coll or Univ
Control: Nonprofit (Private or Religious)
- Occupational Therapy Prgm

Creighton University
Rev John P Schlegel, SJ PhD, President
2500 California Plaza
Omaha, NE 68178-0001
402 280-2770
Type: 4-year Coll or Univ
Control: Nonprofit (Private or Religious)
- Allopathic Medicine Prgm
- Athletic Training Prgm
- Dentistry Prgm
- Emergency Med Tech-Paramedic Prgm
- Nursing Prgm
- Occupational Therapy Prgm (2)
- Pharmacy Prgm
- Physical Therapy Prgm

Kaplan University - Omaha
Michael Ziaisky, BA, President
3350 N 90th St
Omaha, NE 68134
402 572-8500
Type: Junior or Comm Coll
Control: For Profit
- Dental Assistant Prgm
- Medical Assistant Prgm

Metropolitan Community College
JoAnn McDowell, EdD, President
PO Box 3777
Omaha, NE 68103
402 457-2415
Type: Junior or Comm Coll
Control: State, County, or Local Govt
- Dental Assistant Prgm
- Emergency Med Tech-Paramedic Prgm
- Medical Assistant Prgm
- Medical Transcriptionist Prgm
- Respiratory Care Prgm

Nebraska Methodist College
Dennis Joslin, PhD, President
Josie Harper Campus
720 N 87th St
Omaha, NE 68114
402 354-7257
Type: 4-year Coll or Univ
Control: Nonprofit (Private or Religious)
- Diagnostic Med Sonography
  (Gen/Card/Vascular) Prgm
- Medical Assistant Prgm
- Nursing Prgm
- Physical Therapist Assistant Prgm
- Radiography Prgm
- Respiratory Care Prgm
- Surgical Technology Prgm

Nebraska Methodist Hospital
Steve Goeser, President/CEO
8303 Dodge St
Omaha, NE 68114
402 354-4449
Type: Hosp or Med Ctr: 300-499 Beds
Control: Nonprofit (Private or Religious)
- Clin Lab Scientist/Med Technologist Prgm

University of Nebraska - Omaha
Nancy Belck, PhD, Chancellor
EAB 201
Omaha, NE 68182-0108
402 554-3211
Type: 4-year Coll or Univ
Control: State, County, or Local Govt
- Allopathic Medicine Prgm
- Athletic Training Prgm
- Counseling Prgm
- Music Therapy Prgm
- Speech-Language Pathology Prgm

University of Nebraska Medical Center
Harold M Maurer, MD, Chancellor
986605 Nebraska Medical Center
Omaha, NE 68198-6605
402 559-4201
Type: Acad Health Ctr/Med Sch
Control: State, County, or Local Govt
- Clin Lab Scientist/Med Technologist Prgm
- Cytotechnology Prgm
- Dentistry Prgm
- Diagnostic Med Sonography (General) Prgm
- Dietetic Internship Prgm
- Magnetic Resonance Technologist Prgm
- Nuclear Medicine Technology Prgm
- Nursing Prgm
- Perfusion Prgm
- Pharmacy Prgm
- Physical Therapy Prgm
- Physician Assistant Prgm
- Radiation Therapy Prgm
- Radiography Prgm

Vatterott College - Omaha Campus
William J Stuckey, MS, President
225 N 80th St
Omaha, NE 68114-3617
402 392-1300
Type: 4-year Coll or Univ
Control: State, County, or Local Govt
- Dental Assistant Prgm
- Veterinary Technician Prgm

Scottsbluff

Regional West Medical Center
Todd Sorensen, MD, CEO and President
4021 Ave B
Scottsbluff, NE 69361
308 635-3711
Type: Hosp or Med Ctr: 100-299 Beds
Control: Nonprofit (Private or Religious)
- Radiography Prgm

Nevada

Elko

Great Basin College
1500 College Parkway
Elko, NV 89801
Type: 4-year Coll or Univ
Control: State, County, or Local Govt
- Radiography Prgm

Henderson

Nevada State College
Henderson, NV 89002
Type: 4-year Coll or Univ
Control: State, County, or Local Govt
• Nursing Prgm

Roseman University of Health Sciences
Harry Rosenberg, PharmD PhD, President
11 Sunset Way
Henderson, NV 89014
702 990-4433
Type: 4-year Coll or Univ
Control: Nonprofit (Private or Religious)
• Dentistry Prgm
• Pharmacy Prgm

Touro University - Nevada
Michael Harter, PhD, Senior Provost and CEO
874 American Pacific Dr
Henderson, NV 89014
702 777-8687
Type: 4-year Coll or Univ
Control: Nonprofit (Private or Religious)
• Nursing Prgm
• Occupational Therapy Prgm
• Osteopathic Medicine Prgm
• Physician Assistant Prgm

Las Vegas

College of Southern Nevada
Michael D Richards, PhD, President
6375 W Charleston Blvd W3D
Las Vegas, NV 89146-1139
702 651-5600
Type: Junior or Comm Coll
Control: State, County, or Local Govt
• Clin Lab Technician/Med Lab Technician Prgm
• Dental Assistant Prgm
• Dental Hygiene Prgm
• Diagnostic Med Sonography (Gen/Card/Vascular) Prgm
• Emergency Med Tech-Paramedic Prgm
• Massage Therapy Prgm
• Medical Assistant Prgm
• Occupational Therapy Asst Prgm
• Ophthalmic Dispensing Optician Prgm
• Pharmacy Technician Prgm
• Physical Therapist Assistant Prgm
• Respiratory Care Prgm
• Surgical Technology Prgm
• Veterinary Technology Prgm

Nevada Career Institute
Joanne Leming, LPN, Regional Campus Director
3025 E Desert Inn Rd, Ste A
Las Vegas, NV 89121
702 893-3300
Type: Vocational or Tech Sch
Control: For Profit
• Surgical Technology Prgm

Pima Medical Institute
Richard Luebke, Sr, President
3333 E Flamingo Rd
Las Vegas, NV 89121
702 458-9650
Type: Acad Health Ctr/Med Sch
Control: For Profit
• Pharmacy Technician Prgm
• Radiography Prgm
• Respiratory Care Prgm
• Veterinary Technology Prgm

University of Nevada - Las Vegas
David B Ashley, PhD, President
4505 Maryland Pkwy
PO Box 451001
Las Vegas, NV 89154-1001
702 895-3201
Type: 4-year Coll or Univ
Control: State, County, or Local Govt
• Clin Lab Scientist/Med Technologist Prgm
• Counseling Prgm
• Dentistry Prgm
• Dietetic Internship Prgm
• Dietetics-Didactic Prgm
• Music Therapy Prgm
• Nuclear Medicine Technology Prgm
• Nursing Prgm
• Phlebotomy Prgm
• Physical Therapy Prgm
• Psychology (PhD) Prgm
• Radiography Prgm

Reno

Truckee Meadows Community College
Maria Sheehan, PhD, President
7000 Dandini Blvd (R-200)
Reno, NV 89512-3999
702 673-7025
Type: Junior or Comm Coll
Control: State, County, or Local Govt
• Dental Assistant Prgm
• Dental Hygiene Prgm
• Dietetic Technician-AD Prgm
• Veterinary Technology Prgm

University of Nevada - Reno
Milton Glick, PhD, President
Reno, NV 89557-0046
702 784-4805
Type: 4-year Coll or Univ
Control: State, County, or Local Govt
• Allopathic Medicine Prgm
• Counseling Prgm
• Dietetic Internship Prgm
• Dietetics-Didactic Prgm
• Music Therapy Prgm
• Nursing Prgm
• Psychology (PhD) Prgm
• Speech-Language Pathology Prgm

New Brunswick, Canada

Fredericton

University of New Brunswick
Fredericton, NB E3B 6E4
Type: 4-year Coll or Univ
Control: State, County, or Local Govt
• Psychology (PhD) Prgm

New Hampshire

Berlin

White Mountains Community College
Berlin, NH 03570
Type: Junior or Comm Coll
• Medical Assistant Prgm

Claremont

River Valley Community College
Steven Budd, MBA, President
1 College Dr
Claremont, NH 03743-9707
603 542-7744
Type: Junior or Comm Coll
Control: State, County, or Local Govt
• Clin Lab Technician/Med Lab Technician Prgm
• Medical Assistant Prgm
• Occupational Therapy Asst Prgm
• Physical Therapist Assistant Prgm
• Respiratory Care Prgm

Concord

Concord Hospital
Michael Green, BA MS, CEO
250 Pleasant St
Concord, NH 03301
603 225-2711
Type: Hosp or Med Ctr: 100-299 Beds
Control: Nonprofit (Private or Religious)
• Surgical Technology Prgm

NHTI, Concord's Community College
Lynn Kilchenstein, MEd, President
31 College Dr
Concord, NH 03301-7412
603 271-7737
Type: Junior or Comm Coll
Control: State, County, or Local Govt
• Dental Assistant Prgm
• Dental Hygiene Prgm
• Diagnostic Med Sonography (General) Prgm
• Emergency Med Tech-Paramedic Prgm
• Radiation Therapy Prgm
• Radiography Prgm

Durham

University of New Hampshire
Mark Huddleston, PhD, President
204 Thompson Hall, 105 Main Street
Durham, NH 03824-3547
603 862-4296
Type: 4-year Coll or Univ
Control: State, County, or Local Govt
• Athletic Training Prgm
• Clin Lab Scientist/Med Technologist Prgm
• Dietetic Internship Prgm
• Dietetic Technician-AD Prgm
• Dietetics-Didactic Prgm
• Music Therapy Prgm
• Nursing Prgm
• Occupational Therapy Prgm
• Speech-Language Pathology Prgm

Hanover

Dartmouth Medical School
Hanover, NH 03755
Type: Acad Health Ctr/Med Sch
Control: Nonprofit (Private or Religious)
• Allopathic Medicine Prgm

Hudson

New Hampshire Institute for Therapeutic Arts
Patrick Ian Cowan, PhD, Executive Director
153 Lowell Rd
Hudson, NH 03051
603 882-3022
Type: Acad Health Ctr/Med Sch
Control: For Profit
• Massage Therapy Prgm

Keene

Antioch University New England
David Caruso, PhD, President
40 Avon St
Keene, NH 03431-3516
603 357-3122
Type: 4-year Coll or Univ
Control: For Profit
• Counseling Prgm
• Psychology (PsyD) Prgm

Keene State College
Stanley J Yarosewick, PhD, President
229 Main
Keene, NH 03435
603 358-2000
Type: 4-year Coll or Univ
Control: State, County, or Local Govt
• Athletic Training Prgm
• Dietetic Internship Prgm
• Dietetics-Didactic Prgm
• Music Therapy Prgm

Lebanon

Dartmouth Hitchcock Medical Center
Thomas Colachio, MD, President/CEO
One Medical Center Dr
Lebanon, NH 03756-0001
603 650-5000
Type: Hosp or Med Ctr: 300-499 Beds
Control: Nonprofit (Private or Religious)
• Surgical Technology Prgm

Lebanon College
Donald Wenz, PhD, President, CEO
15 Hanover St
Lebanon, NH 03766
603 448-2445
Type: Junior or Comm Coll
Control: Nonprofit (Private or Religious)
• Radiography Prgm

Manchester

Hesser College
Mary Jo Greco, MAT, President
3 Sundial Ave
Manchester, NH 03103
603 668-6660
Type: Junior or Comm Coll
Control: For Profit
• Medical Assistant Prgm
• Physical Therapist Assistant Prgm

Manchester Community College
Manchester, NH 03102
Type: Junior or Comm Coll
• Medical Assistant Prgm

Mass College of Pharmacy & Health Sciences
1260 Elm St
Manchester, NH 03101
Type: Acad Health Ctr/Med Sch
Control: Nonprofit (Private or Religious)
• Physician Assistant Prgm

New England EMS Institute
Doug Dean, CEO
One Elliot Way
Manchester, NH 03103
603 628-2220
Type: Hosp or Med Ctr: 300-499 Beds
Control: Nonprofit (Private or Religious)
• Emergency Med Tech-Paramedic Prgm

Saint Anselm College
Manchester, NH 03102
Type: 4-year Coll or Univ
Control: Nonprofit (Private or Religious)
• Nursing Prgm

New London

Colby-Sawyer College
Thomas Galligan, JD LLM, President
541 Main St
New London, NH 03257
603 526-3737
Type: 4-year Coll or Univ
Control: Nonprofit (Private or Religious)
• Athletic Training Prgm
• Nursing Prgm

Plymouth

Plymouth State University
Sara Jayne Steen, PhD, President
MSC 1
Plymouth, NH 03264
603 535-2211
Type: 4-year Coll or Univ
Control: State, County, or Local Govt
• Athletic Training Prgm
• Counseling Prgm

Portsmouth

Great Bay Community College
Portsmouth, NH 03801
Type: Junior or Comm Coll
• Surgical Technology Prgm

Rindge

Franklin Pierce College
George J Hagerty
20 College Rd
Rindge, NH 03461-0060
800 437-0048
Type: 4-year Coll or Univ
Control: Nonprofit (Private or Religious)
• Physical Therapy Prgm
• Physician Assistant Prgm

Stratham

New Hampshire Comm Tech College - Stratham
Catherine Smith, EdD, President
277 Portsmouth Ave
Stratham, NH 03885
603 772-1194
Type: Junior or Comm Coll
Control: State, County, or Local Govt
• Veterinary Technology Prgm

New Jersey

Blackwood

Camden County College
Raymond A Yannuzzi, PhD, President
PO Box 200 College Drive
Blackwood, NJ 08012
856 227-7200
Type: Junior or Comm Coll
Control: State, County, or Local Govt
• Clin Lab Technician/Med Lab Technician Prgm
• Dental Assistant Prgm
• Dental Hygiene Prgm
• Dietetic Technician-AD Prgm
• Ophthalmic Dispensing Optician Prgm
• Ophthalmic Technician Prgm
• Veterinary Technology Prgm

Bloomfield

Bloomfield College
Bloomfield, NJ 07003
Type: Junior or Comm Coll
Control: Nonprofit (Private or Religious)
• Nursing Prgm

Bridgeton

Cumberland County Technical Education Center
Darlene Barber, Superintendent
601 Bridgeton Ave
Bridgeton, NJ 08302
609 451-9000
Type: Vocational or Tech Sch
Control: State, County, or Local Govt
• Dental Assistant Prgm

Caldwell

Caldwell College
Sister Patrice Werner, OP PhD, President
9 Ryerson Ave
Caldwell, NJ 07006
973 618-3000
Type: Acad Health Ctr/Med Sch
Control: For Profit
• Art Therapy Prgm

Camden

Cooper University Hospital
Christopher Olivia, MD, President
One Cooper Plaza
Camden, NJ 08103
856 342-2000
Type: Hosp or Med Ctr: 300-499 Beds
Control: Nonprofit (Private or Religious)
• Perfusion Prgm
• Radiation Therapy Prgm
• Radiography Prgm

SUNJ Rutgers Camden and UMDNJ
Rutgers University, UM & D
UMDNJ - SHRP, 401 Haddon Ave
Camden, NJ 08103-1506
Type: 4-year Coll or Univ
Control: State, County, or Local Govt
• Nursing Prgm
• Physical Therapy Prgm

Cape May Courthouse

Cape May County Technical Institute
Robert Matthies, Superintendent
188 Crest Haven Rd
Cape May Courthouse, NJ 08210
609 465-2161
Type: Vocational or Tech Sch
Control: State, County, or Local Govt
• Dental Assistant Prgm

Clifton

Dover Business College
Timothy Luing, MBA, President
600 Getty Ave
Clifton, NJ 07011
973 546-0123
Type: Vocational or Tech Sch
Control: For Profit
• Medical Assistant Prgm
• Surgical Technology Prgm

Cranford

Union County College
Thomas H Brown, PhD, President
1033 Springfield Ave
Cranford, NJ 07016-1599
908 709-7100
Type: Junior or Comm Coll
Control: State, County, or Local Govt
• Physical Therapist Assistant Prgm

East Rutherford

Sodexho Health Care Services
405 Murray Hill Pkwy, Ste 2010
East Rutherford, NJ 07073
201 507-5600
Type: Acad Health Ctr/Med Sch
Control: For Profit
• Dietetic Internship Prgm

Edison

JFK Medical Center - Muhlenberg Schools
John P McGee, President
Park Ave and Randolph Rd
Edison, NJ 07061
732 632-1501
Type: Hosp or Med Ctr: 300-499 Beds
Control: Nonprofit (Private or Religious)
• Diagnostic Med Sonography (General) Prgm
• Nuclear Medicine Technology Prgm
• Radiography Prgm

Middlesex County College
Joann LaPerla-Morales, EdD, President
2600 Woodbridge Ave Chambers Hall
PO Box 3050
Edison, NJ 08818-3050
732 906-2515
Type: Junior or Comm Coll
Control: State, County, or Local Govt
• Clin Lab Technician/Med Lab Technician Prgm
• Dental Hygiene Prgm
• Dietetic Technician-AD Prgm
• Radiography Prgm

Egg Harbor

National Massage Therapy Institute
6712 Washington Ave, Ste 302
Egg Harbor, NJ 08234
Type: Acad Health Ctr/Med Sch
Control: For Profit
• Massage Therapy Prgm (2)

Englewood

Englewood Hospital & Medical Center
Douglas Duchak, President/CEO
350 Engle St
Englewood, NJ 07631
201 894-3002
Type: Hosp or Med Ctr: 500 Beds
Control: Nonprofit (Private or Religious)
• Radiography Prgm

Ewing

The College of New Jersey
Barbara Gittenstein, President
2000 Pennington Rd
Ewing, NJ 08628
609 771-1855
Type: 4-year Coll or Univ
Control: State, County, or Local Govt
• Counseling Prgm
• Music Therapy Prgm
• Nursing Prgm

Fairfield

The Institute for Health Education
7 Spielman Rd
Fairfield, NJ 07004
973 808-1110
Type: Vocational or Tech Sch
Control: For Profit
• Dental Assistant Prgm

Glassboro

Rowan University
Donald J Farish, PhD JD, President
Bole Hall
201 Mullica Hill Rd
Glassboro, NJ 08028
856 256-4100
Type: 4-year Coll or Univ
Control: State, County, or Local Govt
• Allopathic Medicine Prgm
• Athletic Training Prgm

Hackensack

Academy of Massage Therapy
Joanna Sechuck-Tringali, NCBTMB BS, Executive
    Director
321 Main St, 2nd Fl
Hackensack, NJ 07601
888 268-7898
Type: Vocational or Tech Sch
Control: For Profit
• Massage Therapy Prgm (2)

Iselin

Sanford-Brown Institute
Dennis Mascali, MEd, President
675 US Hwy 1 South
Iselin, NJ 08830
732 623-5740
Type: Vocational or Tech Sch
Control: For Profit
• Diagnostic Med Sonography (General) Prgm
• Surgical Technology Prgm

Jersey City

Christ Hospital School of Radiography
Peter A Kelly, MBA, President/CEO
176 Palisade Ave
Jersey City, NJ 07306
201 795-8200
Type: Hosp or Med Ctr: 300-499 Beds
Control: Nonprofit (Private or Religious)
• Radiography Prgm

Eastern International College
Jersey City, NJ 07306
• Dental Hygiene Prgm

Jersey City Medical Center EMS
Jersey City, NJ 07302
Type: Consortium
• Emergency Med Tech-Paramedic Prgm

Saint Peter's College
Jersey City, NJ 07306
Type: 4-year Coll or Univ
Control: Nonprofit (Private or Religious)
• Nursing Prgm

Lawrenceville

Rider University
Mordechai Rozanski, President
2083 Lawrenceville Rd
Lawrenceville, NJ 08648-3099
609 896-5000
Type: 4-year Coll or Univ
Control: Nonprofit (Private or Religious)
• Counseling Prgm

Lincroft

Brookdale Community College
Peter F Burnham, PhD, President
765 Newman Springs Rd
Lincroft, NJ 07738-1522
732 224-2204
Type: Junior or Comm Coll
Control: State, County, or Local Govt
• Clin Lab Technician/Med Lab Technician Prgm
• Radiography Prgm
• Respiratory Care Prgm

Livingston

St Barnabas Medical Center
John F Bonamo, MD, Executive Director
Old Short Hill Rd
Livingston, NJ 07039
973 332-5628
Type: Hosp or Med Ctr: 500 Beds
Control: Nonprofit (Private or Religious)
• Radiation Therapy Prgm

Lodi

Felician College
Sr Theresa M Martin, MA, President
262 S Main St
Lodi, NJ 07644
973 778-1190
Type: 4-year Coll or Univ
Control: Nonprofit (Private or Religious)
• Nursing Prgm

Long Branch

Monmouth Medical Center
Frank Vozos, MD, Executive Director
300 Second Ave
Long Branch, NJ 07740
732 923-7504
Type: Hosp or Med Ctr: 500 Beds
Control: Nonprofit (Private or Religious)
• Clin Lab Scientist/Med Technologist Prgm

Mays Landing

Atlantic Cape Community College
Peter Mora, PhD, President
5100 Black Horse Pike
Mays Landing, NJ 08330-9888
609 343-4901
Type: Junior or Comm Coll
Control: State, County, or Local Govt
• Surgical Technology Prgm

Morristown

Atlantic Health - Morristown Memorial Hosp
Joseph Trunfio, Exec VP, COO
100 Madison Ave
Morristown, NJ 07962-1956
973 660-3270
Type: Hosp or Med Ctr: 500 Beds
Control: Nonprofit (Private or Religious)
• Cardiovascular Tech (Invasive/Noninv/Vasc) Prgm
• Clin Lab Scientist/Med Technologist Prgm

College of St Elizabeth
Jacqueline Burns, President
2 Convent Rd
Morristown, NJ 07960
201 292-6300
Type: 4-year Coll or Univ
Control: Nonprofit (Private or Religious)
• Dietetic Internship Prgm
• Dietetics-Didactic Prgm

Mount Holly

Burlington County Institute of Technology
Walter Rudder, EdD, Superintendent
695 Woodlane Rd
Mount Holly, NJ 08060
609 267-4226
Type: Vocational or Tech Sch
Control: State, County, or Local Govt
• Dental Assistant Prgm

Neptune

Jersey Shore University Medical Center
Steve Littleson, FACHE, President
1945 Corlies Ave Administration
Neptune, NJ 07753
732 776-4900
Type: Hosp or Med Ctr: 500 Beds
Control: Nonprofit (Private or Religious)
• Clin Lab Scientist/Med Technologist Prgm

New Brunswick

Rutgers University
Francis L Lawrence, PhD, President
Old Queens
New Brunswick, NJ 08901
732 932-7454
Type: 4-year Coll or Univ
Control: State, County, or Local Govt
• Dietetics-Didactic Prgm
• Medical Librarian Prgm
• Pharmacy Prgm
• Psychology (PhD) Prgm
• Psychology (PsyD) Prgm

Newark

Essex County College
A Zachery Yamba, President
303 University Ave
Newark, NJ 07102
201 877-3021
Type: Hosp or Med Ctr: 100-299 Beds
Control: State, County, or Local Govt
• Ophthalmic Dispensing Optician Prgm
• Physical Therapist Assistant Prgm
• Radiography Prgm

Rutgers - SUNJ
Newark, NJ 07102
Type: 4-year Coll or Univ
Control: Nonprofit (Private or Religious)
• Nursing Prgm

Univ of Medicine & Dent of New Jersey
William F Owen, Jr, MD, President
65 Bergen Street SSB 15
PO Box 1709
Newark, NJ 07107
973 972-4400
Type: 4-year Coll or Univ
Control: State, County, or Local Govt
• Allopathic Medicine Prgm
• Cardiovascular Tech (Vascular) Prgm
• Clin Lab Scientist/Med Technologist Prgm
• Counseling Prgm
• Cytotechnology Prgm
• Dental Assistant Prgm
• Dental Hygiene Prgm
• Dentistry Prgm
• Diagnostic Med Sonography (General) Prgm
• Dietetic Internship Prgm
• Dietetics-Coordinated Prgm
• Nuclear Medicine Technology Prgm
• Nursing Prgm
• Ophthalmic Assistant Prgm
• Osteopathic Medicine Prgm
• Phlebotomy Prgm
• Physical Therapy Prgm
• Physician Assistant Prgm
• Radiologist Assistant Prgm
• Rehabilitation Counseling Prgm
• Respiratory Care Prgm (2)

Newton

Sussex County Community College
Constance Mierendorf, PhD, President
One College Hill
Newton, NJ 07860
973 300-2122
Type: Junior or Comm Coll
Control: State, County, or Local Govt
• Medical Assistant Prgm
• Surgical Technology Prgm

North Brunswick

DeVry University
630 US Hwy One
North Brunswick, NJ 08902
Type: 4-year Coll or Univ
Control: For Profit
• Neurodiagnostic Tech Prgm

Paramus

Bergen Community College
G Jeremiah Ryan, EdD, President/CEO
400 Paramus Rd
Paramus, NJ 07652-1595
201 447-7100
Type: Junior or Comm Coll
Control: State, County, or Local Govt
• Dental Hygiene Prgm
• Diagnostic Med Sonography (General/Cardiac) Prgm
• Medical Assistant Prgm
• Physical Therapist Assistant Prgm
• Radiation Therapy Prgm
• Radiography Prgm
• Respiratory Care Prgm
• Surgical Technology Prgm

Northern NJ Consortium
Judith Winn, PhD, President, Bergen CC
400 Paramus Rd
Paramus, NJ 07652-1595
201 447-7237
Type: Consortium
Control: Nonprofit (Private or Religious)
• Veterinary Technician Prgm

Paterson

Passaic County Community College
Steven M Rose, EdD, President
One College Blvd
Paterson, NJ 07505-1179
201 684-6300
Type: Junior or Comm Coll
Control: State, County, or Local Govt
• Radiography Prgm

Pemberton

Burlington County College
Robert C Messina, Jr, PhD, President
601 Pemberton Browns Mills Rd
Pemberton, NJ 08068-1599
609 894-9311
Type: Junior or Comm Coll
Control: State, County, or Local Govt
• Dental Hygiene Prgm
• Radiography Prgm

Pennsauken

Omega Institute
F Burke, Owner
7050 Rte 38 East
Pennsauken, NJ 08109
856 663-4299
Type: Acad Health Ctr/Med Sch
Control: For Profit
• Massage Therapy Prgm

Piscataway

Cortiva Inst, Somerset Sch of Massage Therapy
Chris Froelich, President
180 Centennial Ave
Piscataway, NJ 08854
212 277-7729
Type: Vocational or Tech Sch
Control: For Profit
• Massage Therapy Prgm (2)

UMDNJ - Robert Wood Johnson Medical School
Piscataway, NJ 08854
Type: Acad Health Ctr/Med Sch
Control: State, County, or Local Govt
• Allopathic Medicine Prgm

Pomona

Richard Stockton College of New Jersey
Herman J Saatkamp, Jr, PhD, President
PO Box 195
Jim Leeds Rd
Pomona, NJ 08240-0195
609 652-4521
Type: 4-year Coll or Univ
Control: State, County, or Local Govt
• Nursing Prgm
• Occupational Therapy Prgm
• Physical Therapy Prgm
• Speech-Language Pathology Prgm

Pompton Lakes

Institute for Therapeutic Massage
Lisa Helbig, LMT, Director
125 Wanaque Ave
Pompton Lakes, NJ 07442
973 839-6131
Type: Acad Health Ctr/Med Sch
Control: For Profit
• Massage Therapy Prgm (5)

Ramsey

Eastwick College
Ramsey, NJ 07446
Type: Junior or Comm Coll
• Surgical Technology Prgm

Randolph

County College of Morris
Edward J Yaw, EdD, President
214 Center Grove Rd
Randolph, NJ 07869
973 328-5370
Type: Junior or Comm Coll
Control: State, County, or Local Govt
• Radiography Prgm

Ridgewood

The Valley Hospital
Audrey Meyers, MBA, President
223 N Van Dien Ave
Ridgewood, NJ 07450
201 447-8021
Type: Hosp or Med Ctr: 300-499 Beds
Control: Nonprofit (Private or Religious)
• Clin Lab Scientist/Med Technologist Prgm
• Radiography Prgm

Sewell

Gloucester County College
Russell Davis, MS, President
1400 Tanyard Rd
Sewell, NJ 08080
856 415-2196
Type: Junior or Comm Coll
Control: State, County, or Local Govt
• Diagnostic Med Sonography (General) Prgm
• Nuclear Medicine Technology Prgm

Somers Point

Shore Memorial Hospital
Al Gutierrez, CHE MBA RT(R), President
1 E New York Ave
Somers Point, NJ 08244-2387
609 653-3924
Type: Hosp or Med Ctr: 300-499 Beds
Control: Nonprofit (Private or Religious)
• Radiography Prgm

Somerville

Raritan Valley Community College
G Jeremiah Ryan, President
PO Box 3300
Somerville, NJ 08876
908 526-1200
Type: Junior or Comm Coll
Control: State, County, or Local Govt
• Medical Assistant Prgm
• Ophthalmic Dispensing Optician Prgm

South Orange

Seton Hall University
Amado Gabriel M Esteban, PhD, President
400 S Orange Ave
South Orange, NJ 07079-2687
973 761-9691
Type: 4-year Coll or Univ
Control: Nonprofit (Private or Religious)
• Athletic Training Prgm
• Nursing Prgm
• Occupational Therapy Prgm
• Physical Therapy Prgm
• Physician Assistant Prgm
• Speech-Language Pathology Prgm

Teaneck

Fairleigh Dickinson University
Francis J Mertz, JD, President
1000 River Rd
Teaneck, NJ 07666
973 692-9170
Type: 4-year Coll or Univ
Control: Nonprofit (Private or Religious)
• Nursing Prgm
• Psychology (PhD) Prgm

Totowa

Fortis Institute - Wayne
Totowa, NJ 07470
Type: Vocational or Tech Sch
• Medical Assistant Prgm

Trenton

Mercer County Community College
Patricia Donohue, PhD, President
PO Box B
Trenton, NJ 08690
609 570-3314
Type: Junior or Comm Coll
Control: State, County, or Local Govt
• Clin Lab Technician/Med Lab Technician Prgm
• Physical Therapist Assistant Prgm
• Radiography Prgm

Mercer County Technical Schools
Patricia Donohue, PhD, Superintendent
1085 Old Trenton Rd
PO Box B
Trenton, NJ 08690
609 570-3613
Type: Vocational or Tech Sch
Control: State, County, or Local Govt
• Medical Assistant Prgm

St Francis Medical Center
Gerard Jablonowski, President/CEO
601 Hamilton Ave
Trenton, NJ 08629-1986
609 599-5000
Type: Hosp or Med Ctr: 100-299 Beds
Control: Nonprofit (Private or Religious)
• Radiography Prgm

Thomas Edison State College
Trenton, NJ 08608
Type: 4-year Coll or Univ
Control: State, County, or Local Govt
• Cytotechnology Prgm
• Nursing Prgm
• Polysomnographic Technology Prgm

Union

Kean University
Dawood Farahi, PhD, President
1000 Morris Ave
Union, NJ 07083-0411
908 737-7000
Type: 4-year Coll or Univ
Control: State, County, or Local Govt
• Athletic Training Prgm
• Counseling Prgm
• Occupational Therapy Prgm
• Speech-Language Pathology Prgm

Upper Montclair

Montclair State University
Susan Cole, PhD, President
Upper Montclair, NJ 07043
973 655-4000
Type: 4-year Coll or Univ
Control: State, County, or Local Govt
• Athletic Training Prgm
• Audiologist Prgm
• Counseling Prgm
• Dietetic Internship Prgm
• Dietetics-Didactic Prgm
• Music Therapy Prgm (2)
• Speech-Language Pathology Prgm

Vineland

Cumberland County College
Roland J Chapdelaine, EdD, President
College Dr, PO Box 517
Vineland, NJ 08362-0517
609 691-8600
Type: Junior or Comm Coll
Control: State, County, or Local Govt
• Radiography Prgm

South Jersey Healthcare Regional Med Center
Vineland, NJ 08360
Type: Acad Health Ctr/Med Sch
Control: State, County, or Local Govt
• Dietetic Internship Prgm

Washington

Northwest NJ Consortium Resp Care Educ
Stephen Serman, Chairman Regl Oper Cncl
c/o Warren County Community College
475 Rte 57 W
Washington, NJ 07882
908 835-2314
Type: Consortium
Control: Nonprofit (Private or Religious)
• Respiratory Care Prgm

Warren County Community College
William Austin, EdD, President
475 Route 57 W
Washington, NJ 07882-4343
908 835-9222
Type: Junior or Comm Coll
Control: State, County, or Local Govt
• Medical Assistant Prgm

Wayne

Fortis Institute
Duncan Anderson, CEO
201 Willowbrook Blvd, 2nd Fl
Wayne, NJ 07470
973 837-1818
Type: Vocational or Tech Sch
Control: For Profit
• Dental Assistant Prgm
• Medical Assistant Prgm

William Paterson Univ of New Jersey
Arnold Speert, PhD, President
300 Pompton Rd
Wayne, NJ 07470
973 720-2222
Type: 4-year Coll or Univ
Control: State, County, or Local Govt
• Athletic Training Prgm
• Counseling Prgm
• Nursing Prgm
• Speech-Language Pathology Prgm

West Long Branch

Monmouth University
West Long Branch, NJ 07764
Type: 4-year Coll or Univ
Control: Nonprofit (Private or Religious)
• Counseling Prgm
• Nursing Prgm

Westwood

Healing Hands Institute for Massage Therapy
Alice Feuerstein, RN LMT, President
41 Bergenline Ave, 2nd Fl
Westwood, NJ 07675
201 722-0099
Type: Vocational or Tech Sch
Control: For Profit
• Massage Therapy Prgm

New Mexico

Albuquerque

Brown Mackie College - Albuquerque
Albuquerque, NM 87123
Type: Vocational or Tech Sch
Control: For Profit
• Occupational Therapy Asst Prgm

Central New Mexico Community College
Katharine Winograd, EdD, President
525 Buena Vista SE
Albuquerque, NM 87106-4096
505 224-4415
Type: Junior or Comm Coll
Control: State, County, or Local Govt
• Clin Lab Technician/Med Lab Technician Prgm
• Dental Assistant Prgm
• Diagnostic Med Sonography (General) Prgm
• Emergency Med Tech-Paramedic Prgm
• Respiratory Care Prgm
• Surgical Technology Prgm
• Veterinary Technology Prgm

Crystal Mountain Sch of Therapeutic Massage
Linda Delker, MS LMT RMTI, Director
4775 Indian School Rd NE, Ste 102
Albuquerque, NM 87110
505 872-2030
Type: Vocational or Tech Sch
Control: For Profit
• Massage Therapy Prgm

National American University-Albuquerque
Albuquerque, NM 87110-3976
Type: Vocational or Tech Sch
• Medical Assistant Prgm

Pima Medical Institute - Albuquerque
Holly Woelber, BS, Campus Director
2201 San Pedro NE Blvd
Building 3, Ste 100
Albuquerque, NM 87110
505 881-1234
Type: Vocational or Tech Sch
Control: For Profit
• Dental Hygiene Prgm
• Radiography Prgm
• Respiratory Care Prgm

Southwestern Indian Polytechnic Institute
Carolyn Elgin, President
9169 Coors NW, Box 10146
Albuquerque, NM 87184
505 897-5347
Type: Junior or Comm Coll
Control: Fed Govt
• Ophthalmic Dispensing Optician Prgm

INSTITUTIONS

University of New Mexico

Paul Roth, President
President's Office
UNM Health Sciences Center / MSC09 5300
Albuquerque, NM 87131-0001
505 272-5849
Type: Acad Health Ctr/Med Sch
Control: State, County, or Local Govt
- Allopathic Medicine Prgm
- Athletic Training Prgm
- Clin Lab Scientist/Med Technologist Prgm
- Clin Lab Technician/Med Lab Technician Prgm
- Counseling Prgm
- Dental Assistant Prgm
- Dental Hygiene Prgm
- Dietetic Internship Prgm
- Dietetics-Didactic Prgm
- Emergency Med Tech-Paramedic Prgm
- Music Therapy Prgm
- Nursing Prgm
- Occupational Therapy Prgm
- Pharmacy Prgm
- Physical Therapy Prgm
- Physician Assistant Prgm
- Psychology (PhD) Prgm
- Speech-Language Pathology Prgm

University of St Francis

Michael Vinciguerra, PhD, President
4401 Silver Ave SE
Ste B
Albuquerque, NM 87108
505 266-5565
Type: 4-year Coll or Univ
Control: Nonprofit (Private or Religious)
- Physician Assistant Prgm

Clovis

Clovis Community College

Jim Turner, Interim President
417 Schepps Blvd
Clovis, NM 88101
505 769-4000
Type: Junior or Comm Coll
Control: State, County, or Local Govt
- Radiography Prgm

Espanola

Northern New Mexico College

Jose Griego, PhD, President
921 Paseo de Onate
Espanola, NM 87532
505 747-2100
Type: 4-year Coll or Univ
Control: State, County, or Local Govt
- Nursing Prgm
- Radiography Prgm

Farmington

San Juan College

Carol Spencer, PhD, President
4601 College Blvd
Farmington, NM 87402
505 566-3209
Type: Junior or Comm Coll
Control: State, County, or Local Govt
- Clin Lab Technician/Med Lab Technician Prgm
- Dental Hygiene Prgm
- Physical Therapist Assistant Prgm
- Surgical Technology Prgm
- Veterinary Technology Prgm

Las Cruces

Dona Ana Community College

Margie Huerta, PhD, President
Box 30001 Dept 3DA
Las Cruces, NM 88003-0001
575 527-7510
Type: Junior or Comm Coll
Control: State, County, or Local Govt
- Dental Assistant Prgm
- Dental Hygiene Prgm
- Diagnostic Med Sonography (General) Prgm
- Emergency Med Tech-Paramedic Prgm
- Radiography Prgm
- Respiratory Care Prgm

New Mexico State University

Barbara Couture, PhD, President
PO Box 30001, MSC 3Z
Las Cruces, NM 88003-0001
505 646-2035
Type: 4-year Coll or Univ
Control: State, County, or Local Govt
- Athletic Training Prgm
- Counseling Prgm
- Dietetics-Didactic Prgm
- Music Therapy Prgm
- Nursing Prgm
- Orientation and Mobility Specialist Prgm
- Speech-Language Pathology Prgm
- Teacher of the Visually Impaired Prgm

Las Vegas

Luna Community College

Lawrence Pino, President
PO Box 1510
Las Vegas, NM 87701-1510
505 454-2500
Type: 4-year Coll or Univ
Control: State, County, or Local Govt
- Dental Assistant Prgm

New Mexico Highlands University

Las Vegas, NM 87701
Type: 4-year Coll or Univ
Control: State, County, or Local Govt
- Nursing Prgm

Roswell

Eastern New Mexico University

John R Madden, PhD, President
52 University Boulevard 88203
PO Box 6000
Roswell, NM 88202-6000
575 624-7112
Type: Junior or Comm Coll
Control: State, County, or Local Govt
- Dental Hygiene Prgm
- Emergency Med Tech-Paramedic Prgm
- Medical Assistant Prgm
- Occupational Therapy Asst Prgm
- Respiratory Care Prgm
- Speech-Language Pathology Prgm

Santa Fe

Santa Fe Community College

Sheila Ortego, PhD, President
6401 Richards Ave
Santa Fe, NM 87509
505 428-1000
Type: Junior or Comm Coll
Control: State, County, or Local Govt
- Dental Assistant Prgm
- Emergency Med Tech-Paramedic Prgm
- Medical Assistant Prgm

Southwestern College

James Nolan, PhD, President
PO Box 4788
Santa Fe, NM 87502-4788
505 471-5756
Type: 4-year Coll or Univ
Control: Nonprofit (Private or Religious)
- Art Therapy Prgm

Silver City

Western New Mexico University

John Counts, PhD, President
PO Box 680
Silver City, NM 88062-0680
505 538-6238
Type: 4-year Coll or Univ
Control: State, County, or Local Govt
- Nursing Prgm
- Occupational Therapy Asst Prgm
- Occupational Therapy Prgm

New York

Albany

Albany College of Pharmacy and Health Science

James Gozzo, President
106 New Scotland Ave
Albany, NY 12208-3492
518 694-7255
Type: 4-year Coll or Univ
Control: Nonprofit (Private or Religious)
- Cytotechnology Prgm
- Pharmacy Prgm

Albany Medical College
Vincent Verdile, MD, Dean
47 New Scotland Ave
Albany, NY 12208
518 262-3830
Type: Acad Health Ctr/Med Sch
Control: Nonprofit (Private or Religious)
• Allopathic Medicine Prgm
• Clin Lab Scientist/Med Technologist Prgm
• Physician Assistant Prgm

Bryant & Stratton College - Albany
Michael Gutierrez, Campus Director
1259 Central Ave
Albany, NY 12205
518 437-1802
Type: Vocational or Tech Sch
Control: For Profit
• Medical Assistant Prgm

College of St Rose
Louis C Vaccaro, PhD, President
432 Western Ave
Albany, NY 12203
518 454-5111
Type: 4-year Coll or Univ
Control: Nonprofit (Private or Religious)
• Speech-Language Pathology Prgm

Maria College
Laureen Fitzgerald, RSM MA MS, President
700 New Scotland Ave
Albany, NY 12208-1798
518 438-3111
Type: Junior or Comm Coll
Control: Nonprofit (Private or Religious)
• Occupational Therapy Asst Prgm

University at Albany/State U of New York
Karen R Hitchcock, President
1400 Washington Ave
Albany, NY 12222
518 442-3300
Type: 4-year Coll or Univ
Control: State, County, or Local Govt
• Medical Librarian Prgm
• Psychology (PhD) Prgm

Alfred

Alfred State College - SUNY
John Clark, PhD, President
10 Upper College Dr
Alfred, NY 14802
607 587-4211
Type: 4-year Coll or Univ
Control: State, County, or Local Govt
• Veterinary Technology Prgm

Alfred University
Charles Edmonson, PhD, President
1 Saxon Dr
Alfred, NY 14802
607 871-2137
Type: 4-year Coll or Univ
Control: Nonprofit (Private or Religious)
• Athletic Training Prgm

Amherst

Daemen College
Martin J Anisman, PhD, President
4380 Main St
Amherst, NY 14226-3592
716 829-8210
Type: 4-year Coll or Univ
Control: Nonprofit (Private or Religious)
• Physical Therapy Prgm
• Physician Assistant Prgm

Batavia

Genesee Community College
Stuart Steiner, JD EdD, President
One College Rd
Batavia, NY 14020-9704
585 343-0055
Type: Junior or Comm Coll
Control: State, County, or Local Govt
• Physical Therapist Assistant Prgm
• Polysomnographic Technology Prgm
• Respiratory Care Prgm

Binghamton

Binghamton University
Joyce Ferrario, PhD RN, Chief Nurse
    Administrator
PO Box 6000
Binghamton, NY 13902
Type: 4-year Coll or Univ
Control: State, County, or Local Govt
• Music Therapy Prgm
• Nursing Prgm
• Psychology (PhD) Prgm

Broome Community College
Danial Hayes, PhD, Interim President
107 Wales Building PO Box 1017
Binghamton, NY 13902
607 778-5100
Type: Junior or Comm Coll
Control: State, County, or Local Govt
• Clin Lab Technician/Med Lab Technician Prgm
• Dental Hygiene Prgm
• Medical Assistant Prgm
• Physical Therapist Assistant Prgm
• Radiography Prgm

Ridley-Lowell Business & Technical Institute
Wilfred T Weymouth, MS, President
116 Front St
Binghamton, NY 13905
607 724-2941
Type: Vocational or Tech Sch
Control: For Profit
• Medical Assistant Prgm (2)

Brockport

SUNY The College at Brockport
John Halstead, PhD, President
350 New Campus Dr
Brockport, NY 14420-2914
585 395-2211
Type: 4-year Coll or Univ
Control: State, County, or Local Govt
• Athletic Training Prgm
• Counseling Prgm
• Nursing Prgm

Bronx

Bronx Community College
Carolyn Williams, President
2155 University Ave and W 181st St
Bronx, NY 10453
718 289-5151
Type: Junior or Comm Coll
Control: State, County, or Local Govt
• Nuclear Medicine Technology Prgm
• Radiography Prgm

Bronx Lebanon Hospital
Steven Anderman, MBA MS, CEO
1650 Grand Concourse
Bronx, NY 10457
718 518-5586
Type: Hosp or Med Ctr: 500 Beds
Control: Nonprofit (Private or Religious)
• Surgical Technology Prgm

CUNY Herbert H Lehman College
Ricardo R Fernandez, President
Bedford Park Blvd W
Bronx, NY 10468
718 960-8000
Type: 4-year Coll or Univ
Control: State, County, or Local Govt
• Dietetic Internship Prgm
• Dietetics-Didactic Prgm
• Nursing Prgm
• Speech-Language Pathology Prgm

Eugenio Maria De Hostos Community College
475 Grand Concourse
Bronx, NY 10451
Type: Junior or Comm Coll
Control: State, County, or Local Govt
• Dental Hygiene Prgm

Fordham University
Bronx, NY 10458
Type: 4-year Coll or Univ
Control: Nonprofit (Private or Religious)
• Psychology (PhD) Prgm

Hostos Community College of CUNY
Dolores Fernandez, PhD, President
475 Grand Concourse
Bronx, NY 10451
718 518-4300
Type: Junior or Comm Coll
Control: State, County, or Local Govt
• Radiography Prgm

James J Peters VA Medical Center
130 W Kingsbridge Rd
Bronx, NY 10468-3904
718 579-1640
Type: Dept of Veterans Affairs
Control: Fed Govt
• Dietetic Internship Prgm

Bronxville

Concordia College New York
Bronxville, NY 10708
Type: 4-year Coll or Univ
Control: Nonprofit (Private or Religious)
• Nursing Prgm

Sarah Lawrence College
Michele Myers, President
One Mead Way
Bronxville, NY 10708
914 337-0700
Type: 4-year Coll or Univ
Control: Nonprofit (Private or Religious)
• Genetic Counseling Prgm

Brooklyn

ASA Institute of Business & Computer Tech
Alex Shchegol, MS, President
81 Willoughby St
Brooklyn, NY 11201
718 522-9073
Type: Vocational or Tech Sch
Control: For Profit
• Medical Assistant Prgm

CUNY Brooklyn College
Christoph M Kimmich, President
2900 Bedford Ave
Brooklyn, NY 11210
718 951-5000
Type: 4-year Coll or Univ
Control: State, County, or Local Govt
• Dietetic Internship Prgm
• Dietetics-Didactic Prgm
• Speech-Language Pathology Prgm

Kingsborough Community College
Regina Peruggi, EdD, President
2001 Oriental Blvd
Brooklyn, NY 11235
718 368-5109
Type: Junior or Comm Coll
Control: State, County, or Local Govt
• Physical Therapist Assistant Prgm
• Surgical Technology Prgm

Long Island University
Gale Steven Hynes, JD, Provost
1 University Plaza
Rm M-315
Brooklyn, NY 11201
718 488-3438
Type: 4-year Coll or Univ
Control: Nonprofit (Private or Religious)
• Art Therapy Prgm
• Athletic Training Prgm
• Clin Lab Scientist/Med Technologist Prgm
• Counseling Prgm
• Diagnostic Med Sonography (Vascular) Prgm
• Dietetic Internship Prgm
• Dietetics-Didactic Prgm
• Genetic Counseling Prgm
• Medical Librarian Prgm
• Nursing Prgm (2)
• Occupational Therapy Prgm
• Pharmacy Prgm
• Physical Therapy Prgm
• Physician Assistant Prgm
• Psychology (PsyD) Prgm (2)
• Radiography Prgm
• Respiratory Care Prgm
• Speech-Language Pathology Prgm (2)
• Surgical Technology Prgm

New York City College of Technology
Russ Hotzler, PhD, President
300 Jay St
Brooklyn, NY 11201-2983
718 260-5400
Type: 4-year Coll or Univ
Control: State, County, or Local Govt
• Dental Hygiene Prgm
• Dental Lab Technician Prgm
• Ophthalmic Dispensing Optician Prgm
• Radiography Prgm

New York Methodist Hospital
Mark J Mundy, MSHA, President
506 Sixth St
Brooklyn, NY 11215
718 780-3101
Type: Hosp or Med Ctr: 500 Beds
Control: Nonprofit (Private or Religious)
• Clin Lab Scientist/Med Technologist Prgm
• Diagnostic Med Sonography (General) Prgm
• Emergency Med Tech-Paramedic Prgm
• Radiation Therapy Prgm
• Radiography Prgm

Pratt Institute
Thomas F Schutte, President
200 Willoughby Ave
Brooklyn, NY 11205
718 636-3600
Type: 4-year Coll or Univ
Control: Nonprofit (Private or Religious)
• Art Therapy Prgm
• Dance/Movement Therapy Prgm
• Medical Librarian Prgm

SUNY Downstate Medical Center
John LaRosa, MD, President
450 Clarkson Ave Box 1
Brooklyn, NY 11203-2098
718 270-2611
Type: Acad Health Ctr/Med Sch
Control: State, County, or Local Govt
• Allopathic Medicine Prgm
• Diagnostic Med Sonography (General/Cardiac) Prgm
• Nursing Prgm
• Occupational Therapy Prgm
• Physical Therapy Prgm
• Physician Assistant Prgm

SUNY Downstate University Hospital Brooklyn @
Debra Carey, Interim CEO
339 Hicks St
Brooklyn, NY 11201
718 780-1134
Type: Hosp or Med Ctr: 500 Beds
Control: State, County, or Local Govt
• Radiography Prgm

Brooklyn Heights

St Francis College
Brooklyn Heights, NY 11201
Type: 4-year Coll or Univ
Control: Nonprofit (Private or Religious)
• Nursing Prgm

Buffalo

Bryant & Stratton College - Buffalo
Jeffrey P Tredo, Campus Director
465 Main St, Ste 400
Buffalo, NY 14203
716 884-9120
Type: Junior or Comm Coll
Control: For Profit
• Medical Assistant Prgm

Buffalo State, SUNY
Muriel Howard, PhD, President
1300 Elmwood Ave
Buffalo, NY 14222
716 878-4000
Type: 4-year Coll or Univ
Control: State, County, or Local Govt
• Dietetics-Coordinated Prgm
• Dietetics-Didactic Prgm
• Speech-Language Pathology Prgm

Canisius College
Vincent M Cooke, SJ PhD, President
2001 Main St
Buffalo, NY 14208-1098
716 888-2100
Type: 4-year Coll or Univ
Control: Nonprofit (Private or Religious)
• Athletic Training Prgm
• Counseling Prgm

D'Youville College
Sister Denise A Roche, GNSH PhD, President
320 Porter Ave
Buffalo, NY 14201-1084
716 829-7673
Type: 4-year Coll or Univ
Control: Nonprofit (Private or Religious)
• Chiropractic Prgm
• Dietetics-Coordinated Prgm
• Nursing Prgm
• Occupational Therapy Prgm
• Pharmacy Prgm
• Physical Therapy Prgm
• Physician Assistant Prgm

Erie Community College
Jack F Quinn, Jr, MA, President
121 Ellicott St
Buffalo, NY 14203
716 851-1200
Type: Junior or Comm Coll
Control: State, County, or Local Govt
• Clin Lab Technician/Med Lab Technician Prgm
• Dental Hygiene Prgm
• Dental Lab Technician Prgm
• Dietetic Technician-AD Prgm
• Medical Assistant Prgm
• Occupational Therapy Asst Prgm
• Ophthalmic Dispensing Optician Prgm
• Radiation Therapy Prgm
• Respiratory Care Prgm

Medaille College
Richard T Jurasek, PhD, President
18 Agassiz Cr
Rm M115
Buffalo, NY 14214
716 880-2201
Type: 4-year Coll or Univ
Control: For Profit
• Veterinary Technology Prgm

Roswell Park Cancer Institute
Elm Street
Buffalo, NY 14263
Type: Nonhosp HC Facil, BB, or Lab
Control: Nonprofit (Private or Religious)
• Medical Dosimetry Prgm

SUNY Educational Opportunity Center
Sherryl Weems, PhD
465 Washington St
Buffalo, NY 14203
716 849-6725
Type: Acad Health Ctr/Med Sch
Control: State, County, or Local Govt
• Dental Assistant Prgm

Trocaire College
Paul B Hurley, Jr, PhD, President
340 Choate St
Buffalo, NY 14220-2094
716 826-1200
Type: Junior or Comm Coll
Control: Nonprofit (Private or Religious)
• Dietetic Technician-AD Prgm
• Medical Assistant Prgm
• Phlebotomy Prgm
• Radiography Prgm
• Surgical Technology Prgm

University at Buffalo - SUNY
Satish K Tripathi, PhD, Officer
507 Capen Hall
Buffalo, NY 14260-0001
716 645-2901
Type: 4-year Coll or Univ
Control: State, County, or Local Govt
• Allopathic Medicine Prgm
• Audiologist Prgm
• Clin Lab Scientist/Med Technologist Prgm
• Dentistry Prgm
• Dietetic Internship Prgm
• Medical Librarian Prgm
• Nuclear Medicine Technology Prgm
• Nursing Prgm
• Occupational Therapy Prgm
• Orthoptist Prgm
• Pharmacy Prgm
• Physical Therapy Prgm
• Psychology (PhD) Prgm
• Rehabilitation Counseling Prgm
• Speech-Language Pathology Prgm

Villa Maria College of Buffalo
Sr Marcella Marie Garus, President
240 Pine Ridge Rd
Buffalo, NY 14225-3999
716 896-0700
Type: Junior or Comm Coll
Control: Nonprofit (Private or Religious)
• Physical Therapist Assistant Prgm

Canton

SUNY at Canton
Joseph L Kennedy, PhD, President
FOB 616, 34 Cornell Dr
Canton, NY 13617-1096
315 386-7204
Type: Junior or Comm Coll
Control: State, County, or Local Govt
• Dental Hygiene Prgm
• Physical Therapist Assistant Prgm
• Veterinary Technology Prgm

Cobleskill

State University of New York at Cobleskill
Donald Zingale, PhD, President
Knapp Hall 202, SUNY Cobleskill
106 Suffolk Circle
Cobleskill, NY 12043
518 255-5111
Type: 4-year Coll or Univ
Control: State, County, or Local Govt
• Histotechnician Prgm

Cooperstown

SUNY Cobleskill
Cooperstown, NY 13326
Type: Hosp or Med Ctr d Beds
• Emergency Med Tech-Paramedic Prgm

Cortland

SUNY College at Cortland
Erik Bitterbaum, PhD, President
PO Box 2000
Cortland, NY 13045
607 753-2201
Type: 4-year Coll or Univ
Control: State, County, or Local Govt
• Athletic Training Prgm

Dansville

Nicholas H Noyes Memorial Hospital
James Wissler, CEO
111 Clara Barton St
Dansville, NY 14437
585 335-4212
Type: Hosp or Med Ctr: 100-299 Beds
Control: Nonprofit (Private or Religious)
• Phlebotomy Prgm

Delhi

SUNY - Delhi
Candace S Vancko, PhD, President
156 Farnsworth Hall
Delhi, NY 13753
Type: 4-year Coll or Univ
Control: State, County, or Local Govt
• Veterinary Technology Prgm

Dix Hills

Western Suffolk BOCES
Michael Mensch, PhD, COO
507 Deer Park Rd
Dix Hills, NY 11746
631 549-4900
Type: Vocational or Tech Sch
Control: Nonprofit (Private or Religious)
• Diagnostic Med Sonography
  (Gen/Card/Vascular) Prgm
• Surgical Technology Prgm

Dobbs Ferry

Mercy College
Kimberly R Cline, EdD, JD, President
555 Broadway
Dobbs Ferry, NY 10522-1134
914 674-7307
Type: 4-year Coll or Univ
Control: Nonprofit (Private or Religious)
• Nursing Prgm
• Occupational Therapy Asst Prgm
• Occupational Therapy Prgm
• Physical Therapy Prgm
• Physician Assistant Prgm
• Speech-Language Pathology Prgm
• Veterinary Technology Prgm

Elmira

Arnot Ogden Medical Center
Anthony J Cooper, CHE, President/CEO
600 Roe Ave
Elmira, NY 14905-1676
607 737-4231
Type: Hosp or Med Ctr: 100-299 Beds
Control: Nonprofit (Private or Religious)
• Radiography Prgm

Elmira Business Institute
Brad C Phillips, BS, President
303 N Main St
Elmira, NY 14901
607 733-7177
Type: Vocational or Tech Sch
Control: For Profit
• Medical Assistant Prgm

Farmingdale

Farmingdale State College, SUNY
W Hubert Keen, PhD, President
2350 Broadhollow Rd
Horton 241
Farmingdale, NY 11735
631 420-2145
Type: 4-year Coll or Univ
Control: State, County, or Local Govt
• Clin Lab Technician/Med Lab Technician Prgm
• Dental Hygiene Prgm

Flushing

CUNY Queens College
James Muyskens, PhD, President
65-30 Kissena Blvd
Flushing, NY 11367
718 997-5000
Type: 4-year Coll or Univ
Control: State, County, or Local Govt
• Dietetic Internship Prgm
• Dietetics-Didactic Prgm
• Medical Librarian Prgm
• Speech-Language Pathology Prgm

Fredonia

SUNY Fredonia
Dennis L Hefner, PhD, President
Fenton Hall 138
Fredonia, NY 14063
716 673-3456
Type: 4-year Coll or Univ
Control: State, County, or Local Govt
• Music Therapy Prgm
• Speech-Language Pathology Prgm

Fresh Meadows

St. John's University
Niels Schmidt, Director of Allied Health
175-05 Horace Harding Expwy
Fresh Meadows, NY 11365
718 357-0500
Type: Hosp or Med Ctr: 300-499 Beds
Control: Nonprofit (Private or Religious)
• Emergency Med Tech-Paramedic Prgm

Garden City

Adelphi University
Robert Scott, President
1 South Ave
Garden City, NY 11530
516 877-3000
Type: 4-year Coll or Univ
Control: Nonprofit (Private or Religious)
• Audiologist Prgm
• Nursing Prgm
• Psychology (PhD) Prgm
• Speech-Language Pathology Prgm

Nassau Community College
Sean A Fanelli, PhD, President
One Education Dr
President, Tower 10th Floor, Nassau Comm
Garden City, NY 11530
516 572-7205
Type: Junior or Comm Coll
Control: State, County, or Local Govt
• Clin Lab Technician/Med Lab Technician Prgm
• Emergency Med Tech-Paramedic Prgm
• Physical Therapist Assistant Prgm
• Radiation Therapy Prgm
• Respiratory Care Prgm
• Surgical Technology Prgm

Sanford-Brown Institute - Garden City
Garden City, NY 11530
Type: Vocational or Tech Sch
• Diagnostic Med Sonography (General) Prgm

Geneseo

SUNY College of Geneseo
Christopher C Dahl, Interim President
One College Circle
Geneseo, NY 14454
716 245-5211
Type: 4-year Coll or Univ
Control: State, County, or Local Govt
• Speech-Language Pathology Prgm

Glens Falls

Glens Falls Hospital
David Kruczlnicki, CEO
100 Park St
Glens Falls, NY 12801
518 792-3151
Type: Hosp or Med Ctr: 300-499 Beds
Control: Nonprofit (Private or Religious)
• Radiography Prgm

Hempstead

Hofstra University
Stuart Rabinowitz, PhD, President
West Library Wing
Hempstead, NY 11550
516 463-6800
Type: 4-year Coll or Univ
Control: Nonprofit (Private or Religious)
• Allopathic Medicine Prgm
• Art Therapy Prgm
• Athletic Training Prgm
• Physician Assistant Prgm
• Rehabilitation Counseling Prgm
• Speech-Language Pathology Prgm

Herkimer

Herkimer County Community College
Ronald F Williams, EdD, President
100 Reservoir Rd
Herkimer, NY 13350
315 866-0300
Type: Junior or Comm Coll
Control: State, County, or Local Govt
• Physical Therapist Assistant Prgm

Hornell

St James Mercy Health System
Mary LeRowe, MBA, President/CEO
411 Canisteo St
Hornell, NY 14843
607 324-8110
Type: Hosp or Med Ctr: 100-299 Beds
Control: Nonprofit (Private or Religious)
• Radiography Prgm

Ithaca

Cornell University
Hunter R Rawlings, President
Ithaca, NY 14853
607 255-2000
Type: 4-year Coll or Univ
Control: Nonprofit (Private or Religious)
• Allopathic Medicine Prgm
• Dietetic Internship Prgm
• Dietetics-Didactic Prgm
• Veterinary Medicine Prgm

Ithaca College
Peggy Ryan Williams, EdD, President
953 Danby Rd
Ithaca, NY 14850-7001
607 274-3111
Type: 4-year Coll or Univ
Control: Nonprofit (Private or Religious)
• Athletic Training Prgm
• Music Therapy Prgm
• Occupational Therapy Prgm
• Physical Therapy Prgm
• Speech-Language Pathology Prgm

Jackson Heights

Plaza College
74-09 37th Ave
Jackson Heights, NY 11372
Type: 4-year Coll or Univ
Control: State, County, or Local Govt
• Medical Assistant Prgm

Jamaica

York College, CUNY
Marcia Keizs, EdD, President
94-20 Guy R Brewer Blvd
Jamaica, NY 11451-9902
718 262-2350
Type: 4-year Coll or Univ
Control: State, County, or Local Govt
• Occupational Therapy Prgm
• Physician Assistant Prgm

Jamestown

Jamestown Community College
Gregory T DeCinque, PhD, President
525 Falconer St
PO Box 20
Jamestown, NY 14702-0020
716 338-1060
Type: Junior or Comm Coll
Control: State, County, or Local Govt
• Occupational Therapy Asst Prgm

Woman's Christian Association Hospital
Betsy Wright, President/CEO
PO Box 840
207 Foote Avenue
Jamestown, NY 14701-0840
716 664-8300
Type: Hosp or Med Ctr: 300-499 Beds
Control: Nonprofit (Private or Religious)
• Clin Lab Scientist/Med Technologist Prgm
• Radiography Prgm

Latham

A&H Training
4 British American Blvd
Latham, NY 12110
Type: Acad Health Ctr/Med Sch
Control: For Profit
• Medical Transcriptionist Prgm

Lewiston

Niagara University
Lewiston, NY 14019
Type: 4-year Coll or Univ
Control: For Profit
• Nursing Prgm

Long Island City

LaGuardia Community College
Gail Mellow, PhD, President
31-10 Thomson Ave
Long Island City, NY 11101-3083
718 482-5050
Type: Junior or Comm Coll
Control: State, County, or Local Govt
• Dietetic Technician-AD Prgm
• Occupational Therapy Asst Prgm
• Physical Therapist Assistant Prgm
• Veterinary Technology Prgm

Manhasset

North Shore University Hospital
Dennis Dowling, CEO
145 Community Dr
Manhasset, NY 11030
516 465-8130
Type: Hosp or Med Ctr: 500 Beds
Control: Nonprofit (Private or Religious)
• Perfusion Prgm

North Shore-Long Island Jewish Hlth System
Manhasset, NY 11030
Type: Acad Health Ctr/Med Sch
Control: Nonprofit (Private or Religious)
• Dietetic Internship Prgm

Middletown

Orange County Community College
William Richards, PhD, President
115 South St
Middletown, NY 10940-6404
845 341-4701
Type: Junior or Comm Coll
Control: State, County, or Local Govt
• Clin Lab Technician/Med Lab Technician Prgm
• Dental Hygiene Prgm
• Occupational Therapy Asst Prgm
• Phlebotomy Prgm
• Physical Therapist Assistant Prgm
• Radiography Prgm

Morrisville

SUNY at Morrisville
Frederick W Woodward, President
Morrisville, NY 13408
315 684-6000
Type: 4-year Coll or Univ
Control: State, County, or Local Govt
• Dietetic Technician-AD Prgm

New Paltz

SUNY at New Paltz
Steven Poskanzer, JD, President
1 Hawk Drive
New Paltz, NY 12561
845 257-2121
Type: 4-year Coll or Univ
Control: State, County, or Local Govt
• Music Therapy Prgm
• Nursing Prgm
• Speech-Language Pathology Prgm

New Rochelle

College of New Rochelle
Steve Sweeny, PhD, President
29 Castle Pl
New Rochelle, NY 10805
914 632-5300
Type: 4-year Coll or Univ
Control: Nonprofit (Private or Religious)
• Art Therapy Prgm
• Nursing Prgm

New York

American University of Beirut
New York, NY 10017
Type: 4-year Coll or Univ
Control: For Profit
• Nursing Prgm

Bellevue Hospital Center
Lynda Curtis, MS, Exec Director
First Ave and 27th St
New York, NY 10016
212 562-4132
Type: Hosp or Med Ctr: 500 Beds
Control: State, County, or Local Govt
• Radiography Prgm

City University of New York, The City College
Gregory Williams, PhD, President
Administration Bldg A-300
138th St and Convent Ave
New York, NY 10031
212 650-7285
Type: Acad Health Ctr/Med Sch
Control: State, County, or Local Govt
• Physician Assistant Prgm
• Psychology (PhD) Prgm

Columbia University
Lee C Bollinger, JD, President
Morningside Campus
411 Low Library
New York, NY 10027
212 854-9970
Type: 4-year Coll or Univ
Control: Nonprofit (Private or Religious)
• Allopathic Medicine Prgm
• Dentistry Prgm
• Nursing Prgm
• Occupational Therapy Prgm
• Physical Therapy Prgm

Columbia University Teachers College
Susan Fuhrman, PhD, President
525 W 120th St
124 Zankel Bldg
New York, NY 10027
212 678-3000
Type: 4-year Coll or Univ
Control: Nonprofit (Private or Religious)
• Dietetic Internship Prgm
• Psychology (PhD) Prgm
• Speech-Language Pathology Prgm

CUNY Borough of Manhattan Community Coll
Antonio Perez, PhD, President
199 Chambers St
New York, NY 10007
212 346-8800
Type: Junior or Comm Coll
Control: State, County, or Local Govt
• Emergency Med Tech-Paramedic Prgm
• Respiratory Care Prgm

CUNY Hunter College
Jennifer Raab, President
365 Fifth Ave
New York, NY 10021
212 772-4000
Type: 4-year Coll or Univ
Control: State, County, or Local Govt
• Audiologist Prgm
• Dietetic Internship Prgm
• Dietetics-Didactic Prgm
• Nursing Prgm
• Orientation and Mobility Specialist Prgm
• Physical Therapy Prgm
• Rehabilitation Counseling Prgm
• Speech-Language Pathology Prgm
• Vision Rehabilitation Therapy Prgm

Harlem Hospital Center
John Palmer, PhD, Exec Director
506 Lenox Ave
New York, NY 10037
212 939-1340
Type: Hosp or Med Ctr: 500 Beds
Control: State, County, or Local Govt
• Radiography Prgm

Memorial Sloan-Kettering Cancer Ctr
Harold Varmus, MD, President
1275 York Ave
New York, NY 10065
212 639-6561
Type: Hosp or Med Ctr: 500 Beds
Control: Nonprofit (Private or Religious)
• Cytotechnology Prgm
• Radiation Therapy Prgm

Mt Sinai School of Medicine
K Davis, MD, President
One Gustave Levy Pl
New York, NY 10029
Type: Acad Health Ctr/Med Sch
Control: Nonprofit (Private or Religious)
• Allopathic Medicine Prgm
• Genetic Counseling Prgm

New York College of Podiatric Medicinie
Louis L Levin, President
1800 Park Ave
New York, NY 10035
212 410-8000
Type: 4-year Coll or Univ
Control: Nonprofit (Private or Religious)
• Podiatric Medicine Prgm

New York Eye & Ear Infirmary
Joseph P Corcoran, President
310 E 14th St
New York, NY 10003
212 979-4300
Type: Hosp or Med Ctr: 100-299 Beds
Control: Nonprofit (Private or Religious)
• Orthoptist Prgm

New York University
John Sexton, PhD, President
70 Washington Square S
Room 216
New York, NY 10012-1172
212 998-2345
Type: 4-year Coll or Univ
Control: Nonprofit (Private or Religious)
• Allopathic Medicine Prgm
• Art Therapy Prgm
• Dental Hygiene Prgm
• Dentistry Prgm
• Diagnostic Med Sonography (General/Cardiac) Prgm
• Dietetic Internship Prgm
• Dietetics-Didactic Prgm
• Music Therapy Prgm
• Nursing Prgm
• Occupational Therapy Prgm
• Physical Therapist Assistant Prgm
• Physical Therapy Prgm
• Psychology (PhD) Prgm
• Speech-Language Pathology Prgm

New York-Presbyterian Hospital
David B Skinner, MD, President/CEO
525 E 68th St
New York, NY 10021
212 746-4000
Type: Hosp or Med Ctr: 500 Beds
Control: Nonprofit (Private or Religious)
• Dietetic Internship Prgm

NYU Langone Medical Center
Theresa Bischoff, EVP Deputy Provost
560 First Ave
New York, NY 10016
212 263-7300
Type: 4-year Coll or Univ
Control: Nonprofit (Private or Religious)
• Surgical Technology Prgm

Pace University - Lenox Hill Hospital
David A Caputo, PhD, President
1 Pace Plaza
New York, NY 10038
212 346-1098
Type: 4-year Coll or Univ
Control: Nonprofit (Private or Religious)
• Physician Assistant Prgm

Sanford-Brown Institute
New York, NY 10003
Type: Vocational or Tech Sch
• Diagnostic Med Sonography (General) Prgm

School of Visual Arts
David Rhodes, BA, President
209 E 23rd St
New York, NY 10010
212 592-2000
Type: Vocational or Tech Sch
Control: For Profit
• Art Therapy Prgm

SUNY - State College of Optometry
David A Bowers, MBA
33 W 10th Ave
New York, NY 10036
212 938-4900
Type: Junior or Comm Coll
Control: Nonprofit (Private or Religious)
• Optometry Prgm

TCI College of Technology
Bruce R Kalisch, President
320 W 31st St
New York, NY 10001
212 399-0091
Type: Junior or Comm Coll
Control: For Profit
• Ophthalmic Dispensing Optician Prgm

The New School
New York, NY 10003
Type: Acad Health Ctr/Med Sch
Control: For Profit
• Psychology (PhD) Prgm

Touro College
Alan Kadish, MD, Senior Provost and CEO
Executive Offices
27-33 W 23rd St
New York, NY 10010-4202
212 463-0400
Type: 4-year Coll or Univ
Control: Nonprofit (Private or Religious)
• Occupational Therapy Asst Prgm
• Occupational Therapy Prgm (2)
• Osteopathic Medicine Prgm
• Pharmacy Prgm
• Physical Therapist Assistant Prgm
• Physical Therapy Prgm
• Physician Assistant Prgm (2)
• Speech-Language Pathology Prgm

Weill Cornell Graduate School of Medical Sci
Antonio Gotto, Jr, MD, Dean
1300 York Ave, Rm F-105
New York, NY 10021
212 746-6005
Type: Acad Health Ctr/Med Sch
Control: Nonprofit (Private or Religious)
• Physician Assistant Prgm

Wood Tobe'-Coburn School
Sandi Gruninger, President
8 E 40th St
New York, NY 10016
212 686-9040
Type: Junior or Comm Coll
Control: For Profit
• Medical Assistant Prgm

Yeshiva University
Richard M Joel, JD
500 W 185th St
New York, NY 10033
212 960-5300
Type: 4-year Coll or Univ
Control: State, County, or Local Govt
• Allopathic Medicine Prgm
• Psychology (PhD) Prgm
• Psychology (PsyD) Prgm

Newburgh

Mt St Mary College
Sr Ann Sakac, OP PhD, President
330 Powell Ave
Newburgh, NY 12550
914 561-0800
Type: 4-year Coll or Univ
Control: Nonprofit (Private or Religious)
• Nursing Prgm

Oceanside

Robt J Hochstime Sch Rad/S Nassau Comm Hosp
Joseph Quagliata, MA MSHA MSHyg, President and CEO
One Healthy Way
PO Box 9007
Oceanside, NY 11572
516 632-3939
Type: Hosp or Med Ctr: 300-499 Beds
Control: Nonprofit (Private or Religious)
• Radiography Prgm

Old Westbury

New York Institute of Technology
Edward Guiliano, PhD, President
Northern Blvd PO Box 8000
Old Westbury, NY 11568-8000
516 686-7658
Type: 4-year Coll or Univ
Control: Nonprofit (Private or Religious)
• Dietetics-Didactic Prgm
• Nursing Prgm
• Occupational Therapy Prgm
• Osteopathic Medicine Prgm
• Physical Therapy Prgm
• Physician Assistant Prgm

Oneonta

Hartwick College
Oneonta, NY 13820
Type: 4-year Coll or Univ
Control: Nonprofit (Private or Religious)
• Nursing Prgm

SUNY College at Oneonta
Alan B Donovan, President
Oneonta, NY 13820
607 436-3500
Type: 4-year Coll or Univ
Control: State, County, or Local Govt
• Dietetic Internship Prgm
• Dietetics-Didactic Prgm

Orangeburg

Dominican College
Mary Eileen O'Brien, OP PhD, President
470 Western Hwy
Orangeburg, NY 10962-1299
845 848-7801
Type: 4-year Coll or Univ
Control: Nonprofit (Private or Religious)
• Athletic Training Prgm
• Nursing Prgm
• Occupational Therapy Prgm
• Physical Therapy Prgm

Patchogue

Briarcliffe College
Patchogue, NY 11772
• Dental Hygiene Prgm

Plattsburgh

CVPH Medical Center
Mundy Stephens, JD, President
75 Beekman St
Plattsburgh, NY 12901
518 561-2000
Type: Hosp or Med Ctr: 300-499 Beds
Control: Nonprofit (Private or Religious)
• Radiography Prgm

SUNY College at Plattsburgh
Plattsburgh, NY 12901
Type: 4-year Coll or Univ
Control: State, County, or Local Govt
• Nursing Prgm

SUNY College at Plattsburgh
Horace A Judson, President
Plattsburgh, NY 12901
518 564-2000
Type: 4-year Coll or Univ
Control: State, County, or Local Govt
• Counseling Prgm
• Dietetics-Didactic Prgm
• Nursing Prgm
• Speech-Language Pathology Prgm

Pleasantville

Pace University
Pleasantville, NY 10570
Type: 4-year Coll or Univ
Control: Nonprofit (Private or Religious)
• Nursing Prgm

Port Ewen

Ulster County Board of Cooperative Ed Service
Martin Ruglis, SDA, District Superintendent
PO Box 601
Rte GW
Port Ewen, NY 12466
845 331-6680
Type: Vocational or Tech Sch
Control: State, County, or Local Govt
• Surgical Technology Prgm

Potsdam

Clarkson University
Dennis G Brown, President
Potsdam, NY 13699-5557
315 268-6400
Type: 4-year Coll or Univ
Control: Nonprofit (Private or Religious)
• Physical Therapy Prgm
• Physician Assistant Prgm

Poughkeepsie

Dutchess Community College
D David Conklin, PhD, President
53 Pendell Rd
Poughkeepsie, NY 12601
845 431-8980
Type: Junior or Comm Coll
Control: State, County, or Local Govt
• Clin Lab Technician/Med Lab Technician Prgm
• Emergency Med Tech-Paramedic Prgm

Marist College
Dennis J Murray, PhD, President
3399 North Rd
Graystone
Poughkeepsie, NY 12601
845 575-3000
Type: 4-year Coll or Univ
Control: Nonprofit (Private or Religious)
• Athletic Training Prgm
• Clin Lab Scientist/Med Technologist Prgm

Queens

St John's University
Donald J Harrington, CM, President
8000 Utopia Pkwy Newman Hall Rm 318
175-05 Horace Harding Exp
Queens, NY 11439
718 990-6301
Type: 4-year Coll or Univ
Control: Nonprofit (Private or Religious)
• Clin Lab Scientist/Med Technologist Prgm
• Counseling Prgm
• Medical Librarian Prgm
• Pharmacy Prgm
• Physician Assistant Prgm
• Psychology (PhD) Prgm
• Radiography Prgm
• Speech-Language Pathology Prgm

Riverdale

College of Mount St Viencent
Charles L Flynn, Jr, PhD, President
6301 Riverdale Ave
Riverdale, NY 10471
718 405-3267
Type: Acad Health Ctr/Med Sch
Control: For Profit
• Nursing Prgm

Riverhead

Peconic Bay Medical Center
Andrew J Mitchell, MBA FACHE, President
1300 Roanoke Ave
Riverhead, NY 11901
631 548-6000
Type: Hosp or Med Ctr: 100-299 Beds
Control: Nonprofit (Private or Religious)
• Radiography Prgm

Rochester

Bryant & Stratton College - Rochester
Beth Tarquino, MS Ed, Market Director
Henrietta Campus
1225 Jefferson Rd
Rochester, NY 14623-3136
716 292-5627
Type: Vocational or Tech Sch
Control: For Profit
• Medical Assistant Prgm

Everest Institute
Carl A Silvio, BA, President
1630 Portland Ave
Rochester, NY 14621
585 266-0430
Type: Junior or Comm Coll
Control: For Profit
• Medical Assistant Prgm

Monroe Community College
Lawrence Tyree, PhD, President
1000 E Henrietta Rd
Rochester, NY 14623
585 292-2100
Type: Junior or Comm Coll
Control: State, County, or Local Govt
• Dental Assistant Prgm
• Dental Hygiene Prgm
• Emergency Med Tech-Paramedic Prgm
• Radiography Prgm

Nazareth College of Rochester
Daan Braveman, PhD, President
4245 East Ave
Rochester, NY 14618-2790
585 586-2525
Type: 4-year Coll or Univ
Control: Nonprofit (Private or Religious)
• Art Therapy Prgm
• Music Therapy Prgm
• Nursing Prgm
• Physical Therapy Prgm
• Speech-Language Pathology Prgm

Roberts Wesleyan College
2301 Westside Dr
Rochester, NY 14624
Type: Junior or Comm Coll
Control: State, County, or Local Govt
• Music Therapy Prgm
• Nursing Prgm

Rochester General Hospital
Mark Clements, MPHA, President and CEO
1425 Portland Ave
Rochester, NY 14621
585 922-4000
Type: Hosp or Med Ctr: 500 Beds
Control: Nonprofit (Private or Religious)
• Clin Lab Scientist/Med Technologist Prgm
• Phlebotomy Prgm

Rochester Institute of Technology
William Destler, PhD, President
One Lomb Memorial Dr
Rochester, NY 14623
585 475-2394
Type: 4-year Coll or Univ
Control: Nonprofit (Private or Religious)
• Diagnostic Med Sonography (General) Prgm
• Dietetics-Didactic Prgm
• Physician Assistant Prgm

St John Fisher College
Rochester, NY 14618
Type: 4-year Coll or Univ
Control: Nonprofit (Private or Religious)
• Counseling Prgm
• Nursing Prgm
• Pharmacy Prgm

University of Rochester
Joel Seligman, PhD, President
Rochester, NY 14627
Type: 4-year Coll or Univ
Control: Nonprofit (Private or Religious)
• Allopathic Medicine Prgm
• Counseling Prgm
• Nursing Prgm
• Psychology (PhD) Prgm

Rockville Centre

Mercy Medical Center
Alan Guerci, MD, President/CEO
PO Box 9024
1000 N Village Ave
Rockville Centre, NY 11571-9024
516 705-2525
Type: Hosp or Med Ctr: 300-499 Beds
Control: Nonprofit (Private or Religious)
• Radiography Prgm

Molloy College
Drew Bogner, PhD, President
1000 Hempstead Ave
PO Box 5002
Rockville Centre, NY 11571-5002
516 678-5000
Type: 4-year Coll or Univ
Control: Nonprofit (Private or Religious)
• Cardiovascular Tech (Invasive/Noninv/Vasc)
  Prgm
• Nuclear Medicine Technology Prgm
• Nursing Prgm
• Respiratory Care Prgm
• Speech-Language Pathology Prgm

Sanborn

Keuka College
James Klyczek, PhD, President
3113 Saunders Settlement Road
Sanborn, NY 14132-9487
716 614-5905
Type: 4-year Coll or Univ
Control: Nonprofit (Private or Religious)
• Nursing Prgm
• Occupational Therapy Prgm

Niagara County Community College
James Klyczek, PhD, President
3111 Saunders Settlement Rd
Sanborn, NY 14132
716 614-6222
Type: Junior or Comm Coll
Control: State, County, or Local Govt
• Medical Assistant Prgm
• Physical Therapist Assistant Prgm
• Radiography Prgm
• Surgical Technology Prgm

Saranac Lake

North Country Community College
Gail Rogers Rice, EdD, President
20 Winona Ave
PO Box 89
Saranac Lake, NY 12983
518 891-2915
Type: Junior or Comm Coll
Control: State, County, or Local Govt
• Radiography Prgm

Saratoga Springs

SUNY Empire State College
Saratoga Springs, NY 12866
Type: 4-year Coll or Univ
Control: State, County, or Local Govt
• Nursing Prgm

Selden

Suffolk County Community College
Shirley Robinson Pippins, EdD, President
533 College Rd
Bldg NFL 37
Selden, NY 11784-2899
631 451-4111
Type: Junior or Comm Coll
Control: State, County, or Local Govt
• Dietetic Technician-AD Prgm
• Occupational Therapy Asst Prgm
• Physical Therapist Assistant Prgm
• Veterinary Technology Prgm

Seneca Falls

New York Chiropractic College
2360 State Route 89
Seneca Falls, NY 13148
Type: Acad Health Ctr/Med Sch
Control: Nonprofit (Private or Religious)
• Chiropractic Prgm

Staten Island

CUNY College of Staten Island
Marlene Springer, PhD, President
2800 Victory Blvd
Staten Island, NY 10314
718 982-2400
Type: 4-year Coll or Univ
Control: State, County, or Local Govt
• Clin Lab Scientist/Med Technologist Prgm
• Physical Therapy Prgm

Wagner College/Staten Island University
Norman R Smith, EdD, President
631 Howard Ave
Staten Island, NY 10301
718 390-3131
Type: Consortium
Control: Nonprofit (Private or Religious)
• Physician Assistant Prgm

Stone Ridge

SUNY Ulster
Donald C Katt, EdD, President
Cottekill Rd
Stone Ridge, NY 12484
845 687-5279
Type: Junior or Comm Coll
Control: State, County, or Local Govt
• Veterinary Technology Prgm

Stony Brook

State University at Stony Brook
Shirley Strum Kenny, PhD, President
310 Administration Bldg
Stony Brook, NY 11794-0701
631 632-6265
Type: 4-year Coll or Univ
Control: State, County, or Local Govt
• Dentistry Prgm
• Psychology (PhD) Prgm

Stony Brook University

Shirley Strum Kenny, PhD, President
Nicolls Rd
Admin Bldg Third Fl
Stony Brook, NY 11794-0701
631 632-6255
Type: 4-year Coll or Univ
Control: State, County, or Local Govt
• Athletic Training Prgm
• Clin Lab Scientist/Med Technologist Prgm
• Dietetic Internship Prgm
• Nursing Prgm
• Occupational Therapy Prgm
• Physical Therapy Prgm
• Physician Assistant Prgm
• Polysomnographic Technology Prgm
• Respiratory Care Prgm

University at Stony Brook
Michael Maffetone, DA, CEO
University Hospital and Medical Center
Health Sciences Center-Level 4, Rm 215
Stony Brook, NY 11794-8410
631 444-2701
Type: 4-year Coll or Univ
Control: State, County, or Local Govt
• Allopathic Medicine Prgm

Suffern

Rockland Community College
Cliff Wood, PhD, President
145 College Rd
Suffern, NY 10901-3699
845 574-4575
Type: Junior or Comm Coll
Control: State, County, or Local Govt
• Occupational Therapy Asst Prgm

Syracuse

Bryant & Stratton College - Syracuse
Michael Sattler, Campus Director
953 James St
Syracuse, NY 13203
315 472-6603
Type: Vocational or Tech Sch
Control: For Profit
• Medical Assistant Prgm

Le Moyne College
Charles Beirne, SJ PhD, President
Le Moyne Heights
Syracuse, NY 13214-1399
315 445-4120
Type: 4-year Coll or Univ
Control: Nonprofit (Private or Religious)
• Nursing Prgm
• Physician Assistant Prgm

Onondaga Community College
Deborah Sydow, PhD, President
4941 Onondaga Rd
Syracuse, NY 13215
315 498-2211
Type: Junior or Comm Coll
Control: State, County, or Local Govt
• Physical Therapist Assistant Prgm
• Respiratory Care Prgm
• Surgical Technology Prgm

SUNY Upstate Medical University
David Smith, MD, President
750 E Adams St
1154 Weiskotten Hall
Syracuse, NY 13210
315 464-4513
Type: Acad Health Ctr/Med Sch
Control: State, County, or Local Govt
• Allopathic Medicine Prgm
• Clin Lab Scientist/Med Technologist Prgm
• Diagnostic Molecular Scientist Prgm
• Nursing Prgm
• Perfusion Prgm
• Physical Therapy Prgm
• Physician Assistant Prgm
• Radiation Therapy Prgm
• Radiography Prgm
• Respiratory Care Prgm

Syracuse University
Kenneth A Shaw, Chancellor & President
Syracuse, NY 13244
315 443-1870
Type: 4-year Coll or Univ
Control: Nonprofit (Private or Religious)
• Audiologist Prgm
• Counseling Prgm
• Dietetic Internship Prgm
• Dietetics-Didactic Prgm
• Medical Librarian Prgm
• Psychology (PhD) Prgm
• Speech-Language Pathology Prgm

Troy

Hudson Valley Community College
Drew Matonak, PhD, President
80 Vandenburgh Ave
Troy, NY 12180-6096
518 629-4822
Type: Junior or Comm Coll
Control: State, County, or Local Govt
• Dental Hygiene Prgm
• Diagnostic Med Sonography (General/Cardiac) Prgm
• Emergency Med Tech-Paramedic Prgm
• Respiratory Care Prgm

The Sage Colleges
Susan Scrimshaw, PhD, President
65 First Street
Troy, NY 12180-4115
518 244-2214
Type: 4-year Coll or Univ
Control: Nonprofit (Private or Religious)
• Dietetic Internship Prgm
• Dietetics-Didactic Prgm
• Nursing Prgm
• Occupational Therapy Prgm
• Physical Therapy Prgm

Utica

Faxton - St Luke's Healthcare
Andrew E Peterson, MS, Exec Director
Champlin Ave, PO Box 479
Utica, NY 13503-0479
315 798-6001
Type: Hosp or Med Ctr: 300-499 Beds
Control: Nonprofit (Private or Religious)
• Emergency Med Tech-Paramedic Prgm
• Radiography Prgm

Mohawk Valley Community College
Michael I Schafer, EdD, President
Payne Hall 305
1101 Sherman Dr
Utica, NY 13501
315 792-5333
Type: Junior or Comm Coll
Control: State, County, or Local Govt
• Respiratory Care Prgm

St Elizabeth Medical Center
Sr M Johanna Deleys, OSF, President, CEO
2209 Genesee St
Utica, NY 13501
315 798-8123
Type: Hosp or Med Ctr: 100-299 Beds
Control: Nonprofit (Private or Religious)
• Radiography Prgm

SUNY Institute of Tech - Utica/Rome
Peter Spina, PhD, President
PO Box 3050
Utica, NY 13504-3050
315 792-7400
Type: 4-year Coll or Univ
Control: State, County, or Local Govt
• Nursing Prgm

Utica College
Todd S Hutton, PhD, President
1600 Burrstone Rd
Utica, NY 13502-4892
315 792-3222
Type: 4-year Coll or Univ
Control: Nonprofit (Private or Religious)
• Nursing Prgm
• Occupational Therapy Prgm
• Physical Therapy Prgm

Valhalla

New York Medical College
Harry C Barrett, DMin MPH, President, CEO
Sunshine Administration Building
Valhalla, NY 10595
914 993-4000
Type: 4-year Coll or Univ
Control: Nonprofit (Private or Religious)
• Allopathic Medicine Prgm
• Physical Therapy Prgm
• Speech-Language Pathology Prgm

Westchester Community College
Joseph N Hankin, EdD, President
75 Grasslands Rd
Valhalla, NY 10595
914 606-6706
Type: Junior or Comm Coll
Control: State, County, or Local Govt
• Dietetic Technician-AD Prgm
• Radiography Prgm
• Respiratory Care Prgm

White Plains

Sanford-Brown Institute - White Plains
White Plains, NY 10604
Type: Vocational or Tech Sch
• Diagnostic Med Sonography (General) Prgm

Yonkers

St Joseph's Medical Center
Michael J Spicer, FACHE, President
127 S Broadway
Yonkers, NY 10701
914 378-7000
Type: Hosp or Med Ctr: 100-299 Beds
Control: Nonprofit (Private or Religious)
• Radiography Prgm

New Zealand

Palmerston North

Massey University
Steven La Grow, MA EdD COMS, Professor, Head of School
School of Health Sciences
Private Bag 11222
Palmerston North, NZ
646 350-5799
Type: 4-year Coll or Univ
Control: State, County, or Local Govt
• Orientation and Mobility Specialist Prgm

Newfoundland, Canada

St John's

Memorial University of Newfoundland
St John's, NF A1C 5S7
Type: Acad Health Ctr/Med Sch
Control: State, County, or Local Govt
• Allopathic Medicine Prgm

North Carolina

Albemarle

Stanly Community College
Michael R Taylor, EdD, President
141 College Dr
Albemarle, NC 28001-9402
704 991-0220
Type: Junior or Comm Coll
Control: State, County, or Local Govt
• Clin Lab Technician/Med Lab Technician Prgm
• Medical Assistant Prgm
• Respiratory Care Prgm

Asheville

Asheville-Buncombe Technical Comm College
Richard Mauney, President
340 Victoria Rd
Asheville, NC 28801
828 254-1921
Type: Junior or Comm Coll
Control: State, County, or Local Govt
- Clin Lab Technician/Med Lab Technician Prgm
- Dental Assistant Prgm
- Dental Hygiene Prgm
- Diagnostic Med Sonography (General/Vascular) Prgm
- Medical Assistant Prgm
- Phlebotomy Prgm
- Radiography Prgm
- Surgical Technology Prgm
- Veterinary Technology Prgm

South College - Asheville
Robert Davis, MSL, Executive Director
29 Turtle Creek Dr
Asheville, NC 28803
828 398-2500
Type: 4-year Coll or Univ
Control: For Profit
- Medical Assistant Prgm
- Physical Therapist Assistant Prgm
- Radiography Prgm
- Surgical Technology Prgm

Banner Elk

Lees-McRae College
David Bushman, PhD, President
PO Box 128
191 Main St
Banner Elk, NC 28604
828 898-8785
Type: 4-year Coll or Univ
Control: Nonprofit (Private or Religious)
- Athletic Training Prgm
- Nursing Prgm

Boiling Springs

Gardner-Webb University
Frank Bonner, PhD, President
Boiling Springs, NC 28017
704 406-4236
Type: 4-year Coll or Univ
Control: State, County, or Local Govt
- Athletic Training Prgm
- Counseling Prgm

Boone

Appalachian State University
Kenneth Peacock, PhD, Chancellor
Boone, NC 28608
828 262-2040
Type: 4-year Coll or Univ
Control: State, County, or Local Govt
- Athletic Training Prgm
- Counseling Prgm
- Dietetic Internship Prgm
- Dietetics-Didactic Prgm
- Music Therapy Prgm
- Nursing Prgm
- Speech-Language Pathology Prgm

Buies Creek

Campbell University
Jerry M Wallace, PhD, President
PO Box 127
143 Main St
Buies Creek, NC 27506
910 893-1205
Type: 4-year Coll or Univ
Control: Nonprofit (Private or Religious)
- Athletic Training Prgm
- Pharmacy Prgm
- Physician Assistant Prgm

Chapel Hill

University of North Carolina
Holden Thorp, President
Campus Box 3100
205 South Building
Chapel Hill, NC 27599-9100
919 962-3082
Type: 4-year Coll or Univ
Control: State, County, or Local Govt
- Allopathic Medicine Prgm
- Athletic Training Prgm (4)
- Audiologist Prgm
- Clin Lab Scientist/Med Technologist Prgm
- Counseling Prgm (2)
- Dental Assistant Prgm
- Dental Hygiene Prgm
- Diagnostic Molecular Scientist Prgm
- Dietetic Internship Prgm
- Dietetics-Coordinated Prgm
- Dietetics-Didactic Prgm (2)
- Genetic Counseling Prgm
- Medical Librarian Prgm (2)
- Nursing Prgm (4)
- Occupational Therapy Prgm
- Physical Therapy Prgm
- Psychology (PhD) Prgm (2)
- Radiography Prgm
- Radiologist Assistant Prgm
- Rehabilitation Counseling Prgm
- Speech-Language Pathology Prgm (2)

University of North Carolina Hospitals
Todd Peterson, MBA, President
101 Manning Dr
Chapel Hill, NC 27514
919 966-5111
Type: Hosp or Med Ctr: 500 Beds
Control: State, County, or Local Govt
- Dentistry Prgm
- Medical Dosimetry Prgm
- Nuclear Medicine Technology Prgm
- Pharmacy Prgm
- Radiation Therapy Prgm

Charlotte

Brookstone College of Business
F Jack Henderson, MBA, President
10125 Berkeley Place Dr
Charlotte, NC 28262
704 547-8600
Type: Vocational or Tech Sch
Control: For Profit
- Medical Assistant Prgm

Carolinas College of Health Sciences
Ellen Sheppard, PhD, President
1200 Blythe Boulevard
PO Box 32861
Charlotte, NC 28203
704 355-5316
Type: Acad Health Ctr/Med Sch
Control: Nonprofit (Private or Religious)
- Clin Lab Scientist/Med Technologist Prgm
- Phlebotomy Prgm
- Radiography Prgm
- Surgical Technology Prgm

Central Piedmont Community College
P Anthony Zeiss, EdD, President
PO Box 35009
Charlotte, NC 28235-5009
704 330-6566
Type: Junior or Comm Coll
Control: State, County, or Local Govt
- Cardiovascular Tech (Invasive/Echo) Prgm
- Clin Lab Technician/Med Lab Technician Prgm
- Cytotechnology Prgm
- Dental Assistant Prgm
- Dental Hygiene Prgm
- Medical Assistant Prgm
- Physical Therapist Assistant Prgm
- Respiratory Care Prgm
- Surgical Technology Prgm

King's College
Barbara Rockecharlie, MBA, Chief Acad Officer, Dir
322 Lamar Ave
Charlotte, NC 28204
704 688-3613
Type: Junior or Comm Coll
Control: For Profit
- Medical Assistant Prgm

Presbyterian Healthcare
Tim Billings, President/COO
200 Hawthorne Ln
PO Box 33549
Charlotte, NC 28204
704 384-4942
Type: Hosp or Med Ctr: 500 Beds
Control: Nonprofit (Private or Religious)
- Radiography Prgm

Queens University of Charlotte
Pamela Lewis Davies, EdD, President
1900 Selwyn Ave
Charlotte, NC 28274-0001
704 337-2200
Type: 4-year Coll or Univ
Control: Nonprofit (Private or Religious)
- Music Therapy Prgm
- Nursing Prgm

Univ of North Carolina at Charlotte
Phil Dubois, PhD, Chancellor
9201 University Blvd
Charlotte, NC 28223-0001
704 687-2000
Type: 4-year Coll or Univ
Control: State, County, or Local Govt
- Athletic Training Prgm
- Counseling Prgm
- Exercise Physiology - Clinical Prgm
- Exercise Science Prgm
- Nursing Prgm

Clyde

Haywood Community College
Nathan Hodges, EdD, President
Freedlander Dr
Clyde, NC 28721-9454
704 627-4515
Type: Junior or Comm Coll
Control: State, County, or Local Govt
• Medical Assistant Prgm

Concord

Cabarrus College of Health Sciences
Dianne O Snyder, RN DHA, Chancellor
401 Medical Park Dr
Concord, NC 28025
704 783-1521
Type: 4-year Coll or Univ
Control: Nonprofit (Private or Religious)
• Medical Assistant Prgm
• Nursing Prgm
• Occupational Therapy Asst Prgm
• Surgical Technology Prgm

Cullowhee

Western Carolina University
John W Bardo, PhD, Chancellor
511 HF Robinson Admin Bldg
Cullowhee, NC 28723
828 227-7100
Type: 4-year Coll or Univ
Control: State, County, or Local Govt
• Athletic Training Prgm
• Counseling Prgm
• Dietetic Internship Prgm
• Dietetics-Didactic Prgm
• Emergency Med Tech-Paramedic Prgm
• Nursing Prgm
• Physical Therapy Prgm
• Recreational Therapy Prgm
• Speech-Language Pathology Prgm

Dallas

Gaston College
Patricia A Skinner, PhD, President
201 Hwy 321 S
Dallas, NC 28034-1499
704 922-6475
Type: Junior or Comm Coll
Control: State, County, or Local Govt
• Dietetic Technician-AD Prgm
• Medical Assistant Prgm
• Veterinary Technology Prgm

Dobson

Surry Community College
G Frank Sells, EdD, President
630 S Main St
Dobson, NC 27017-8432
336 386-3213
Type: Junior or Comm Coll
Control: State, County, or Local Govt
• Medical Assistant Prgm
• Physical Therapist Assistant Prgm

Durham

Duke University
Richard H Brodhead, PhD, President
1202 Spring Garden St
Durham, NC 27708
Type: 4-year Coll or Univ
Control: State, County, or Local Govt
• Nursing Prgm
• Psychology (PhD) Prgm

Duke University Medical Center
Victor Dzau, MD, Chancellor
Health Affairs
PO Box 3701 M106A Davison Bldg
Durham, NC 27710
919 684-2255
Type: Acad Health Ctr/Med Sch
Control: Nonprofit (Private or Religious)
• Allopathic Medicine Prgm
• Ophthalmic Technician Prgm
• Pathologists' Assistant Prgm
• Physical Therapy Prgm
• Physician Assistant Prgm

Durham Technical Community College
William Ingram, EdD, President
1637 Lawson St
Durham, NC 27703
919 536-7250
Type: Junior or Comm Coll
Control: State, County, or Local Govt
• Dental Lab Technician Prgm
• Medical Assistant Prgm
• Occupational Therapy Asst Prgm
• Ophthalmic Dispensing Optician Prgm
• Pharmacy Technician Prgm
• Respiratory Care Prgm
• Surgical Technology Prgm

North Carolina Central University
James H Ammons, PhD, Chancellor
1801 Fayetteville St
113 Hoey Administration Bldg
Durham, NC 27707
919 530-6104
Type: 4-year Coll or Univ
Control: State, County, or Local Govt
• Athletic Training Prgm
• Counseling Prgm
• Dietetic Internship Prgm
• Dietetics-Didactic Prgm
• Medical Librarian Prgm
• Orientation and Mobility Specialist Prgm
• Speech-Language Pathology Prgm

Elizabeth City

College of The Albemarle
Lynne M Bunch, MA, President
PO Box 2327
1208 N Road St
Elizabeth City, NC 27909
252 335-0821
Type: Junior or Comm Coll
Control: State, County, or Local Govt
• Clin Lab Technician/Med Lab Technician Prgm
• Medical Assistant Prgm
• Surgical Technology Prgm

Elon

Elon University
Leo Lambert, PhD, President
Campus Box 2185
Elon, NC 27244
336 278-7900
Type: 4-year Coll or Univ
Control: Nonprofit (Private or Religious)
• Physical Therapy Prgm

Fayetteville

Fayetteville State University
Fayetteville, NC 28301
Type: 4-year Coll or Univ
Control: State, County, or Local Govt
• Nursing Prgm (2)

Fayetteville Technical Community College
Dr. J. Larry Keen, EdD, President
PO Box 35236
Fayetteville, NC 28303-0236
910 678-8400
Type: Junior or Comm Coll
Control: State, County, or Local Govt
• Dental Hygiene Prgm
• Phlebotomy Prgm
• Physical Therapist Assistant Prgm
• Radiography Prgm
• Respiratory Care Prgm
• Surgical Technology Prgm

Methodist University
Elton Hendricks, PhD, President
5400 Ramsey St
Fayetteville, NC 28311
910 630-7005
Type: 4-year Coll or Univ
Control: Nonprofit (Private or Religious)
• Athletic Training Prgm
• Physician Assistant Prgm

Flat Rock

Blue Ridge Community College
David W Sink, Jr, EdD, President
College Dr
Flat Rock, NC 28737-9624
828 692-3572
Type: Junior or Comm Coll
Control: State, County, or Local Govt
• Emergency Med Tech-Paramedic Prgm
• Surgical Technology Prgm

Fort Bragg

Joint Special Operations Medical Training Ctr
Jeffrey L Kingsbury, MD MPH, Dean
CDR, SWMG(A)
AOJK-MED (attn: EMT Coord)
Fort Bragg, NC 28310-5200
910 396-7775
Type: Dept of Defense
Control: Fed Govt
• Emergency Med Tech-Paramedic Prgm

INSTITUTIONS

Goldsboro

Wayne Community College
Kay Albertson, EdD, President
Caller Box 8002
Goldsboro, NC 27530
919 735-5151
Type: Junior or Comm Coll
Control: State, County, or Local Govt
• Dental Assistant Prgm
• Dental Hygiene Prgm
• Medical Assistant Prgm

Graham

Alamance Community College
Martin H Nadelman, EdD, President
PO Box 8000
1247 Jimmie Kerr Road
Graham, NC 27253-8000
336 506-4100
Type: Junior or Comm Coll
Control: State, County, or Local Govt
• Clin Lab Technician/Med Lab Technician Prgm
• Dental Assistant Prgm
• Medical Assistant Prgm

Grantsboro

Pamlico Community College
Marion Altman, EdD, President
PO Box 185
Grantsboro, NC 28529-0185
252 249-1851
Type: Junior or Comm Coll
Control: State, County, or Local Govt
• Medical Assistant Prgm
• Neurodiagnostic Tech Prgm

Greensboro

Greensboro College
Craven E Williams, DMin, President
815 W Market St
Greensboro, NC 27401
336 272-7102
Type: 4-year Coll or Univ
Control: State, County, or Local Govt
• Athletic Training Prgm

North Carolina A&T State University
Edward B Fort, Chancellor
1601 E Market St
Greensboro, NC 27411
910 334-7500
Type: 4-year Coll or Univ
Control: State, County, or Local Govt
• Counseling Prgm
• Dietetics-Didactic Prgm
• Music Therapy Prgm
• Rehabilitation Counseling Prgm

TRS Institute
628 Green Valley Rd
Ste 300
Greensboro, NC 27408
Type: Acad Health Ctr/Med Sch
Control: For Profit
• Medical Transcriptionist Prgm

Greenville

East Carolina University
Steven Ballard, PhD, Chancellor
Spillman Building
Office of the Chancellor
Greenville, NC 27858-4353
252 328-6212
Type: 4-year Coll or Univ
Control: State, County, or Local Govt
• Allopathic Medicine Prgm
• Athletic Training Prgm
• Audiologist Prgm
• Clin Lab Scientist/Med Technologist Prgm
• Dentistry Prgm
• Dietetic Internship Prgm
• Dietetics-Didactic Prgm
• Music Therapy Prgm
• Occupational Therapy Prgm
• Physical Therapy Prgm
• Physician Assistant Prgm
• Rehabilitation Counseling Prgm
• Speech-Language Pathology Prgm

Pitt Community College
Dennis Massey, PhD, President
PO Drawer 7007
Greenville, NC 27835-7007
252 493-7220
Type: Junior or Comm Coll
Control: State, County, or Local Govt
• Diagnostic Med Sonography (General/Cardiac) Prgm
• Medical Assistant Prgm
• Medical Dosimetry Prgm
• Occupational Therapy Asst Prgm
• Polysomnographic Technology Prgm
• Radiation Therapy Prgm
• Radiography Prgm
• Respiratory Care Prgm

Hamlet

Richmond Community College
Diane Honeycutt, EdD, President
PO Box 1189
Hamlet, NC 28345
910 582-7000
Type: Junior or Comm Coll
Control: State, County, or Local Govt
• Medical Assistant Prgm

Henderson

Vance-Granville Community College
Randy Parker, MEd, President
PO Box 917
Popular Creek Rd
Henderson, NC 27536
252 492-2061
Type: Junior or Comm Coll
Control: State, County, or Local Govt
• Medical Assistant Prgm
• Radiography Prgm

Hickory

Catawba Valley Community College
Garrett Hinshaw, EdD, President
2550 Hwy 70 SE
Hickory, NC 28602
828 327-7000
Type: Junior or Comm Coll
Control: State, County, or Local Govt
• Dental Hygiene Prgm
• Emergency Med Tech-Paramedic Prgm
• Neurodiagnostic Tech Prgm
• Polysomnographic Technology Prgm
• Radiography Prgm
• Respiratory Care Prgm
• Surgical Technology Prgm

Lenoir - Rhyne University
Wayne Powell, PhD, President
Box 7163
Hickory, NC 28603
828 328-7334
Type: 4-year Coll or Univ
Control: Nonprofit (Private or Religious)
• Athletic Training Prgm
• Dietetic Internship Prgm
• Nursing Prgm
• Occupational Therapy Prgm

High Point

High Point University
Nido Qubein, LLD, President
833 Montlieu Ave
High Point, NC 27262
336 841-9201
Type: 4-year Coll or Univ
Control: Nonprofit (Private or Religious)
• Athletic Training Prgm

Hudson

Caldwell Comm College & Tech Institute
Kenneth A Boham, EdD, President
2855 Hickory Blvd
Hudson, NC 28638-1399
828 726-2200
Type: Junior or Comm Coll
Control: State, County, or Local Govt
• Diagnostic Med Sonography (General/Cardiac) Prgm
• Nuclear Medicine Technology Prgm
• Ophthalmic Assistant Prgm
• Physical Therapist Assistant Prgm
• Radiography Prgm

Jacksonville

Coastal Carolina Community College
Ronald K Lingle, PhD, President
444 Western Blvd
Jacksonville, NC 28546-6816
910 938-6210
Type: Junior or Comm Coll
Control: State, County, or Local Govt
• Clin Lab Technician/Med Lab Technician Prgm
• Dental Assistant Prgm
• Dental Hygiene Prgm
• Surgical Technology Prgm

Jamestown

Guilford Technical Community College
Donald C Cameron, EdD, President
PO Box 309
601 High Point Rd
Jamestown, NC 27282
336 334-4822
Type: Junior or Comm Coll
Control: State, County, or Local Govt
• Dental Assistant Prgm
• Dental Hygiene Prgm
• Medical Assistant Prgm
• Medical Transcriptionist Prgm
• Physical Therapist Assistant Prgm
• Radiography Prgm
• Surgical Technology Prgm

Kenansville

James Sprunt Community College
Mary T Wood, EdD, President
PO Box 398, James Sprunt Dr
Kenansville, NC 28349
910 296-2450
Type: Junior or Comm Coll
Control: State, County, or Local Govt
• Medical Assistant Prgm

Kinston

Lenoir Community College
Brantley Briley, EdD, President
PO Box 188
231 Hwy 58S
Kinston, NC 28502
252 527-6223
Type: Junior or Comm Coll
Control: State, County, or Local Govt
• Medical Assistant Prgm
• Polysomnographic Technology Prgm
• Radiography Prgm
• Surgical Technology Prgm

Lumberton

Robeson Community College
Charles Chrestman, EdD, President
PO Box 1420
Lumberton, NC 28359
910 272-3230
Type: Junior or Comm Coll
Control: State, County, or Local Govt
• Respiratory Care Prgm
• Surgical Technology Prgm

Mars Hill

Mars Hill College
Dan G Lunsford, EdD, President
PO Box 6748
Mars Hill, NC 28754
828 689-1141
Type: 4-year Coll or Univ
Control: State, County, or Local Govt
• Athletic Training Prgm

Morehead City

Carteret Community College
Joseph T Barwick, PhD, President
3505 Arendell St
Morehead City, NC 28557
252 222-6140
Type: Junior or Comm Coll
Control: State, County, or Local Govt
• Medical Assistant Prgm
• Radiography Prgm
• Respiratory Care Prgm

Morganton

Western Piedmont Community College
Jim Burnett, EdD, President
1001 Burkemont Ave
Morganton, NC 28655
828 448-3100
Type: Junior or Comm Coll
Control: State, County, or Local Govt
• Clin Lab Technician/Med Lab Technician Prgm
• Dental Assistant Prgm
• Medical Assistant Prgm

Murphy

Tri-County Community College
Norman Oglesby, PhD, President
2300 Hwy 64 E
Murphy, NC 28906
704 837-6810
Type: Junior or Comm Coll
Control: State, County, or Local Govt
• Medical Assistant Prgm

New Bem

Craven Community College
R Scott Ralls, PhD, President
800 College Court
New Bem, NC 28562
252 638-4131
Type: Junior or Comm Coll
Control: State, County, or Local Govt
• Medical Assistant Prgm

North Wilkesboro

Wilkes Regional Medical Center
Fred Brown, Interim CEO
PO Box 609
North Wilkesboro, NC 28659
336 651-8100
Type: Hosp or Med Ctr: 100-299 Beds
Control: State, County, or Local Govt
• Radiography Prgm

Pinehurst

Sandhills Community College
John R Dempsey, PhD, President
3395 Airport Rd
Pinehurst, NC 28374
910 695-3700
Type: Junior or Comm Coll
Control: State, County, or Local Govt
• Clin Lab Technician/Med Lab Technician Prgm
• Polysomnographic Technology Prgm
• Radiography Prgm
• Respiratory Care Prgm
• Surgical Technology Prgm

Polkton

South Piedmont Community College
John McKay, EdD, President
PO Box 126
Polkton, NC 28135
704 272-7635
Type: Junior or Comm Coll
Control: State, County, or Local Govt
• Diagnostic Med Sonography (General) Prgm
• Medical Assistant Prgm
• Surgical Technology Prgm

Raleigh

Meredith College
John E Weems, President
Raleigh, NC 27607
919 829-8600
Type: 4-year Coll or Univ
Control: Nonprofit (Private or Religious)
• Dietetic Internship Prgm
• Dietetics-Didactic Prgm
• Music Therapy Prgm

North Carolina State University
James Oblinger, PhD, Chancellor
Holladay Hall A, Box 7001
Raleigh, NC 27695
919 515-2191
Type: 4-year Coll or Univ
Control: State, County, or Local Govt
• Counseling Prgm
• Veterinary Medicine Prgm

Shaw University
Clarence G Newsome, PhD, President
118 E South St
Raleigh, NC 27601
919 546-8330
Type: 4-year Coll or Univ
Control: Nonprofit (Private or Religious)
• Athletic Training Prgm
• Kinesiotherapy Prgm

Wake Technical Community College
Stephen Scott, EdD, President
9191 Fayetteville Rd
Raleigh, NC 27603
919 866-5141
Type: Junior or Comm Coll
Control: State, County, or Local Govt
• Clin Lab Technician/Med Lab Technician Prgm
• Dental Assistant Prgm
• Dental Hygiene Prgm
• Medical Assistant Prgm
• Phlebotomy Prgm
• Radiography Prgm
• Surgical Technology Prgm

Rocky Mount

Nash Community College
William Carver II, MBA, President
522 N Old Carriage Rd
PO Box 7488
Rocky Mount, NC 27804-0488
252 443-4011
Type: Junior or Comm Coll
Control: State, County, or Local Govt
• Medical Assistant Prgm
• Phlebotomy Prgm
• Physical Therapist Assistant Prgm

Roxboro

Piedmont Community College
Roxboro, NC 27573
Type: Junior or Comm Coll
• Medical Assistant Prgm

Salisbury

Catawba College
Craig Turner, PhD, President
2300 W Innes St
Salisbury, NC 28144
704 637-4414
Type: 4-year Coll or Univ
Control: Nonprofit (Private or Religious)
• Athletic Training Prgm

Rowan-Cabarrus Community College
Richard L Brownell, EdD, President
PO Box 1595
1333 Jake Alexander Blvd
Salisbury, NC 28145-1595
704 637-0760
Type: Junior or Comm Coll
Control: State, County, or Local Govt
• Dental Assistant Prgm
• Radiography Prgm

Sanford

Central Carolina Community College
Trelawney 'Bud' Marchant, EdD, President
1105 Kelly Dr
Sanford, NC 27330
919 775-5401
Type: Junior or Comm Coll
Control: State, County, or Local Govt
• Dental Assistant Prgm
• Dental Hygiene Prgm
• Medical Assistant Prgm (2)
• Polysomnographic Technology Prgm
• Veterinary Technology Prgm

Shelby

Cleveland Community College
L Steve Thornburg, EdD, President
137 S Post Rd
Shelby, NC 28152
704 484-4000
Type: Junior or Comm Coll
Control: State, County, or Local Govt
• Radiography Prgm

Foothills Surgical Technology Consortium
Shelby, NC 28152
Type: Junior or Comm Coll
• Surgical Technology Prgm

Siler City

Body Therapy Institute
Rick Rosen, MA LMT, Codirector
300 Southwind Rd
Siler City, NC 27344
919 663-3111
Type: Vocational or Tech Sch
Control: For Profit
• Massage Therapy Prgm

Smithfield

Johnston Community College
Donald Reichard, President
PO Box 2350
Smithfield, NC 27577
919 209-2050
Type: Junior or Comm Coll
Control: State, County, or Local Govt
• Diagnostic Med Sonography
  (Gen/Card/Vascular) Prgm
• Medical Assistant Prgm
• Radiography Prgm

Spruce Pine

Mayland Community College
Thomas Williams, EdD, President
PO Box 547
Spruce Pine, NC 28777
828 765-7351
Type: Junior or Comm Coll
Control: State, County, or Local Govt
• Medical Assistant Prgm

Statesville

Mitchell Community College
Douglas O Eason, PhD, President
West Broad St
Statesville, NC 28677
704 878-3200
Type: Junior or Comm Coll
Control: State, County, or Local Govt
• Medical Assistant Prgm

Supply

Brunswick Community College
Steven Greiner, EdD, President
PO Box 30
50 College Rd
Supply, NC 28462
910 755-7302
Type: Junior or Comm Coll
Control: State, County, or Local Govt
• Phlebotomy Prgm

Sylva

Southwestern Community College
Cecil Groves, PhD, President
447 College Dr
Sylva, NC 28779
828 586-4091
Type: Junior or Comm Coll
Control: State, County, or Local Govt
• Clin Lab Technician/Med Lab Technician Prgm
• Diagnostic Med Sonography (General) Prgm
• Emergency Med Tech-Paramedic Prgm
• Medical Assistant Prgm
• Phlebotomy Prgm
• Physical Therapist Assistant Prgm
• Radiography Prgm
• Respiratory Care Prgm

Tarboro

Edgecombe Community College
Deborah L Lamm, EdD, President
2009 W Wilson St
Tarboro, NC 27886
252 823-5166
Type: Junior or Comm Coll
Control: State, County, or Local Govt
• Medical Assistant Prgm
• Radiography Prgm
• Respiratory Care Prgm
• Surgical Technology Prgm

Thomasville

Davidson County Community College
Mary Rittling, EdD, President
PO Box 1287, 297 DCCC Road
President - Administration Bldg
Thomasville, NC 27360
336 249-8186
Type: Junior or Comm Coll
Control: State, County, or Local Govt
• Cancer Registrar Prgm
• Clin Lab Technician/Med Lab Technician Prgm
  (2)
• Histotechnician Prgm
• Medical Assistant Prgm

Troy

Montgomery Community College
Mary Kirk, EdD, President
1011 Page St
Troy, NC 27371
910 576-6222
Type: Junior or Comm Coll
Control: State, County, or Local Govt
• Dental Assistant Prgm
• Medical Assistant Prgm

Washington

Beaufort County Community College
David McLawhorn, EdD, President
PO Box 1069
Highway 264 East
Washington, NC 27889
252 940-6201
Type: Junior or Comm Coll
Control: State, County, or Local Govt
• Clin Lab Technician/Med Lab Technician Prgm

Weldon

Halifax Community College
Ervin Griffin, Interim President
PO Box 809
100 College Drive
Weldon, NC 27890
252 536-7217
Type: Junior or Comm Coll
Control: State, County, or Local Govt
• Clin Lab Technician/Med Lab Technician Prgm
• Dental Hygiene Prgm
• Phlebotomy Prgm

Wentworth

Rockingham Community College
Robert C Keys, PhD, President
PO Box 38
Rockingham Community College
Wentworth, NC 27375-0038
336 342-4261
Type: Junior or Comm Coll
Control: State, County, or Local Govt
- Phlebotomy Prgm
- Respiratory Care Prgm
- Surgical Technology Prgm

Whiteville

Southeastern Community College
Kathy Matlock, PhD, President
PO Box 151
Whiteville, NC 28472-0151
910 642-7141
Type: Junior or Comm Coll
Control: State, County, or Local Govt
- Clin Lab Technician/Med Lab Technician Prgm
- Phlebotomy Prgm

Wilkesboro

Wilkes Community College
Gordon Burns, PhD, President
1328 S Collegiate Dr
PO Box 120
Wilkesboro, NC 28697-0120
336 838-6100
Type: Junior or Comm Coll
Control: State, County, or Local Govt
- Dental Assistant Prgm
- Medical Assistant Prgm

Williamston

Martin Commuity College
Ann R Britt, EdD, President
1161 Kehukee Park Rd
Williamston, NC 27892
919 792-1521
Type: Junior or Comm Coll
Control: State, County, or Local Govt
- Dental Assistant Prgm
- Medical Assistant Prgm
- Physical Therapist Assistant Prgm

Wilmington

Cape Fear Community College
Eric B McKeithan, EdD, President
411 N Front St
Wilmington, NC 28401-3993
910 362-7555
Type: Junior or Comm Coll
Control: State, County, or Local Govt
- Dental Assistant Prgm
- Dental Hygiene Prgm
- Diagnostic Med Sonography (General) Prgm
- Occupational Therapy Asst Prgm
- Pharmacy Technician Prgm
- Phlebotomy Prgm
- Radiography Prgm
- Surgical Technology Prgm

Miller-Motte College
Ruth Hodge, BS, Executive Director
5000 Market St
Wilmington, NC 28405
910 392-4660
Type: 4-year Coll or Univ
Control: For Profit
- Dental Assistant Prgm (2)
- Medical Assistant Prgm (3)
- Surgical Technology Prgm (2)

Wilson

Barton College
Norval C Kneten, PhD, President
PO Box 5000
Wilson, NC 27893
252 399-6309
Type: 4-year Coll or Univ
Control: Nonprofit (Private or Religious)
- Athletic Training Prgm

Wilson Technical Community College
Frank L Eagles, EdD, President
904 Herring Ave
Wilson, NC 27893
252 291-1195
Type: Junior or Comm Coll
Control: State, County, or Local Govt
- Surgical Technology Prgm

Wingate

Wingate University
Jerry McGee, EdD, President
PO Box 3055
Wingate, NC 28714
704 233-8013
Type: 4-year Coll or Univ
Control: Nonprofit (Private or Religious)
- Athletic Training Prgm
- Pharmacy Prgm
- Physician Assistant Prgm

Winston-Salem

Forsyth Technical Community College
Gary M Green, EdD, President
2100 Silas Creek Pky
Winston-Salem, NC 27103
336 734-7414
Type: Junior or Comm Coll
Control: State, County, or Local Govt
- Dental Assistant Prgm
- Dental Hygiene Prgm
- Diagnostic Med Sonography (General) Prgm
- Medical Assistant Prgm
- Nuclear Medicine Technology Prgm
- Radiation Therapy Prgm
- Radiography Prgm
- Respiratory Care Prgm

Living Arts Institute at School of Comm Arts
Winston-Salem, NC 27103-3217
Type: Vocational or Tech Sch
- Medical Assistant Prgm

Wake Forest University
Nathan Hatch, PhD, President
7622 Reynolda Station
Winston-Salem, NC 27109
910 759-5000
Type: 4-year Coll or Univ
Control: Nonprofit (Private or Religious)
- Counseling Prgm

Wake Forest University Baptist Medical Center
Donny Lambeth
Medical Center Blvd
Winston-Salem, NC 27157-1072
336 716-3003
Type: Acad Health Ctr/Med Sch
Control: Nonprofit (Private or Religious)
- Clin Lab Scientist/Med Technologist Prgm

Wake Forest University School of Medicine
William Applegate, MD MPH, Interim
President/Dean
Medical Center Blvd
Winston-Salem, NC 27157
336 716-4424
Type: Acad Health Ctr/Med Sch
Control: Nonprofit (Private or Religious)
- Allopathic Medicine Prgm
- Physician Assistant Prgm

Winston-Salem State University
Donald J Reaves, PhD, Interim Chancellor
601 Martin Luther King Jr Dr
Blair Hall 200
Winston-Salem, NC 27100
336 750-2000
Type: 4-year Coll or Univ
Control: State, County, or Local Govt
- Clin Lab Scientist/Med Technologist Prgm
- Nursing Prgm
- Occupational Therapy Prgm
- Physical Therapy Prgm
- Rehabilitation Counseling Prgm

North Dakota

Belcourt

Turtle Mountain Community College
Gerald Monette, EdD, President
PO Box 340
Belcourt, ND 58316
701 477-5605
Type: Junior or Comm Coll
Control: Nonprofit (Private or Religious)
- Clin Lab Technician/Med Lab Technician Prgm
- Phlebotomy Prgm

Bismarck

Bismarck State College
Larry Skogen, PhD, President
PO Box 5587
1500 Edwards Ave
Bismarck, ND 58506-5587
701 224-5431
Type: Junior or Comm Coll
Control: State, County, or Local Govt
- Clin Lab Technician/Med Lab Technician Prgm
- Phlebotomy Prgm
- Surgical Technology Prgm

Medcenter One
James Cooper, President/CEO
300 N Seventh St
Bismarck, ND 58506-5525
701 323-6104
Type: Hosp or Med Ctr: 100-299 Beds
Control: Nonprofit (Private or Religious)
• Nursing Prgm
• Radiography Prgm

St Alexius Med Ctr/Bismarck State College
Bismarck, ND 58506-5587
Type: Consortium
Control: Other
• Emergency Med Tech-Paramedic Prgm

University of Mary
Sister Thomas Welder, OSB MM, President
7500 University Dr
Bismarck, ND 58504-9652
701 355-8100
Type: 4-year Coll or Univ
Control: Nonprofit (Private or Religious)
• Athletic Training Prgm
• Exercise Science Prgm
• Nursing Prgm
• Occupational Therapy Prgm
• Physical Therapy Prgm

University of Mary/St Alexius Medical Ctr
Richard A Tschider, MA, Administrator
PO Box 5510
Bismarck, ND 58506-5510
701 224-7600
Type: Hosp or Med Ctr: 100-299 Beds
Control: Nonprofit (Private or Religious)
• Respiratory Care Prgm

Fargo

NDSU/Sanford Health Consortium
Gary Lee, BA RRT, CEO
MeritCare Hospital
PO Box MC
Fargo, ND 58122-0118
701 234-5190
Type: Consortium
Control: State, County, or Local Govt
• Phlebotomy Prgm
• Respiratory Care Prgm

North Dakota State University
Joseph Chapman, PhD, President
PO Box 5167
Fargo, ND 58105-5167
701 231-8011
Type: 4-year Coll or Univ
Control: State, County, or Local Govt
• Athletic Training Prgm
• Counseling Prgm
• Dietetics-Coordinated Prgm
• Dietetics-Didactic Prgm
• Exercise Science Prgm
• Nursing Prgm
• Pharmacy Prgm
• Veterinary Technology Prgm

Sanford Medical Center/Sanford Health
Roger Gilbertson, MD, President
801 N Broadway
PO Box MC
Fargo, ND 58122
701 234-6954
Type: Hosp or Med Ctr: 500 Beds
Control: Nonprofit (Private or Religious)
• Clin Lab Scientist/Med Technologist Prgm
• Radiography Prgm

Grand Forks

University of North Dakota
Robert Kelley, PhD, President
300 Twamley Hall
264 Centennial Dr Stop 8193
Grand Forks, ND 58202-8193
701 777-2121
Type: 4-year Coll or Univ
Control: State, County, or Local Govt
• Allopathic Medicine Prgm
• Athletic Training Prgm
• Clin Lab Scientist/Med Technologist Prgm
• Cytotechnology Prgm
• Dietetics-Coordinated Prgm
• Histotechnician Prgm
• Music Therapy Prgm
• Nursing Prgm
• Occupational Therapy Prgm
• Physical Therapy Prgm
• Physician Assistant Prgm
• Psychology (PhD) Prgm
• Speech-Language Pathology Prgm

Minot

Minot State University
David Fuller, President
500 University Ave W
Minot, ND 58707
701 858-3031
Type: 4-year Coll or Univ
Control: State, County, or Local Govt
• Music Therapy Prgm
• Speech-Language Pathology Prgm

Trinity Health
Terry G Hoff, FCHA, President
1 Burdick Expwy West
Minot, ND 58701
701 857-5000
Type: Hosp or Med Ctr: 100-299 Beds
Control: Nonprofit (Private or Religious)
• Radiography Prgm

Wahpeton

F-M Ambulance-North Dakota State
Wahpeton, ND 58076
Type: Consortium
Control: Other
• Emergency Med Tech-Paramedic Prgm

North Dakota State College of Science
John Richman, PhD, President
800 N Sixth St
Wahpeton, ND 58076-0002
701 671-2221
Type: Junior or Comm Coll
Control: State, County, or Local Govt
• Dental Assistant Prgm
• Dental Hygiene Prgm
• Occupational Therapy Asst Prgm
• Pharmacy Technician Prgm

Williston

Williston State College
Joseph McCann, PhD, President
1410 University Ave
PO Box 1326
Williston, ND 58802-1326
701 774-4200
Type: Junior or Comm Coll
Control: State, County, or Local Govt
• Physical Therapist Assistant Prgm

Northwest Territories, Canada

Yellowknife

Stanton Territorial Health Authority
Goga Cho Building, 47th Street
P.O. Box 10
Yellowknife, NT X1A 2N1
Type: Acad Health Ctr/Med Sch
Control: For Profit
• Ophthalmic Med Technologist Prgm

Nova Scotia, Canada

Halifax

Dalhousie University
Tom Traves, President
Halifax, NS B3H 3J5
902 424-2511
Type: 4-year Coll or Univ
Control: State, County, or Local Govt
• Allopathic Medicine Prgm
• Medical Librarian Prgm

IWK Health Centre
5850 University Ave
PO Box 3070
Halifax, NS B3J 3G9
Type: Hosp or Med Ctr: 500 Beds
Control: State, County, or Local Govt
• Ophthalmic Med Technologist Prgm
• Orthoptist Prgm

Ohio

Ada

Ohio Northern University
Kendall Baker, PhD, President
525 S Main St
Ada, OH 45810
419 772-2000
Type: 4-year Coll or Univ
Control: Nonprofit (Private or Religious)
• Athletic Training Prgm
• Clin Lab Scientist/Med Technologist Prgm
• Exercise Science Prgm
• Nursing Prgm
• Pharmacy Prgm

Akron

Akron Children's Hospital
William H Considine, MHA, President
One Perkins Square
Akron, OH 44308-1062
330 543-8293
Type: Hosp or Med Ctr: 100-299 Beds
Control: Nonprofit (Private or Religious)
• Clin Lab Scientist/Med Technologist Prgm
• Radiography Prgm

Akron General Medical Center
Alan Bleyer, MHA, President
400 Wabash Ave
Akron, OH 44307
330 846-6548
Type: Hosp or Med Ctr: 500 Beds
Control: Nonprofit (Private or Religious)
• Emergency Med Tech-Paramedic Prgm

Akron Institute of Herzing College
David LaRue, Campus President
1600 S Arlington Ste 100
Akron, OH 44306
330 724-1600
Type: Vocational or Tech Sch
Control: For Profit
• Clin Lab Technician/Med Lab Technician Prgm
• Medical Assistant Prgm

Brown Mackie College - Akron
Kimberly Ames, MA, Campus President
755 White Pond Drive
Akron, OH 44320
330 869-3600
• Occupational Therapy Asst Prgm
• Surgical Technology Prgm

Summa Health System
Thomas Strauss, PhD, President and CEO
525 E Market St
PO Box 2090
Akron, OH 44309-2090
330 375-3000
Type: Hosp or Med Ctr: 500 Beds
Control: Nonprofit (Private or Religious)
• Emergency Med Tech-Paramedic Prgm

The University of Akron
Luis M Proenza, PhD, President
Buchtel Hall 114
Akron, OH 44325-4702
330 972-7074
Type: 4-year Coll or Univ
Control: State, County, or Local Govt
• Athletic Training Prgm
• Counseling Prgm
• Dietetics-Coordinated Prgm
• Dietetics-Didactic Prgm
• Medical Assistant Prgm
• Music Therapy Prgm
• Nursing Prgm
• Respiratory Care Prgm
• Speech-Language Pathology Prgm
• Surgical Technology Prgm

Alliance

University of Mount Union
Richard F Giese, PhD, President
1972 Clark Ave
Alliance, OH 44601
330 823-6050
Type: 4-year Coll or Univ
Control: Nonprofit (Private or Religious)
• Athletic Training Prgm
• Physician Assistant Prgm

Archbold

Northwest State Community College
Betty Young, PhD, President
22600 State Route 34
Archbold, OH 43502
419 267-1365
Type: Junior or Comm Coll
Control: State, County, or Local Govt
• Medical Assistant Prgm

Ashland

Ashland County - West Holmes Career Center
Michael McDaniel, BS MS, Superintendent
1783 State Rte 60
Ashland, OH 44805
419 289-3313
Type: Vocational or Tech Sch
Control: For Profit
• Medical Assistant Prgm

Ashland University
Fred Finks, DMin, President
205 Founders Hall
Ashland, OH 44805
419 289-5050
Type: 4-year Coll or Univ
Control: Nonprofit (Private or Religious)
• Athletic Training Prgm
• Dietetics-Didactic Prgm
• Nursing Prgm

Athens

Ohio University
Roderick McDavis, PhD, President
Cutler Hall 108
Athens, OH 45701
740 593-1804
Type: 4-year Coll or Univ
Control: State, County, or Local Govt
• Athletic Training Prgm
• Audiologist Prgm
• Counseling Prgm
• Dietetics-Didactic Prgm
• Medical Assistant Prgm
• Music Therapy Prgm
• Nursing Prgm
• Osteopathic Medicine Prgm
• Physical Therapy Prgm
• Psychology (PhD) Prgm
• Rehabilitation Counseling Prgm
• Speech-Language Pathology Prgm

Batavia

Univ of Cincinnati - Clermont College
David H Devier, PhD, Dean
4200 Clermont College Dr
Batavia, OH 45103
513 732-5209
Type: Junior or Comm Coll
Control: State, County, or Local Govt
• Medical Assistant Prgm
• Surgical Assistant Prgm
• Surgical Technology Prgm

Berea

Baldwin-Wallace College
Dick Durst, MFA, President
275 Eastland Rd
Berea, OH 44017
440 826-2424
Type: 4-year Coll or Univ
Control: For Profit
• Athletic Training Prgm
• Music Therapy Prgm

Bluffton

Bluffton College
Elmer Neufeld, President
280 W College Ave
Bluffton, OH 45817
419 358-3000
Type: 4-year Coll or Univ
Control: Nonprofit (Private or Religious)
• Dietetics-Didactic Prgm

Bowling Green

Bowling Green State University
Carol Cartwright, President
220 McFall Ctr
Bowling Green, OH 43403
419 372-2211
Type: 4-year Coll or Univ
Control: State, County, or Local Govt
• Athletic Training Prgm
• Clin Lab Scientist/Med Technologist Prgm
• Dietetic Internship Prgm
• Dietetics-Didactic Prgm
• Music Therapy Prgm
• Nursing Prgm
• Psychology (PhD) Prgm
• Rehabilitation Counseling Prgm
• Respiratory Care Prgm
• Speech-Language Pathology Prgm

Canfield

Mahoning County Career & Technical Center
Roan Craig, PhD, Superintendent
7300 N Palmyra Rd
Canfield, OH 44406-9710
330 729-4100
Type: Vocational or Tech Sch
Control: State, County, or Local Govt
• Medical Assistant Prgm

Canton

Aultman College of Nursing and Health Science
Edward Roth, MBA, President
2600 Sixth St SW
Canton, OH 44710
330 438-6241
Type: Hosp or Med Ctr: 500 Beds
Control: Nonprofit (Private or Religious)
• Radiography Prgm

Canton City Schools
Dianne Talarico, Superintendent
617 McKinley Ave SW
Canton, OH 44707
330 438-2530
Type: Vocational or Tech Sch
Control: State, County, or Local Govt
• Medical Assistant Prgm

Malone College
Canton, OH 44709
Type: 4-year Coll or Univ
Control: Nonprofit (Private or Religious)
• Nursing Prgm

Mercy Medical Center
Thomas E Cecconi, President/CEO
1320 Mercy Dr NW
Canton, OH 44708
330 489-1001
Type: Hosp or Med Ctr: 500 Beds
Control: Nonprofit (Private or Religious)
• Diagnostic Med Sonography (General) Prgm
• Radiography Prgm

Cedarville

Cedarville University
William Brown, PhD, President
251 N Main St
Cedarville, OH 45314
937 766-7900
Type: 4-year Coll or Univ
Control: Nonprofit (Private or Religious)
• Athletic Training Prgm
• Nursing Prgm
• Pharmacy Prgm

Centerville

Fortis College- Centerville
Centerville, OH 45459
Type: Vocational or Tech Sch
• Medical Assistant Prgm

Chesapeake

Collins Career Center
Steve Dodgion, BA MSEd, Superintendent
11627 St Rte 243
Chesapeake, OH 45619
740 867-6641
Type: Vocational or Tech Sch
Control: Nonprofit (Private or Religious)
• Diagnostic Med Sonography (General/Vascular) Prgm
• Pharmacy Technician Prgm
• Phlebotomy Prgm
• Radiography Prgm
• Respiratory Care Prgm
• Surgical Technology Prgm

Chillicothe

Pickaway Ross Joint Vocational School
Brett Smith, Superintendent
895 Crouse Chapel Rd
Chillicothe, OH 45601-9010
740 642-2111
Type: Vocational or Tech Sch
Control: State, County, or Local Govt
• Medical Assistant Prgm

Cincinnati

Brown Mackie College
Richard Thome, MS, President
2791 Mogadore Rd
Cincinnati, OH 45215
513 771-2424
Type: Junior or Comm Coll
Control: For Profit
• Medical Assistant Prgm (3)
• Occupational Therapy Asst Prgm
• Surgical Technology Prgm

Christ Hospital
Susan Croushore, Senior Executive Officer
2139 Auburn Ave
Cincinnati, OH 45219
513 585-1399
Type: Hosp or Med Ctr: 300-499 Beds
Control: Nonprofit (Private or Religious)
• Dietetic Internship Prgm

Cincinnati Children's Hospital Medical Center
Nancy L Zimpher, President
3333 Burnet Ave
Cincinnati, OH 45229
513 556-2201
Type: Hosp or Med Ctr: 300-499 Beds
Control: Nonprofit (Private or Religious)
• Genetic Counseling Prgm

Cincinnati School of Medical Massage
111250 Cornell Park Dr, Ste 203
Cincinnati, OH 45242
Type: Vocational or Tech Sch
Control: For Profit
• Massage Therapy Prgm

Cincinnati State Tech & Comm College
O'dell Owens, MD, President
3520 Central Pkwy
Cincinnati, OH 45223
513 569-1515
Type: Junior or Comm Coll
Control: State, County, or Local Govt
• Clin Lab Technician/Med Lab Technician Prgm
• Diagnostic Med Sonography (Gen/Card/Vascular) Prgm
• Dietetic Technician-AD Prgm
• Medical Assistant Prgm
• Occupational Therapy Asst Prgm
• Respiratory Care Prgm
• Surgical Technology Prgm

Good Samaritan Hospital
375 Dixmyth Ave
Cincinnati, OH 45220-2489
513 872-1983
Type: Hosp or Med Ctr: 500 Beds
Control: Nonprofit (Private or Religious)
• Dietetic Internship Prgm

National College - Cincinnati
Cincinnati, OH 45237
Type: Junior or Comm Coll
• Surgical Technology Prgm

UC Raymond Walters College
Nancy Zimpher, PhD, President
PO Box 210063
Cincinnati, OH 45221-0063
513 745-5600
Type: Junior or Comm Coll
Control: State, County, or Local Govt
• Veterinary Technology Prgm

University of Cincinnati
Monica Rimai, President
PO Box 210063
Cincinnati, OH 45221-0063
513 556-2201
Type: 4-year Coll or Univ
Control: State, County, or Local Govt
- Allopathic Medicine Prgm
- Athletic Training Prgm
- Audiologist Prgm
- Clin Lab Scientist/Med Technologist Prgm
- Counseling Prgm
- Dental Hygiene Prgm
- Dietetics-Coordinated Prgm
- Dietetics-Didactic Prgm
- Emergency Med Tech-Paramedic Prgm
- Medical Assistant Prgm
- Nuclear Medicine Technology Prgm
- Nursing Prgm
- Pharmacy Prgm
- Physical Therapist Assistant Prgm
- Physical Therapy Prgm
- Psychology (PhD) Prgm
- Radiation Therapy Prgm
- Radiography Prgm
- Speech-Language Pathology Prgm

University of Cincinnati Medical Center
Nancy Zimpher, PhD, President
Admin Bldg
Cincinnati, OH 45221-0063
513 558-2201
Type: Acad Health Ctr/Med Sch
Control: State, County, or Local Govt
- Specialist in BB Tech Prgm

Xavier University
Michael J Graham, SJ PhD, President
3800 Victory Pkwy
Cincinnati, OH 45207-4511
513 745-3501
Type: 4-year Coll or Univ
Control: Nonprofit (Private or Religious)
- Athletic Training Prgm
- Counseling Prgm
- Music Therapy Prgm
- Nursing Prgm
- Occupational Therapy Prgm
- Psychology (PsyD) Prgm
- Radiography Prgm

Clayton

Miami Valley Career Technology Center
John Boggess, PhD, Superintendent
6800 Hoke Rd
Clayton, OH 45315
937 854-6272
Type: Vocational or Tech Sch
Control: State, County, or Local Govt
- Medical Assistant Prgm

Cleveland

Case Western Reserve University
Edward Hundert, President
University Circle
Cleveland, OH 44106
216 368-2000
Type: Acad Health Ctr/Med Sch
Control: Nonprofit (Private or Religious)
- Allopathic Medicine Prgm
- Anesthesiologist Asst Prgm
- Dentistry Prgm
- Dietetic Internship Prgm
- Dietetics-Didactic Prgm
- Genetic Counseling Prgm
- Music Therapy Prgm
- Psychology (PhD) Prgm
- Speech-Language Pathology Prgm

Cleveland Clinic Foundation
Delos M Cosgrove, MD, Chairman
9500 Euclid Ave H18
Cleveland, OH 44195-5108
216 445-2500
Type: Hosp or Med Ctr: 500 Beds
Control: Nonprofit (Private or Religious)
- Clin Lab Scientist/Med Technologist Prgm
- Dietetic Internship Prgm
- Medical Dosimetry Prgm
- Perfusion Prgm

Cleveland State University
Ronald Berkman, PhD, President
2121 Euclid Ave
Administration Center 302
Cleveland, OH 44115-2440
216 687-3544
Type: 4-year Coll or Univ
Control: State, County, or Local Govt
- Counseling Prgm
- Music Therapy Prgm
- Nursing Prgm
- Occupational Therapy Prgm
- Physical Therapy Prgm
- Speech-Language Pathology Prgm

Cuyahoga Community College
Jerry Sue Thornton, PhD, President
700 Carnegie Ave
CCC District Office
Cleveland, OH 44115-3196
216 987-4850
Type: Junior or Comm Coll
Control: State, County, or Local Govt
- Clin Lab Technician/Med Lab Technician Prgm
- Dental Hygiene Prgm
- Diagnostic Med Sonography (Gen/Card/Vascular) Prgm
- Dietetic Technician-AD Prgm
- Medical Assistant Prgm
- Neurodiagnostic Tech Prgm
- Nuclear Medicine Technology Prgm
- Occupational Therapy Asst Prgm
- Pharmacy Technician Prgm
- Phlebotomy Prgm
- Physical Therapist Assistant Prgm
- Physician Assistant Prgm
- Polysomnographic Technology Prgm
- Radiography Prgm
- Respiratory Care Prgm
- Surgical Technology Prgm
- Veterinary Technology Prgm

John Carroll University
20700 N Park Blvd
Cleveland, OH 44118-4581
216 397-1886
Type: 4-year Coll or Univ
Control: Nonprofit (Private or Religious)
- Counseling Prgm

Louis Stokes Cleveland VA Med Ctr
10701 East Blvd
Cleveland, OH 44106-1702
216 421-3028
Type: Acad Health Ctr/Med Sch
Control: Fed Govt
- Dietetic Internship Prgm

MetroHealth Medical Center
Terry R White, MBA, President/CEO
2500 Metro Health Dr
Cleveland, OH 44109-1998
216 459-5700
Type: Hosp or Med Ctr: 500 Beds
Control: State, County, or Local Govt
- Dietetic Internship Prgm

Ohio College of Podiatric Medicine
Thomas V Melitto, DPM
10515 Carnegie Ave
Cleveland, OH 44106
216 231-3300
Type: Acad Health Ctr/Med Sch
Control: Nonprofit (Private or Religious)
- Podiatric Medicine Prgm

University Hospitals Case Medical Center
Farah M Walters, MS, President/CEO
11100 Euclid Ave
Cleveland, OH 44106
216 844-7565
Type: Hosp or Med Ctr: 500 Beds
Control: Nonprofit (Private or Religious)
- Dietetic Internship Prgm

Columbus

American Red Cross Blood Services
Ambrose Ng, MD, Chief Executive Officer
995 E Broad St
Columbus, OH 43205
614 253-2740
Type: Nonhosp HC Facil, BB, or Lab
Control: Nonprofit (Private or Religious)
- Specialist in BB Tech Prgm

American School of Technology
Susan Stella, BS BA, Director
2100 Morse Rd
Columbus, OH 43229
614 436-4820
Type: Vocational or Tech Sch
Control: For Profit
- Medical Assistant Prgm

Bradford School
Dennis Bartels, President
2469 Stelzer Rd
Columbus, OH 43219
614 416-6200
Type: Vocational or Tech Sch
Control: For Profit
- Medical Assistant Prgm
- Veterinary Technology Prgm

Capital University
Denvy Bowman, PhD, President
Yochum Hall
1 College & Main
Columbus, OH 43209
614 236-6908
Type: 4-year Coll or Univ
Control: Nonprofit (Private or Religious)
• Athletic Training Prgm
• Music Therapy Prgm
• Nursing Prgm

Columbus State Community College
David T Harrison, PhD, President
550 E Spring St, 120 Franklin Hall
PO Box 1609
Columbus, OH 43216-1609
614 287-2402
Type: Junior or Comm Coll
Control: State, County, or Local Govt
• Clin Lab Technician/Med Lab Technician Prgm
• Dental Hygiene Prgm
• Dietetic Technician-AD Prgm
• Emergency Med Tech-Paramedic Prgm
• Histotechnician Prgm
• Medical Assistant Prgm
• Phlebotomy Prgm
• Radiography Prgm
• Respiratory Care Prgm
• Surgical Technology Prgm
• Veterinary Technology Prgm

Mt Carmel College of Nursing
Ann E Schiele, President
127 S Davis Ave
Columbus, OH 43222
614 234-5032
Type: 4-year Coll or Univ
Control: Nonprofit (Private or Religious)
• Dietetic Internship Prgm
• Nursing Prgm

Sleep Care Inc
Craig Pickerill, RPSGT, President
7634 Rivers Edge Dr
Columbus, OH 43235
614 901-8989
Type: Nonhosp HC Facil, BB, or Lab
Control: For Profit
• Polysomnographic Technology Prgm

The Ohio State University
Gordon E Gee, JD EdD, President
190 N Oval Mall
205 Bricker Hall
Columbus, OH 43210-1357
614 292-2424
Type: 4-year Coll or Univ
Control: State, County, or Local Govt
• Allopathic Medicine Prgm
• Athletic Training Prgm
• Audiologist Prgm
• Clin Lab Scientist/Med Technologist Prgm
• Dental Hygiene Prgm
• Dentistry Prgm
• Dietetic Internship Prgm (2)
• Dietetics-Coordinated Prgm
• Dietetics-Didactic Prgm
• Nursing Prgm
• Occupational Therapy Prgm
• Optometry Prgm
• Pharmacy Prgm
• Physical Therapy Prgm
• Psychology (PhD) Prgm
• Radiation Therapy Prgm
• Radiologist Assistant Prgm
• Respiratory Care Prgm
• Speech-Language Pathology Prgm
• Veterinary Medicine Prgm

Wexner Medical Center at Ohio State Univ
Wiley "Chip" Souba, MD ScD, CEO - Interim
370 West 9th Ave
370 West 9th Ave
Columbus, OH 43210
614 292-2600
Type: Hosp or Med Ctr: 300-499 Beds
Control: State, County, or Local Govt
• Nuclear Medicine Technology Prgm

Cuyahoga Falls

Fortis College
Cuyahoga Falls, OH 44221
• Dental Assistant Prgm

Dayton

Community Blood Center/Community Tissue Svc
David Smith, MD, CEO
349 South Main St
Dayton, OH 45402
937 461-3610
Type: Nonhosp HC Facil, BB, or Lab
Control: Nonprofit (Private or Religious)
• Specialist in BB Tech Prgm

Dayton School of Medical Message
4457 Far Hills Ave
Dayton, OH 45429
Type: Vocational or Tech Sch
Control: Nonprofit (Private or Religious)
• Massage Therapy Prgm (2)

Kaplan College - Dayton
Dayton, OH 45439
Type: Vocational or Tech Sch
• Medical Assistant Prgm

Miami Valley Hospital
Karl R Tague, President/CEO
One Wyoming St
Dayton, OH 45409
513 223-6192
Type: Hosp or Med Ctr: 500 Beds
Control: Nonprofit (Private or Religious)
• Dietetic Internship Prgm

Miami-Jacobs Career College
Darlene Waite, MBA, President
110 N Patterson Ave
PO Box 1433
Dayton, OH 45402
937 461-5174
Type: Junior or Comm Coll
Control: For Profit
• Dental Assistant Prgm
• Medical Assistant Prgm
• Surgical Technology Prgm

Ohio Institute of Photography & Technology
Robert A Martin, BS, Executive Director
2029 Edgefield Rd
Dayton, OH 45439
937 294-6155
Type: Vocational or Tech Sch
Control: For Profit
• Medical Assistant Prgm

Sinclair Community College
Steven Lee Johnson, PhD, President
444 W Third St
Dayton, OH 45402-1460
937 512-2525
Type: Junior or Comm Coll
Control: State, County, or Local Govt
• Dental Hygiene Prgm
• Dietetic Technician-AD Prgm
• Medical Assistant Prgm
• Occupational Therapy Asst Prgm
• Personal Fitness Training Prgm
• Physical Therapist Assistant Prgm
• Radiography Prgm
• Respiratory Care Prgm
• Surgical Technology Prgm

University of Dayton
Raymond Fitz, PhD SM, President
300 College Pk
Dayton, OH 45469-1624
937 229-1000
Type: 4-year Coll or Univ
Control: Nonprofit (Private or Religious)
• Counseling Prgm
• Dietetics-Didactic Prgm
• Music Therapy Prgm
• Physical Therapy Prgm

Wright State University
David Hopkins, PhD, President
3640 Colonel Glenn Hwy
University Hall 260A, Wright State Unive
Dayton, OH 45435
937 775-2312
Type: 4-year Coll or Univ
Control: State, County, or Local Govt
• Allopathic Medicine Prgm
• Athletic Training Prgm
• Clin Lab Scientist/Med Technologist Prgm
• Counseling Prgm
• Nursing Prgm
• Psychology (PsyD) Prgm
• Rehabilitation Counseling Prgm

Defiance

Defiance College
Charles O Warren, PhD, Interim President
701 N Clinton St
Defiance, OH 43512
419 783-2300
Type: 4-year Coll or Univ
Control: Nonprofit (Private or Religious)
• Athletic Training Prgm
• Nursing Prgm

East Liverpool

Ohio Valley College of Technology
Debra A Sanford, BS, President
16808 St Clair Ave
PO Box 7000
East Liverpool, OH 43920
330 385-1070
Type: Vocational or Tech Sch
Control: For Profit
• Medical Assistant Prgm

Elyria

Lorain County Community College
Roy A Church, EdD, President
1005 N Abbe Rd
Elyria, OH 44035
440 366-4050
Type: Junior or Comm Coll
Control: State, County, or Local Govt
• Clin Lab Technician/Med Lab Technician Prgm
• Dental Hygiene Prgm
• Diagnostic Med Sonography (General) Prgm
• Medical Assistant Prgm
• Phlebotomy Prgm
• Physical Therapist Assistant Prgm
• Radiography Prgm
• Surgical Technology Prgm

Fairlawn

Medical Transcription Education Center, Inc.
3634 W Market St
Ste 103
Fairlawn, OH 44333
Type: Acad Health Ctr/Med Sch
Control: For Profit
• Medical Transcriptionist Prgm

Findlay

Brown Mackie College - Findlay
Wayne Korpics, MA, Campus President
1700 Fostoria Avenue
Findlay, OH 45840
419 429-8616
• Occupational Therapy Asst Prgm
• Surgical Technology Prgm

The University of Findlay
Katherine Fell, PhD, President
1000 North Main St
Findlay, OH 45840
419 434-4510
Type: 4-year Coll or Univ
Control: Nonprofit (Private or Religious)
• Athletic Training Prgm
• Nuclear Medicine Technology Prgm
• Occupational Therapy Prgm
• Pharmacy Prgm
• Physical Therapy Prgm
• Physician Assistant Prgm

Granville

Denison University
Dale T Knobel, PhD, President
Doane Hall
Granville, OH 43023
740 587-6281
Type: 4-year Coll or Univ
Control: Nonprofit (Private or Religious)
• Athletic Training Prgm

Green

Portage Lakes Career Center
Mark Lukens, MA, Superintendent
4401 Shriver Rd
PO Box 248
Green, OH 44232-0248
330 896-8200
Type: Vocational or Tech Sch
Control: State, County, or Local Govt
• Medical Assistant Prgm

Groveport

Fairfield Career Center (EVSD)
Mark Weedy, MEd, Superintendent
4465 S Hamilton Rd
Groveport, OH 43125
614 836-5725
Type: Vocational or Tech Sch
Control: State, County, or Local Govt
• Medical Assistant Prgm

Hillsboro

Southern State Community College
Lawrence N Dukes, EdD, President
100 Hobart Dr
Hillsboro, OH 45133
937 393-3431
Type: Junior or Comm Coll
Control: State, County, or Local Govt
• Medical Assistant Prgm

Hiram

Hiram College
Hiram, OH 44234
Type: 4-year Coll or Univ
Control: Nonprofit (Private or Religious)
• Nursing Prgm

Kent

Kent State University
Lester Lefton, PhD, President
Executive Office, Second Floor
Kent, OH 44242-0001
330 672-2210
Type: 4-year Coll or Univ
Control: State, County, or Local Govt
• Athletic Training Prgm
• Audiologist Prgm
• Counseling Prgm
• Dietetic Internship Prgm
• Dietetics-Didactic Prgm
• Exercise Science Prgm
• Medical Librarian Prgm
• Music Therapy Prgm
• Nuclear Medicine Technology Prgm
• Nursing Prgm
• Occupational Therapy Asst Prgm (2)
• Physical Therapist Assistant Prgm (2)
• Psychology (PhD) Prgm
• Radiation Therapy Prgm
• Radiography Prgm (2)
• Rehabilitation Counseling Prgm
• Speech-Language Pathology Prgm

Kettering

Kettering College of Medical Arts
Charles Scriven, PhD, President
3737 Southern Blvd
Kettering, OH 45429
937 298-3399
Type: 4-year Coll or Univ
Control: For Profit
• Diagnostic Med Sonography
  (Gen/Card/Vascular) Prgm
• Physician Assistant Prgm
• Radiography Prgm
• Respiratory Care Prgm

Kirtland

Lakeland Community College
Morris Beverage, Jr, EdM, President
7700 Clocktower Dr
Kirtland, OH 44094
440 525-7177
Type: Junior or Comm Coll
Control: State, County, or Local Govt
• Clin Lab Technician/Med Lab Technician Prgm
• Dental Hygiene Prgm
• Histotechnician Prgm
• Medical Assistant Prgm
• Radiography Prgm
• Respiratory Care Prgm
• Surgical Technology Prgm

LaGrange

Life Care EMS Training Academy
LaGrange, OH 44050
Type: Consortium
• Emergency Med Tech-Paramedic Prgm

Lima

Apollo Career Center
J Chris Pfister, Superintendent
3325 Shawnee Rd
Lima, OH 45806
479 998-2911
Type: Vocational or Tech Sch
Control: State, County, or Local Govt
• Medical Assistant Prgm

Rhodes State College
Debra McCurdy, PhD, President
4240 Campus Dr
Lima, OH 45804
419 995-8200
Type: Junior or Comm Coll
Control: State, County, or Local Govt
• Dental Hygiene Prgm
• Occupational Therapy Asst Prgm
• Physical Therapist Assistant Prgm
• Radiography Prgm
• Respiratory Care Prgm

University of Northwestern Ohio
Loren R Jarvis, LLD, President
1441 N Cable Rd
Lima, OH 45805
419 227-3141
Type: 4-year Coll or Univ
Control: Nonprofit (Private or Religious)
• Medical Assistant Prgm

Lucasville

Scioto County Career Technical Center
Stan Jennings, MS, Superintendent
951 Vern Riffe Dr
Lucasville, OH 45648
740 259-5526
Type: Vocational or Tech Sch
Control: State, County, or Local Govt
• Surgical Technology Prgm

Mansfield

North Central State College
Don Plotts, ME, President
2441 Kenwood Circle
PO Box 698
Mansfield, OH 44901-0698
419 755-4758
Type: Vocational or Tech Sch
Control: State, County, or Local Govt
• Occupational Therapy Asst Prgm
• Physical Therapist Assistant Prgm
• Radiography Prgm
• Respiratory Care Prgm

Marietta

Marietta College
Jean Scott, PhD, President
215 Fifth St
Marietta, OH 45750
740 376-4701
Type: 4-year Coll or Univ
Control: Nonprofit (Private or Religious)
• Athletic Training Prgm
• Physician Assistant Prgm

Marietta Memorial Hospital
Larry J Unroe, MHA, President
401 Matthew St
Marietta, OH 45750
740 374-1411
Type: Hosp or Med Ctr: 100-299 Beds
Control: Nonprofit (Private or Religious)
• Radiography Prgm

Washington County Career Center
DeWayne O Poling, MA, Director
1750 Lancaster St
Marietta, OH 45750
740 373-6283
Type: Vocational or Tech Sch
Control: State, County, or Local Govt
• Medical Assistant Prgm
• Surgical Technology Prgm

Washington State Community College
Charlotte Hatfield, PhD, President
710 Colegate Dr
Marietta, OH 45750
740 374-8716
Type: Junior or Comm Coll
Control: State, County, or Local Govt
• Clin Lab Technician/Med Lab Technician Prgm
• Physical Therapist Assistant Prgm
• Respiratory Care Prgm

Marion

Marion Technical College
J Richard Bryson, PhD, President
1467 Mt Vernon Ave
Marion, OH 43302-5694
740 389-4636
Type: Vocational or Tech Sch
Control: Nonprofit (Private or Religious)
• Clin Lab Technician/Med Lab Technician Prgm
• Medical Assistant Prgm
• Occupational Therapy Asst Prgm
• Physical Therapist Assistant Prgm
• Radiography Prgm

Maumee

Stautzenberger College
George Simon, President
1796 Indian Wood Circle
Maumee, OH 43537
800 552-5099
Type: Vocational or Tech Sch
Control: For Profit
• Medical Assistant Prgm
• Veterinary Technology Prgm (2)

Mayfield Heights

Cleveland Clinic Health System
Fred DeGrandis, CEO, Western Region
6803 Mayfield Rd
Ste 500, Bldg 1
Mayfield Heights, OH 44124
440 312-8720
Type: Hosp or Med Ctr: 500 Beds
Control: Nonprofit (Private or Religious)
• Radiography Prgm

Medina

Medina County Career Center
Thomas Horwedel, MEd, Superintendent
1101 W Liberty St
Medina, OH 44256-9969
216 725-8461
Type: Vocational or Tech Sch
Control: State, County, or Local Govt
• Medical Assistant Prgm

Middleburg Heights

Cleveland Institute of Medical Massage
18334-D E Bagley Rd
Middleburg Heights, OH 44130
Type: Vocational or Tech Sch
Control: Nonprofit (Private or Religious)
• Massage Therapy Prgm

Polaris Career Center
Bob Timmons, MA, Superintendent
7285 Old Oak Blvd
Middleburg Heights, OH 44130
440 891-7600
Type: Vocational or Tech Sch
Control: Nonprofit (Private or Religious)
• Medical Assistant Prgm

Sanford-Brown College
Christine Smith, BS, President
17535 Rosbough Dr
Ste 100
Middleburg Heights, OH 44130
440 202-3223
Type: Vocational or Tech Sch
Control: For Profit
• Cardiovascular Tech (Echocardiography) Prgm
• Diagnostic Med Sonography (General) Prgm
• Radiography Prgm

Southwest General Health Center
Thomas Seldon, MA, President, CEO
18697 Bagley Rd
Middleburg Heights, OH 44130
440 816-8000
Type: Hosp or Med Ctr: 300-499 Beds
Control: Nonprofit (Private or Religious)
• Clin Lab Scientist/Med Technologist Prgm

Milan

EHOVE Ghrist Adult Career Center
Sharon Mastroianni, Superintendent
316 W Mason Rd
Milan, OH 44846
419 499-4663
Type: Vocational or Tech Sch
Control: State, County, or Local Govt
• Medical Assistant Prgm
• Surgical Technology Prgm

Mount St Joseph

College of Mt St Joseph
Tony Aretz, PhD, President
5701 Delhi
Mount St Joseph, OH 45233
513 244-4232
Type: 4-year Coll or Univ
Control: Nonprofit (Private or Religious)
• Athletic Training Prgm
• Nursing Prgm
• Physical Therapy Prgm

Mount Vernon

Knox County Career Center
Ray Richardson, Superintendent
306 Martinsburg Rd
Mount Vernon, OH 43050
614 397-5820
Type: Vocational or Tech Sch
Control: State, County, or Local Govt
• Medical Assistant Prgm

Mount Vernon Nazarene University
Mount Vernon, OH 43050
Type: 4-year Coll or Univ
Control: Nonprofit (Private or Religious)
• Medical Assistant Prgm
• Nursing Prgm

Nelsonville

Hocking College
John J Light, PhD, President
3301 Hocking Pkwy
Nelsonville, OH 45764
740 753-3591
Type: Junior or Comm Coll
Control: Nonprofit (Private or Religious)
• Medical Assistant Prgm
• Physical Therapist Assistant Prgm

New Concord

Muskingum University
New Concord, OH 43762
Type: 4-year Coll or Univ
Control: Nonprofit (Private or Religious)
• Nursing Prgm

Newark

Central Ohio Technical College
Bonnie Coe, PhD, President
1179 University Dr
Newark, OH 43055-1767
740 364-9509
Type: Junior or Comm Coll
Control: State, County, or Local Govt
• Diagnostic Med Sonography
  (Gen/Card/Vascular) Prgm
• Radiography Prgm
• Surgical Technology Prgm

North Canton

Stark State College
John O'Donnell, EdD, President
6200 Frank Ave NW
North Canton, OH 44720-7299
330 494-6170
Type: Vocational or Tech Sch
Control: State, County, or Local Govt
• Clin Lab Technician/Med Lab Technician Prgm
• Dental Hygiene Prgm
• Medical Assistant Prgm
• Occupational Therapy Asst Prgm
• Ophthalmic Assistant Prgm
• Physical Therapist Assistant Prgm
• Respiratory Care Prgm

Walsh University
Richard Jusseaume, President
2020 E Maple St
North Canton, OH 44720-3396
330 490-7102
Type: 4-year Coll or Univ
Control: Nonprofit (Private or Religious)
• Counseling Prgm
• Physical Therapy Prgm

Oberlin

Lorain Cnty Joint Voc School - Adult Career
William B Randall, MS, Superintendent
15181 St Rte 58
Oberlin, OH 44074
440 774-1056
Type: Vocational or Tech Sch
Control: State, County, or Local Govt
• Medical Assistant Prgm

Oxford

Miami University
David Hodge, PhD, President
201 Roudebush
Oxford, OH 45056
513 529-2345
Type: 4-year Coll or Univ
Control: State, County, or Local Govt
• Athletic Training Prgm
• Dietetics-Didactic Prgm
• Nursing Prgm
• Psychology (PhD) Prgm
• Speech-Language Pathology Prgm

Parma

Bryant & Stratton College - Parma
Lisa Mason, Campus Director
12955 Snow Rd
Parma, OH 44130
216 265-3151
Type: Junior or Comm Coll
Control: For Profit
• Medical Assistant Prgm

Pepper Pike

Ursuline College
Anne Marie Diederich, President
2550 Lander Rd
Pepper Pike, OH 44124
216 449-4200
Type: 4-year Coll or Univ
Control: Nonprofit (Private or Religious)
• Art Therapy Prgm
• Nursing Prgm

Piqua

Edison Community College
Kenneth A Yowell, President
1973 Edison Dr
Piqua, OH 45356
937 778-7802
Type: Junior or Comm Coll
Control: State, County, or Local Govt
• Clin Lab Technician/Med Lab Technician Prgm
• Medical Assistant Prgm
• Phlebotomy Prgm

Portsmouth

Shawnee State University
Rita Rice Morris, PhD, President
940 Second St
Portsmouth, OH 45662-4303
740 351-3208
Type: 4-year Coll or Univ
Control: State, County, or Local Govt
• Athletic Training Prgm
• Clin Lab Technician/Med Lab Technician Prgm
• Dental Hygiene Prgm
• Occupational Therapy Asst Prgm
• Occupational Therapy Prgm
• Physical Therapist Assistant Prgm
• Radiography Prgm
• Respiratory Care Prgm

Rio Grande

Buckeye Hills Career Center
D Kent Lewis, BS MS, Superintendent
PO Box 157
Rio Grande, OH 45674
740 245-5334
Type: Vocational or Tech Sch
Control: State, County, or Local Govt
• Surgical Technology Prgm

University of Rio Grande
Barry M Dorsey, PhD, President
218 N College Ave
PO Box 500
Rio Grande, OH 45674-0500
740 245-7204
Type: 4-year Coll or Univ
Control: Nonprofit (Private or Religious)
• Diagnostic Med Sonography (General) Prgm
• Radiography Prgm

Rootstown

Northeast Ohio Medical University
Lois Margaret Nora, MD JD, President
4209 St Rte 44
PO Box 95
Rootstown, OH 44272
Type: 4-year Coll or Univ
Control: State, County, or Local Govt
• Allopathic Medicine Prgm
• Pharmacy Prgm

Sheffield Village

Ohio Business College
Sheffield Village, OH 44035
Type: Junior or Comm Coll
• Medical Assistant Prgm (2)

Smithville

Wayne County Schools Career Center
Smithville, OH 44677
Type: Vocational or Tech Sch
• Medical Assistant Prgm

South Euclid

Notre Dame College
Robert E Karsten, Interim President
4545 College Rd
South Euclid, OH 44121
216 381-1680
Type: 4-year Coll or Univ
Control: Nonprofit (Private or Religious)
• Nursing Prgm

Springfield

Clark State Community College
Karen Rafinski, PhD, President
570 E Leffel Ln
Springfield, OH 45501-0570
937 328-6001
Type: Junior or Comm Coll
Control: State, County, or Local Govt
• Clin Lab Technician/Med Lab Technician Prgm
• Medical Assistant Prgm
• Physical Therapist Assistant Prgm

St Clairsville

Belmont Technical College
Joseph Bukowski, EdD, President
120 Fox-Shannon Pl
St Clairsville, OH 43950
740 695-9500
Type: Vocational or Tech Sch
Control: State, County, or Local Govt
• Medical Assistant Prgm

Steubenville

Eastern Gateway Community College
Laura M Meeks, PhD, President
4000 Sunset Blvd
Steubenville, OH 43952
740 264-5591
Type: Junior or Comm Coll
Control: State, County, or Local Govt
• Clin Lab Technician/Med Lab Technician Prgm
• Dental Assistant Prgm
• Medical Assistant Prgm
• Radiography Prgm
• Respiratory Care Prgm

Stow

National College - Stow
Stow, OH 44224-4305
Type: Junior or Comm Coll
• Medical Assistant Prgm (2)
• Surgical Technology Prgm

Sylvania

Lourdes College
George Matthews, PhD, President
6832 Convent Blvd
Sylvania, OH 43560-2898
419 885-3211
Type: 4-year Coll or Univ
Control: Nonprofit (Private or Religious)
• Nursing Prgm

Tiffin

Heidelberg University
Dominic Dottavio, PhD, President
310 E Market St
Tiffin, OH 44883
419 448-2202
Type: 4-year Coll or Univ
Control: Nonprofit (Private or Religious)
• Athletic Training Prgm

Toledo

Davis College
Diane Brunner, MEd, President/CEO
4747 Monroe St
Toledo, OH 43623
419 473-2700
Type: Junior or Comm Coll
Control: For Profit
• Medical Assistant Prgm

Mercy College of Northwest Ohio
Paul Kessler, EdD, President
2221 Madison Ave
Toledo, OH 43624-1133
419 259-1279
Type: 4-year Coll or Univ
Control: Nonprofit (Private or Religious)
• Nursing Prgm
• Ophthalmic Assistant Prgm
• Polysomnographic Technology Prgm
• Radiography Prgm

Owens Community College
Larry McDougle, PhD, Interim President
Oregon Rd, PO Box 10000
Toledo, OH 43699
567 661-7210
Type: Junior or Comm Coll
Control: State, County, or Local Govt
• Cancer Registrar Prgm
• Dental Hygiene Prgm
• Diagnostic Med Sonography (General) Prgm
• Dietetic Technician-AD Prgm
• Emergency Med Tech-Paramedic Prgm
• Medical Assistant Prgm
• Occupational Therapy Asst Prgm
• Physical Therapist Assistant Prgm
• Radiography Prgm
• Surgical Technology Prgm

Professional Skills Institute
Patricia A Finch, RN, President
20 Arco Dr
Toledo, OH 43607
419 531-9610
Type: Acad Health Ctr/Med Sch
Control: For Profit
• Physical Therapist Assistant Prgm

St Vincent Mercy Medical Center
Imran Andrabi, President
2213 Cherry St
Toledo, OH 43608
419 251-4675
Type: Hosp or Med Ctr: 500 Beds
Control: Nonprofit (Private or Religious)
• Clin Lab Scientist/Med Technologist Prgm

University of Toledo

Lloyd Jacobs, MD, President
2801 W Bancroft St
Toledo, OH 43606-3390
419 530-2211
Type: 4-year Coll or Univ
Control: State, County, or Local Govt
• Allopathic Medicine Prgm
• Athletic Training Prgm
• Clin Lab Scientist/Med Technologist Prgm
• Counseling Prgm
• Kinesiotherapy Prgm
• Music Therapy Prgm
• Nursing Prgm
• Occupational Therapy Prgm
• Pharmacy Prgm
• Physical Therapy Prgm
• Physician Assistant Prgm
• Psychology (PhD) Prgm
• Respiratory Care Prgm
• Speech-Language Pathology Prgm

Urbana

Urbana University
Robert L Head, PhD, President
579 College Way
Urbana, OH 43078
937 484-1300
Type: 4-year Coll or Univ
Control: Nonprofit (Private or Religious)
• Athletic Training Prgm
• Nursing Prgm

Warren

Trumbull Career & Technical Center
Wayne McClain, PhD, Superintendent
528 Educational Hwy
Warren, OH 44483
330 847-0503
Type: Vocational or Tech Sch
Control: State, County, or Local Govt
• Medical Assistant Prgm

Trumbull Memorial Hospital
Kris Hoce, MBA, President and CEO
1350 E Market St
Warren, OH 44482
216 841-9117
Type: Hosp or Med Ctr: 300-499 Beds
Control: Nonprofit (Private or Religious)
• Phlebotomy Prgm

Westerville

Fortis College-Westerville
Westerville, OH 43081
Type: Vocational or Tech Sch
• Radiography Prgm
• Surgical Technology Prgm

Otterbein College
C Brent DeVore, PhD, President
Roush Hall 302
Westerville, OH 43081
614 823-1410
Type: 4-year Coll or Univ
Control: Nonprofit (Private or Religious)
• Athletic Training Prgm
• Nursing Prgm

Wilmington

Wilmington College
Daniel DiBiasio, PhD, President
1870 Quaker Way
Pyle Center Box 1246
Wilmington, OH 45177
937 382-6661
Type: 4-year Coll or Univ
Control: Nonprofit (Private or Religious)
• Athletic Training Prgm

Wooster

College of Wooster
R Stanton Hales, Director
1189 Beall Ave
Wooster, OH 44691
330 263-2311
Type: 4-year Coll or Univ
Control: State, County, or Local Govt
• Music Therapy Prgm

Youngstown

Choffin Career & Technical Center
Wendy Webb, PhD, Superintendent
20 W Wood St
Youngstown, OH 44501
330 744-6915
Type: Vocational or Tech Sch
Control: State, County, or Local Govt
• Dental Assistant Prgm
• Surgical Technology Prgm

National College - Youngstown
Youngstown, OH 44505
Type: Junior or Comm Coll
• Surgical Technology Prgm

Youngstown State University
David C Sweet, PhD, President
One University Plaza
Tod Hall
Youngstown, OH 44555
330 941-3101
Type: 4-year Coll or Univ
Control: State, County, or Local Govt
• Clin Lab Technician/Med Lab Technician Prgm
• Counseling Prgm
• Dental Hygiene Prgm
• Dietetic Technician-AD Prgm
• Dietetics-Coordinated Prgm
• Dietetics-Didactic Prgm
• Emergency Med Tech-Paramedic Prgm
• Histotechnician Prgm
• Medical Assistant Prgm
• Physical Therapy Prgm
• Respiratory Care Prgm

Zanesville

Zane State College
Paul R Brown, EdD, President
1555 Newark Rd
Zanesville, OH 43701-2694
740 588-1200
Type: Junior or Comm Coll
Control: State, County, or Local Govt
• Clin Lab Technician/Med Lab Technician Prgm
• Medical Assistant Prgm
• Occupational Therapy Asst Prgm
• Phlebotomy Prgm
• Physical Therapist Assistant Prgm
• Radiography Prgm

Oklahoma

Ada

East Central University
Richard Rafes, PhD JD, President
1100 E 14th St
Ada, OK 74820
405 332-8000
Type: 4-year Coll or Univ
Control: State, County, or Local Govt
• Athletic Training Prgm
• Rehabilitation Counseling Prgm

Valley View Regional Hospital
Bob Thompson, President
Health Administration
430 N Monta Vista
Ada, OK 74820
580 421-6195
Type: Hosp or Med Ctr: 100-299 Beds
Control: Nonprofit (Private or Religious)
• Clin Lab Scientist/Med Technologist Prgm

Altus

Western Oklahoma State College
Randy Cumby, MEd, President
2801 N Main
Altus, OK 73521-1397
580 477-2000
Type: Junior or Comm Coll
Control: State, County, or Local Govt
• Radiography Prgm

Bartlesville

Oklahoma Wesleyan University
Bartlesville, OK 74006
Type: 4-year Coll or Univ
Control: Nonprofit (Private or Religious)
• Nursing Prgm

Bethany

Southern Nazarene University
Loren P Gresham, PhD, President
6729 NW 39th Expwy
Bethany, OK 73008
405 491-6300
Type: 4-year Coll or Univ
Control: Nonprofit (Private or Religious)
• Athletic Training Prgm
• Nursing Prgm

Drumright

Central Technology Center
Phil Waul, MA, Superintendent
3 CT Circle
Drumright, OK 74030
918 352-2551
Type: Vocational or Tech Sch
Control: State, County, or Local Govt
• Surgical Technology Prgm

Edmond

Oklahoma Christian University
2501 E Memorial Rd
Edmond, OK 73013
Type: 4-year Coll or Univ
Control: Nonprofit (Private or Religious)
• Music Therapy Prgm
• Nursing Prgm

University of Central Oklahoma
W Roger Webb, President
100 N University Dr
Edmond, OK 73034
405 974-2000
Type: 4-year Coll or Univ
Control: State, County, or Local Govt
• Athletic Training Prgm
• Dietetic Internship Prgm
• Dietetics-Didactic Prgm
• Exercise Science Prgm
• Speech-Language Pathology Prgm

El Reno

Canadian Valley Technology Center
Greg Winters, EdD, Superintendent
6505 E Hwy 66
El Reno, OK 73036
405 262-2629
Type: Vocational or Tech Sch
Control: State, County, or Local Govt
• Surgical Technology Prgm

Enid

Autry Technology Center
James Strate, EdD, Superintendent
1201 W Willow
Enid, OK 73703
405 242-2750
Type: Vocational or Tech Sch
Control: State, County, or Local Govt
• Radiography Prgm
• Surgical Technology Prgm

Fort Cobb

SW Oklahoma St Univ/Caddo Kiowa Tech Ctr
Dennis Ruttman, MEd, Superintendent/CEO
PO Box 190
Fort Cobb, OK 73038
405 643-3230
Type: Vocational or Tech Sch
Control: Nonprofit (Private or Religious)
• Occupational Therapy Asst Prgm
• Physical Therapist Assistant Prgm

Langston

Langston University
Ernest L Holloway, President
Langston, OK 73050
405 466-2231
Type: 4-year Coll or Univ
Control: State, County, or Local Govt
• Dietetics-Didactic Prgm
• Physical Therapy Prgm
• Rehabilitation Counseling Prgm

Lawton

Comanche County Memorial Hospital
Randy Segler, MHA, Chief Executive Officer
3401 W Gore Blvd, Box 129
Lawton, OK 73505
580 355-8699
Type: Hosp or Med Ctr: 100-299 Beds
Control: State, County, or Local Govt
• Clin Lab Scientist/Med Technologist Prgm

Great Plains Technology Center
James Nisbett, MSEd, Superintendent
4500 W Lee Blvd
Lawton, OK 73505
580 355-6371
Type: Vocational or Tech Sch
Control: State, County, or Local Govt
• Emergency Med Tech-Paramedic Prgm
• Radiography Prgm
• Respiratory Care Prgm
• Surgical Technology Prgm

Miami

Northeastern Oklahoma A&M College
Jeffrey Hale, President
200 I Street
PO Box 3841
Miami, OK 74354
918 540-6201
Type: Junior or Comm Coll
Control: State, County, or Local Govt
• Clin Lab Technician/Med Lab Technician Prgm
• Physical Therapist Assistant Prgm

Midwest City

Rose State College
Terry Britton, PhD, President
6420 SE 15th
Health Sciences Division
Midwest City, OK 73110-2797
405 733-7300
Type: Junior or Comm Coll
Control: State, County, or Local Govt
• Clin Lab Technician/Med Lab Technician Prgm
• Dental Assistant Prgm
• Dental Hygiene Prgm
• Radiography Prgm
• Respiratory Care Prgm

Muskogee

Bacone College
Robert Duncan, DMin, President
Office of the President
Muskogee, OK 74403-1568
888 682-5514
Type: 4-year Coll or Univ
Control: Nonprofit (Private or Religious)
• Radiography Prgm

Indian Capital Technology Center
Tom Stiles, Superintendent
2403 N 41st St East
Muskogee, OK 74403
918 687-7565
Type: Vocational or Tech Sch
Control: State, County, or Local Govt
• Radiography Prgm
• Surgical Technology Prgm

Norman

Moore Norman Technology Center
John Hunter, MEd, Superintendent
4701 12th Ave NW
Norman, OK 73070-4701
405 364-5763
Type: Vocational or Tech Sch
Control: State, County, or Local Govt
• Dental Assistant Prgm
• Diagnostic Med Sonography (General) Prgm
• Medical Assistant Prgm
• Surgical Technology Prgm

University of Oklahoma
David L Boren, President
660 Parrington Oval
Norman, OK 73019
405 325-3916
Type: 4-year Coll or Univ
Control: State, County, or Local Govt
• Allopathic Medicine Prgm
• Genetic Counseling Prgm
• Medical Librarian Prgm
• Music Therapy Prgm
• Pharmacy Prgm
• Physician Assistant Prgm

Oklahoma City

Francis Tuttle Technology Center
Kay Martin, PhD, Superintendent/CEO
12777 N Rockwell Ave
Oklahoma City, OK 73142
405 717-4266
Type: Vocational or Tech Sch
Control: State, County, or Local Govt
• Dental Assistant Prgm
• Medical Assistant Prgm
• Respiratory Care Prgm

Metro Tech Health Careers Center
James Branscum, EdD, Superintendent
1900 Springlake Dr
Oklahoma City, OK 73111
405 605-4400
Type: Vocational or Tech Sch
Control: State, County, or Local Govt
• Dental Assistant Prgm
• Medical Assistant Prgm
• Radiography Prgm
• Surgical Technology Prgm

Oklahoma City Community College
Paul W Sechrist, PhD, President
7777 S May Ave
Oklahoma City, OK 73159-4444
405 682-7502
Type: Junior or Comm Coll
Control: State, County, or Local Govt
• Emergency Med Tech-Paramedic Prgm
• Occupational Therapy Asst Prgm
• Physical Therapist Assistant Prgm

Platt College
Micheal A Pugliese, President
309 S Ann Arbor
Oklahoma City, OK 73128
405 946-7799
Type: Vocational or Tech Sch
Control: For Profit
• Clin Lab Technician/Med Lab Technician Prgm
  (4)
• Surgical Technology Prgm

Univ of Oklahoma Health Sciences Center
Joseph J Ferretti, PhD, SVP/Provost
1000 Stanton L Young, Ste 221
Oklahoma City, OK 73117
405 271-2332
Type: Acad Health Ctr/Med Sch
Control: State, County, or Local Govt
• Audiologist Prgm
• Dental Hygiene Prgm
• Diagnostic Med Sonography (General/Cardiac)
  Prgm
• Dietetic Internship Prgm
• Dietetics-Coordinated Prgm
• Dietetics-Didactic Prgm
• Nuclear Medicine Technology Prgm
• Occupational Therapy Prgm (2)
• Physical Therapy Prgm
• Physician Assistant Prgm
• Radiation Therapy Prgm
• Radiography Prgm
• Speech-Language Pathology Prgm

University of Oklahoma Health Sciences Center
940 NE 13th St
Oklahoma City, OK 73104
Type: Hosp or Med Ctr: 300-499 Beds
Control: Nonprofit (Private or Religious)
• Dentistry Prgm
• Medical Dosimetry Prgm

Poteau

Carl Albert State College
Joe E White, PhD, President
1507 S McKenna
Poteau, OK 74953-5208
918 647-1210
Type: Junior or Comm Coll
Control: Nonprofit (Private or Religious)
• Physical Therapist Assistant Prgm
• Radiography Prgm

Kiamichi Technical Center
Poteau, OK 74953
Type: Vocational or Tech Sch
• Emergency Med Tech-Paramedic Prgm

Seminole

Seminole State College
James W Utterback, PhD, President
2701 Boren Blvd
PO Box 351
Seminole, OK 74818-0351
405 382-9200
Type: Junior or Comm Coll
Control: State, County, or Local Govt
• Clin Lab Technician/Med Lab Technician Prgm
• Phlebotomy Prgm

Shawnee

Gordon Cooper Technology Center
Shawnee, OK 74804
Type: Vocational or Tech Sch
• Emergency Med Tech-Paramedic Prgm

Oklahoma Baptist University
500 West University Avenue
Shawnee, OK 74804
Type: 4-year Coll or Univ
Control: Nonprofit (Private or Religious)
• Nursing Prgm

Stillwater

Meridian Technology Center
Andrea Kelly, EdD, Superintendent
1312 S Sangre St
Stillwater, OK 74074
405 377-3333
Type: Vocational or Tech Sch
Control: State, County, or Local Govt
• Radiography Prgm

Oklahoma State University
Marlene Strathe, Interim President and CEO
Stillwater, OK 74078
405 744-5000
Type: 4-year Coll or Univ
Control: State, County, or Local Govt
• Athletic Training Prgm
• Counseling Prgm
• Diagnostic Med Sonography (Cardiac) Prgm
• Dietetic Internship Prgm
• Dietetic Technician-AD Prgm
• Dietetics-Didactic Prgm
• Music Therapy Prgm
• Osteopathic Medicine Prgm
• Psychology (PhD) Prgm
• Speech-Language Pathology Prgm
• Veterinary Medicine Prgm
• Veterinary Technology Prgm

Tahlequah

Northeastern State University
W Roger Webb, President
Tahlequah, OK 74464
918 456-5511
Type: 4-year Coll or Univ
Control: State, County, or Local Govt
• Clin Lab Scientist/Med Technologist Prgm
• Dietetics-Didactic Prgm
• Music Therapy Prgm
• Optometry Prgm
• Speech-Language Pathology Prgm

Tishomingo

Murray State College
Noble Jobe III, PhD, Interim President
One Murray Campus
NAH 116
Tishomingo, OK 73460
580 371-2371
Type: Junior or Comm Coll
Control: State, County, or Local Govt
• Occupational Therapy Asst Prgm
• Physical Therapist Assistant Prgm
• Veterinary Technology Prgm

Tulsa

Community Care College
Teresa Knox, CEO
4242 S Sheridan
Tulsa, OK 74145
918 610-0027
Type: Vocational or Tech Sch
Control: For Profit
• Surgical Technology Prgm

Oral Roberts University
Tulsa, OK 74171
Type: 4-year Coll or Univ
Control: Nonprofit (Private or Religious)
• Nursing Prgm

Orthoptic Teaching Program of Tulsa
4606 E 67th St
Ste 400
Tulsa, OK 74136
918 481-2781
Control: Nonprofit (Private or Religious)
• Orthoptist Prgm

Saint Francis Hospital
Jake Henry, MD, CEO
6161 S Yale Ave
Tulsa, OK 74136
918 494-6342
Type: Hosp or Med Ctr: 500 Beds
Control: Nonprofit (Private or Religious)
• Clin Lab Scientist/Med Technologist Prgm

Tulsa Community College
Thomas McKeon, EdD, President, CEO
Central Office
6111 E Skelly Dr
Tulsa, OK 74135-6198
918 595-7868
Type: Junior or Comm Coll
Control: State, County, or Local Govt
• Clin Lab Technician/Med Lab Technician Prgm
• Dental Hygiene Prgm
• Medical Assistant Prgm
• Occupational Therapy Asst Prgm
• Phlebotomy Prgm
• Physical Therapist Assistant Prgm
• Radiography Prgm
• Respiratory Care Prgm
• Veterinary Technology Prgm

Tulsa Technology Center
Barbara Hagy, Superintendent
3550 S Memorial Dr
Tulsa, OK 74147
918 828-1201
Type: Vocational or Tech Sch
Control: State, County, or Local Govt
• Ophthalmic Assistant Prgm
• Radiography Prgm
• Surgical Technology Prgm

University of Tulsa
Steadman Upham, PhD, President
600 S College Ave
Tulsa, OK 74104
918 631-2000
Type: 4-year Coll or Univ
Control: Nonprofit (Private or Religious)
• Athletic Training Prgm
• Psychology (PhD) Prgm
• Speech-Language Pathology Prgm

Weatherford

Southwestern Oklahoma State University
John Hays, EdD, President
100 Campus Dr
Weatherford, OK 73096
580 774-3766
Type: 4-year Coll or Univ
Control: State, County, or Local Govt
• Athletic Training Prgm
• Music Therapy Prgm
• Pharmacy Prgm
• Radiography Prgm

Western Technology Center
Weatherford, OK 73096
• Dental Assistant Prgm

Wetumka

Wes Watkins Technology Center District 25
James R Moore, MS, Superintendent
7892 Hwy 9
Wetumka, OK 74883
405 452-5500
Type: Vocational or Tech Sch
Control: State, County, or Local Govt
• Surgical Technology Prgm

Wilburton

Eastern Oklahoma State College
1301 West Main St.
Wilburton, OK 74578
Type: Junior or Comm Coll
Control: State, County, or Local Govt
• Clin Lab Technician/Med Lab Technician Prgm

Ontario, Canada

Brantford

Mohawk College
411 Elgin St
Brantford, ON N3T 5V2
Type: 4-year Coll or Univ
Control: State, County, or Local Govt
• Orientation and Mobility Specialist Prgm
• Vision Rehabilitation Therapy Prgm

INSTITUTIONS

Guelph

University of Guelph
Alastair Summerlee, President
50 Stone Rd E
Guelph, ON N1G 2W1
519 824-4120
Type: 4-year Coll or Univ
Control: State, County, or Local Govt
• Veterinary Medicine Prgm
• Veterinary Technology Prgm

Hamiliton

McMaster University
1400 Main St W
IAHS - 403
Hamiliton, ON L8N 3Z5
905 525-9140
Type: 4-year Coll or Univ
Control: Nonprofit (Private or Religious)
• Allopathic Medicine Prgm

Kingston

Kingston Ophthalmic Training Centre
Kingston, ON K7L 5G2
Type: Nonhosp HC Facil, BB, or Lab
• Ophthalmic Technician Prgm

Queen's University
Kingston, ON K7L 3N6
Type: Acad Health Ctr/Med Sch
Control: State, County, or Local Govt
• Allopathic Medicine Prgm

London

University of Western Ontario
London, ON N6G 1H1
Type: 4-year Coll or Univ
Control: Nonprofit (Private or Religious)
• Allopathic Medicine Prgm
• Medical Librarian Prgm
• Pathologists' Assistant Prgm
• Physical Therapy Prgm

Ottawa

University of Ottawa
501 Smyth Rd
Ottawa, ON K1H 8M5
Type: 4-year Coll or Univ
Control: Nonprofit (Private or Religious)
• Allopathic Medicine Prgm
• Ophthalmic Med Technologist Prgm
• Psychology (PhD) Prgm

Scarborough

Centennial College
941 Progress Avenue
Scarborough, ON M1G 3T8
416 289-5000
Type: Junior or Comm Coll
Control: Other
• Ophthalmic Assistant Prgm

Thunder Bay, Sudbury

Northern Ontario Medical School
Thunder Bay, Sudbury, ON P7B 5E1
Type: Acad Health Ctr/Med Sch
Control: State, County, or Local Govt
• Allopathic Medicine Prgm

Toronto

Hospital for Sick Children
Mary Jo Haddad
555 University Ave
Toronto, ON M5G 1X8
416 813-5798
Type: Hosp or Med Ctr: 100-299 Beds
Control: Nonprofit (Private or Religious)
• Orthoptist Prgm

University of Toronto
David Naylor, MD DPhil, President
Simcoe Hall, Room 206
27 King's College Circle
Toronto, ON M5S 1A1
416 978-2121
Type: 4-year Coll or Univ
Control: Nonprofit (Private or Religious)
• Allopathic Medicine Prgm
• Genetic Counseling Prgm
• Medical Illustrator Prgm
• Medical Librarian Prgm
• Physical Therapy Prgm

York University
Toronto, ON M3J 1P3
Type: 4-year Coll or Univ
Control: Nonprofit (Private or Religious)
• Psychology (PhD) Prgm

Waterloo

University of Waterloo
Thomas Freddo, OD PhD, Director
Waterloo, ON N2L 3G1
519 888-4567
Type: 4-year Coll or Univ
Control: Nonprofit (Private or Religious)
• Optometry Prgm
• Psychology (PhD) Prgm

Windsor

University of Windsor
Windsor, ON N9B 3P4
519 253-3000
Type: 4-year Coll or Univ
Control: Nonprofit (Private or Religious)
• Music Therapy Prgm

Oregon

Albany

Linn-Benton Community College
Greg Hamann, Ed D, President
6500 SW Pacific Blvd
Albany, OR 97321
541 917-4200
Type: Junior or Comm Coll
Control: State, County, or Local Govt
• Dental Assistant Prgm
• Medical Assistant Prgm
• Occupational Therapy Asst Prgm
• Polysomnographic Technology Prgm

Bend

Central Oregon Community College
James Middleton, EdD, President
2600 NW College Way
Bend, OR 97701
541 383-7201
Type: Junior or Comm Coll
Control: State, County, or Local Govt
• Dental Assistant Prgm
• Medical Assistant Prgm

Corvallis

Oregon State University
Edward Ray, PhD, President
646 Kerr Administration Bldg
Corvallis, OR 97331
541 737-4133
Type: 4-year Coll or Univ
Control: State, County, or Local Govt
• Athletic Training Prgm
• Counseling Prgm
• Dietetic Internship Prgm
• Dietetics-Didactic Prgm
• Pharmacy Prgm
• Veterinary Medicine Prgm

Eugene

Lane Community College
Mary Spilde, PhD, President
4000 E 30th Ave
Eugene, OR 97405-0640
541 463-3000
Type: Junior or Comm Coll
Control: State, County, or Local Govt
• Dental Assistant Prgm
• Dental Hygiene Prgm
• Emergency Med Tech-Paramedic Prgm
• Medical Assistant Prgm
• Respiratory Care Prgm

University of Oregon
David B Frohnmayer, President
Eugene, OR 97403
503 346-3111
Type: 4-year Coll or Univ
Control: State, County, or Local Govt
• Music Therapy Prgm
• Psychology (PhD) Prgm
• Speech-Language Pathology Prgm

Forest Grove

Pacific University
Lesley M Hallick, PhD, President
2043 College Way
Forest Grove, OR 97116-1797
503 352-2123
Type: 4-year Coll or Univ
Control: Nonprofit (Private or Religious)
• Dental Hygiene Prgm
• Occupational Therapy Prgm
• Optometry Prgm
• Pharmacy Prgm
• Physical Therapy Prgm
• Physician Assistant Prgm
• Psychology (PsyD) Prgm

Gresham

Mt Hood Community College
John Sygielski, EdD, President
26000 SE Stark St
Gresham, OR 97030-3300
503 491-7212
Type: Junior or Comm Coll
Control: State, County, or Local Govt
• Dental Hygiene Prgm
• Medical Assistant Prgm
• Physical Therapist Assistant Prgm
• Respiratory Care Prgm
• Surgical Technology Prgm

Klamath Falls

Oregon Institute of Technology
Christopher Maples, PhD, President
3201 Campus Dr
Klamath Falls, OR 97601-8801
541 885-1103
Type: 4-year Coll or Univ
Control: State, County, or Local Govt
• Dental Hygiene Prgm
• Polysomnographic Technology Prgm
• Respiratory Care Prgm

Marylhurst

Marylhurst University
Nancy Wilgenbusch, PhD, President
17600 Pacific Hwy
Marylhurst, OR 97036-0261
503 636-8141
Type: 4-year Coll or Univ
Control: Nonprofit (Private or Religious)
• Art Therapy Prgm
• Music Therapy Prgm

McMinnville

Linfield College
Thomas Hellie, PhD, President
900 SE Baker St
McMinnville, OR 97128
503 434-2234
Type: 4-year Coll or Univ
Control: Nonprofit (Private or Religious)
• Athletic Training Prgm
• Music Therapy Prgm
• Nursing Prgm

Milwaukie

National College of Technical Instruction
Milwaukie, OR 97222
Type: Vocational or Tech Sch
• Emergency Med Tech-Paramedic Prgm

Monmouth

Western Oregon University
John Minahan, PhD, President
345 N Monmouth Ave
Monmouth, OR 97361
503 838-8888
Type: 4-year Coll or Univ
Control: State, County, or Local Govt
• Rehabilitation Counseling Prgm

Newberg

George Fox University
Robin Baker, PhD, President
414 N Meridian St #6246
Newberg, OR 97132
503 554-2142
Type: 4-year Coll or Univ
Control: Nonprofit (Private or Religious)
• Athletic Training Prgm
• Nursing Prgm
• Psychology (PsyD) Prgm

Oregon City

Clackamas Community College
Joanne Truesdell, PhD, President
19600 S Molalla Ave
Oregon City, OR 97045
503 657-6958
Type: Junior or Comm Coll
Control: State, County, or Local Govt
• Clinical Assisting Prgm
• Medical Assistant Prgm

Pendleton

Blue Mountain Community College
John Turner, President
2411 NW Carden
PO Box 100
Pendleton, OR 97801
541 278-5950
Type: Junior or Comm Coll
Control: State, County, or Local Govt
• Dental Assistant Prgm

Portland

Carrington College Portland
Portland, OR 97232
• Dental Hygiene Prgm

Concorde Career College - Portland
Al Short, School Director
1425 NE Irving
Bldg 300
Portland, OR 97232
503 281-4181
Type: Vocational or Tech Sch
Control: For Profit
• Dental Assistant Prgm
• Medical Assistant Prgm
• Surgical Technology Prgm

East-West Coll of the Healing Arts
David Slawson
525 NE Oregon St
Portland, OR 97232
503 233-6500
Type: Vocational or Tech Sch
Control: For Profit
• Massage Therapy Prgm

Everest College
Mickey Sieracki, MA MT(ASCP), President
425 SW Washington St
Portland, OR 97204
503 222-3225
Type: Vocational or Tech Sch
Control: For Profit
• Medical Assistant Prgm

Heald College
Amy McCombs, BA MA, President
625 SW Broadway
Ste 200
Portland, OR 97205
415 808-1400
Type: Vocational or Tech Sch
Control: For Profit
• Medical Assistant Prgm

Oregon Health & Science University
Joseph E Robertson, MD MBA, President
3181 SW Sam Jackson Pk Rd, L101
Portland, OR 97239
503 494-8252
Type: Acad Health Ctr/Med Sch
Control: State, County, or Local Govt
• Allopathic Medicine Prgm
• Clin Lab Scientist/Med Technologist Prgm
• Dentistry Prgm
• Dietetic Internship Prgm
• Emergency Med Tech-Paramedic Prgm
• Nursing Prgm
• Orthoptist Prgm
• Physician Assistant Prgm
• Radiation Therapy Prgm

Portland Community College
Preston Pulliams, EdD, District President
PO Box 19000
Portland, OR 97280-0990
503 244-6111
Type: Junior or Comm Coll
Control: State, County, or Local Govt
• Clin Lab Technician/Med Lab Technician Prgm
• Dental Assistant Prgm
• Dental Hygiene Prgm
• Dental Lab Technician Prgm
• Emergency Med Tech-Paramedic Prgm
• Medical Assistant Prgm
• Ophthalmic Technician Prgm
• Radiography Prgm
• Veterinary Technology Prgm

Portland State University
Daniel Bernstine, President
Portland, OR 97207-0751
503 725-3000
Type: 4-year Coll or Univ
Control: State, County, or Local Govt
• Counseling Prgm
• Music Therapy Prgm
• Rehabilitation Counseling Prgm
• Speech-Language Pathology Prgm

University of Portland
Portland, OR 97203
Type: 4-year Coll or Univ
Control: State, County, or Local Govt
• Nursing Prgm

Western State Chiropractic College
2900 NE 132nd Ave
Portland, OR 97230
Type: Acad Health Ctr/Med Sch
Control: For Profit
• Chiropractic Prgm

Salem

Chemeketa Community College
Gretchen Schuette, PhD, President
4000 Lancaster Dr NE
PO Box 14007
Salem, OR 97309-7070
503 399-6591
Type: Junior or Comm Coll
Control: State, County, or Local Govt
• Dental Assistant Prgm
• Emergency Med Tech-Paramedic Prgm
• Pharmacy Technician Prgm

Mid Willamette Valley Dietetic Internship
Capital Manor Retirement Community
1955 Dallas Hwy NW, Ste 1200
Salem, OR 97304
503 362-4101
Control: For Profit
• Dietetic Internship Prgm

Pennsylvania

Abington

Abington Memorial Hospital
Richard Jones, MS, President CEO
1200 Old York Rd
Abington, PA 19001
215 576-2000
Type: Hosp or Med Ctr: 500 Beds
Control: Nonprofit (Private or Religious)
• Radiography Prgm

Allentown

Cedar Crest College
Carmen Ambar, PhD, President
100 College Dr
Allentown, PA 18104-6196
610 606-4666
Type: 4-year Coll or Univ
Control: Nonprofit (Private or Religious)
• Dietetic Internship Prgm
• Dietetics-Didactic Prgm
• Nuclear Medicine Technology Prgm

Lehigh Valley Hospital
Elliot J Sussman, MD MBA, President/CEO
Cedar Crest and I-78
PO Box 689
Allentown, PA 18105-1556
610 402-2204
Type: Hosp or Med Ctr: 500 Beds
Control: Nonprofit (Private or Religious)
• Emergency Med Tech-Paramedic Prgm

Sodexho Health Care Services
Allentown, PA 18106
Type: Acad Health Ctr/Med Sch
Control: For Profit
• Dietetic Internship Prgm (2)

Altoona

Altoona Regional Health System
Jerry Murray, President/CEO
620 Howard Ave
Altoona, PA 16601-4899
814 889-2223
Type: Hosp or Med Ctr: 500 Beds
Control: Nonprofit (Private or Religious)
• Clin Lab Scientist/Med Technologist Prgm

Greater Altoona Career & Technology Center
Lanny F Ross, DEd, Executive Director
1500 Fourth Ave
Altoona, PA 16602
814 946-8450
Type: Vocational or Tech Sch
Control: State, County, or Local Govt
• Medical Assistant Prgm

Annville

Lebanon Valley College
Stephen C MacDonald, President
Humanities 102
Annville, PA 17003-0501
717 867-6211
Type: Acad Health Ctr/Med Sch
Control: Nonprofit (Private or Religious)
• Physical Therapy Prgm

Aston

Neumann University
Rosalie Mirenda, DNSC, President
One Neumann Dr
Aston, PA 19014
610 558-5501
Type: 4-year Coll or Univ
Control: Nonprofit (Private or Religious)
• Athletic Training Prgm
• Clin Lab Scientist/Med Technologist Prgm
• Counseling Prgm
• Physical Therapy Prgm

Beaver Falls

Geneva College
John H White, PhD, President
3200 College Ave
Beaver Falls, PA 15010-3599
724 846-5100
Type: 4-year Coll or Univ
Control: Nonprofit (Private or Religious)
• Cardiovascular Tech (Invasive) Prgm
• Counseling Prgm

Bethlehem

Moravian College
Bethlehem, PA 18018
Type: 4-year Coll or Univ
Control: Nonprofit (Private or Religious)
• Nursing Prgm

Northampton Community College
Arthur Scott, EdD, President
3835 Green Pond Rd
Bethlehem, PA 18020
610 861-5458
Type: Junior or Comm Coll
Control: State, County, or Local Govt
• Dental Hygiene Prgm
• Diagnostic Med Sonography (General) Prgm
• Radiography Prgm
• Surgical Technology Prgm

St Luke's Hospital
Richard Anderson, President
801 Ostrum St
Bethlehem, PA 18015
610 954-4900
Type: Hosp or Med Ctr: 300-499 Beds
Control: Nonprofit (Private or Religious)
• Surgical Technology Prgm

Bloomsburg

Bloomsburg University
Jessica S Kozloff, PhD, President
Bloomsburg, PA 17815
570 389-4000
Type: 4-year Coll or Univ
Control: State, County, or Local Govt
• Athletic Training Prgm
• Audiologist Prgm
• Exercise Physiology - Applied Prgm
• Exercise Science Prgm
• Music Therapy Prgm
• Nursing Prgm
• Speech-Language Pathology Prgm

Blue Bell

Montgomery County Community College
Karen Stout, EdD, President
340 DeKalb Pike, PO Box 400
East House
Blue Bell, PA 19422
215 641-6500
Type: Junior or Comm Coll
Control: State, County, or Local Govt
• Clin Lab Technician/Med Lab Technician Prgm
• Dental Hygiene Prgm
• Medical Assistant Prgm
• Phlebotomy Prgm
• Radiography Prgm
• Surgical Technology Prgm

Blue Ridge Summit

Synergy Healting Arts Center & Massage School
13593 Monterey Ln
Blue Ridge Summit, PA 17214
Type: Vocational or Tech Sch
Control: Nonprofit (Private or Religious)
• Massage Therapy Prgm

Bradford

Bradford Regional Medical Center
George E Leonhardt, President/CEO
116 Interstate Pkwy
PO Box 0218
Bradford, PA 16701-0218
814 368-4143
Type: Hosp or Med Ctr: 100-299 Beds
Control: Nonprofit (Private or Religious)
• Radiography Prgm

Bryn Mawr

Harcum College
Jon Jay DeTemple, PhD, President
750 Montgomery Ave
Bryn Mawr, PA 19010
610 526-6001
Type: Junior or Comm Coll
Control: Nonprofit (Private or Religious)
• Clin Lab Technician/Med Lab Technician Prgm
• Dental Assistant Prgm
• Dental Hygiene Prgm
• Histotechnician Prgm
• Neurodiagnostic Tech Prgm
• Occupational Therapy Asst Prgm
• Physical Therapist Assistant Prgm
• Radiography Prgm
• Veterinary Technology Prgm

Butler

Butler County Community College
Nicholas Neupauer, EdD, President
PO Box 1203
College Drive
Butler, PA 16003-1203
412 287-8711
Type: Junior or Comm Coll
Control: State, County, or Local Govt
• Medical Assistant Prgm
• Physical Therapist Assistant Prgm

California

California University of Pennsylvania
Angelo Armenti, Jr, PhD, President
250 University Ave
California, PA 15419
412 938-4400
Type: 4-year Coll or Univ
Control: Nonprofit (Private or Religious)
• Athletic Training Prgm
• Counseling Prgm
• Nursing Prgm
• Physical Therapist Assistant Prgm
• Speech-Language Pathology Prgm

Camp Hill

Holy Spirit Hospital
Romaine Niemeyer, MHA, President
503 N 21st St
Camp Hill, PA 17011-2288
717 763-2106
Type: Hosp or Med Ctr: 300-499 Beds
Control: Nonprofit (Private or Religious)
• Radiography Prgm

Center Valley

DeSales University
Bernard O'Connor, OSFS PhD, President
2755 Station Ave
Center Valley, PA 18034-9568
610 282-1100
Type: 4-year Coll or Univ
Control: Nonprofit (Private or Religious)
• Physician Assistant Prgm

Chambersburg

Wilson College
Lorna Duphiney Edmundson, President
1015 Philadelphia Ave
Chambersburg, PA 17204
717 264-3226
Type: 4-year Coll or Univ
Control: For Profit
• Veterinary Technology Prgm

Chester

Widener University
James T Harris, EdD, President
One University Pl
Chester, PA 19013
610 499-4102
Type: 4-year Coll or Univ
Control: Nonprofit (Private or Religious)
• Nursing Prgm
• Physical Therapy Prgm
• Psychology (PsyD) Prgm

Clarion

Clarion University of Pennsylvania
Joseph Grunenwald, President
Clarion, PA 16214
814 393-2000
Type: 4-year Coll or Univ
Control: State, County, or Local Govt
• Medical Librarian Prgm
• Speech-Language Pathology Prgm

Clearfield

Clearfield Hospital
David McConnell, CHE NHA, President/CEO
PO Box 992
Clearfield, PA 16830
814 768-2497
Type: Hosp or Med Ctr d Beds
Control: Nonprofit (Private or Religious)
• Radiography Prgm

Cresson

Mount Aloysius College
Mary Ann Dillon, MD RSM
7373 Admiral Peary Hwy
Cresson, PA 16630
814 886-4131
Type: 4-year Coll or Univ
Control: Nonprofit (Private or Religious)
• Clin Lab Technician/Med Lab Technician Prgm
• Diagnostic Med Sonography (General) Prgm
• Medical Assistant Prgm
• Physical Therapist Assistant Prgm
• Surgical Technology Prgm

Dallas

Misericordia University
Michael MacDowell, EdD, President
301 Lake St
Dallas, PA 18612-1098
570 674-6265
Type: 4-year Coll or Univ
Control: Nonprofit (Private or Religious)
• Diagnostic Med Sonography (General) Prgm
• Nuclear Medicine Technology Prgm
• Nursing Prgm
• Occupational Therapy Prgm
• Physical Therapy Prgm
• Radiography Prgm
• Speech-Language Pathology Prgm

Danville

Geisinger Medical Center
Glenn Steele, MD, President
100 N Academy Ave
Danville, PA 17822-2201
570 271-5200
Type: Hosp or Med Ctr: 300-499 Beds
Control: Nonprofit (Private or Religious)
• Cardiovascular Tech (Invasive) Prgm
• Dietetic Internship Prgm
• Radiography Prgm

East Stroudsburg

East Stroudsburg University
Robert J Dillman, PhD, President
200 Prospect St
East Stroudsburg, PA 18301
717 422-3546
Type: 4-year Coll or Univ
Control: State, County, or Local Govt
• Athletic Training Prgm
• Exercise Physiology - Applied Prgm
• Exercise Physiology - Clinical Prgm
• Exercise Science Prgm
• Speech-Language Pathology Prgm

Pocono Medical Center Laboratory
206 East Brown Street
East Stroudsburg, PA 18301
Type: Nonhosp HC Facil, BB, or Lab
Control: Other
• Clin Lab Scientist/Med Technologist Prgm

Edinboro

Edinboro University of Pennsylvania
Jeremy D Brown, President
219 Meadville St
Edinboro, PA 16444
814 732-2711
Type: 4-year Coll or Univ
Control: State, County, or Local Govt
• Counseling Prgm
• Nursing Prgm
• Rehabilitation Counseling Prgm
• Speech-Language Pathology Prgm

Elizabethtown

Elizabethtown College
Theodore E Long, PhD, President
One Alpha Dr
Elizabethtown, PA 17022-2298
717 361-1193
Type: 4-year Coll or Univ
Control: Nonprofit (Private or Religious)
• Music Therapy Prgm
• Occupational Therapy Prgm

Elkins Park

Salus University
8360 Old York Rd
Elkins Park, PA 19027-1598
Type: Acad Health Ctr/Med Sch
Control: Nonprofit (Private or Religious)
• Audiologist Prgm
• Optometry Prgm
• Orientation and Mobility Specialist Prgm
• Physician Assistant Prgm
• Teacher of the Visually Impaired Prgm
• Vision Rehabilitation Therapy Prgm

Erie

Fortis Institute-Erie
Erie, PA 16506-1013
Type: Vocational or Tech Sch
• Clin Lab Technician/Med Lab Technician Prgm
• Medical Assistant Prgm
• Radiography Prgm

Gannon University
Phillip Kelly, DA, Interim President
109 University Square
Erie, PA 16541-0001
814 871-5800
Type: 4-year Coll or Univ
Control: Nonprofit (Private or Religious)
• Counseling Prgm
• Nursing Prgm
• Occupational Therapy Prgm
• Physical Therapy Prgm
• Physician Assistant Prgm
• Radiography Prgm
• Respiratory Care Prgm

Great Lakes Institute of Technology
Tony Piccirillo, President/CEO
5100 Peach St
Erie, PA 16509
814 864-6666
Type: Vocational or Tech Sch
Control: For Profit
• Diagnostic Med Sonography (General) Prgm
• Pharmacy Technician Prgm
• Surgical Technology Prgm

Lake Erie Coll of Osteopathic Medicine - Erie
1858 W Grandview Blvd
Erie, PA 16509
Type: Acad Health Ctr/Med Sch
Control: Nonprofit (Private or Religious)
• Osteopathic Medicine Prgm
• Pharmacy Prgm

Mercyhurst University
Thomas Gamble, PhD, President
501 E 38th St
Glenwood Hills
Erie, PA 16546
814 824-2000
Type: 4-year Coll or Univ
Control: Nonprofit (Private or Religious)
• Athletic Training Prgm
• Clin Lab Technician/Med Lab Technician Prgm
• Occupational Therapy Asst Prgm
• Physical Therapist Assistant Prgm

Saint Vincent Health Center
Angela Bontempo, President
232 W 25th St
Erie, PA 16544
814 452-5111
Type: Hosp or Med Ctr: 300-499 Beds
Control: Nonprofit (Private or Religious)
• Clin Lab Scientist/Med Technologist Prgm

Tri-State Business Institute
Guy Euliano, President
5757 W 26th St
Erie, PA 16506
814 838-7673
Type: Vocational or Tech Sch
Control: For Profit
• Dental Hygiene Prgm

Glenside

Arcadia University
Jerry M Greiner, PhD, President
450 S Easton Rd
Glenside, PA 19038
215 572-2908
Type: 4-year Coll or Univ
Control: Nonprofit (Private or Religious)
• Genetic Counseling Prgm
• Physical Therapy Prgm
• Physician Assistant Prgm

Grantham

Messiah College
Kim Phipps, PhD, President
Grantham, PA 17027
717 766-2511
Type: 4-year Coll or Univ
Control: Nonprofit (Private or Religious)
• Athletic Training Prgm
• Dietetics-Didactic Prgm
• Music Therapy Prgm
• Nursing Prgm

Greensburg

Seton Hill University
JoAnne W Boyle, MA PhD, President
Box 231K
Greensburg, PA 15601
724 838-4212
Type: 4-year Coll or Univ
Control: Nonprofit (Private or Religious)
• Art Therapy Prgm
• Dietetics-Coordinated Prgm
• Physician Assistant Prgm

Gwynedd Valley

Gwynedd-Mercy College
Kathleen Cieplak Owens, PhD, President
1325 Sumneytown Pike
PO Box 901
Gwynedd Valley, PA 19437-0901
610 641-5560
Type: 4-year Coll or Univ
Control: Nonprofit (Private or Religious)
• Cardiovascular Tech (Invasive/Noninvasive) Prgm
• Radiation Therapy Prgm
• Respiratory Care Prgm

Harrisburg

Harrisburg Area Community College
Edna V Baehre, PhD, President
One HACC Dr
Harrisburg, PA 17110-2999
717 780-2341
Type: Junior or Comm Coll
Control: State, County, or Local Govt
• Cardiovascular Tech (Invasive/Noninvasive) Prgm
• Clin Lab Technician/Med Lab Technician Prgm
• Dental Assistant Prgm
• Dental Hygiene Prgm
• Diagnostic Med Sonography (General) Prgm
• Emergency Med Tech-Paramedic Prgm
• Medical Assistant Prgm
• Radiography Prgm
• Respiratory Care Prgm
• Surgical Technology Prgm

Kaplan Career Institute - Harrisburg
Harrisburg, PA 17111
Type: Vocational or Tech Sch
• Medical Assistant Prgm

Immaculata

Immaculata University
Sr R Patricia Fadden, IHM EdD, President
1145 King Rd
Immaculata, PA 19345
610 647-4400
Type: 4-year Coll or Univ
Control: State, County, or Local Govt
• Dietetic Internship Prgm
• Dietetics-Didactic Prgm
• Music Therapy Prgm
• Nursing Prgm
• Psychology (PsyD) Prgm

Indiana

Indiana University of Pennsylvania
Tony Atwater, PhD, President
201 Sutton Hall
1011 South Dr
Indiana, PA 15705
724 357-2200
Type: 4-year Coll or Univ
Control: State, County, or Local Govt
• Athletic Training Prgm
• Counseling Prgm
• Dietetic Internship Prgm
• Dietetics-Didactic Prgm
• Exercise Science Prgm
• Music Therapy Prgm
• Nursing Prgm
• Psychology (PsyD) Prgm
• Respiratory Care Prgm
• Speech-Language Pathology Prgm

Jenkintown

Manor College
Sr Mary Cecilia Jurasinski, OSBM, President
700 Fox Chase Rd
Jenkintown, PA 19046
215 885-2360
Type: Junior or Comm Coll
Control: Nonprofit (Private or Religious)
• Dental Assistant Prgm
• Dental Hygiene Prgm
• Veterinary Technology Prgm

Johnstown

Commonwealth Tech Inst at Hiram G Andrews Ctr
Donald Rullman, BA, Director
727 Goucher St
Johnstown, PA 15905
814 255-8231
Type: Vocational or Tech Sch
Control: State, County, or Local Govt
• Dental Assistant Prgm

Conemaugh Valley Memorial Hospital
Steven Tucker, CEO
1086 Franklin St
Johnstown, PA 15905
814 539-9712
Type: Hosp or Med Ctr: 500 Beds
Control: Nonprofit (Private or Religious)
• Clin Lab Scientist/Med Technologist Prgm
• Emergency Med Tech-Paramedic Prgm
• Histotechnician Prgm
• Radiography Prgm
• Surgical Technology Prgm

Kittanning

Armstrong County Memorial Hospital
Jack Hoard, President/CEO
One Nolte Dr
Kittanning, PA 16201
412 543-8404
Type: Hosp or Med Ctr: 100-299 Beds
Control: Nonprofit (Private or Religious)
• Radiography Prgm

Lancaster

Lancaster Gen Coll of Nursing & Hlth Sciences
Mary Grace Simcox, EdD, President
410 N Lime St
Lancaster, PA 17602
717 544-4787
Type: Junior or Comm Coll
Control: Nonprofit (Private or Religious)
• Cardiovascular Tech (Invasive) Prgm
• Clin Lab Scientist/Med Technologist Prgm
• Diagnostic Med Sonography (General) Prgm
• Nuclear Medicine Technology Prgm
• Nursing Prgm
• Radiography Prgm
• Surgical Technology Prgm

Lock Haven

Lock Haven University
Keith Miller, PhD, President
Sullivan 202
Lock Haven, PA 17745
570 484-2000
Type: 4-year Coll or Univ
Control: State, County, or Local Govt
• Athletic Training Prgm
• Physician Assistant Prgm

Loretto

St Francis University
Rev Gabriel Zeis, TOR, President
PO Box 600
Loretto, PA 15940-0600
814 472-3001
Type: 4-year Coll or Univ
Control: Nonprofit (Private or Religious)
• Nursing Prgm
• Occupational Therapy Prgm
• Physical Therapy Prgm
• Physician Assistant Prgm

Mansfield

Mansfield University
Maravene Loeschke, PhD, President
500 North Hall
Mansfield, PA 16933
570 662-4046
Type: 4-year Coll or Univ
Control: State, County, or Local Govt
• Dietetics-Didactic Prgm
• Music Therapy Prgm
• Radiography Prgm
• Respiratory Care Prgm

McKees Rock

Ohio Valley General Hospital
William F Provenzano, FACHE, President
25 Heckel Rd
McKees Rock, PA 15136
Type: Hosp or Med Ctr: 100-299 Beds
Control: Nonprofit (Private or Religious)
• Radiography Prgm

Media

Delaware County Community College
Jerome Parker, PhD, President
901 S Media Line Rd
Media, PA 19603-1094
610 359-5100
Type: Junior or Comm Coll
Control: State, County, or Local Govt
• Medical Assistant Prgm
• Surgical Technology Prgm

Millersville

Millersville University of Pennsylvania
Francine McNairey, PhD, President
Biemesderfer Executive Ctr
Millersville, PA 17551
717 872-3592
Type: 4-year Coll or Univ
Control: State, County, or Local Govt
• Respiratory Care Prgm

Monaca

Community College of Beaver County
Joe D Forrester, EdD, President
One Campus Dr
Monaca, PA 15061
724 775-8561
Type: Junior or Comm Coll
Control: State, County, or Local Govt
• Phlebotomy Prgm

Moon Township

Robert Morris University
Edward A Nicholson, PhD, President
Narrows Run Rd
Moon Township, PA 15108
Type: Consortium
Control: Nonprofit (Private or Religious)
• Nuclear Medicine Technology Prgm
• Nursing Prgm

Nanticoke

Luzerne County Community College
Thomas Leary, MA, President
1333 S Prospect St
Nanticoke, PA 18634-3899
570 740-0384
Type: Junior or Comm Coll
Control: State, County, or Local Govt
• Dental Assistant Prgm
• Dental Hygiene Prgm
• Respiratory Care Prgm
• Surgical Technology Prgm

New Castle

Jameson Health System
Thomas White, FACHE, President and CEO
1000 S Mercer St
South Campus
New Castle, PA 16101
724 658-9001
Type: Hosp or Med Ctr: 100-299 Beds
Control: Nonprofit (Private or Religious)
• Nuclear Medicine Technology Prgm

Jameson Hospital
Thomas White, FACHE, President/CEO
1211 Wilmington Ave
New Castle, PA 16105
412 658-3511
Type: Hosp or Med Ctr: 100-299 Beds
Control: Nonprofit (Private or Religious)
• Radiography Prgm

Newton

Bucks County Community College
James J Linksz, EdD, President
275 Swamp Rd
Tyler Hall 220
Newton, PA 18940
215 968-8222
Type: Junior or Comm Coll
Control: State, County, or Local Govt
• Radiography Prgm

Oakdale

Pittsburgh Technical Institute
1111 McKee Rd
Oakdale, PA 15071
Type: Vocational or Tech Sch
Control: For Profit
• Medical Assistant Prgm
• Surgical Technology Prgm

Oaks

Cortiva Inst - Penn School of Muscle Therapy
Jeff Mann, PDMT NCBTMB, President
1173 Egypt Rd
PO Box 400
Oaks, PA 19456-0400
610 666-9060
Type: Vocational or Tech Sch
Control: For Profit
• Massage Therapy Prgm

Philadelphia

Albert Einstein Medical Center
Barry Freedman, MBA, President
5501 Old York Rd
Philadelphia, PA 19141-3098
215 456-7010
Type: Hosp or Med Ctr: 500 Beds
Control: Nonprofit (Private or Religious)
• Radiography Prgm

ARAMARK Healthcare
1717 Arch St, 42nd Fl
Philadelphia, PA 19103
Control: For Profit
• Dietetic Internship Prgm

Chestnut Hill College
Philadelphia, PA 19118
Type: 4-year Coll or Univ
Control: Nonprofit (Private or Religious)
• Psychology (PsyD) Prgm

Community College of Philadelphia
Stephen M Curtis, PhD, President
1700 Spring Garden St
Philadelphia, PA 19130
215 751-8028
Type: Junior or Comm Coll
Control: State, County, or Local Govt
• Clin Lab Technician/Med Lab Technician Prgm
• Dental Hygiene Prgm
• Medical Assistant Prgm
• Phlebotomy Prgm
• Radiography Prgm
• Respiratory Care Prgm

Drexel University College of Medicine
Richard Homan, M D, President
245 N 15th Street New College Building M
Philadelphia, PA 19102-1192
215 762-3500
Type: 4-year Coll or Univ
Control: Nonprofit (Private or Religious)
• Allopathic Medicine Prgm
• Art Therapy Prgm
• Dietetics-Didactic Prgm
• Histotechnology Prgm
• Medical Librarian Prgm
• Music Therapy Prgm
• Nursing Prgm
• Pathologists' Assistant Prgm
• Physical Therapy Prgm
• Physician Assistant Prgm
• Psychology (PhD) Prgm
• Radiography Prgm

Holy Family University
Sr M Francesca Onley, PhD CSFN, President
Grant & Frankford Aves
Philadelphia, PA 19114
215 637-7700
Type: 4-year Coll or Univ
Control: Nonprofit (Private or Religious)
• Nursing Prgm
• Radiography Prgm

Kaplan Institute - Philadelphia
Philadelphia, PA 19104
Type: Vocational or Tech Sch
• Medical Assistant Prgm

La Salle University
Michael McGinniss, President
1900 W Olney Ave
Philadelphia, PA 19141-1108
Type: 4-year Coll or Univ
Control: State, County, or Local Govt
• Dietetics-Coordinated Prgm
• Dietetics-Didactic Prgm
• Nursing Prgm
• Psychology (PhD) Prgm
• Speech-Language Pathology Prgm

National Massage Therapy Insitute
Division of PSB
10050 Roosevelt Blvd
Philadelphia, PA 19116
Type: Acad Health Ctr/Med Sch
Control: For Profit
• Massage Therapy Prgm

Penn Medicine - Hospital of the U of Penn
Ralph Muller
3400 Spruce St
21 Penn Tower
Philadelphia, PA 19104
215 662-2203
Type: Hosp or Med Ctr: 500 Beds
Control: Nonprofit (Private or Religious)
• Radiography Prgm

Pennsylvania Hospital
Kathleen Kinslow, RN BSN MBA, CEO
800 Spruce St
Pennsylvania Hospital
Philadelphia, PA 19107
215 829-7191
Type: Hosp or Med Ctr: 300-499 Beds
Control: Nonprofit (Private or Religious)
• Clin Lab Scientist/Med Technologist Prgm

Philadelphia College of Osteopathic Medicine
Matthew Schure, PhD, President, CEO
4170 City Ave
Evans Hall - President's Office
Philadelphia, PA 19131-1694
215 871-6800
Type: Acad Health Ctr/Med Sch
Control: Nonprofit (Private or Religious)
• Osteopathic Medicine Prgm
• Pharmacy Prgm
• Physician Assistant Prgm
• Psychology (PhD) Prgm

Philadelphia University
Stephen Spinelli, PhD, President
School House Ln and Henry Ave
Philadelphia, PA 19144
215 951-2970
Type: 4-year Coll or Univ
Control: Nonprofit (Private or Religious)
• Occupational Therapy Asst Prgm
• Occupational Therapy Prgm
• Physician Assistant Prgm

St Christopher Hospital School of Rad Tech
Jill Tillman, MBA, Interim CEO
Erie Ave at Front
Philadelphia, PA 19134
215 427-5480
Type: Hosp or Med Ctr: 100-299 Beds
Control: For Profit
• Radiography Prgm

St Christopher's Hospital for Children
Bernadette Mangan
E Erie Ave at N Front St
3601 A St
Philadelphia, PA 19134
215 427-5000
Type: Hosp or Med Ctr: 300-499 Beds
Control: For Profit
• Clin Lab Scientist/Med Technologist Prgm

Temple University
Ann Weaver Hart, PhD, President
President's Office
2nd Fl, Sullivan Hall
Philadelphia, PA 19122
215 204-7405
Type: 4-year Coll or Univ
Control: State, County, or Local Govt
- Allopathic Medicine Prgm
- Athletic Training Prgm
- Dentistry Prgm
- Music Therapy Prgm
- Nursing Prgm
- Occupational Therapy Prgm
- Pharmacy Prgm
- Physical Therapy Prgm
- Podiatric Medicine Prgm
- Psychology (PhD) Prgm
- Speech-Language Pathology Prgm

Thomas Jefferson University
Robert L Barchi, MD PhD, President
1020 Walnut St, Room 641 Scott Bldg
Philadelphia, PA 19107-5587
215 955-6617
Type: Acad Health Ctr/Med Sch
Control: Nonprofit (Private or Religious)
- Allopathic Medicine Prgm
- Clin Lab Scientist/Med Technologist Prgm
- Cytotechnology Prgm
- Diagnostic Med Sonography (Gen/Card/Vascular) Prgm
- Magnetic Resonance Technologist Prgm
- Medical Dosimetry Prgm
- Nuclear Medicine Technology Prgm
- Nursing Prgm
- Occupational Therapy Prgm
- Pharmacy Prgm
- Physical Therapy Prgm
- Radiation Therapy Prgm
- Radiography Prgm

Univ of Penn School of Dental Medicine
Marjorie K Jeffcoat, DMD, Dean
240 S 40th St
Robert Shattner Center
Philadelphia, PA 19104
215 898-8961
Type: Acad Health Ctr/Med Sch
Control: Nonprofit (Private or Religious)
- Dentistry Prgm

University of Pennsylvania
Amy Gutmann, President
100 College Hall
Philadelphia, PA 19104
215 898-7221
Type: 4-year Coll or Univ
Control: Nonprofit (Private or Religious)
- Allopathic Medicine Prgm
- Nursing Prgm
- Psychology (PhD) Prgm
- Veterinary Medicine Prgm

University of the Sciences
Philip P Gerbino, PhD, President
600 S 43rd St
Philadelphia, PA 19104-4495
215 596-8970
Type: 4-year Coll or Univ
Control: Nonprofit (Private or Religious)
- Occupational Therapy Prgm
- Pharmacy Prgm
- Physical Therapy Prgm

Pittsburgh

Adagio Health
960 Penn Ave, Ste 600
Pittsburgh, PA 15222
412 288-9039
Type: Acad Health Ctr/Med Sch
Control: Nonprofit (Private or Religious)
- Dietetic Internship Prgm

Bidwell Training Center
William E Strickland, Jr, President and CEO
1815 Metropolitan St
Pittsburgh, PA 15233-2200
412 323-4000
Type: Vocational or Tech Sch
Control: Nonprofit (Private or Religious)
- Pharmacy Technician Prgm

Bradford School - Pittsburgh
Vincent Graziano, MBA, President
125 West Station Square Dr, Ste 129
Pittsburgh, PA 15219
412 391-6710
Type: Vocational or Tech Sch
Control: For Profit
- Dental Assistant Prgm
- Medical Assistant Prgm

Brown Mackie College - Tulsa
Todd Nelson, Chief Executive Officer
Education Management Corporation
210 6th Avenue, 33rd Floor
Pittsburgh, PA 15222
412 995-7340
- Occupational Therapy Asst Prgm

Carlow University
Mary Hines, PhD, President
3333 Fifth Ave
Pittsburgh, PA 15213
Type: 4-year Coll or Univ
Control: Nonprofit (Private or Religious)
- Nursing Prgm

Chatham University
Esther L Barazzone, PhD, President
Woodland Rd
Pittsburgh, PA 15232-2826
412 365-1160
Type: 4-year Coll or Univ
Control: Nonprofit (Private or Religious)
- Nursing Prgm
- Occupational Therapy Prgm
- Physical Therapy Prgm
- Physician Assistant Prgm

Community College of Allegheny County
Alex Johnson, PhD, President
800 Allegheny Ave
Pittsburgh, PA 15233
412 323-2323
Type: Junior or Comm Coll
Control: State, County, or Local Govt
- Clin Lab Technician/Med Lab Technician Prgm
- Clinical Assisting Prgm
- Diagnostic Med Sonography (General/Cardiac) Prgm
- Dietetic Technician-AD Prgm
- Medical Assistant Prgm
- Nuclear Medicine Technology Prgm
- Occupational Therapy Asst Prgm
- Pharmacy Technician Prgm
- Physical Therapist Assistant Prgm
- Radiation Therapy Prgm
- Radiography Prgm
- Respiratory Care Prgm
- Surgical Technology Prgm

Ctr for Emer Med of Western Pennsylvania
Douglas Garretson, BA NREMT-P, President
230 McKee Pl, Ste 500
Pittsburgh, PA 15213
412 647-5300
Type: Consortium
Control: Nonprofit (Private or Religious)
- Emergency Med Tech-Paramedic Prgm

Duquesne University
Charles Dougherty, PhD, President
600 Forbes Ave
Administration Bldg Rm 510
Pittsburgh, PA 15282
412 396-6060
Type: 4-year Coll or Univ
Control: Nonprofit (Private or Religious)
- Athletic Training Prgm
- Counseling Prgm
- Music Therapy Prgm
- Nursing Prgm
- Occupational Therapy Prgm
- Pharmacy Prgm
- Physical Therapy Prgm
- Physician Assistant Prgm
- Psychology (PhD) Prgm
- Speech-Language Pathology Prgm

Everest Institute
James Callahan, President
100 Forbes Ave, Ste 1200
Pittsburgh, PA 15222
412 261-4520
Type: Vocational or Tech Sch
Control: For Profit
- Medical Assistant Prgm

Kaplan Career Institute - ICM Campus
Hunter H Hopkins, President
10 Wood St
Pittsburgh, PA 15222-1977
412 261-2647
Type: Vocational or Tech Sch
Control: For Profit
- Medical Assistant Prgm
- Occupational Therapy Asst Prgm

Sanford-Brown Institute
Patti Yakshe, MA, President
421 7th Ave
Pittsburgh, PA 15219
412 281-2600
Type: Vocational or Tech Sch
Control: For Profit
• Anesthesia Technologist/Technician Prgm
• Diagnostic Med Sonography (General) Prgm
• Pharmacy Technician Prgm
• Radiography Prgm
• Surgical Technology Prgm
• Veterinary Technology Prgm

Univ Health Center of Pittsburgh
Leslie Davis, MS, CEO
300 Halket St
Pittsburgh, PA 15213
412 641-4664
Type: Hosp or Med Ctr: 300-499 Beds
Control: Nonprofit (Private or Religious)
• Cytotechnology Prgm

University of Pittsburgh
Mark A Nordenberg, JD, Chancellor
Rm 107 Cathedral of Learning
Pittsburgh, PA 15260
412 624-4200
Type: 4-year Coll or Univ
Control: State, County, or Local Govt
• Allopathic Medicine Prgm
• Athletic Training Prgm (2)
• Audiologist Prgm
• Dental Hygiene Prgm
• Dentistry Prgm
• Dietetics-Coordinated Prgm
• Dietetics-Didactic Prgm
• Genetic Counseling Prgm
• Histotechnician Prgm
• Medical Librarian Prgm
• Nursing Prgm
• Occupational Therapy Prgm
• Orientation and Mobility Specialist Prgm
• Orthotist/Prosthetist Prgm
• Pharmacy Prgm
• Physical Therapist Assistant Prgm
• Physical Therapy Prgm
• Physician Assistant Prgm
• Psychology (PhD) Prgm
• Rehabilitation Counseling Prgm
• Respiratory Care Prgm
• Speech-Language Pathology Prgm

UPMC Presbyterian Shadyside
Liz Concordia, CEO
5230 Centre Ave
Pittsburgh, PA 15232
412 622-2010
Type: Hosp or Med Ctr: 500 Beds
Control: Nonprofit (Private or Religious)
• Perfusion Prgm

Vet Tech Institute
125 Seventh St
Pittsburgh, PA 15222
Type: Vocational or Tech Sch
Control: For Profit
• Veterinary Technology Prgm

Pottsville

McCann School of Business and Technology
Linda Walinsky, MPA, Regional Exec Director
2650 Woodglen Rd
Pottsville, PA 17901
570 622-3293
Type: Vocational or Tech Sch
Control: For Profit
• Clin Lab Technician/Med Lab Technician Prgm (6)
• Medical Assistant Prgm (4)
• Surgical Technology Prgm (3)

Reading

Alvernia University
Thomas F Flynn, PhD, President
400 Saint Bernardine St
Reading, PA 19607-1799
610 796-8324
Type: 4-year Coll or Univ
Control: Nonprofit (Private or Religious)
• Athletic Training Prgm
• Nursing Prgm
• Occupational Therapy Prgm

Reading Area Community College
Anna Weitz, EdD, President
10 S Second St
PO Box 1706
Reading, PA 19603
610 372-4721
Type: Junior or Comm Coll
Control: State, County, or Local Govt
• Clin Lab Technician/Med Lab Technician Prgm
• Respiratory Care Prgm

Reading Hospital & Medical Center
Scott Wolfe, MS, CEO
PO Box 16052
Reading, PA 19612-6052
610 988-8428
Type: Hosp or Med Ctr: 500 Beds
Control: Nonprofit (Private or Religious)
• Clin Lab Scientist/Med Technologist Prgm
• Radiography Prgm
• Surgical Technology Prgm

Sayre

Robert Packer Hospital
Marie Droege, President and COO
One Guthrie Square
Sayre, PA 18840
570 888-6666
Type: Hosp or Med Ctr: 300-499 Beds
Control: Nonprofit (Private or Religious)
• Clin Lab Scientist/Med Technologist Prgm

Schnecksville

Lehigh Carbon Community College
Donald W Snyder, MBA JD LLM, President
4525 Education Pk Dr
Schnecksville, PA 18078-2598
610 799-2121
Type: Junior or Comm Coll
Control: State, County, or Local Govt
• Medical Assistant Prgm
• Occupational Therapy Asst Prgm
• Physical Therapist Assistant Prgm
• Veterinary Technology Prgm

Scranton

Fortis Institute
Scranton, PA 18509
• Dental Hygiene Prgm

Johnson College
Ann L Pipinski, EdD, President and CEO
3427 N Main Ave
Scranton, PA 18508-1495
570 702-8901
Type: Vocational or Tech Sch
Control: Nonprofit (Private or Religious)
• Radiography Prgm
• Veterinary Technology Prgm

Lackawanna College
Raymond S Angeli, MS, President
501 Vine St
Scranton, PA 18509
570 961-7850
Type: Junior or Comm Coll
Control: Nonprofit (Private or Religious)
• Diagnostic Med Sonography (General/Vascular) Prgm
• Surgical Technology Prgm

Marywood University
Sr Anne Munley, PhD, President
2300 Adams Ave
Scranton, PA 18509
570 348-6231
Type: 4-year Coll or Univ
Control: Nonprofit (Private or Religious)
• Art Therapy Prgm
• Athletic Training Prgm
• Counseling Prgm
• Dietetic Internship Prgm
• Dietetics-Coordinated Prgm
• Dietetics-Didactic Prgm
• Music Therapy Prgm
• Physician Assistant Prgm
• Psychology (PhD) Prgm
• Speech-Language Pathology Prgm

The Commonwealth Medical College
Scranton, PA 18509
Type: 4-year Coll or Univ
Control: Nonprofit (Private or Religious)
• Allopathic Medicine Prgm

University of Scranton
Rev Scott J Pilarz, SJ PhD, President
Scranton, PA 18510-4622
570 941-7500
Type: 4-year Coll or Univ
Control: Nonprofit (Private or Religious)
• Counseling Prgm
• Nursing Prgm
• Occupational Therapy Prgm
• Physical Therapy Prgm
• Rehabilitation Counseling Prgm

Seneca

UPMC Northwest
Neil E Todhunter, CHE NHA, President/CEO
100 Fairfield Dr
Seneca, PA 16346
814 676-7140
Type: Hosp or Med Ctr: 100-299 Beds
Control: Nonprofit (Private or Religious)
• Radiography Prgm

Sharon

Laurel Technical Institute
200 Stering Avenue
Sharon, PA 16146
Type: Vocational or Tech Sch
Control: For Profit
• Clin Lab Technician/Med Lab Technician Prgm

Sharon Regional Health System
John A Zidansek, MHA, President/CEO
740 E State St
Sharon, PA 16146
412 983-3911
Type: Hosp or Med Ctr: 100-299 Beds
Control: Nonprofit (Private or Religious)
• Radiography Prgm

Shippensburg

Shippensburg University
Shippensburg, PA 17257-2210
717 532-9121
Type: 4-year Coll or Univ
Control: State, County, or Local Govt
• Counseling Prgm

Slippery Rock

Slippery Rock University of Pennsylvania
G Warren Smith, PhD, President
300 Old Main
Slippery Rock, PA 16057
412 738-2000
Type: 4-year Coll or Univ
Control: State, County, or Local Govt
• Athletic Training Prgm
• Counseling Prgm
• Exercise Science Prgm
• Music Therapy Prgm
• Physical Therapy Prgm

Spring Mills

Central Pennsylvania Institute of Sci & Tech
Henry Yeagley, Chairman
198 Pennfield Lane
Spring Mills, PA 16875
814 422-8446
Type: Vocational or Tech Sch
Control: State, County, or Local Govt
• Medical Assistant Prgm

St David

Eastern University
David Black, President
1300 Eagle Rd
St David, PA 19087
Type: 4-year Coll or Univ
Control: State, County, or Local Govt
• Athletic Training Prgm
• Exercise Science Prgm
• Nursing Prgm

State College

Mount Nittany Medical Center
Rich Wisniewski, Interim President and CEO
1800 E Park Ave
State College, PA 16803
814 234-6148
Type: Acad Health Ctr/Med Sch
Control: For Profit
• Clin Lab Scientist/Med Technologist Prgm

South Hills School of Business & Technology
S Paul Mazza, JD, President
480 Waupelani Dr
State College, PA 16801
814 234-7755
Type: Vocational or Tech Sch
Control: For Profit
• Diagnostic Med Sonography
  (Gen/Card/Vascular) Prgm

Summerdale

Central Pennsylvania College
Todd A Milano, BS, President
College Hill and Valley Rds
Summerdale, PA 17093-0309
800 759-2727
Type: 4-year Coll or Univ
Control: For Profit
• Medical Assistant Prgm
• Physical Therapist Assistant Prgm

Uniontown

Laurel Business Institute
Christopher D Decker, MEd BS, President
11-15 Penn St
PO Box 877
Uniontown, PA 15401
412 439-4900
Type: Vocational or Tech Sch
Control: For Profit
• Clin Lab Technician/Med Lab Technician Prgm

University Park

Penn State University
Graham Spanier, President
201 Old Main
University Park, PA 16802
814 865-4700
Type: 4-year Coll or Univ
Control: State, County, or Local Govt
• Allopathic Medicine Prgm
• Athletic Training Prgm
• Clin Lab Technician/Med Lab Technician Prgm
• Counseling Prgm
• Dietetic Internship Prgm
• Dietetic Technician-AD Prgm
• Dietetics-Didactic Prgm
• Music Therapy Prgm
• Nursing Prgm
• Occupational Therapy Asst Prgm (3)
• Physical Therapist Assistant Prgm (4)
• Psychology (PhD) Prgm
• Radiography Prgm (2)
• Rehabilitation Counseling Prgm
• Speech-Language Pathology Prgm

Upland

Crozer-Keystone Medical Center
Joseph Saunders, President
One Medical Center Blvd
Upland, PA 19013
610 447-2766
Type: Hosp or Med Ctr: 300-499 Beds
Control: Nonprofit (Private or Religious)
• Diagnostic Med Sonography (General) Prgm
• Neurodiagnostic Tech Prgm
• Radiography Prgm
• Respiratory Care Prgm

Villanova

Villanova University
Villanova, PA 19085
Type: 4-year Coll or Univ
Control: Nonprofit (Private or Religious)
• Nursing Prgm

Washington

Penn Commercial Inc
Robert S Bazant, BS, Director
242 Oak Spring Rd
Washington, PA 15301
724 222-5330
Type: Vocational or Tech Sch
Control: For Profit
• Medical Assistant Prgm

Washington Hospital
Telford W Thomas, MHA, President/CEO
155 Wilson Ave
Washington, PA 15301
724 223-3007
Type: Hosp or Med Ctr: 300-499 Beds
Control: Nonprofit (Private or Religious)
• Radiography Prgm

Waynesburg

Waynesburg University
Timothy R Thyreen, LHD, President
51 W College St
Waynesburg, PA 15370
724 852-3212
Type: 4-year Coll or Univ
Control: Nonprofit (Private or Religious)
• Athletic Training Prgm
• Nursing Prgm

West Chester

West Chester University
Madeleine Wing Adler, PhD, President
102 Phillips Hall
West Chester, PA 19383
610 436-2471
Type: 4-year Coll or Univ
Control: State, County, or Local Govt
• Athletic Training Prgm
• Counseling Prgm
• Dietetics-Didactic Prgm
• Exercise Science Prgm
• Nursing Prgm
• Respiratory Care Prgm
• Speech-Language Pathology Prgm

Wilkes-Barre

King's College
Rev Thomas J O'Hara, CSC PhD, President
133 N River St
Wilkes-Barre, PA 18711
570 208-5899
Type: 4-year Coll or Univ
Control: Nonprofit (Private or Religious)
• Athletic Training Prgm
• Physician Assistant Prgm

Wilkes University
Wilkes-Barre, PA 18766
Type: 4-year Coll or Univ
Control: Nonprofit (Private or Religious)
• Nursing Prgm
• Pharmacy Prgm

Wilkes-Barre General Hospital
William Host, MD, CEO
575 N River St
Wilkes-Barre, PA 18764
570 552-3006
Type: Hosp or Med Ctr: 300-499 Beds
Control: Nonprofit (Private or Religious)
• Diagnostic Med Sonography (General) Prgm

Williamsport

Pennsylvania College of Technology
Davie Jane Gilmour, PhD, President
One College Ave
Williamsport, PA 17701-5799
570 326-3761
Type: 4-year Coll or Univ
Control: State, County, or Local Govt
• Dental Hygiene Prgm
• Emergency Med Tech-Paramedic Prgm
• Occupational Therapy Asst Prgm
• Physician Assistant Prgm
• Radiography Prgm
• Surgical Technology Prgm

Susquehanna Health / Williamsport Hospital
Steven P Johnson, MBA, President
c/o Williamsport Hospital
777 Rural Ave
Williamsport, PA 17701
570 321-3170
Type: Hosp or Med Ctr: 300-499 Beds
Control: Nonprofit (Private or Religious)
• Music Therapy Prgm

Williamsport Hosp & Medical Center
Steve Johnson, President
777 Rural Ave
Williamsport, PA 17701
570 321-3170
Type: Hosp or Med Ctr: 100-299 Beds
Control: Nonprofit (Private or Religious)
• Clin Lab Scientist/Med Technologist Prgm

Wyomissing

Berks Technical Institute
Kenneth S Snyder, President
Four Park Plaza
Wyomissing, PA 19610
610 372-1722
Type: Vocational or Tech Sch
Control: For Profit
• Medical Assistant Prgm

York

Baltimore School of Massage
170 Red Rock Rd
York, PA 17402
Type: Vocational or Tech Sch
Control: For Profit
• Massage Therapy Prgm

York College of Pennsylvania
George W Waldner, PhD, President
Country Club Rd
York, PA 17405-7199
717 846-7788
Type: 4-year Coll or Univ
Control: Nonprofit (Private or Religious)
• Nursing Prgm
• Respiratory Care Prgm

York Hospital/WellSpan Health
Richard L Seim, MBA, President
1001 S George St
York, PA 17405
717 851-2650
Type: Hosp or Med Ctr: 500 Beds
Control: Nonprofit (Private or Religious)
• Clin Lab Scientist/Med Technologist Prgm
• Radiography Prgm

YTI Career Institute
Timothy E Foster, BA, CEO
1405 Williams Rd
York, PA 17402
717 757-1100
Type: Vocational or Tech Sch
Control: Nonprofit (Private or Religious)
• Dental Assistant Prgm
• Medical Assistant Prgm

Youngwood

Westmoreland County Community College
Steven C Ender, EdD, President
145 Pavilion Lane
Youngwood, PA 15697-1895
724 925-4000
Type: Junior or Comm Coll
Control: State, County, or Local Govt
• Dental Assistant Prgm
• Dental Hygiene Prgm
• Medical Assistant Prgm

Prince Edward Island, Canada

Charlottetown

University of Prince Edward Island
H Wade MacLauchlan, President
550 University Ave
Charlottetown, PE C1A 4P3
Type: 4-year Coll or Univ
Control: State, County, or Local Govt
• Veterinary Medicine Prgm

Puerto Rico

Bayamon

Universidad Central del Caribe
Jose Ginel Rodriguez, MD, Interim President
PO Box 60-327
Bayamon, PR 00960-6032
787 798-3001
Type: 4-year Coll or Univ
Control: Nonprofit (Private or Religious)
• Allopathic Medicine Prgm
• Radiography Prgm

Caguas

San Juan Bautista School of Medicine
Caguas, PR 00726
Type: Acad Health Ctr/Med Sch
Control: For Profit
• Allopathic Medicine Prgm

Gurabo

Universidad Del Turabo
Gurabo, PR 00778
Type: 4-year Coll or Univ
Control: Nonprofit (Private or Religious)
• Dietetics-Coordinated Prgm
• Nursing Prgm
• Speech-Language Pathology Prgm

Humacao

University of Puerto Rico at Humacao
Angel M Gierbolini, EdD, Chancellor
CUH Postal Station 100, Carr 908
Humacao, PR 00791-4300
787 850-9374
Type: 4-year Coll or Univ
Control: State, County, or Local Govt
• Occupational Therapy Asst Prgm
• Physical Therapist Assistant Prgm

Ponce

Ponce School of Medicine
Ponce, PR 00732
Type: Acad Health Ctr/Med Sch
Control: Nonprofit (Private or Religious)
• Allopathic Medicine Prgm
• Psychology (PsyD) Prgm

Ponce Technological University College
University of Puerto Rico
PO Box 7186
Ponce, PR 00732
Type: Vocational or Tech Sch
Control: Nonprofit (Private or Religious)
• Physical Therapist Assistant Prgm

Pontifical Catholic University of Puerto Rico
Marcelina Velez de Santiago, MS CHEM,
  President
2250 Las Americas Ave, Ste 564
Ponce, PR 00717-9997
787 841-2000
Type: 4-year Coll or Univ
Control: Nonprofit (Private or Religious)
• Clin Lab Scientist/Med Technologist Prgm
• Rehabilitation Counseling Prgm

San Juan

Carlos Albizu University
San Juan, PR 00902
Type: 4-year Coll or Univ
Control: Nonprofit (Private or Religious)
• Psychology (PhD) Prgm
• Psychology (PsyD) Prgm
• Speech-Language Pathology Prgm

Inter American University of Puerto Rico
Manuel Fernos, Esq, President
PO Box 363255
San Juan, PR 00936-3255
787 766-1912
Type: 4-year Coll or Univ
Control: Nonprofit (Private or Religious)
• Clin Lab Scientist/Med Technologist Prgm (2)
• Optometry Prgm
• Radiography Prgm

Puerto Rico Department of Health
PO Box 70184
San Juan, PR 00936
787 274-6831
Type: Acad Health Ctr/Med Sch
Control: State, County, or Local Govt
• Dietetic Internship Prgm

University of Puerto Rico
Rafael Rodriguez Mercado, MD FACS, Acting
   Chancellor
PO Box 365067
Medical Sciences' Chancellor
San Juan, PR 00956-5067
787 785-2525
Type: 4-year Coll or Univ
Control: State, County, or Local Govt
• Allopathic Medicine Prgm
• Clin Lab Scientist/Med Technologist Prgm
• Cytotechnology Prgm
• Dental Assistant Prgm
• Dentistry Prgm
• Dietetic Internship Prgm
• Dietetics-Didactic Prgm
• Medical Librarian Prgm
• Nuclear Medicine Technology Prgm
• Nursing Prgm
• Occupational Therapy Prgm
• Ophthalmic Technician Prgm
• Pharmacy Prgm
• Physical Therapy Prgm
• Radiography Prgm
• Rehabilitation Counseling Prgm
• Speech-Language Pathology Prgm
• Veterinary Technology Prgm

VA Caribbean Healthcare System
10 Calle Casia
San Juan, PR 00921
Type: Dept of Veterans Affairs
Control: Fed Govt
• Dietetic Internship Prgm

Qatar

Doha, Qatar

Qatar University
Doha, Qatar, QA
• Clin Lab Scientist/Med Technologist Prgm

Quebec, Canada

Montreal

McGill University
Jennifer Fitzpatrick, MS, Director, GC program
Human Genetics, Stewart Biology N5/13
1205 Dr Penfield Ave
Montreal, QC H3G 1Y5
514 398-3600
Type: 4-year Coll or Univ
Control: Nonprofit (Private or Religious)
• Allopathic Medicine Prgm
• Genetic Counseling Prgm
• Medical Librarian Prgm
• Psychology (PhD) Prgm

University de Montreal
Pavillon Marguerite-D'Youville
CP 6128-Succ Centreville
Montreal, QC H3C 3J7
Type: 4-year Coll or Univ
Control: Nonprofit (Private or Religious)
• Allopathic Medicine Prgm
• Medical Librarian Prgm
• Optometry Prgm
• Veterinary Medicine Prgm

Quebec City

University Laval
Pavillon Vandry
Quebec City, QC G1K 7P4
Type: 4-year Coll or Univ
Control: Nonprofit (Private or Religious)
• Allopathic Medicine Prgm

Sherbrooke

University of Sherbrooke
Sherbrooke, QC J1K 2R1
Type: Acad Health Ctr/Med Sch
Control: State, County, or Local Govt
• Allopathic Medicine Prgm

West Montreal

Concordia University
Frederick H Lowy, MD
1455 de Maisonneuve Blvd
West Montreal, QC H3G 1M8
514 848-4850
Type: 4-year Coll or Univ
Control: Nonprofit (Private or Religious)
• Art Therapy Prgm
• Psychology (PhD) Prgm

Rhode Island

Kingston

University of Rhode Island
David Dooley, President
35 Campus Ave
Presidents Office, Green Hall
Kingston, RI 02881-1303
401 874-4462
Type: 4-year Coll or Univ
Control: State, County, or Local Govt
• Cytotechnology Prgm
• Dietetic Internship Prgm
• Dietetics-Didactic Prgm
• Medical Librarian Prgm
• Music Therapy Prgm
• Nursing Prgm
• Pharmacy Prgm
• Physical Therapy Prgm
• Psychology (PhD) Prgm
• Speech-Language Pathology Prgm

Newport

Salve Regina University
M Therese Antone, EdD RSM, President
100 Ochre Point Ave
Newport, RI 02840
Type: Acad Health Ctr/Med Sch
Control: Nonprofit (Private or Religious)
• Rehabilitation Counseling Prgm

North Providence

Our Lady of Fatima Hospital
John Fogarty, MHA, Acting President
200 High Service Ave
North Providence, RI 02904
401 456-3000
Type: Hosp or Med Ctr: 100-299 Beds
Control: Nonprofit (Private or Religious)
• Clin Lab Scientist/Med Technologist Prgm

Providence

Johnson & Wales University
Morris J Gaebe, Chancellor
8 Abbott Park Palace
Providence, RI 02903-3703
401 598-1000
Type: 4-year Coll or Univ
Control: Nonprofit (Private or Religious)
• Dietetics-Didactic Prgm

Rhode Island College
Providence, RI 02908
Type: 4-year Coll or Univ
Control: State, County, or Local Govt
• Music Therapy Prgm
• Nursing Prgm

INSTITUTIONS

Rhode Island Hospital
Timothy Babineau, MD, President/CEO
593 Eddy St
Providence, RI 02903
401 444-5724
Type: Hosp or Med Ctr: 500 Beds
Control: For Profit
• Clin Lab Scientist/Med Technologist Prgm
• Diagnostic Med Sonography (General) Prgm
• Magnetic Resonance Technologist Prgm
• Nuclear Medicine Technology Prgm
• Radiography Prgm

Warren Alpert Medical School of Brown Univ
Providence, RI 02912
Type: Acad Health Ctr/Med Sch
Control: Nonprofit (Private or Religious)
• Allopathic Medicine Prgm

Warwick

Community College of Rhode Island
Ray M Di Pasquale, MA, President
400 East Ave
Warwick, RI 02886
401 825-2188
Type: Junior or Comm Coll
Control: State, County, or Local Govt
• Clin Lab Technician/Med Lab Technician Prgm
• Dental Assistant Prgm
• Dental Hygiene Prgm
• Diagnostic Med Sonography
  (Gen/Card/Vascular) Prgm
• Histotechnician Prgm
• Massage Therapy Prgm
• Occupational Therapy Asst Prgm
• Physical Therapist Assistant Prgm
• Radiography Prgm
• Respiratory Care Prgm

New England Institute of Technology
Richard I Gouse, BA, President
2500 Post Rd
Warwick, RI 02886-2251
401 739-5000
Type: 4-year Coll or Univ
Control: Nonprofit (Private or Religious)
• Occupational Therapy Asst Prgm
• Surgical Technology Prgm

Saskatchewan, Canada

Saskatoon

Saskatoon Health Region Orthoptic Program
Maura Davies
701 Queen St
Saskatoon, SK S7K 0M7
306 655-8058
Type: Hosp or Med Ctr: 100-299 Beds
Control: State, County, or Local Govt
• Orthoptist Prgm

University of Saskatchewan
1121 College Dr
Saskatoon, SK S7N 0W3
Type: 4-year Coll or Univ
Control: Nonprofit (Private or Religious)
• Allopathic Medicine Prgm
• Psychology (PhD) Prgm
• Veterinary Medicine Prgm

Saudi Arabia

Riyadh

King Khaled Eye Specialist Hospital
Riyadh, SA 11462
• Ophthalmic Assistant Prgm

South Carolina

Anderson

AnMed Health Medical Center
John Miller, MHA, President
800 N Fant St
Anderson, SC 29621
864 261-1109
Type: Hosp or Med Ctr: 500 Beds
Control: Nonprofit (Private or Religious)
• Radiography Prgm

Forrest College
John Re, PhD, President
601 E River St
Anderson, SC 29624
864 225-7653
Type: Junior or Comm Coll
Control: For Profit
• Medical Assistant Prgm

Beaufort

Technical College of the Lowcountry
Anne McNutt, PhD, President
PO Box 1288
Beaufort, SC 29901
843 525-8211
Type: Vocational or Tech Sch
Control: For Profit
• Radiography Prgm
• Surgical Technology Prgm

Bluffton

University of South Carolina Beaufort
1 University Boulevard
Bluffton, SC 29909
Type: 4-year Coll or Univ
Control: State, County, or Local Govt
• Nursing Prgm

Charleston

Charleston Southern University
Jairy C Hunter, PhD, President
PO Box 118087
Charleston, SC 29423-8087
803 863-7000
Type: 4-year Coll or Univ
Control: Nonprofit (Private or Religious)
• Athletic Training Prgm
• Music Therapy Prgm

College of Charleston
Leo I Higdon, Jr, President
66 George St
Charleston, SC 29424-0001
843 953-5500
Type: 4-year Coll or Univ
Control: State, County, or Local Govt
• Athletic Training Prgm
• Music Therapy Prgm

Medical University of South Carolina
Raymond S Greenberg, MD, President
179 Ashley Ave
MSC 001
Charleston, SC 29425-0010
843 792-2211
Type: Acad Health Ctr/Med Sch
Control: State, County, or Local Govt
• Allopathic Medicine Prgm
• Dentistry Prgm
• Dietetic Internship Prgm
• Histotechnology Prgm
• Nursing Prgm
• Occupational Therapy Prgm
• Perfusion Prgm
• Physical Therapy Prgm
• Physician Assistant Prgm

Miller-Motte Technical College
James Weaver, MS, Campus Director
8085 Rivers Ave
Charleston, SC 29406
843 574-0101
Type: Vocational or Tech Sch
Control: For Profit
• Medical Assistant Prgm
• Surgical Technology Prgm

South Carolina College of Pharmacy
Joseph T DiPiro, PharmD, Executive Dean
280 Calhoun St
Charleston, SC 29425
843 792-8450
Type: Acad Health Ctr/Med Sch
Control: Nonprofit (Private or Religious)
• Pharmacy Prgm

Trident Technical College
Mary D Thornley, EdD, President
PO Box 118067
7000 Rivers Avenue
Charleston, SC 29423-8067
843 574-6241
Type: Vocational or Tech Sch
Control: State, County, or Local Govt
• Clin Lab Technician/Med Lab Technician Prgm
• Dental Assistant Prgm
• Dental Hygiene Prgm
• Emergency Med Tech-Paramedic Prgm
• Medical Assistant Prgm
• Medical Transcriptionist Prgm
• Occupational Therapy Asst Prgm
• Ophthalmic Assistant Prgm
• Pharmacy Technician Prgm
• Physical Therapist Assistant Prgm
• Radiography Prgm
• Respiratory Care Prgm
• Veterinary Technology Prgm

Clemson

Clemson University
Constantine W Curris, President
201 Sikes Hall
Clemson, SC 29634
803 656-3311
Type: 4-year Coll or Univ
Control: State, County, or Local Govt
• Counseling Prgm
• Dietetics-Didactic Prgm
• Nursing Prgm

Clinton

Presbyterian College
Clinton, SC 29325
Type: 4-year Coll or Univ
Control: Nonprofit (Private or Religious)
• Pharmacy Prgm

Columbia

Midlands Technical College
Marshall (Sonny) White, PhD, President
PO Box 2408
Columbia, SC 29202-2408
803 738-7600
Type: Junior or Comm Coll
Control: State, County, or Local Govt
• Clin Lab Technician/Med Lab Technician Prgm
• Dental Assistant Prgm
• Dental Hygiene Prgm
• Medical Assistant Prgm
• Nuclear Medicine Technology Prgm
• Pharmacy Technician Prgm
• Physical Therapist Assistant Prgm
• Radiography Prgm
• Respiratory Care Prgm
• Surgical Technology Prgm

Palmetto Health Baptist
James Bridges, President
Taylor at Marion St
Columbia, SC 29220
803 296-5174
Type: Hosp or Med Ctr: 300-499 Beds
Control: Nonprofit (Private or Religious)
• Clin Lab Scientist/Med Technologist Prgm

SC Dept of Health & Environmental Control
Mills Complex, PO Box 101106
Columbia, SC 29211-0106
803 737-3954
Type: Acad Health Ctr/Med Sch
Control: State, County, or Local Govt
• Dietetic Internship Prgm

Sister of Charity Providence Hospital
Stephen Purves, MHA, President
2435 Forest Dr
Columbia, SC 29204
803 256-5313
Type: Hosp or Med Ctr: 300-499 Beds
Control: Nonprofit (Private or Religious)
• Cardiovascular Tech (Invasive/Noninv/Vasc) Prgm

South University
Anne F Patton, BBA, President
3810 Main St
Columbia, SC 29203
803 799-9082
Type: Junior or Comm Coll
Control: For Profit
• Medical Assistant Prgm

University of South Carolina
Harris Pastides, PhD, President
Osborne 203
Columbia, SC 29208
803 777-2001
Type: 4-year Coll or Univ
Control: State, County, or Local Govt
• Allopathic Medicine Prgm (2)
• Athletic Training Prgm
• Counseling Prgm
• Genetic Counseling Prgm
• Medical Librarian Prgm
• Music Therapy Prgm
• Nursing Prgm (2)
• Physical Therapy Prgm
• Psychology (PhD) Prgm
• Rehabilitation Counseling Prgm
• Speech-Language Pathology Prgm

Conway

Horry - Georgetown Technical College
H Neyle Wilson, BS MEd, President
PO Box 261966
2050 Highway 501 E
Conway, SC 29528
843 349-5201
Type: Vocational or Tech Sch
Control: State, County, or Local Govt
• Dental Assistant Prgm
• Dental Hygiene Prgm
• Diagnostic Med Sonography (General) Prgm
• Emergency Med Tech-Paramedic Prgm
• Pharmacy Technician Prgm
• Radiography Prgm
• Surgical Technology Prgm

Due West

Erskine College
Randy T Ruble, PhD, President
2 Washington St
Due West, SC 29639
864 379-8833
Type: 4-year Coll or Univ
Control: Nonprofit (Private or Religious)
• Athletic Training Prgm

Florence

Florence-Darlington Technical College
Charles W Gould, PhD, President
PO Box 100548
Florence, SC 29501-0548
843 661-8000
Type: Vocational or Tech Sch
Control: State, County, or Local Govt
• Clin Lab Technician/Med Lab Technician Prgm
• Dental Assistant Prgm
• Dental Hygiene Prgm
• Radiography Prgm
• Respiratory Care Prgm
• Surgical Technology Prgm

McLeod Regional Medical Center
Marie Segars, President and CEO
555 E Cheves St
PO Box 100551
Florence, SC 29501
843 777-5333
Type: Hosp or Med Ctr: 300-499 Beds
Control: Nonprofit (Private or Religious)
• Clin Lab Scientist/Med Technologist Prgm

Gaffney

Limestone College
Walt Griffin, PhD, President
1115 College Dr
Gaffney, SC 29340
864 488-4616
Type: 4-year Coll or Univ
Control: Nonprofit (Private or Religious)
• Athletic Training Prgm

Graniteville

Aiken Technical College
Susan Winsor, PhD, President
2276 Jefferson Davis Hwy
PO Box 400
Graniteville, SC 29829
803 593-9954
Type: Vocational or Tech Sch
Control: State, County, or Local Govt
• Dental Assistant Prgm
• Medical Assistant Prgm
• Pharmacy Technician Prgm
• Radiography Prgm
• Surgical Technology Prgm

Greenville

Greenville Technical College
Keith Miller, EdD, President
PO Box 5616
620 South Pleasantburg Drive
Greenville, SC 29607
864 250-8111
Type: Junior or Comm Coll
Control: State, County, or Local Govt
• Clin Lab Technician/Med Lab Technician Prgm
• Dental Assistant Prgm
• Dental Hygiene Prgm
• Diagnostic Med Sonography (General) Prgm
• Emergency Med Tech-Paramedic Prgm
• Medical Assistant Prgm
• Occupational Therapy Asst Prgm
• Pharmacy Technician Prgm
• Physical Therapist Assistant Prgm
• Radiography Prgm
• Respiratory Care Prgm
• Surgical Technology Prgm

Virginia College of Greenville
Greenville, SC 29607
Type: 4-year Coll or Univ
• Surgical Technology Prgm

Greenwood

Lander University
Daniel Ball, EdD, President
320 Stanley Ave
Greenwood, SC 29649
864 388-8300
Type: 4-year Coll or Univ
Control: State, County, or Local Govt
• Athletic Training Prgm
• Nursing Prgm

Piedmont Technical College
Lex D Walters, PhD, President
PO Box 1467
Emerald Rd
Greenwood, SC 29647-1467
864 941-8324
Type: Vocational or Tech Sch
Control: State, County, or Local Govt
- Medical Assistant Prgm
- Radiography Prgm
- Respiratory Care Prgm
- Surgical Technology Prgm

Newberry

Newberry College
2100 College Street
Newberry, SC 29108-2126
Type: 4-year Coll or Univ
Control: Nonprofit (Private or Religious)
- Nursing Prgm

Piedmont Technical College
Mitchell Zais, PhD, President
2100 College St
Holland Hall-101
Newberry, SC 29108
803 321-5102
Type: Acad Health Ctr/Med Sch
Control: For Profit
- Pharmacy Technician Prgm
- Veterinary Technology Prgm

Orangeburg

Orangeburg Calhoun Technical College
Anne Crook, PhD, President
3250 St Matthews Rd
Orangeburg, SC 29118
803 536-0311
Type: Junior or Comm Coll
Control: State, County, or Local Govt
- Medical Assistant Prgm
- Radiography Prgm

South Carolina State University
Andrew Hugine, PhD, President
300 College St NE
Orangeburg, SC 29117
803 536-7014
Type: 4-year Coll or Univ
Control: State, County, or Local Govt
- Counseling Prgm
- Dietetics-Didactic Prgm
- Nursing Prgm
- Orientation and Mobility Specialist Prgm
- Rehabilitation Counseling Prgm
- Speech-Language Pathology Prgm

Pendleton

Tri-County Technical College
Ronnie L Booth, PhD, President
PO Box 587
7900 Hwy 76
Pendleton, SC 29670
864 646-8361
Type: Junior or Comm Coll
Control: State, County, or Local Govt
- Clin Lab Technician/Med Lab Technician Prgm
- Dental Assistant Prgm
- Medical Assistant Prgm
- Respiratory Care Prgm
- Surgical Technology Prgm
- Veterinary Technology Prgm

Rock Hill

Winthrop University
Anthony J Digiorgio, PhD, President
701 Oakland Ave
Rock Hill, SC 29733
803 323-2225
Type: 4-year Coll or Univ
Control: State, County, or Local Govt
- Athletic Training Prgm
- Counseling Prgm
- Dietetic Internship Prgm
- Dietetics-Didactic Prgm

York Technical College
Greg F Rutherford, PhD, President
452 S Anderson Rd
Rock Hill, SC 29730
803 327-8050
Type: Junior or Comm Coll
Control: State, County, or Local Govt
- Clin Lab Technician/Med Lab Technician Prgm
- Dental Assistant Prgm
- Dental Hygiene Prgm
- Radiography Prgm
- Surgical Technology Prgm

Spartanburg

Sherman College of Straight Chiropractic
2020 Springfield Rd
Spartanburg, SC 29304
Type: Acad Health Ctr/Med Sch
Control: For Profit
- Chiropractic Prgm

Spartanburg Community College
Dan L Terhune, EdD, President
PO Drawer 4386
Bus I-85 & New Cut Rd
Spartanburg, SC 29305-4386
864 592-4610
Type: Junior or Comm Coll
Control: State, County, or Local Govt
- Clin Lab Technician/Med Lab Technician Prgm
- Dental Assistant Prgm
- Medical Assistant Prgm
- Pharmacy Technician Prgm
- Radiography Prgm
- Respiratory Care Prgm
- Surgical Technology Prgm

University of South Carolina Upstate
Spartanburg, SC 29303
Type: 4-year Coll or Univ
Control: State, County, or Local Govt
- Nursing Prgm

Sumter

Central Carolina Technical College
Kay Raffield, President
506 N Guignard Dr
Sumter, SC 29150
803 778-1961
Type: Vocational or Tech Sch
Control: State, County, or Local Govt
- Medical Assistant Prgm
- Surgical Technology Prgm

West Columbia

Lexington Medical Center
Mike Biedeger, President
2720 Sunset Blvd
West Columbia, SC 29169
803 791-2000
Type: Hosp or Med Ctr: 300-499 Beds
Control: State, County, or Local Govt
- Clin Lab Scientist/Med Technologist Prgm

South Dakota

Aberdeen

Presentation College
Lorraine Hale, PhD, President
1500 N Main St
Aberdeen, SD 57401-1299
605 229-8405
Type: 4-year Coll or Univ
Control: Nonprofit (Private or Religious)
- Medical Assistant Prgm
- Radiography Prgm
- Surgical Technology Prgm

Brookings

South Dakota State University
David Chicoine, PhD, President
Office of the President - AD 222
Brookings, SD 57007
605 688-4151
Type: 4-year Coll or Univ
Control: State, County, or Local Govt
- Athletic Training Prgm
- Clin Lab Scientist/Med Technologist Prgm
- Counseling Prgm
- Dietetics-Didactic Prgm
- Nursing Prgm
- Pharmacy Prgm

Madison

Dakota State University
Douglas Knowlton, PhD, President
314 Heston Hall
Madison, SD 57042-1799
605 256-5112
Type: 4-year Coll or Univ
Control: State, County, or Local Govt
- Respiratory Care Prgm

Mitchell

Dakota Wesleyan University
Robert Duffet, PhD, President
1200 W University
Box 911
Mitchell, SD 57301
605 995-2601
Type: 4-year Coll or Univ
Control: Nonprofit (Private or Religious)
• Athletic Training Prgm

Mitchell Technical Institute
Greg Von Wald, MA, President
821 N Capital St
Mitchell, SD 57301
605 995-3023
Type: Vocational or Tech Sch
Control: State, County, or Local Govt
• Clin Lab Technician/Med Lab Technician Prgm
• Medical Assistant Prgm
• Radiography Prgm

Rapid City

National American University
Jerry L Gallentine, PhD, President
14 St Joseph St
Rapid City, SD 57709
605 394-4900
Type: 4-year Coll or Univ
Control: For Profit
• Athletic Training Prgm
• Medical Assistant Prgm
• Nursing Prgm
• Pharmacy Technician Prgm
• Veterinary Technology Prgm

Rapid City Regional Hospital
Timothy Sughrue, MBA, President/CEO
353 Fairmont Blvd
Rapid City, SD 57701
605 719-8162
Type: Hosp or Med Ctr: 300-499 Beds
Control: Nonprofit (Private or Religious)
• Radiography Prgm

Western Dakota Technical Institute
Rich Gross, MEd PhD, Director
800 Mickelson Dr
Rapid City, SD 57703
605 394-4034
Type: Vocational or Tech Sch
Control: Nonprofit (Private or Religious)
• Pharmacy Technician Prgm
• Surgical Technology Prgm

Sioux Falls

Augustana College
Robert Oliver, PhD, President
2001 S Summit Ave
Sioux Falls, SD 57197
605 336-4111
Type: 4-year Coll or Univ
Control: State, County, or Local Govt
• Athletic Training Prgm
• Nursing Prgm

Avera McKennan Hospital
Fred Slunecka, MHA, President/CEO
800 E 21st St
PO Box 5045
Sioux Falls, SD 57117-5045
605 322-7808
Type: Hosp or Med Ctr: 300-499 Beds
Control: Nonprofit (Private or Religious)
• Emergency Med Tech-Paramedic Prgm
• Radiography Prgm

Colorado Technical University
David Heflin, President
3901 W 59th St
Sioux Falls, SD 57108
605 361-0200
Type: 4-year Coll or Univ
Control: For Profit
• Medical Assistant Prgm

Sanford USD Medical Center
Charles O'Brien, President
1305 W 18th St
Sioux Falls, SD 57117-5039
605 333-6437
Type: Hosp or Med Ctr: 300-499 Beds
Control: Nonprofit (Private or Religious)
• Clin Lab Scientist/Med Technologist Prgm
• Radiography Prgm

Southeast Technical Institute
Jeff Holcomb, MBA, Director and CEO
2320 N Career Ave
Sioux Falls, SD 57107
605 367-7485
Type: Vocational or Tech Sch
Control: Nonprofit (Private or Religious)
• Cardiovascular Tech (Invasive/Noninv/Vasc) Prgm
• Diagnostic Med Sonography (General) Prgm
• Neurodiagnostic Tech Prgm
• Nuclear Medicine Technology Prgm
• Pharmacy Technician Prgm
• Surgical Technology Prgm

University of Sioux Falls
1101 West 22nd Street
Sioux Falls, SD 57105-1699
Type: 4-year Coll or Univ
Control: State, County, or Local Govt
• Nursing Prgm

Vermillion

University of South Dakota
Jim Abbott, JD, President
414 E Clark St
Vermillion, SD 57069-2390
605 677-5641
Type: 4-year Coll or Univ
Control: State, County, or Local Govt
• Allopathic Medicine Prgm
• Audiologist Prgm
• Counseling Prgm
• Dental Hygiene Prgm
• Dietetic Internship Prgm
• Music Therapy Prgm
• Occupational Therapy Prgm
• Physical Therapy Prgm
• Physician Assistant Prgm
• Psychology (PhD) Prgm
• Rehabilitation Counseling Prgm
• Speech-Language Pathology Prgm

Watertown

Lake Area Technical Institute
Deb Shehard, President
230 11th St NE
PO Box 730
Watertown, SD 57201-0730
605 882-5284
Type: Vocational or Tech Sch
Control: State, County, or Local Govt
• Clin Lab Technician/Med Lab Technician Prgm
• Dental Assistant Prgm
• Emergency Med Tech-Paramedic Prgm
• Medical Assistant Prgm
• Occupational Therapy Asst Prgm
• Physical Therapist Assistant Prgm

Yankton

Avera Sacred Heart Hospital
Pamela J Rezac, PhD, CEO
501 Summit St
Yankton, SD 57078
605 668-8000
Type: Hosp or Med Ctr: 100-299 Beds
Control: Nonprofit (Private or Religious)
• Radiography Prgm

Mt Marty College
Sr Jacquelyn Ernster, PhD, President
Yankton, SD 57078
605 668-1514
Type: 4-year Coll or Univ
Control: Nonprofit (Private or Religious)
• Nursing Prgm

Tennessee

Blountville

Northeast State Community College
William W Locke, PhD, President
PO Box 246
2425 Hwy 75
Blountville, TN 37617-0246
423 323-0201
Type: Junior or Comm Coll
Control: State, County, or Local Govt
• Cardiovascular Tech (Invasive) Prgm
• Clin Lab Technician/Med Lab Technician Prgm
• Dental Assistant Prgm
• Emergency Med Tech-Paramedic Prgm
• Surgical Technology Prgm

Bristol

King College
Bristol, TN 37620
Type: 4-year Coll or Univ
Control: Nonprofit (Private or Religious)
• Athletic Training Prgm
• Nursing Prgm

National College of Business and Technology
Frank E Longaker, MBA, President
1328 Highway 11W
Bristol, TN 37620
540 986-1800
Type: Junior or Comm Coll
Control: For Profit
• Medical Assistant Prgm (4)
• Surgical Technology Prgm

Chattanooga

Chattanooga State Community College
James L Catanzaro, PhD, President
4501 Amnicola Hwy
Chattanooga, TN 37406-1097
423 697-4455
Type: Junior or Comm Coll
Control: State, County, or Local Govt
- Dental Assistant Prgm
- Dental Hygiene Prgm
- Diagnostic Med Sonography (Gen/Card/Vascular) Prgm
- Emergency Med Tech-Paramedic Prgm
- Medical Assistant Prgm
- Nuclear Medicine Technology Prgm
- Pharmacy Technician Prgm
- Physical Therapist Assistant Prgm
- Radiation Therapy Prgm
- Radiography Prgm
- Respiratory Care Prgm
- Surgical Technology Prgm

Miller-Motte Technical College - Chattanooga
Faron Boreham, EdD, Campus Director
6020 Shallowford Rd
Chattanooga, TN 37421
423 510-9675
Type: Vocational or Tech Sch
Control: For Profit
- Medical Assistant Prgm
- Surgical Technology Prgm

University of Tennessee - Chattanooga
Roger G Brown, PhD, Chancellor
615 McCallie Ave
101 Founders Hall, Dept 5605
Chattanooga, TN 37403-2598
423 425-4141
Type: 4-year Coll or Univ
Control: State, County, or Local Govt
- Athletic Training Prgm
- Counseling Prgm
- Dietetics-Didactic Prgm
- Music Therapy Prgm
- Nursing Prgm
- Physical Therapy Prgm

Clarksville

Austin Peay State University
Tim Hall, JD, President
Office of the President
Clarksville, TN 37044
931 221-7566
Type: 4-year Coll or Univ
Control: State, County, or Local Govt
- Clin Lab Scientist/Med Technologist Prgm
- Music Therapy Prgm
- Radiography Prgm

Miller-Motte Technical College - Clarksville
Virginia Castleberry, BA MS, Campus Director
1820 Business Park Dr
Clarksville, TN 37040
931 553-0071
Type: Vocational or Tech Sch
Control: For Profit
- Medical Assistant Prgm
- Polysomnographic Technology Prgm
- Surgical Technology Prgm

Cleveland

Cleveland State Community College
Carl Hite, PhD, President
3535 Adkisson Dr
PO Box 3570
Cleveland, TN 37320-3570
423 472-7141
Type: Junior or Comm Coll
Control: State, County, or Local Govt
- Medical Assistant Prgm

Lee University
Carolyn Dirksen, PhD, VP Academic Affairs
1120 N Ocoee St
Cleveland, TN 37320-3450
423 614-8118
Type: 4-year Coll or Univ
Control: Nonprofit (Private or Religious)
- Athletic Training Prgm

Columbia

Columbia State Community College
O Rebecca Hawkins, PhD, President
Hwy 412 PO Box 1315
Columbia, TN 38401
615 540-2722
Type: Junior or Comm Coll
Control: State, County, or Local Govt
- Emergency Med Tech-Paramedic Prgm
- Medical Transcriptionist Prgm
- Radiography Prgm
- Respiratory Care Prgm
- Veterinary Technology Prgm

Cookeville

Fortis Institute
John Hopkins, BS, President
1025 Highway 111
Cookeville, TN 38501
615 586-3660
Type: Vocational or Tech Sch
Control: For Profit
- Clin Lab Technician/Med Lab Technician Prgm
- Radiography Prgm (2)
- Surgical Technology Prgm

Tennessee Technological University
Robert R Bell, President
1000 N Dixie Ave
Cookeville, TN 38505-0001
931 372-3101
Type: 4-year Coll or Univ
Control: State, County, or Local Govt
- Dietetics-Didactic Prgm
- Emergency Med Tech-Paramedic Prgm
- Music Therapy Prgm
- Nursing Prgm

Crossville

Tennessee Technology Center - Crossville
James Purcell, Director
910 Miller Ave
PO Box 2959
Crossville, TN 38557
931 484-7502
Type: Vocational or Tech Sch
Control: State, County, or Local Govt
- Surgical Technology Prgm

Dickson

Tennessee Technology Center - Dickson
Warner Taylor, MS, Interim Director
740 Hwy 46 South
Dickson, TN 37055
615 441-6220
Type: Vocational or Tech Sch
Control: State, County, or Local Govt
- Dental Assistant Prgm

Gallatin

Volunteer State Community College
Warren Nichols, EdD, President
1480 Nashville
Gallatin, TN 37066-3188
615 452-8600
Type: Junior or Comm Coll
Control: State, County, or Local Govt
- Clin Lab Technician/Med Lab Technician Prgm
- Dental Assistant Prgm
- Diagnostic Med Sonography (General) Prgm
- Emergency Med Tech-Paramedic Prgm
- Ophthalmic Technician Prgm
- Physical Therapist Assistant Prgm
- Polysomnographic Technology Prgm
- Radiography Prgm
- Respiratory Care Prgm

Greenville

Tusculum College
Russell Nichols, PhD, President
106 McCormick
60 Old Shiloh Rd
Greenville, TN 37743
800 729-0256
Type: 4-year Coll or Univ
Control: Nonprofit (Private or Religious)
- Athletic Training Prgm

Harriman

Roane State Community College
Gary Goff, EdD, President
276 Patton Ln
Harriman, TN 37748-5011
865 882-4501
Type: Junior or Comm Coll
Control: State, County, or Local Govt
- Dental Hygiene Prgm
- Emergency Med Tech-Paramedic Prgm
- Massage Therapy Prgm
- Medical Transcriptionist Prgm
- Occupational Therapy Asst Prgm
- Ophthalmic Dispensing Optician Prgm
- Physical Therapist Assistant Prgm
- Polysomnographic Technology Prgm
- Radiography Prgm
- Respiratory Care Prgm

Harrogate

Lincoln Memorial University
C Warren Neel, President
PO Box 2028
6965 Cumberland Gap Parkway
Harrogate, TN 37752
423 869-7091
Type: 4-year Coll or Univ
Control: Nonprofit (Private or Religious)
• Athletic Training Prgm
• Clin Lab Scientist/Med Technologist Prgm
• Osteopathic Medicine Prgm
• Physician Assistant Prgm
• Veterinary Technology Prgm

Hohenwald

Tennessee Technology Center - Hohenwald
Rick C Brewer, MEd ED SPEC, Director
813 W Main St
Hohenwald, TN 38462
931 796-5351
Type: Vocational or Tech Sch
Control: Nonprofit (Private or Religious)
• Surgical Technology Prgm

Jackson

Jackson State Community College
Bruce Blanding, PhD, President
2046 N Parkway St
Administration Building
Jackson, TN 38301-3797
731 424-3520
Type: Junior or Comm Coll
Control: State, County, or Local Govt
• Clin Lab Technician/Med Lab Technician Prgm
• Emergency Med Tech-Paramedic Prgm
• Physical Therapist Assistant Prgm
• Radiography Prgm
• Respiratory Care Prgm

Tennessee Technology Center - Jackson
Don Williams, PhD, Director
2468 Technology Center Dr
Jackson, TN 38301
731 424-0691
Type: Vocational or Tech Sch
Control: State, County, or Local Govt
• Pharmacy Technician Prgm
• Surgical Technology Prgm

Union University
David S Dockery, PhD, President
1050 Union University Dr
Jackson, TN 38305
731 661-5180
Type: 4-year Coll or Univ
Control: Nonprofit (Private or Religious)
• Athletic Training Prgm
• Music Therapy Prgm
• Nursing Prgm
• Pharmacy Prgm

Jefferson City

Carson-Newman College
J Cordell Maddox, President
1646 Russell Ave
Jefferson City, TN 37760
615 471-4000
Type: 4-year Coll or Univ
Control: Nonprofit (Private or Religious)
• Athletic Training Prgm
• Dietetics-Didactic Prgm
• Nursing Prgm

Joelton

Meridian Institute of Surgical Assisting
Dennis A Stover, CST SA-C, President
PO Box 758
Joelton, TN 37080
615 298-1416
Type: Hosp or Med Ctr: 100-299 Beds
Control: For Profit
• Surgical Assistant Prgm

Johnson City

East Tennessee State University
Paul E Stanton, Jr, MD, President
College of Public and Allied Health
Box 70734
Johnson City, TN 37614
423 439-4211
Type: 4-year Coll or Univ
Control: State, County, or Local Govt
• Allopathic Medicine Prgm
• Audiologist Prgm
• Counseling Prgm
• Dental Hygiene Prgm
• Dietetic Internship Prgm
• Dietetics-Didactic Prgm
• Music Therapy Prgm
• Nursing Prgm
• Pharmacy Prgm
• Physical Therapy Prgm
• Polysomnographic Technology Prgm
• Radiography Prgm
• Respiratory Care Prgm
• Speech-Language Pathology Prgm

Knoxville

South College
Stephen A South, BS, President
3904 Lonas Dr
Knoxville, TN 37909
865 251-1800
Type: 4-year Coll or Univ
Control: For Profit
• Medical Assistant Prgm
• Nuclear Medicine Technology Prgm
• Pharmacy Prgm
• Physical Therapist Assistant Prgm
• Physician Assistant Prgm
• Radiography Prgm

Tennessee Technology Center - Knoxville
David Esa, MSEd, Director
1100 Liberty St
Knoxville, TN 37919
615 546-5567
Type: Vocational or Tech Sch
Control: For Profit
• Dental Assistant Prgm
• Medical Assistant Prgm
• Surgical Technology Prgm

Tennessee Wesleyan College
Knoxville, TN 37932
Type: 4-year Coll or Univ
Control: Nonprofit (Private or Religious)
• Nursing Prgm

University of Tennessee - Knoxville
Loren Crabtree, PhD, Chancellor
810 Andy Holt Tower
Knoxville, TN 37996
865 974-3265
Type: 4-year Coll or Univ
Control: State, County, or Local Govt
• Audiologist Prgm
• Counseling Prgm
• Dietetic Internship Prgm
• Dietetics-Didactic Prgm
• Medical Librarian Prgm
• Music Therapy Prgm
• Nursing Prgm
• Psychology (PhD) Prgm
• Rehabilitation Counseling Prgm
• Speech-Language Pathology Prgm

University of Tennessee Medical Center
Joseph Landsman, BS, President and CEO
1520 Cherokee Trail, Ste 200
Knoxville, TN 37920-6999
865 305-9430
Type: Hosp or Med Ctr: 500 Beds
Control: Nonprofit (Private or Religious)
• Clin Lab Scientist/Med Technologist Prgm
• Radiography Prgm
• Veterinary Medicine Prgm

Lebanon

Cumberland University
Harvill C Eaton, PhD, President
One Cumberland Square
Lebanon, TN 37087-3408
615 547-1234
Type: 4-year Coll or Univ
Control: Nonprofit (Private or Religious)
• Athletic Training Prgm

Madisonville

Hiwassee College
Madisonville, TN 37354
• Dental Hygiene Prgm

Martin

University of Tennessee - Martin
Tom Rakes, EdD, Chancellor
325 Adminstration Bldg
Martin, TN 38238
731 881-7500
Type: 4-year Coll or Univ
Control: State, County, or Local Govt
• Dietetic Internship Prgm
• Dietetics-Didactic Prgm

McKenzie

Bethel University
Rev Robert D Prosser, President
325 Cherry St
McKenzie, TN 38201-1705
901 352-4000
Type: 4-year Coll or Univ
Control: Nonprofit (Private or Religious)
• Nursing Prgm
• Physician Assistant Prgm

McMinnville

Tennessee Technology Center - McMinnville
Andy Forrester, MS, Director
241 Vo-Tech Dr
McMinnville, TN 37110
931 473-5587
Type: Vocational or Tech Sch
Control: State, County, or Local Govt
• Medical Assistant Prgm

Memphis

Baptist College of Health Sciences
Betty Sue McGarvey, DSN, President
1003 Monroe Ave
Memphis, TN 38104-3199
901 572-2468
Type: 4-year Coll or Univ
Control: Nonprofit (Private or Religious)
• Clin Lab Scientist/Med Technologist Prgm
• Diagnostic Med Sonography (General/Vascular) Prgm
• Nuclear Medicine Technology Prgm
• Nursing Prgm
• Radiation Therapy Prgm
• Radiography Prgm
• Respiratory Care Prgm

Christian Brothers College
Br Theodore Drahmann, FCS EdS, President
650 E Parkway S
Memphis, TN 38104
901 278-0100
Type: 4-year Coll or Univ
Control: Nonprofit (Private or Religious)
• Physician Assistant Prgm

Concorde Career College - Memphis
Tommy Stewart, AAS, Director
5100 Poplar Ave, Ste 132
Memphis, TN 38137
901 761-9494
Type: Vocational or Tech Sch
Control: For Profit
• Dental Assistant Prgm
• Dental Hygiene Prgm
• Pharmacy Technician Prgm
• Radiography Prgm
• Respiratory Care Prgm
• Surgical Technology Prgm

Hamilton Eye Institute
UTHSC 956 Court Ave, Room D-222
Memphis, TN 38163
901 866-8864
• Orthoptist Prgm

Memphis VA Medical Center
Memphis, TN 38104
Type: Dept of Defense
Control: Fed Govt
• Dietetic Internship Prgm

Methodist Le Bonheur Healthcare
Peggy Troy, RN MSN, CEO
Methodist Professional Bldg
1211 Union Ave, Ste 700
Memphis, TN 38104
901 516-0546
Type: Hosp or Med Ctr: 500 Beds
Control: Nonprofit (Private or Religious)
• Diagnostic Med Sonography (General) Prgm

Methodist University Hospital
Cecelia Sawyer, CEO
1265 Union Ave
Memphis, TN 38104
901 516-0543
Type: Hosp or Med Ctr: 500 Beds
Control: Nonprofit (Private or Religious)
• Nuclear Medicine Technology Prgm
• Radiography Prgm

Southern College of Optometry
Richard W Phillips, OD FAAO, President
1245 Madison Ave
Memphis, TN 38104
901 722-3200
Type: Junior or Comm Coll
Control: Nonprofit (Private or Religious)
• Optometry Prgm

Southwest Tennessee Community College
Nathan L Essex, President
5983 Macon Cove
Memphis, TN 38134-7693
901 333-4462
Type: Junior or Comm Coll
Control: State, County, or Local Govt
• Clin Lab Technician/Med Lab Technician Prgm
• Dietetic Technician-AD Prgm
• Emergency Med Tech-Paramedic Prgm
• Phlebotomy Prgm
• Physical Therapist Assistant Prgm
• Radiography Prgm

Tennessee Technology Center - Memphis
Lana Pierce, Director
550 Alabama Ave
Memphis, TN 38105-3799
901 543-6156
Type: Vocational or Tech Sch
Control: State, County, or Local Govt
• Dental Assistant Prgm
• Pharmacy Technician Prgm

University of Memphis
Shirley C Raines, President
Memphis, TN 38152
901 678-2000
Type: 4-year Coll or Univ
Control: State, County, or Local Govt
• Audiologist Prgm
• Counseling Prgm
• Dietetic Internship Prgm
• Dietetics-Didactic Prgm
• Music Therapy Prgm
• Nursing Prgm
• Psychology (PhD) Prgm
• Rehabilitation Counseling Prgm
• Speech-Language Pathology Prgm

University of Tennessee Health Science Ctr
Hershel P Wall, MD, Chancellor
62 South Dunlap, Room 219
Hyman Admin Bldg, Suite 219
Memphis, TN 38163-4901
901 448-4796
Type: Acad Health Ctr/Med Sch
Control: State, County, or Local Govt
• Allopathic Medicine Prgm
• Clin Lab Scientist/Med Technologist Prgm
• Cytotechnology Prgm
• Dental Hygiene Prgm
• Dentistry Prgm
• Histotechnology Prgm
• Occupational Therapy Prgm
• Pharmacy Prgm
• Physical Therapy Prgm

Milligan College

Milligan College
William B Greer, PhD, President
PO Box 1
Milligan College, TN 37682
423 461-8710
Type: 4-year Coll or Univ
Control: Nonprofit (Private or Religious)
• Nursing Prgm
• Occupational Therapy Prgm

Morristown

Walters State Community College
Wade B McCamey, EdD, President
500 S Davy Crockett Pkwy
Morristown, TN 37813-6899
423 585-2600
Type: Junior or Comm Coll
Control: State, County, or Local Govt
• Emergency Med Tech-Paramedic Prgm
• Pharmacy Technician Prgm
• Physical Therapist Assistant Prgm
• Respiratory Care Prgm

Murfreesboro

Middle Tennessee State University
Sydney McPhee, PhD, President
Cope Administration Bldg 110
Murfreesboro, TN 37132
615 898-2622
Type: 4-year Coll or Univ
Control: State, County, or Local Govt
• Athletic Training Prgm
• Counseling Prgm
• Dietetics-Didactic Prgm
• Music Therapy Prgm
• Nursing Prgm

National HealthCare LP
PO Box 1398
Murfreesboro, TN 37133-1398
615 890-2020
Control: For Profit
• Dietetic Internship Prgm

Tennessee Technology Center - Murfreesboro
Carol Puryear, BS MS, Director
1303 Old Fort Pkwy
Murfreesboro, TN 37130
615 898-8010
Type: Vocational or Tech Sch
Control: State, County, or Local Govt
- Dental Assistant Prgm
- Pharmacy Technician Prgm
- Surgical Technology Prgm

Nashville

Belmont U/Trevecca Nazarene U Consortium
1900 Belmont Boulevard
Nashville, TN 37212-3757
Type: Consortium
Control: Nonprofit (Private or Religious)
- Nursing Prgm

Belmont University
Robert C Fisher, PhD, President
1900 Belmont Blvd
Nashville, TN 37212
615 460-6793
Type: 4-year Coll or Univ
Control: Nonprofit (Private or Religious)
- Music Therapy Prgm
- Nursing Prgm
- Occupational Therapy Prgm
- Pharmacy Prgm
- Physical Therapy Prgm

Fortis Institute
3354 Perimeter Hill Drive, Suite 105
Nashville, TN 37211-4149
615 320-5917
Type: Vocational or Tech Sch
Control: For Profit
- Clin Lab Technician/Med Lab Technician Prgm
- Surgical Technology Prgm

Kaplan Career Institute
Nashville, TN 37217
- Dental Assistant Prgm

Lipscomb University
L Randolph Lowry III, BA MPA JD, President
3901 Granny White Pike
Nashville, TN 37204
615 279-6194
Type: 4-year Coll or Univ
Control: Nonprofit (Private or Religious)
- Dietetic Internship Prgm
- Dietetics-Didactic Prgm
- Music Therapy Prgm
- Pharmacy Prgm

Meharry Medical College
1005 Dr D B Todd Jr Blvd
Nashville, TN 37208
615 327-6000
Type: Acad Health Ctr/Med Sch
Control: Nonprofit (Private or Religious)
- Allopathic Medicine Prgm
- Dentistry Prgm

Nashville General Hospital
Reginald Coopwood, MD, CEO
1818 Albion St
Nashville, TN 37208
615 341-4490
Type: Hosp or Med Ctr: 500 Beds
Control: State, County, or Local Govt
- Radiography Prgm

Nashville State Community College
George H Van Allen, EdD, President
120 White Bridge Rd
PO Box 90285
Nashville, TN 37209-4515
615 353-3236
Type: Junior or Comm Coll
Control: State, County, or Local Govt
- Occupational Therapy Asst Prgm
- Surgical Technology Prgm

Remington College - Nashville Campus
Nashville, TN 37214
- Dental Hygiene Prgm

Tennessee State University
Melvin Johnson, DBA, President
3500 John A Merritt Blvd
Nashville, TN 37209-1561
615 963-7406
Type: 4-year Coll or Univ
Control: State, County, or Local Govt
- Dental Hygiene Prgm
- Dietetics-Didactic Prgm
- Music Therapy Prgm
- Occupational Therapy Prgm
- Physical Therapy Prgm
- Respiratory Care Prgm
- Speech-Language Pathology Prgm

Tennessee Technology Center - Nashville
Charles F Malin, Director
100 White Bridge Rd
Nashville, TN 37209
Type: Vocational or Tech Sch
Control: For Profit
- Pharmacy Technician Prgm

Trevecca Nazarene University
Dan Boone, DMin, President
333 Murfreesboro Rd
Nashville, TN 37210
615 248-1251
Type: 4-year Coll or Univ
Control: Nonprofit (Private or Religious)
- Nursing Prgm
- Physician Assistant Prgm

Vanderbilt Eye Institute
2311 Pierce Ave
Nashville, TN 37232
615 936-1034
- Orthoptist Prgm

Vanderbilt University
Nicholas S Zeppos, Interim Chancellor
Nashville, TN 37240-0001
615 322-7311
Type: 4-year Coll or Univ
Control: Nonprofit (Private or Religious)
- Allopathic Medicine Prgm
- Counseling Prgm
- Psychology (PhD) Prgm
- Teacher of the Visually Impaired Prgm

Vanderbilt University Medical Center
Jeffrey Balser, Vice Chancellor, Hlth Aff
1211 Medical Center Drive
D-3300 MCN
Nashville, TN 37232-2104
615 936-3030
Type: Acad Health Ctr/Med Sch
Control: Nonprofit (Private or Religious)
- Audiologist Prgm
- Clin Lab Scientist/Med Technologist Prgm
- Diagnostic Med Sonography (General) Prgm
- Dietetic Internship Prgm
- Nuclear Medicine Technology Prgm
- Perfusion Prgm
- Radiation Therapy Prgm
- Speech-Language Pathology Prgm

Pulaski

Martin Methodist College
Pulaski, TN 38478
Type: 4-year Coll or Univ
Control: For Profit
- Nursing Prgm

Texas

Abilene

Abilene Christian University
Royce L Money, PhD, President
ACU Box 29100
Abilene, TX 79699
325 674-2000
Type: 4-year Coll or Univ
Control: Nonprofit (Private or Religious)
- Dietetics-Didactic Prgm
- Music Therapy Prgm
- Nursing Prgm
- Speech-Language Pathology Prgm

Hardin-Simmons University
William Ellis, PhD, Interim Co-COO
2200 Hickory
HSU Box 16000
Abilene, TX 79698
325 670-1210
Type: 4-year Coll or Univ
Control: Nonprofit (Private or Religious)
- Athletic Training Prgm
- Nursing Prgm
- Physical Therapy Prgm

Hendrick Medical Center
Tim Lancaster, FACHE, President
1900 Pine
Abilene, TX 79601-2316
325 670-2364
Type: Hosp or Med Ctr: 300-499 Beds
Control: Nonprofit (Private or Religious)
- Radiography Prgm

McMurry University
1400 Sayles Boulevard
Abilene, TX 79697
Type: 4-year Coll or Univ
Control: Nonprofit (Private or Religious)
- Nursing Prgm

INSTITUTIONS

Patty Hanks Shelton School of Nursing
Abilene, TX 79601
Type: Acad Health Ctr/Med Sch
Control: Nonprofit (Private or Religious)
• Nursing Prgm

SWT/HMC Respiratory Care School Consortium
Jeff Lawrence, Program Director
1900 N Pine St
Abilene, TX 79601
915 670-2368
Type: Consortium
Control: Nonprofit (Private or Religious)
• Respiratory Care Prgm

Alpine

Sul Ross State University
R Vic Morgan, PhD, President
SR Box C-114
Alpine, TX 79830
432 837-8032
Type: 4-year Coll or Univ
Control: State, County, or Local Govt
• Veterinary Technology Prgm

Alvin

Alvin Community College
A Rodney Allbright, JD, President
3110 Mustang Rd
Alvin, TX 77511
281 756-3598
Type: Junior or Comm Coll
Control: State, County, or Local Govt
• Neurodiagnostic Tech Prgm
• Polysomnographic Technology Prgm
• Respiratory Care Prgm

Amarillo

Amarillo College
J Paul Matney, EdD, Acting President
2011 South Washington
PO Box 447
Amarillo, TX 79178
806 371-5123
Type: Junior or Comm Coll
Control: State, County, or Local Govt
• Clin Lab Technician/Med Lab Technician Prgm
• Dental Hygiene Prgm
• Nuclear Medicine Technology Prgm
• Occupational Therapy Asst Prgm
• Physical Therapist Assistant Prgm
• Radiation Therapy Prgm
• Radiography Prgm
• Respiratory Care Prgm
• Surgical Technology Prgm

Angleton

Med-Line School of Medical Transcription
12006 Annette Rd
Angleton, TX 77515
Type: Vocational or Tech Sch
Control: For Profit
• Medical Transcriptionist Prgm

Arlington

Concorde Career Institute - Arlington
Rebecca Zielinski, RN, Campus President
600 East Lamar Blvd, Ste 200
Ste 200
Arlington, TX 76011
817 267-1594
Type: Vocational or Tech Sch
Control: For Profit
• Surgical Technology Prgm

Iverson Business School
Arlington, TX 76010
Type: Vocational or Tech Sch
• Surgical Technology Prgm

University of Texas at Arlington
James D Spaniolo, President
321 Davis Hall, Box 19125
Arlington, TX 76019-0125
817 272-2101
Type: 4-year Coll or Univ
Control: State, County, or Local Govt
• Athletic Training Prgm
• Music Therapy Prgm
• Nursing Prgm

Athens

Trinity Valley Community College
Glendon Forgey, MBA EdD, President
100 Cardinal Dr
Athens, TX 75751
903 675-6211
Type: Junior or Comm Coll
Control: State, County, or Local Govt
• Surgical Technology Prgm

Austin

Austin Community College
Richard Rhodes, PhD, President
5930 Middle Fiskville Rd
Austin, TX 78752-4390
512 223-4390
Type: Junior or Comm Coll
Control: State, County, or Local Govt
• Clin Lab Technician/Med Lab Technician Prgm
• Dental Hygiene Prgm
• Diagnostic Med Sonography (Gen/Card/Vascular) Prgm
• Emergency Med Tech-Paramedic Prgm
• Occupational Therapy Asst Prgm
• Pharmacy Technician Prgm
• Phlebotomy Prgm
• Physical Therapist Assistant Prgm
• Radiography Prgm
• Surgical Technology Prgm

Austin State Hospital
Carl Schock, Superintendent
4110 Guadalupe St
Austin, TX 78751
512 419-2100
Type: Hosp or Med Ctr: 500 Beds
Control: State, County, or Local Govt
• Clin Lab Scientist/Med Technologist Prgm

Texas WIC
1100 W 49th St
Austin, TX 78756
Type: Acad Health Ctr/Med Sch
Control: State, County, or Local Govt
• Dietetic Internship Prgm

University of St Augustine for Health Science
5401 LaCrosse Avenue
Austin, TX 78739
• Physical Therapy Prgm

University of Texas at Austin
William Powers, PhD, President
1 University Station
Austin, TX 78712
512 471-3434
Type: 4-year Coll or Univ
Control: State, County, or Local Govt
• Athletic Training Prgm
• Audiologist Prgm
• Dietetics-Coordinated Prgm
• Dietetics-Didactic Prgm
• Medical Librarian Prgm
• Music Therapy Prgm
• Nursing Prgm
• Pharmacy Prgm
• Psychology (PhD) Prgm
• Rehabilitation Counseling Prgm
• Speech-Language Pathology Prgm

Virginia College at Austin
Harvey Giblin, MEd, Campus President
6301 E Hwy 290
Austin, TX 78723
512 279-2802
Type: Vocational or Tech Sch
Control: For Profit
• Surgical Technology Prgm

Beaumont

Baptist Hospitals of Southeast Texas
David Parmer, MS, President
Hospital Admin and Accounting
PO Drawer 1591
Beaumont, TX 77704
409 212-5012
Type: Hosp or Med Ctr: 300-499 Beds
Control: Nonprofit (Private or Religious)
• Radiography Prgm

CHRISTUS Hospital - St Elizabeth
Ellen Jones, Administrator
2830 Calder St
PO Box 5405
Beaumont, TX 77726-5405
409 899-7171
Type: Hosp or Med Ctr: 300-499 Beds
Control: Nonprofit (Private or Religious)
• Clin Lab Scientist/Med Technologist Prgm

Lamar Institute of Technology
Paul J Szuch, EdD, President
855 E Lavaca
PO Box 10043
Beaumont, TX 77705
409 880-8405
Type: Vocational or Tech Sch
Control: State, County, or Local Govt
• Dental Hygiene Prgm
• Diagnostic Med Sonography (General) Prgm
• Radiography Prgm
• Respiratory Care Prgm

Lamar University
James Simmons, President
PO Box 10001
Beaumont, TX 77710
409 880-8405
Type: 4-year Coll or Univ
Control: State, County, or Local Govt
• Audiologist Prgm
• Dietetic Internship Prgm
• Dietetics-Didactic Prgm
• Speech-Language Pathology Prgm

Beeville

Coastal Bend College
Thomas Baynum, PhD, President
3800 Charco Rd
Beeville, TX 78102
361 354-2200
Type: Junior or Comm Coll
Control: State, County, or Local Govt
• Dental Hygiene Prgm
• Radiography Prgm

Belton

University of Mary Hardin-Baylor
Jerry Bawcom, PhD, President
900 Colllege St
Belton, TX 76502
254 295-8642
Type: 4-year Coll or Univ
Control: Nonprofit (Private or Religious)
• Athletic Training Prgm
• Counseling Prgm
• Nursing Prgm

Big Spring

Howard College
Cheryl T Sparks, EdD, President
1001 Birdwell Ln
Big Spring, TX 79720
432 264-5000
Type: Junior or Comm Coll
Control: State, County, or Local Govt
• Dental Hygiene Prgm
• Radiography Prgm
• Surgical Technology Prgm

Brenham

Blinn College
Dan Holt, PhD, President
902 College Ave
Brenham, TX 77833
979 830-4112
Type: Dept of Defense
Control: State, County, or Local Govt
• Dental Hygiene Prgm
• Emergency Med Tech-Paramedic Prgm
• Physical Therapist Assistant Prgm
• Radiography Prgm

Brownsville

Univ TX at Brownsville/TX Southmost Coll
Juliet Garcia, PhD, President
83 Ft Brown
Brownsville, TX 78520
956 882-8201
Type: Consortium
Control: State, County, or Local Govt
• Clin Lab Technician/Med Lab Technician Prgm
• Diagnostic Med Sonography (General) Prgm
• Emergency Med Tech-Paramedic Prgm
• Respiratory Care Prgm

Canyon

West Texas A&M University
J Patrick O'Brien, President/CEO
Office of the President, WTAMU Box 60247
Canyon, TX 79016
806 656-2000
Type: 4-year Coll or Univ
Control: State, County, or Local Govt
• Athletic Training Prgm
• Music Therapy Prgm
• Nursing Prgm
• Speech-Language Pathology Prgm

Carthage

Panola College
Gregory S Powell, EdD, President
1109 W Panola
Carthage, TX 75633-2397
903 693-2022
Type: Junior or Comm Coll
Control: State, County, or Local Govt
• Occupational Therapy Asst Prgm

Cisco

Cisco College
Colleen Smith, PhD, President
101 College Heights Drive
Cisco, TX 76437
254 442-2567
Type: Junior or Comm Coll
Control: State, County, or Local Govt
• Medical Assistant Prgm
• Surgical Technology Prgm

College Station

Baylor College of Dentistry, Texas A&M HSC
Nancy Dickey, MD, President
TAMU 1364
College Station, TX 77843-1364
979 458-7200
Type: Consortium
Control: State, County, or Local Govt
• Dental Hygiene Prgm
• Dentistry Prgm

Texas A&M University
Robert Gates, President
College Station, TX 77843
409 845-3211
Type: 4-year Coll or Univ
Control: State, County, or Local Govt
• Allopathic Medicine Prgm
• Athletic Training Prgm
• Clin Lab Scientist/Med Technologist Prgm
• Counseling Prgm (2)
• Dietetic Internship Prgm (2)
• Dietetics-Didactic Prgm (2)
• Nursing Prgm (3)
• Psychology (PhD) Prgm
• Speech-Language Pathology Prgm
• Veterinary Medicine Prgm

Commerce

Texas A&M University - Commerce
Keith McFarland, PhD, President/CEO
295 McDowell Administration Bldg
Commerce, TX 75429-3011
903 886-5104
Type: 4-year Coll or Univ
Control: State, County, or Local Govt
• Counseling Prgm
• Music Therapy Prgm

Conroe

Montgomery College
Thomas E Butler, EdD, President
3200 College Park Dr
Conroe, TX 77384
936 273-7222
Type: Junior or Comm Coll
Control: State, County, or Local Govt
• Physical Therapist Assistant Prgm
• Radiography Prgm

Corpus Christi

Del Mar College
Mark Escamilla, PhD, President
101 Baldwin Blvd
Corpus Christi, TX 78404
361 698-1203
Type: Junior or Comm Coll
Control: State, County, or Local Govt
• Clin Lab Technician/Med Lab Technician Prgm
• Dental Assistant Prgm
• Dental Hygiene Prgm
• Diagnostic Med Sonography (General/Cardiac) Prgm
• Music Therapy Prgm
• Nuclear Medicine Technology Prgm
• Occupational Therapy Asst Prgm
• Physical Therapist Assistant Prgm
• Radiography Prgm
• Respiratory Care Prgm
• Surgical Technology Prgm

Texas A&M University - Corpus Christi
Flavious Killebrew, PhD, President
6300 Ocean Dr
Office of the President, Texas A&M Unive
Corpus Christi, TX 78412
361 825-5700
Type: 4-year Coll or Univ
Control: State, County, or Local Govt
• Athletic Training Prgm
• Counseling Prgm

Corsicana

Navarro College
Richard Sanchez, EdD, President
3200 W 7th Ave
Corsicana, TX 75110-4818
903 875-7308
Type: Junior or Comm Coll
Control: State, County, or Local Govt
• Clin Lab Technician/Med Lab Technician Prgm
• Occupational Therapy Asst Prgm

Cypress

Lone Star College-CyFair
Diane K Troyer, PhD, President
9191 Barker-Cyress Rd
Cypress, TX 77433
281 290-3940
Type: Junior or Comm Coll
Control: State, County, or Local Govt
• Diagnostic Med Sonography (General/Vascular) Prgm
• Emergency Med Tech-Paramedic Prgm
• Medical Assistant Prgm
• Radiography Prgm

Dallas

ATI Health Education Centers
Joe Mehlmann, President
2777 Stemmons Freeway
Dallas, TX 75207
214 630-5651
Type: Vocational or Tech Sch
Control: For Profit
• Respiratory Care Prgm

ATI-Career Training
Gerald Parr, BS, Executive Director
10003 Technology Blvd W
Dallas, TX 75220
214 902-8191
Type: Vocational or Tech Sch
Control: For Profit
• Respiratory Care Prgm

Baylor University Med Center
John McWhorter, MHA, President/CEO
3500 Gaston Ave
3535 Worth St
Dallas, TX 75204
214 820-4642
Type: Hosp or Med Ctr: 500 Beds
Control: Nonprofit (Private or Religious)
• Dietetic Internship Prgm
• Nuclear Medicine Technology Prgm
• Radiography Prgm

Concorde Career College - Dallas
Dallas, TX 75243
• Dental Assistant Prgm
• Dental Hygiene Prgm

El Centro College
Paul McCarthy, PhD, President
801 Main St
Dallas, TX 75202-3604
214 860-2010
Type: Junior or Comm Coll
Control: State, County, or Local Govt
• Cardiovascular Tech (Invasive) Prgm
• Clin Lab Technician/Med Lab Technician Prgm
• Diagnostic Med Sonography (General) Prgm
• Medical Assistant Prgm
• Radiography Prgm
• Respiratory Care Prgm
• Surgical Technology Prgm

Parker College of Chiropractic
2500 Walnut Hill Lane
Dallas, TX 75229
Type: Acad Health Ctr/Med Sch
Control: For Profit
• Chiropractic Prgm

Presbyterian Hospital of Dallas
8200 Walnut Hill Ln
Dallas, TX 75231-4402
214 345-7558
Type: Hosp or Med Ctr: 300-499 Beds
Control: Nonprofit (Private or Religious)
• Dietetic Internship Prgm

Richland College
Stephen Mittelstet, PhD, President
12800 Abrams Rd
Dallas, TX 75243
214 238-6364
Type: Junior or Comm Coll
Control: State, County, or Local Govt
• Medical Assistant Prgm
• Pharmacy Technician Prgm

Sanford-Brown College - Dallas
Dallas, TX 75247
• Dental Assistant Prgm
• Dental Hygiene Prgm

Sanford-Brown College - Dallas
Gary C Jack, BS MS, Executive Director
2998 N Stemmons Frwy
Dallas, TX 75247
214 638-6400
Type: Vocational or Tech Sch
Control: For Profit
• Cardiovascular Tech (Echocardiography) Prgm
• Diagnostic Med Sonography (General) Prgm

Southern Methodist University
R Gerald Turner, President
6425 Boaz St
PO Box 296
Dallas, TX 75275
214 768-2000
Type: 4-year Coll or Univ
Control: Nonprofit (Private or Religious)
• Music Therapy Prgm

Univ of Texas Southwestern Med Ctr
Daniel Podolsky, MD, President
5323 Harry Hines Blvd, B12.100
Dallas, TX 75390-9082
214 648-2508
Type: Acad Health Ctr/Med Sch
Control: State, County, or Local Govt
• Allopathic Medicine Prgm
• Clin Lab Scientist/Med Technologist Prgm
• Dietetics-Coordinated Prgm
• Emergency Med Tech-Paramedic Prgm
• Medical Illustrator Prgm
• Orthotist/Prosthetist Prgm
• Physical Therapy Prgm
• Physician Assistant Prgm
• Psychology (PhD) Prgm
• Radiation Therapy Prgm
• Rehabilitation Counseling Prgm
• Specialist in BB Tech Prgm

Westwood College
Paul Kepic, BS MBA, Executive Director
8390 LBJ Freeway, Suite 100
Dallas, TX 75243
214 570-0100
Type: Vocational or Tech Sch
Control: For Profit
• Medical Assistant Prgm (3)

Denison

Grayson County College
Alan Scheibmeir, PhD, President
6101 Grayson Dr
Denison, TX 75020
903 465-6030
Type: Junior or Comm Coll
Control: State, County, or Local Govt
• Clin Lab Technician/Med Lab Technician Prgm
• Dental Assistant Prgm
• Emergency Med Tech-Paramedic Prgm

Denton

Texas Woman's University
Ann Stuart, PhD, President and Chancellor
PO Box 425587
TWU Station (ACT-15)
Denton, TX 76204-3587
940 898-3201
Type: 4-year Coll or Univ
Control: State, County, or Local Govt
• Counseling Prgm
• Dental Hygiene Prgm
• Dietetic Internship Prgm (2)
• Dietetics-Didactic Prgm
• Medical Librarian Prgm
• Music Therapy Prgm
• Nursing Prgm
• Occupational Therapy Prgm (3)
• Physical Therapy Prgm
• Speech-Language Pathology Prgm

University of North Texas

Lee Jackson, Chancellor
Denton, TX 76203-5008
940 565-2000
Type: 4-year Coll or Univ
Control: State, County, or Local Govt
- Audiologist Prgm
- Counseling Prgm
- Medical Librarian Prgm
- Music Therapy Prgm
- Psychology (PhD) Prgm (2)
- Rehabilitation Counseling Prgm
- Speech-Language Pathology Prgm

Edinburg

Univ of Texas - Pan American

Robert S Nelsen, PhD, President
1201 W University Dr
Edinburg, TX 78539-2999
956 381-2100
Type: 4-year Coll or Univ
Control: State, County, or Local Govt
- Clin Lab Scientist/Med Technologist Prgm
- Dietetics-Coordinated Prgm
- Nursing Prgm
- Occupational Therapy Prgm
- Physician Assistant Prgm
- Rehabilitation Counseling Prgm
- Speech-Language Pathology Prgm

El Paso

Anamarc College

El Paso, TX 79930
- Occupational Therapy Asst Prgm

El Paso Community College

Richard M Rhodes, PhD, President
PO Box 20500
El Paso, TX 79998-0500
915 831-6511
Type: Junior or Comm Coll
Control: State, County, or Local Govt
- Clin Lab Technician/Med Lab Technician Prgm
- Dental Assistant Prgm
- Dental Hygiene Prgm
- Diagnostic Med Sonography (General) Prgm
- Medical Assistant Prgm
- Pharmacy Technician Prgm
- Physical Therapist Assistant Prgm
- Radiography Prgm
- Surgical Technology Prgm

Kaplan College

El Paso, TX 79907
Type: Vocational or Tech Sch
- Medical Assistant Prgm

University of Texas at El Paso

Diana Natalicio, PhD, President
500 W University Ave
El Paso, TX 79902
915 747-5555
Type: 4-year Coll or Univ
Control: State, County, or Local Govt
- Clin Lab Scientist/Med Technologist Prgm
- Music Therapy Prgm
- Nursing Prgm
- Occupational Therapy Prgm
- Physical Therapy Prgm
- Speech-Language Pathology Prgm

Vista College

El Paso, TX 79925
Type: Vocational or Tech Sch
- Medical Assistant Prgm

Farmers Branch

Brookhaven College

Sharon L Blackman, EdD, President
3939 Valley View Ln
Farmers Branch, TX 75244
972 860-4809
Type: Junior or Comm Coll
Control: State, County, or Local Govt
- Emergency Med Tech-Paramedic Prgm
- Radiography Prgm

Fort Sam Houston

Medical Education and Training Campus (METC)

David Rubenstein, DC, US Army, Commanding General
2250 Stanley Rd, Ste 301
Fort Sam Houston, TX 78234-6100
210 221-6325
Type: Dept of Defense
Control: Fed Govt
- Cardiovascular Tech (Invasive) Prgm
- Clin Lab Technician/Med Lab Technician Prgm
- Cytotechnology Prgm
- Dental Assistant Prgm
- Dental Lab Technician Prgm (2)
- Histotechnician Prgm
- Neurodiagnostic Tech Prgm
- Occupational Therapy Asst Prgm
- Ophthalmic Assistant Prgm
- Pharmacy Technician Prgm
- Physician Assistant Prgm
- Radiography Prgm
- Respiratory Care Prgm
- Surgical Technology Prgm

US Army-Baylor University

MCCS-HMT, Physical Therapy Branch
3151 Scott Rd
Fort Sam Houston, TX 78234-6138
Type: Dept of Defense
Control: Fed Govt
- Physical Therapy Prgm

Fort Worth

Texas Christian University

Victor Boschini, EdD, Chancellor
TCU 297080
Fort Worth, TX 76129
817 257-7783
Type: 4-year Coll or Univ
Control: Nonprofit (Private or Religious)
- Athletic Training Prgm
- Dietetics-Coordinated Prgm
- Dietetics-Didactic Prgm
- Music Therapy Prgm
- Nursing Prgm
- Speech-Language Pathology Prgm

Texas Wesleyan University

Harold G Jeffcoat, EdD, President
1201 Wesleyan St
Fort Worth, TX 76105
817 531-4401
Type: 4-year Coll or Univ
Control: State, County, or Local Govt
- Athletic Training Prgm
- Music Therapy Prgm

Univ of North Texas Hlth Sci Ctr at Ft Worth

Scott Ransom, DO, President
3500 Camp Bowie Blvd
Fort Worth, TX 76107
817 735-2555
Type: Acad Health Ctr/Med Sch
Control: State, County, or Local Govt
- Osteopathic Medicine Prgm
- Physician Assistant Prgm

Friendswood

Texas School of Business

Kevin Green, JD, Executive Director
3208 FM 528
Friendswood, TX 77546
281 443-8900
Type: Vocational or Tech Sch
Control: For Profit
- Medical Assistant Prgm (4)

Gainesville

North Central Texas College

Eddie Hadlock, EdD, President
1525 W California St
Gainesville, TX 76240
940 668-7731
Type: Junior or Comm Coll
Control: State, County, or Local Govt
- Surgical Technology Prgm

Galveston

Galveston College

Myles Shelton, EdD, President
4015 Ave Q
Galveston, TX 77550-2782
409 944-1665
Type: Junior or Comm Coll
Control: State, County, or Local Govt
- Emergency Med Tech-Paramedic Prgm
- Nuclear Medicine Technology Prgm
- Radiation Therapy Prgm
- Radiography Prgm
- Surgical Technology Prgm

University of Texas Medical Branch

David Callender, MD, President
301 University Blvd
Galveston, TX 77555-0129
409 772-1902
Type: Acad Health Ctr/Med Sch
Control: State, County, or Local Govt
- Allopathic Medicine Prgm
- Clin Lab Scientist/Med Technologist Prgm
- Nursing Prgm
- Occupational Therapy Prgm
- Pharmacy Technician Prgm
- Physical Therapy Prgm
- Physician Assistant Prgm
- Respiratory Care Prgm
- Specialist in BB Tech Prgm

Grand Prairie

MedVance Institute
401 E Palace Parkway, Suite 100
Grand Prairie, TX 75050
Type: Vocational or Tech Sch
Control: For Profit
• Radiography Prgm

Houston

Academy of Health Care Professions
A John Emerald, BA, CEO
240 Northwest Mall
Houston, TX 77092
713 425-3100
Type: Vocational or Tech Sch
Control: For Profit
• Surgical Technology Prgm

Baylor College of Medicine
Peter Traber, MD, President/CEO
BCMC 143A, One Baylor Plaza
Houston, TX 77030
713 798-4433
Type: Acad Health Ctr/Med Sch
Control: Nonprofit (Private or Religious)
• Allopathic Medicine Prgm
• Physician Assistant Prgm

Case Western Reserve University
Houston, TX 77030
Type: Acad Health Ctr/Med Sch
• Anesthesiologist Asst Prgm

Fortis Institute
Deborah Schwarzberg, PhD, President
6220 Westpark
Houston, TX 77057
Type: Vocational or Tech Sch
Control: For Profit
• Surgical Technology Prgm (3)

Gulf Coast School of Blood Bank Technology
Brian Gannon, MBA, President/CEO
1400 La Concha Ln
Houston, TX 77054-1802
713 791-6303
Type: Nonhosp HC Facil, BB, or Lab
Control: Nonprofit (Private or Religious)
• Specialist in BB Tech Prgm

Harris County Hosp Dist/Ben Taub Gen Hosp
David Lopez, MS, CEO/President
2525 Holly Hall
Houston, TX 77266
713 566-6400
Type: Hosp or Med Ctr: 500 Beds
Control: State, County, or Local Govt
• Diagnostic Med Sonography (General) Prgm
• Radiography Prgm

Houston Comm College System - Southeast Coll
Bruce Leslie, PhD, Chancellor
3100 Main St, 12th Flr
PO Box 667517
Houston, TX 77266
713 718-2000
Type: Junior or Comm Coll
Control: State, County, or Local Govt
• Dental Hygiene Prgm

Houston Community College
Betty Young, Chancellor
3100 Main, Ste 12D
PO Box 667517 1900 Pressler
Houston, TX 77030
713 718-7378
Type: Junior or Comm Coll
Control: State, County, or Local Govt
• Clin Lab Technician/Med Lab Technician Prgm
• Dental Assistant Prgm
• Diagnostic Med Sonography (General) Prgm
• Emergency Med Tech-Paramedic Prgm
• Histotechnician Prgm
• Medical Assistant Prgm
• Nuclear Medicine Technology Prgm
• Occupational Therapy Asst Prgm
• Physical Therapist Assistant Prgm
• Radiography Prgm
• Respiratory Care Prgm
• Surgical Technology Prgm

Lone Star College-North Harris
Stephen Head, PhD, President
2700 W W Thorne Drive
Houston, TX 77073-3499
281 618-5444
Type: Junior or Comm Coll
Control: Nonprofit (Private or Religious)
• Emergency Med Tech-Paramedic Prgm
• Medical Assistant Prgm
• Pharmacy Technician Prgm

Michael E DeBakey VA Medical Center
Robert F Stott, MPH, Hospital Director
2002 Holcombe Blvd 00/580
Houston, TX 77030
713 794-7100
Type: Dept of Veterans Affairs
Control: Fed Govt
• Dietetic Internship Prgm

Pima Medical Institute - Houston
Richard L Luebke, Jr, CEO
10201 Katy Freeway
Houston, TX 77024
Type: Vocational or Tech Sch
Control: For Profit
• Radiography Prgm

San Jacinto College North
Allatia Harris, PhD, President
5800 Uvalde Rd
Houston, TX 77049-4599
281 459-7100
Type: Junior or Comm Coll
Control: State, County, or Local Govt
• Emergency Med Tech-Paramedic Prgm
• Medical Assistant Prgm
• Pharmacy Technician Prgm

San Jacinto College South
Linda Watkins, PhD, President
13735 Beamer Rd
Houston, TX 77089
281 922-3400
Type: Junior or Comm Coll
Control: State, County, or Local Govt
• Cancer Registrar Prgm
• Pharmacy Technician Prgm
• Physical Therapist Assistant Prgm

Sanford-Brown College - Houston
James Garrett, BS, Executive Director
10500 Forum Pl, Ste 200
Houston, TX 77036
713 779-1110
Type: Vocational or Tech Sch
Control: For Profit
• Clin Lab Technician/Med Lab Technician Prgm
• Diagnostic Med Sonography (General) Prgm
• Surgical Technology Prgm

Sanford-Brown College - North Loop
Houston, TX 77008
Type: Vocational or Tech Sch
• Radiography Prgm
• Surgical Technology Prgm

Texas Heart Institute
Denton A Cooley, MD, President
PO Box 20345, MC 1-224
Houston, TX 77225
832 355-4026
Type: Hosp or Med Ctr d Beds
Control: Nonprofit (Private or Religious)
• Perfusion Prgm

Texas Southern University
John Rudley, President
3100 Cleburne St
Houston, TX 77004
713 313-7035
Type: 4-year Coll or Univ
Control: State, County, or Local Govt
• Clin Lab Scientist/Med Technologist Prgm
• Dietetics-Didactic Prgm
• Pharmacy Prgm
• Respiratory Care Prgm

The Methodist Hospital
Ron Girotto, CEO, President
6565 Fannin, D 200
Houston, TX 77030
713 441-3366
Type: Hosp or Med Ctr: 500 Beds
Control: Nonprofit (Private or Religious)
• Clin Lab Scientist/Med Technologist Prgm

Univ of Texas M D Anderson Cancer Ctr
John Mendelsohn, MD, President
1515 Holcombe Blvd, Box 213
Unit 91 R11 2339
Houston, TX 77030
713 792-6000
Type: Hosp or Med Ctr: 500 Beds
Control: State, County, or Local Govt
• Clin Lab Scientist/Med Technologist Prgm
• Cytogenetic Technology Prgm
• Cytotechnology Prgm
• Diagnostic Molecular Scientist Prgm
• Histotechnician Prgm
• Histotechnology Prgm
• Medical Dosimetry Prgm
• Radiation Therapy Prgm
• Radiography Prgm

Univ of Texas Medical School at Houston
PO Box 20708
Houston, TX 77225
Type: Acad Health Ctr/Med Sch
Control: State, County, or Local Govt
• Allopathic Medicine Prgm
• Genetic Counseling Prgm

University of Houston
Thomas M Stauffer, PhD, President
2700 Bay Area Blvd
Houston, TX 77058-1098
713 488-9336
Type: 4-year Coll or Univ
Control: State, County, or Local Govt
- Dietetic Internship Prgm
- Dietetics-Didactic Prgm
- Music Therapy Prgm
- Optometry Prgm
- Pharmacy Prgm
- Psychology (PsyD) Prgm
- Speech-Language Pathology Prgm

University of Texas Health Sci Ctr Houston
James Willerson, MD, President
PO Box 20036
Houston, TX 77225-0708
713 500-3000
Type: Acad Health Ctr/Med Sch
Control: State, County, or Local Govt
- Dental Hygiene Prgm
- Dentistry Prgm
- Dietetic Internship Prgm
- Nursing Prgm

Huntsville

Sam Houston State University
James Gaertner, PhD, President
Box 2026
Huntsville, TX 77341
936 294-1013
Type: 4-year Coll or Univ
Control: State, County, or Local Govt
- Counseling Prgm
- Dietetic Internship Prgm
- Dietetics-Didactic Prgm
- Music Therapy Prgm
- Psychology (PhD) Prgm

Hurst

Tarrant County College
Larry Darlage, PhD, President, NE Campus
828 W Harwood Rd
Hurst, TX 76054-3219
817 515-6200
Type: Junior or Comm Coll
Control: State, County, or Local Govt
- Dental Hygiene Prgm
- Dietetic Technician-AD Prgm
- Emergency Med Tech-Paramedic Prgm
- Physical Therapist Assistant Prgm
- Radiography Prgm
- Respiratory Care Prgm
- Surgical Technology Prgm

Keene

Southwestern Adventist University
Keene, TX 76059
Type: 4-year Coll or Univ
Control: Nonprofit (Private or Religious)
- Nursing Prgm

Kilgore

Kilgore College
William M Holda, EdD, President
1100 Broadway
Kilgore, TX 75662
903 983-8100
Type: Junior or Comm Coll
Control: State, County, or Local Govt
- Physical Therapist Assistant Prgm
- Surgical Technology Prgm

Killeen

Central Texas College
James R Anderson, PhD, Chancellor
US Hwy 190 W
PO Box 1800
Killeen, TX 76540
254 526-1214
Type: Junior or Comm Coll
Control: State, County, or Local Govt
- Clin Lab Technician/Med Lab Technician Prgm
- Emergency Med Tech-Paramedic Prgm
- Medical Transcriptionist Prgm

Kingsville

Texas A&M University - Kingsville
Rumaldo Juarez, President
MSC 101, 700 University Blvd
Kingsville, TX 78363
361 593-3207
Type: 4-year Coll or Univ
Control: State, County, or Local Govt
- Pharmacy Prgm

Kingwood

Lone Star College
Linda Stegall, EdD, President
20000 Kingwood Dr
Kingwood, TX 77339
281 312-1640
Type: Junior or Comm Coll
Control: State, County, or Local Govt
- Dental Hygiene Prgm
- Occupational Therapy Asst Prgm
- Respiratory Care Prgm
- Surgical Technology Prgm

Lackland AFB

US Military Dietetic Internship Consortium
Lackland AFB, TX 78236-5300
Type: Dept of Defense
Control: Fed Govt
- Dietetic Internship Prgm (2)

Lake Jackson

Brazosport College
Millicent Valek, PhD, President
500 College Dr
Lake Jackson, TX 77568
979 230-3200
Type: Junior or Comm Coll
Control: State, County, or Local Govt
- Emergency Med Tech-Paramedic Prgm

Lancaster

Cedar Valley College
Jennifer Wimbish, PhD, President
3030 N Dallas Ave
Lancaster, TX 75134
Type: Acad Health Ctr/Med Sch
Control: For Profit
- Veterinary Technology Prgm

Laredo

Laredo Community College
Juan L Maldonado, PhD, President
West End Washington St
Laredo, TX 78040-4395
956 721-5101
Type: Junior or Comm Coll
Control: State, County, or Local Govt
- Clin Lab Technician/Med Lab Technician Prgm
- Occupational Therapy Asst Prgm
- Physical Therapist Assistant Prgm
- Radiography Prgm

Levelland

South Plains College
Kelvin Sharp, EdD, President
1401 S College Ave
Levelland, TX 79336
806 894-9611
Type: Junior or Comm Coll
Control: State, County, or Local Govt
- Emergency Med Tech-Paramedic Prgm (2)
- Respiratory Care Prgm
- Surgical Technology Prgm

Lubbock

Covenant Medical Center
Melinda Clark, President, CEO
3615 19th St PO Box 1201
Lubbock, TX 79410
806 725-0447
Type: Hosp or Med Ctr: 500 Beds
Control: Nonprofit (Private or Religious)
- Radiography Prgm
- Surgical Technology Prgm

Texas Tech Univ Health Sciences Center
Tedd L. Mitchell, MD, President
3601 4th St, Stop 6258
Lubbock, TX 79430
806 743-3223
Type: Acad Health Ctr/Med Sch
Control: State, County, or Local Govt
- Allopathic Medicine Prgm (2)
- Athletic Training Prgm
- Audiologist Prgm
- Clin Lab Scientist/Med Technologist Prgm
- Diagnostic Molecular Scientist Prgm
- Occupational Therapy Prgm
- Pharmacy Prgm
- Physical Therapy Prgm
- Physician Assistant Prgm
- Speech-Language Pathology Prgm

Texas Tech University
David Schmidly, PhD, President
PO Box 2005
Lubbock, TX 79409
806 742-2121
Type: 4-year Coll or Univ
Control: State, County, or Local Govt
• Counseling Prgm
• Dietetic Internship Prgm
• Dietetics-Didactic Prgm
• Music Therapy Prgm
• Nursing Prgm
• Orientation and Mobility Specialist Prgm
• Psychology (PhD) Prgm
• Rehabilitation Counseling Prgm

Lufkin

Angelina College
Larry M Phillips, EdD, President
PO Box 1768
3500 South First
Lufkin, TX 75902-1768
936 639-1301
Type: Junior or Comm Coll
Control: State, County, or Local Govt
• Diagnostic Med Sonography (General) Prgm
• Pharmacy Technician Prgm
• Radiography Prgm
• Respiratory Care Prgm
• Surgical Technology Prgm

Marshall

East Texas Baptist University
Bob Riley, EdD, President
1209 N Grove
Marshall, TX 75670
903 923-2222
Type: 4-year Coll or Univ
Control: Nonprofit (Private or Religious)
• Athletic Training Prgm
• Nursing Prgm

McAllen

South Texas College
Shirley Reed, EdD, President
3201 W Pecan Blvd
PO Box 9701
McAllen, TX 78501-9701
956 872-8366
Type: Junior or Comm Coll
Control: State, County, or Local Govt
• Occupational Therapy Asst Prgm
• Pharmacy Technician Prgm
• Physical Therapist Assistant Prgm

McKinney

Collin College
Cary A Israel, JD, President
2200 W University Dr
McKinney, TX 75071
972 758-3801
Type: Junior or Comm Coll
Control: State, County, or Local Govt
• Dental Hygiene Prgm
• Respiratory Care Prgm

Collin County Community College District
McKinney, TX 75070
Type: Junior or Comm Coll
• Emergency Med Tech-Paramedic Prgm
• Surgical Technology Prgm

Midland

Midland College
Steve Thomas, Ed D, President
3600 N Garfield
Midland, TX 79705
432 685-4520
Type: Junior or Comm Coll
Control: State, County, or Local Govt
• Diagnostic Med Sonography (General) Prgm
• Respiratory Care Prgm
• Veterinary Technology Prgm

Mt Pleasant

Northeast Texas Community College
Mt Pleasant, TX 75456
Type: Junior or Comm Coll
Control: State, County, or Local Govt
• Clin Lab Technician/Med Lab Technician Prgm
• Dental Hygiene Prgm
• Medical Assistant Prgm
• Radiography Prgm

Nacogdoches

Stephen F Austin State University
Baker Patillo, PhD, President
1936 North St
Austin Bldg
Nacogdoches, TX 75962
936 468-2011
Type: 4-year Coll or Univ
Control: State, County, or Local Govt
• Athletic Training Prgm
• Counseling Prgm
• Dietetic Internship Prgm
• Dietetics-Didactic Prgm
• Music Therapy Prgm
• Orientation and Mobility Specialist Prgm
• Rehabilitation Counseling Prgm
• Speech-Language Pathology Prgm

Odessa

Odessa College
Greg Wilson, PhD, President
201 W University
Odessa, TX 79764-8299
915 335-6410
Type: Junior or Comm Coll
Control: State, County, or Local Govt
• Physical Therapist Assistant Prgm
• Radiography Prgm

Orange

Lamar State College - Orange
J Michael Shahan, PhD, President
410 Front St
Orange, TX 77630-5802
409 882-3314
Type: Junior or Comm Coll
Control: State, County, or Local Govt
• Clin Lab Technician/Med Lab Technician Prgm
• Pharmacy Technician Prgm

Paris

Paris Junior College
Pamela Anglin, EdD, President
2400 Clarksville St
Paris, TX 75460
903 782-0330
Type: Junior or Comm Coll
Control: State, County, or Local Govt
• Emergency Med Tech-Paramedic Prgm
• Radiography Prgm
• Surgical Technology Prgm

Pasadena

San Jacinto College Central
Brenda Hellyer, President
8060 Spencer Hwy
PO Box 2007
Pasadena, TX 77505
281 998-6100
Type: Junior or Comm Coll
Control: State, County, or Local Govt
• Clin Lab Technician/Med Lab Technician Prgm
• Emergency Med Tech-Paramedic Prgm
• Ophthalmic Technician Prgm
• Radiography Prgm
• Respiratory Care Prgm
• Surgical Technology Prgm

Texas Chiropractic College
5912 Spencer Hwy
Pasadena, TX 77505
Type: Acad Health Ctr/Med Sch
Control: For Profit
• Chiropractic Prgm

Port Arthur

Lamar State College - Port Arthur
W Sam Monroe, LLD, President
PO Box 310
Port Arthur, TX 77641-0310
409 984-7101
Type: Junior or Comm Coll
Control: State, County, or Local Govt
• Surgical Technology Prgm

Prairie View

Prairie View A&M University
Charles A Hines, President
Prairie View, TX 77446
409 857-3311
Type: 4-year Coll or Univ
Control: State, County, or Local Govt
• Dietetic Internship Prgm
• Dietetics-Didactic Prgm
• Nursing Prgm

Richardson

University of Texas at Dallas
Franklyn G Jenifer, President
PO Box 8630688
Richardson, TX 75083
214 883-2111
Type: 4-year Coll or Univ
Control: State, County, or Local Govt
• Audiologist Prgm
• Speech-Language Pathology Prgm

San Angelo

Angelo State University
Joseph Rallo, PhD, President
2601 W Ave N
ASU Station #11007
San Angelo, TX 76909-0001
325 942-2555
Type: 4-year Coll or Univ
Control: State, County, or Local Govt
- Athletic Training Prgm
- Music Therapy Prgm
- Physical Therapy Prgm

San Antonio

Baptist Health System
Trip Pilgrim, MBA, President/CEO
215 E Quincy
San Antonio, TX 78215
210 297-1140
Type: Hosp or Med Ctr: 500 Beds
Control: For Profit
- Dietetic Internship Prgm
- Radiography Prgm
- Surgical Technology Prgm

Concorde Career College - San Antonio
San Antonio, TX 78229
- Dental Assistant Prgm
- Dental Hygiene Prgm

Hallmark College of Technology
Joe Fisher, PhD, President
10401 IH - 10 West
San Antonio, TX 78230
210 690-9000
Type: Vocational or Tech Sch
Control: For Profit
- Medical Assistant Prgm

Kaplan College - San Antonio
San Antonio, TX 78216-6255
Type: Vocational or Tech Sch
- Medical Assistant Prgm

Northwest Vista College
Jacqueline Claunch, President
3535 N Ellison Dr
San Antonio, TX 78251-4217
210 348-2001
Type: Junior or Comm Coll
Control: State, County, or Local Govt
- Pharmacy Technician Prgm

Our Lady of the Lake University
Elizabeth A Sueltenfuss, President
411 SW 24th St
San Antonio, TX 78207
210 434-6711
Type: 4-year Coll or Univ
Control: Nonprofit (Private or Religious)
- Speech-Language Pathology Prgm

Palo Alto College
Ana Cha Guzman, EdD, President
1400 W Villaret Blvd
San Antonio, TX 78224
210 921-5260
Type: Junior or Comm Coll
Control: State, County, or Local Govt
- Veterinary Technology Prgm

San Antonio College
Robert E Zeigler, PhD, President
1300 San Pedro Ave
San Antonio, TX 78212-4299
210 733-2190
Type: Junior or Comm Coll
Control: State, County, or Local Govt
- Dental Assistant Prgm
- Dental Lab Technician Prgm
- Emergency Med Tech-Paramedic Prgm
- Medical Assistant Prgm

St Mary's University
One Camino Santa Maria
San Antonio, TX 78228
210 436-3011
Type: 4-year Coll or Univ
Control: Nonprofit (Private or Religious)
- Counseling Prgm

St Philip's College
Adena Loston, PhD, President
1801 Martin Luther King Dr
San Antonio, TX 78203-2098
210 486-2900
Type: Junior or Comm Coll
Control: State, County, or Local Govt
- Clin Lab Technician/Med Lab Technician Prgm
- Histotechnician Prgm
- Occupational Therapy Asst Prgm
- Physical Therapist Assistant Prgm
- Radiography Prgm
- Surgical Technology Prgm

The University of the Incarnate Word
Louis J Agnese, Jr, PhD, President
4301 Broadway
San Antonio, TX 78209
210 829-3900
Type: 4-year Coll or Univ
Control: Nonprofit (Private or Religious)
- Athletic Training Prgm
- Dietetic Internship Prgm
- Dietetics-Didactic Prgm
- Music Therapy Prgm
- Nuclear Medicine Technology Prgm
- Nursing Prgm
- Optometry Prgm
- Pharmacy Prgm

TSSMT/STRC Consortium for Polysom Edu
San Antonio, TX 78229
Type: Consortium
- Polysomnographic Technology Prgm

UT Health Science Center - San Antonio
Francisco Cigarroa, MD, President
7703 Floyd Curl Dr
San Antonio, TX 78229-3900
210 567-2050
Type: Vocational or Tech Sch
Control: State, County, or Local Govt
- Allopathic Medicine Prgm
- Clin Lab Scientist/Med Technologist Prgm
- Cytogenetic Technology Prgm
- Dental Hygiene Prgm
- Dentistry Prgm
- Dietetics-Coordinated Prgm
- Emergency Med Tech-Paramedic Prgm
- Histotechnician Prgm
- Medical Dosimetry Prgm
- Nursing Prgm
- Occupational Therapy Prgm
- Physical Therapy Prgm
- Physician Assistant Prgm
- Respiratory Care Prgm
- Specialist in BB Tech Prgm

San Marcos

Texas State University - San Marcos
Denise M Trauth, PhD, President
601 University Dr
313 Village West Drive
San Marcos, TX 78666
512 245-2121
Type: 4-year Coll or Univ
Control: State, County, or Local Govt
- Athletic Training Prgm
- Clin Lab Scientist/Med Technologist Prgm
- Counseling Prgm
- Dietetic Internship Prgm
- Dietetics-Didactic Prgm
- Music Therapy Prgm
- Physical Therapy Prgm
- Radiation Therapy Prgm
- Respiratory Care Prgm
- Speech-Language Pathology Prgm

Seguin

Texas Lutheran University
Ann Svennungsen, MDiv, President
1000 W Court St
Seguin, TX 78155
830 372-8001
Type: 4-year Coll or Univ
Control: Nonprofit (Private or Religious)
- Athletic Training Prgm

Sheppard AFB

USAF School of Health Care Sciences
COL Nancy Dezell, RN BAN MSN, Group
  Commander
882 TRG/CC
939 Missile Rd
Sheppard AFB, TX 76311
940 676-2700
Type: Dept of Defense
Control: Fed Govt
- Pharmacy Technician Prgm
- Respiratory Care Prgm

INSTITUTIONS

Stephenville

Tarleton State University
F Domnic Dottavio, PhD, President
Tarleton Station
Box T-0001
Stephenville, TX 76104
817 968-9100
Type: 4-year Coll or Univ
Control: State, County, or Local Govt
• Clin Lab Scientist/Med Technologist Prgm
• Clin Lab Technician/Med Lab Technician Prgm
• Histotechnician Prgm
• Music Therapy Prgm
• Nursing Prgm

Temple

Scott & White Hospital
Alfred Knight, President
2401 S 31st St
Temple, TX 76508
254 724-1912
Type: Hosp or Med Ctr: 500 Beds
Control: Nonprofit (Private or Religious)
• Clin Lab Scientist/Med Technologist Prgm

Temple College
Glenda Barron, PhD, President
2600 S First St
Temple, TX 76504
254 298-8600
Type: Junior or Comm Coll
Control: State, County, or Local Govt
• Dental Hygiene Prgm
• Diagnostic Med Sonography (General) Prgm
• Emergency Med Tech-Paramedic Prgm
• Respiratory Care Prgm
• Surgical Technology Prgm

Texas City

College of the Mainland
Larry Durrence, PhD, President
1200 Amburn Rd
Texas City, TX 77591
409 938-1211
Type: Junior or Comm Coll
Control: State, County, or Local Govt
• Emergency Med Tech-Paramedic Prgm
• Medical Assistant Prgm

Tomball

Lone Start College - Tomball
Raymond M Hawkins, PhD, President
30555 Tomball Pkwy
Tomball, TX 77375-4036
281 351-3333
Type: Junior or Comm Coll
Control: State, County, or Local Govt
• Occupational Therapy Asst Prgm
• Veterinary Technology Prgm

Tyler

Tyler Junior College
L Michael Metke, PhD, President
PO Box 9020
Tyler, TX 75711
903 510-2380
Type: Junior or Comm Coll
Control: State, County, or Local Govt
• Clin Lab Technician/Med Lab Technician Prgm
• Dental Hygiene Prgm
• Diagnostic Med Sonography (General) Prgm
• Ophthalmic Assistant Prgm
• Ophthalmic Dispensing Optician Prgm
• Radiography Prgm
• Respiratory Care Prgm
• Surgical Technology Prgm

University of Texas at Tyler
Rodney Maybry, PhD, President
3900 University Blvd
Tyler, TX 75799
903 566-7100
Type: 4-year Coll or Univ
Control: State, County, or Local Govt
• Nursing Prgm

Vernon

Vernon College
Steve Thomas, PhD, President
4400 College Dr
Vernon, TX 76384
940 552-6291
Type: Junior or Comm Coll
Control: State, County, or Local Govt
• Pharmacy Technician Prgm
• Surgical Technology Prgm

Victoria

Citizens Medical Center
David Brown, FACHE, Administrator
2701 Hospital Dr
Victoria, TX 77901
512 573-9181
Type: Hosp or Med Ctr: 100-299 Beds
Control: State, County, or Local Govt
• Radiography Prgm

Victoria College
Tom Butler, President
2200 E Red River
Victoria, TX 77901
361 582-2560
Type: Junior or Comm Coll
Control: State, County, or Local Govt
• Clin Lab Technician/Med Lab Technician Prgm
• Respiratory Care Prgm

Waco

Baylor University
John Lilley, PhD, President/CEO
1 Bear Pl #97096
Waco, TX 76798
254 710-3555
Type: 4-year Coll or Univ
Control: Nonprofit (Private or Religious)
• Athletic Training Prgm
• Dietetics-Didactic Prgm
• Nursing Prgm
• Psychology (PsyD) Prgm
• Speech-Language Pathology Prgm

McLennan Community College
Dennis F Michaelis, PhD, President
1400 College Dr
Waco, TX 76708
254 299-8601
Type: Junior or Comm Coll
Control: State, County, or Local Govt
• Clin Lab Technician/Med Lab Technician Prgm
• Neurodiagnostic Tech Prgm
• Physical Therapist Assistant Prgm
• Radiography Prgm
• Surgical Technology Prgm
• Veterinary Technology Prgm

Texas State Technical College
Bill Segura, PhD, Chancellor
3801 Campus Dr
Waco, TX 76705
254 867-4836
Type: Junior or Comm Coll
Control: State, County, or Local Govt
• Dental Assistant Prgm
• Dental Hygiene Prgm
• Emergency Med Tech-Paramedic Prgm
• Medical Assistant Prgm
• Surgical Technology Prgm

Weatherford

Weatherford College
Joe Birmingham, EdD, President
225 College Park
Weatherford, TX 76086-5699
817 594-5471
Type: Junior or Comm Coll
Control: State, County, or Local Govt
• Diagnostic Med Sonography (General/Vascular) Prgm
• Emergency Med Tech-Paramedic Prgm
• Pharmacy Technician Prgm
• Phlebotomy Prgm
• Radiography Prgm
• Respiratory Care Prgm

Wharton

Wharton County Junior College
Betty McCrohan, MS, President
911 Boling Hwy
Wharton, TX 77488
979 532-6400
Type: Junior or Comm Coll
Control: State, County, or Local Govt
• Dental Hygiene Prgm
• Emergency Med Tech-Paramedic Prgm
• Physical Therapist Assistant Prgm
• Radiography Prgm
• Surgical Technology Prgm

Wichita Falls

882d Training Group, 382 Training Squadron
Nancy Dezell, COL USAF, CEO
939 Missile Rd
Sheppard AFB
Wichita Falls, TX 76311-2245
940 676-2700
Type: Dept of Defense
Control: Fed Govt
• Clin Lab Technician/Med Lab Technician Prgm (2)

Midwestern State University
Jesse Rogers, PhD, President
3410 Taft Blvd
Wichita Falls, TX 76308-2099
940 397-4211
Type: 4-year Coll or Univ
Control: State, County, or Local Govt
• Athletic Training Prgm
• Dental Hygiene Prgm
• Nursing Prgm
• Radiography Prgm
• Radiologist Assistant Prgm
• Respiratory Care Prgm

United Regional Health Care Systems
Phyllis Cowling, CEO
1600 10th St
Wichita Falls, TX 76301
940 764-3035
Type: Hosp or Med Ctr: 300-499 Beds
Control: State, County, or Local Govt
• Clin Lab Scientist/Med Technologist Prgm

United Kingdom

Garthdee Aberdeen

Robert Gordon University
William Stevely, Vice Chancellor/President
Garthdee Rd
Garthdee Aberdeen, UK AB107QG
Type: 4-year Coll or Univ
Control: State, County, or Local Govt
• Physical Therapy Prgm

Utah

Cedar City

Southern Utah University
Michael T Benson, PhD, President
351 W University Blvd
Cedar City, UT 84720
435 586-7702
Type: 4-year Coll or Univ
Control: State, County, or Local Govt
• Athletic Training Prgm
• Nursing Prgm

Kaysville

Davis Applied Technology College
Michael J Bouwhuis, MEd, Campus President
550 East 300 South
Kaysville, UT 84037
801 593-2500
Type: Junior or Comm Coll
Control: State, County, or Local Govt
• Dental Assistant Prgm
• Medical Assistant Prgm
• Surgical Technology Prgm

Logan

Bridgerland Applied Technology College
Richard L Maughan, MS PhD, Campus President
1301 West 600 North
Logan, UT 84321
435 753-6780
Type: Vocational or Tech Sch
Control: State, County, or Local Govt
• Dental Assistant Prgm
• Medical Assistant Prgm

Utah State University
Stan Albrecht, President
Logan, UT 84322
435 797-1000
Type: 4-year Coll or Univ
Control: State, County, or Local Govt
• Audiologist Prgm
• Dietetic Internship Prgm
• Dietetics-Coordinated Prgm
• Dietetics-Didactic Prgm
• Music Therapy Prgm
• Rehabilitation Counseling Prgm
• Speech-Language Pathology Prgm

Ogden

Ogden-Weber Applied Technology College
Collette Mercier, MA, President
200 N Washington Blvd
Ogden, UT 84404
801 627-8304
Type: Vocational or Tech Sch
Control: State, County, or Local Govt
• Dental Assistant Prgm
• Medical Assistant Prgm

Stevens-Henager College
Vicky Dewsnup, President, Regional Dir
1890 South 1350 West
PO Box 9428
Ogden, UT 84409-0428
801 394-7791
Type: 4-year Coll or Univ
Control: For Profit
• Medical Assistant Prgm (3)
• Respiratory Care Prgm
• Surgical Technology Prgm

Weber State University

F Ann Milner, EdD, President
1001 University Circle
Ogden, UT 84408-1001
801 626-6001
Type: 4-year Coll or Univ
Control: State, County, or Local Govt
• Athletic Training Prgm
• Clin Lab Scientist/Med Technologist Prgm
• Clin Lab Technician/Med Lab Technician Prgm
• Dental Hygiene Prgm
• Emergency Med Tech-Paramedic Prgm
• Radiologist Assistant Prgm
• Respiratory Care Prgm

Orem

The Utah College of Dental Hygiene
Orem, UT 84058
• Dental Hygiene Prgm

Utah Valley University
William A Sederburg, PhD, President
800 W University Pkwy
Orem, UT 84058-5999
801 863-8550
Type: 4-year Coll or Univ
Control: State, County, or Local Govt
• Dental Hygiene Prgm
• Emergency Med Tech-Paramedic Prgm

Provo

Ameritech College
Ken Bentley, BS CDA, CEO Administrator
1675 N Freedom Blvd, Ste 5A
Provo, UT 84604
801 377-2900
Type: Vocational or Tech Sch
Control: For Profit
• Surgical Technology Prgm

Brigham Young University
Cecil O Samuelson, MD, President
D 346 ASB
Provo, UT 84602
801 422-2521
Type: 4-year Coll or Univ
Control: Nonprofit (Private or Religious)
• Athletic Training Prgm
• Clin Lab Scientist/Med Technologist Prgm
• Dietetic Internship Prgm
• Dietetics-Didactic Prgm
• Music Therapy Prgm
• Nursing Prgm
• Psychology (PhD) Prgm
• Speech-Language Pathology Prgm

Provo College
Gordon C Peters, MBA, Campus President
1450 W North
Provo, UT 84601-1305
801 818-8912
Type: Junior or Comm Coll
Control: For Profit
• Physical Therapist Assistant Prgm

Salt Lake City

Fortis College - Salt Lake City
Salt Lake City, UT 84107
• Dental Hygiene Prgm

Latter Day Saints Business College
Steven K Woodhouse, MBA, President
411 E South Temple
Salt Lake City, UT 84111
801 524-8101
Type: Vocational or Tech Sch
Control: Nonprofit (Private or Religious)
• Medical Assistant Prgm

Salt Lake Community College
Cynthia Bioteau, PhD, President
4600 S Redwood Rd
PO Box 30808
Salt Lake City, UT 84130-0808
801 957-4226
Type: Junior or Comm Coll
Control: State, County, or Local Govt
• Dental Hygiene Prgm
• Medical Assistant Prgm
• Occupational Therapy Asst Prgm
• Physical Therapist Assistant Prgm
• Radiography Prgm
• Surgical Technology Prgm

Unified Fire Authority/Utah Valley University
Don Berry, Fire Chief
3380 South 900 West
Salt Lake City, UT 84119
801 743-7200
Type: Junior or Comm Coll
Control: State, County, or Local Govt
• Emergency Med Tech-Paramedic Prgm

University of Phoenix - Utah
Brian Mueller, CEO
Salt Lake City, UT 84123
Type: 4-year Coll or Univ
Control: State, County, or Local Govt
• Counseling Prgm

University of Utah
Michael K Young, JD, President
201 S President Circle, Rm 203
Park Building
Salt Lake City, UT 84112
801 581-5701
Type: 4-year Coll or Univ
Control: State, County, or Local Govt
• Allopathic Medicine Prgm
• Athletic Training Prgm
• Audiologist Prgm
• Dietetics-Coordinated Prgm
• Emergency Med Tech-Paramedic Prgm
• Music Therapy Prgm
• Nursing Prgm
• Occupational Therapy Prgm
• Pharmacy Prgm
• Physical Therapy Prgm
• Psychology (PhD) Prgm
• Speech-Language Pathology Prgm

University of Utah Health Science Center
Michael K Young, JD, President
203 Park Bldg
Salt Lake City, UT 84112
801 581-5701
Type: Acad Health Ctr/Med Sch
Control: State, County, or Local Govt
• Clin Lab Scientist/Med Technologist Prgm
• Cytotechnology Prgm
• Genetic Counseling Prgm
• Nuclear Medicine Technology Prgm
• Physician Assistant Prgm

Western Governors University
Salt Lake City, UT 84107-2533
Type: 4-year Coll or Univ
Control: Nonprofit (Private or Religious)
• Nursing Prgm

Westminster College
Salt Lake City, UT 84105
Type: 4-year Coll or Univ
Control: Nonprofit (Private or Religious)
• Nursing Prgm

Springville

Career Step
1220 N Main St
Ste 6
Springville, UT 84663
Type: Acad Health Ctr/Med Sch
Control: For Profit
• Medical Transcriptionist Prgm

St George

Dixie State College of Utah
Stephen Nadauld, PhD, President
225 South 700 East
St George, UT 84770-3876
435 652-7501
Type: Junior or Comm Coll
Control: State, County, or Local Govt
• Clin Lab Scientist/Med Technologist Prgm
• Dental Hygiene Prgm
• Emergency Med Tech-Paramedic Prgm
• Radiography Prgm
• Surgical Technology Prgm

West Jordan

Broadview University
West Jordan, UT 840884721
• Medical Assistant Prgm

Utah Career College
Terry Myhre, CEO
1902 West 7800 South
West Jordan, UT 84088
801 304-4224
Type: Vocational or Tech Sch
Control: For Profit
• Veterinary Technology Prgm

West Valley City

Everest College
Larry Banks, President
3280 West 3500 South
West Valley City, UT 84119
801 840-4800
Type: Junior or Comm Coll
Control: For Profit
• Medical Assistant Prgm
• Pharmacy Technician Prgm
• Surgical Technology Prgm

Bennington

Southern Vermont College
982 Mansion Drive
Bennington, VT 05201
Type: 4-year Coll or Univ
Control: Nonprofit (Private or Religious)
• Radiography Prgm

Burlington

Champlain College
David F Finney, PhD, President
163 S Willard St
PO Box 670
Burlington, VT 05402
802 865-2700
Type: 4-year Coll or Univ
Control: Nonprofit (Private or Religious)
• Radiography Prgm

Fletcher Allen Health Care
Melinda Estes, MD, CEO and President
111 Colchester Ave
Burlington, VT 05401-1429
802 847-5959
Type: Hosp or Med Ctr: 300-499 Beds
Control: Nonprofit (Private or Religious)
• Cytotechnology Prgm

University of Vermont
Daniel Fogel, PhD, President
349 Waterman Bldg
83 South Prospect Street
Burlington, VT 05405
802 656-3186
Type: 4-year Coll or Univ
Control: State, County, or Local Govt
• Allopathic Medicine Prgm
• Athletic Training Prgm
• Clin Lab Scientist/Med Technologist Prgm
• Counseling Prgm
• Dietetics-Coordinated Prgm
• Dietetics-Didactic Prgm
• Nuclear Medicine Technology Prgm
• Nursing Prgm
• Physical Therapy Prgm
• Psychology (PhD) Prgm
• Radiation Therapy Prgm
• Speech-Language Pathology Prgm

Castleton

Castleton State College
David Wolk, MS, President
Woodruff Hall
Castleton, VT 05735
802 468-1201
Type: 4-year Coll or Univ
Control: State, County, or Local Govt
• Athletic Training Prgm

Essex Junction

Center for Technology - Essex
Kathy Finck, Director
Three Educational Dr
Essex Junction, VT 05452
802 879-5562
Type: Vocational or Tech Sch
Control: State, County, or Local Govt
• Dental Assistant Prgm
• Ophthalmic Assistant Prgm

Lyndonville

Lyndon State College
Lyndonville, VT 05851
Type: 4-year Coll or Univ
• Exercise Science Prgm

Northfield

Norwich University
Richard W Schneider, PhD, President
158 Harmon Dr
Northfield, VT 05663
802 485-2065
Type: 4-year Coll or Univ
Control: Nonprofit (Private or Religious)
• Athletic Training Prgm

Randolph Center

Vermont Technical College
Ty Handy, MBA, President
PO Box 500
Randolph Center, VT 05061
802 728-1258
Type: Junior or Comm Coll
Control: State, County, or Local Govt
• Dental Hygiene Prgm
• Respiratory Care Prgm
• Veterinary Technology Prgm

Virginia

Annandale

Northern Virginia Community College
Robert G Templin, Jr, PhD, President
4001 Wakefield Chapel Rd
Annandale, VA 22003-3796
703 323-3101
Type: Junior or Comm Coll
Control: State, County, or Local Govt
• Clin Lab Technician/Med Lab Technician Prgm
• Dental Hygiene Prgm
• Diagnostic Med Sonography (General) Prgm
• Emergency Med Tech-Paramedic Prgm
• Physical Therapist Assistant Prgm
• Respiratory Care Prgm
• Veterinary Technology Prgm

Arlington

ACT College
Jeffrey Moore, MBA, President and CEO
1100 Wilson Blvd
Arlington, VA 22209
Type: 4-year Coll or Univ
Control: State, County, or Local Govt
• Radiography Prgm

Argosy University
Arlington, VA 22209
Type: 4-year Coll or Univ
Control: For Profit
• Counseling Prgm
• Psychology (PsyD) Prgm

Marymount University
James Bundschuh, President
2807 N Glebe Rd
Arlington, VA 22207-4299
703 522-5600
Type: 4-year Coll or Univ
Control: Nonprofit (Private or Religious)
• Counseling Prgm
• Nursing Prgm
• Physical Therapy Prgm

Big Stone Gap

Mountain Empire Community College
Terrance Suarez, PhD, President
3441 Mountain Empire Rd
Big Stone Gap, VA 24219
540 523-2400
Type: Junior or Comm Coll
Control: State, County, or Local Govt
• Respiratory Care Prgm

Blacksburg

Edward Via Virginia Coll of Opteopathic Med
2265 Kraft Dr
Blacksburg, VA 24060
Type: Acad Health Ctr/Med Sch
Control: Nonprofit (Private or Religious)
• Osteopathic Medicine Prgm

Virginia Polytechnic Inst & State Univ
Charles W Steger, President
Blacksburg, VA 24061
540 231-6000
Type: 4-year Coll or Univ
Control: State, County, or Local Govt
• Counseling Prgm
• Dietetic Internship Prgm
• Dietetics-Didactic Prgm
• Music Therapy Prgm
• Psychology (PhD) Prgm
• Veterinary Medicine Prgm

Bridgewater

Bridgewater College
Phillip C Stone, JD, President
402 E College St
Bridgewater, VA 22812
540 828-5605
Type: 4-year Coll or Univ
Control: State, County, or Local Govt
• Athletic Training Prgm

Charlottesville

Piedmont Virginia Community College
Frank Friedman, PhD, President
501 College Dr
Charlottesville, VA 22902
434 961-5200
Type: Junior or Comm Coll
Control: State, County, or Local Govt
• Emergency Med Tech-Paramedic Prgm
• Radiography Prgm
• Surgical Technology Prgm

University of Virginia
John Casteen, President
PO Box 400224
Charlottesville, VA 22904-4224
434 924-3337
Type: 4-year Coll or Univ
Control: State, County, or Local Govt
• Allopathic Medicine Prgm
• Counseling Prgm
• Nursing Prgm (2)
• Psychology (PhD) Prgm
• Psychology (PsyD) Prgm
• Speech-Language Pathology Prgm

University of Virginia Health System
Edward R Howell, MS, VP and CEO, Hlth Systems
PO Box 800809
Charlottesville, VA 22908
434 243-9308
Type: Hosp or Med Ctr: 500 Beds
Control: State, County, or Local Govt
• Dietetic Internship Prgm
• Radiation Therapy Prgm

Virginia School of Massage
Charlottesville, VA 22903
Type: Acad Health Ctr/Med Sch
Control: For Profit
• Massage Therapy Prgm

Chester

Richmond School of Health and Technology
Chester, VA
Type: Vocational or Tech Sch
Control: For Profit
• Radiography Prgm

Danville

Averett University
Richard A Pfau, PhD, President
420 W Main St
Danville, VA 24541
434 791-5670
Type: 4-year Coll or Univ
Control: Nonprofit (Private or Religious)
• Athletic Training Prgm

Danville Regional Medical Center
Warren E Callaway, FACHE, President
142 S Main St
Danville, VA 24541
804 799-3700
Type: Hosp or Med Ctr: 300-499 Beds
Control: Nonprofit (Private or Religious)
• Radiography Prgm

Emory

Emory & Henry College
Rosalind Reichard, PhD, President
PO Box 947
Emory, VA 24327-0947
276 944-6107
Type: 4-year Coll or Univ
Control: Nonprofit (Private or Religious)
• Athletic Training Prgm

INSTITUTIONS

Fairfax

George Mason University
Alan G Merten, PhD, President
4400 University Dr
Fairfax, VA 22030-4444
703 993-8700
Type: 4-year Coll or Univ
Control: State, County, or Local Govt
• Athletic Training Prgm
• Music Therapy Prgm
• Nursing Prgm
• Psychology (PhD) Prgm

Falls Church

Inova Fairfax Hospital
Reuven Pasternak, Administrator
3300 Gallows Rd
Falls Church, VA 22042
703 776-3230
Type: Hosp or Med Ctr: 500 Beds
Control: State, County, or Local Govt
• Clin Lab Scientist/Med Technologist Prgm

National Massage Therapy Institute
803 W Board St
Falls Church, VA 22046
Type: Acad Health Ctr/Med Sch
Control: For Profit
• Massage Therapy Prgm

Farmville

Longwood University
Patricia Cormier, PhD, President
201 High St
Farmville, VA 23909-1899
804 395-2000
Type: 4-year Coll or Univ
Control: State, County, or Local Govt
• Athletic Training Prgm
• Music Therapy Prgm
• Speech-Language Pathology Prgm

Fredericksburg

Mary Washington Hospital
Fred M Rankin III, MPH, President/CEO
1001 Sam Perry Blvd
Fredericksburg, VA 22401
540 741-1414
Type: Hosp or Med Ctr: 300-499 Beds
Control: Nonprofit (Private or Religious)
• Radiography Prgm

Grundy

University of Appalachia College of Pharmacy
Eleanor Sue Cantrell, MD, President
PO Box 2858
Grundy, VA 24614
Type: Acad Health Ctr/Med Sch
Control: Nonprofit (Private or Religious)
• Pharmacy Prgm

Hampton

Hampton University
William R Harvey, President
Hampton, VA 23668
804 727-5000
Type: 4-year Coll or Univ
Control: Nonprofit (Private or Religious)
• Nursing Prgm
• Pharmacy Prgm
• Physical Therapy Prgm
• Speech-Language Pathology Prgm

Thomas Nelson Community College
Charles Taylor, EdD, President
PO Box 9407
Hampton, VA 23670
757 825-2711
Type: Junior or Comm Coll
Control: State, County, or Local Govt
• Dental Hygiene Prgm

Harrisonburg

Eastern Mennonite University
Loren E Swartzendruber, President
Swartzendruber
Harrisonburg, VA 22802
540 432-4000
Type: Acad Health Ctr/Med Sch
Control: For Profit
• Counseling Prgm
• Nursing Prgm

James Madison University
Linwood Rose, EdD, President
Office of the President, MSC 7608
Harrisonburg, VA 22807
540 568-6868
Type: 4-year Coll or Univ
Control: State, County, or Local Govt
• Athletic Training Prgm
• Audiologist Prgm
• Counseling Prgm
• Dietetics-Didactic Prgm
• Music Therapy Prgm
• Nursing Prgm
• Occupational Therapy Prgm
• Physician Assistant Prgm
• Speech-Language Pathology Prgm

Rockingham Memorial Hospital
James Krauss, MHA, President
235 Cantrell Ave
Harrisonburg, VA 22801
540 564-5620
Type: Hosp or Med Ctr: 100-299 Beds
Control: Nonprofit (Private or Religious)
• Clin Lab Scientist/Med Technologist Prgm
• Radiography Prgm

Leesburg

Loudoun County Dept of Fire-Rescue
Joseph Pozzo, MA, Chief
16600 Courage Court
Leesburg, VA 20175
703 777-0333
Type: Vocational or Tech Sch
Control: State, County, or Local Govt
• Emergency Med Tech-Paramedic Prgm

Locust Grove

Germanna Community College
Locust Grove, VA 22508
• Dental Assistant Prgm

Lynchburg

Centra Health Systems of Lynchburg
George W Dawson, MHA, President/CEO
1920 Atherholt Rd
Lynchburg, VA 24501
434 200-4705
Type: Hosp or Med Ctr: 500 Beds
Control: Other
• Clin Lab Technician/Med Lab Technician Prgm

Central Virginia Community College
Darrel W Staat, DA, President
3506 Wards Rd
Lynchburg, VA 24502
804 832-7601
Type: Junior or Comm Coll
Control: State, County, or Local Govt
• Emergency Med Tech-Paramedic Prgm
• Radiography Prgm
• Respiratory Care Prgm

Liberty University
Ronald Godwin, PhD, CEO
1971 University Blvd
Lynchburg, VA 24502
434 582-7600
Type: 4-year Coll or Univ
Control: Nonprofit (Private or Religious)
• Athletic Training Prgm
• Exercise Science Prgm
• Nursing Prgm

Lynchburg College
Kenneth R Garren, President
1501 Lakeside Dr
Lynchburg, VA 24501-3199
804 544-8100
Type: 4-year Coll or Univ
Control: Nonprofit (Private or Religious)
• Athletic Training Prgm
• Counseling Prgm
• Exercise Science Prgm
• Nursing Prgm

Miller-Motte Technical College
Ned Snyder, MA, Campus Director
1011 Creekside Lane
Lynchburg, VA 24502
434 239-5222
Type: Vocational or Tech Sch
Control: For Profit
• Medical Assistant Prgm
• Surgical Technology Prgm

Newport News

ECPI University
Barbara Larar, Director
1001 Omni Blvd, Ste 200
Newport News, VA 23606
757 873-2423
Type: Vocational or Tech Sch
Control: For Profit
• Radiography Prgm

Riverside School of Health Careers
Tracee Carmean, VP Education
316 Main St
Newport News, VA 23601
757 240-2202
Type: Vocational or Tech Sch
Control: Nonprofit (Private or Religious)
• Radiography Prgm
• Surgical Technology Prgm

Norfolk

Centura College
Norfolk, VA 23518
• Dental Assistant Prgm

Eastern Virginia Medical School
Harry T Lester, MD, President
PO Box 1980
Norfolk, VA 23507
757 446-5600
Type: Acad Health Ctr/Med Sch
Control: Nonprofit (Private or Religious)
• Allopathic Medicine Prgm
• Art Therapy Prgm
• Physician Assistant Prgm
• Surgical Assistant Prgm

Norfolk State University
Carolyn Meyers, PhD, President
700 Park Ave
Echols Hall Rm 165
Norfolk, VA 23504
757 823-8670
Type: 4-year Coll or Univ
Control: State, County, or Local Govt
• Clin Lab Scientist/Med Technologist Prgm
• Dietetics-Didactic Prgm
• Kinesiotherapy Prgm

Old Dominion University
John Broderick, PhD, Acting President
200 Koch Hall
Norfolk, VA 23529-0001
757 683-3159
Type: 4-year Coll or Univ
Control: State, County, or Local Govt
• Clin Lab Scientist/Med Technologist Prgm
• Counseling Prgm
• Cytotechnology Prgm
• Dental Hygiene Prgm
• Exercise Science Prgm
• Histotechnician Prgm
• Nuclear Medicine Technology Prgm
• Nursing Prgm
• Ophthalmic Med Technologist Prgm
• Ophthalmic Technician Prgm
• Physical Therapy Prgm
• Speech-Language Pathology Prgm

Sentara Norfolk General Hospital
Rodney Hochman, MD, CEO
600 Gresham Dr
Norfolk, VA 23507
757 668-3361
Type: Hosp or Med Ctr: 500 Beds
Control: Nonprofit (Private or Religious)
• Cardiovascular Tech (Invasive/Noninv/Vasc) Prgm
• Surgical Technology Prgm

Tidewater Community College
Deborah M DiCroce, EdD, President
121 College Place
Norfolk, VA 23510
757 822-1050
Type: Junior or Comm Coll
Control: State, County, or Local Govt
• Diagnostic Med Sonography (General) Prgm
• Emergency Med Tech-Paramedic Prgm
• Medical Assistant Prgm
• Occupational Therapy Asst Prgm
• Physical Therapist Assistant Prgm
• Radiography Prgm
• Respiratory Care Prgm

Petersburg

Southside Regional Medical Center
David J Fikse, MBA, CEO
200 Medical Park Blvd
Petersburg, VA 23805
804 765-5902
Type: Hosp or Med Ctr: 300-499 Beds
Control: Nonprofit (Private or Religious)
• Diagnostic Med Sonography (General) Prgm
• Radiography Prgm

Virginia State University
Eddie N Moore, Jr, President
Petersburg, VA 23806
804 524-5000
Type: 4-year Coll or Univ
Control: State, County, or Local Govt
• Dietetic Internship Prgm
• Dietetics-Didactic Prgm

Portsmouth

Naval School of Health Sciences
Susan E Herron, CAPT NC USN, Commanding
   Officer
1001 Holcomb Rd
Portsmouth, VA 23708-5200
757 953-5040
Type: Dept of Defense
Control: Fed Govt
• Pharmacy Technician Prgm

Radford

Radford University
Penelope Kyle, MBA JD, President
PO Box 6890
Martin Hall
Radford, VA 24142
540 831-5401
Type: 4-year Coll or Univ
Control: State, County, or Local Govt
• Athletic Training Prgm
• Counseling Prgm
• Dietetics-Didactic Prgm
• Music Therapy Prgm
• Nursing Prgm
• Occupational Therapy Prgm
• Speech-Language Pathology Prgm

Richlands

Southwest Virginia Community College
J Mark Estepp, PhD, President
PO Box SVCC
Richlands, VA 24641-1101
276 964-7315
Type: Junior or Comm Coll
Control: State, County, or Local Govt
• Emergency Med Tech-Paramedic Prgm
• Occupational Therapy Asst Prgm (2)
• Radiography Prgm
• Respiratory Care Prgm

Richmond

Bon Secours St Mary's Hospital
Joey S Battles, MA Ed RT(R), Association
   Directorr
8550 Magellan Pkwy, Ste 700
Richmond, VA 23227
Type: Hosp or Med Ctr: 300-499 Beds
Control: Nonprofit (Private or Religious)
• Radiography Prgm

Bryant & Stratton College - Richmond
John Staschak, President
8141 Hull St Road
Richmond, VA 23235
804 745-2444
Type: Junior or Comm Coll
Control: For Profit
• Medical Assistant Prgm

Fortis College - Richmond
Richmond, VA 23230
Type: Vocational or Tech Sch
• Dental Assistant Prgm
• Surgical Technology Prgm

J Sargeant Reynolds Community College
Gary Rhodes, EdD, President
PO Box 85622
Richmond, VA 23285-5622
804 523-5200
Type: Junior or Comm Coll
Control: State, County, or Local Govt
• Clin Lab Technician/Med Lab Technician Prgm
• Dental Assistant Prgm
• Dental Lab Technician Prgm
• Emergency Med Tech-Paramedic Prgm
• Ophthalmic Dispensing Optician Prgm
• Polysomnographic Technology Prgm
• Respiratory Care Prgm

Virginia Commonwealth Univ/Health System
Michael Rao, PhD, President
PO Box 842512
Richmond, VA 23284-2512
804 828-1200
Type: Acad Health Ctr/Med Sch
Control: State, County, or Local Govt
• Dentistry Prgm
• Dietetic Internship Prgm
• Emergency Med Tech-Paramedic Prgm
• Genetic Counseling Prgm
• Pharmacy Prgm
• Physical Therapy Prgm

Virginia Commonwealth University
Eugene P Trani, PhD, President
910 W Franklin St
PO Box 842512
Richmond, VA 23284-2512
804 828-1200
Type: 4-year Coll or Univ
Control: State, County, or Local Govt
• Allopathic Medicine Prgm
• Athletic Training Prgm
• Clin Lab Scientist/Med Technologist Prgm
• Counseling Prgm
• Dental Hygiene Prgm
• Nuclear Medicine Technology Prgm
• Occupational Therapy Prgm
• Radiation Therapy Prgm
• Radiography Prgm
• Radiologist Assistant Prgm
• Rehabilitation Counseling Prgm

Virginia Department of Health
Div of Public Health Nutrition
1500 E Main St Rm 132
Richmond, VA 23219
804 786-5420
Type: Acad Health Ctr/Med Sch
Control: State, County, or Local Govt
• Dietetic Internship Prgm

Roanoke

Carilion Medical Center
Edward Murphy, Senior Vice President
Carilion Roanoke Memorial Hospital
101 Elm Ave SE Belleview at Jefferson
Roanoke, VA 24014
540 981-7831
Type: Hosp or Med Ctr: 500 Beds
Control: Nonprofit (Private or Religious)
• Clin Lab Scientist/Med Technologist Prgm

Jefferson College of Health Sciences
Nathaniel L Bishop, DMin, Interim President
920 S Jefferson St
PO Box 13186
Roanoke, VA 24031-3186
540 985-8484
Type: 4-year Coll or Univ
Control: Nonprofit (Private or Religious)
• Emergency Med Tech-Paramedic Prgm
• Nursing Prgm
• Occupational Therapy Asst Prgm
• Occupational Therapy Prgm
• Physical Therapist Assistant Prgm
• Respiratory Care Prgm

National College
Frank E Longaker, MBA, President
PO Box 6400
Roanoke, VA 24017
540 986-1800
Type: Junior or Comm Coll
Control: For Profit
• Emergency Med Tech-Paramedic Prgm
• Medical Assistant Prgm (7)
• Surgical Technology Prgm

National College - Danville
Frank Longaker, MBA, President
PO Box 6400
1813 E Main St
Roanoke, VA 24017
540 986-1800
Type: Junior or Comm Coll
Control: For Profit
• Surgical Technology Prgm

Virginia Tech Carilion School of Medicine and
2 Riverside Circle Suite M140
Roanoke, VA 24016
• Allopathic Medicine Prgm

Virginia Western Community College
Robert Sandel, PhD, President
3097 Colonial Ave SW
PO Box 14007
Roanoke, VA 24015
540 857-7311
Type: Junior or Comm Coll
Control: State, County, or Local Govt
• Dental Hygiene Prgm
• Radiation Therapy Prgm
• Radiography Prgm

Salem

National College
Frank Longaker, MBA, President
1813 E Main St
Salem, VA 24153
540 986-1800
Type: Junior or Comm Coll
Control: For Profit
• Medical Assistant Prgm (2)
• Surgical Technology Prgm

Roanoke College
Michael Maxey, MS, President
221 College Lane
Salem, VA 24153
540 375-2200
Type: 4-year Coll or Univ
Control: Nonprofit (Private or Religious)
• Athletic Training Prgm

Stuarts Draft

Augusta Medical Center
Mary Mannix, COO
PO Box 1000
78 Medical Center Dr
Stuarts Draft, VA 22939
540 332-4820
Type: Hosp or Med Ctr: 100-299 Beds
Control: Nonprofit (Private or Religious)
• Clin Lab Scientist/Med Technologist Prgm

Virginia Beach

Bryant & Stratton College - Virginia Beach
Lee E Hicklin, Director
301 Centre Pointe Dr
Virginia Beach, VA 23462
757 499-7900
Type: Junior or Comm Coll
Control: For Profit
• Medical Assistant Prgm

Cayce/Reilly School of Massotherapy
215 67th St
Virginia Beach, VA 23451
Type: Acad Health Ctr/Med Sch
Control: For Profit
• Massage Therapy Prgm

Regent University
Rosemarie Hughes, PhD, Dean
School of Psychology and Counseling
1000 Regent University Dr, CRB 174
Virginia Beach, VA 23464-9800
757 226-4000
Type: 4-year Coll or Univ
Control: Nonprofit (Private or Religious)
• Counseling Prgm
• Psychology (PsyD) Prgm

Virginia Consortium Program in Clinical Psych
Virginia Beach, VA 23453
Type: Acad Health Ctr/Med Sch
Control: For Profit
• Psychology (PsyD) Prgm

Weyers Cave

Blue Ridge Community College
James Perkins, PhD, President
PO Box 80
Weyers Cave, VA 24486
540 234-9261
Type: 4-year Coll or Univ
Control: State, County, or Local Govt
• Veterinary Technology Prgm

Williamsburg

College of William & Mary
Timothy J Sullivan, President
PO Box 8795
Williamsburg, VA 23187-8794
757 221-4000
Type: 4-year Coll or Univ
Control: State, County, or Local Govt
• Counseling Prgm

Winchester

Shenandoah University
Tracy Fitzsimmons, PhD, President
1460 University Drive
Winchester, VA 22601
540 665-4505
Type: 4-year Coll or Univ
Control: Nonprofit (Private or Religious)
• Athletic Training Prgm
• Music Therapy Prgm
• Nursing Prgm
• Occupational Therapy Prgm
• Pharmacy Prgm
• Physical Therapy Prgm
• Physician Assistant Prgm
• Respiratory Care Prgm

Winchester Medical Center Inc
1840 Amherst St
PO Box 3340
Winchester, VA 22601
Type: Hosp or Med Ctr: 300-499 Beds
Control: Nonprofit (Private or Religious)
• Radiography Prgm

Wytheville

Wytheville Community College
Charlie White, PhD, President
1000 E Main St
Wytheville, VA 24382
276 223-4848
Type: Junior or Comm Coll
Control: State, County, or Local Govt
- Clin Lab Technician/Med Lab Technician Prgm
- Dental Hygiene Prgm
- Physical Therapist Assistant Prgm

Yorktown

Tri-Service Optician School (TOPS)
CDR Lee Cornforth, USN OD MBA, Training
   Officer
Naval Ophthalmic Support & Trng Activity
160 Main Rd, Ste 360
Yorktown, VA 23691-9984
757 887-7329
Type: Dept of Defense
Control: Fed Govt
- Ophthalmic Laboratory Technician Prgm

Washington

Auburn

Green River Community College
Eileen Ely, PhD, President
12401 SE 320th St
Auburn, WA 98002-3622
253 833-9111
Type: Junior or Comm Coll
Control: State, County, or Local Govt
- Occupational Therapy Asst Prgm
- Physical Therapist Assistant Prgm

Bellevue

Bellevue College
B Jean Floten, MS, President
3000 Landerholm Circle SE
Bellevue, WA 98007-6484
425 564-2301
Type: Junior or Comm Coll
Control: State, County, or Local Govt
- Diagnostic Med Sonography (General/Cardiac) Prgm
- Medical Dosimetry Prgm
- Nuclear Medicine Technology Prgm
- Radiation Therapy Prgm
- Radiologist Assistant Prgm

Bellingham

Bellingham Technical College
Thomas Eckert, EdD, President
3028 Lindbergh Ave
Bellingham, WA 98225
360 752-8333
Type: Vocational or Tech Sch
Control: State, County, or Local Govt
- Dental Assistant Prgm
- Dental Hygiene Prgm
- Surgical Technology Prgm

Western Washington University
Karen W Morse, PhD, President
516 High St
Old Main 450, MS 9000
Bellingham, WA 98225
360 650-3480
Type: 4-year Coll or Univ
Control: State, County, or Local Govt
- Counseling Prgm
- Music Therapy Prgm
- Rehabilitation Counseling Prgm
- Speech-Language Pathology Prgm

Whatcom Community College
Harold G Heiner, PhD, President
237 W Kellogg Rd
Bellingham, WA 98226
360 676-2170
Type: Junior or Comm Coll
Control: State, County, or Local Govt
- Medical Assistant Prgm
- Physical Therapist Assistant Prgm

Whatcom Medic One/Bellingham Fire Dept
Bellingham, WA 98225
Type: Consortium
- Emergency Med Tech-Paramedic Prgm

Bremerton

Everest College
Janet O'Connell, EdC, President
155 Washington Ave
Ste 200
Bremerton, WA 98337
360 473-1120
Type: Vocational or Tech Sch
Control: For Profit
- Medical Assistant Prgm (4)

Olympic College
David Mitchell, PhD, President
1600 Chester Ave
Bremerton, WA 98337-1699
360 792-6050
Type: Junior or Comm Coll
Control: State, County, or Local Govt
- Medical Assistant Prgm
- Nursing Prgm

Cheney

Eastern Washington University
Rodolfo Arevalo, PhD, President
214 Showalter Hall
526 5th St
Cheney, WA 99004-2431
509 359-2371
Type: 4-year Coll or Univ
Control: State, County, or Local Govt
- Athletic Training Prgm
- Counseling Prgm
- Dental Hygiene Prgm
- Nursing Prgm
- Occupational Therapy Prgm
- Physical Therapy Prgm
- Speech-Language Pathology Prgm

Des Moines

Highline Community College
Jack Bermingham, Interim President
PO Box 98000
Des Moines, WA 98198-9800
206 878-3710
Type: Junior or Comm Coll
Control: State, County, or Local Govt
- Medical Assistant Prgm
- Polysomnographic Technology Prgm
- Respiratory Care Prgm

Ellensburg

Central Washington University
Jerilyn McIntyre, PhD, President
400 E University Way
Ellensburg, WA 98926-7501
509 963-2111
Type: 4-year Coll or Univ
Control: State, County, or Local Govt
- Counseling Prgm
- Dietetic Internship Prgm
- Dietetics-Didactic Prgm
- Emergency Med Tech-Paramedic Prgm
- Music Therapy Prgm

Everett

Everett Community College
David Beyer, President
2000 Tower St
Everett, WA 98201
425 388-9572
Type: Junior or Comm Coll
Control: State, County, or Local Govt
- Medical Assistant Prgm
- Medical Transcriptionist Prgm

Kirkland

Lake Washington Institute of Technology
David woodall, PhD, Interm President
11605 132nd Ave NE
Kirkland, WA 98034
425 739-8100
Type: Vocational or Tech Sch
Control: State, County, or Local Govt
- Dental Assistant Prgm
- Dental Hygiene Prgm
- Medical Assistant Prgm
- Occupational Therapy Asst Prgm

Northwest University
Kirkland, WA 98033
Type: 4-year Coll or Univ
Control: Nonprofit (Private or Religious)
- Nursing Prgm

Lakewood

Clover Park Technical College
John Walstrum, PhD, President
4500 Steilacoom Blvd SW
Lakewood, WA 98499-4098
253 589-5500
Type: Junior or Comm Coll
Control: State, County, or Local Govt
• Clin Lab Technician/Med Lab Technician Prgm
• Dental Assistant Prgm
• Histotechnician Prgm
• Medical Assistant Prgm
• Surgical Technology Prgm

Pierce College
Michele Johnson, PhD, President
9401 Farwest Dr SW
Lakewood, WA 98498-1999
253 964-6500
Type: Junior or Comm Coll
Control: State, County, or Local Govt
• Dental Hygiene Prgm
• Veterinary Technology Prgm

Longview

Lower Columbia College
James McLaughlin, PhD, President
1600 Maple St
Longview, WA 98632
360 577-2320
Type: Junior or Comm Coll
Control: State, County, or Local Govt
• Medical Assistant Prgm

Lynwood

Edmonds Community College
Lynwood, WA 98036
• Clinical Assisting Prgm

Mount Vernon

Skagit Valley College
Gary Tollefson, EdD, President
2405 E College Way
Mount Vernon, WA 98273
360 416-7997
Type: Junior or Comm Coll
Control: State, County, or Local Govt
• Medical Assistant Prgm

Olympia

South Puget Sound Community College
Gerald Pumphrey, PhD, President
2011 Mottman Rd SW
Olympia, WA 98512-6292
360 596-5206
Type: Junior or Comm Coll
Control: State, County, or Local Govt
• Dental Assistant Prgm
• Medical Assistant Prgm

Pasco

Columbia Basin College
Richard Cummins, PhD, President
2600 N 20th Ave
Pasco, WA 99301
509 547-0511
Type: Junior or Comm Coll
Control: State, County, or Local Govt
• Dental Hygiene Prgm
• Emergency Med Tech-Paramedic Prgm
• Medical Assistant Prgm
• Surgical Technology Prgm

Pullman

Washington State University
Elson S. Floyd, PhD, President
PO Box 641067
PO Box 641048
Pullman, WA 99164-1048
888 468-6978
Type: 4-year Coll or Univ
Control: State, County, or Local Govt
• Athletic Training Prgm
• Dietetics-Coordinated Prgm (2)
• Dietetics-Didactic Prgm
• Music Therapy Prgm
• Nursing Prgm
• Pharmacy Prgm
• Psychology (PhD) Prgm
• Speech-Language Pathology Prgm
• Veterinary Medicine Prgm

Renton

Renton Technical College
Donald E Bressler, PhD, President
3000 NE 4th Street
Renton, WA 98056
425 235-2352
Type: Vocational or Tech Sch
Control: State, County, or Local Govt
• Dental Assistant Prgm
• Medical Assistant Prgm
• Ophthalmic Assistant Prgm
• Pharmacy Technician Prgm
• Surgical Technology Prgm

Seattle

Antioch University - Seattle
Toni Murdock, President
2326 Sixth Ave
Seattle, WA 98121-1814
Type: 4-year Coll or Univ
Control: State, County, or Local Govt
• Art Therapy Prgm

Bastyr University
Joseph E Pizzorno, Jr, President
144 NE 54th St
Seattle, WA 98105
206 523-9585
Type: 4-year Coll or Univ
Control: Nonprofit (Private or Religious)
• Dietetic Internship Prgm
• Dietetics-Didactic Prgm

Cortiva Institute - Seattle
Dina Boon, LMP, President
425 Pontius Ave N, Ste 100
Seattle, WA 98109
206 282-1233
Type: Vocational or Tech Sch
Control: For Profit
• Massage Therapy Prgm

North Seattle Community College
Ron LaFayette, PhD, President
9600 College Way N
Seattle, WA 98103
206 527-3602
Type: Junior or Comm Coll
Control: State, County, or Local Govt
• Medical Assistant Prgm

Pima Medical Institute - Seattle
Richard Luebke, Sr, BS, President
9709 Third Ave NE, #400
Seattle, WA 98115
206 322-6100
Type: Vocational or Tech Sch
Control: For Profit
• Dental Hygiene Prgm
• Radiography Prgm
• Veterinary Technology Prgm

Sea Mar Community Health Center
8720 14th Ave S
Seattle, WA 98108-4807
206 726-3730
Type: Acad Health Ctr/Med Sch
Control: Nonprofit (Private or Religious)
• Dietetic Internship Prgm

Seattle Central Community College
Mildred Ollee, EdD, President
1701 Broadway, 2BE4180
Seattle, WA 98122
206 587-4144
Type: Junior or Comm Coll
Control: State, County, or Local Govt
• Ophthalmic Dispensing Optician Prgm
• Respiratory Care Prgm
• Surgical Technology Prgm

Seattle Pacific University
3307 Third Ave W
Seattle, WA 98119
206 281-2050
Type: 4-year Coll or Univ
Control: Nonprofit (Private or Religious)
• Dietetics-Didactic Prgm
• Nursing Prgm
• Psychology (PhD) Prgm

Seattle University
Stephen Sundborg, SJ STD, President
901 12th Ave
PO Box 222000
Seattle, WA 98122-4460
206 296-5960
Type: 4-year Coll or Univ
Control: Nonprofit (Private or Religious)
• Diagnostic Med Sonography
  (Gen/Card/Vascular) Prgm
• Nursing Prgm

Seattle Vocational Institute
Norward J Brooks, PhD, Director
2120 S Jackson
Seattle, WA 98144
206 587-4940
Type: Vocational or Tech Sch
Control: State, County, or Local Govt
• Dental Assistant Prgm
• Medical Assistant Prgm

Shoreline Community College
Lee Lambert, JD, President
16101 Greenwood Ave N
Administration, Shoreline Community Coll
Seattle, WA 98133
206 546-4551
Type: Junior or Comm Coll
Control: State, County, or Local Govt
• Clin Lab Technician/Med Lab Technician Prgm
• Dental Hygiene Prgm

University of Washington
Mark Emmert, PhD, President
301 Gerberding Hall
Box 351230
Seattle, WA 98195-1230
206 543-5010
Type: 4-year Coll or Univ
Control: State, County, or Local Govt
• Allopathic Medicine Prgm
• Audiologist Prgm
• Clin Lab Scientist/Med Technologist Prgm
• Dentistry Prgm
• Emergency Med Tech-Paramedic Prgm
• Medical Librarian Prgm
• Music Therapy Prgm
• Nursing Prgm
• Occupational Therapy Prgm
• Orthotist/Prosthetist Prgm
• Pharmacy Prgm
• Physical Therapy Prgm
• Physician Assistant Prgm
• Psychology (PhD) Prgm
• Speech-Language Pathology Prgm

Spokane

Apollo College
George Montgomery, BA, President and CEO
10102 E Knox, Ste 200
Spokane, WA 99206
509 532-8888
Type: Junior or Comm Coll
Control: For Profit
• Radiography Prgm

Gonzaga University
Spokane, WA 99258
Type: 4-year Coll or Univ
Control: Nonprofit (Private or Religious)
• Counseling Prgm
• Nursing Prgm

Providence Sacred Heart Medical Center
Elaine Couture, President/CEO
W 101 Eighth Ave
PO Box 2555 Providence Sacred Heart Medi
Spokane, WA 99220-2555
509 474-3040
Type: Hosp or Med Ctr: 500 Beds
Control: Nonprofit (Private or Religious)
• Clin Lab Scientist/Med Technologist Prgm

Spokane Community College
Joe Dunlap, EdD, President
N 1810 Greene St MS 2150
Spokane, WA 99217
509 533-7042
Type: Junior or Comm Coll
Control: State, County, or Local Govt
• Cardiovascular Tech (Invasive/Noninvasive) Prgm
• Dental Assistant Prgm
• Diagnostic Med Sonography (General) Prgm
• Emergency Med Tech-Paramedic Prgm
• Medical Assistant Prgm
• Pharmacy Technician Prgm
• Radiography Prgm
• Respiratory Care Prgm
• Surgical Technology Prgm

Spokane Falls Community College
Mark Palek, President
3410 W Fort George Wright Dr, MS3160
Spokane, WA 99224-5288
509 533-3535
Type: Junior or Comm Coll
Control: State, County, or Local Govt
• Physical Therapist Assistant Prgm

Whitworth University
William P Robinson, PhD, President
300 W Hawthorne Rd
Spokane, WA 99251
509 777-1000
Type: 4-year Coll or Univ
Control: Nonprofit (Private or Religious)
• Athletic Training Prgm
• Nursing Prgm

Tacoma

Bates Technical College
Lyle Quasim, MS, President
1101 S Yakima Ave
Tacoma, WA 98405
253 680-7100
Type: Vocational or Tech Sch
Control: State, County, or Local Govt
• Dental Assistant Prgm
• Dental Lab Technician Prgm
• Occupational Therapy Asst Prgm

Pacific Lutheran University
Tacoma, WA 98447
Type: 4-year Coll or Univ
Control: Nonprofit (Private or Religious)
• Music Therapy Prgm
• Nursing Prgm

St Joseph Medical Center
Joseph W Wilezek, President and CEO
1717 South J St
Tacoma, WA 98401-2197
Type: Acad Health Ctr/Med Sch
Control: For Profit
• Pharmacy Technician Prgm

Tacoma Community College
Pamela Transue, PhD, President
6501 S 19th St
Tacoma, WA 98466
253 566-5100
Type: Junior or Comm Coll
Control: State, County, or Local Govt
• Diagnostic Med Sonography (General) Prgm
• Emergency Med Tech-Paramedic Prgm
• Radiography Prgm
• Respiratory Care Prgm

Tacoma Fire Department
Ron Stephens, Fire Chief
901 Fawcett Ave
Tacoma, WA 98402
253 591-5737
Type: Consortium
Control: State, County, or Local Govt
• Emergency Med Tech-Paramedic Prgm

University of Puget Sound
Ronald R Thomas, PhD, President
1500 N Warner St, CMB 1094
Tacoma, WA 98416-0510
253 879-3201
Type: 4-year Coll or Univ
Control: Nonprofit (Private or Religious)
• Music Therapy Prgm
• Occupational Therapy Prgm
• Physical Therapy Prgm

Vancouver

Clark College
Robert Knight, MA, President
1933 Fort Vancouver Way
Vancouver, WA 98663-3598
360 992-2000
Type: Junior or Comm Coll
Control: State, County, or Local Govt
• Dental Hygiene Prgm
• Medical Assistant Prgm

Wenatchee

Wenatchee Valley College
James Richardson, MSEd, President
1300 Fifth St
Wenatchee, WA 98801
509 680-6800
Type: Junior or Comm Coll
Control: State, County, or Local Govt
• Clin Lab Technician/Med Lab Technician Prgm
• Medical Assistant Prgm

Yakima

Heritage University
Rick Garnier, CEO
1120 W Spruce St
Yakima, WA 98902
Type: 4-year Coll or Univ
Control: Nonprofit (Private or Religious)
• Clin Lab Scientist/Med Technologist Prgm

Pacific Northwest Univ of Hlth Sci
111 University Parkway, Ste 202
Yakima, WA 98901
Type: Acad Health Ctr/Med Sch
Control: For Profit
• Osteopathic Medicine Prgm

INSTITUTIONS

Yakima Valley Community College
Linda J Kaminski, EdD, President
PO Box 22520
Yakima, WA 98907
509 574-4635
Type: Junior or Comm Coll
Control: State, County, or Local Govt
- Dental Hygiene Prgm
- Medical Assistant Prgm
- Surgical Technology Prgm
- Veterinary Technology Prgm

West Virginia

Athens

Concord University
Jerry Beasley, PhD, President
PO Box 1000
Campus Box Wall
Athens, WV 24712
304 384-9188
Type: 4-year Coll or Univ
Control: State, County, or Local Govt
- Athletic Training Prgm

Beckley

Mountain State University
Charles H Polk, EdD, President
PO Box 9003
Beckley, WV 25802
304 253-7351
Type: 4-year Coll or Univ
Control: Nonprofit (Private or Religious)
- Diagnostic Med Sonography (General) Prgm
- Medical Assistant Prgm
- Occupational Therapy Asst Prgm
- Physical Therapist Assistant Prgm
- Physician Assistant Prgm
- Radiography Prgm

Bluefield

Bluefield Regional Medical Center
Leland Farnel, CEO
500 Cherry St
Bluefield, WV 24701
304 327-1100
Type: Hosp or Med Ctr: 100-299 Beds
Control: Nonprofit (Private or Religious)
- Clin Lab Technician/Med Lab Technician Prgm

Bluefield State College
Albert Walker, EdD, President
219 Rock St
Bluefield, WV 24701
304 327-4030
Type: 4-year Coll or Univ
Control: State, County, or Local Govt
- Nursing Prgm
- Radiography Prgm

Buckhannon

West Virginia Wesleyan College
Pamela Balch, MA, President
59 College Ave
Buckhannon, WV 26201-2995
304 473-8181
Type: 4-year Coll or Univ
Control: Nonprofit (Private or Religious)
- Athletic Training Prgm

Charleston

Carver Career Center
Jim Casdorph, MA, Principal
4799 Midland Dr
Charleston, WV 25306
304 348-1965
Type: Vocational or Tech Sch
Control: State, County, or Local Govt
- Pharmacy Technician Prgm
- Respiratory Care Prgm
- Surgical Technology Prgm

Mountain State School of Massage
Robert Rogers, LMTNCTMB, Executive Director
601 50th St
Charleston, WV 25304
304 926-8822
Type: Vocational or Tech Sch
Control: For Profit
- Massage Therapy Prgm

University of Charleston
Edwin H Welch, PhD, President
2300 McCorkle Ave SE
Charleston, WV 25304
304 357-4713
Type: 4-year Coll or Univ
Control: Nonprofit (Private or Religious)
- Athletic Training Prgm
- Pharmacy Prgm
- Radiography Prgm

Clarksburg

United Hospital Center
Bruce C Carter, MS, President
Three Hospital Plaza
Clarksburg, WV 26301
304 624-2332
Type: Hosp or Med Ctr: 300-499 Beds
Control: Nonprofit (Private or Religious)
- Radiography Prgm

Dunbar

Benjamin Franklin Career & Technical Ed Ctr
Alvin L Brown, BA MA MS, Principal
500 28th St
Dunbar, WV 25064
304 766-0369
Type: Vocational or Tech Sch
Control: State, County, or Local Govt
- Medical Assistant Prgm

Fairmont

Fairmont State Univ
Blair Montgomery, MS, President
230 Hardway Building
1201 Locust Ave
Fairmont, WV 26554
304 367-4692
Type: Junior or Comm Coll
Control: State, County, or Local Govt
- Clin Lab Technician/Med Lab Technician Prgm
- Nursing Prgm
- Physical Therapist Assistant Prgm
- Veterinary Technology Prgm

Fayetteville

Bridgemont Community and Technical College
Fayetteville, WV 25840
- Dental Hygiene Prgm

Huntington

Cabell Huntington Hospital
Brent Marstellar, BS, President
1340 Hal Greer Blvd
Huntington, WV 25701
304 526-2111
Type: Hosp or Med Ctr: 300-499 Beds
Control: Nonprofit (Private or Religious)
- Cytotechnology Prgm

Huntington Junior College
Carolyn Smith, BA, President
900 Fifth Ave
Huntington, WV 25701
304 697-7550
Type: Junior or Comm Coll
Control: For Profit
- Medical Assistant Prgm

Marshall University
Stephen Kopp, PhD, President
One John Marshall Dr
Office of the President
Huntington, WV 25755
304 696-3977
Type: 4-year Coll or Univ
Control: State, County, or Local Govt
- Allopathic Medicine Prgm
- Athletic Training Prgm
- Clin Lab Scientist/Med Technologist Prgm
- Clin Lab Technician/Med Lab Technician Prgm
- Dietetic Internship Prgm
- Dietetics-Didactic Prgm
- Music Therapy Prgm
- Psychology (PhD) Prgm
- Speech-Language Pathology Prgm

Mountwest Community & Technical College
Dan D Angel, President
One John Marshall Dr
Huntington, WV 25755
304 696-2300
Type: Vocational or Tech Sch
Control: State, County, or Local Govt
- Medical Assistant Prgm
- Physical Therapist Assistant Prgm

St Mary's Medical Center
Michael Sellards, BS MHA, Exec Director/CEO
2900 First Ave
Huntington, WV 25702
304 526-1270
Type: Hosp or Med Ctr: 300-499 Beds
Control: Nonprofit (Private or Religious)
• Radiography Prgm

Institute

Kanawha Valley Community & Technical College
Ervin V Griffin, PhD, President
PO Box 1000
105 Cole Complex
Institute, WV 25112
304 766-3111
Type: Junior or Comm Coll
Control: State, County, or Local Govt
• Nuclear Medicine Technology Prgm

Lewisburg

West Virginia of Osteopathic Medicine
400 N Lee St
Lewisburg, WV 24901
Type: Acad Health Ctr/Med Sch
Control: Nonprofit (Private or Religious)
• Osteopathic Medicine Prgm

Martinsburg

Blue Ridge Community & Technical College
Martinsburg, WV 25401
Type: Junior or Comm Coll
• Emergency Med Tech-Paramedic Prgm

James Rumsey Technical Institute
Vicki Jenkins, BA MS, Director
3274 Hedgesville Rd
Martinsburg, WV 25403
304 754-7925
Type: Vocational or Tech Sch
Control: State, County, or Local Govt
• Surgical Technology Prgm

Morgantown

Monongalia County Tech Education Center
John George, MA, Director/Principal
1000 Mississippi St
Morgantown, WV 26505
304 291-9240
Type: Vocational or Tech Sch
Control: State, County, or Local Govt
• Surgical Technology Prgm

West Virginia University
C Peter Magrath, President
102A Stewart Hall, PO Box 6201
Morgantown, WV 26506-6201
304 293-5531
Type: 4-year Coll or Univ
Control: State, County, or Local Govt
• Allopathic Medicine Prgm
• Athletic Training Prgm
• Audiologist Prgm
• Clin Lab Scientist/Med Technologist Prgm
• Counseling Prgm
• Dental Hygiene Prgm
• Dentistry Prgm
• Dietetic Internship Prgm
• Dietetics-Didactic Prgm
• Histotechnology Prgm
• Nursing Prgm
• Occupational Therapy Prgm
• Pathologists' Assistant Prgm
• Pharmacy Prgm
• Physical Therapy Prgm
• Psychology (PhD) Prgm
• Rehabilitation Counseling Prgm
• Speech-Language Pathology Prgm

West Virginia University Hospitals
Bruce McClymonds, President
Ruby Memorial Hospital
PO Box 8136
Morgantown, WV 26505
304 598-4355
Type: Hosp or Med Ctr: 300-499 Beds
Control: Nonprofit (Private or Religious)
• Diagnostic Med Sonography (General) Prgm
• Dietetic Internship Prgm
• Magnetic Resonance Technologist Prgm
• Nuclear Medicine Technology Prgm
• Radiation Therapy Prgm
• Radiography Prgm

Mount Gay

Southern West Virginia Comm & Tech College
Joanne C Tomblin, MA, President
PO Box 2900
Dempsey Branch Road
Mount Gay, WV 25637
304 896-7439
Type: Junior or Comm Coll
Control: State, County, or Local Govt
• Clin Lab Technician/Med Lab Technician Prgm
• Dental Hygiene Prgm
• Radiography Prgm
• Surgical Technology Prgm

Parkersburg

West Virginia University - Parkersburg
Marie Foster Gnage, PhD, President
300 Campus Dr
Parkersburg, WV 26104
304 424-8200
Type: Junior or Comm Coll
Control: State, County, or Local Govt
• Surgical Technology Prgm

Philippi

Alderson-Broaddus College
J Michael Clyburn, EdD, President
Box 2065
Philippi, WV 26416
304 457-6201
Type: 4-year Coll or Univ
Control: Nonprofit (Private or Religious)
• Athletic Training Prgm
• Physician Assistant Prgm

Princeton

Mercer County Technical Education Center
1397 Stafford Dr
Princeton, WV 24720
Type: Vocational or Tech Sch
Control: Nonprofit (Private or Religious)
• Dental Assistant Prgm

Shepherdstown

Shepherd University
Shepherdstown, WV 25443-5000
Type: 4-year Coll or Univ
Control: State, County, or Local Govt
• Nursing Prgm

West Liberty

West Liberty State College
robin capehart, Interim President
Main Hall West Liberty University
Office of the President
West Liberty, WV 26074
304 336-8000
Type: 4-year Coll or Univ
Control: State, County, or Local Govt
• Clin Lab Scientist/Med Technologist Prgm
• Dental Hygiene Prgm
• Nursing Prgm

Wheeling

Ohio Valley Medical Center
Brian Felici, MS, President
2000 Eoff St
Wheeling, WV 26003
304 234-8294
Type: Hosp or Med Ctr: 100-299 Beds
Control: Nonprofit (Private or Religious)
• Radiography Prgm

West Virginia Northern Community College
Martin Olshinsky, PhD, President
1704 Market St
Wheeling, WV 26003
304 214-8800
Type: Junior or Comm Coll
Control: State, County, or Local Govt
• Medical Assistant Prgm
• Radiography Prgm
• Respiratory Care Prgm
• Surgical Technology Prgm

Wheeling Jesuit University
Rev Julio Giuletti, SJ, President
316 Washington Ave
Wheeling, WV 26003
304 243-2233
Type: 4-year Coll or Univ
Control: Nonprofit (Private or Religious)
• Athletic Training Prgm
• Nuclear Medicine Technology Prgm
• Nursing Prgm
• Physical Therapy Prgm
• Respiratory Care Prgm

Wisconsin

Appleton

Affinity Health System - St Elizabeth Hosp
Travis Anderson, MS, COO
St Elizabeth Hospital
1506 S Oneida St
Appleton, WI 54915
920 831-8912
Type: Hosp or Med Ctr: 100-299 Beds
Control: Nonprofit (Private or Religious)
• Clin Lab Scientist/Med Technologist Prgm

Fox Valley Technical College
Susan A May, EdD, President
1825 N Bluemound Dr
PO Box 2277
Appleton, WI 54913-2277
920 735-5731
Type: Vocational or Tech Sch
Control: State, County, or Local Govt
• Dental Assistant Prgm
• Dental Hygiene Prgm
• Medical Assistant Prgm
• Occupational Therapy Asst Prgm

Cleveland

Lakeshore Technical College
Michael Lanser, EdD, Director
1290 North Ave
Cleveland, WI 53015
920 693-1000
Type: Vocational or Tech Sch
Control: State, County, or Local Govt
• Emergency Med Tech-Paramedic Prgm
• Medical Transcriptionist Prgm
• Radiography Prgm

Eau Claire

Chippewa Valley Technical College
Bruce Barker, JD, President
620 W Clairemont Ave
Eau Claire, WI 54701
715 833-6211
Type: Vocational or Tech Sch
Control: State, County, or Local Govt
• Clin Lab Technician/Med Lab Technician Prgm
• Dental Hygiene Prgm
• Diagnostic Med Sonography (General) Prgm
• Medical Assistant Prgm
• Radiography Prgm
• Respiratory Care Prgm
• Surgical Technology Prgm

Sacred Heart Hospital
Steve Ronstrom, MHA, Administrator
900 W Clairemont Ave
Eau Claire, WI 54701
715 717-4232
Type: Hosp or Med Ctr: 300-499 Beds
Control: Nonprofit (Private or Religious)
• Clin Lab Scientist/Med Technologist Prgm

University of Wisconsin - Eau Claire
Brian Levin-Stankevich, PhD, Chancellor
Schofield 204
105 Garfield Ave
Eau Claire, WI 54702-4004
715 836-2327
Type: 4-year Coll or Univ
Control: State, County, or Local Govt
• Athletic Training Prgm
• Music Therapy Prgm
• Nursing Prgm
• Speech-Language Pathology Prgm

Fennimore

Southwest Wisconsin Technical College
Karen Knox, EdD, President
1800 Bronson Blvd
Fennimore, WI 53809
608 288-3262
Type: Vocational or Tech Sch
Control: State, County, or Local Govt
• Clin Lab Technician/Med Lab Technician Prgm
• Medical Assistant Prgm

Fond du Lac

Marian College
Fond du Lac, WI 54935
Type: 4-year Coll or Univ
Control: State, County, or Local Govt
• Nursing Prgm

Moraine Park Technical College
Gayle Hytrek, PhD, President
235 N National Ave
PO Box 1940
Fond du Lac, WI 54936-1940
920 929-2127
Type: Vocational or Tech Sch
Control: State, County, or Local Govt
• Clin Lab Technician/Med Lab Technician Prgm
• Medical Assistant Prgm
• Radiography Prgm
• Surgical Technology Prgm

Glendale

Columbia College of Nursing
Glendale, WI 53212
Type: Junior or Comm Coll
Control: Nonprofit (Private or Religious)
• Nursing Prgm

Grafton

Blue Sky School of Professional Massage
Karen Lewis, Dean, Co-Founder
220 Oak St
Manchester Mall
Grafton, WI 53024
262 376-1011
Type: Vocational or Tech Sch
Control: Nonprofit (Private or Religious)
• Massage Therapy Prgm (3)

Green Bay

Bellin College/Bellin Health Systems Inc
George Kerwin, MBA, President and CEO
744 S Webster Ave
PO Box 23400
Green Bay, WI 54305-3400
414 433-7898
Type: Hosp or Med Ctr: 100-299 Beds
Control: Nonprofit (Private or Religious)
• Nursing Prgm
• Radiography Prgm

Northeast Wisconsin Technical College
H Jeffrey Rafn, PhD, President
2740 W Mason St
PO Box 19042
Green Bay, WI 54307-9042
920 498-5444
Type: Vocational or Tech Sch
Control: State, County, or Local Govt
• Clin Lab Technician/Med Lab Technician Prgm
• Dental Assistant Prgm
• Dental Hygiene Prgm
• Diagnostic Med Sonography (General) Prgm
• Medical Assistant Prgm
• Physical Therapist Assistant Prgm
• Radiography Prgm
• Respiratory Care Prgm
• Surgical Technology Prgm

Rasmussen College - Green Bay
Green Bay, WI 54302-2349
Type: 4-year Coll or Univ
• Medical Assistant Prgm

University of Wisconsin - Green Bay
Mark L Perkins, Chancellor
Green Bay, WI 54311
414 465-2000
Type: 4-year Coll or Univ
Control: State, County, or Local Govt
• Dietetic Internship Prgm
• Dietetics-Didactic Prgm
• Nursing Prgm

Hayward

Lac Courte Oreills Ojibwa Community College
Danielle Hornett, PhD, President
13466 Trepania Rd
Hayward, WI 54843
715 634-4790
Type: Junior or Comm Coll
Control: State, County, or Local Govt
• Medical Assistant Prgm

Janesville

Blackhawk Technical College
Eric Larson, EdD, President
6004 County Road G
PO Box 5009
Janesville, WI 53547-5009
608 756-4121
Type: Vocational or Tech Sch
Control: State, County, or Local Govt
• Clin Lab Technician/Med Lab Technician Prgm
• Dental Assistant Prgm
• Diagnostic Med Sonography (General/Vascular) Prgm
• Medical Assistant Prgm
• Physical Therapist Assistant Prgm
• Radiography Prgm

Kenosha

Carthage College
F Gregory Campbell, President
2001 Alford Park Dr
Kenosha, WI 53140-1994
262 551-5858
Type: 4-year Coll or Univ
Control: State, County, or Local Govt
- Athletic Training Prgm
- Music Therapy Prgm

Gateway Technical College
Bryan Albrecht, PhD, President
3520 30th Ave
Kenosha, WI 53144
262 564-2200
Type: Vocational or Tech Sch
Control: State, County, or Local Govt
- Dental Assistant Prgm
- Medical Assistant Prgm
- Physical Therapist Assistant Prgm
- Surgical Technology Prgm

La Crosse

University of Wisconsin - La Crosse
Joe Gow, PhD, Chancellor
1725 State St
135 Main Hall
La Crosse, WI 54601
608 785-8004
Type: 4-year Coll or Univ
Control: State, County, or Local Govt
- Athletic Training Prgm
- Medical Dosimetry Prgm
- Music Therapy Prgm
- Occupational Therapy Prgm
- Physical Therapy Prgm
- Physician Assistant Prgm
- Radiation Therapy Prgm

Viterbo University
Robert E Gibbons, PhD, President
818 S 9th St
La Crosse, WI 54601
608 784-0040
Type: 4-year Coll or Univ
Control: State, County, or Local Govt
- Dietetic Internship Prgm
- Dietetics-Coordinated Prgm
- Nursing Prgm

Western Technical College
Lee Rasch, EdD, President/District Dir
400 N Seventh St
PO Box C-0908
La Crosse, WI 54601
608 785-9210
Type: Vocational or Tech Sch
Control: State, County, or Local Govt
- Clin Lab Technician/Med Lab Technician Prgm
- Dental Assistant Prgm
- Dental Hygiene Prgm
- Medical Assistant Prgm
- Occupational Therapy Asst Prgm
- Physical Therapist Assistant Prgm
- Radiography Prgm
- Respiratory Care Prgm
- Surgical Technology Prgm

Madison

Edgewood College
Daniel J Carey, PhD, President
1000 Edgewood College Dr
Madison, WI 53711
Type: 4-year Coll or Univ
Control: Nonprofit (Private or Religious)
- Nursing Prgm

Madison Area Technical College
Bettsey Barhorst, PhD, President
3550 Anderson St
Madison, WI 53704-2599
608 246-6676
Type: Vocational or Tech Sch
Control: State, County, or Local Govt
- Clin Lab Technician/Med Lab Technician Prgm
- Dental Hygiene Prgm
- Medical Assistant Prgm
- Occupational Therapy Asst Prgm
- Ophthalmic Assistant Prgm
- Radiography Prgm
- Respiratory Care Prgm
- Surgical Technology Prgm
- Veterinary Technology Prgm

University of Wisconsin - Madison
Catherine Martin, PhD, Chancellor
500 Lincoln Dr
161 Bascom Hall
Madison, WI 53706-1380
608 262-9946
Type: 4-year Coll or Univ
Control: State, County, or Local Govt
- Allopathic Medicine Prgm
- Athletic Training Prgm
- Audiologist Prgm
- Clin Lab Scientist/Med Technologist Prgm
- Dietetics-Didactic Prgm
- Genetic Counseling Prgm
- Medical Librarian Prgm
- Music Therapy Prgm
- Nursing Prgm
- Occupational Therapy Prgm
- Pharmacy Prgm
- Physical Therapy Prgm
- Physician Assistant Prgm
- Psychology (PhD) Prgm
- Rehabilitation Counseling Prgm
- Speech-Language Pathology Prgm
- Veterinary Medicine Prgm

University of Wisconsin Hospital and Clinics
Donna Katen-Bahensky, MD, President and CEO
600 Highland Ave
Dept of Administration
Madison, WI 53792-8310
608 263-8025
Type: Hosp or Med Ctr: 500 Beds
Control: State, County, or Local Govt
- Diagnostic Med Sonography (General/Cardiac) Prgm
- Dietetic Internship Prgm
- Orthoptist Prgm
- Radiography Prgm

Wisconsin State Laboratory of Hygiene
Charles Brokopp, DPh, Director
Center for Health Studies - UW Madison
465 Henry Hall
Madison, WI 53706
608 890-1569
Type: Nonhosp HC Facil, BB, or Lab
Control: State, County, or Local Govt
- Cytotechnology Prgm

Manitowoc

Silver Lake College of the Holy Family
Manitowoc, WI 54220
Type: 4-year Coll or Univ
Control: Nonprofit (Private or Religious)
- Nursing Prgm

Marshfield

Marshfield Clinic
Reed Hall, MS JD, Executive Director
1000 N Oak Ave
Marshfield, WI 54449
715 387-5218
Type: Nonhosp HC Facil, BB, or Lab
Control: Nonprofit (Private or Religious)
- Cytotechnology Prgm

Saint Joseph's Hospital
Karl J Ulrich, CEO
1000 North Oak Avenue
Marshfield, WI 54449
715 387-5253
Type: Hosp or Med Ctr: 500 Beds
Control: Nonprofit (Private or Religious)
- Clin Lab Scientist/Med Technologist Prgm
- Histotechnician Prgm
- Nuclear Medicine Technology Prgm
- Radiography Prgm

Menasha

Mercy Medical Center/Affinity Health System
Daniel Neufelder, MS, President
1570 Midway Place
Menasha, WI 54952
920 720-1713
Type: Hosp or Med Ctr: 100-299 Beds
Control: Nonprofit (Private or Religious)
- Radiography Prgm

Menomonie

University of Wisconsin - Stout
Charles W Sorensen, Chancellor
Menomonie, WI 54751
715 232-1123
Type: 4-year Coll or Univ
Control: State, County, or Local Govt
- Dietetic Internship Prgm
- Dietetics-Didactic Prgm
- Rehabilitation Counseling Prgm

INSTITUTIONS

593

Mequon

Concordia University Wisconsin
Patrick Ferry, PhD, President
12800 N Lake Shore Dr
Mequon, WI 53097
262 243-4368
Type: 4-year Coll or Univ
Control: Nonprofit (Private or Religious)
• Athletic Training Prgm
• Medical Assistant Prgm
• Nursing Prgm
• Occupational Therapy Prgm
• Pharmacy Prgm
• Physical Therapy Prgm

Milwaukee

Alverno College
Mary Meehan, President
3401 S 39th St, Box 343922
Milwaukee, WI 53234-3922
414 382-6000
Type: 4-year Coll or Univ
Control: Nonprofit (Private or Religious)
• Music Therapy Prgm
• Nursing Prgm

Aurora St Luke's Medical Center
Nick Turkal, MD, President
2900 W Oklahoma Ave
PO Box 2901
Milwaukee, WI 53201-2901
414 649-7500
Type: Hosp or Med Ctr: 500 Beds
Control: Nonprofit (Private or Religious)
• Diagnostic Med Sonography (General/Vascular) Prgm
• Nuclear Medicine Technology Prgm
• Radiography Prgm

BloodCenter of Wisconsin
Jacquelyn Fredrick, President
PO Box 2178
638 N 18th Street
Milwaukee, WI 53201-2178
414 937-6390
Type: Nonhosp HC Facil, BB, or Lab
Control: Nonprofit (Private or Religious)
• Specialist in BB Tech Prgm

Bryant & Stratton College - Milwaukee
Peter Pavone, MS, Dir, Milwaukee Colleges
310 W Wisconsin Ave, Ste 500 E
Milwaukee, WI 53203
414 276-5200
Type: Junior or Comm Coll
Control: For Profit
• Medical Assistant Prgm

Cardinal Stritch University
Sister Mary Lea Schneider, President
6801 N Yates Rd
Milwaukee, WI 53217
414 410-4001
Type: 4-year Coll or Univ
Control: Nonprofit (Private or Religious)
• Nursing Prgm

Clement J Zablocki VA Medical Center
Robert Beller, Director
5000 W National Ave
Milwaukee, WI 53295
414 384-2000
Type: Dept of Veterans Affairs
Control: Fed Govt
• Clin Lab Scientist/Med Technologist Prgm

Columbia St Mary's Hospitals
Leo Brideau, President, CEO
2025 E Newport Ave
Milwaukee, WI 53211
414 961-3638
Type: Hosp or Med Ctr: 300-499 Beds
Control: Nonprofit (Private or Religious)
• Diagnostic Med Sonography (General/Vascular) Prgm
• Radiography Prgm

Froedtert Hospital
William D Petasnick, MHA, President
9200 W Wisconsin Ave
PO Box 26099
Milwaukee, WI 53226
414 805-3000
Type: Hosp or Med Ctr: 300-499 Beds
Control: Nonprofit (Private or Religious)
• Nuclear Medicine Technology Prgm
• Radiography Prgm

Lakeside School of Massage Therapy
Carole Ostendorf, PhD PT, Chief Executive Officer
1726 N 1st St, Ste 200
Milwaukee, WI 53212
414 372-4345
Type: Vocational or Tech Sch
Control: Nonprofit (Private or Religious)
• Massage Therapy Prgm

Marquette University
Rev Robert A Wild, SJ, President
O'Hara Hall
PO Box 1881
Milwaukee, WI 53201-1881
414 288-7223
Type: 4-year Coll or Univ
Control: Nonprofit (Private or Religious)
• Athletic Training Prgm
• Clin Lab Scientist/Med Technologist Prgm
• Dentistry Prgm
• Nursing Prgm
• Physical Therapy Prgm
• Physician Assistant Prgm
• Psychology (PhD) Prgm
• Speech-Language Pathology Prgm

Medical College of Wisconsin
T Michael Bolger, JD, President
8701 Watetown Plank Rd
Milwaukee, WI 53226
414 257-8225
Type: Acad Health Ctr/Med Sch
Control: Nonprofit (Private or Religious)
• Allopathic Medicine Prgm

Milwaukee Area Technical College
Michael L Burke, PhD, President
700 W State St
Milwaukee, WI 53233-1443
414 297-7269
Type: Vocational or Tech Sch
Control: State, County, or Local Govt
• Cardiovascular Tech (Invasive) Prgm
• Clin Lab Technician/Med Lab Technician Prgm
• Dental Hygiene Prgm
• Dietetic Technician-AD Prgm
• Medical Assistant Prgm
• Occupational Therapy Asst Prgm
• Pharmacy Technician Prgm
• Phlebotomy Prgm
• Physical Therapist Assistant Prgm
• Radiography Prgm
• Respiratory Care Prgm
• Surgical Technology Prgm

Milwaukee School of Engineering
Hermann Viets, PhD, President
1025 N Broadway
Milwaukee, WI 53202-3109
414 277-7100
Type: 4-year Coll or Univ
Control: Nonprofit (Private or Religious)
• Nursing Prgm
• Perfusion Prgm

Mount Mary College
Eileen Schwalbach, PhD, President
2900 N Menomonee River Pkwy
Milwaukee, WI 53222-4597
414 256-1207
Type: 4-year Coll or Univ
Control: Nonprofit (Private or Religious)
• Art Therapy Prgm
• Dietetic Internship Prgm
• Dietetics-Coordinated Prgm
• Occupational Therapy Prgm

University of Wisconsin - Milwaukee
Michael R Lovell, PhD, Interm Chancellor
PO Box 413, Chapman Hall 202
Milwaukee, WI 53201
414 229-4331
Type: 4-year Coll or Univ
Control: State, County, or Local Govt
• Athletic Training Prgm
• Clin Lab Scientist/Med Technologist Prgm
• Cytotechnology Prgm
• Medical Librarian Prgm
• Nursing Prgm
• Occupational Therapy Prgm
• Psychology (PhD) Prgm
• Speech-Language Pathology Prgm

University of Wisconsin-Milwaukee
PO Box 413
Milwaukee, WI 53201-1041
• Physical Therapy Prgm

Wheaton Franciscan Healthcare - St Francis
Debra Standridge, MBA, President
3237 S 16th St
Milwaukee, WI 53215
414 647-5106
Type: Hosp or Med Ctr: 100-299 Beds
Control: Nonprofit (Private or Religious)
• Diagnostic Med Sonography (General) Prgm

Wheaton Franciscan Healthcare - St Joseph
Ronald Groepper, RN MBA FACHE,
    President/CEO
5000 West Chambers St
Milwaukee, WI 53210
414 447-2847
Type: Hosp or Med Ctr: 300-499 Beds
Control: Nonprofit (Private or Religious)
• Radiography Prgm

Neenah

Theda Clark Regional Medical Center
John Toiusant, MD, President
130 Second St
PO Box 2021
Neenah, WI 54957-2021
920 729-3100
Type: Hosp or Med Ctr: 300-499 Beds
Control: Nonprofit (Private or Religious)
• Radiography Prgm

Oshkosh

University of Wisconsin - Oshkosh
Richard Wells, Chancellor
800 Algoma Blvd
Oshkosh, WI 54901
920 424-0200
Type: 4-year Coll or Univ
Control: State, County, or Local Govt
• Athletic Training Prgm
• Counseling Prgm
• Music Therapy Prgm
• Nursing Prgm

Pewaukee

Waukesha County Technical College
Barbara Prindiville, PhD, President
800 Main St
Pewaukee, WI 53072
414 691-5435
Type: Vocational or Tech Sch
Control: State, County, or Local Govt
• Dental Hygiene Prgm
• Emergency Med Tech-Paramedic Prgm
• Medical Assistant Prgm
• Surgical Technology Prgm

Racine

Wheaton Franciscan Healthcare - All Saints
Kenneth R Buser, FACHE, President and CEO
3801 Spring St
Racine, WI 53405
262 687-4285
Type: Hosp or Med Ctr: 300-499 Beds
Control: Nonprofit (Private or Religious)
• Radiography Prgm

Rhinelander

Nicolet Area Technical College
Adrian Lorbetske, JD, President
PO Box 518
Rhinelander, WI 54501
715 365-4410
Type: Vocational or Tech Sch
Control: State, County, or Local Govt
• Medical Assistant Prgm

River Falls

University of Wisconsin - River Falls
Gary A Thibodeau, Chancellor
River Falls, WI 54022
715 425-3911
Type: 4-year Coll or Univ
Control: State, County, or Local Govt
• Music Therapy Prgm
• Speech-Language Pathology Prgm

Shell Lake

Wisconsin Indianhead Technical College
Charles Levine, PhD, Interim President
505 Pine Ridge Dr
Shell Lake, WI 54871-9300
715 468-2815
Type: Vocational or Tech Sch
Control: State, County, or Local Govt
• Medical Assistant Prgm (2)
• Occupational Therapy Asst Prgm

Stevens Point

University of Wisconsin - Stevens Point
Mark Nook, Provost & Vice Chancellor
2100 Main
Stevens Point, WI 54481
715 346-4686
Type: 4-year Coll or Univ
Control: State, County, or Local Govt
• Athletic Training Prgm
• Clin Lab Scientist/Med Technologist Prgm
• Dietetics-Didactic Prgm
• Music Therapy Prgm
• Speech-Language Pathology Prgm

Superior

University of Wisconsin - Superior
Julius E Erlenbach, Chancellor
1800 Grand Ave
Superior, WI 54880-2898
715 394-8101
Type: 4-year Coll or Univ
Control: State, County, or Local Govt
• Counseling Prgm
• Music Therapy Prgm

Waukesha

Carroll University
Douglas N Hastad, DEd, President
100 N East Ave
Waukesha, WI 53186-5593
414 547-1211
Type: 4-year Coll or Univ
Control: Nonprofit (Private or Religious)
• Athletic Training Prgm
• Nursing Prgm
• Physical Therapy Prgm
• Physician Assistant Prgm

Wausau

Aspirus Wausau Hospital
Diane Postler-Slattery, PhD, President and COO
333 Pine Ridge Blvd
Wausau, WI 54401
715 847-2988
Type: Hosp or Med Ctr: 300-499 Beds
Control: Nonprofit (Private or Religious)
• Clin Lab Scientist/Med Technologist Prgm

Northcentral Technical College
Lori A Weyers, PhD, President
1000 W Campus Drive
Wausau, WI 54401-1899
715 675-3331
Type: Vocational or Tech Sch
Control: State, County, or Local Govt
• Clin Lab Technician/Med Lab Technician Prgm
• Dental Hygiene Prgm
• Emergency Med Tech-Paramedic Prgm
• Medical Assistant Prgm
• Phlebotomy Prgm
• Radiography Prgm
• Surgical Technology Prgm

West Allis

Sanford-Brown College
6737 West Washington Street #2355
West Allis, WI 53214
Type: Vocational or Tech Sch
Control: For Profit
• Radiography Prgm

Whitewater

University of Wisconsin - Whitewater
Richard Telfer, Interim Chancellor
800 W Main
Hyer 421
Whitewater, WI 53190-1791
262 472-1918
Type: 4-year Coll or Univ
Control: State, County, or Local Govt
• Counseling Prgm
• Music Therapy Prgm
• Speech-Language Pathology Prgm

Wisconsin Rapids

Mid-State Technical College
John Clark, PhD, President
500 32nd St N
Wisconsin Rapids, WI 54494
715 422-5320
Type: Vocational or Tech Sch
Control: State, County, or Local Govt
• Medical Assistant Prgm
• Phlebotomy Prgm
• Respiratory Care Prgm
• Surgical Technology Prgm

Wyoming

Casper

Casper College
Walter Nolte, PhD, President
125 College Dr
Casper, WY 82601
307 268-2100
Type: Junior or Comm Coll
Control: State, County, or Local Govt
• Clin Lab Technician/Med Lab Technician Prgm
• Emergency Med Tech-Paramedic Prgm
• Occupational Therapy Asst Prgm
• Radiography Prgm

University of North Dakota at Casper College
Walter Nolte, President
125 College Dr
Casper, WY 82601-9958
Type: 4-year Coll or Univ
Control: State, County, or Local Govt
• Occupational Therapy Prgm

Cheyenne

Laramie County Community College
Darrel L Hammon, PhD, President
1400 E College Dr
Cheyenne, WY 82007
307 778-5222
Type: Junior or Comm Coll
Control: State, County, or Local Govt
• Dental Hygiene Prgm
• Diagnostic Med Sonography (General) Prgm
• Emergency Med Tech-Paramedic Prgm
• Radiography Prgm
• Surgical Technology Prgm

Laramie

University of Wyoming
Thomas Buchanan, PhD, President
Dept 3434
1000 E University Ave
Laramie, WY 82071
307 766-4121
Type: 4-year Coll or Univ
Control: State, County, or Local Govt
• Counseling Prgm
• Dietetics-Didactic Prgm
• Music Therapy Prgm
• Nursing Prgm
• Pharmacy Prgm
• Psychology (PhD) Prgm
• Speech-Language Pathology Prgm

Powell

Northwest College
John Dewitt, President
231 W Sixth St
Powell, WY 82435
307 754-6200
Type: Junior or Comm Coll
Control: State, County, or Local Govt
• Music Therapy Prgm

Sheridan

Sheridan College
Kevin Drumm, EdD, President
3059 Coffeen Ave
Box 1500
Sheridan, WY 82801
307 674-6446
Type: Junior or Comm Coll
Control: State, County, or Local Govt
• Dental Hygiene Prgm

Torrington

Eastern Wyoming College
Jack Bottenfield, PhD, President
3200 West C St
Torrington, WY 82240
307 532-8202
Type: Junior or Comm Coll
Control: State, County, or Local Govt
• Veterinary Technology Prgm